Handbook of Cardiac Anatomy, Physiology, and Devices

Paul A. Iaizzo

Editor

Handbook of Cardiac Anatomy, Physiology, and Devices

Second Edition

Foreword by Timothy G. Laske

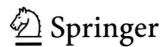 Springer

Editor
Paul A. Iaizzo
University of Minnesota
Department of Surgery
B172 Mayo, MMC 195
420 Delaware St. SE.,
Minneapolis, MN 55455
USA
iaizz001@umn.edu

Additional material to this book can be downloaded from http://extras.springer.com

ISBN 978-1-60327-371-8   e-ISBN 978-1-60327-372-5
DOI 10.1007/978-1-60327-372-5

Library of Congress Control Number: 2009920269

Printed on acid-free paper

Springer is part of Springer Science+Business Media (www.springer.com)

Foreword

A revolution began in my professional career and education in 1997. In that year, I visited the University of Minnesota to discuss collaborative opportunities in cardiac anatomy, physiology, and medical device testing. The meeting was with a faculty member of the Department of Anesthesiology, Professor Paul Iaizzo. I didn't know what to expect but, as always, I remained open minded and optimistic. Little did I know that my life would never be the same. . . .

During the mid to late 1990s, Paul Iaizzo and his team were performing anesthesia research on isolated guinea pig hearts. We found the work appealing, but it was unclear how this research might apply to our interest in tools to aid in the design of implantable devices for the cardiovascular system. As discussions progressed, we noted that we would be far more interested in reanimation of large mammalian hearts, in particular, human hearts. Paul was confident this could be accomplished on large hearts, but thought that it would be unlikely that we would ever have access to human hearts for this application. We shook hands and the collaboration was born in 1997. In the same year, Paul and the research team at the University of Minnesota (including Bill Gallagher and Charles Soule) reanimated several swine hearts. Unlike the previous work on guinea pig hearts which were reanimated in Langendorff mode, the intention of this research was to produce a fully functional working heart model for device testing and cardiac research. Such a model would allow engineers and scientists easy access to the epicardium and the chambers through transmural ports. It took numerous attempts to achieve the correct osmotic balance and an adequately oxygenated perfusate, and to avoid poisoning the preparation with bacteria (which we found were happy to lurk anywhere and everywhere in the plumbing of the apparatus). This project required a combination of art, science, and dogged persistence.

In addition to the breakthrough achieved in the successful animation of numerous swine hearts, bigger and better things were in store. Serendipitously, when faced with a need to see inside the heart, the research team found a fiberoptic scope on an upper shelf in the laboratory. The scope was inserted into the heart and a whole new world was observed. Due to the clear nature of the perfusate, we immediately saw the flashing of the tricuspid valve upon insertion of the scope. We were in awe as we viewed the first images ever recorded inside of a working heart. This is the moment when my personal revolution began.

The years that have followed have included numerous achievements which I attribute to the vision and persistence of Paul and the team. The human hearts that Paul initially considered impossible to access and reanimate were soon functioning in the apparatus due to a collaboration with LifeSource. Indeed, the team's "never say never" attitude is at the heart of their pursuit of excellence in education and research.

The Visible Heart Laboratory has evolved into a dream for engineers, educators, and cardiac physiologists as scientific equipment has been added (echocardiography, electrical mapping systems, hemodynamic monitors, etc.) and endoscopic video capabilities have improved (the lab is currently using video endoscopes with media quality recording equipment). The lab produces educational images, conducts a wide spectrum of cardiac research, and evaluates current and future medical device concepts each week. Hundreds of engineers and students have worked and studied in the lab, countless physicians have assisted with procedures, and thousands of educational CDs/DVDs have been distributed (free of charge).

Eleven years after the beginning of our collaborative effort, the Visible Heart Laboratory remains the only place in the world where a human heart can be reanimated outside of the body and made to work for an extended period of time. This is a tribute to the efforts of Paul and his team in managing the difficulty it takes to make this happen. Interestingly, the team currently works in the laboratory in which Lillehei and Bakken first tested the battery-powered pacemaker; the "good karma" lives on.

This book is a result of Paul's passion for excellence in teaching and for innovation in the medical device field. I am confident that the reader will find this book an invaluable resource. It is a testament to Paul's dedication to both education, collaboration, and the ongoing development of his current and past students.

By the way.... The personal revolution I referred to, fueled by my collaboration with Paul, has included numerous patents, countless device concepts accepted and/or rejected, several scientific articles, a PhD in Biomedical Engineering, and a collaboration in black bear hibernation physiology. None of this would have happened had I not met Paul that day in 1997, and benefited from his friendship and mentoring over the years. I can only imagine what the future will bring, but you can be rest assured that success is sure to come to those that associate themselves with Paul Iaizzo.

Minneapolis, MN   Timothy G. Laske, Ph. D.

Preface

Worldwide, the medical device industry continues to grow at an incredibly rapid pace. Our overall understanding of the molecular basis of disease continues to increase, in addition to the number of available therapies to treat specific health problems. This remains particularly true in the field of cardiovascular care. Hence, with this rapid growth rate, the biomedical engineer has been challenged to both retool and continue to seek out sources of concise information.

The major impetus for the second edition of this text was to update this resource textbook for interested students, residents, and/or practicing biomedical engineers. A secondary motivation was to promote the expertise, past and present, in the area of cardiovascular sciences at the University of Minnesota. As Director of Education for The Lillehei Heart Institute and the Associate Director for Education of the Institute for Engineering in Medicine at the University of Minnesota, I feel that this book also represents a unique outreach opportunity to carry on the legacies of C. Walton Lillehei and Earl Bakken through the 21st century. Interestingly, the completion of the textbook also coincides with two important anniversaries in cardiovascular medicine and engineering at the University of Minnesota. First, it was 50 years ago, in 1958, that the first wearable, battery-powered pacemaker, built by Earl Bakken (and Medtronic) at the request of Dr. Lillehei, was first used on a patient. Second, 30 years ago, in 1978, the first human heart transplantation was performed at the University of Minnesota.

For the past 10 years, the University of Minnesota has presented the week-long short course, Advanced Cardiac Physiology and Anatomy, which was designed specifically for the biomedical engineer working in industry; this is the course textbook. As this course has evolved, there was a need to update the textbook. For example, six new chapters were added to this second edition, and all other chapters were either carefully updated and/or greatly expanded. One last historical note that I feel is interesting to mention is that my current laboratory, where isolated heart studies are performed weekly (the Visible Heart® laboratory), is the same laboratory in which C. Walton Lillehei and his many esteemed colleagues conducted a majority of their cardiovascular research studies in the late 1950s and early 1960s.

As with the first edition of this book, I have included electronic files on the companion DVD that will enhance this textbook's utility. Part of the companion DVD, the "The Visible Heart® Viewer," was developed as a joint venture between my laboratory at the University of Minnesota and the Cardiac Rhythm Management Division at Medtronic, Inc. Importantly, this electronic textbook also includes functional images of human hearts. These images were obtained from hearts made available via LifeSource, more specifically through the generosity of families and individuals who made the final gift of organ donation (these hearts were not deemed viable for transplantation). Furthermore, the companion

DVD contains various additional color images and movies that were provided by the various authors to supplement their chapters. Since the first printing of this textbook, my laboratory has also developed the free-access website, "The Atlas of Human Cardiac Anatomy," that readers of this text should also find valuable as a complementary resource (http://www.vhlab.umn.edu/atlas).

I would especially like to acknowledge the exceptional efforts of our lab coordinator, Monica Mahre, who for a second time: (1) assisted me in coordinating the efforts of the contributing authors; (2) skillfully incorporated my editorial changes; (3) verified the readability and formatting of each chapter; (4) pursued requested additions or missing materials for each chapter; (5) contributed as a co-author; and (6) kept a positive outlook throughout. I would also like to thank Gary Williams for his computer expertise and assistance with numerous figures; William Gallagher and Charles Soule who made sure the laboratory kept running smoothly while many of us were busy writing or editing; Dick Bianco for his support of our lab and this book project; the chairman of the Department of Surgery, Dr. Selwyn Vickers, for his support and encouragement; and the Institute for Engineering in Medicine at the University of Minnesota, headed by Dr. Jeffrey McCullough, who supported this project by funding the Cardiovascular Physiology Interest Group (many group members contributed chapters).

I would like to thank Medtronic, Inc. for their continued support of the Visible Heart® Laboratory for the past 12 years, and I especially acknowledge the commitments, partnerships, and friendships of Drs. Tim Laske, Alex Hill, and Nick Skadsberg for making our collaborative research possible. In addition, I would like to thank Jilean Welch and Mike Leners for their creative efforts in producing many of the movie and animation clips that are on the DVD.

It is also my pleasure to thank the past and present graduate students or residents who have worked in my laboratory and who were contributors to this second edition, including Sara Anderson, James Coles, Anthony Dupre, Michael Eggen, Kevin Fitzgerald, Alexander Hill, Jason Johnson, Ryan Lahm, Timothy Laske, Anna Legreid Dopp, Michael Loushin, Jason Quill, Maneesh Shrivastav, Daniel Sigg, Eric Richardson, Nicholas Skadsberg, and Sarah Vieau. I feel extremely fortunate to have the opportunity to work with such a talented group of scientists and engineers, and I have learned a great deal from each of them.

Finally, I would like to thank my family and friends for their continued support of my career and their assistance over the years. Specifically, I would like to thank my wife, Marge, my three daughters, Maria, Jenna, and Hanna, my mom Irene, and siblings Mike, Chris, Mark, and Susan for always being there for me. On a personal note, some of my inspiration for working on this project comes from the memory of my father, Anthony, who succumbed to a sudden cardiac event, and from the memory of my Uncle Tom Halicki, who passed away 9 years after a heart transplantation.

Minneapolis, MN   Paul A. Iaizzo

Contents

Contributors

Sara E. Anderson, PhD University of Minnesota, Departments of Biomedical Engineering and Surgery and University of Minnesota, Covidien, 5920 Longbow Dr., Boulder, CO 80301, USA, sara.e.anderson1@gmail.com

Robert J. Bache, MD University of Minnesota, Cardiovascular Division, Center for Magnetic Resonance Research, MMC 508, 420 Delaware St. SE, Minneapolis, MN 55455, USA, bache001@umn.edu

Vincent A. Barnett, PhD University of Minnesota, Department of Integrative Biology and Physiology, 6-125 Jackson Hall, 321 Church St, SE, Minneapolis, MN 55455, USA, barne014@umn.edu

John L. Bass, MD University of Minnesota, Department of Pediatric Cardiology, MMC 94, 420 Delaware St. SE, Minneapolis, MN 55455, USA, bassx001@umn.edu

Gregory J. Beilman, MD University of Minnesota, Department of Surgery, MMC 11, 420 Delaware St. SE, Minneapolis, MN 55455, USA, beilm001@umn.edu

Richard W. Bianco University of Minnesota, Experimental Surgical Services, Department of Surgery, MMC 220, 420 Delaware St. SE, Minneapolis, MN 55455, USA, bianc001@umn.edu

George Bojanov, MD University of Minnesota, Department of Anesthesiology, MMC 294, 420 Delaware St. SE, Minneapolis, MN 55455, USA, boja0003@umn.edu

James A. Coles, Jr., PhD Medtronic, Inc., 8200 Coral Sea St. NE, MNV41, Mounds View, MN 55112, USA, james.coles@medtronic.com

Mark S. Cook, PT, PhD University of Minnesota, Department of Integrative Biology and Physiology, 6-125 Jackson Hall, 321 Church St. SE, Minneapolis, MN 55455, USA, cookx072@umn.edu

Agustin P. Dalmasso, MD University of Minnesota, Departments of Surgery, Laboratory Medicine, and Pathology, MMC 220, 420 Delaware St. SE, Minneapolis, MN 55455, USA, dalma001@umn.edu

Anna Legreid Dopp, PharmD University of Wisconsin-Madison, School of Pharmacy, 777 Highland Avenue, Madison, WI 58705, USA, alegreiddopp@pharmacy.wisc.edu

Anthony Dupre, MS Boston Scientific Scimed, 1 Scimed Place, Osseo, MN 55311, USA, tony.dupre@gmail.com

Michael D. Eggen, PhD University of Minnesota, Departments of Biomedical Engineering and Surgery, B 172 Mayo, MMC 195, 420 Delaware St. SE, Minneapolis, MN 55455, USA, egge0075@umn.edu

Kevin Fitzgerald, MS Medtronic, Inc., 1129 Jasmine St., Denver, CO 80220, USA, kevin.fitzgerald@medtronic.com

Arthur H.L. From, MD University of Minnesota, Cardiovascular Division, Center for Magnetic Resonance Research, 2021 6th St. SE, Minneapolis, MN 55455, USA, fromx001@umn.edu

Robert P. Gallegos, MD, PhD Brigham and Women's Hospital, Division of Cardiac Surgery, 75 Francis St., Boston, MA 02115, USA, rgallegos@partners.org

Daniel J. Garry, MD, PhD University of Minnesota, Division of Cardiology, Department of Medicine, MMC 508, 420 Delaware St. SE, Minneapolis, MN 55455, USA, garry@umn.edu

Daniel H. Gruenstein, MD University of Minnesota, Department of Pediatric Cardiology, MMC 94, 420 Delaware St. SE, Minneapolis, MN 55455, USA, gruen040@umn.edu

Bin He, PhD University of Minnesota, Department of Biomedical Engineering, 7-105 BSBE, 312 Church St. SE, Minneapolis, MN 55455, USA, binhe@umn.edu

Ayala Hezi-Yamit, PhD Medtronic, Inc., 3576 Unocal Place, Santa Rosa, CA 95403, USA, ayala.hezi-yamit@medtronic.com

Alexander J. Hill, PhD University of Minnesota, Departments of Biomedical Engineering and Surgery, Medtronic, Inc., 8200 Coral Sea St. NE, MVS84, Mounds View, MN 55112, USA, alex.hill@medtronic.com

Paul A. Iaizzo, PhD University of Minnesota, Department of Surgery, B172 Mayo, MMC 195, 420 Delaware St. SE, Minneapolis, MN 55455, USA, iaizz001@umn.edu

Mohammad N. Jameel, MD University of Minnesota, Department of Medicine, MMC 508, 420 Delaware St. SE, Minneapolis, MN 55455, USA, jamee001@umn.edu

Ranjit John, MD University of Minnesota, Division of Cardiovascular and Thoracic Surgery, Department of Surgery, MMC 207, 420 Delaware St. SE, Minneapolis, MN 55455, USA, johnx008@umn.edu

Jason S. Johnson, MD University of Minnesota, Department of Anesthesiology, MMC 294, 420 Delaware St. SE, Minneapolis, MN 55455, USA, john6578@umn.edu

Ryan Lahm, MS Medtronic, Inc., 8200 Coral Sea St. NE, Mail Stop: MVN51, Mounds View, MN 55112, USA, ryan.lahm@medtronic.com

Timothy G. Laske, PhD University of Minnesota, Department of Surgery and Medtronic, Inc., 8200 Coral Sea St. NE, MVS84, Mounds View, MN 55112, USA, tim.g.laske@medtronic.com

Joseph Lee, MD, PhD University of Minnesota, MMC 293, 420 Delaware St. SE, Minneapolis, MN 55455, USA, joelee@umn.edu

Xiao-huan Li, MD University of Minnesota, Department of Surgery, MMC 195, 420 Delaware St. SE, Minneapolis, MN 55455, USA, lixxx475@umn.edu

Kenneth K. Liao, MD University of Minnesota, Division of Cardiovascular and Thoracic Surgery, Department of Surgery, MMC 207, 420 Delaware St. SE, Minneapolis, MN 55455, USA, liaox014@umn.edu

Jamie L. Lohr, MD University of Minnesota, Division of Pediatric Cardiology, Department of Pediatrics, MMC 94, 420 Delaware St. SE, Minneapolis, MN 55455, USA, lohrx003@umn.edu

Michael K. Loushin, MD University of Minnesota, Department of Anesthesiology, MMC 294, 420 Delaware St. SE, Minneapolis, MN 55455, USA, loush001@umn.edu

Fei Lü, MD, PhD, FACC University of Minnesota, Department of Medicine, MMC 508, 420 Delaware St. SE, Minneapolis, MN, 55455, USA, luxxx074@umn.edu

Keith Lurie, MD University of Minnesota, Department of Emergency Medicine, HCMC, 701 Park Ave. S., Minneapolis, MN 55415, USA, lurie002@umn.edu

Monica A. Mahre, BS University of Minnesota, Department of Surgery, B172 Mayo, MMC 195, 420 Delaware St. SE, Minneapolis, MN 55455, USA, mahre002@umn.edu

Brad J. Martinsen, PhD University of Minnesota, Division of Pediatric Cardiology, Department of Pediatrics, 1-140 MoosT, 515 Delaware St. SE, Minneapolis, MN 55455, USA, marti198@umn.edu

Anja Metzger, PhD University of Minnesota, Department of Emergency Medicine, 13683 47th St. N., Minneapolis, MN 55455, USA, ametzger@advancedcirculatory.com or kohl0005@umn.edu

J. Ernesto Molina, MD, PhD University of Minnesota, Division of Cardiothoracic Surgery, MMC 207, 420 Delaware St. SE, Minneapolis, MN 55455, USA, molin001@umn.edu

Jason L. Quill, PhD University of Minnesota, Departments of Biomedical Engineering and Surgery, B172 Mayo, MMC 195, 420 Delaware St. SE, Minneapolis, MN 55455, USA, quill010@umn.edu

Eric S. Richardson, PhD University of Minnesota, Departments of Biomedical Engineering and Surgery, B172 Mayo, MMC 195, 420 Delaware St. SE, Minneapolis, MN 55455, USA, richa483@umn.edu

Andrew L. Rivard, MD University of Florida, College of Medicine, Department of Radiology, PO Box 100374, Gainesville, FL 32610-0374, USA, andrewrivard@hotmail.com

Kenneth P. Roberts, PhD Washington State University-Spokane, WWAMI Medical Educational Program, 320N Health Sciences Building, PO Box 1495, Spokane, WA 99210, USA, kenroberts@wsu.edu

Maneesh Shrivastav, PhD Medtronic, Inc., 8200 Coral Sea St. NE, MVN42, Mounds View, MN 55112, USA, paricay@yahoo.com

Daniel C. Sigg, MD, PhD University of Minnesota, Department of Integrative Biology and Physiology, 1485 Hoyt Ave W, Saint Paul, MN 55108, siggx001@umn.edu

J. Jason Sims, PharmD Medtronic, Inc., 135 Highpoint Pass, Fayettville, GA 30215, USA, j.jason.sims@medtronic.com

Shanthi Sivanandam, MD University of Minnesota, Division of Pediatric Cardiology, Department of Pediatrics, MMC 94, 420 Delaware St. SE, Minneapolis, MN 55455, USA, silv0099@umn.edu

Nicholas D. Skadsberg, PhD Medtronic, Inc., 8200 Coral Sea St. NE, Mounds View, MN 55112, USA, nick.skadsberg@medtronic.com

James D. St. Louis, MD University of Minnesota, Departments of Surgery and Pediatrics, MMC 495, 420 Delaware St. SE, Minneapolis, MN 55455, USA, stlou012@umn.edu

Cory M. Swingen, PhD University of Minnesota, Department of Medicine, MMC 508, 420 Delaware St. SE, Minneapolis, MN 55455, USA, swing001@umn.edu

Michael Ujhelyi, PharmD, FCCP Medtronic, Inc., 7000 Central Ave., MS CW330, Minneapolis, MN 55432, USA, michael.ujhelyi@medtronic.com

Sarah A. Vieau, MS Medtronic, Inc., 8200 Coral Sea St. NE, MVS41, Mounds View, MN 55112, USA, sarah.a.vieau@medtronic.com

Anthony J. Weinhaus, PhD University of Minnesota, Department of Integrative Biology and Physiology, 6-130 Jackson Hall, 321 Church St. SE, Minneapolis, MN 55455, USA, weinh001@umn.edu

Robert F. Wilson, MD University of Minnesota, Department of Medicine, MMC 508, 420 Delaware St. SE, Minneapolis, MN 55455, USA, wilso008@umn.edu

Yong-Fu Xiao, MD, PhD Medtronic, Inc., 8200 Coral Sea St. NE, MVN42, Mounds View, MN 55112, USA, yong-fu.xiao@medtronic.com

Jianyi Zhang, MD, PhD University of Minnesota, Department of Medicine, 268 Variety Club Research Center, 401 East River Rd., Minneapolis, MN 55455, USA, zhang047@umn.edu

Part I
Introduction

Chapter 1
General Features of the Cardiovascular System

Paul A. Iaizzo

Abstract The purpose of this chapter is to provide a general overview of the cardiovascular system, to serve as a quick reference on the underlying physiological composition of this system. The rapid transport of molecules over long distances between internal cells, the body surface, and/or various specialized tissues and organs is the primary function of the cardiovascular system. This body-wide transport system is composed of several major components: blood, blood vessels, the heart, and the lymphatic system. When functioning normally, this system adequately provides for the wide-ranging activities that a human can accomplish. Failure in any of these components can lead to grave consequence. Subsequent chapters will cover, in greater detail, the anatomical, physiological, and/or pathophysiological features of the cardiovascular system.

Keywords Cardiovascular system · Blood · Blood vessels · Blood flow · Heart · Coronary circulation · Lymphatic system

1.1 Introduction

Currently, approximately 80 million individuals in the United States alone have some form of cardiovascular disease. More specifically, heart attacks continue to be an increasing problem in our society. Coronary bypass surgery, angioplasty, stenting, the implantation of pacemakers and/or defibrillators, and valve replacement are currently routine treatment procedures, with growing numbers of such procedures being performed each year. However, such treatments often provide only temporary relief of the progressive symptoms of cardiac disease. Optimizing therapies and/or the development of new treatments continues to dominate the cardiovascular biomedical industry (e.g., coated vascular or coronary stents, left ventricular assist devices, biventricular pacing, and transcatheter-delivered valves).

The purpose of this chapter is to provide a general overview of the cardiovascular system, to serve as a quick reference on the underlying physiological composition of this system. More details concerning the pathophysiology of the cardiovascular system and state-of-the-art treatments can be found in subsequent chapters. In addition, the reader should note that a list of source references is provided at the end of this chapter.

1.2 Components of the Cardiovascular System

The principle components considered to make up the cardiovascular system include blood, blood vessels, the heart, and the lymphatic system.

1.2.1 Blood

Blood is composed of formed elements (cells and cell fragments) which are suspended in the liquid fraction known as plasma. Blood, considered as the only liquid connective tissue in the body, has three general functions: (1) transportation (e.g., O_2, CO_2, nutrients, waste, and hormones); (2) regulation (e.g., pH, temperature, and osmotic pressures); and (3) protection (e.g., against foreign molecules and diseases, as well as for clotting to prevent excessive loss of blood). Dissolved within the plasma are many proteins, nutrients, metabolic waste products, and various other molecules being transported between the various organ systems.

The formed elements in blood include red blood cells (erythrocytes), white blood cells (leukocytes), and the cell

P.A. Iaizzo (✉)
University of Minnesota, Department of Surgery, B172 Mayo, MMC 195, 420 Delaware St. SE, Minneapolis, MN 55455, USA
e-mail: iaizz001@umn.edu

P.A. Iaizzo (ed.), *Handbook of Cardiac Anatomy, Physiology, and Devices*, DOI 10.1007/978-1-60327-372-5_1,

fragments known as platelets; all are formed in bone marrow from a common stem cell. In a healthy individual, the majority of bloods cells are red blood cells (∼99%) which have a primary role in O_2 exchange. Hemoglobin, the iron-containing heme protein which binds oxygen, is concentrated within the red cells; hemoglobin allows blood to transport 40–50 times the amount of oxygen that plasma alone could carry. The white cells are required for the immune process to protect against infections and also cancers. The platelets play a primary role in blood clotting. In a healthy cardiovascular system, the constant movement of blood helps keep these cells well dispersed throughout the plasma of the larger diameter vessels.

The *hematocrit* is defined as the percentage of blood volume that is occupied by the red cells (erythrocytes). It can be easily measured by centrifuging (spinning at high speed) a sample of blood, which forces these cells to the bottom of the centrifuge tube. The leukocytes remain on the top and the platelets form a very thin layer between the cell fractions (other more sophisticated methods are also available for such analyses). Normal hematocrit is approximately 45% in men and 42% in women. The total volume of blood in an average-sized individual (70 kg) is approximately 5.5 l; hence the average red cell volume would be roughly 2.5 l. Since the fraction containing both leukocytes and platelets is normally relatively small or negligible, in such an individual, the plasma volume can be estimated to be 3.0 l. Approximately 90% of plasma is water which acts: (1) as a solvent; (2) to suspend the components of blood; (3) in the absorption of molecules and their transport; and (4) in the transport of thermal energy. Proteins make up 7% of the plasma (by weight) and exert a colloid osmotic pressure. Protein types include albumins, globulins (antibodies and immunoglobulins), and fibrinogen. To date, more than 100 distinct plasma proteins have been identified, and each presumably serves a specific function. The other main solutes in plasma include electrolytes, nutrients, gases (some O_2, large amounts of CO_2 and N_2), regulatory substances (enzymes and hormones), and waste products (urea, uric acid, creatine, creatinine, bilirubin, and ammonia).

1.2.2 Blood Vessels

Blood flows throughout the body tissues in blood vessels via bulk flow (i.e., all constituents together and in one direction). An extraordinary degree of blood vessel branching exists within the human body, which ensures that nearly every cell in the body lies within a short distance from at least one of the smallest branches of this system—a capillary. Nutrients and metabolic end products move between the capillary vessels and the surroundings of the cell through the interstitial fluid by diffusion. Subsequent movement of these molecules into a cell is accomplished by both diffusion and mediated transport. Nevertheless, blood flow through all organs can be considered as passive and occurs only because arterial pressure is kept higher than venous pressure via the pumping action of the heart.

In an individual at rest at a given moment, approximately only 5% of the total circulating blood is actually in capillaries. Yet, this volume of blood can be considered to perform the primary functions of the entire cardiovascular system, specifically the supply of nutrients and removal of metabolic end products. The cardiovascular system, as reported by the British physiologist William Harvey in 1628, is a closed loop system, such that blood is pumped out of the heart through one set of vessels (arteries) and then returns to the heart in another (veins).

More specifically, one can consider that there are two closed loop systems which both originate and return to the heart—the pulmonary and systemic circulations (Fig. 1.1). The pulmonary circulation is composed of the

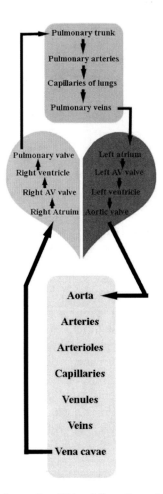

Fig. 1.1 The major paths of blood flow through pulmonary and systemic circulatory systems. AV, atrioventricular

right heart pump and the lungs, whereas the systemic circulation includes the left heart pump which supplies blood to the systemic organs (i.e., all tissues and organs except the gas exchange portions of the lungs). Because the right and left heart pumps function in a series arrangement, both will circulate an identical volume of blood in a given minute (cardiac output, normally expressed in liters per minute).

In the systemic circuit, blood is ejected out of the left ventricle via a single large artery—the aorta. All arteries of the systemic circulation branch from the aorta (this is the largest artery of the body, with a diameter of 2–3 cm) and divide into progressively smaller vessels. The aorta's four principle divisions are the ascending aorta (begins at the aortic valve where, close by, the two coronary artery branches have their origin), arch of the aorta, thoracic aorta, and abdominal aorta.

The smallest of the arteries eventually branch into arterioles. They, in turn, branch into an extremely large number of the smallest diameter vessels—the capillaries (with an estimated 10 billion in the average human body). Next, blood exits the capillaries and begins its return to the heart via the venules. "Microcirculation" is a term coined to collectively describe the flow of blood through arterioles, capillaries, and the venules (Fig. 1.2).

Importantly, blood flow through an individual vascular bed is profoundly regulated by changes in activity of

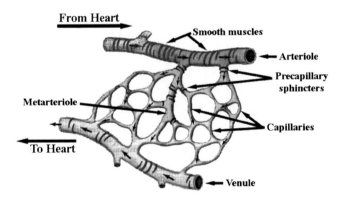

Fig. 1.2 The microcirculation including arterioles, capillaries, and venules. The capillaries lie between, or connect, the arterioles and venules. They are found in almost every tissue layer of the body, but their distribution varies. Capillaries form extensive branching networks that dramatically increase the surface areas available for the rapid exchange of molecules. A metarteriole is a vessel that emerges from an arteriole and supplies a group of 10–100 capillaries. Both the arteriole and the proximal portion of the metarterioles are surrounded by smooth muscle fibers whose contractions and relaxations regulate blood flow through the capillary bed. Typically, blood flows intermittently through a capillary bed due to the periodic contractions of the smooth muscles (5–10 times per minute, vasomotion), which is regulated both locally (metabolically) and by sympathetic control. (Figure modified from Tortora and Grabowski, 2000)

the sympathetic nerves innervating the arterioles. In addition, arteriolar smooth muscle is very responsive to changes in local chemical conditions within an organ (i.e., those changes associated with increases or decreases in the metabolic rates within a given organ).

Capillaries, which are the smallest and most numerous blood vessels in the human body (ranging from 5 to 10 μm in diameter) are also the thinnest walled vessels; an inner diameter of 5 μm is just wide enough for an erythrocyte (red blood cell) to squeeze through. Furthermore, it is estimated that there are 25,000 miles of capillaries in an adult, each with an individual length of about 1 mm.

Most capillaries are little more than a single cell layer thick, consisting of a layer of endothelial cells and a basement membrane. This minimal wall thickness facilitates the capillary's primary function, which is to permit the exchange of materials between cells in tissues and the blood. As mentioned above, small molecules (e.g., O_2, CO_2, sugars, amino acids, and water) are relatively free to enter and leave capillaries readily, promoting efficient material exchange. Nevertheless, the relative permeability of capillaries varies from region to region with regard to the physical properties of these formed walls.

Based on such differences, capillaries are commonly grouped into two major classes: continuous and fenestrated capillaries. In the continuous capillaries, which are more common, the endothelial cells are joined together such that the spaces between them are relatively narrow (i.e., tight intercellular gaps). These capillaries are permeable to substances having small molecular sizes and/or high lipid solubilities (e.g., O_2, CO_2, and steroid hormones) and are somewhat less permeable to small water-soluble substances (e.g., Na^+, K^+, glucose, and amino acids). In fenestrated capillaries, the endothelial cells possess relatively large pores that are wide enough to allow proteins and other large molecules to pass through. In some such capillaries, the gaps between the endothelial cells are even wider than usual, enabling quite large proteins (or even small cells) to pass through. Fenestrated capillaries are primarily located in organs whose functions depend on the rapid movement of materials across capillary walls, e.g., kidneys, liver, intestines, and bone marrow.

If a molecule cannot pass between capillary endothelial cells, then it must be transported across the cell membrane. The mechanisms available for transport across a capillary wall differ for various substances depending on their molecular size and degree of lipid solubility. For example, certain proteins are selectively transported across endothelial cells by a slow, energy-requiring process known as *transcytosis*. In this process, the endothelial cells initially engulf the proteins in the plasma within capillaries by *endocytosis*. The molecules are then ferried across the cells by vesicular transport and released by *exocytosis* into the interstitial fluid on the other side. Endothelial cells generally contain large numbers of endocytotic and exocytotic vesicles, and sometimes these fuse to form continuous vesicular channels across the cell.

The capillaries within the heart normally prevent excessive movement of fluids and molecules across their walls, but several clinical situations have been noted where they may become "leaky." For example, "capillary leak syndrome," which may be induced following cardiopulmonary bypass, may last from hours up to days. More specifically, in such cases, the inflammatory response in the vascular endothelium can disrupt the "gatekeeper" function of capillaries; their increased permeability will result in myocardial edema.

From capillaries, blood throughout the body then flows into the venous system. It first enters the venules which then coalesce to form larger vessels—the veins (Fig. 1.2). Then veins from the various systemic tissues and organs (minus the gas exchange portion of the lungs) unite to produce two major veins—the inferior vena cava (lower body) and superior vena cava (above the heart). By way of these two great vessels, blood is returned to the right heart pump, specifically into the right atrium.

Like capillaries, the walls of the smallest venules are very porous and are the sites where many phagocytic white blood cells emigrate from the blood into inflamed or infected tissues. Venules and veins are also richly innervated by sympathetic nerves and smooth muscles which constrict when these nerves are activated. Thus, increased sympathetic nerve activity is associated with a decreased venous volume, which results in increased cardiac filling and therefore an increased cardiac output (via Starling's Law of the Heart).

Many veins, especially those in the limbs, also feature abundant valves (which are notably also found in the cardiac venous system) which are thin folds of the inter-vessel lining that form flap-like cusps. The valves project into the vessel lumen and are directed toward the heart (promoting unidirectional flow of blood). Because blood pressure is normally low in veins, these valves are important in aiding in venous return by preventing the backflow of blood, which is especially true in the upright individual. In addition, contractions of skeletal muscles (e.g., in the legs) also play a role in decreasing the size of the venous reservoir and thus the return of blood volume to the heart (Fig. 1.3).

The pulmonary circulation is comprised of a similar circuit. Blood leaves the right ventricle in a single great vessel, the pulmonary artery (trunk) which, within a short distance (centimeters), divides into the two main pulmonary arteries, one supplying the right lung and

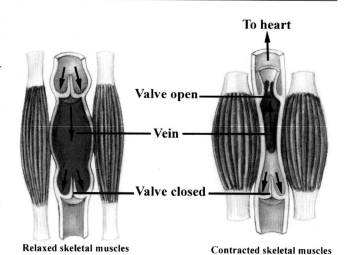

Fig. 1.3 Contractions of the skeletal muscles aid in returning blood to the heart—skeletal muscle pump. While standing at rest, the relaxed vein acts as a reservoir for blood; contractions of limb muscles not only decrease this reservoir size (venous diameter), but also actively force the return of more blood to the heart. Note that the resulting increase in blood flow due to the contractions is only toward the heart due to the valves in the veins

another the left. Once within the lung proper, the arteries continue to branch down to arterioles and then ultimately form capillaries. From there, the blood flows into venules, eventually forming four main pulmonary veins which empty into the left atrium. As blood flows through the lung capillaries, it picks up oxygen supplied to the lungs by breathing air; hemoglobin within the red blood cells is loaded up with oxygen (oxygenated blood).

1.2.3 Blood Flow

The task of maintaining an adequate interstitial homeostasis (the nutritional environment surrounding cells) requires that blood flows almost continuously through each of the millions of capillaries in the body. The following is a brief description of the parameters that govern flow through a given vessel. All blood vessels have certain lengths (L) and internal radii (r) through which blood flows when the pressure in the inlet and outlet is unequal (P_i and P_o, respectively); in other words there is a pressure difference (ΔP) between the vessel ends, which supplies the driving force for flow. Because friction develops between moving blood and the stationary vessels' walls, this fluid movement has a given resistance (vascular), which is the measure of how difficult it is to create blood flow through a vessel. One can then describe a relative relationship between vascular flow, the pressure difference, and resistance (i.e., the basic flow equation):

$$\text{Flow} = \frac{\text{Pressure difference}}{\text{resistance}} \quad \text{or} \quad Q = \frac{\Delta P}{R}$$

where Q is the flow rate (volume/time), ΔP the pressure difference (mmHg), and R the resistance to flow (mmHg × time/volume).

This equation not only may be applied to a single vessel, but can also be used to describe flow through a network of vessels (i.e., the vascular bed of an organ or the entire systemic circulatory system). It is known that the resistance to flow through a cylindrical tube or vessel depends on several factors (described by Poiseuille) including: (1) radius; (2) length; (3) viscosity of the fluid (blood); and (4) inherent resistance to flow, as follows:

$$R = \frac{8L\eta}{\pi r^4}$$

where r is the inside radius of the vessel, L the vessel length, and η the blood viscosity.

It is important to note that a small change in vessel radius will have a very large influence (fourth power) on its resistance to flow; e.g., decreasing vessel diameter by 50% will increase its resistance to flow by approximately 16-fold. If one combines the preceding two equations into one expression, which is commonly known as the Poiseuille equation, it can be used to better approximate the factors that influence flow though a cylindrical vessel:

$$Q = \frac{\Delta P \pi r^4}{8L\eta}$$

Nevertheless, flow will only occur when a pressure difference exists. Hence, it is not surprising that arterial blood pressure is perhaps the most regulated cardiovascular variable in the human body, and this is principally accomplished by regulating the radii of vessels (e.g., primarily within the arterioles and metarterioles) within a given tissue or organ system. Whereas vessel length and blood viscosity are factors that influence vascular resistance, they are not considered variables that can be easily regulated for the purpose of the moment-to-moment control of blood flow. Regardless, the primary function of the heart is to keep pressure within arteries higher than those in veins, hence a pressure gradient to induce flow. Normally, the average pressure in systemic arteries is approximately 100 mmHg, and this decreases to near 0 mmHg in the great caval veins.

The volume of blood that flows through any tissue in a given period of time (normally expressed as ml/min) is called the *local blood flow*. The velocity (speed) of blood flow (expressed as cm/s) can generally be considered to be inversely related to the vascular cross-sectional area, such

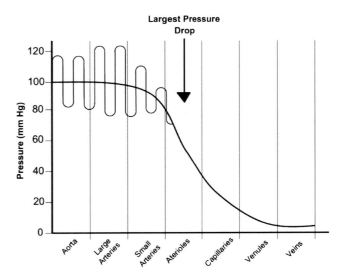

Fig. 1.4 Shown here are the relative pressure changes one could record in the various branches of the human vascular system due to contractions and relaxation of the heart (pulsatile pressure changes). Note that pressure may be slightly higher in the large arteries than that leaving the heart into the aorta due to their relative compliance and diameter properties. The largest drops in pressures occur within the arterioles which are the active regulatory vessels. The pressures in the large veins that return blood to the heart are near zero

that velocity is slowest where the total cross-sectional area is largest. Shown in Fig. 1.4 are the relative pressure drops one can detect through the vasculature; the pressure varies in a given vessel also relative to the active and relaxation phases of the heart function (see below).

1.2.4 Heart

The heart lies in the center of the thoracic cavity and is suspended by its attachment to the great vessels within a fibrous sac known as the *pericardium*; note that humans have relatively thick-walled pericardiums compared to those of the commonly studied large mammalian cardiovascular models (i.e., canine, porcine, or ovine; see also Chapter 8). A small amount of fluid is present within the sac, *pericardial fluid*, which lubricates the surface of the heart and allows it to move freely during function (contraction and relaxation). The pericardial sac extends upward enclosing the proximal portions of the great vessels (see also Chapters 4 and 5).

The pathway of blood flow through the chambers of the heart is indicated in Fig. 1.5. Recall that venous blood returns from the systemic organs to the right atrium via the superior and inferior venae cavae. It next passes through the tricuspid valve into the right ventricles and from there is pumped through the pulmonary valve into the pulmonary artery. After passing through the

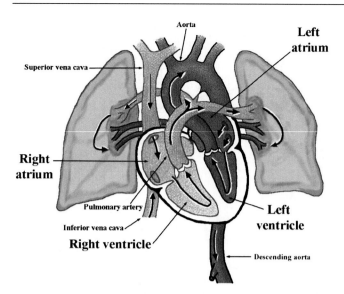

Fig. 1.5 Pathway of blood flow through the heart and lungs. Note that the pulmonary artery (trunk) branches into left and right pulmonary arteries. There are commonly four main pulmonary veins that return blood from the lungs to the left atrium. (Modified from Tortora and Grabowski, 2000)

pulmonary capillary beds, the oxygenated pulmonary venous blood returns to the left atrium through the pulmonary veins. The flow of blood then passes through the mitral valve into the left ventricle and is pumped through the aortic valve into the aorta.

In general, the gross anatomy of the right heart pump is considerably different from that of the left heart pump, yet the pumping principles of each are primarily the same. The ventricles are closed chambers surrounded by muscular walls, and the valves are structurally designed to allow flow in only one direction. The cardiac valves passively open and close in response to the direction of the pressure gradient across them.

The myocytes of the ventricles are organized primarily in a circumferential orientation; hence when they contract, the tension generated within the ventricular walls causes the pressure within the chamber to increase. As soon as the ventricular pressure exceeds the pressure in the pulmonary artery (right) and/or aorta (left), blood is forced out of the given ventricular chamber. This active contractile phase of the cardiac cycle is known as *systole*. The pressures are higher in the ventricles than the atria during systole; hence the tricuspid and mitral (atrioventricular) valves are closed. When the ventricular myocytes relax, the pressure in the ventricles falls below that in the atria, and the atrioventricular valves open; the ventricles refill and this phase is known as *diastole*. The aortic and pulmonary (semilunar or outlet) valves are closed during diastole because the arterial pressures (in the aorta and pulmonary artery) are greater than the intraventricular pressures. Shown in Fig. 1.6 are the average pressures within the

various chambers and great vessels of the heart. For more details on the cardiac cycle, see Chapter 18.

The effective pumping action of the heart requires that there be a precise coordination of the myocardial contractions (millions of cells), and this is accomplished via the conduction system of the heart. Contractions of each cell are normally initiated when electrical excitatory impulses (action potentials) propagate along their surface membranes. The myocardium can be viewed as a functional syncytium; action potentials from one cell conduct to the next cell via the gap junctions. In the healthy heart, the normal site for initiation of a heartbeat is within the sinoatrial node, located in the right atrium. For more details on this internal electrical system, refer to Chapter 11.

The heart normally functions in a very efficient fashion and the following properties are needed to maintain this effectiveness: (1) the contractions of the individual myocytes must occur at regular intervals and be synchronized (not arrhythmic); (2) the valves must fully open (not stenotic); (3) the valves must not leak (not insufficient or regurgitant); (4) the ventricular contractions must be forceful (not failing or lost due to an ischemic event); and (5) the ventricles must fill adequately during diastole (no arrhythmias or delayed relaxation).

1.2.5 Regulation of Cardiovascular Function

Cardiac output in a normal individual at rest ranges between 4 and 6 l/min, but during severe exercise the heart may be required to pump three to four times this amount. There are two primary modes by which the blood volume pumped by the heart, at any given moment, is regulated: (1) intrinsic cardiac regulation, in response to changes in the volume of blood flowing into the heart; and (2) control of heart rate and cardiac contractility by the autonomic nervous system. The intrinsic ability of the heart to adapt to changing volumes of inflowing blood is known as the *Frank–Starling* mechanism (law) of the heart, named after two great physiologists of a century ago.

In general, the Frank–Starling response can simply be described—the more the heart is stretched (an increased blood volume), the greater will be the subsequent force of ventricular contraction and, thus, the amount of blood ejected through the aortic valve. In other words, within its physiological limits, the heart will pump out nearly all the blood that enters it without allowing excessive damming of blood in veins. The underlying basis for this phenomenon is related to the optimization of the lengths of "sarcomeres," the functional subunits of striate muscle; there is optimization in the potential for the contractile

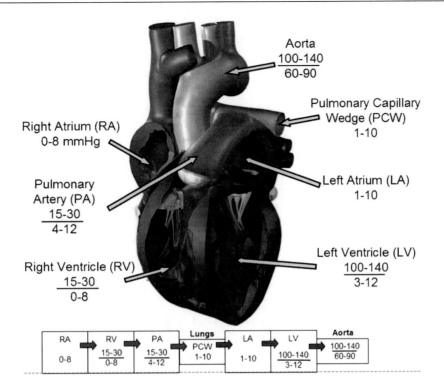

Fig. 1.6 Average relative pressures within the various chambers and great vessels of the heart. During filling of the ventricles the pressures are much lower and, upon the active contraction, they will increase dramatically. Relative pressure ranges that are normally elicited during systole (active contraction; ranges noted above lines) and during diastole (relaxation; ranges noted below lines) are shown for the right and left ventricles, right and left atria, the pulmonary artery and pulmonary capillary wedge, and aorta. Shown at the *bottom* of this figure are the relative pressure changes one can detect in a normal healthy heart as one moves from the right heart through the left heart and into the aorta; this flow pattern is the series arrangement of the two-pump system

proteins (actin and myosin) to form "crossbridges". It should also be noted that "stretch" of the right atrial wall (e.g., because of an increased venous return) can directly increase the rate of the sinoatrial node by 10–20%; this also aids in the amount of blood that will ultimately be pumped per minute by the heart. For more details on the contractile function of heart, refer to Chapter 10.

The pumping effectiveness of the heart is also effectively controlled by the sympathetic and parasympathetic components of the autonomic nervous system. There is extensive innervation of the myocardium by such nerves (for more details on innervation see Chapter 12). To get a feel for how effective the modulation of the heart by this innervation is, investigators have reported that cardiac output often can be increased by more than 100% by sympathetic stimulation and, by contrast, output can be nearly terminated by strong parasympathetic (vagal) stimulation.

Cardiovascular function is also modulated through reflex mechanisms that involve baroreceptors, the chemical composition of the blood, and via the release of various hormones. More specifically, "baroreceptors," which are located in the walls of some arteries and veins, exist to monitor the relative blood pressure. Those specifically located in the carotid sinus help to reflexively maintain normal blood pressure in the brain, whereas those located in the area of the ascending arch of the aorta help to govern general systemic blood pressure (for more details, see Chapters 12, 13, and 19).

Chemoreceptors that monitor the chemical composition of blood are located close to the baroreceptors of the carotid sinus and arch of the aorta, in small structures known as the carotid and aortic bodies. The chemoreceptors within these bodies detect changes in blood levels of O_2, CO_2, and H^+. Hypoxia (a low availability of O_2), acidosis (increased blood concentrations of H^+), and/or hypercapnia (high concentrations of CO_2) stimulate the chemoreceptors to increase their action potential firing frequencies to the brain's cardiovascular control centers. In response to this increased signaling, the central nervous system control centers (hypothalamus), in turn, cause an increased sympathetic stimulation to arterioles and veins, producing vasoconstriction and a subsequent increase in blood pressure. In addition, the chemoreceptors simultaneously send neural input to the respiratory control centers in the brain, to induce the appropriate control of respiratory function (e.g., increase O_2 supply and reduce CO_2 levels). Features of this hormonal regulatory system include: (1) the renin–angiotensin–aldosterone system; (2) the release of epinephrine and norepinephrine; (3) antidiuretic hormones; and (4) atrial natriuretic peptides (released from the atrial heart cells). For details on this complex regulation, refer to Chapter 13.

The overall functional arrangement of the blood circulatory system is shown in Fig. 1.7. The role of the heart needs to be considered in three different ways: as the right pump, as the left pump, and as the heart muscle tissue which has its own metabolic and flow requirements. As described above, the pulmonary (right heart) and system (left heart) circulations are arranged in a series (see also Fig. 1.6). Thus, cardiac output increases in each at the same rate; hence an increased systemic need for a greater cardiac output will automatically lead to a greater flow of blood through the lungs (simultaneously producing a greater potential for O_2 delivery).

In contrast, the systemic organs are functionally arranged in a parallel arrangement; hence, (1) nearly all systemic organs receive blood with an identical composition (arterial blood) and (2) the flow through each organ can be and is controlled independently. For example, during exercise, the circulatory response is an increase in blood flow through some organs (e.g., heart, skeletal muscle, brain) but not others (e.g., kidney and gastrointestinal system). The brain, heart, and skeletal muscles typify organs in which blood flows solely to supply the metabolic needs of the tissue; they do not recondition the blood.

The blood flow to the heart and brain is normally only slightly greater than that required for their metabolism; hence small interruptions in flow are not well tolerated. For example, if coronary flow to the heart is interrupted, electrical and/or functional (pumping ability) activities will noticeably be altered within a few beats. Likewise, stoppage of flow to the brain will lead to unconsciousness within a few seconds and permanent brain damage can occur in as little as 4 min without flow. The flow to skeletal muscles can dramatically change (flow can increase from 20 to 70% of total cardiac output) depending on use, and thus their metabolic demand.

Many organs in the body perform the task of continually reconditioning the circulating blood. Primary organs performing such tasks include: (1) the lungs (O_2 and CO_2 exchange); (2) the kidneys (blood volume and electrolyte composition, Na^+, K^+, Ca^{2+}, Cl^-, and phosphate ions); and (3) the skin (temperature). Blood-conditioning organs can often withstand, for short periods of time, significant reductions of blood flow without subsequent compromise.

1.2.6 The Coronary Circulation

In order to sustain viability, it is not possible for nutrients to diffuse from the chambers of the heart through all the layers of cells that make up the heart tissue. Thus, the coronary circulation is responsible for delivering blood to the heart tissue itself (the myocardium). The normal heart functions almost exclusively as an aerobic organ with little capacity for anaerobic metabolism to produce energy. Even during resting conditions, 70–80% of the oxygen available within the blood circulating through the coronary vessels is extracted by the myocardium.

It then follows that because of the limited ability of the heart to increase oxygen availability by further increasing oxygen extraction, increases in myocardial demand for oxygen (e.g., during exercise or stress) must be met by equivalent increases in coronary blood flow. Myocardial ischemia results when the arterial blood supply fails to meet the needs of the heart muscle for oxygen and/or metabolic substrates. Even mild cardiac ischemia can result in anginal pain, electrical changes (detected on an electrocardiogram), and the cessation of regional cardiac contractile function. Sustained ischemia within a given myocardial region will most likely result in an infarction.

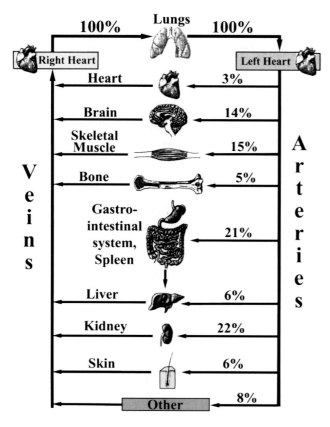

Fig. 1.7 A functional representation of the blood circulatory system. The percentages indicate the approximate relative percentage of the cardiac output that is delivered, at a given moment in time, to the major organ systems within the body

As noted above, as in any microcirculatory bed, the greatest resistance to coronary blood flow occurs in the arterioles. Blood flow through such vessels varies approximately with the fourth power of these vessels' radii; hence, the key regulated variable for the control of coronary blood flow is the degree of constriction or dilatation of coronary arteriolar vascular smooth muscle. As with all systemic vascular beds, the degree of coronary arteriolar smooth muscle tone is normally controlled by multiple independent negative feedback loops. These mechanisms include various neural, hormonal, local non-metabolic, and local metabolic regulators.

It should be noted that the local metabolic regulators of arteriolar tone are usually the most important for coronary flow regulation; these feedback systems involve oxygen demands of the local cardiac myocytes. In general, at any point in time, coronary blood flow is determined by integrating all the different controlling feedback loops into a single response (i.e., inducing either arteriolar smooth muscle constriction or dilation). It is also common to consider that some of these feedback loops are in opposition to one another. Interestingly, coronary arteriolar vasodilation from a resting state to one of intense exercise can result in an increase of mean coronary blood flow from approximately 0.5–4.0 ml/min/g. For more details on metabolic control of flow, see Chapters 13 and 19.

As with all systemic circulatory vascular beds, the aortic and/or arterial pressures (perfusion pressures) are vital for driving blood through the coronaries, and thus need to be considered as additional important determinants of coronary flow. More specifically, coronary blood flow varies directly with the pressure across the coronary microcirculation, which can be essentially considered as the immediate aortic pressure, since coronary venous pressure is near zero. However, since the coronary circulation perfuses the heart, some very unique determinants for flow through these capillary beds may also occur; during systole, myocardial extravascular compression causes coronary flow to be near zero, yet it is relatively high during diastole (note that this is the opposite of all other vascular beds in the body). For more details on the coronary vasculature and its function, refer to Chapter 7.

1.2.7 Lymphatic System

The lymphatic system represents an accessory pathway by which large molecules (proteins, long-chain fatty acids, etc.) can reenter the general circulation and thus not accumulate in the interstitial space. If such particles accumulate in the interstitial space, then filtration forces exceed reabsorptive forces and edema occurs. Almost all tissues in the body have lymph channels that drain excessive fluids from the interstitial space (exceptions include portions of skin, the central nervous system, the endomysium of muscles, and bones which have pre-lymphatic channels).

The lymphatic system begins in various tissues with blind-end-specialized lymphatic capillaries that are roughly the size of regular circulatory capillaries, but they are less numerous (Fig. 1.8). However, the lymphatic capillaries are very porous and, thus, can easily collect the large particles within the interstitial fluid known as lymph. This fluid moves through the converging lymphatic vessels and is filtered through lymph nodes where bacteria and other particulate matter are removed. Foreign particles that are trapped in the lymph nodes can then be destroyed (phagocytized) by tissue macrophages which line a meshwork of sinuses that lie within. Lymph nodes also contain T and B lymphocytes which can destroy foreign substances by a variety of immune responses. There are approximately 600 lymph nodes located along the lymphatic vessels; they are 1–25 mm long (bean shaped) and covered by a capsule of dense connective tissue. Lymph flow is typically unidirectional through the nodes (Fig. 1.8).

The lymphatic system is also one of the major routes for absorption of nutrients from the gastrointestinal tract (particularly for the absorption of fat- and lipid-soluble vitamins A, D, E, and K). For example, after a fatty meal, lymph in the thoracic duct may contain as much as 1–2% fat.

The majority of lymph then reenters the circulatory system in the thoracic duct which empties into the venous

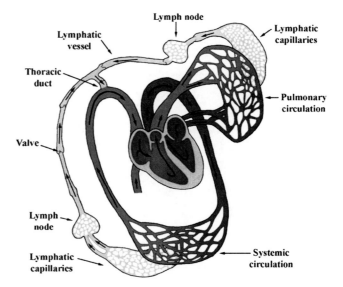

Fig. 1.8 Schematic diagram showing the relationship between the lymphatic system and the cardiopulmonary system. The lymphatic system is unidirectional, with fluid flowing from interstitial space back to the general circulatory system. The sequence of flow is from blood capillaries (systemic and pulmonary) to the interstitial space, to the lymphatic capillaries (lymph), to the lymphatic vessels, to the thoracic duct, into the subclavian veins (back to the right atrium). (Modified from Tortora and Grabowski, 2000)

system at the juncture of the left internal jugular and subclavian veins (which then enters into the right atrium; see Chapters 4 and 5). The flow of lymph from tissues toward the entry point into the circulatory system is induced by two main factors: (1) higher tissue interstitial pressure and (2) the activity of the lymphatic pump (contractions within the lymphatic vessels themselves, contractions of surrounding muscles, movement of parts of the body, and/or pulsations of adjacent arteries). In the largest lymphatic vessels (e.g., thoracic duct), the pumping action can generate pressures as high as 50–100 mmHg. Valves located in the lymphatic vessel, like in veins, aid in the prevention of the backflow of lymph.

Approximately 2.5 l of lymphatic fluid enters the general blood circulation (cardiopulmonary system) each day. In the steady state, this indicates a total body net transcapillary fluid filtration rate of 2.5 l/day. When compared with the total amount of blood that circulates each day (approximately 7,000 l/day), this seems almost insignificant; however, blockage of such flow will quickly cause serious edema. Therefore, the lymphatic circulation plays a critical role in keeping the interstitial protein concentration low and also in removing excess capillary filtrate from tissues throughout the body.

1.2.8 Summary

The rapid transport of molecules over long distances between internal cells, the body surface, and/or various specialized tissues and organs is the primary function of the cardiovascular system. This body-wide transport system is composed of several major components: blood, blood vessels, the heart, and the lymphatic system. When functioning normally, this system adequately provides for the wide-ranging activities that a human can accomplish. Failure in any of these components can lead to grave consequence. Many of the subsequent chapters in this book will cover, in greater detail, the anatomical, physiological, and pathophysiological features of the cardiovascular system. Furthermore, the normal and abnormal performance of the heart and various clinical treatments to enhance function will be discussed.

General References and Suggested Reading

Alexander RW, Schlant RC, Fuster V, eds. Hurst's the heart, arteries and veins. 9th ed. New York, NY: McGraw-Hill, 1998.

Germann WJ, Stanfield CL, eds. Principles of human physiology. San Francisco, CA: Pearson Education, Inc./Benjamin Cummings, 2002.

Guyton AC, Hall JE, eds. Textbook of medical physiology. 10th ed. Philadelphia, PA: W.B. Saunders Co., 2000.

Mohrman DE, Heller LJ, eds. Cardiovascular physiology. 5th ed. New York, NY: McGraw-Hill, 2003.

Tortora GJ, Grabowski SR, eds. Principles of anatomy and physiology. 9th ed. New York, NY: John Wiley & Sons, Inc., 2000.

http://www.vhlab.umn.edu/atlas

Part II
Anatomy

Chapter 2
Attitudinally Correct Cardiac Anatomy

Alexander J. Hill

Abstract Anatomy is one of the oldest branches of medicine. Throughout time, the discipline has been served well by a universal system for describing structures based on the "anatomic position." Unfortunately, cardiac anatomy has been a detractor from this long-standing tradition, and has been incorrectly described using confusing and inappropriate nomenclature. This is most likely due to the examination of the heart in the "valentine position," in which the heart stands on its apex as opposed to how it is actually oriented in the body. The description of the major coronary arteries, such as the "anterior descending" and "posterior descending," is attitudinally incorrect; as the heart is oriented in the body, the surfaces are actually superior and inferior. An overview of attitudinally correct human anatomy, the problem areas, and the comparative aspects of attitudinally correct anatomy will be presented in this chapter.

Keywords Cardiac anatomy · Attitudinally correct nomenclature · Comparative anatomy

2.1 Introduction

Anatomy is one of the oldest branches of medicine, with historical records dating back at least as far as the 3rd century BC. Cardiac anatomy has been a continually explored topic throughout this time, and there are still publications on new facets of cardiac anatomy being researched and reported today. One of the fundamental tenets of the study of anatomy has been the description of the structure based on the universal orientation, otherwise termed the "anatomic position" which depicts the subject facing the observer, and is then divided into three orthogonal planes (Fig. 2.1). Each plane divides the body or individual structure within the body (such as the heart) into two portions. Thus, using all three planes, each portion of the anatomy can be localized precisely within the body. These three planes are called: (1) the *sagittal* plane, which divides the body into right and left portions; (2) the *coronal* plane, which divides the body into anterior and posterior portions; and (3) the *transverse* plane, which divides the body into superior and inferior portions. Each plane can then be viewed as a slice through a body or organ and will also have specific terms that can be used to define the structures within. If one is looking at a sagittal cut through a body, the observer would be able to describe structures as being anterior or posterior and superior or inferior. On a coronal cut, the structures would be able to be described as superior or inferior and right or left. Finally, on a transverse cut, anterior or posterior and right or left would be used to describe the structures. This terminology should be used regardless of the actual position of the body. For example, assume an observer is looking down at a table and does not move. If a body is lying on its back on this table, the anterior surface would be facing upwards toward the observer. Now, if the body is lying on its left side, the right surface of the body would be facing upwards toward the observer, and the anterior surface would be facing toward the right. Regardless of how the body is moved, the orthogonal planes used to describe it move with the body and do not stay fixed in space. The use of this position and universal terms to describe structure have served anatomists well and have led to easier discussion and translation of findings amongst different investigators.

2.2 The Problem: Cardiac Anatomy Does Not Play by the Rules

As described above, the use of the "anatomic position" has stood the test of time and is still used to describe the position of structures within the body. However, within

A.J. Hill (✉)
Universitty of Minnesota, Departments of Biomedical Engineering and Surgery, and Medtronic, Inc.,
8200 Coral Sea St. NE, MVS84, Mounds View, MN 55112, USA
e-mail: alex.hill@medtronic.com

P.A. Iaizzo (ed.), *Handbook of Cardiac Anatomy, Physiology, and Devices*, DOI 10.1007/978-1-60327-372-5_2,

Fig. 2.1 Illustration showing the anatomic position. Regardless of the position of the body or organ upon examination, the anatomy of an organ or the whole should be described as if observed from this vantage point. The anatomic position can be divided by three separate orthogonal planes: (1) the sagittal plane, which divides the body into right and left portions; (2) the coronal plane, which divides the body into anterior and posterior portions; and (3) the transverse plane, which divides the body into superior and inferior portions

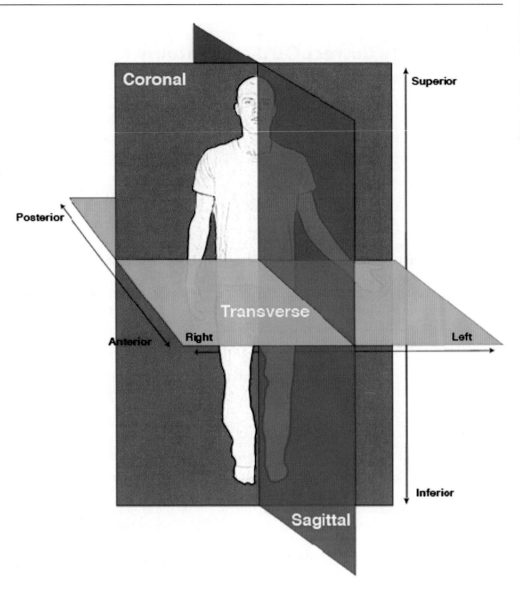

approximately the last 50 years, descriptions of cardiac anatomy have not adhered to the proper use of these terms, and rather have been replaced with inappropriate descriptors. There are two major reasons for this: (1) many descriptions of heart anatomy have been done with the heart removed from the body and incorrectly positioned during examination and (2) a "heart-centric" orientation has been preferred to describe the structures. These two reasons are interrelated and negatively affect the proper description of cardiac anatomy. Typically, when the heart is examined outside the body it has been placed on its apex into the so-called "valentine position," which causes the heart to appear similar to the common illustration of the heart used routinely in everything from greeting cards to instant messenger icons (Fig. 2.2). It is this author's opinion that this problem has been confounded by the comparative positional differences seen between humans and large mammalian cardiac models used to help understand human cardiac anatomy and physiology. As you will see in the following sections, the position of the heart within a sheep thorax is very similar to the valentine position used to examine human hearts. I will point out that I have been guilty of describing structures in such a manner, as is evidenced by some of the images available in the Visible Heart® Viewer CD (Fig. 2.2), as have countless others as seen in the scientific literature and many textbooks (even including this one). Regardless, it is a practice I have since given up and have reverted to the time-honored method using the "anatomic position."

Fig. 2.2 A human heart viewed from the so-called anterior position, demonstrating the "valentine" heart orientation used by many to incorrectly describe anatomy. The *red line* surrounding the heart is the characteristic symbol, which was theoretically derived from observing the heart in the orientation

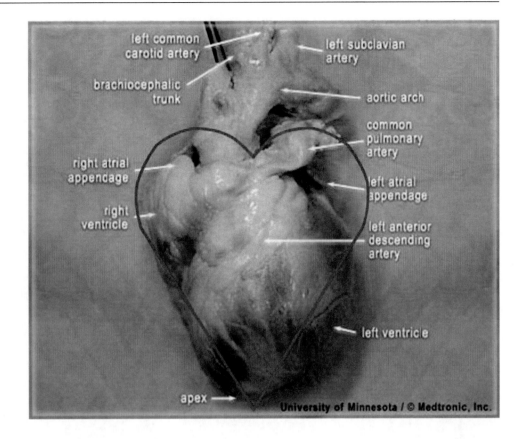

Further impacting the incorrect description of cardiac anatomy is the structure of the heart itself. A common practice in examining the heart is to cut the ventricular chambers in the short axis, which is perpendicular to the long axis of the heart which runs from the base to the apex. This practice is useful in the examination of the ventricular chambers, but the cut plane is typically confused as actually being transverse to the body when it is, in most cases, an oblique plane. The recent explosion of tomographic imaging techniques, such as magnetic resonance imaging (MRI) and computed tomography (CT), in which cuts such as the one just described are commonly made, have further fueled the confusion.

Nevertheless, this incorrect use of terminology to describe the heart can be considered to impact a large and diverse group of individuals. Practitioners of medicine, such as interventional cardiologists and electrophysiologists are affected, as are scientists investigating the heart and engineers designing medical devices. It is considered here that describing terms in a more consistent manner, and thus using the appropriate terminology, would greatly increase the efficiency of interactions between these groups.

It should be noted that there have been a few exceptions to this rule, in that attempts have been made to promote proper use of anatomic terminology. Most notable are the works of Professor Robert Anderson [1–4],

although he will also admit that he has been guilty of using incorrect terminology in the past. Other exceptions to this rule are Wallace McAlpine's landmark cardiac anatomy textbook [5] and an excellent textbook by Walmsley and Watson [6].

In addition to these exceptions, a small group of scientists and physicians has begun to correct the many misnomers that have been used to describe the heart in the recent past; this is the major goal of this chapter. A description of the correct position of the body within the heart will be presented as well as specific problem areas, such as the coronary arteries where terms such as left anterior descending artery are most obviously incorrect and misleading.

2.3 The Attitudinally Correct Position of the Human Heart

The following set of figures used to describe the correct position of the heart within the body was created from 3D volumetric reconstructions of magnetic resonance images of healthy humans with normal cardiac anatomy. In Fig. 2.3, the anterior surfaces of two human hearts are shown. Note that in this view of the heart, the major structures visible are the right atrium and right ventricle. In reality, the right ventricle is positioned anteriorly and to the right of the left ventricle. Also, note that the apex of the heart is positioned to the left and is not inferior, as in the valentine position. Furthermore, note that the so-called anterior interventricular sulcus (shown with a red star), in fact, begins superiorly and travels to the left and only slightly anteriorly. Figure 2.4 shows the posterior surfaces of two human hearts, in which the first visible structure is the descending aorta. Anterior to that are the right and left atria. Figure 2.5 shows the inferior or diaphragmatic surfaces of two human hearts, commonly referred to as the posterior surface, based on valentine positioning. The

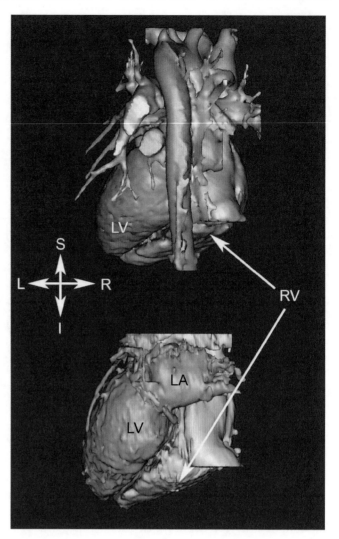

Fig. 2.4 Volumetric reconstructions from magnetic resonance imaging showing the posterior surfaces of two human hearts. The major structures visible are the right and left atrium and the descending aorta (*top image* only). The apex of the heart is positioned to the left and is not inferior as in the valentine position. I, inferior; L, left; LA, left atrium; LV, left ventricle; R, right; RV, right ventricle; S, superior

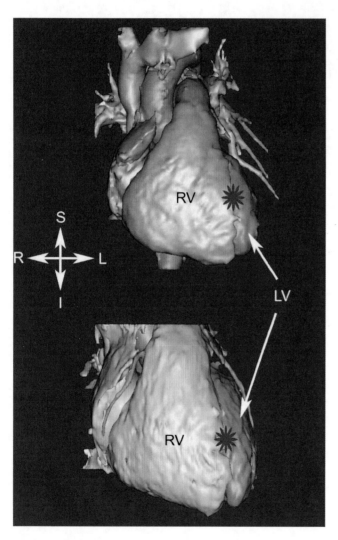

Fig. 2.3 Volumetric reconstructions from magnetic resonance imaging showing the anterior surfaces of two human hearts. The major structures visible are the right atrium and right ventricle. The apex of the heart is positioned to the left and is not inferior as in the valentine position. The so-called anterior interventricular sulcus (shown with a *red star*) in fact begins superiorly and travels to the left and only slightly anteriorly. I, inferior; L, left; LV, left ventricle; R, right; RV, right ventricle; S, superior

inferior caval vein and descending aorta are cut in the short axis; in this region of the thorax, they tend to travel parallel to the long axis of the body. Note that the so-called posterior interventricular sulcus is actually positioned inferiorly (shown with a red star). Figure 2.6 shows a superior view of two human hearts. In this view, the following structures are visible: (1) the superior caval vein; (2) aortic arch and the major arteries arising from it; (3) the free portion of the right atrial appendage; and (4) the pulmonary trunk which, after arising from the right ventricle, runs in the transverse plane before bifurcating into the right and left pulmonary arteries. Also, note that the position of the "anterior" interventricular

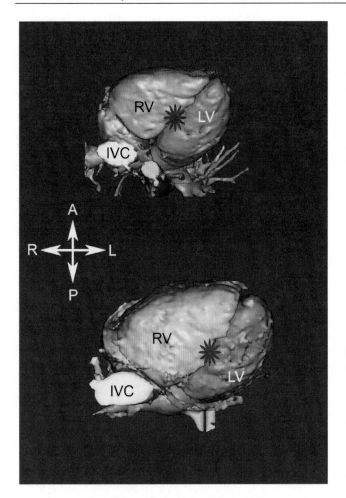

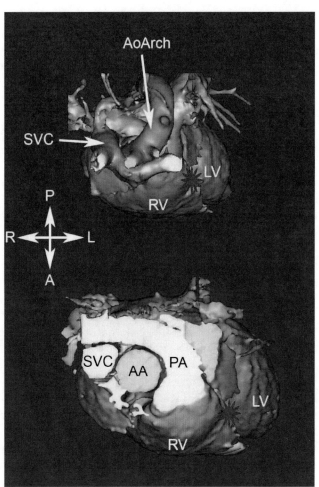

Fig. 2.5 Volumetric reconstructions from magnetic resonance imaging showing the inferior or diaphragmatic surfaces of two human hearts. This surface is commonly, and incorrectly, referred to as the posterior surface, based on valentine positioning. The inferior caval vein (IVC) and descending aorta are cut in the short axis; in this region of the thorax, they tend to travel parallel to the long axis of the body. The so-called posterior interventricular sulcus is actually positioned inferiorly and is denoted by a *red star*. A, anterior; L, left; LV, left ventricle; P, posterior; R, right; RV, right ventricle

Fig. 2.6 Volumetric reconstructions from magnetic resonance imaging showing the superior surfaces of two human hearts. In this view the following structures are visible: the superior caval vein (SVC), aortic arch (AoArch) and the major arteries arising from it, the free portion of the right atrial appendage, and the pulmonary trunk (PA) which, after arising from the right ventricle, runs in the transverse plane before bifurcating into the right and left pulmonary arteries. Also, note that the position of the "anterior" interventricular sulcus (shown with a *red star*) is more correctly termed superior. A, anterior; AA, ascending aorta; L, left; LV, left ventricle; P, posterior; R, right; RV, right ventricle

sulcus (shown with a red star) is more correctly termed "superior."

2.4 Commonly Used Incorrect Terms

This section will specifically describe a few obvious problem areas in which attitudinally incorrect nomenclature is commonly used: the coronary arteries, myocardial segmentation for depiction of infarcts, and cardiac valve nomenclature.

In the normal case, there are two coronary arteries which arise from the aortic root, specifically from two of the three sinuses of Valsalva. These two coronary arteries

supply the right and left halves of the heart, although there is considerable overlap in supply, especially in the interventricular septum. Nevertheless, the artery which supplies the right side of the heart is aptly termed the "right coronary artery," and the corresponding artery which supplies the left side of the heart is termed the "left coronary artery." Therefore, the sinuses in which these arteries arise can be similarly named the right coronary sinus, left coronary sinus, and for the sinus with no coronary artery, the noncoronary sinus; this convention is commonly used. These arteries then branch as they continue their paths along the heart, with the major arteries commonly following either the atrioventricular or interventricular grooves, with smaller branches extending from them. It is beyond the scope of this chapter to fully engage in a description of the nomenclature for the entire coronary arterial system. However, there are two glaring problems which persist in the nomenclature used to describe the coronary arteries, both of which involve the interventricular grooves. First, shortly after the left coronary artery arises from the left coronary sinus, it bifurcates into the left "anterior descending" and the "left circumflex" arteries. The left "anterior descending" artery follows the so-called "anterior" interventricular groove, which was described previously as being positioned superiorly and to the left and only slightly anteriorly (Fig. 2.3). Second, depending on the individual, either the right coronary artery (80–90%) or the left circumflex supplies the opposite side of the interventricular septum as the left "anterior" descending. Regardless of the parent artery, this artery is commonly called the "posterior" descending artery. However, similar to the so-called "anterior" descending artery, the position of this artery is not posterior but rather inferior (Fig. 2.5).

Now that the courses of the two main coronary arteries are clear, the description of myocardial segmentation needs to be addressed. It is rather interesting that, although clinicians typically call the inferior interventricular artery the posterior descending artery, they often correctly term an infarction caused by blockage in this artery as an inferior infarct. Current techniques used to assess the location and severity of myocardial infarctions include MRI, CT, and 2D, 3D, or 4D cardiac ultrasound. These techniques allow for the clinician to view the heart in any plane or orientation; due to this, a similar confusion in terminology arises. Recently, an American Heart Association working group issued a statement in an attempt to standardize nomenclature for use with these techniques [7]. Upon close examination, this publication correctly terms areas supplied by the inferior interventricular artery as inferior, but incorrectly terms the opposite aspect of the heart as anterior.

Finally, nomenclatures commonly used to describe the leaflets of the atrioventricular valves, the tricuspid, and mitral valves are typically not attitudinally correct. For example, the tricuspid valve is situated between the right atrium and right ventricle, and is so named because, in the majority of cases, there are three major leaflets or cusps. These are currently referred to as the anterior, posterior, and septal leaflets, and were most likely termed in this manner due to examination of the heart in the "valentine" position. Figure 2.7 shows an anterior view of a human heart in an attitudinally correct orientation, with the tricuspid annulus shown in orange. The theorized

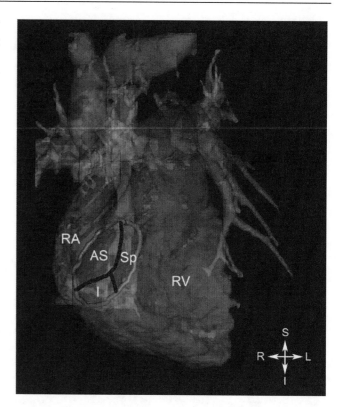

Fig. 2.7 Volumetric reconstruction from magnetic resonance imaging (MRI) showing the anterior surfaces of the right ventricle and atrium of a human heart. The tricuspid annulus is highlighted in *orange*, and was traced on the MRI images. The theorized positions of the commissures between the leaflets are drawn in *red*, and the leaflets are labeled appropriately. AS, anterosuperior; I, inferior; L, left; R, right; RA, right atrium; RV, right ventricle; RV, right ventricle; S, superior; Sp, septal

locations of the commissures between the leaflets are shown in red. In order for the "anterior" leaflet to be truly anterior, the tricuspid annulus would need to be orthogonal to the image. However, the actual location of the annulus is in an oblique plane as shown in the figure, and therefore the leaflets would be more correctly termed anterosuperior, inferior, and septal.

The same is true for the mitral valve, although the terms used to describe it are a bit closer to reality than the tricuspid valve. The mitral valve has two leaflets, commonly referred to as the anterior and posterior. However, Fig. 2.8 shows that the leaflets are not strictly anterior or posterior, or else the plane of the annulus (shown in orange) would be perpendicular to the screen. Therefore, based on attitudinal terms, one would prefer to define these leaflets as anterosuperior and posteroinferior. It should be noted that these leaflets have also been described as aortic and mural, which is less dependent on orientational terms and also technically correct.

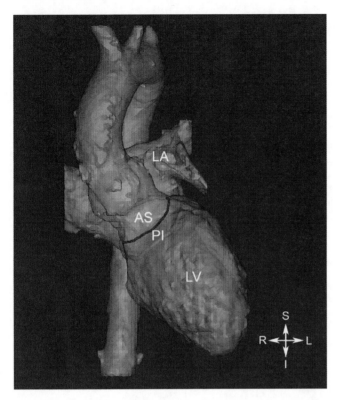

Fig. 2.8 Volumetric reconstruction from magnetic resonance imaging (MRI) showing the anterior surfaces of the left ventricle and atrium of a human heart. The mitral annulus is highlighted in *orange*, and was traced on the MRI images. The theorized positions of the commissures between the leaflets are drawn in *red*, and the leaflets are labeled appropriately. AS, anterosuperior; I, inferior; L, left; LA, left atrium; LV, left ventricle; PI, posteroinferior; R, right; S, superior

2.5 Comparative Aspects of Attitudinally Correct Cardiac Anatomy

In addition to the incorrect terminology used to describe the human heart, translation of cardiac anatomy between human and other species is often further complicated due to differences in the orientation of the heart within the thorax. Compared to the human heart, the commonly used large mammalian heart is rotated so that the apex is aligned with the long axis of the body. Furthermore, the apex of the heart is oriented anteriorly, and is commonly attached to the posterior (dorsal) aspect of the sternum. Further confounding the differences is a different nomenclature. The terms inferior and superior are rarely used and are rather replaced by cranial and caudal. Likewise,

the terms anterior and posterior are commonly replaced with ventral and dorsal. Also see Figs. 6.10 and 6.11 for more information on the relative position of a sheep heart compared to a human heart.

2.6 Summary

As the field of cardiac anatomy continues to play an important role in the practice of medicine and the development of medical devices, it behooves all involved to adopt commonly used terminologies to describe the heart and its proper location in the body. Furthermore, it may be of great utility to describe the cardiac anatomy of major animal models using the same terminology as that of humans, at least when comparisons are being made between species. Finally, due to advances in 3D and 4-D imaging and their growing use in the cardiac arena, a sound foundation of attitudinally correct terms will benefit everyone involved.

References

1. Anderson RH, Becker AE, Allwork SP, et al. Cardiac anatomy: An integrated text and colour atlas. London Edinburgh; New York: Gower Medical Pub; Churchill Livingston, 1980.
2. Anderson RH, Razavi R, Taylor AM. Cardiac anatomy revisited. J Anat 2004;205:159–77.
3. Cook AC, Anderson RH. Attitudinally correct nomenclature. Heart 2002;87:503–6.
4. Cosio FG, Anderson RH, Kuck KH, et al. Living anatomy of the atrioventricular junctions. A guide to electrophysiologic mapping. A Consensus Statement from the Cardiac Nomenclature Study Group, Working Group of Arrhythmias, European Society of Cardiology, and the Task Force on Cardiac Nomenclature from NASPE. Circulation 1999;100:e31–7.
5. McAlpine WA. Heart and coronary arteries: An anatomical atlas for clinical diagnosis, radiological investigation, and surgical treatment. Berlin; New York: Springer-Verlag, 1975.
6. Walmsley R, Watson H. Clinical anatomy of the heart. New York, NY: Edinburgh, Churchill Livingstone (distributed by Longman), 1978.
7. Cerqueira MD, Weissman NJ, Dilsizian V, et al. Standardized myocardial segmentation and nomenclature for tomographic imaging of the heart: A statement for healthcare professionals from the Cardiac Imaging Committee of the Council on Clinical Cardiology of the American Heart Association. Circulation 2002;105:539–42.

Chapter 3
Cardiac Development

Brad J. Martinsen and Jamie L. Lohr

Abstract The primary heart field, secondary heart field, cardiac neural crest, and proepicardial organ are the four major embryonic regions involved in vertebrate heart development. They each make an important contribution to cardiac development with complex developmental timing and regulation. This chapter describes how these regions interact to form the final structure of the heart in relationship to the developmental timeline of human embryology.

Keywords Human heart embryology · Primary heart field · Secondary heart field · Cardiac neural crest · Proepicardial organ · Cardiac development

3.1 Introduction to Human Heart Embryology and Development

The primary heart field, secondary heart field, cardiac neural crest, and the proepicardial organ are the four major embryonic regions involved in the process of vertebrate heart development (Fig. 3.1). They each make an important contribution to cardiac development with their own complex developmental timing and regulation (Table 3.1). The heart is the first internal organ to form and function during vertebrate development and many of the mechanisms are molecularly and developmentally conserved [1]. The description presented here is based on development research from the chick, mouse, frog, and human model systems. Recent research has redefined the primary heart field that gives rise to the main structure of the heart (atria and ventricles); furthermore, it has led to the exciting discovery of the secondary heart field

which gives rise to the outflow tract of the mature heart [2–4]. These discoveries were a critical step in helping us to understand how the outflow tract of the heart forms, a cardiac structure where many congenital heart defects arise, and thus which has important implications for the understanding and prevention of human congenital heart disease [5]. Great strides have also been made in understanding the contribution of the cardiac neural crest and the proepicardial organ to heart development.

3.2 Primary Heart Field and Linear Heart Tube Formation

The cells that will become the heart are among the first cell lineages formed in the vertebrate embryo [6, 7]. By day 15 of human development, the primitive streak has formed [8] and the first mesodermal cells to migrate (gastrulate) through the primitive streak are also the cells fated to become myocytes, or heart cells [9, 10] (Fig. 3.2). These mesodermal cells dedicated for heart development migrate to an anterior and lateral position where they initially form bilateral primary heart fields [11] (Fig. 3.1A). Observations from recent studies in the chick have been reported to dispute the previously held notion of a medial cardiac crescent that bridges the two bilateral primary heart fields [12]. Thus, complete comparative molecular and developmental studies between the chick and mouse will be required to confirm these results. Specifically, the posterior border of the bilateral primary heart field reaches down to the first somite in the lateral mesoderm on both sides of the midline [3, 12] (Fig. 3.1A). At day 18 of human development, the lateral plate mesoderm is split into two layers—somatopleuric and splanchnopleuric [8]. It is the splanchnopleuric mesoderm layer that contains the myocardial and endocardial cardiogenic precursors in the region of the primary heart

B.J. Martinsen (✉)
University of Minnesota, Division of Pediatric Cardiology, Department of Pediatrics, 1-140 MoosT, 515 Delaware St. SE, Minneapolis, MN 55455, USA
e-mail: marti198@umn.edu

Fig. 3.1 The four major
contributors to heart
development illustrated in the
chick model system: primary
heart field, secondary heart
field, cardiac neural crest, and
the proepicardial organ. (**A**)
Day 1 chick embryo (equivalent
to day 20 of human
development). *Red* denotes
primary heart field cells. (**B**)
Day 2.5 chick embryo
(equivalent to approximately 5
weeks of human development).
Color code: *green*=cardiac
neural crest cells;
yellow=secondary heart field
cells; *blue*=proepicardial cells.
(**C**) Day 8 chick heart
(equivalent to approximately 9
weeks of human development).
Color code: *green*=derivatives
of the cardiac neural crest;
yellow=derivatives of the
secondary heart field;
red=derivatives of the primary
heart fields; *blue*=derivatives of
the proepicardial organ.
Ao=aorta; APP=anterior
parasympathetic plexis;
Co=coronary vessels; E=eye;
H=heart; IFT=inflow tract;
LA=left atrium; LV=left
ventricle; Mb=midbrain;
NF=neural folds;
OFT=outflow tract; Otc=otic
vesicle; P=pulmonary artery;
RA=right atrium; RV=right
ventricle; T=trunk

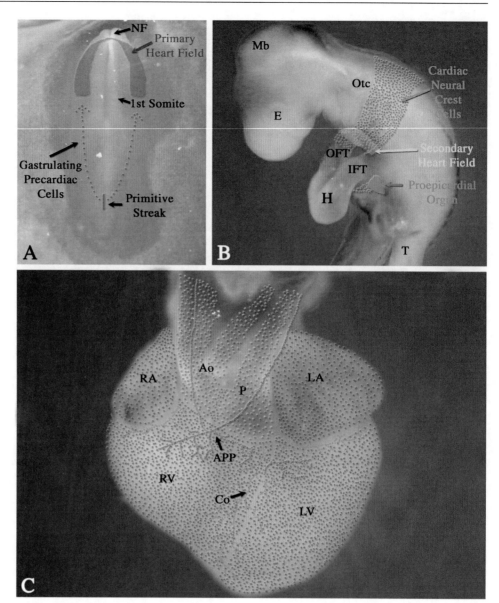

fields, as defined above. Presumptive endocardial cells delaminate from the splanchnopleuric mesoderm and coalesce via vasculogenesis to form two lateral endocardial tubes [13]. During the third week of human development, two bilateral layers of myocardium surrounding the endocardial tubes are brought into the ventral midline during closure of the ventral foregut via cephalic and lateral folding of the embryo [8] (Fig. 3.2A). The lateral borders of the myocardial mesoderm layers are the first heart structures to fuse, followed by the fusion of the two endocardial tubes which then form one endocardial tube surrounded by splanchnopleuric-derived myocardium (Fig. 3.2B, C). The medial borders of the myocardial mesoderm layers are the last to fuse [14]. Thus, the early heart is continuous with noncardiac splanchnopleuric

mesoderm across the dorsal mesocardium (Fig. 3.2C). This will eventually partially break down to form the ventral aspect of the linear heart tube with a posterior inflow (venous pole) and anterior outflow (arterial pole), as well as the dorsal wall of the pericardial cavity [5, 14]. During the fusion of the endocardial tubes, the myocardium secretes an acellular matrix, forming the cardiac jelly layer separating the myocardium and endocardium. By day 22 of human development, the linear heart tube begins to beat. As the human heart begins to fold and loop from day 22 to day 28 (described below), epicardial cells will invest the outer layer of the heart tube (Figs. 3.1B and 3.3A), resulting in a heart tube with four primary layers: endocardium, cardiac jelly, myocardium, and epicardium [8] (Fig. 3.3B).

Table 3.1 Developmental timeline of human heart embryology. Most of the human developmental timing information is from Larson [8], except for the human staging of the secondary heart field and proepicardium which was correlated from other model systems [2–4, 14]

Human development (days)	Developmental process
0	Fertilization
1–4	Cleavage and movement down the oviduct to the uterus
5–12	Implantation of the embryo into the uterus
13–14	Primitive streak formation (midstreak level contains precardiac cells)
15–17	Formation of the three primary germ layers (gastrulation): ectoderm, mesoderm, and endoderm; midlevel primitive streak cells that migrate to an anterior and lateral position form the bilateral *primary heart field*
17–18	Lateral plate mesoderm splits into the somatopleuric mesoderm and splanchnopleuric mesoderm; splanchnopleuric mesoderm contains the myocardial and endocardial cardiogenic precursors in the region of the *primary heart field*
18–26	Neurulation (formation of the neural tube)
20	Cephalocaudal and lateral folding brings the bilateral endocardial tubes into the ventral midline of the embryo
21–22	Heart tube fusion
22	Heart tube begins to beat
22–28	Heart looping and the accretion of cells from the primary and *secondary heart fields*; *proepicardial cells* invest the outer layer of the heart tube and eventually form the epicardium and coronary vasculature; neural crest migration starts
32–37	*Cardiac neural crest* migrates through the aortic arches and enters the outflow tract of the heart
57 +	Outflow tract and ventricular septation complete
Birth	Functional septation of the atrial chambers, as well as the pulmonary and systemic circulatory systems

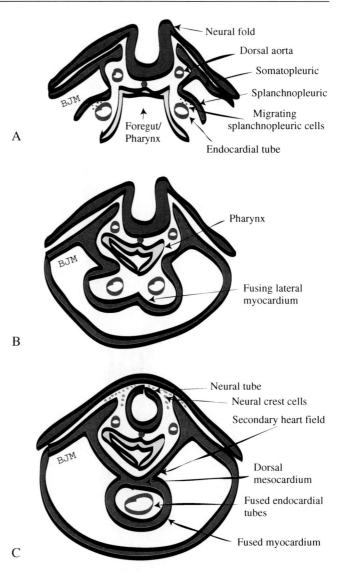

Fig. 3.2 Cross-sectional view of human heart tube fusion. (**A**) Day 20, cephalocaudal and lateral folding brings bilateral endocardial tubes into the ventral midline of the embryo. (**B**) Day 21, start of heart tube fusion. (**C**) Day 22, complete fusion, resulting in the beating primitive heart tube. Color code of the embryonic primary germ layer origin: *blue/purple* = ectoderm; *red* = mesoderm; *yellow* = endoderm

3.3 Secondary Heart Field, Outflow Tract Formation, and Cardiac Looping

A cascade of signals identifying the left and right sides of the embryo is thought to initiate the process of primary linear heart tube looping [15]. The primary heart tube loops to the right of the embryo and bends to allow convergence of the inflow (venous) and outflow (arterial) ends between day 22 and day 28 of human development (Fig. 3.4). This process occurs prior to the division of the heart tube into four chambers and is required for proper alignment and septation of the mature cardiac chambers.

During the looping process, the primary heart tube increases dramatically in length (by four- to five-fold) and this process displaces atrial myocardium posteriorly and superiorly, i.e., dorsal to the forming ventricular chambers [5, 8, 15]. During the looping process, the inflow (venous) pole, atria, and atrioventricular region are added to or accreted from the posterior region of the paired primary heart fields, while the myocardium of proximal outflow tract (conus) and distal outflow tract (truncus) is added to the arterial pole from a recently discovered secondary heart field [2, 3, 16, 17]. The secondary heart field (Figs. 3.1B and 3.2C) is located along the

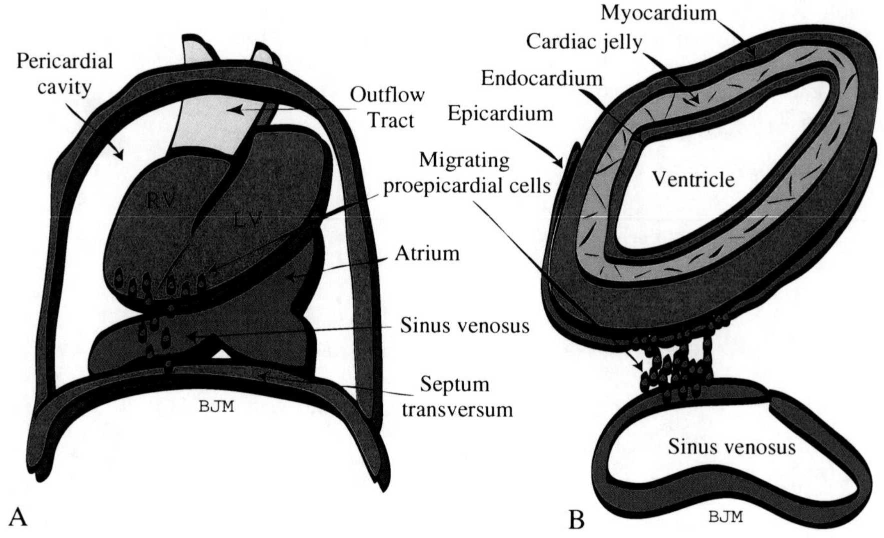

Fig. 3.3 Origin and migration of proepicardial cells. (**A**) Whole mount view of the looping human heart within the pericardial cavity at day 28. Proepicardial cells (*blue dots*) emigrate from the sinus venosus and possibly the septum transversum and then migrate out over the outer surface of the ventricles, eventually surrounding the entire heart. (**B**) Cross-sectional view of the looping heart showing the four layers of the heart: epicardium, myocardium, cardiac jelly, and endocardium. LV=left ventricle; RV=right ventricle

Fig. 3.4 Looping and septation of the human primary linear heart tube. *Blue* and *yellow* regions represent tissue added during the looping process from the primary heart field and secondary heart field, respectively. AO=aorta; AV=atrioventricular; LA=left atrium; LV=left ventricle; RA=right atrium; RV=right ventricle

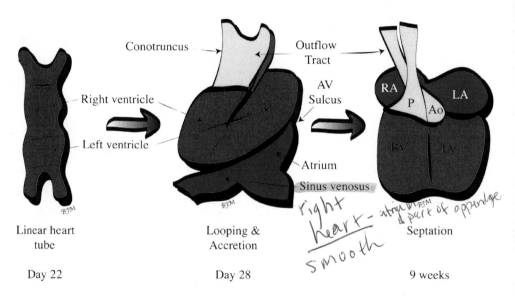

splanchnopleuric mesoderm (beneath the floor of the foregut) at the attachment site of the dorsal mesocardium [2, 3, 14, 16, 17]. During looping, the secondary heart field cells undergo epithelial-to-myocardial transformation at the outflow (arterial) pole and add additional myocardial cells onto the then developing outflow tract. This lengthening of the primary heart tube appears to be an important process for the proper alignment of the inflow and outflow tracts prior to septation. If this process does not occur normally, ventricular septal defects and malpositioning of the aorta may occur [14]. Recent evidence suggests that the secondary heart field may also contribute to the inflow tract, leading some scientists to hypothesize that the secondary heart field contains two regions: (1) an anterior region that contributes to the outflow tract and (2) a posterior region that contributes to the inflow tract, as well as the proepicardial organ

[18–20]. By day 28 of human development, the chambers of the heart are in position and are demarcated by visible constrictions and expansions which denote the sinus venosus, common atrial chamber, atrioventricular sulcus, ventricular chamber, and conotruncus (proximal and distal outflow tracts) [8, 14] (Fig. 3.4).

3.4 Cardiac Neural Crest and Outflow Tract, Atrial, and Ventricular Septation

Once the chambers are in the correct position after looping, extensive remodeling of the primitive vasculature and septation of the heart can occur. The cardiac neural crest is an extracardiac (from outside of the primary or secondary heart field) population of cells that arise from the

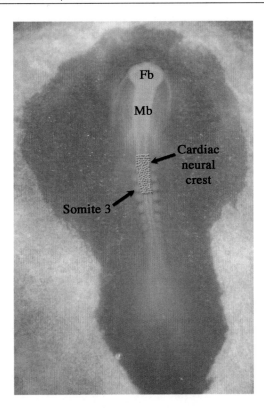

Fig. 3.5 Origin of the cardiac neural crest within a 34-h chick embryo. *Green dots* represent cardiac neural crest cells in the neural folds of hindbrain rhombomeres 6, 7, and 8 (the region of the first three somites up to the midotic placode level). Fb = forebrain; Mb = midbrain

neural tube in the region of the first three somites up to the midotic placode level (rhombomeres 6, 7, and 8) (Fig. 3.5). Cardiac neural crest cells leave the neural tube during weeks 3–4 of human development, then migrate through aortic arches 3, 4, and 6 (Fig. 3.1B) and eventually into the developing outflow tract of the heart (during weeks 5–6). These cells are necessary for complete septation of the outflow tract and ventricles (completed by week 8 of human development), as well as the formation of the anterior parasympathetic plexis which contributes to cardiac innervation and regulation of heart rate [8, 21–25]. Recent evidence also shows that cardiac neural crest cells migrate to the venous pole of the heart as well, and that their role is in the development of the parasympathetic innervation, the leaflets of the atrioventricular valves, and possibly the cardiac conduction system [26–28]. The primitive vasculature of the heart is bilaterally symmetrical but, during weeks 4–8 of human development, there is remodeling of the inflow end of the heart so that all systemic blood flows into the future right atrium [8]. In addition, there is also extensive remodeling of the initially bilaterally symmetrical aortic arch arteries into the great arteries (septation of the aortic and pulmonary vessels) that is dependent on the presence of the

cardiac neural crest [14, 29]. The distal outflow tract (truncus) septates into the aorta and pulmonary trunk via the fusion of two streams or prongs of cardiac neural crest that migrate into the distal outflow tract. In contrast, the proximal outflow tract septates by fusion of the endocardial cushions and eventually joins proximally with the atrioventricular endocardial cushion tissue and the ventricular septum [16, 30]. The endocardial cushions are formed by both atrioventricular canal and outflow tract endocardial cells that migrate into the cardiac jelly, forming bulges or cushions.

Despite its clinical importance, to this date almost nothing is known about the molecular pathways that determine cell lineages in the cardiac neural crest or regulate outflow tract septation [14]. However, it is known that if the cardiac neural crest is removed before it begins to migrate, conotruncal septa completely fail to develop, and blood leaves both the ventricles through what is termed a "persistent truncus arteriosus," a rare congenital heart anomaly that can be seen in humans. Failure of outflow tract septation may also be responsible for other forms of congenital heart disease including transposition of the great vessels, high ventricular septal defects, and tetralogy of Fallot [8, 21, 23]. Additional information on these congenital defects can be found in Chapter 9.

The septation of the outflow tract (conotruncus) is tightly coordinated with the septation of the ventricles and atria to produce a functional heart. All of these septa eventually fuse with the atrioventricular (AV) cushions that also divide the left and right AV canals and serve as a source of cells for the AV valves. Prior to septation, the right atrioventricular canal and right ventricle expand to the right, causing a realignment of the atria and ventricles so that they are directly over each other. This allows venous blood entering from the sinus venosus to flow directly from the right atrium to the presumptive right ventricle without flowing through the presumptive left atrium and ventricle [8, 14]. The new alignment also simultaneously provides the left ventricle with a direct outflow path to the truncus arteriosus and subsequently to the aorta.

Between weeks 4 and 7 of human development, the left and right atria undergo extensive remodeling and are eventually septated. Yet, during the septation process, a right-to-left shunting of oxygenated blood (oxygenated by the placenta) is created via a series of shunts, ducts, and foramens (Fig. 3.6). Prior to birth, the use of the pulmonary system is not necessary, but eventually a complete separation of the systemic and pulmonary circulatory systems will be required for normal cardiac and systemic function [8]. Initially, the right sinus horn is incorporated into the right posterior wall of the primitive atrium, and the trunk of the pulmonary venous system is incorporated

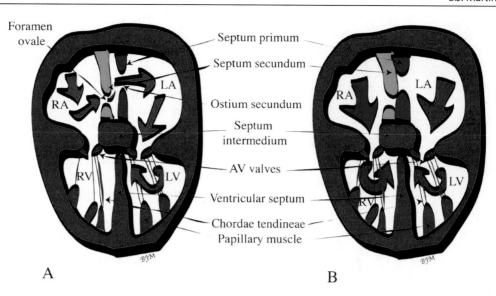

Fig. 3.6 Transition from fetal dependence on the placenta for oxygenated blood to self-oxygenation via the lungs. (**A**) Circulation in the fetal heart before birth. *Pink arrows* show right-to-left shunting of placentally oxygenated blood through the foramen ovale and ostium secundum. (**B**) Circulation in the infant heart after birth. The first breath of the infant and cessation of blood flow from the placenta cause final septation of the heart chambers (closure of the foramen ovale and ostium secundum) and thus separation of the pulmonary and systemic circulatory systems. *Blue arrows* show the pulmonary circulation and the *red arrows* show the systemic circulation within the heart. AV = atrioventricular; LA = left atrium; LV = left ventricle; RA = right atrium; RV = right ventricle

into the posterior wall of the left atrium via a process called "intussusception." At day 26 of human development, a crescent-shaped wedge of tissue called the septum primum begins to extend into the atrium from the mesenchyme of the dorsal mesocardium. As it grows, the septum primum diminishes the ostium primum, a foramen allowing shunting of blood from the right to left atrium. However, programmed cell death near the superior edge of the septum primum creates a new foramen, the ostium secundum, which continues the right-to-left shunting of oxygenated blood. An incomplete, ridged septum secundum with a foramen ovale near the floor of the right atrium forms next to the septum primum, both of which fuse with the septum intermedium of the AV cushions [8]. At the same time as atrial septation is beginning, about the end of the fourth week of human development, the muscular ventricular septum begins to grow toward the septum intermedium (created by the fusion of the atrioventricular cushions), creating a partial ventricular septum. By the end of the ninth week of human development, the outflow tract septum has grown down onto the upper ridge of this muscular ventricular septum and onto the inferior endocardial cushion, completely separating the right and left ventricular chambers.

It is not until after birth, however, that the heart is functionally septated in the atrial region. At birth, dramatic changes in the circulatory system occur due to the transition from fetal dependence on the placenta for oxygenated blood to self-oxygenation via the lungs. During

fetal life, only small amounts of blood are flowing through the pulmonary system because the fluid-filled lungs create high flow resistance, resulting in low pressure and low volume flow into the left atrium from the pulmonary veins. This allows the high volume blood flow coming from the placenta to pass through the inferior vena cava into the right atrium, where it is then directed across the foramen ovale into the left atrium. The oxygenated blood then flows into the left ventricle and directly out to the body via the aorta. At birth, the umbilical blood flow is interrupted, stopping the high volume flow from the placenta. In addition, the alveoli and pulmonary vessels open when the infant takes its first breath, dropping the resistance in the lungs and allowing more flow into the left atrium from the lungs. This reverse in pressure difference between the atria pushes the flexible septum primum against the ridged septum secundum and closes off the foramen ovale and ostium secundum, ideally resulting in the complete septation of the heart chambers [8] (Fig. 3.6).

3.5 Proepicardial Organ and Coronary Artery Development

The last major contributor to vertebrate heart development discussed in this chapter is the proepicardial organ. Prior to heart looping, the primary heart tube consists of endocardium, cardiac jelly, and myocardium. It is not until the start of heart looping that the epicardium surrounds the myocardium, forming the fourth layer of the primary heart tube [31] (Fig. 3.3). This population of cells will eventually give rise to the coronary vasculature. A neural crest origin of the coronary vessels was originally hypothesized, but recent lineage tracing studies have shown that the neural crest gives rise to cells of the tunica media of the aortic and pulmonary trunks, but not the coronary arteries [13, 32]. These experiments eventually showed that the coronary vasculature is derived from the proepicardial organ, a nest of cells in the dorsal mesocardium of the sinus venosus or septum transversum. These cells, which are derived from an independent population of splanchnopleuric mesoderm cells, migrate onto the primary heart tube (Fig. 3.3) between days 22 and 28 of human development, just as the heart initiates looping [8, 14]. Prior to migration, these cells are collectively called the proepicardial organ (or proepicardium). Interestingly, three lineages of the coronary vessel cells (smooth muscle, endothelial, and connective tissue cells) are segregated in the proepicardial organ prior to migration into the heart tube [13, 33]. These cells will coalesce to form coronary vessels de novo via the process of vasculogenesis [34]. Recently, it has also been shown that the epicardium provides a factor needed for normal myocardial development and is a source of cells forming the interstitial myocardium and cushion mesenchyme [14, 19]. It is considered that understanding the embryological origin of the vascular system and its molecular regulation may help to explain the varying susceptibility of different components of the vascular system to atherosclerosis [13, 35].

3.6 Cardiac Maturation

Although the embryonic heart is fully formed and functional by the 11th week of pregnancy, the fetal and neonatal heart continues to grow and mature rapidly, with many clinically relevant changes taking place after birth. During fetal development, or from the time after the embryo is completely formed in the first trimester of pregnancy until birth, the heart grows primarily by the process of cell division [36–39]. Within a few weeks after birth, the predominant mechanism of cardiac growth is cell hypertrophy, so that most existing cardiac cells become larger, rather than increasing significantly in number [36–38]. The exact timing of this process and the mechanisms regulating this change are not yet completely elucidated. It has classically been thought that mature cardiac cells lose the ability to divide; however, recent work suggests that limited amounts of cell division do

occur in adult hearts that have been damaged by ischemia [40]. This finding has led to a renewed interest in understanding the regulation of cell division during cardiac maturation. Additional maturational changes in the fetal and neonatal heart include: (1) alteration in the composition of cardiac muscle; (2) differences in energy production; and (3) maturation of the contractile function. These changes, along with physiologic changes in the transitional circulation, as discussed earlier, significantly affect the treatment of newborns with congenital heart disease, particularly those requiring interventional procedures or cardiac surgery.

The hemodynamic changes associated with birth include a significant increase in left ventricular cardiac output to meet the increased metabolic needs of the newborn infant. This improvement in cardiac output occurs despite the fact that the neonatal myocardium has less muscle mass and less cellular organization than the mature myocardium. The newborn myocardium consists of 30% contractile proteins (mass) and 70% noncontractile mass (membranes, connective tissues, and organelles), in contrast to the adult myocardium which is 60% contractile mass [38]. The myocardial cells of the fetus are rounded, and both the myocardial cells and myofibrils within them are oriented randomly. As the fetal heart matures, these myofibrils increase in size and number, and also orient themselves to the long axis of the rows of cells, which is likely to contribute to improved myocardial function [36]. The fetal myocardial cell contains higher amounts of glycogen than the mature myocardium, suggesting an increased dependence on glucose for energy production. In experiments in nonprimate model systems, the fetal myocardium is able to meet metabolic needs, with lactate and glucose as the primary fuel [41]. In contrast, the preferred substrate for energy metabolism in the adult heart is long-chain fatty acids, although the adult heart is able to utilize carbohydrates as well [41, 42]. This change is presumably triggered in the first few days or weeks of life by an increase in serum long-chain fatty acids with feeding, yet the timing and clinical impact of this change in ill or nonfeeding neonates with cardiovascular disease remain unknown.

In addition to the changes described above, maturing myocardial cells undergo changes in the expression of many innate contractile proteins, which may be responsible for some of the maturational differences in cardiovascular function. For example, the gradual increase in expression of myosin light chain 2 (MLC 2) in the ventricle from the neonatal period through adolescence is considered to be important in humans. In the fetal ventricle, two myosin light-chain forms, MLC 1 and MLC 2, are expressed in equal amounts [38, 43]; MLC 1 is associated with increased contractility and has been documented to increase contractility in isolated muscle from patients with tetralogy of Fallot [44]. After birth, there is a gradual increase in the amount of MLC 2, or the "regulatory" myosin light chain, which has a slower rate of force development but can be phosphorylated to increase calcium-dependent force development in mature cardiac muscle [38, 45]. There is also variability in actin isoform expression during cardiac development. More specifically, the human fetal heart predominantly expresses cardiac alpha-actin, while the more mature human heart expresses skeletal alpha-actin [36, 46]. Furthermore, actin is responsible for interacting with myosin cross bridges and regulating ATPase activity, and work done in the mouse model system suggests that the change to skeletal actin may be one of the mechanisms of enhanced contractility in the mature heart [36, 47, 48]. There are also developmental changes of potential functional significance in the regulatory proteins of the sarcomere. Initially, the fetal heart expresses both alpha- and beta-tropomyosin, a regulatory filament, in nearly equal amounts. After birth, the proportion of beta-tropomyosin decreases and alpha-tropomyosin increases, possibly optimizing diastolic relaxation [36, 49, 50]. In contrast, expression of high levels of beta-tropomyosin in the neonatal heart is associated with early death due to myocardial dysfunction [51]. Lastly, the isoform of the inhibitory troponin, troponin I, changes after birth. The fetal myocardium contains mostly the skeletal isoform of troponin I [36, 52]. After birth, the myocardium begins to express cardiac troponin I, and by approximately 9 months of age only cardiac troponin I is present [36, 53, 54]. Importantly, cardiac troponin I can be phosphorylated to improve calcium responsivity and contractility, which correlates with improved function in the more mature heart. It is thought that the skeletal form of troponin I may serve to protect the fetal and neonatal myocardium from acidosis [38, 47, 55]. The full impact of these developmental changes in contractile proteins and their effect on cardiac function or perioperative treatment of the newborn with heart disease remains unclear at the present time.

Two of the most clinically relevant features of the immature myocardium are its requirement for high levels of extracellular calcium and a decreased sensitivity to beta-adrenergic inotropic agents. The neonatal heart has a decrease in both volume and amounts of functionally mature sarcoplasmic reticulum, which is the intercellular storage site for calcium [36]. The paucity of intracellular calcium storage and release via the sarcoplasmic reticulum in the fetal and neonatal myocardium increases the requirement of the fetal myocardium for extracellular calcium, so that exogenous administration of calcium can be used to augment cardiac contractility in the appropriate

clinical setting. In addition, neonates and infants are significantly more sensitive to calcium channel blocking drugs than older children or adults, and thus may be at risk for severe depression of myocardial contractility with the administration of these agents [36, 38, 56]. Lastly, although data in humans are limited, there appears to be significantly decreased sensitivity to beta-agonist agents in the immature myocardium and also in older children with congenital heart disease [38, 57–59]. This may be due to: (1) a paucity of receptors; (2) sensitization to endogenous catecholamines at birth or with heart failure; or (3) some combination of these or additional factors. Due to this decreased responsiveness to beta-agonists, there is a common requirement for higher doses of beta-agonist inotropic agents in newborns and infants. Note that alternative medications, including phosphodiesterase inhibitors, are often useful adjuncts to improve contractility in newborns with myocardial dysfunction [38].

Although the structure of the heart is complete in the first trimester of pregnancy, cardiac growth and maturation continue to occur in the fetus, newborn, and child. Many of these developmental changes, particularly decreased intracellular calcium stores in the immature sarcoplasmic reticulum and a decreased responsiveness to beta-agonist inotropic agents, significantly impact the care of newborns, infants, and children with congenital heart disease, particularly those requiring surgical intervention early in life.

3.7 Summary of Embryonic Contribution to Heart Development

The contribution of the four major embryonic regions to heart development—primary heart field, secondary heart field, cardiac neural crest, and proepicardial organ—illustrates the complexity of human heart development. Each of these regions has a unique contribution to the heart, but they ultimately depend on each other for the creation of a fully functional organ. Furthermore, a better understanding of the mechanisms of human heart development will provide clues to the etiology of congenital heart disease. The genetic regulatory mechanisms of these developmental processes are just beginning to be characterized. A molecular review of heart development is outside the scope of this chapter, but several wonderful molecular heart reviews have been recently published [14, 60, 61]. A better understanding of the embryological origins of the heart, combined with the characterization of the genes that control heart development [62], will most likely lead to many new clinical applications to treat congenital and/or adult heart disease.

References

1. Srivastava D, Olson EN. A genetic blueprint for cardiac development. Nature 2000;407:221–6.
2. Kelly RG, Brown NA, Buckingham ME. The arterial pole of the mouse heart forms from Fgf10-expressing cells in pharyngeal mesoderm. Dev Cell 2001;1:435–40.
3. Mjaatvedt CH, Nakaoka T, Moreno-Rodriguez R, et al. The outflow tract of the heart is recruited from a novel heart-forming field. Dev Biol 2001;238:97–109.
4. Waldo KL, Kumiski DH, Wallis KT, et al. Conotruncal myocardium arises from a secondary heart field. Development 2001;128:3179–88.
5. Kelly RG, Buckingham ME. The anterior heart-forming field: Voyage to the arterial pole of the heart. Trends Genet 2002;18:210–6.
6. Hatada Y, Stern CD. A fate map of the epiblast of the early chick embryo. Development 1994;120:2879–89.
7. Yutzey KE, Kirby ML. Wherefore heart thou? Embryonic origins of cardiogenic mesoderm. Dev Dyn 2002;223:307–20.
8. Sherman LS, Potter SS, Scott WJ, eds. Human embryology. 3rd ed. New York: Churchill Livingstone, 2001.
9. Garcia-Martinez V, Schoenwolf GC. Primitive streak origin of the cardiovascular system in avian embryos. Dev Biol 1993;159:706–19.
10. Psychoyos D, Stern CD. Fates and migratory routes of primitive streak cells in the chick embryo. Development 1996;122:1523–34.
11. DeHaan RL. Organization of the cardiogenic plate in the early chick embryo. Acta Embryol Morphol Exp 1963;6:26–38.
12. Ehrman LA, Yutzey KE. Lack of regulation in the heart forming region of avian embryos. Dev Biol 1999;207:163–75.
13. Harvey RP, Rosenthal N. Heart development. 1st ed. San Diego: Academic Press, 1999.
14. Kirby ML. Molecular embryogenesis of the heart. Pediatr Dev Pathol 2002;23:537–44.
15. Lohr JL, Yost JH. Vertebrate model systems in the study of early heart development: Xenopus and Zebrafish. Am J Med Genet Semin Med Genet 2000;97:248–57.
16. Waldo K, Miyagawa-Tomita S, Kumiski D, Kirby ML. Cardiac neural crest cells provide new insight into septation of the cardiac outflow tract: Aortic sac to ventricular septal closure. Dev Biol 1998;196:129–44.
17. Abu-Issa R, Kirby ML. Heart field: From mesoderm to heart tube. Annu Rev Cell Dev Biol 2007;23:45–68.
18. Kelly RG. Molecular inroads into the anterior heart field. Trends Cardiovasc Med 2005;15:51–6.
19. Gittenberger-de Groot AC, Vrancken Peeters MP, Bergwerff M, Mentink MM, Poelmann RE. Epicardial outgrowth inhibition leads to compensatory mesothelial outflow tract collar and abnormal cardiac septation and coronary formation. Circ Res 2000;87:969–71.
20. Lie-Venema H, van den Akker NMS, Bax NAM, et al. Origin, fate, and function of epicardium-derived cells (EPDCs) in normal and abnormal cardiac development. Sci World J TSW Develop Embryol 2007;7:1777–98. DOI 10.1100/tsw.2007.294.
21. Kirby ML, Gale TF, Stewart DE. Neural crest cells contribute to normal aorticopulmonary septation. Science 1983;220:1059–61.
22. Kirby ML, Stewart DE. Neural crest origin of cardiac ganglion cells in the chick embryo: Identification and extirpation. Dev Biol 1983;97:433–43.
23. Kirby ML, Turnage KL III, Hays BM. Characterization of conotruncal malformations following ablation of "cardiac" neural crest. Anat Rec 1985;213:87–93.
24. O'Rahilly R, Muller F. The development of the neural crest in the human. J Anat 2007;211:335–51.
25. Porras D, Brown CB. Temporal–spatial ablation of neural crest in the mouse results in cardiovascular defects. Dev Dyn 2008;237:153–62.
26. Hildreth V, Webb S, Bradshaw L, Brown NA, Anderson RH, Henderson DJ. Cells migrating from the neural crest contribute to the innervation of the venous pole of the heart. J Anat 2008;212:1–11.
27. Poelmann RE, Jongbloed MR, Molin DG, et al. The neural crest is contiguous with the cardiac conduction system in the mouse embryo: A role in induction? Anat Embryol 2004;208:389–93.
28. Poelmann RE, Gittenberger-de Groot AC. A sub-population of apoptosis prone cardiac neural crest cells targets the venous pole: Multiple functions in heart development? Dev Biol 1999;207:271–86.
29. Bockman DE, Redmond ME, Kirby ML. Alteration of early vascular development after ablation of cranial neural crest. Anat Rec 1989;225:209–17.
30. Waldo KL, Lo CW, Kirby ML. Connexin 43 expression reflects neural crest patterns during cardiovascular development. Dev Biol 1999;208:307–23.
31. Komiyama M, Ito K, Shimada Y. Origin and development of epicardium in the mouse embryo. Anat Embryol 1996;176:183–9.
32. Noden DM, Poelmann RE, Gittenberger-de Groot AC. Cell origins and tissue boundaries during outflow tract development. Trends Cardiovasc Med 1995;5:69–75.
33. Mikawa T, Gourdie RG. Pericardial mesoderm generates a population of coronary smooth muscle cells migrating into the heart along with ingrowth of the epicardial organ. Dev Biol 1996;173:221–32.
34. Noden DM. Origins and assembly of avian embryonic blood vessels. Ann NY Acad Sci 1990;588:236–49.
35. Hood LA, Rosenquist TH. Coronary artery development in the chick: Origin and development of smooth muscle cells, and effects of neural crest ablation. Anat Rec 1992;234:291–300.
36. Anderson PAW. Developmental cardiac physiology and myocardial function. In: Moller JH, Hoffman JIE, eds. Pediatric cardiovascular medicine. New York: Churchill Livingstone, 2000:35–57.
37. Huttenbach YL, Ostrowski ML, Thaller D, Kim HS. Cell proliferation in the growing human heart: MIB-1 immunostaining in preterm and term infants at autopsy. Cardiovasc Pathol 2001;10:119–23.
38. Kern FH, Bengur AR, Bello EA. Developmental cardiac physiology. In: Rogers MC, ed. Textbook of pediatric intensive care. 3rd ed. Baltimore: Lippincott, Williams and Wilkins, 1996:397–423.
39. Kim HD, Kim DJ, Lee IJ, Rah BJ, Sawa Y, Schaper J. Human fetal heart development after mid-term: Morphometry and ultrastructural study. J Mol Cell Cardiol 1992;24:949–65.
40. Beltrami AP, Urbanek K, Kajstura J, et al. Evidence that human cardiac myocytes divide after myocardial infarction. N Engl J Med 2001;344:1750–7.
41. Vick GW, Fisher DA. Cardiac metabolism. In: Garson AJ, Bricker TJ, Timothy J, Fisher DJ, Neish SR, eds. The science and practice of pediatric cardiology. Baltimore: Williams and Wilkens, 1998:155–69.
42. Opie LH. Carbohydrates and lipids. In: Lionel H. Opie, ed. The heart: Physiology and metabolism. New York: Raven Press, 1991:208–46.
43. Price KM, Littler WA, Cummins P. Human atrial and ventricular myosin light-chains subunits in the adult and during development. Biochem J 1980;191:571–80.

44. Morano M, Zacharzowski U, Maier M, et al. Regulation of human heart contractility by essential myosin light chain isoforms. J Clin Invest 1996;98:467–73.

45. Morano I. Tuning the human heart molecular motors by myosin light chains. J Mol Med 1999;77:544–55.

46. Boheler KR, Carrier L, de la Bastie D, et al. Skeletal actin mRNA increases in the human heart during ontogenic development and is the major isoform of control and failing adult hearts. J Clin Invest 1991;88:323–30.

47. Anderson PAW, Kleinman CS, Lister G, Talner N. Cardiovascular function during normal fetal and neonatal development and with hypoxic stress. In: Polin RA, Fox WW, eds. Fetal and neonatal physiology. 2nd ed. Philadelphia: WB Saunders Company, 1998:837–90.

48. Hewett TE, Grupp IL, Grupp G, Robbins J. Alpha-skeletal actin is associated with increased contractility in the mouse heart. Circ Res 1994;74:740–6.

49. Muthuchamy M, Grupp IL, Grupp G, et al. Molecular and physiological effects of overexpressing striated muscle beta-tropomyosin in the adult murine heart. J Biol Chem 1995;270:30593–603.

50. Palmiter KA, Kitada Y, Muthuchamy M, Wieczorek DF, Solaro RJ. Exchange of beta- for alpha-tropomyosin in hearts of transgenic mice induces changes in thin filament response to Ca2 +, strong cross-bridge binding, and protein phosphorylation. J Biol Chem 1996;271:11611–4.

51. Muthuchamy M, Boivin GP, Grupp IL, Wieczorek DF. Beta-tropomyosin overexpression induces severe cardiac abnormalities. J Mol Cell Cardiol 1998;30:1545–57.

52. Kim SH, Kim HS, Lee MM. Re-expression of fetal troponin isoforms in the postinfarction failing heart of the rat. Circ J 2002;66:959–64.

53. Hunkeler NM, Kullman J, Murphy AM. Troponin I isoform expression in human heart. Circ Res 1991;69:1409–14.

54. Purcell IF, Bing W, Marston SB. Functional analysis of human cardiac troponin by the in vitro motility assay: Comparison of adult, fetal and failing hearts. Cardiovasc Res 1999;43:884–91.

55. Morimoto S, Goto T. Role of troponin I isoform switching in determining the pH sensitivity of Ca(2 +) regulation in developing rabbit cardiac muscle. Biochem Biophys Res Commun 2000;267:912–7.

56. Tanaka H, Sekine T, Nishimaru K, Shigenobu K. Role of sarcoplasmic reticulum in myocardial contraction of neonatal and adult mice. Comp Biochem Physiol A Mol Integr Physiol 1998;120:431–8.

57. Buchorn R, Hulpke-Wette M, Ruschewski W, et al. Beta-receptor downregulation in congenital heart disease: A risk factor for complications after surgical repair? Ann Thorac Surg 2002;73:610–3.

58. Schiffmann H, Flesch M, Hauseler C, Pfahlberg A, Bohm M, Hellige G. Effects of different inotropic interventions on myocardial function in the developing rabbit heart. Basic Res Cardiol 2002;97:76–87.

59. Sun LS. Regulation of myocardial beta-adrenergic receptor function in adult and neonatal rabbits. Biol Neonate 1999;76:181–92.

60. Dees E, Baldwin HS. New frontiers in molecular pediatric cardiology. Curr Opin Pediatr 2002;14:627–33.

61. McFadden DG, Olson EN. Heart development: Learning from mistakes. Curr Opin Genet Dev 2002;12:328–35.

62. Martinsen BJ, Groebner NJ, Frasier AJ, Lohr JL. Expression of cardiac neural crest and heart genes isolated by modified differential display. Gene Expr Patterns 2003;3:407–11.

Chapter 4
Anatomy of the Thoracic Wall, Pulmonary Cavities, and Mediastinum

Mark S. Cook, Kenneth P. Roberts, and Anthony J. Weinhaus

Abstract This chapter will review the anatomy of the mediastinum and pulmonary cavities within the thorax and their contents. The wall of the thorax and its associated muscles, nerves, and vessels will be covered in relationship to respiration. The surface anatomical landmarks that designate deeper anatomical structures and sites of access and auscultation will be reviewed. The goal of this chapter is to provide a complete picture of the thorax and its contents, with detailed anatomic descriptions of thoracic structures excluding the heart.

Keywords Thorax · Cardiac anatomy · Thoracic wall · Superior mediastinum · Middle mediastinum · Anterior mediastinum · Posterior mediastinum · Plura · Lungs

4.1 Introduction

The thorax is the body cavity, surrounded by the bony rib cage, that contains the heart and the lungs, the great vessels, the esophagus and trachea, the thoracic duct, and the autonomic innervation for these structures. The inferior boundary of the thoracic cavity is the respiratory diaphragm, which separates the thoracic and abdominal cavities. Superiorly, the thorax communicates with the root of the neck and the upper extremity. The wall of the thorax contains the muscles that assist with respiration and those connecting the upper extremity to the axial skeleton. The wall of the thorax is responsible for protecting the contents of the thoracic cavity and for generating the negative pressure required for respiration. The thorax is covered by muscle, superficial fascia containing the mammary tissue, and skin. A detailed description of cardiac anatomy is the subject of Chapters 5 and 6.

4.2 Overview of the Thorax

Anatomically, the thorax is typically divided into compartments; there are two pulmonary cavities bilaterally, containing the two lungs with their pleural coverings (Fig. 4.1). The space between the pleural cavities is the mediastinum which contains all the other structures found in the thorax. The mediastinum is divided into the superior and inferior compartments by a plane referred to as the "transverse thoracic plane," passing through the mediastinum at the level of the sternal angle and the junction of the T4 and T5 vertebrae (Fig. 4.1). The superior mediastinum contains the major vessels supplying the upper extremity, the neck, and the head. The inferior mediastinum, the space between the transverse thoracic plane and the diaphragm, is further divided into the anterior, middle, and posterior mediastinum. The middle mediastinum is the space containing the heart and pericardium. The anterior mediastinum is the space between the pericardium and the sternum. The posterior mediastinum extends from the posterior pericardium to the posterior wall of the thorax.

The inferior aperture of the thorax is formed by the lower margin of the ribs and costal cartilages and is closed off from the abdomen by the respiratory diaphragm (Fig. 4.1). The superior aperture of the thorax leads to the neck and the upper extremity. It is formed by the 1st ribs and their articulation with the manubrium and 1st thoracic vertebra. The superior aperture of the thorax, or root of the neck, allows for the passage of structures from the neck to the thoracic cavity. The clavicle crosses the 1st rib at its anterior edge close to its articulation with the manubrium. Structures exiting the superior thoracic aperture and communicating with the upper extremity pass between the 1st rib and clavicle.

M.S. Cook (✉)
University of Minnesota, Department of Integrative Biology and Physiology, 6-125 Jackson Hall, 321 Church St. SE, Minneapolis, MN 55455, USA
e-mail: cookx072@umn.edu

P.A. Iaizzo (ed.), *Handbook of Cardiac Anatomy, Physiology, and Devices*, DOI 10.1007/978-1-60327-372-5_4,
© Springer Science+Business Media, LLC 2009

Fig. 4.1 The *left panel* is a diagrammatic representation of pulmonary cavities on each side of the thorax with the mediastinum in between. The *right panel* illustrates the divisions of the mediastinum. Figure adapted from Grant's Dissector, 12th ed. (Figs. 1.14 (*left*) and 1.24)

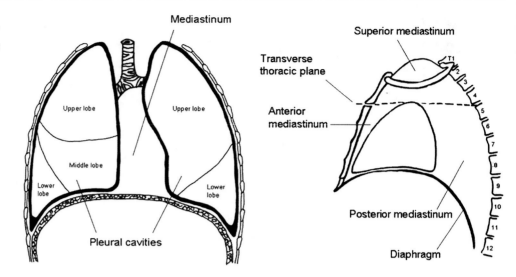

4.3 Bones of the Thoracic Wall

4.3.1 The Thoracic Cage

The skeleton of the thoracic wall is comprised of the 12 ribs, the thoracic vertebrae and intervertebral discs, and the sternum. Articulating with the thorax are the bones of the pectoral girdle, the clavicle, and the scapula (Fig. 4.2). Of these, the clavicle is particularly important because it forms, with the 1st rib, the thoracic outlet to the upper extremity.

The thoracic vertebrae comprise the middle portion of the posterior wall of the thorax. Each thoracic vertebra has a body anteriorly, two pedicles and two lamina (which together form an arch creating the vertebral foramen), a relatively long spinous process projecting posteriorly and inferiorly, and two transverse processes projecting laterally and somewhat posteriorly (Fig. 4.3). Each thoracic

vertebra articulates with at least one rib. The 1st through 9th thoracic vertebrae have a set of costal facets on their bodies for articulation with the head of the rib. These costal facets are also called "demifacets." The superior demifacet articulates with the head of the rib of the same number as the vertebra. The inferior demifacet articulates with the head of the rib below. The head of rib 1 articulates only with the T1 vertebra. Thus, this vertebra has a single facet for articulation with rib 1 and a demifacet for articulation with rib 2. The heads of ribs 10, 11, and 12 articulate only with the vertebra of the same number. The articular facets on vertebrae T10, T11, and T12 are located at the junction of the body and pedicle (T10) or fully on the pedicle (T11 and T12). The first 10 thoracic vertebrae also have costal facets on their transverse processes for articulation with the tubercles of the ribs of the same number. The transverse processes of the thoracic

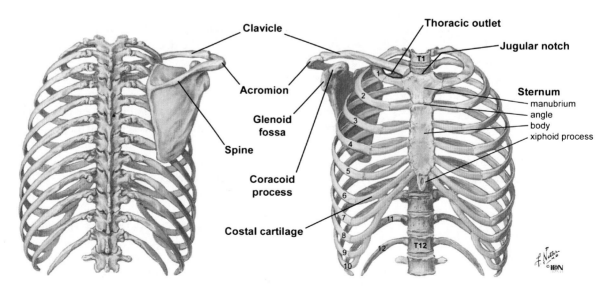

Fig. 4.2 The *left panel* illustrates the bones of the thorax from an anterior view. The *right panel* is a posterior view of the bony thorax. Figure adapted from Atlas of Human Anatomy, 2nd ed. (Plate 170)

Fig. 4.3 The T6 vertebra as viewed from above (*upper left*) and laterally (*upper right*), and a typical rib (*lower*). Figure adapted from Atlas of Human Anatomy, 2nd ed. (Plates 143 and 171)

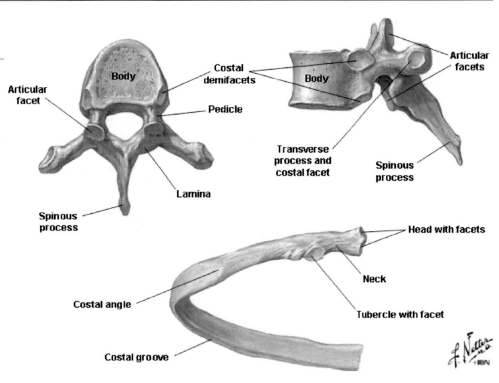

vertebrae get progressively shorter and the transverse processes of T11 and T12 do not articulate with the tubercles of their respective ribs.

The ribs form the largest part of the bony wall of the thorax (Fig. 4.2). Each rib articulates with one or two thoracic vertebrae and the upper 10 ribs articulate directly or indirectly with the sternum anteriorly. The upper seven ribs are referred to as "true" ribs because each connects to the sternum via its own costal cartilage. Ribs 8–10 are referred to as "false" ribs because they connect indirectly to the sternum. Each of these ribs is connected to the rib immediately above via its costal cartilage and ultimately to the sternum via the costal cartilage of the 7th rib. Ribs 11 and 12 are referred to as "floating" ribs because they do not connect to the sternum, but end in the musculature of the abdominal wall. Each rib has a head that articulates with the thoracic vertebra and a relatively thin flat shaft that is curved (Fig. 4.3). The costal angle, the sharpest part of the curved shaft, is located where the rib turns anteriorly. At the inferior margin of the shaft, the internal surface of each rib is recessed to form a costal groove. This depression provides some protection to the intercostal neurovascular bundle, something that must be considered when designing devices for intercostal access to the thorax. The heads of ribs 2–9 have two articular facets for articulation with the vertebrae of the same level and the vertebrae above. The heads of ribs 1, 10, 11, and 12 only articulate with the vertebrae of the same number and, consequently, have only one articular facet. In ribs 1–10, the head is connected to the shaft by a narrowing called the "neck." At the junction of

the head and the neck is a tubercle that has an articular surface for articulation with the costal facet of the transverse process. Ribs 11 and 12 do not articulate with the transverse process of their respective vertebrae and do not have a tubercle or, therefore, a neck portion.

The sternum is the flat bone making up the median anterior part of the thoracic cage (Fig. 4.2). It is comprised of three parts—the manubrium, body, and xiphoid process. The manubrium (from the Latin word for "handle" like the handle of a sword) is the superior part of the sternum; it is the widest and thickest part of the sternum. The manubrium alone articulates with the clavicle and the 1st rib. The sternal heads of the clavicle can be readily seen and palpated at their junction with the manubrium. The depression between the sternal heads of the clavicle above the manubrium is the suprasternal, or jugular, notch. The manubrium and the body of the sternum lie in slightly different planes and thus form a noticeable and easily palpated angle, the sternal angle (of Louis), at the point where they articulate. The 2nd rib articulates with both the body of the sternum and the manubrium and can easily be identified just lateral to the sternal angle. The body of the sternum is formed from the fusion of segmental bones (the sternebrae). The remnants of this fusion can be seen in the transverse ridges of the sternal body, especially in young people. The 3rd through 6th ribs articulate with the body of the sternum and the 7th rib articulates at the junction of the sternum and xiphoid process. The xiphoid process is the inferior most part of the sternum and is easily palpated. It lies at the level of thoracic vertebra 10 and marks the inferior boundary of the thoracic cavity anteriorly. It also lies at the level even with the central tendon of the diaphragm and the inferior border of the heart.

4.3.2 The Pectoral Girdle

Many of the muscles encountered on the wall of the anterior thorax are attached to the bones of the pectoral girdle and the upper extremity. Since movement of these bones can impact the anatomy of vascular structures communicating between the thorax and upper extremity, it is important to include these structures in a discussion of the thorax.

The clavicle is a somewhat "S-shaped" bone that articulates at its medial end with the manubrium of the sternum and at its lateral end with the acromion of the scapula (Fig. 4.2). It is convex medially and concave laterally. The scapula is a flat triangular bone, concave anteriorly, that rests upon the posterior thoracic wall. It has a raised ridge posteriorly called the "spine" that ends in a projection of bone called the "acromion" that articulates with the clavicle. The coracoid process is an anterior projection of bone from the superior border of the clavicle that serves as an attachment point for muscles that act on the scapula and upper extremity. The head of the humerus articulates

with the glenoid fossa of the scapula, forming the glenohumeral joint. The clavicle serves as a strut to hold the scapula in position away from the lateral aspect of the thorax. It is a highly mobile bone, with a high degree of freedom at the sternoclavicular joint that facilitates movement of the shoulder girdle against the thorax. The anterior extrinsic muscles of the shoulder pass from the wall of the thorax to the bones of the shoulder girdle.

4.4 Muscles of the Thoracic Wall

4.4.1 The Pectoral Muscles

Several muscles of the thoracic wall, including the most superficial ones that create some of the contours of the thoracic wall, are muscles that act upon the upper extremity. Some of these muscles form important surface landmarks on the thorax and others have relationships to vessels that communicate with the thorax. In addition to moving the upper extremity, some of these muscles also can play a role in movement of the thoracic wall and participate in respiration. The pectoralis major muscle forms the surface contour of the upper lateral part of the thoracic wall (Fig. 4.4). It originates on the clavicle (clavicular head), the sternum, and ribs

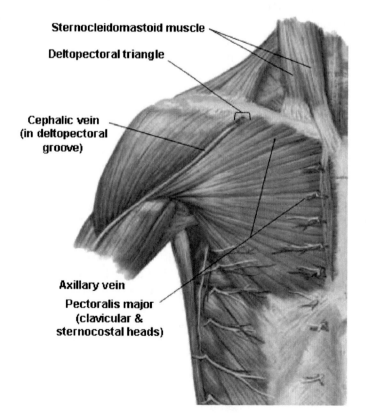
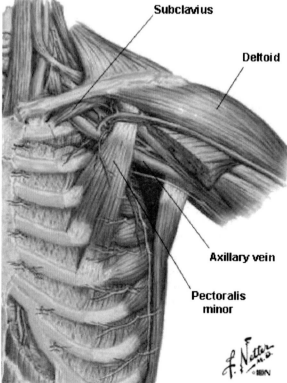

Fig. 4.4 The musculature of the anterior thoracic wall. The *left panel* shows the superficial muscles intact. The *right panel* shows structures deep to the pectoralis major muscle. Figure adapted from Atlas of Human Anatomy, 2nd ed. (Plate 174 and 175)

(sternocostal head) and inserts on the greater tubercle of the humerus. The lower margin of this muscle, passing from the thorax to the humerus, forms the major part of the anterior axillary fold. The pectoralis major muscle is a powerful adductor and medial rotator of the arm.

The pectoralis minor muscle is a much smaller muscle and lies directly below, deep to the pectoralis major muscle (Fig. 4.4). It originates on ribs 3–5 and inserts upon the coracoid process of the scapula. This muscle forms part of the anterior axillary fold medially. It acts to depress the scapula and stabilizes the scapula when upward force is exerted on the shoulder.

The anterior part of the deltoid muscle also forms a small aspect of the anterior thoracic wall. This muscle has its origin on the lateral part of the clavicle and the acromion and spine of the scapula (Fig. 4.4). It inserts upon the deltoid tubercle of the humerus and is the most powerful abductor of the arm. The anterior deltoid muscle borders the superior aspect of the pectoralis major muscle. The depression found at the junction of these two muscles is called the "deltopectoral groove." Importantly, within this groove the cephalic vein can consistently be found. The muscles diverge at their origins on the clavicle, creating an opening bordered by these two muscles and the clavicle known as the "deltopectoral triangle." Through this space the cephalic vein passes to join the axillary vein.

The subclavius is a small muscle originating on the lateral inferior aspect of the clavicle and inserting on the sternal end of the 1st rib (Fig. 4.4). This muscle depresses the clavicle and exerts a medial traction on the clavicle that stabilizes the

sternoclavicular joint. In addition to these actions, the subclavius muscle provides a soft surface on the inferior aspect of the clavicle that serves to cushion the contact of this bone with structures passing under the clavicle (i.e., nerves of the brachial plexus and the subclavian artery) when the clavicle is depressed during movement of the shoulder girdle, and especially when the clavicle is fractured.

The serratus anterior muscle originates on the lateral aspect of the first eight ribs and passes laterally to insert upon the medial aspect of the scapula (Fig. 4.5). This muscle forms the "serrated" contour of the lateral thoracic wall in individuals with good muscle definition. The serratus anterior forms the medial border of the axilla and acts to pull the scapula forward (protraction), stabilize the scapula against a posterior force on the shoulder, and assist with cranial rotation of the scapula with elevation.

4.4.2 The Intercostal Muscles

Each rib is connected to the one above and below by a series of three intercostal muscles. The external intercostal muscles are the most superficial (Fig. 4.5). These muscles course in an obliquely medial direction as they pass from superior to inferior between the ribs. Near the anterior end of the ribs, the external intercostal muscle fibers are replaced by the external intercostal membrane. Deep to the external intercostals are the internal intercostals

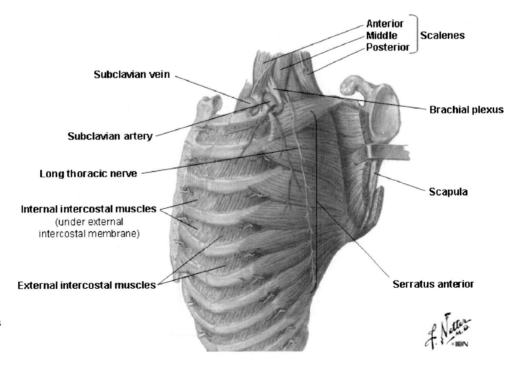

Fig. 4.5 A lateral view of the musculature of the thoracic wall. Figure adapted from Atlas of Human Anatomy, 2nd ed. (Plate 177)

(Figs. 4.5 and 4.6). The direction of the internal intercostal muscle fibers is perpendicular to the external intercostals. Near the posterior end of the ribs, the internal intercostal muscle fibers are replaced by the internal intercostal membrane. The deepest layer of intercostal muscles is the innermost intercostal muscles (Fig. 4.6). These muscles have a fiber direction similar to the internal intercostals, but form a separate plane. The connective tissues of the innermost intercostal muscles form a fibrous membrane near the anterior and posterior ends of the ribs. The intercostal nerves and vessels pass between the internal and innermost intercostal muscles. There are two additional sets of muscles in the same layer as the innermost intercostals—the subcostals and the transversus thoracis muscles. The subcostal muscles are located posteriorly and span more than one rib. The transverus thoracis muscles are found anteriorly and are continuous with the innermost muscle layer of the abdomen, the transversus abdominus, inferiorly. The transversus thoracis muscles pass from the internal surface of the sternum to ribs 2 through 6 (Fig. 4.6).

The intercostal muscles, especially the external and internal intercostals, are involved with respiration by elevating or depressing the ribs. The external intercostal muscles and the anterior interchondral part of the internal intercostals act to elevate the ribs. The lateral parts of the internal intercostal muscles depress the ribs. The innermost intercostals most likely have an action similar to the internal intercostals. The subcostal muscles probably help to elevate the ribs. The transversus thoracis muscles have little, if any, effect on respiration.

4.4.3 Respiratory Diaphragm

The respiratory diaphragm is the musculotendinous sheet separating the abdominal and thoracic cavities (Figs. 4.6 and 4.7). It is also considered a primary muscle of respiration. The diaphragm originates along the inferior border of the rib cage, the xiphoid process of the sternum, the posterior abdominal wall musculature, and the upper lumbar vertebrae. The medial and lateral arcuate ligaments are thickenings of the investing fascia over the quadratus lumborum (lateral) and the psoas major (medial) muscles of the posterior abdominal wall that serve as attachments for the diaphragm (Fig. 4.7). The vertebral origins of the diaphragm are the right and left crura. The crura originate on the bodies of lumbar vertebra 1 through 3, their intervertebral discs, and the anterior longitudinal ligament spanning these vertebrae. The diaphragm ascends from its origin to form a right and left dome, the right dome being typically higher than the left. The muscular part of the diaphragm contracts during respiration, causing the dome of the diaphragm to flatten downward, and increasing the volume of the thoracic cavity. The aponeurotic central part of the diaphragm, called the "central tendon," contains the opening for the inferior vena cava (Fig. 4.7). The esophagus also passes through the diaphragm, and the hiatus for the esophagus is created by a muscular slip originating from the right crus of the diaphragm. The aorta passes from the thorax to the abdomen behind the diaphragm, under the median arcuate ligament created by the intermingling of fibers from the right and left crura of the diaphragm. The inferior vena cava, esophagus, and

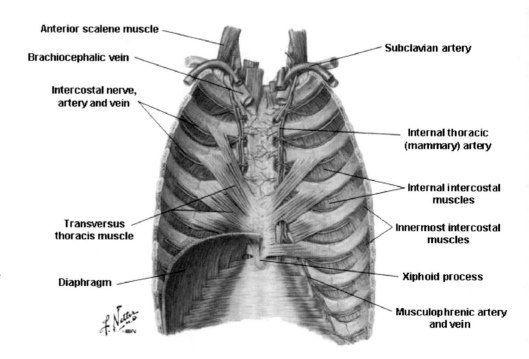

Fig. 4.6 The deep musculature of the anterior thoracic wall viewed from the posterior side. Figure adapted from Atlas of Human Anatomy, 2nd ed. (Plate 176)

Anterior scalene muscle

Brachiocephalic vein

Intercostal nerve, artery and vein

Transversus thoracis muscle

Diaphragm

Subclavian artery

Internal thoracic (mammary) artery

Internal intercostal muscles

Innermost intercostal muscles

Xiphoid process

Musculophrenic artery and vein

Fig. 4.7 The abdominal side of the respiratory diaphragm illustrating the origins of the muscle. Figure adapted from Atlas of Human Anatomy, 2nd ed. (Plate 181)

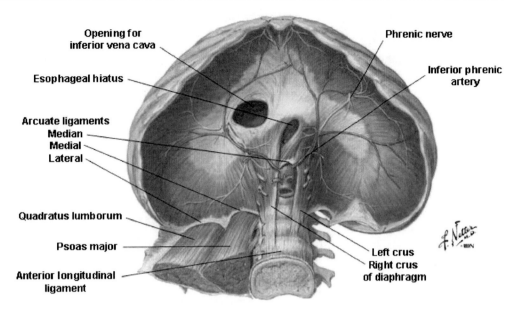

Opening for inferior vena cava

Esophageal hiatus

Arcuate ligaments
Median
Medial
Lateral

Quadratus lumborum

Psoas major

Anterior longitudinal ligament

Phrenic nerve

Inferior phrenic artery

Left crus
Right crus of diaphragm

aorta pass from the thorax to the abdomen at thoracic vertebral levels 8, 10, and 12, respectively.

4.4.4 Other Muscles of Respiration

The scalene muscles and the sternocleidomastoid muscle in the neck also contribute to respiration, especially during deep respiration (Figs. 4.4 and 4.5). Collectively, the scalene muscles have their origin on the transverse processes of cervical vertebrae 2–7. The anterior and middle scalenes insert on the 1st rib and the posterior scalene on the 2nd rib. As its name suggests, the sternocleidomastoid has its origin on the mastoid process of the skull and inserts upon the medial aspect of the clavicle and the manubrium of the sternum. When contracting with the head and neck fixed, these muscles exert an upward pull on the thorax and assist in respiration. The muscles of the anterior abdominal wall are also involved with respiration. These muscles, the rectus abdominus, external and internal abdominal obliques, and the transversus abdominus act together during forced expiration to pull down on the rib cage and to increase intra-abdominal pressure forcing the diaphragm to expand upward, reducing the volume of the pulmonary cavities. The mechanics of respiration are explained in detail in Section 4.11.2.

4.5 Nerves of the Thoracic Wall

The wall of the thorax receives its innervation from intercostal nerves (Fig. 4.8). These nerves are the ventral rami of segmental nerves leaving the spinal cord at the thoracic vertebral levels. Intercostal nerves are mixed nerves carrying both somatic motor and sensory nerves, as well as autonomics to the skin. The intercostal nerves pass out of the intervertebral foramina and run inferior to the rib. As they reach the costal angle, the nerves pass between the innermost and the internal intercostal muscles. The motor innervation to all the intercostal muscles comes from the intercostal nerves. These nerves give off lateral and anterior cutaneous branches that provide cutaneous sensory innervation to the skin of the thorax (Fig. 4.8). The intercostal nerves also carry sympathetic nerve fibers to the sweat glands, smooth muscle, and blood vessels. However, the first two intercostal nerves are considered atypical. The 1st intercostal nerve divides shortly after it emerges from the intervertebral foramen. The larger superior part of this nerve joins the brachial plexus to provide innervation to the upper extremity. The lateral cutaneous branch of the 2nd intercostal nerve is large and typically pierces the serratus anterior muscle to provide sensory innervation to the floor of the axilla and medial aspect of the arm. The nerve associated with the 12th rib is the subcostal nerve, since there is no rib below this level; it is a nerve of the abdominal wall.

The pectoral muscles receive motor innervation from branches of the brachial plexus of nerves (derived from cervical levels 5–8 and thoracic level 1) which supply the muscles of the shoulder and upper extremity. The lateral and medial pectoral nerves, branches of the lateral and medial cords of the brachial plexus, supply the pectoralis major and minor muscles (Fig. 4.9). The pectoralis major muscle is innervated by both nerves and the pectoralis minor muscle by only the medial pectoral nerve, which

Fig. 4.8 A typical set of intercostal arteries and nerves. Figure adapted from Atlas of Human Anatomy, 2nd ed. (Plate 179)

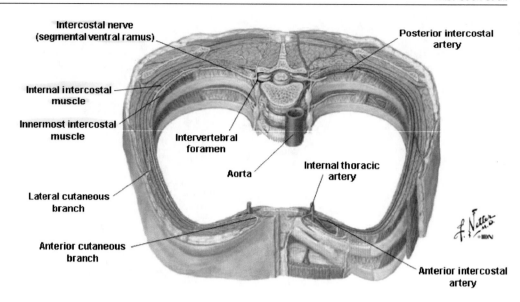

Intercostal nerve (segmental ventral ramus)

Posterior intercostal artery

Internal intercostal muscle

Innermost intercostal muscle

Intervertebral foramen

Aorta

Internal thoracic artery

Lateral cutaneous branch

Anterior cutaneous branch

Anterior intercostal artery

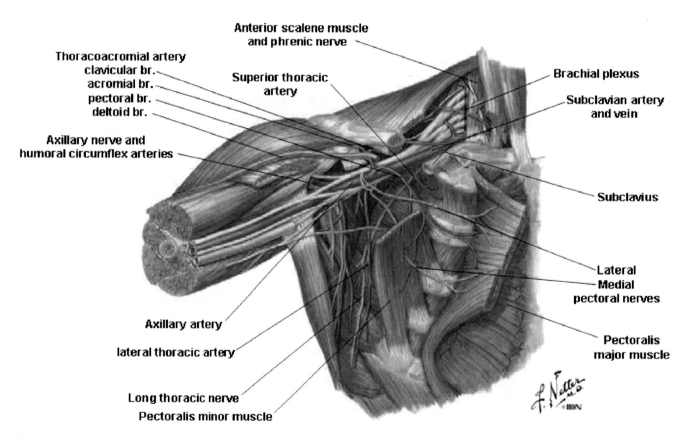

Anterior scalene muscle and phrenic nerve

Thoracoacromial artery
clavicular br.
acromial br.
pectoral br.
deltoid br.

Superior thoracic artery

Brachial plexus

Subclavian artery and vein

Axillary nerve and humoral circumflex arteries

Subclavius

Lateral
Medial
pectoral nerves

Axillary artery

lateral thoracic artery

Pectoralis major muscle

Long thoracic nerve
Pectoralis minor muscle

Fig. 4.9 Nerves and arteries of the axilla viewed with the pectoralis major and minor muscles reflected. Figure adapted from Atlas of Human Anatomy, 2nd ed. (Plate 400)

pierces this muscle before entering the pectoralis major muscle. The serratus anterior muscle is innervated by the long thoracic nerve which originates from the ventral rami of C5, C6, and C7 (Figs. 4.5 and 4.9). The deltoid muscle is innervated by the axillary nerve, a branch of the posterior cord of the brachial plexus (Fig. 4.9). Finally, the subclavius muscle is innervated by its own nerve from the superior trunk of the brachial plexus.

4.6 Vessels of the Thoracic Wall

The intercostal muscles and the skin of the thorax receive their blood supply from both the intercostal arteries and the internal thoracic artery (Figs. 4.6 and 4.8). Intercostal arteries 3 through 11 (and the subcostal artery) are branches directly from the thoracic descending aorta. The first two intercostal arteries are branches of the supreme intercostal artery, which is a branch of the costocervical trunk from the subclavian artery. The posterior intercostals run with the intercostal nerve and pass with the nerve between the innermost and internal intercostal muscles. The intercostals then anastomose with anterior intercostal branches arising from the internal thoracic artery, descending immediately lateral to the sternum. The internal thoracic arteries are anterior branches from the subclavian arteries. The anterior and posterior intercostal anastomoses create an anastomotic network around the thoracic wall. The intercostal arteries are accompanied by intercostal veins (Fig. 4.6). These veins drain to the azygos system of veins in the posterior mediastinum. The anatomy of the azygos venous system is described in detail in Section 4.10.2. Anteriorly the intercostal veins drain to the internal thoracic veins which, in turn, drain to the subclavian veins in the superior mediastinum (Fig. 4.7).

The intercostal nerves, arteries, and veins run together in each intercostal space, just inferior to each rib. They are characteristically found in this order (vein, artery, nerve) with the vein closest to the rib.

The diaphragm receives blood from the musculophrenic artery, a terminal branch of the internal thoracic artery, which runs along the anterior superior surface of the diaphragm (Fig. 4.6). There is also a substantial blood supply to the inferior aspect of the diaphragm from the inferior phrenic arteries, the superior most branches from the abdominal aorta that branch along the inferior surface of the diaphragm (Fig. 4.7).

The muscles of the pectoral region get their blood supply from branches of the axillary artery. This artery is the continuation of the subclavian artery emerging from the thorax and passing under the clavicle (Fig. 4.9). The first branch of the axillary artery, the superior (supreme) thoracic artery, gives blood supply to the first two intercostal spaces. The second branch forms the thoracoacromial artery or trunk. Subsequently, this artery gives off four sets of branches (pectoral, deltoid, clavicular, acromial) that supply blood to the pectoral muscles, the deltoid muscle, the clavicle, and subclavius muscle. The lateral thoracic artery, the third branch from the subclavian artery, participates along with the intercostal arteries in supplying the serratus anterior muscle. Additional distal branches from the axillary artery, the humeral circumflex arteries, also participate in blood supply to the deltoid muscle. Venous blood returns through veins of the same names to the axillary vein.

4.7 The Superior Mediastinum

The superior mediastinum is the space behind the manubrium of the sternum (Fig. 4.1). It is bounded by parietal (mediastinal) pleura on each side and the first four thoracic vertebrae behind. It is continuous with the root of the neck at the top of the first ribs and with the inferior mediastinum below the transverse thoracic plane, a horizontal plane that passes from the sternal angle through the space between the T4 and T5 vertebrae. Due to the inferior sloping of the first ribs, the superior mediastinum is wedge shaped, being longer posteriorly. The superior mediastinum contains several important structures including the branches of the aortic arch, the veins that coalesce to form the superior vena cava, the trachea, the esophagus, the vagus and phrenic nerves, the cardiac plexus of autonomic nerves, the thoracic duct, and the thymus (Fig. 4.10).

4.7.1 Arteries in the Superior Mediastinum

As the aorta emerges from the pericardial sac, it begins to arch posteriorly (Fig. 4.11). At the level of the T4 vertebra, the aorta has become vertical again, descending through the posterior mediastinum. The intervening segment is the arch of the aorta and it courses from right to left as it arches posteriorly. It passes over the right pulmonary artery and ends by passing posterior to the left pulmonary artery. The trachea and esophagus pass posterior and to the right of the aortic arch. The arch of the aorta gives off the major arteries that supply blood to the head and to the upper extremity. This branching is asymmetrical. The first and most anterior branch from the aorta is the brachiocephalic trunk. This arterial trunk bends toward the right as it ascends and, as it reaches the upper limit of the superior mediastinum, bifurcates into the right common carotid and right subclavian arteries. The next two branches from the aortic arch, from anterior to posterior, are the left common carotid and the left subclavian arteries. These two arteries ascend almost vertically to the left of the trachea. The common carotid arteries supply the majority of the blood to the head and neck. The subclavian arteries continue as the axillary and brachial arteries, and supply the upper extremity. The arch of the aorta and its branches make contact with the upper lobe of the right lung, and their

Fig. 4.10 Contents of the superior and middle mediastinum. Figure adapted from Atlas of Human Anatomy, 2nd ed. (Plate 200)

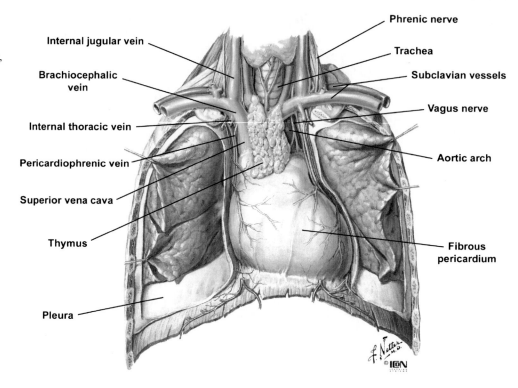

Fig. 4.11 Vessels of the superior and middle mediastinum. Figure adapted from Atlas of Human Anatomy, 2nd ed. (Plate 195)

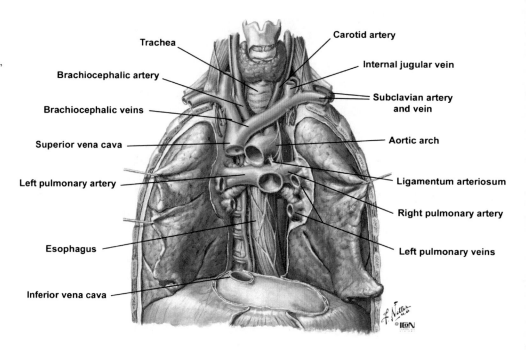

impressions are normally seen on the fixed lung after removal. Neither the brachiocephalic trunk, left common carotid, nor the left subclavian give off consistent branches in the superior mediastinum. However, the subclavian arteries at the root of the neck give off the internal thoracic arteries which re-enter the superior mediastinum and descend along each side of the sternum. On occasion, there will be an artery branching from the aortic arch, the right common carotid, or one of the subclavian arteries, and supplying the thyroid gland in the midline. This variant artery is called a thyroid ima. Since this artery is often found crossing the region where a tracheostomy is performed, it is important to remember that this artery is present in ∼10% of individuals.

4.7.2 Brachiocephalic Veins

The bilateral brachiocephalic veins are formed by the merging of the internal jugular vein and the subclavian vein on both sides at the base of the neck (Fig. 4.11). The right brachiocephalic vein descends nearly vertically, while the left crosses obliquely behind the manubrium to join the right and form the superior vena cava. The superior vena cava continues inferiorly into the middle mediastinum, entering the pericardial sac. The brachiocephalic veins run anterior in the superior mediastinum. The left brachiocephalic vein passes anterior to the three branches of the aortic arch and is separated from the manubrium only by the thymus (Fig. 4.10). The brachiocephalic veins receive the internal thoracic veins, the inferior thyroid veins, and the small pericardiacophrenic veins. They also receive the superior intercostal veins from behind.

4.7.3 The Trachea and Esophagus

The trachea is a largely cartilaginous tube that runs from the larynx inferiorly through the superior mediastinum and ends by branching into the main bronchi (Fig. 4.11). It serves as a conduit for air to the lungs. The trachea can be palpated at the root of the neck, superior to the manubrium in the midline. The esophagus is a muscular tube that connects the pharynx with the stomach. The upper part of the esophagus descends behind the trachea and, in contact with it, through the superior mediastinum (Fig. 4.11). The esophagus continues through the posterior mediastinum behind the heart, pierces the diaphragm at the level of T10, and enters the stomach at the cardia. Both the trachea and esophagus are crossed on the left by the arch of the aorta. The impression of the aorta on the esophagus can usually be seen on a posterior to anterior radiograph of the esophagus coated with barium contrast. The trachea and esophagus are crossed on the right side by the azygos vein at the lower border of the superior mediastinum. Both the trachea and esophagus come into contact with the upper lobe of the right lung. The esophagus also contacts the upper lobe of the left lung. The arch of the aorta and its branches shield the trachea from the left lung.

4.7.4 Nerves of the Superior Mediastinum

Both the vagus nerve (cranial nerve 10; CN X) and the phrenic nerve pass through the superior mediastinum. The phrenic nerve originates from the ventral rami from cervical levels 3, 4, and 5. This nerve travels inferiorly in the neck on the surface of the anterior scalene muscle, entering the superior mediastinum behind the subclavian vein and passing under the internal thoracic artery (Fig. 4.12). On the right, the phrenic nerve passes through the superior mediastinum lateral to the subclavian artery and the arch of the aorta. On the left, the phrenic nerve passes lateral to the brachiocephalic vein and the superior vena cava. The phrenic nerves then enter the middle mediastinum where they pass anterior to the root of the lung, across the pericardium, finally piercing the diaphragm lateral to the base of the pericardium. Throughout their course, the phrenic nerves pass under the mediastinal pleura. The phrenic nerve is the motor innervation to the diaphragm ("C-3-4-5 keeps your diaphragm alive") and it also provides sensory innervation to the pericardium, mediastinal and diaphragmatic pleura, and to the diaphragmatic peritoneum on the inferior surface of the diaphragm. The course of the phrenic nerve behind the subclavian vein makes it susceptible to stimulation if current leaks from a pacing lead with the vessel.

The bilateral vagus nerves pass out of the skull via the jugular foramen and descend through the neck in the carotid sheath, just lateral to the common carotid arteries. These nerves are the parasympathetic supply to the thorax and most of the abdomen. On the right, the vagus crosses

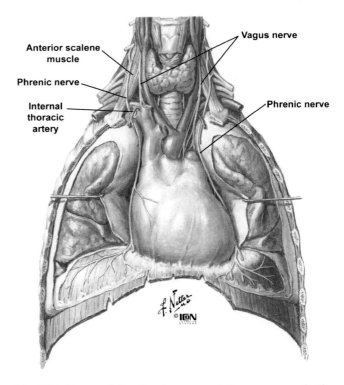

Fig. 4.12 Course of the phrenic nerve and the vagus nerve in the superior and middle mediastinum. Figure adapted from Atlas of Human Anatomy, 2nd ed. (Plate 182)

anterior to the subclavian artery and then turns posterior to pass behind the root of the lung and onto the esophagus. Before the right vagus enters the superior mediastinum, it gives off a recurrent laryngeal branch that passes behind the subclavian artery and ascends into the neck. On the left, the vagus passes lateral to the arch of the aorta, then turns posterior to pass behind the root of the lung and onto the esophagus (Fig. 4.12). At the level of the aortic arch, it gives off the left recurrent laryngeal nerve that passes under the aorta, just posterior to the ligamentum arteriosum, and ascends into the neck. The recurrent laryngeal nerves provide motor innervation to most of the muscles of the larynx. It should be noted that an aneurism in the arch of the aorta can injure the left recurrent laryngeal nerve and manifest as hoarseness of the voice due to unilateral paralysis of the laryngeal musculature. The right and left vagus nerves contribute to the esophageal plexus of nerves in the middle mediastinum. They give off cardiac branches in the neck (superior and inferior cardiac nerves) and a variable number of small cardiac nerves in the superior mediastinum (thoracic cardiac branches) that provide parasympathetic innervation to the heart via the cardiac nerve plexus.

Sympathetic innervation to the heart is also found in the superior mediastinum. The heart receives postganglionic branches from the superior, middle, and inferior cardiac nerves, each branching from their respective sympathetic ganglia in the neck (Fig. 4.13). There are also thoracic cardiac nerves emanating from the upper four or five thoracic sympathetic ganglia. The uppermost

thoracic ganglion and the inferior cervical ganglion are often fused to form an elongated ganglion called the "stellate ganglion" which will give off the inferior cardiac nerve.

The cardiac plexus is located between the trachea, the arch of the aorta, and the pulmonary trunk (Fig. 4.13). It is a network of sympathetic and parasympathetic nerves derived from the branches described above and provides autonomic innervation to the heart. Nerves from the plexus reach the heart by traveling along the vasculature and primarily innervate the conduction system and the atria. The sympathetic components cause the strength and pace of the heartbeats to increase; the parasympathetics counter this effect. Pain afferents from the heart travel with the sympathetic nerves to the upper thoracic and lower cervical levels. This distribution accounts for the pattern of referred heart pain to the upper thorax, shoulder, and arm.

4.7.5 The Thymus

The thymus is found in the most anterior part of the superior mediastinum (Fig. 4.10). It is considered an endocrine gland, but is actually more important as a lymphoid organ. The thymus produces lymphocytes that populate the lymphatic system and bloodstream. It is particularly active in young individuals and becomes much less prominent with aging. The thymus is located directly behind the manubrium and may extend up into the neck and inferiorly into the anterior mediastinum. It lies in contact with the aorta, the left brachiocephalic vein, and trachea.

4.8 The Middle Mediastinum

4.8.1 The Pericardium

The middle mediastinum is the central area of the inferior mediastinum occupied by the heart and a portion of the great vessels (Fig. 4.14). Within this space, the heart is situated with the right atrium on the right, the right ventricle anterior, the left ventricle to the left and posterior, and the left atrium entirely posterior. The apex, a part of the left ventricle, is projected inferiorly and to the left. The pericardium is the closed sac that contains the heart and the proximal portion of the great vessels; it is attached to the diaphragm inferiorly. The pericardium is a serous membrane, with a visceral and parietal layer, into which the heart projects such that there is a potential space

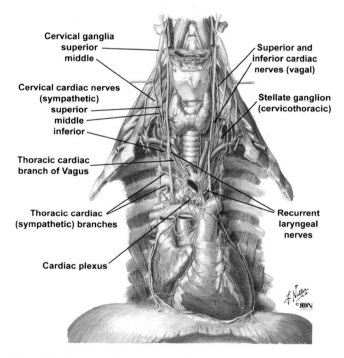

Fig. 4.13 Pattern of innervation in the superior mediastinum. Figure adapted from Atlas of Human Anatomy, 2nd ed. (Plate 228)

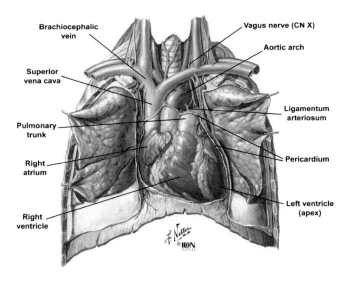

Fig. 4.14 The position of the heart in the middle mediastinum and the relationship of the pericardium to the heart and great vessels. Figure adapted from Atlas of Human Anatomy, 2nd ed. (Plate 201)

within pericardial sac called the "pericardial cavity." The visceral pericardium, also called the "epicardium," covers the entire surface of the heart and base of the great vessels, reflecting from the great vessels to become the parietal pericardium. The parietal pericardium is characterized by a thickened, strong outer layer called the fibrous pericardium. The fibrous pericardium is fused to the layer of parietal serous pericardium, creating a single layer with two surfaces. The fibrous pericardium has little elasticity and, by its fusion with the base of the great vessels, effectively creates a closed space in which the heart

beats. The pericardial cavity can accumulate fluids under pathological conditions and create pressure within the pericardium, a condition known as "cardiac tamponade." For a complete description of the pericardium and its features, see Chapter 8.

4.8.2 The Great Vessels

"Great vessels" is a composite term for the large arteries and veins directly entering and exiting the heart (Figs. 4.11 and 4.15). They include the superior and inferior vena cavae, the aorta, pulmonary trunk, and pulmonary veins; these vessels are found mostly in the superior mediastinum. The inferior vena cava and the pulmonary vein are the shortest of the great vessels. The inferior vena cava enters the right atrium from below, almost immediately after passing through the diaphragm. The pulmonary veins (there are normally two emerging from each lung) enter the left atrium with a very short intrapericardial portion. The superior vena cava is formed from the confluence of the right and left brachiocephalic veins. It also receives the azygos vein from behind and empties into the superior aspect of the right atrium. The pulmonary trunk ascends from the right ventricle on the anterior surface of the heart at an oblique angle to the left and posterior, passing anterior to the base of the aorta in its course. As the pulmonary trunk emerges from the pericardium, it bifurcates into left and right pulmonary arteries which enter the hilum of each lung (Fig. 4.11). The right pulmonary artery passes under

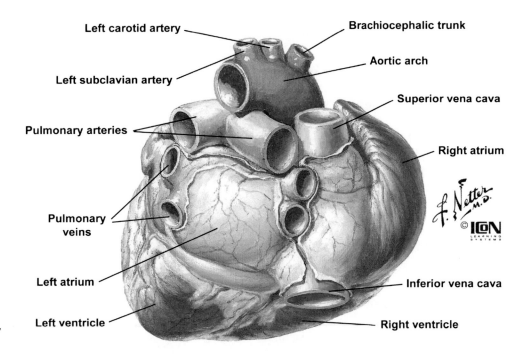

Fig. 4.15 The great vessels as viewed from the posterior side of the heart. Figure adapted from Atlas of Human Anatomy, 2nd ed. (Plate 202)

the arch of the aorta to reach the right lung. The left pulmonary artery is connected to the arch of the aorta by the ligamentum arteriosum, the remnant of the ductus arteriosus (the connection between the aorta and pulmonary trunk present in the fetus). The aorta ascends from the left ventricle at an angle to the right and curves back to the left and posterior as it becomes the aortic arch. As the aorta exits the pericardium, it arches over the right pulmonary trunk, passing to the left of the trachea and esophagus and entering the posterior mediastinum as the descending aorta (Fig. 4.15). Backflow of blood from both the aorta and the pulmonary trunk is prevented by semilunar valves. The semilunar valves, each with a set of three leaflets, are found at the base of each of these great vessels. Immediately above these valves are the "aortic and pulmonary sinuses," which are regions where the arteries are dilated. The coronary arteries branch from the right and left aortic sinuses (see Chapter 5).

Also passing through the middle mediastinum are the phrenic nerves and the pericardiacophrenic vessels (Fig. 4.10). The phrenic nerves pass out of the neck and through the superior mediastinum. They travel through the middle mediastinum on the lateral surfaces of the fibrous pericardium and under the mediastinal pleura to reach the diaphragm. The phrenic nerve on each side is accompanied by a pericardiacophrenic artery, a branch from the proximal internal thoracic artery, and a pericardiacophrenic vein, which empties into the subclavian vein. These vessels, as their name implies, supply the pericardium and the diaphragm, as well as the mediastinal pleura.

4.9 The Anterior Mediastinum

The anterior mediastinum is the subdivision of the inferior mediastinum bounded by the sternum anteriorly and the pericardium posteriorly (Fig. 4.1). It contains sternopericardial ligaments, made up of loose connective tissue, the internal thoracic vessels and their branches, lymphatic vessels and nodes, and fat. In children, the thymus often extends from the superior mediastinum into the anterior mediastinum.

4.10 The Posterior Mediastinum

The posterior mediastinum is the division of the inferior mediastinum bounded by the pericardium anteriorly and the posterior thoracic wall posteriorly (Fig. 4.1). Structures found in the posterior mediastinum include the descending aorta, azygos system of veins, thoracic duct, esophagus, esophageal plexus, thoracic sympathetic trunk, and thoracic splanchnic nerves.

4.10.1 The Esophagus and Esophageal Plexus

The esophagus descends into the posterior mediastinum, passing along the right side of the descending aorta (Fig. 4.11). It courses directly behind the left atrium and veers to the left before passing through the esophageal hiatus of the diaphragm at the level of T10. Because of the juxtaposition of the esophagus to the heart, high-resolution ultrasound images of the heart can be obtained via the esophagus. As the bilateral vagus nerves approach the esophagus, they divide into several commingling branches, forming the esophageal plexus (Fig. 4.16). Toward the distal end of the esophagus, the plexus begins

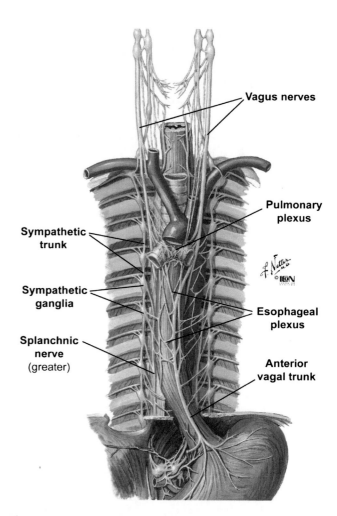

Fig. 4.16 Course of the esophagus in the posterior mediastinum and the esophageal plexus of nerves. Figure adapted from Atlas of Human Anatomy, 2nd ed. (Plate 228)

to coalesce into an anterior and a posterior vagal trunk that pass with the esophagus into the abdomen. The left side of the esophageal plexus from the left vagus nerve contributes preferentially to the anterior vagal trunk and likewise for the right vagus and the posterior vagal trunk, reflecting the normal rotation of the gut (during development). The parasympathetic branches of the anterior and posterior vagal trunks comprise the innervation to the abdominal viscera as far as the splenic flexure.

4.10.2 The Azygos System of Veins

The azygos venous system in the thorax is responsible primarily for draining venous blood from the thoracic wall to the superior vena cava (Fig. 4.17). The azygos veins also receive venous blood from the viscera of the thorax, such as the esophagus, bronchi, and pericardium. The term azygos means "unpaired" and describes the asymmetry in this venous system. The system consists of the azygos vein on the right and the hemiazygos and accessory hemiazygos veins on the left. Both the azygos vein and the hemiazygos vein are formed from the lumbar veins ascending from the abdomen uniting with the subcostal vein. On the right, the azygos vein is continuous, collecting blood from the right intercostal veins before arching over the root of the lung to join the superior vena cava. On the left, the hemiazygos vein ends typically at the level of T8 by crossing over to communicate with the azygos vein on the right. Above

the hemiazygos vein, the accessory hemiazygos vein collects blood from the posterior intercostal veins. It typically communicates with the hemiazygos vein and crosses over to communicate with the azygos vein. On both sides, the 2nd and 3rd intercostal spaces are drained to a superior intercostal vein that drains directly to the subclavian vein, but also communicates with the azygos and accessory hemiazygos veins on their respective sides. The first intercostal vein drains directly to the subclavian vein. There is a tremendous amount of variation in the azygos system of veins, all of which is functionally inconsequential. However, it should be noted that the azygos system can be quite different in some of the large animal models used to study cardiac function (see Chapter 6).

4.10.3 The Thoracic Duct and Lymphatics

The thoracic duct is the largest lymphatic vessel in the body (Fig. 4.18). It conveys lymph from the cisterna chyli, which is the collection site for all lymph from the abdomen, pelvis, and lower extremities, back to the venous system. The thoracic duct enters the posterior mediastinum through the aortic hiatus and travels between the thoracic aorta and the azygos vein behind the esophagus. It ascends through the superior mediastinum to the left and empties into the venous system at or close to the junction of the internal jugular and subclavian veins. The thoracic duct often appears white due to presence of

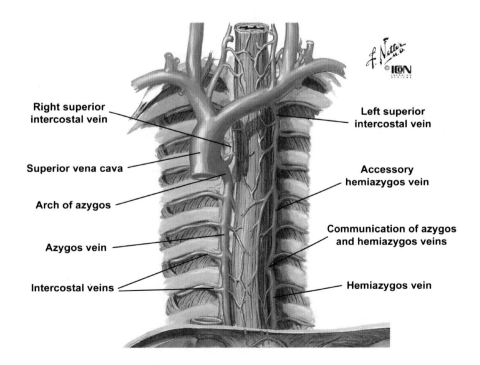

Fig. 4.17 The azygos venous system in the posterior mediastinum. This figure illustrates a "typical" pattern of the azygos and hemiazygos veins. Figure adapted from Atlas of Human Anatomy, 2nd ed. (Plate 226)

Right superior intercostal vein

Superior vena cava

Arch of azygos

Azygos vein

Intercostal veins

Left superior intercostal vein

Accessory hemiazygos vein

Communication of azygos and hemiazygos veins

Hemiazygos vein

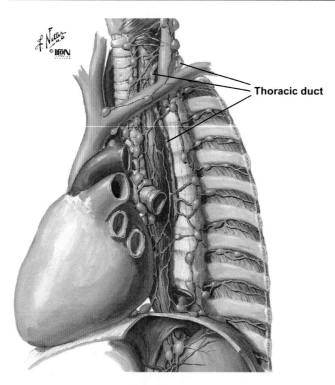

Fig. 4.18 The course of the thoracic duct in the posterior mediastinum through the superior mediastinum and ending at the junction of the internal jugular and subclavian veins. Figure adapted from Atlas of Human Anatomy, 2nd ed. (Plate 227)

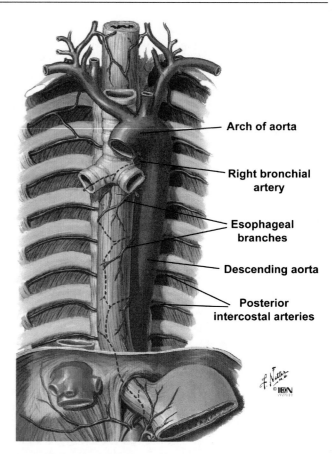

Fig. 4.19 Course of the descending aorta in the posterior mediastinum with posterior intercostal branches and branches to the esophagus and bronchi. Figure adapted from Atlas of Human Anatomy, 2nd ed. (Plate 225)

chyle in the lymph and beaded due to the many valves within the duct. The thoracic duct also receives lymphatic drainage from posterior mediastinal lymph nodes that collect lymph from the esophagus, posterior intercostal spaces, and posterior parts of the pericardium and diaphragm.

4.10.4 The Descending Thoracic Aorta

The descending thoracic aorta is the continuation of the aortic arch through the posterior mediastinum (Fig. 4.19). It begins to the left of the T5 vertebra and gradually moves to the middle of the vertebral column as it descends. It passes behind the diaphragm, under the median arcuate ligament (the aortic hiatus), and into the abdomen at the level of T12. The thoracic aorta gives off the 3rd through 11th posterior intercostal arteries and the subcostal artery. It also supplies blood to the proximal bronchi and the esophagus via bronchial and esophageal branches. The superior phrenic arteries supply the posterior aspect of the diaphragm and anastomose with the musculophrenic and pericardiacophrenic branches of the internal thoracic artery.

4.10.5 The Thoracic Sympathetic Nerves

The sympathetic chain of ganglia, or "sympathetic trunk," extends from the lower lumbar region to the cervical spine. It is also called the thoracolumbar division of the autonomic nervous system because preganglionic neurons of this system have their cell bodies in the thoracic and lumbar segments of the spinal cord, from T1 to L2. The thoracic portion of the sympathetic trunk is found in the posterior mediastinum (Fig. 4.16). It is composed of sympathetic ganglia, located along the spine at the junction of the vertebrae and the heads of the ribs and the intervening nerve segments that connect the ganglia. These sympathetic ganglia are also called "paravertebral sympathetic ganglia" due to their position alongside the vertebral column.

There is approximately one sympathetic chain ganglion for each spinal nerve. There are fewer ganglia than nerves because some adjacent ganglia fuse during embryologic development. Such fusion is most evident in the cervical region where there are eight spinal nerves but only three sympathetic ganglia—the superior, middle, and inferior cervical ganglia (Fig. 4.13). The inferior cervical ganglion and the first thoracic (T1) ganglion are often fused, forming the cervicothoracic or stellate ("star-shaped") ganglion.

An axon of the sympathetic nervous system that emerges from the spinal cord in the thorax travels with the ventral nerve root to a ventral ramus (in the thorax, this would be an intercostal nerve) (Fig. 4.20). After traveling a short distance on this nerve, this presynaptic (preganglionic) neuron enters the chain ganglion at its level (Fig. 4.21). Within the ganglion, it either synapses or travels superiorly or inferiorly to synapse at another spinal cord level (C_1 to S_4). After synapsing, the postsynaptic (postganglionic) neuron travels out of the ganglion and onto the ventral ramus to its target structure or organ. Presynaptic sympathetic nerves travel from the ventral ramus to the chain ganglion, and postsynaptic nerves travel back to the ventral ramus via small nerve fibers called rami communicantes (so named because they communicate between the ventral ramus and the sympathetic ganglion). The presynaptic neuron has a myelin protective coating and the postsynaptic neuron does not. This pattern of myelination is true of all nerves in the autonomic system. The myelin coating appears white and thus the presynaptic (myelinated) rami

communicantes form "white rami communicantes," and the postsynaptic (unmyelinated) neurons form "gray rami communicantes." The gray and white rami communicantes can be seen spanning the short distance between the intercostal nerves and the sympathetic ganglia in the posterior mediastinum (Fig. 4.8).

Also present in the posterior mediastinum are the thoracic splanchnic nerves which are seen leaving the sympathetic trunk and running inferiorly toward the midline (Fig. 4.20). Splanchnic nerves are preganglionic sympathetic neurons that emerge from the spine and pass through the chain ganglion, but do not synapse (Fig. 4.21). In the thorax, these preganglionic splanchnic nerves emerge from spinal cord segments T_5 to T_{12} and travel into the abdomen where they synapse in collateral ganglia called "prevertebral ganglia," located along the aorta. The postganglionic fibers then innervate the abdominal organs. There are three splanchnic nerves that arise from the sympathetic trunk in the thorax and travel down to the abdomen. The greater splanchnic nerves emerge from spinal cord segments T_5 to T_9, although a few studies report that they can emerge from T_2 to T_{10}. The axons of the lesser and least splanchnic nerves emerge from segments T_{10}, T_{11}, and T_{12}, respectively.

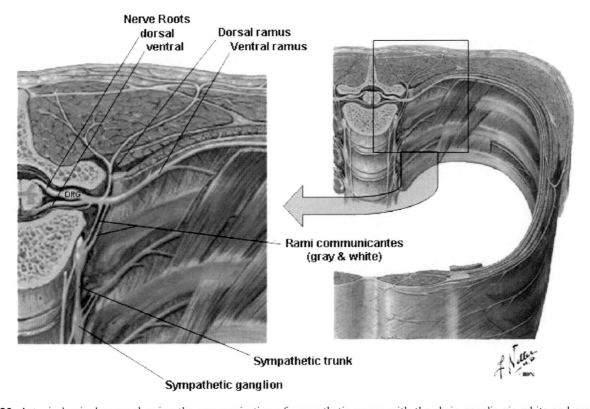

Fig. 4.20 A typical spinal nerve showing the communication of sympathetic nerves with the chain ganglia via white and gray rami communicantes. Figure adapted from Atlas of Human Anatomy, 2nd ed. (Plate 241)

Fig. 4.21 The three options taken by presynaptic sympathetic fibers are illustrated. All presynaptic nerves enter the sympathetic trunk via white rami communicantes. They can synapse at their level and exit via gray rami communicantes, travel up or down the chain before synapsing, or exit before synapsing in the splanchnic nerves. Figure adapted from Clinically Oriented Anatomy, 4th ed. (Fig. 1.32)

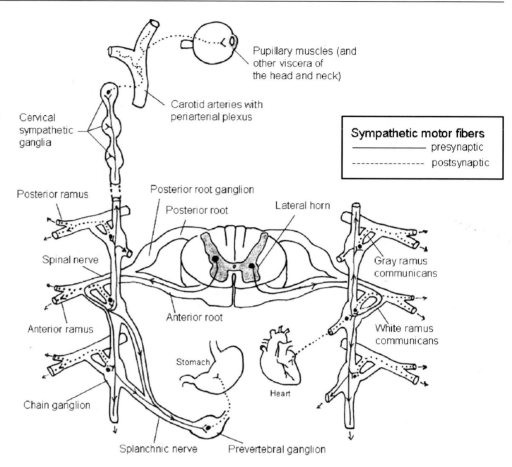

4.11 Pleura and Lungs

4.11.1 The Pleura

The bilateral pulmonary cavities contain the lungs and the pleural membranes (Fig. 4.1). The pleural membrane is a continuous serous membrane forming a closed pleural cavity within (Fig. 4.10). The relationship of the lung to this membrane is the same as a fist (representing the lung) pushed into an underinflated balloon (representing the pleural membrane). The fist becomes covered by the membrane of the balloon, but it is not "inside" the balloon. In the case of the lung, the pleura that is in contact with the lung is the parietal pleura and the outer layer, which is in contact with the inner wall of the thorax and the mediastinum, is the parietal pleura (Fig. 4.22). The space within the pleural sac is the pleural cavity. Under normal conditions, the pleural cavity contains only a small amount of serous fluid and has no open space at all. It is referred to as a "potential space" because a real space can be created if outside material, such as blood, pathologic fluids, or air, is introduced into this area.

The parietal pleura is subdivided into specific parts based on the part of the thorax it contacts (Figs. 4.10

and 4.22). Costal pleura overlies the ribs and intercostal spaces. In this region, the pleura is in contact with the endothoracic fascia, the fascial lining of the thoracic cavity. The mediastinal and diaphragmatic pleura are named for their contact with these structures. The cervical pleura extends over the cupola of the lung, above the 1st rib into the root of the neck; it is strengthened by the suprapleural

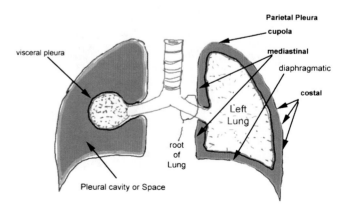

Fig. 4.22 Relationship of the lungs and walls of the thoracic cavity to the pleural membrane. Figure adapted from Grant's Dissector, 12th ed. (Fig. 1.15)

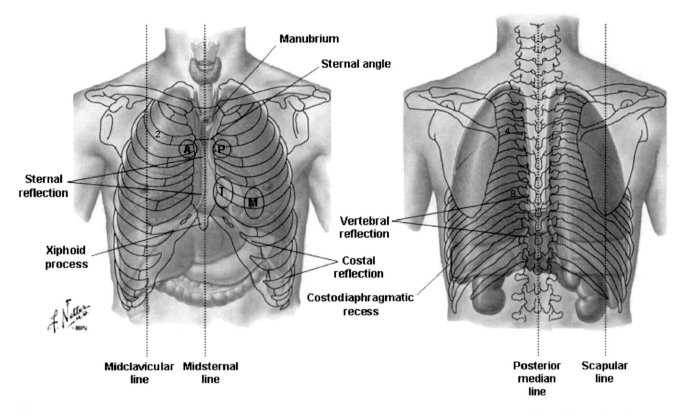

Fig. 4.23 Surface anatomy and important surface landmarks on the anterior and posterior thorax. Figure adapted from Atlas of Human Anatomy, 2nd ed. (Plates 184 and 185)

membrane, an extension of the endothoracic fascia over the cupola of lung.

The lines of pleural reflection are the lines along which the parietal pleura transitions from one region to the next (Fig. 4.23). The sternal line of reflection is the point where costal pleura transitions to mediastinal pleura on the anterior side of the thorax. The costal line of pleural reflection lies along the origin of the diaphragm where the costal pleura transitions to diaphragmatic pleura. Both the costal and sternal lines of reflection are very abrupt. The vertebral line of pleural reflection lies along the line where costal pleura becomes mediastinal pleura posteriorly. This angle of reflection is shallower than the other two. The surface projections of the parietal pleura are discussed in Section 4.12.2.

The parietal pleura reflects onto the lung to become the visceral pleura at the root of the lung. A line of reflection descends from the root of the lung, much like the sleeve of a loose robe hangs from the forearm, forming the pulmonary ligament (Fig. 4.24). The visceral pleura covers the entire surface of each lung including the surfaces in the fissures, where the visceral pleura on one lobe is in direct contact with the visceral pleura of the other lobe. On the surface of the lung, the parietal pleura is in contact with the parietal pleura.

The pleural cavity is the space inside the pleural membrane (Fig. 4.22). It is a potential space that, under normal conditions, contains only a small amount of serous fluid that lubricates the movement of the visceral pleura against the parietal pleura during respiration. During expiration, the lungs do not entirely fill the inferiormost aspect of the pulmonary cavity. This creates a region, along the costal line of reflection, where the diaphragmatic and costal pleura come into contact with each other with no intervening lung tissue. This space is the costodiaphragmatic recess.

4.11.2 The Lungs

The primary function of the lungs is to acquire O_2, required for metabolism in tissues, and to release CO_2, a metabolic waste product from tissues. The lungs fill the pulmonary cavities and are separated from each other by structures in the mediastinum. In the living, the lung tissue is soft, light, and elastic, filling the pulmonary cavity and accommodating surrounding structures that impinge on the lungs. In the fixed cadaveric lung, the imprint of structures adjacent to the lungs is easily seen.

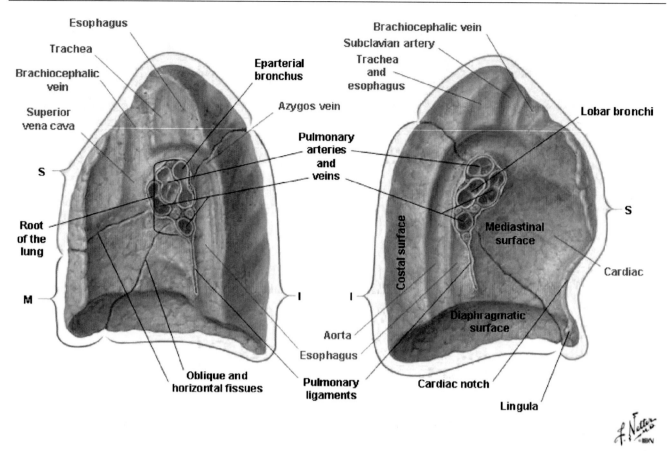

Fig. 4.24 Surface anatomy of the right (*right*) and left (*left*) lungs. Figure adapted from Atlas of Human Anatomy, 2nd ed. (Plate 187)

Blood and air enter and exit the lung at the hilum or root of the lung via the pulmonary vessels and the bronchi.

Each lung is divided into a superior and inferior lobe by an oblique (major) fissure (Fig. 4.24). The right lung has a second, horizontal (minor) fissure that creates a third lobe called the "middle lobe." Each lung has three surfaces—costal, mediastinal, and diaphragmatic—and an apex extending into the cupula at the root of the neck. The costal surface is smooth and convex, and diaphragmatic surfaces are smooth and concave. The mediastinal surface is concave and is the site of the root of the lung, where the primary bronchi and pulmonary vessels enter and exit the lungs. The mediastinal surface has several impressions created by structures in the mediastinum. The left lung has a deep impression accommodating the apex of the heart called the "cardiac impression." There is also a deep impression of the aortic arch and the descending thoracic aorta behind the root of the lung. At the superior end of the mediastinal surface, there are impressions from the brachiocephalic vein and the subclavian artery, and a shallow impression from the esophagus and trachea. On the right side, there are prominent impressions of the esophagus, behind the root of the lung,

and the arch of the azygos vein, extending over the root of the lung. An impression of the superior vena cava and the brachiocephalic vein appears anterior and above the root of the lung. An impression of both the trachea and the esophagus is seen close to the apex of the lung. Descending from the root of both lungs, the pulmonary ligament can be seen.

The lungs also have three borders where the three surfaces meet. The posterior border is where the costal and mediastinal surfaces meet posteriorly. The inferior border is where the diaphragmatic and costal surfaces meet; the inferior border of the lung does not extend to the costal pleural reflection. The anterior border is where the costal and mediastinal surfaces meet anteriorly. On the left lung, the cardiac impression creates a visible curvature on the anterior border called the "cardiac notch." Below the cardiac notch, a segment of lung called the "lingula" protrudes around the apex of the heart.

The main bronchi are the initial right and left branches from the bifurcation of the trachea that enter the lung at the hilum (Fig. 4.25). They, like the trachea, are held open by "C-shaped" segments of hyaline cartilage. The right main bronchus is wider and shorter and enters the lung

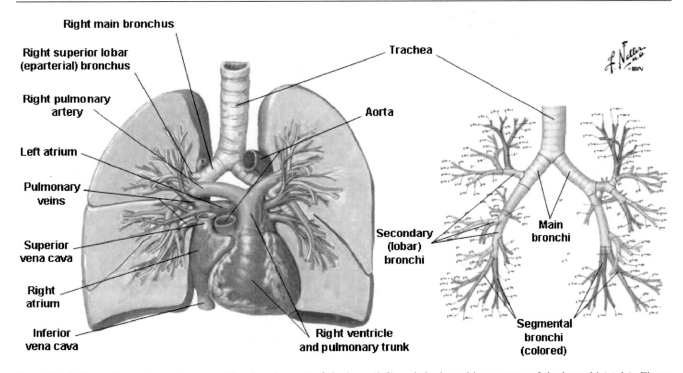

Fig. 4.25 Pattern of structure entering and leaving the root of the lung (*left*) and the branching pattern of the bronchi (*right*). Figure adapted from Atlas of Human Anatomy, 2nd ed. (Plates 191 and 194)

more vertically than the left main bronchus. This is the reason aspirated foreign objects more often enter the right lung than the left. The left main bronchus passes anterior to the esophagus and under the aortic arch to enter the lung. Once in the lung, the main bronchi branch multiple times to form the bronchial tree (Fig. 4.25). The first branching supplies each lobe of the lung. These are the secondary or lobar bronchi. There are three lobar bronchi on the right and two on the left supplying their respective lobes. The lobar bronchi branch into several segmental bronchi, each of which supplies air to a subpart of the lobe called a bronchopulmonary segment. Each bronchopulmonary segment has an independent blood supply and can be resected without impacting the remaining lung. The segmental bronchi then further divide into a series of intersegmental bronchi. The smallest intersegmental bronchi branch to become bronchioles, which can be distinguished from bronchi in that they contain no cartilage in their wall. The terminal bronchioles branch into a series of respiratory bronchioles, each of which contains alveoli. The respiratory bronchioles terminate by branching into alveolar ducts that lead into alveolar sacs, where there are clusters of alveoli. It is in the alveoli where gasses in the air are exchanged with the blood.

Each lung is supplied by a pulmonary artery that carries deoxygenated blood (thus they are typically blue in anatomical atlases) from the right ventricle of the heart (Fig. 4.25). Each pulmonary artery enters the hilum of the

lung and branches with the bronchial tree to supply blood to the capillary bed surrounding the alveoli. The arterial branches have the same names as the bronchial branches. Oxygenated blood is returned to the left atrium of the heart via the paired pulmonary veins emerging from the hilum of both lungs. The pulmonary veins do not run the same course as the pulmonary arteries within the lung. At the hilum of the lung, the pulmonary artery is typically the most superior structure, with the main bronchus immediately below. On the right, the main bronchus is somewhat higher and the superior lobar bronchus crosses superior to the pulmonary artery; it is referred to as the eparterial bronchus. The pulmonary veins exit the hilum of the lung inferior to both the main bronchus and the pulmonary artery.

Lymphatic drainage of the lungs is to tracheobronchial lymph nodes located at the bifurcation of the trachea (Fig. 4.26). A subpleural lymphatic plexus lies under the visceral pleura and drains directly to the tracheobronchial nodes. A deep lymphatic plexus drains along the vasculature of the lungs to pulmonary nodes along the bronchi, which communicate with bronchopulmonary nodes at the hilum, and from there to the tracheobronchial nodes. The lymphatic drainage from the lungs may drain directly to the subclavian veins via the bronchomediastinal trunks or into the thoracic duct.

The lungs receive innervation from the pulmonary plexus (Fig. 4.16). The parasympathetic nerves are from

Fig. 4.26 Pattern of lymphatic drainage from the lungs. Figure adapted from Atlas of Human Anatomy, 2nd ed. (Plate 197)

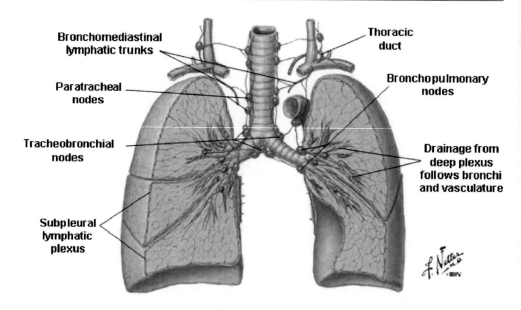

Bronchomediastinal lymphatic trunks

Paratracheal nodes

Tracheobronchial nodes

Subpleural lymphatic plexus

Thoracic duct

Bronchopulmonary nodes

Drainage from deep plexus follows bronchi and vasculature

vagus (CN X) and are responsible for constriction of the bronchi and vasodilatation of the pulmonary vessels; they are also secretomotor to the glands in the bronchial tree. The sympathetics act opposite to the parasympathetics. Pain afferents from the costal pleura and the outer parts of the diaphragmatic pleura are derived from the intercostal nerves. The phrenic nerves contain sensory afferents for the mediastinal pleura and the central part of the diaphragmatic pleura.

4.11.3 Mechanics of Respiration

Respiration is controlled by the muscles of the thoracic wall, the respiratory diaphragm, the muscles of the abdominal wall, and the natural elasticity of the lungs (Fig. 4.27). The diaphragm contracts during inspiration, causing the dome of the diaphragm to descend and the vertical dimension of the thoracic cavity to increase. Simultaneously, the ribs are elevated by contraction of external intercostal muscles and the interchondral parts of the internal intercostals. During deep inspiration, the ribs are further elevated by contraction of muscles in the neck. Elevation of the ribs increases the diameter of the thoracic cavity. The net result is the expansion of the pulmonary cavities. When the walls of the thorax expand, the lungs expand with them due to the negative pressure created in the pleural cavity and the propensity of the visceral pleura to maintain contact with the parietal pleura due to the surface tension of the liquid between these surfaces (somewhat like two plates of glass sticking together with water in between them). The resultant negative pressure in the lungs forces the subsequent intake of air.

Quiet expiration of air is primarily caused by the elastic recoil of the lungs when the muscles of inspiration are relaxed. Further expiration is achieved by contraction of the lateral internal intercostal muscles, depressing the ribs, and the contraction of abdominal muscles causing increased abdominal pressure which pushes up on the diaphragm. At rest, the inward pull of the lungs (trying to deflate further) is at equilibrium with the spring-like outward pull of the thoracic wall.

4.12 Surface Anatomy

4.12.1 Landmarks of the Thoracic Wall

There are several defined vertical lines that demark regions of the anterior and posterior thoracic wall (Fig. 4.23). These lines are used to describe the location of surface landmarks and the locations of injuries or lesions on or within the thorax. The anterior median line runs vertically in the midline; it is also referred to as the "midsternal line." The midclavicular line bisects the clavicle at its midpoint and typically runs through or close to the nipple. Three lines demarcate the axilla. The anterior axillary line runs vertically along the anterior axillary fold and the posterior axillary line runs parallel to it, along the posterior axillary fold. The midaxillary line runs in the midline of the axilla, at its deepest part. The scapular line runs vertically on the posterior thorax, through the inferior angle of the scapula. The posterior median line, also called the "midvertebral or midspinal line," runs vertically in the midline on the posterior thorax.

Muscles of Respiration

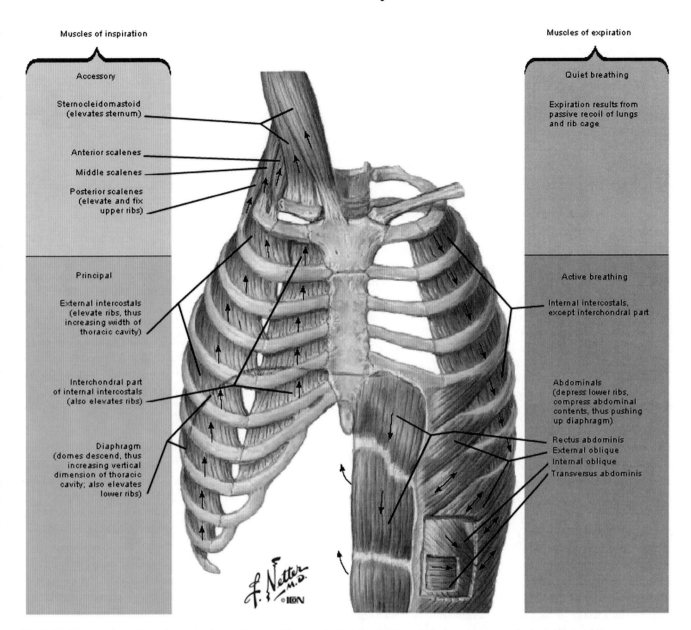

Fig. 4.27 The participation of muscles in respiration. Figure adapted from Atlas of Human Anatomy, 2nd ed. (Plate 183)

The sternum lies subcutaneously in the anterior median line and can be palpated throughout its length. The jugular notch is found at the upper margin of the sternum, between the medial ends of the clavicle. The jugular notch is easily palpated and can usually be seen as a depression on the surface. The jugular notch represents the anterior junction of the superior mediastinum and the root of the neck. It lies at the level of the T2 vertebra posteriorly. The manubrium intersects with the body of the sternum about 4 cm inferior to the jugular notch, at the manubriosternal joint; this joint creates the sternal angle which is normally visible on the surface of the thorax. The sternal angle

demarcates the inferior border of the superior mediastinum and lies at the level of the intervertebral disc between T4 and T5. The 2nd rib articulates with the sternum at the sternal angle, making this site an excellent landmark for determining rib number. Immediately adjacent to the sternal angle is rib 2; the other ribs can be found by counting up or down from rib 2. Intercostal spaces are numbered for the rib above. On the posterior thorax, the 4th rib can be found at the level of the medial end of the spine of the scapula and 8th rib at the inferior angle.

The manubrium overlies the junction of the brachiocephalic veins to form the superior vena cava (Fig. 4.23). The superior vena cava passes at the level of the sternal angle and at (or slightly to the right of) the border of the manubrium. The superior vena cava typically enters the right atrium behind the costal cartilage of the 3rd rib on the right; it is sometimes accessed for various procedures and knowledge of this surface anatomy is critical for such a procedure.

The xiphoid process is the inferior part of the sternum and lies in a depression called the "epigastric fossa" at the apex of the infrasternal angle formed by the convergence of the costal margins at the inferior border of the thorax (Fig. 4.23). The location of the xiphisternal joint is used as a landmark to determine hand position for cardiopulmonary resuscitation.

The breasts are also surface features of the thoracic wall. In women, the breasts vary greatly in size and conformation but the base of the breast usually occupies the space between ribs 2 and 6, from the lateral edge of the sternum to the midaxillary line. The nipples, surrounded by an area of darker pigmented skin called the "areola," are the prominent features of the breast. In men, the nipples are located anterior to the 4th intercostal space in the midclavicular line. Because of the variation in breast anatomy in the female, the location of the nipple is impossible to predict.

4.12.2 The Lungs and Pleura

The pleural sac is outlined by the parietal pleura as it projects onto the surface of the lungs (Fig. 4.23). From the root of the neck, these projections follow the lateral edge of the sternum inferiorly. On the left, the border of the parietal pleura moves laterally at the level of 4th costal cartilage to accommodate the cardiac notch within the mediastinum. The pleura follows a line just superior to the costal margin, reaching the level of the 10th rib at the midaxillary line. Posteriorly, the inferior margin of the plural cavity lies at the level of T12 and the medial margin follows the lateral border of the vertebral column to the root of the neck. In the superior parts of the pleural cavity, the visceral pleura of the lungs is in close contact with the parietal pleura, with the lungs consequently filling the plural cavity. Both lungs and parietal pleura (cervical part) extend above the clavicles into the supraclavicular fossae, at the root of the neck. At the inferior reaches of the pleural cavities, the lungs stop short of filling the plural cavity, reaching only to the level of the 6th rib in the midclavicular line, the 8th rib in the midaxillary line, and the 10th rib posteriorly, creating the costodiaphragmatic recesses. The major (oblique) fissures of the lungs extend along a line from the spinous process of T2 to the costal cartilage of the 6th rib. The minor (horizontal) fissure of the right lung lies under the 4th rib.

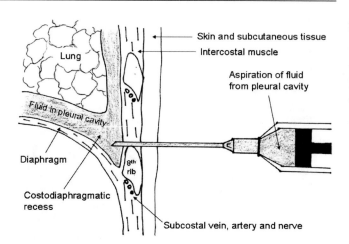

Fig. 4.28 Illustration of thoracocentesis. Figure adapted from Grant's Dissector, 12th ed. (Fig. 1.16)

Under pathologic conditions, fluid can accumulate in the pleural cavity. This fluid normally drains inferiorly and accumulates in the costodiaphragmatic recess. Thoracocentesis refers to the procedure used to drain such fluid (Fig. 4.28). A needle is inserted into the costodiaphragmatic recess by passing it through the middle of the intercostal space, being careful to avoid the primary intercostal neurovascular bundle immediately below the rib above and collaterals above the rib below.

4.12.3 The Heart

The heart and great vessels are covered by the sternum and central part of the thoracic cage (Fig. 4.23). The apex of the heart usually lies in the 5th intercostal space, just medial of the midclavicular line. The upper border of the heart follows a line from the inferior border of the left 2nd costal cartilage to the superior border of the right costal cartilage. The inferior border of the heart lies along a line from the right 6th costal cartilage to the 5th intercostal space, at the midclavicular line where the apex of the heart is located. The right and left borders follow lines connecting the right and left ends of the superior and inferior borders. All four heart valves, the closing of which accounts for the heart sounds, lie well protected behind the sternum. The sounds of the individual valves closing are best heard at ausculatory sites to which their sounds are transmitted. The bicuspid (mitral) valve is heard at the apex of the heart in the region of the 4th or 5th intercostal spaces on the left near the midclavicular line. The tricuspid valve can be heard along the left margin of the sternum at the level of the 4th or 5th intercostal space. The pulmonary valve is heard along the left border of the sternum in the 2nd intercostal space. The aortic valve is heard at the 2nd intercostal space on the right sternal border. For more details on heart sounds see Chapter 16.

4.12.4 Vascular Access

Understanding the surface landmarks relative to the axilla and subclavian region is critical for successful access of the venous system via the subclavian vein. The subclavian vein passes over the 1st rib and under the clavicle at the junction of its middle and medial thirds, it courses through the base of the neck where it passes anterior to the apex of the lung and the pleural cavity (Fig. 4.29). The subclavian vein is immediately anterior to the subclavian artery and is separated from the artery medially by the anterior scalene muscle. To access the subclavian vein, a needle is inserted approximately 1 cm inferior to the clavicle at the junction of its medial and middle thirds, and aimed toward the jugular notch, parallel with the vein to minimize risk of injury to adjacent structures. The most common complication of subclavian venous access is puncture of the apical pleura with resulting pneumothorax or hemopneumothorax. In addition, the subclavian artery, lying behind the vein, also has the potential to be injured by this procedure. If subclavian access is attempted on the left, one must also be aware of the junction of the thoracic duct with the subclavian vein. Injury to the thoracic duct can result in chylothorax, the accumulation of lymph in the plural cavity. This is difficult to treat and has an associated high morbidity. When access of the subclavian is attempted for cardiac lead placement, care must be taken to avoid piercing the subclavius muscle or costoclavicular ligament. Passing the lead through these structures tethers it to the highly mobile clavicle which may cause premature breakage of the lead.

4.12.5 Summary

Options for accessing the heart, in a minimally invasive fashion, are limited by the vascular anatomy of the superior mediastinum and the axilla. Percutaneous access strategies are limited by the bony anatomy of the thoracic cage. How a device interacts with the thorax and accommodates basic thoracic movements and movements of the upper extremity and neck must be understood in order to design devices that will endure in the body. Thus, a thorough understanding of the thoracic anatomy surrounding the heart is important to those seeking to design and deploy devices for placement and use in the heart. With an understanding of the important thoracic anatomical relationships presented in this chapter, the engineer should be able to design devices with an intuition for the anatomical challenges that will be faced for proper use and deployment of the device.

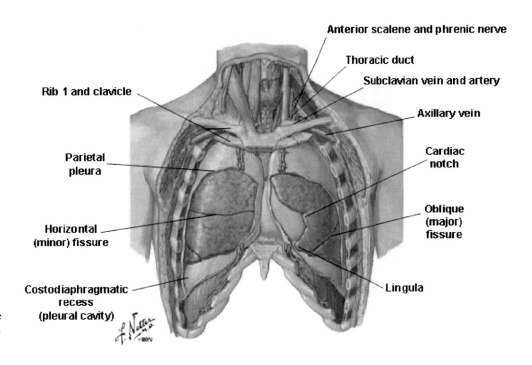

Fig. 4.29 Anatomy of the subclavian veins and surrounding structures. Figure adapted from Atlas of Human Anatomy, 2nd ed. (Plate 186)

General References and Suggested Reading

Hollinshead WH, Rosse C, eds. In: Textbook of anatomy. 4th ed. Philadelphia, PA: Harper & Row, 1985:463–575.

Magney LE, Flynn DM, Parsons JA, et al. Anatomical mechanisms explaining damage to pacemaker leads, defibrillator leads, and failure of central venous catheters adjacent to the sternoclavicular joint. Pacing Clin Electrophysiol 1993;16:445–57.

Moore KL, Dalley AF, eds. In: Clinically oriented anatomy. 4th ed. Philadelphia, PA: Lippincott Williams & Wilkins, 1990:62–173.

Netter FH. In: Atlas of human anatomy. 3rd ed. Teterboro, NJ: Icon Learning Systems, 2003.

Sauerland EK, ed. In: Grant's dissector. 12th ed. Philadelphia, PA: Lippincott Williams & Wilkins, 1999:1–39.

Weinberger SE. In: Principles of pulmonary medicine. 3rd ed. Philadelphia, PA: W. B. Saunders, 1998:1–20.

Chapter 5
Anatomy of the Human Heart

Anthony J. Weinhaus and Kenneth P. Roberts

Abstract This chapter covers the internal and external anatomy and function of the heart, as well as its positioning within the thorax. Briefly, the heart is a muscular pump, located in the protective thorax, which serves two functions: (1) collect blood from the tissues of the body and pump it to the lungs; and (2) collect blood from the lungs and pump it to all the tissues of the body. The heart's two upper chambers (or atria) function primarily as collecting chambers, while two lower chambers (ventricles) are much stronger and function to pump blood. The right atrium and ventricle collect blood from the body and pump it to the lungs, and the left atrium and ventricle collect blood from the lungs and pump it throughout the body. There is a one-way flow of blood through the heart which is maintained by a set of four valves (tricuspid, bicuspid, pulmonary, and aortic). The tissues of the heart are supplied with nourishment and oxygen by a separate vascular supply committed only to the heart; the arterial supply to the heart arises from the base of the aorta as the right and left coronary arteries, and the venous drainage is via cardiac veins that return deoxygenated blood to the right atrium.

Keywords Cardiac anatomy · Mediastinum · Pericardium · Atrium · Ventricle · Valves · Coronary artery · Cardiac veins · Cardiac skeleton · Cardiopulmonary circulation

5.1 Introduction

The heart is a muscular pump which serves two primary functions: (1) collect blood from the tissues of the body and pump it to the lungs; and (2) collect blood from the lungs and pump it to all other tissues other body. The human heart lies in the protective thorax, posterior to the sternum and costal cartilages, and rests on the superior surface of the diaphragm. The heart assumes an oblique position in the thorax, with two-thirds to the left of midline. It occupies a space between the pleural cavities called the *middle mediastinum*, defined as the space inside of the pericardium, the covering around the heart. This serous membrane has an inner and an outer layer, with a lubricating fluid in between. The fluid allows the inner visceral pericardium to "glide" against the outer parietal pericardium.

The internal anatomy of the heart reveals four chambers composed of cardiac muscle or "myocardium". The two upper chambers (or atria) function mainly as collecting chambers; the two lower chambers (ventricles) are much stronger and function to pump blood. The role of the right atrium and ventricle is to collect blood from the body and pump it to the lungs. The role of the left atrium and ventricle is to collect blood from the lungs and pump it throughout the body. There is a one-way flow of blood through the heart; this flow is maintained by a set of four valves. The atrioventricular or AV valves (tricuspid and bicuspid) allow blood to flow only from atria to ventricles. The semilunar valves (pulmonary and aortic) allow blood to flow only from the ventricles out of the heart and through the great arteries.

Various structures that can be observed in the adult heart are remnants of fetal circulation. In the fetus, the lungs do not function as a site for the exchange of oxygen and carbon dioxide, and the fetus receives all of its oxygen from the mother. In the fetal heart, blood arriving to the right side of the heart is passed through specialized structures to the left side. Shortly after birth, these specialized fetal structures normally collapse and the heart takes on the "adult" pattern of circulation. However, in rare cases, some fetal remnants and defects can occur.

A.J. Weinhaus (✉)
University of Minnesota, Department of Integrative Biology and Physiology, 6-130 Jackson Hall, 321 Church St. SE, Minneapolis, MN 55455, USA
e-mail: weinh001@umn.edu

P.A. Iaizzo (ed.), *Handbook of Cardiac Anatomy, Physiology, and Devices*, DOI 10.1007/978-1-60327-372-5_5,
© Springer Science+Business Media, LLC 2009

Although the heart is filled with blood, it provides very little nourishment and oxygen to the tissues of the heart. Instead, the tissues of the heart are supplied by a separate vascular supply committed only to the heart. The arterial supply to the heart arises from the base of the aorta as the right and left coronary arteries (running in the coronary sulcus). The venous drainage is via cardiac veins that return deoxygenated blood to the right atrium. See Chapter 7 for more details on the coronary vascular system.

It is important to note that besides pumping oxygen-rich blood to the tissues of the body for exchange of oxygen for carbon dioxide, the blood also circulates many other important substances. Nutrients from digestion are collected from the small intestine and pumped through the circulatory system to be delivered to all cells of the body. Hormones are produced from one type of tissue and distributed to all cells of the body. The circulatory system also carries waste materials (salts, nitrogenous wastes, and excess water) from cells to the kidneys, where they are extracted and passed to the bladder. The

pumping of interstitial fluid from the blood into the extracellular space is an important function of the heart. Excess interstitial fluid is then returned to the circulatory system via the lymphatic system.

5.2 Position of the Heart in the Thorax

The heart lies in the protective thorax, posterior to the sternum and costal cartilages, and rests on the superior surface of the diaphragm. The thorax is often referred to as the thoracic cage because of its protective function of the delicate structures within. The heart is located between the two lungs which occupy the lateral spaces called the *pleural cavities*. The space between these two cavities is referred to as the *mediastinum* ("that which stands in the middle"; Fig. 5.1).

The mediastinum is divided first into the superior and inferior mediastinum by a mid-sagittal imaginary line called the *transverse thoracic plane*. This plane passes

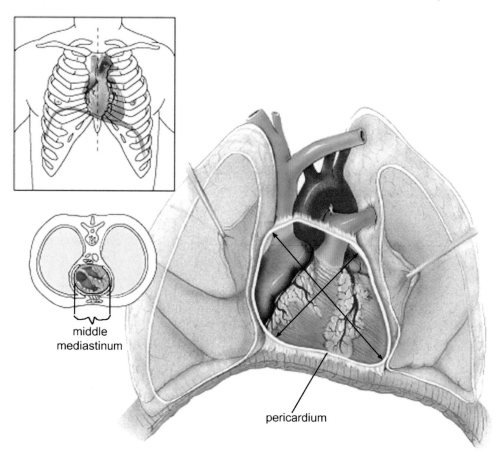

middle mediastinum

pericardium

Fig. 5.1 Position of the heart in the thorax. The heart lies in the protective thorax, posterior to the sternum and costal cartilages, and rests on the superior surface of the diaphragm. The heart assumes an oblique position in the thorax, with two-thirds to the left of midline. It is located between the two lungs which occupy the lateral spaces called the pleural cavities. The space between these

two cavities is referred to as the mediastinum. The heart lies obliquely in a division of this space, the middle mediastinum, surrounded by the pericardium. (Figs. 18.2 a,b,c, p. 523 from HUMAN ANATOMY, 3rd ed. by Elaine N. Marieb and Jon Mallatt. © 2001 by Benjamin Cummings. Reprinted by permission of Pearson Education, Inc.)

through the sternal angle (junction of the manubrium and body of the sternum) and the space between thoracic vertebrae T_4 and T_5. This plane acts as a convenient landmark as it also passes through the following structures: the bifurcation of the trachea; the superior border of the pericardium; the artificial division of the ascending and arch of the aortic artery; and the bifurcation of the pulmonary trunk.

The human heart assumes an oblique position in the thorax, with two-thirds to the left of midline (Figs. 5.2 and 5.3). The heart is roughly in a plane that runs from the right shoulder to the left nipple. The base is located below the 3rd rib as it approaches the sternum (note that the sternal angle occurs at the level of the 2nd rib). The base is directed superiorly, to the right of midline, and posterior. The pointed apex projects to the left of midline and anterior. Thus, the heartbeat can be easily palpated between the 5th and 6th ribs (just inferior to the left nipple) from the apex of the heart where it comes into close proximity of the thoracic wall. Importantly, the heart lies in such an oblique plane that it is often referred to as being horizontal. Thus, the anterior side may be imagined as the superior, and the posterior side as inferior.

The heart is composed of four distinct chambers. There are two atria (left and right) responsible for collecting blood and two ventricles (left and right) responsible for pumping blood. The atria are positioned superior to

(or posterior to) and somewhat to the right of their respective ventricles (Fig. 5.3). From superior to inferior, down the anterior (or superior) surface of the heart runs the anterior interventricular sulcus ("a groove"). This sulcus separates the left and right ventricles. This groove continues around the apex as the posterior interventricular sulcus on the posterior (inferior) surface. Between these sulci, located within the heart, is the interventricular septum ("wall between the ventricles"). The base of the heart is defined by a plane that separates the atria from the ventricles called the *atrioventricular groove or sulcus*. This groove appears like a belt cinched around the heart. Since this groove appears as though it might also be formed by placing a crown atop the heart, the groove is also called the *coronary* (*corona* = "crown") *sulcus*. The plane of this sulcus also contains the AV valves (and the semilunar valves) and a structure that surrounds the valves called the *cardiac skeleton*. The interatrial ("between the atria") septum is represented on the posterior surface of the heart as the atrial sulcus. Also on the posterior (inferior) side of the heart, the crux cordis ("cross of the heart") is formed from the atrial sulcus, posterior interventricular sulcus, and the relatively perpendicular coronary sulcus.

Note that the great arteries, aorta, and pulmonary trunk arise from the base of the heart, and the inferior angle of the heart is referred to as the *apex*; this resembles

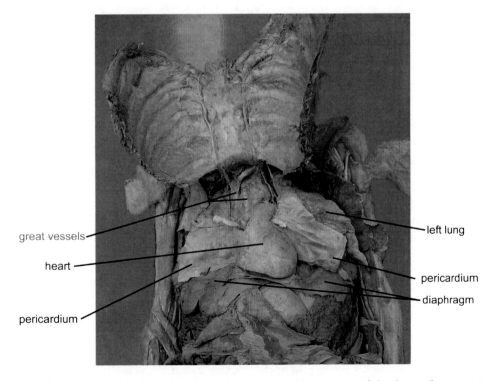

great vessels

heart

pericardium

left lung

pericardium

diaphragm

Fig. 5.2 Human cadaver dissection in which the ribs were cut laterally, and the sternum and ribs reflected superiorly. This dissection exposes the contents of the thorax (heart, great vessels, lungs, and diaphragm)

Fig. 5.3 The anterior surface of the heart. The atria are positioned superior to (posterior to) and to the right of their respective ventricles. From superior to inferior, down the anterior surface of the heart, runs the anterior interventricular sulcus ("a groove"). This sulcus separates the left and right ventricles. The base of the heart is defined by a plane that separates the atria from the ventricles called the atrioventricular groove or sulcus. Note that the great arteries, aorta, and pulmonary trunk arise from the base of the heart. The right and left atrial appendages appear as extensions hanging off each atria. The anterior (superior) surface of the heart is formed primarily by the right ventricle. The right lateral border is formed by the right atrium and the left lateral border by the left ventricle. The posterior surface is formed by the left ventricle and the left atrium which is centered equally upon the midline

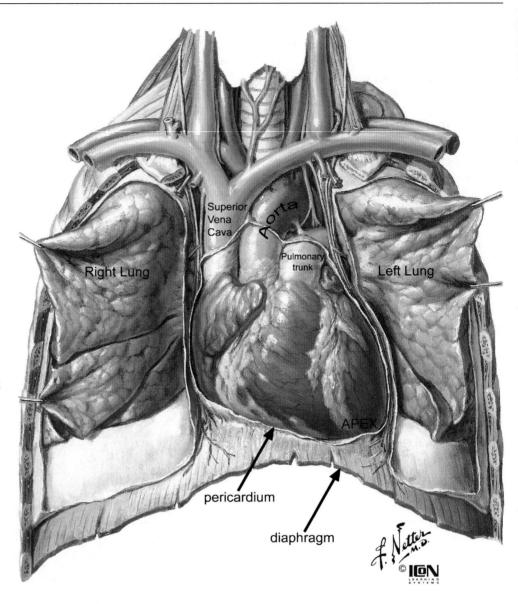

an inverted pyramid. The right and left atrial appendages (or auricles, so named because they look like dog ears, *auricle* = "little ear") appear as extensions hanging off each atrium.

The anterior (superior) surface of the heart is formed primarily by the right ventricle. The right lateral border is formed by the right atrium, and the left lateral border by the left ventricle. The posterior surface is formed by the left ventricle and the left atrium which is centered equally upon the midline.

The acute angle found on the right anterior side of the heart is referred to as the *acute* margin of the heart and continues toward the diaphragmatic surface. The rounded left anterior side is referred to as the *obtuse* margin of the heart and continues posteriorly and anteriorly. Both right

and left ventricles contribute equally to the diaphragmatic surface, lying in the plane of the diaphragm.

5.3 The Pericardium

The pericardium (*peri* = "around" + *cardia* = "heart") is the covering around the heart. It is composed of two distinct but continuous layers that are separated from each other by a potential space containing a lubricating substance called *serous fluid*. During embryological development, the heart moves from a peripheral location into a space called the *celomic cavity*. The cavity has a serous fluid secreting lining. As the heart migrates into the

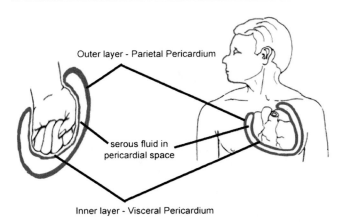

Outer layer - Parietal Pericardium

serous fluid in
pericardial space

Inner layer - Visceral Pericardium

Fig. 5.4 The pericardium is the covering around the heart. It is composed of two distinct but continuous layers that are separated from each other by a potential space containing a lubricating serous fluid. During embryological development, the heart migrates into the celomic cavity and a serous lining wraps around it, a process similar to a fist being pushed into a balloon. Note that the balloon, and the pericardium, is one continuous layer of material. The pericardium can be divided into the visceral pericardium (epicardium) and the parietal pericardium. A small amount of serous fluid is secreted into the pericardial space to lubricate the movement of the epicardium on the parietal pericardium. The parietal pericardium contains an epipericardial layer called the fibrous pericardium

cavity, the serous lining wraps around the heart. This process can be described as being similar to a fist being pushed into a balloon (Fig. 5.4). Note that the fist is surrounded by balloon; however, it does not enter the balloon, and the balloon is still one continuous layer of material. These same properties are true for the pericardium. Furthermore, although it is one continuous layer, the pericardium is divided into two components. The part of the pericardium that is in contact with the heart is called the *visceral pericardium* (*viscus* = "internal organ") or epicardium (epi = "upon" + "heart"). The free surface of the epicardium is covered by a single layer of flat-shaped epithelial cells called *mesothelium*. The mesothelial cells secrete a small amount of serous fluid to lubricate the movement of the epicardium on the parietal pericardium. The epicardium also includes a thin layer of fibroelastic connective tissue which supports the mesothelium, and a broad layer of adipose tissue which serves to connect the fibroelastic layer to the myocardium. The part of the pericardium forming the outer border is called the *parietal pericardium* (parietes = "walls"). The parietal pericardium, in addition to a serous layer, also contains a fibrous or epipericardial layer referred to as the *fibrous pericardium*. These layers contain collagen and elastin fibers to provide strength and some degree of elasticity to the parietal pericardium. The serous portions of

the epicardium and parietal pericardium are often referred to as the *serous pericardium*, with the fibrous portion of the parietal pericardium called the *fibrous pericardium*.

Inferiorly, the parietal pericardium is attached to the diaphragm. Anteriorly, the superior and inferior pericardiosternal ligaments secure the parietal pericardium to the manubrium and the xiphoid process, respectively. Laterally, the parietal pericardium is in contact with the parietal pleura (the covering of the lungs). Between the parietal and fibrous layers of the pericardium are found running together the phrenic nerve (motor innervation to the diaphragm) and the pericardiacophrenic artery and vein (supplying the pericardium and diaphragm). It is important to note, however, that there is no potential space between the parietal and fibrous pericardium.

Under normal circumstances, only serous fluid exists between the visceral and parietal layers in the pericardial space or cavity. However, the accumulation of fluid (blood from trauma, inflammatory exudate following infection) in the pericardial space leads to the compression of the heart. This condition, called *cardiac tamponade* ("heart" + *tampon* = "plug"), occurs when the excess fluid limits the expansion of the heart (the fibrous pericardium resists stretching) between beats and reduces the ability to pump blood, leading to hypoxia (*hypo* = "low" + "oxygen") (see Fig. 8.5).

Superiorly, the parietal pericardium surrounds the aorta and pulmonary trunk (about 3 cm above their departure from the heart) and is referred to as the *arterial reflections* or *arterial mesocardium*; and the superior vena cava, inferior vena cava, and pulmonary veins are surrounded by the venous reflections or venous mesocardium. The outer fibrous epipericardial layer merges with the outer adventitial layer of the great vessels, which is continuous with the visceral pericardium. The result of this reflection is that the heart hangs "suspended" within the pericardial cavity.

Within the parietal pericardium, a blind-ended sac-like recess called the *oblique pericardial sinus* is formed from the venous reflections of the inferior vena cava and pulmonary veins (Fig. 5.5). A space called the *transverse pericardial sinus* is formed between the arterial reflections above, and the venous reflections of the superior vena cava and pulmonary veins below. This sinus is important to cardiac surgeons in various procedures when it is important to stop or divert the circulation of blood from the aorta and pulmonary trunk. By passing a surgical clamp or ligature through the transverse sinus and around the great vessels, the tubes of a circulatory bypass machine can be inserted. Cardiac surgery may then be performed while the patient is on cardiopulmonary bypass (see Chapter 30).

Fig. 5.5 Pericardial sinuses. A blind-ended sac called the oblique pericardial sinus is formed from the venous reflections of the inferior vena cava and pulmonary veins. Another sac, the transverse pericardial sinus, is formed between the arterial reflections above and the venous reflections of the superior vena cava and pulmonary veins below

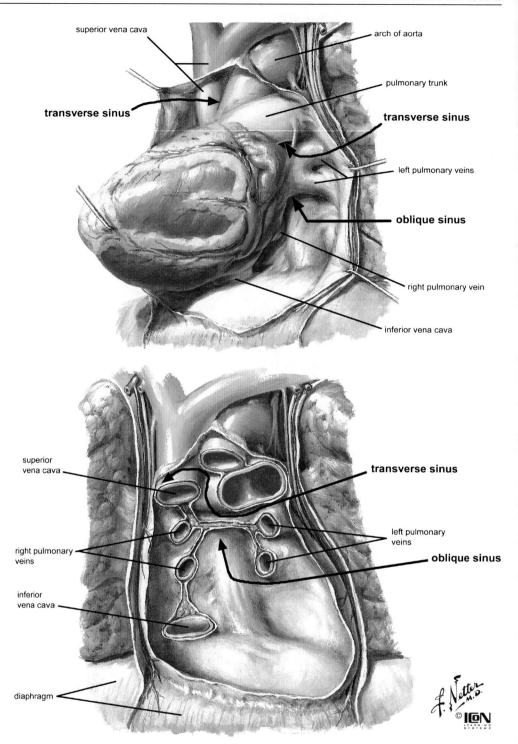

5.4 Internal Anatomy of the Heart

A cross-section cut through the heart reveals a number of layers (Fig. 5.6). From superficial to deep these are: (1) the parietal pericardium with its dense fibrous layer, the fibrous pericardium; (2) the pericardial cavity (containing only serous fluid); (3) a superficial visceral pericardium or epicardium (*epi* = "upon" + "heart"); (4) a middle

myocardium (*myo* = "muscle" + "heart"); and (5) a deep lining called the endocardium (*endo* = "within"). The endocardium is the internal lining of the atrial and ventricular chambers, and is continuous with the endothelium (lining) of the incoming veins and outgoing arteries. It also covers the surfaces of the AV valves, pulmonary and aortic valves, as well as the chordae tendinae and papillary muscles. The endocardium is a sheet of epithelium called

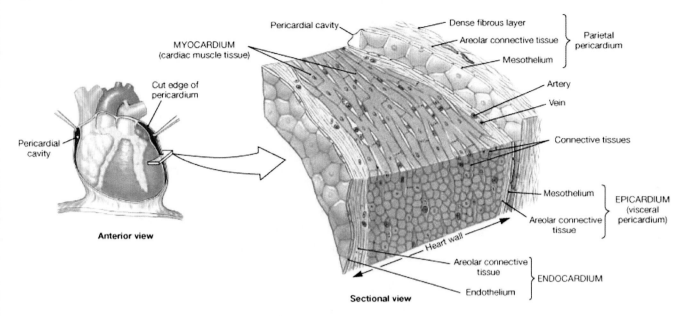

Fig. 5.6 Internal anatomy of the heart. The walls of the heart contain three layers—the superficial epicardium, the middle myocardium composed of cardiac muscle, and the inner endocardium. Note that cardiac muscle cells contain intercalated discs which enable the cells to communicate and allow direct transmission of electrical impulses from one cell to another. (Fig. 21.3a & b, p. 553 from HUMAN ANATOMY, 4th Edition by Frederic H. Martini, Michael J. Timmons, and Robert B. Tallitsch. © 2003 by Frederic H. Martini, Inc. and Michael J. Timmons.)

endothelium that rests on a dense connective tissue layer consisting of elastic and collagen fibers. These fibers also extend into the core of the previously mentioned valves.

The myocardium is the tissue of the heart wall and the layer that actually contracts. The myocardium consists of cardiac muscles which are circularly and spirally arranged networks of muscle cells that squeeze blood through the heart in the proper directions (inferiorly through the atria and superiorly through the ventricles). Unlike all other types of muscle cells: (1) cardiac muscle cells branch; (2) cardiac muscles join together at complex junctions called *intercalated discs*, so that they form cellular networks; and (3) each cell contains single centrally located nuclei. A cardiac muscle cell is typically not called a fiber. The term cardiac muscle fiber, when used, refers to a long row of joined cardiac muscle cells.

Like skeletal muscle, cardiac muscle cells are triggered to contract by Ca^{2+} ions flowing into the cell. Cardiac muscle cells are joined by complex junctions called *intercalated discs*. The discs contain adherans to hold the cells together, and there are gap junctions to allow ions to pass easily between the cells. The free movement of ions between cells allows for the direct transmission of an electrical impulse through an entire network of cardiac muscle cells. This impulse, in turn, signals all the muscle cells to contract at the same time. For more details on the electrical properties of the heart, the reader is referred to Chapter 11.

5.4.1 Cardiopulmonary Circulation

In order to best understand the internal anatomy of the heart, it is desirable to first understand its general function. The heart has two primary functions—collect oxygen-poor blood and pump it to the lungs for release of carbon dioxide in exchange for oxygen and collect oxygen-rich blood from the lungs and pumps it to all tissues in the body to provide oxygen in exchange for carbon dioxide.

The four chambers in the heart can be segregated into the left and the right side, each containing an atrium and a ventricle. The right side is responsible for collecting oxygen-poor blood and pumping it to the lungs. The left side is responsible for collecting oxygen-rich blood from the lungs and pumping it to all tissues in the body. Within each side, the atrium is a site for the collection of blood, before pumping it to the ventricle. The ventricle is much stronger, and it is a site for the pumping of blood out and away from the heart (Fig. 5.7).

The right ventricle is the site for the collection of ALL oxygen-poor blood. The large superior and inferior venae cavae, among other veins, carry oxygen-poor blood from the upper and lower parts of the body to the right atrium. The right ventricle pumps the blood out of the heart, and through the pulmonary trunk. The term *trunk*, when referring to a vessel, is a convention that indicates an artery that bifurcates. The pulmonary trunk bifurcates into the left and right pulmonary arteries that enter the

Fig. 5.7 Cardiopulmonary circulation. The four chambers in the heart can be segregated into the left and the right side, each containing an atrium and a ventricle. The right side is responsible for collecting oxygen-poor blood and pumping it to the lungs. The left side is responsible for collecting oxygen-rich blood from the lungs and pumping it to the body. An artery is a vessel that carries blood away from the heart, while a vein is a vessel that carries blood toward the heart. The pulmonary trunk and arteries carry blood to the lungs. Exchange of carbon dioxide for oxygen occurs in the lung through the smallest of vessels, the capillaries. Oxygenated blood is returned to the heart through the pulmonary veins and collected in the left atrium

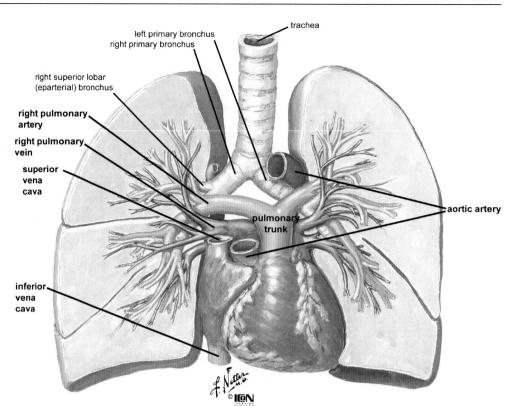

lungs. It is important to note that the term "artery" is always used for a vessel that carries blood AWAY from the heart. This is irrespective of the oxygen content of the blood that flows through the vessel.

Once oxygenated, the oxygen-rich blood returns to the heart from the right and left lung through the right and left pulmonary vein, respectively ("vein"—a vessel carrying blood TOWARD the heart). Each pulmonary vein bifurcates before reaching the heart. Thus, there are four pulmonary veins entering the left atrium. Oxygen-rich blood is pumped out of the heart by the left ventricle and into the aortic artery. The right side of the heart and the pulmonary artery and veins are part of the pulmonary circuit because of their role in getting blood to and from the lungs (*pulmo* = "lungs"). The left side of the heart, the aortic artery, and the venae cavae are part of the systemic circuit because of their role in getting blood to and from all the tissues of the body.

Observing the heart from a superior vantage point, the pulmonary trunk assumes a left-most anterior location projecting upward from the base of the heart, the aorta is located in a central location, and the superior vena cava has the right-most posterior location. The general pattern of blood flow through the heart is shown in Fig. 5.8. Note that the function of the atria is generally to collect, while the function of ventricles is to pump. The right side is involved in pulmonary circulation, while the left side is involved in

the systemic circulation. There is a unidirectional flow of blood through the heart; this is accomplished by valves.

5.4.2 The Right Atrium

The interior of the right atrium has three anatomically distinct regions, each a remnant of embryologic development. The posterior portion of the right atrium has a smooth wall and is referred to as the *sinus venarum* (embryologically derived from the right horn of the sinus venosus). The wall of the anterior portion of the right atrium is lined by horizontal, parallel ridges of muscle bundles that resemble the teeth of a comb, hence the name *pectinate* muscle (*pectin* = "a comb," embryologically derived from the primitive right atrium). Finally, the atrial septum is primarily derived from the embryonic septum primum and septum secundum. For more details on the embryology of the heart, refer to Chapter 3.

The smooth posterior wall of the right atrium holds the majority of the named structures of the right atrium. It receives both the superior and inferior venae cavae and the coronary sinus. It also contains the fossa ovalis, the sinoatrial (SA) node, and the AV node.

The inferior border of the right atrium contains the opening or ostium of the inferior vena cava, and the os or

Fig. 5.8 Cardiac circulation. Blood collected in the right atrium is pumped into the right ventricle. Upon contraction of the right ventricle, blood passes through the pulmonary trunk and arteries to the lungs. Oxygenated blood returns to the left atrium via pulmonary veins. The left atrium pumps the blood into the left ventricle. Contraction of the left ventricle sends the blood through the aortic artery to all tissues in the body. The release of oxygen in exchange for carbon dioxide occurs through capillaries in the tissues. Return of oxygen-poor blood is through the superior and inferior venae cavae which empty into the right atrium. Note that a unidirectional flow of blood through the heart is accomplished by valves

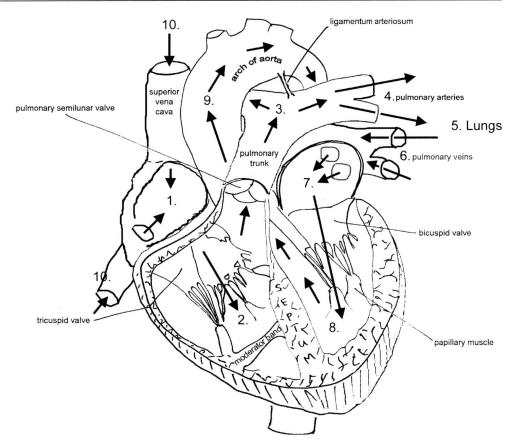

ostium of the coronary sinus (Fig. 5.9). The coronary sinus is located on the posterior (inferior) side of the heart and receives almost all of the deoxygenated blood from the vasculature of the heart. The os of the coronary sinus opens into the right atrium anteriorly and inferiorly to the orifice of the inferior vena cava. A valve of the inferior vena cava (Eustachian valve, a fetal remnant) guards the orifice of the inferior vena cava (Bartolommeo E. Eustachio, Italian anatomist, 1520–1574). The valve of the coronary sinus (Thebesian valve) covers the opening of the coronary sinus to prevent backflow (Adam C. Thebesius, German physician, 1686–1732). Both of these valves vary in size and presence. For more details on these valves of the heart, refer to Chapter 7. These two venous valves insert into a prominent ridge, the Eustachian ridge (sinus septum), that runs medial–lateral across the inferior border of the atrium and separates the os of the coronary sinus and inferior vena cava.

On the medial side of the right atrium, the interatrial septum (atrial septum) has an interatrial and an atrioventricular part. The fossa ovalis (a fetal remnant) is found in the interatrial part of the atrial septum. It appears as a central depression surrounded by a muscular ridge or limbus. The fossa ovalis is positioned anterior and superior to the ostia of both the inferior vena cava and the coronary sinus. A tendinous structure, the tendon of

Todaro, connects the valve of the inferior vena cava to the central fibrous body (the right fibrous trigone) as a fibrous extension of the membranous portion of the interventricular septum. It courses obliquely within the Eustachian ridge and separates the fossa ovalis above from the coronary sinus below. This tendon likely has a structural role to support the inferior vena cava via the Eustachian valve and is a useful landmark in approximating the location of the AV node (conduction system).

To approximate the location of the AV node, found in the floor of the right atrium and the atrial septum, it is necessary to form a triangle (triangle of Koch; Walter Koch, German Surgeon, unknown—1880) using the following structures: (1) the os of the coronary sinus, posteriorly; (2) the right AV opening, anteriorly; and (3) the tendon of Todaro, posteriorly (Fig. 5.10).

In the lateral wall and the septum of the smooth portion of the right ventricle are numerous small openings in the endocardial surface. These openings are the ostia of the smallest cardiac (Thebesian) veins. These veins function to drain deoxygenated blood from the myocardium to empty into the right atrium which is the collecting site for all deoxygenated blood.

In the anterior-superior portion of the right atrium, the smooth wall of the interior becomes pectinate. The

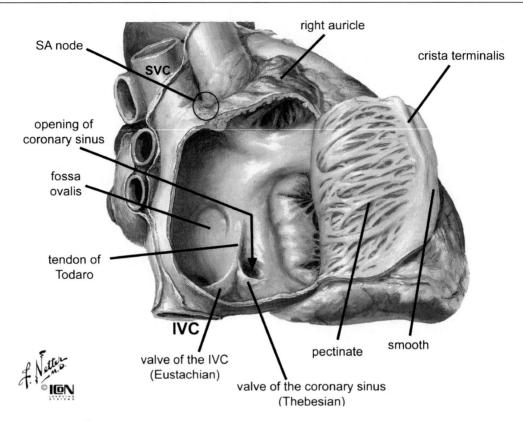

Fig. 5.9 Internal anatomy of the right atrium. The interior of the right atrium has three anatomically distinct regions: (1) the posterior portion (sinus venarum) which has a smooth wall; (2) the wall of the anterior portion which is lined by horizontal, parallel ridges of muscle referred to as pectinate; and (3) the atrial septum. IVC = inferior vena cava; SA=sinoatrial; SVC=superior vena cava

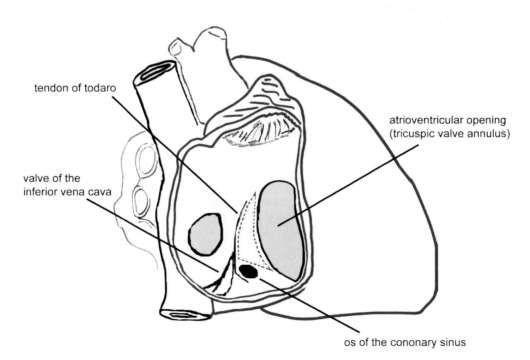

Fig. 5.10 Koch's triangle. Three landmarks are used to triangulate (*dotted red lines*) the location of the atrioventricular node (Taware's node) of the conduction system: (1) coronary sinus; (2) atrioventricular opening; and (3) tendon of Todaro

smooth and pectinate regions are separated by a ridge, the *crista terminalis* (*crista* = "crest" + "terminal"). The ridge represents the end of the smooth wall and the beginning of the pectinate wall. It begins at the junction of the right auricle with the atrium and passes inferiorly over the "roof" of the atrium. The crista runs inferiorly and parallel to the openings of the superior and inferior venae cavae. Recall that the crista terminalis separates the sinus venosus and the primitive atrium in the embryo and remains to separate the smooth and the pectinate portion of the right atrium after fetal development. The crista terminalis on the internal side results in a groove on the external side of the atrium, the sulcus terminalis.

The SA node is the "pacemaker" of the conduction system. This structure spontaneously produces a regular impulse for contraction of the atria and is located between the myocardium and epicardium in the superior portion of the right atrium. The intersection of three lines indicates the location of the SA node: (1) the sulcus terminalis; (2) the lateral border of the superior vena cava; and (3) the superior border of the right auricle (Fig. 5.11). The name of the SA node is derived from its location between the sinus venarum and primitive atrium. The crista terminalis is the division between these two components in the fetus and adult. It seems logical that the sulcus terminalis is a useful landmark for the approximation of the location of the SA node.

On the "floor" of the right atrium is the AV portion of the atrial septum which has muscular and membranous components. At the anterior and inferior aspect of the atrial septum, the tricuspid valve annulus (*annulus* = "ring") is attached to the membranous septum. As a result, a portion of the membranous septum lies superior to the annulus and therefore functions as a membranous atrial and a membranous ventricular septum.

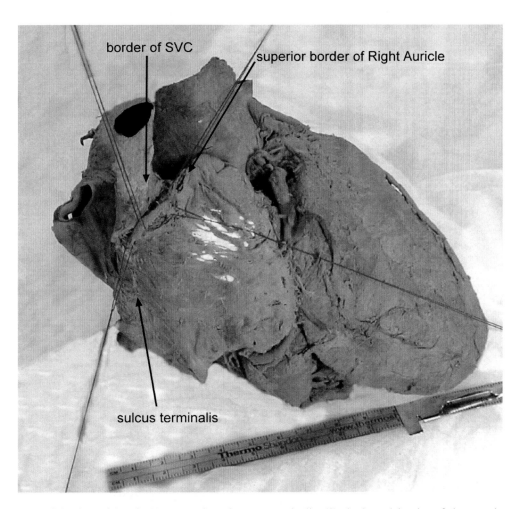

Fig. 5.11 The location of the sinoatrial node. Human cadaver heart demonstrating that the intersection of three lines indicates the position of the sinoatrial node (pacemaker of the conduction system) in the smooth muscle portion of the right atrium: (1) the sulcus terminalis; (2) the lateral border of the superior vena cava; and (3) the superior border of the right auricle. Note the muscle fiber bundles in the wall of the pectinate portion of right atrium. IVC = inferior vena cava; SVC = superior vena cava

5.4.3 The Right Ventricle

The right ventricle receives blood from the right atrium and pumps it to the lungs through the pulmonary trunk and arteries. Most of the anterior surface of the heart is formed by the right ventricle (Fig. 5.12). Abundant, coarse trabeculae carnae ("beams of meat") characterize the walls of the right ventricle. Trabeculae carnae are analogous to pectinate muscle of the right atrium (being bundles of myocardium) and are found in both the right and left ventricles. The outflow tract, conus arteriosus ("arterial cone") or infundibulum ("funnel"), carries blood out of the ventricle in an anterior-superior direction and is relatively smooth walled. A component of the conus arteriosus forms part of the interventricular septum. This small septum, the infundibular (conal) septum, separates the left and right ventricular outflow tracts and is located just inferior to both semilunar valves. Four distinct muscle bundles, collectively known as the *semicircular arch*, separate the outflow tract from the rest of the right atrium. These muscle bundles are also known as the *supraventricular crest* and the *septomarginal trabeculae*.

5.4.3.1 Tricuspid Valve

Blood is pumped from the right atrium through the AV orifice into the right ventricle. When the right ventricle contracts, blood is prevented from flowing back into the atrium by the right AV valve or tricuspid ("three cusps") valve. The valve consists of the annulus, three valvular leaflets, three papillary muscles, and three sets of chordae tendinae (Figs. 5.12 and 5.13).

The AV orifice is reinforced by the annulus fibrosus of the cardiac skeleton (dense connective tissue). Medially, the annulus is attached to the membranous ventricular septum.

The tricuspid valve has three leaflets—anterior (superior), posterior (inferior), and septal. The anterior leaflet is the largest, and extends from the medial border of the ventricular septum to the anterior free wall. This, in effect, forms a partial separation between the inflow and outflow tracts of the right ventricle. The posterior leaflet extends from the lateral free wall to the posterior portion of the ventricular septum. The septal leaflet tends to be somewhat oval in shape and extends from the annulus of the

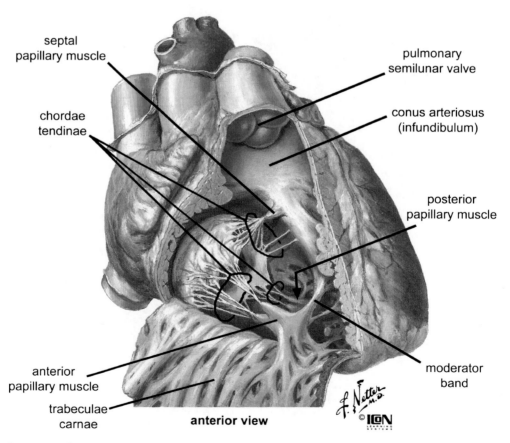

septal
papillary muscle

chordae
tendinae

pulmonary
semilunar valve

conus arteriosus
(infundibulum)

posterior
papillary muscle

anterior
papillary muscle

trabeculae
carnae

moderator
band

anterior view

Fig. 5.12 Internal anatomy of the right ventricle. Coarse trabeculae carnae characterize the walls of the right ventricle. The conus arteriosus makes up most of the outflow tract. The right atrioventricular or tricuspid valve is made up of three sets of cusps, chordae tendinae, and papillary muscles

Fig. 5.13 Valves of the heart. During ventricular systole, atrioventricular (AV) valves close in order to prevent the regurgitation of blood from the ventricles into the atria. The right AV valve is the tricuspid valve, the left is the bicuspid valve. During ventricular diastole, the AV valves open as the ventricles relax, and the semilunar valves close. The semilunar valves prevent the backflow of blood from the great arteries into the resting ventricles. The valve of the pulmonary trunk is the pulmonary semilunar valve, and the aortic artery has the aortic semilunar valve. To the *right* of each figure are human cadaveric hearts

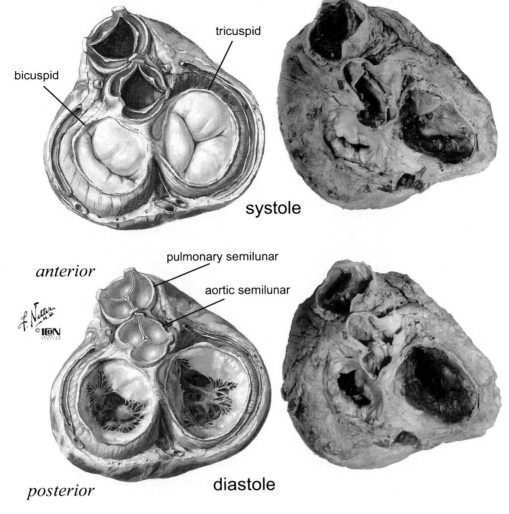

Papillary ("nipple") muscles contract and "tug" down on chordae tendinae ("tendinous cords") that are attached to the leaflets in order to secure them in place in preparation for the contraction of the ventricle. This is done to prevent the prolapse of the leaflets up into the atrium. This is somewhat analogous to the tightening of the sails on a yacht, in preparation for a big wind. Note that the total surface area of the cusps of the AV valve is approximately twice that of the respective orifice, so that considerable overlap of the leaflets occurs when the valves are in the closed position. The leaflets remain relatively close together even during ventricular filling. The partial approximation of the valve surfaces is caused by eddy currents that prevail behind the leaflets and by tension that is exerted by the chordae tendinae and papillary muscle. As the filling of the ventricle reduces, the valve leaflets float toward each other, but the valve does not

close. The valve is closed by ventricular contractions, and the valve leaflets, which bulge toward the atrium but do not prolapse, stay pressed together throughout ventricular contraction. The junction between two leaflets is called a *commissure* and is named by the two adjoining leaflets (anteroseptal, anteroposterior, and posteroseptal). Each commissure contains a relatively smooth arc of valvular tissue that is delineated by the insertion of the chordae tendinae.

There are three papillary muscles, just as there are three leaflets or cusps. The anterior papillary muscle is located in the apex of the right ventricle. This is the largest of the papillary muscles in the right ventricle, and it may have one or two heads. When this papillary muscle contracts, it pulls on chordae tendinae that are attached to the margins of the anterior and posterior leaflets. The posterior papillary muscle is small and located in the posterior lateral free wall. When this papillary contracts, it pulls on chordae tendinae that are attached to posterior and septal leaflets. The septal papillary muscle (including the variable papillary of the conus) arises from the muscular interventricular septum near the outflow tract (conus arteriosus). This papillary muscle may consist of a collection of small muscles in close proximity and has attachments to the anterior and septal valve leaflets. In addition, chordae tendinae in this region may extend simply from the myocardium and attach to the valve leaflets directly without a papillary muscle. The most affected is the septal leaflet which has restricted mobility due to extensive chordae tendinae attachment directly to the myocardium. In addition, there is a variable set of papillary muscles that should be considered. The medial papillary muscle complex is a collection of small papillary muscles with chordae attachments to septal and anterior cusps. This complex is located in the uppermost posterior edge of the septomarginal trabeculae, just inferior to the junction of the septal and anterior leaflets of the tricuspid valve, and is superior and distinct from the septal papillary muscles. An important feature of this complex is that it serves as an important landmark for identification of the right bundle branch as it runs posterior to it, deep to the endocardium [1].

Near the anterior free wall of the right ventricle is a muscle bundle of variable size, the *moderator band*, which is occasionally absent. This muscle bundle extends from the interventricular septum to the anterior papillary muscle and contains the right bundle branch of the conduction system. It seems logical that the anterior papillary muscle, with its remote location away from the septum, would need special conduction fibers in order for it to contract with the other papillary muscles and convey control of the valve leaflets equal to the other valve leaflets. The moderator band is a continuation of another muscle bundle, the septal band (septal trabeculae). Together they are called *septomarginal trabeculae* and are components of the semicircular arch (delineation of the outflow tract).

5.4.3.2 Pulmonary Semilunar Valve

During ventricular systole, blood is pumped from the right ventricle into the pulmonary trunk and arteries toward the lungs. When the right ventricle relaxes, in diastole, blood is prevented from flowing back into the ventricle by the pulmonary semilunar valve (Figs. 5.12 and 5.13). The semilunar valve is composed of three symmetric, semilunar-shaped cusps. Each cusp looks like a cup composed of a thin membrane. Each cusp acts like an upside-down parachute facing into the pulmonary trunk, opening as it fills with blood. This filled space or recess of each cusp is called the *sinus of Valsalva*. Upon complete filling, the three cusps contact each other and block the flow of blood. Each of the three cusps is attached to an annulus ("ring") such that the cusp opens into the lumen

forming a U-shape. The annulus is anchored to both the right ventricular infundibulum and the pulmonary trunk. The cusps are named according to their orientation in the body—anterior, left (septal), and right.

During ventricular systole, the cusps collapse against the arterial wall as the right ventricle contracts, sending blood flowing past them. When the ventricle rests (diastole), the cusps meet in the luminal center. There is a small thickening on the center of the free edge of each cusp, at the point where the cusps meet. This nodule (of Arantius or Morgagni) ensures central valve closure (Giulio C. (Aranzi) Arantius, Italian anatomist and physician, 1530–1589, Giovanni B. Morgagni, Italian anatomist and pathologist, 1682–1771). Radiating from this nodule around the free edge of the cusp is a ridge, the *linea alba* ("line" + "white").

5.4.4 The Left Atrium

The left atrium (Fig. 5.14) receives oxygenated blood from the lungs via the left and right pulmonary veins. The pulmonary veins enter the heart as two pairs of veins inserting posteriorly and laterally into the left atrium.

The left atrium is found midline, posterior to the right atrium and superior to the left ventricle. Anteriorly, a left atrial appendage (auricle) extends over the atrioventricular (coronary) sulcus. The walls of the atrial appendage are pectinate, and the walls of the left atrium are smooth, reflecting their embryological origin. The atrial appendage is derived from the primitive atrium (a strong pumping structure), and the atrium is derived from the fetal pulmonary vein as a connection with the embryonic pulmonary venous plexus. The venous structures are absorbed into the left atrium, resulting in the posteriolateral connections of the right and left pulmonary veins.

The atrial septum of the left atrium is derived from the embryonic septum primum. In the left atrium, the resulting structure in the adult is called the *valve of the foramen ovale* (a sealed valve flap).

5.4.5 The Left Ventricle

The left ventricle receives blood from the left atrium and pumps it through the aortic artery to all the tissues of the body (Fig. 5.14). Most of the left lateral surface of the heart is formed by the left ventricle, also forming part of the inferior and posterior surface. As with the right ventricle, abundant trabeculae carnae ("beams of meat") characterize the walls of the left. However, in contrast to the right

Fig. 5.14 Internal anatomy of the left atrium and ventricle. The left atrium receives oxygenated blood from the lungs via the left and right pulmonary veins. The pulmonary veins enter the heart as two pairs of veins inserting posteriorly and laterally. Anteriorly, the pectinate left auricle extends over the smooth-walled atrium. Most of the left lateral surface of the heart is formed by the left ventricle. Trabeculae carnae characterize the walls and the myocardium is much thicker than the left ventricle. The interventricular septum bulges into the right ventricle creating a barrel-shaped left ventricle

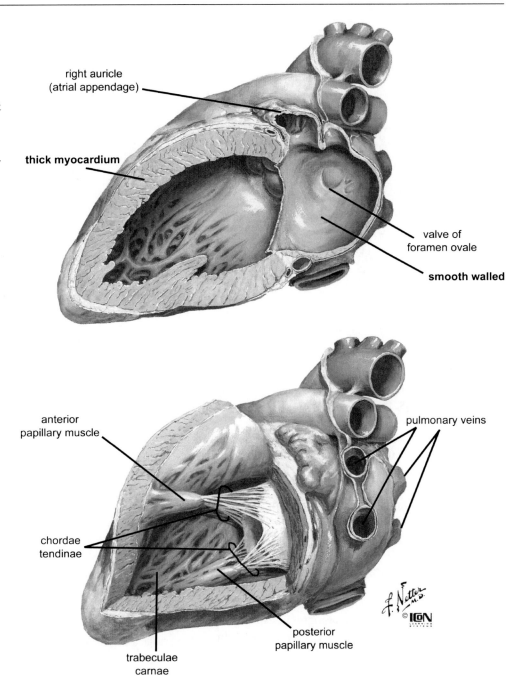

ventricle, the muscular ridges tend to be relatively fine. Also in contrast to the right ventricle, the myocardium in the wall of the left ventricle is much thicker. The interventricular septum appears from within the left ventricle to bulge into the right ventricle. This creates a barrel-shaped left ventricle.

5.4.5.1 Bicuspid (Mitral) Valve

Blood is pumped from the left atrium through the left AV orifice into the left ventricle. When the left ventricle contracts, blood is prevented from flowing back into the atrium

by the left AV valve or bicuspid ("two cusps") valve (Figs. 5.13 and 5.14). The valve consists of the annulus, two leaflets, two papillary muscles, and two sets of chordae tendinae.

The atrioventricular orifice is partly reinforced by the annulus fibrosus of the cardiac skeleton. The annulus fibrosus supports the posterior and lateral two-thirds of the annulus. The remaining medial third is supported by attachment to the left atrium and by fibrous support to the aortic semilunar valve.

The bicuspid valve has two leaflets—anterior (medial or aortic) and posterior (inferior or mural, "wall"). The

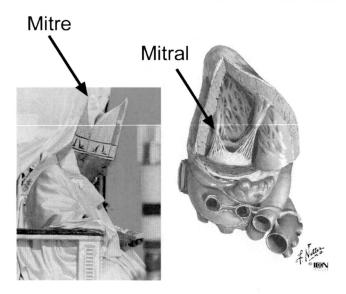

Fig. 5.15 The mitral valve. The mitral (left atrioventricular or bicuspid) valve is so named because of its resemblance to a cardinal's hat, known as a mitre. *Left*: Photo of Pope John Paul II from the Vatican web site

two apposing leaflets of the valve resemble a cardinal's hat or mitre. Thus, the bicuspid valve is often referred to as the mitral valve (Fig. 5.15).

The anterior leaflet is trapezoidal shaped. The distance from its attachment on the annulus to its free edge is longer than the length of attachment across the annulus. In contrast, the posterior leaflet is relatively narrow, with a very long attachment distance across the annulus. The distance from annulus to free edge in the anterior cusp is twice as long as the posterior cusp. The posterior cusp is so long and narrow that the free edge is often subdivided into the anterior, central, and posterior crescent shapes.

Papillary muscles, in conjunction with chordae tendinae, attach to the leaflets in order to secure them in place. This is done in preparation for the contraction of the ventricle to prevent the prolapse of the leaflets up into the atrium. As with the other AV valve, the total surface area of the two cusps of the valve is significantly greater than the area described by the orifice. There is considerable overlap of the leaflets when the valves are in the closed position (Fig. 5.13).

As with the tricuspid valve, the leaflets remain relatively close together even when the atrium is contracting and the ventricle is filling. The partial approximation of the valve surfaces is caused by eddy currents that prevail behind the leaflets and by tension that is exerted by the chordae tendinae and papillary muscle. In the open position, the leaflets and commissures are in an oblique plane of orientation that is roughly parallel to the ventricular septum. The valve is closed by ventricular contractions. The valve leaflets, which bulge toward the atrium, stay

pressed together throughout the contraction and do not prolapse. The junctions of the two leaflets are called the *anterolateral* and the *posteromedial* commissures. The line of apposition of the leaflets during valvular closure is indicated by a fibrous ridge.

There are two papillary muscles of the left ventricle that extend from the ventricular free wall toward and perpendicular to the atrioventricular orifice. The anterior papillary muscle is slightly larger than the posterior, and each papillary muscle consists of a major trunk that often has multiple heads from which extend the chordae tendinae. The chordae tendinae of each papillary muscle extend to the two valvular commissures, and to the multiple crescent shapes of the posterior cusp. Thus, each papillary muscle pulls on chordae from both leaflets. In addition, the posterior leaflet has occasionally chordae that extend simply from the ventricular myocardium without a papillary muscle.

5.4.5.2 Aortic Semilunar Valve

During ventricular systole, blood is pumped from the left ventricle into the aortic artery to all of the tissues of the body. When the left ventricle relaxes in diastole, blood is prevented from flowing back into the ventricle by the aortic semilunar valve (Figs. 5.13 and 5.14). Like the pulmonary semilunar valve, the aortic valve is composed of three symmetric, semilunar-shaped cusps, and each cusp acts like an upside-down parachute facing into the aortic artery, opening as it fills with blood. The filled space or recess of each cusp is called the *sinus of Valsalva* (Antonio M. Valsalva, 1666–1723). Upon complete filling, the three cusps contact each other and block the flow of blood. Each of the three cusps is attached to an annulus ("ring") such that the cusp opens into the lumen forming a U-shape. The cusps are firmly anchored to the fibrous skeleton within the root of the aorta (Fig. 5.16). A circular ridge on the innermost aspect of the aortic wall, at the upper margin of each sinus, is the sinotubular ridge—the junction of the sinuses and the aorta.

At the sinotubular ridge, the wall of the aorta is thin, bulges slightly, and is the narrowest portion of the aortic artery. The cusps are named according to their orientation in the body—left and right (both facing the pulmonary valve) and posterior. Within the sinuses of Valsalva, there are openings or ostia (*ostium* = "door or mouth") into the blood supply of the heart called *coronary arteries*. These ostia are positioned below the sinotubular junction near the center of the sinuses. Only the two sinuses facing the pulmonary valve (left and right) have ostia that open into the left and right coronary arteries, respectively. Coronary arteries carry oxygenated blood to the myocardium of the heart. During ventricular diastole, the aortic

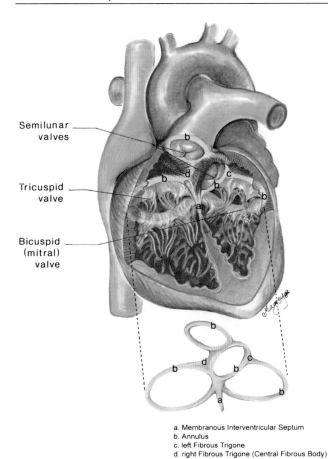

a. Membranous Interventricular Septum
b. Annulus
c. left Fibrous Trigone
d. right Fibrous Trigone (Central Fibrous Body)

Fig. 5.16 The cardiac skeleton. A dense connective tissue that functions to attach the atrial and ventricular myocardium, support and reinforce the openings of the four valves of the heart, and electrically separate the ventricles from the atria. Courtesy of Jean Magney, University of Minnesota

valve snaps shut as pressure in the aorta increases. Under such pressure, the walls of the great artery distend, the sinuses fill, and blood is sent under great pressure through the coronary ostia into the coronary arteries. The posterior (noncoronary) sinus is in a position that it abuts the fibrous skeleton and the annuli of both AV valves (Fig. 5.13).

When the left ventricle contracts, the cusps collapse against the arterial wall as blood flows past them. When the ventricle rests (diastole), the cusps meet in the luminal center. As with the pulmonary valve, there is a small thickening on the center of the free edge of each cusp, at the point where the cusps meet. This nodule (of Arantius or Morgagni) ensures central valve closure. Radiating from this nodule around the free edge of the cusp is a ridge, the *linea alba* ("line" + "white"). This valve is exposed to a greater degree of hemodynamic stress than the pulmonary valve. The aortic cusps can thicken and the linea alba can become more pronounced. For this and other reasons, the aortic pulmonary valve is the most likely valve to be surgically repaired or replaced.

5.5 The Cardiac Skeleton

Passing transversely through the base of the heart is a fibrous framework or "skeleton" made of dense connective tissue, not bone as the name might suggest. The purpose of this tough, immobile scaffold is to (1) provide an attachment for the atrial and ventricular myocardium; (2) anchor the four valves of the heart; and (3) electrically insulate the myocardium of the ventricles from the atria.

The supporting framework of the cardiac skeleton (Figs. 5.13 and 5.16) provides immobile support for the AV openings during atrial and ventricular contractions, and support for the semilunar valves against the high pressures generated during and after ventricular contractions. The skeleton is a formation of four attached rings with the opening for the aortic semilunar valve in the central position and the other valve rings attached to it.

The triangular formation between the aortic semilunar valve and the medial parts of the tricuspid and bicuspid valve openings is the right *fibrous trigone* ("triangle") or the central fibrous body, the strongest portion of the cardiac skeleton. The smaller left fibrous trigone is formed between the aortic semilunar valve and the anterior cusp of the mitral valve. Continuations of fibroelastic tissue from the right and left fibrous trigone partially encircle the AV openings to form the tricuspid and bicuspid annulus or annulus fibrosus. The annuli serve as attachment sites for the AV valves as well as atrial and ventricular myocardium. Strong collagenous tissue passes anteriorly from the right and left fibrous trigones to encircle and support the aortic and pulmonary semilunar valve annuli. The membranous interventricular septum is an inferior extension of the central fibrous body that attaches to the muscular interventricular septum. The membranous septum provides support for the medial (right and posterior) cusps of the aortic semilunar valve and continues superiorly to form part of the atrial septum. The tendon of Todaro is a fibrous extension of the membranous septum that is continuous with the valve (Eustachian) of the inferior vena cava. The AV bundle of conduction fibers from the AV node penetrates the central fibrous body, passes through the membranous septum, and splits into left and right bundle branches at the apex of the muscular septum (or the junction of the right and posterior cusps of the aortic semilunar valve).

5.6 The Fetal Heart

By the third month of fetal development, the heart and all major blood vessels are basically formed and the blood flow is generally the same direction as the adult. However, there are some major differences between fetal and post-natal circulation (Fig. 5.17). First, oxygenated blood flows

Fig. 5.17 Fetal circulation. The fetal heart has unique features to shunt blood away from the relatively nonfunctional lungs: (1) foramen ovale; (2) ductus arteriosus; and (3) valve (Eustachian) of the inferior vena cava

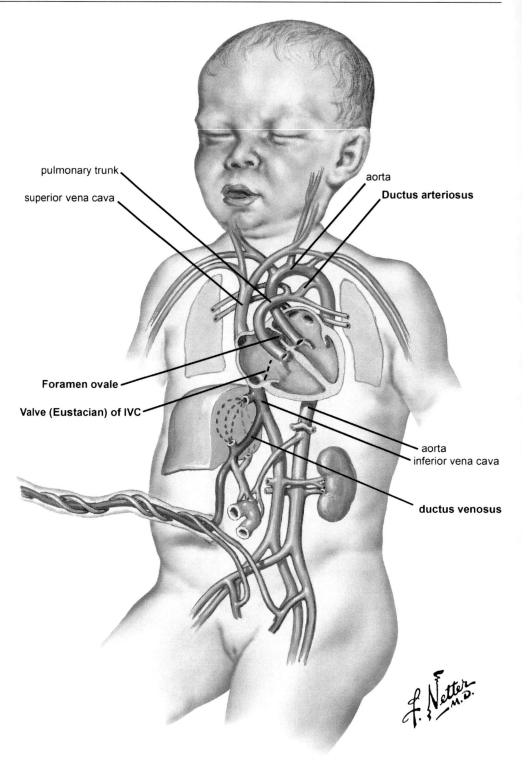

toward the fetus and into the heart in umbilical veins, and deoxygenated blood flows away from the fetus in umbilical arteries. Second, the fetus obtains oxygen from the uterus through the placenta, and the fetal lungs are essentially nonfunctional. Therefore, fetal circulation has a number of features to direct most of the blood away from the lungs.

In fetal circulation, oxygenated blood from the placenta flows toward the heart. Most of it is diverted away

from entering the liver (through the ductus venosus) and into the inferior vena cava. Thus, unlike the adult heart, oxygenated blood mixes with deoxygenated blood and collects in the right atrium. Because very little of this blood is required in the lungs, the fetus has three unique features to ensure that the blood is shunted from the right (pulmonary) side of the heart to the left (systemic) side. The first is an oval hole in the interatrial septum called the foramen ovale (the foramen ovale is not really a hole, but rather a valve composed of two flaps that prevent the regurgitation of blood). For more information on this topic, the reader is referred to Chapter 3.

Before birth, pressure is higher in the right atrium than in the left because of the large vasculature from the placenta. The foramen ovale is a passage for blood to flow from the right atrium into the left. A second feature of the fetal heart is the ligament of the inferior vena cava. This ligament is located inferior to the opening of the vena cava, and extends medially to the atrial septum, passing inferior to the foramen ovale. It is much more prominent in the fetus than in the adult and functions in fetal circulation to direct, in a laminar flow, the blood coming into the right ventricle toward the foramen ovale, to pass into the left atrium.

The third feature of fetal circulation is a way for oxygenated blood that has been pumped from the right atrium to the right ventricle to be diverted from the pulmonary circulation into the systemic circulation. Despite the shunt from the right atrium to the left, much of the oxygenated blood that enters the right atrium gets pumped into the right ventricle. The ductus arteriosus ("duct of the artery") is a connection between the left pulmonary artery and the aortic artery so that very little blood reaches the immature lungs. Because the pulmonary vascular resistance of the fetus is large, only one-tenth of right ventricular output passes through the lungs. The remainder passes from the pulmonary artery through the

ductus arteriosus to the aorta. In the fetus, the diameter of the ductus arteriosus can be as large as the aorta.

Shortly after birth, the umbilical cord is cut and the newborn takes its first breath. Rising concentrations of the hormone prostaglandin are believed to result in the closure of the ductus arteriosus (ligamentum arteriosum), and the lungs receive much more blood. The increase in pressure is translated to the left atrium. This pressure pushes together the two valve flaps of the foramen ovale, closing it to form the fossa ovalis, and preventing the flow of blood from the right to the left atrium.

5.7 Other Fetal Remnants: Chiari Network

Between 3 and 4 weeks of fetal development, the openings of the superior and inferior venae cavae and future coronary sinus are incorporated into the posterior wall of the right atrium, becoming the sinus venarum (smooth) portion of the right atrium. A pair of tissue flaps, the left and right venous valves, develop on either side of the three ostia.

The left valve eventually becomes part of the septum secundum (which becomes the definitive interatrial septum). The right valve remains intact and forms the valve of the inferior vena cava (Eustachian), the crista terminalis, and the valve of the coronary sinus (Thebesian) (Fig. 5.18).

Infrequently, incomplete resorption of the right valve of the sinus venarum may lead to the presence of a

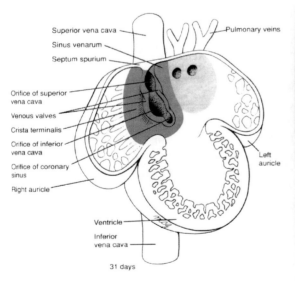
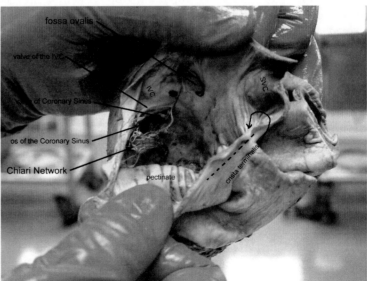

Fig. 5.18 Chiari network. *Left*: The ostia of the superior and inferior venae cavae, as well as the coronary sinus, incorporate into the smooth wall of the definitive right atrium. Two tissue flaps develop on the sides of the ostia as the left and right venous valves. The left valve eventually gives rise to the septum secundum (definitive interatrial septum); the right valve gives rise to the valve of the inferior vena cava (Eustachian), the valve of the coronary sinus (Thebesian), and the crista terminalis. Incomplete resorption of the right valve of the embryonic sinus

venarum leads to the presence of a meshwork of fibrous strands attached to the edges of the Eustachian valve, or the Thebesian valve inferiorly and the crista terminalis superiorly. *Right*: Human cadaveric heart. IVC = inferior vena cava; SVC = superior vena cava. (Left: from Human Embryology, 2nd Edition (1997), W. J. Larsen (ed.), Churchill Livingstone, Inc., New York, NY, p. 163, Fig. 7-12. © 1997, with permission from Elsevier.)

meshwork of fibrous strands attached to the edges of the Eustachian valve or Thebesian valve inferiorly and the crista terminalis superiorly. This is called a Chiari net or network (Fig. 5.18). Remnants of the other valve, the left sinus venarum valve, may be found adherent to the superior portion of the atrial septum or the fossa ovalis. For more information on this topic, see Chapter 3.

5.8 Other Fetal Remnants: Atrial Septal Defect

The first step in the separation of the systemic and pulmonary circulation in the fetal heart is the separation of the definitive atrium. The adult interatrial septum is formed by the fusion of two embryonic septa. However, note that right-to-left shunting of oxygenated blood remains.

Between 3 and 4 weeks of development, the roof of the atrium becomes depressed and produces a wedge of tissue called the *septum primum* ("first partition") that extends inferiorly. During the fifth week, the crescent-shaped septum reaches the "floor," thus separating the right and left atria and forming along its free edge a foramen, ostium primum ("first mouth/opening"). At the end of the sixth week, the growing edge of the septum primum reduces the ostium primum to nothing. At the same time, the septum primum grows perforations that coalesce to form a new foramen, the ostium secundum ("second opening"). Thus, a new channel for right-to-left blood flow opens before the old one closes. At the same time, a second crescent-shaped wedge of tissue, the septum secundum ("second partition"), grows from the roof of the atrium. It is located adjacent to the septum primum on the side of the right atrium. Unlike the septum primum, the secundum is thick and muscular as it grows posteroinferiorly. It completely extends to the floor of the right atrium and leaves a hole in the inferior portion called the *foramen ovale* ("oval hole"). Throughout the rest of fetal development, blood shunts from the right to the left atrium to pump out of the heart through the aortic artery. This shunt closes at birth due to the abrupt dilation of the pulmonary vasculature, combined with the loss of flow through the umbilical vein. The increase in pressure in the left atrium and the loss of pressure in the right pushes the flexible septum primum against the septum secundum.

If the septum secundum is too short to cover the ostium secundum completely, an atrial septal defect allows left-to-right atrial flow after the septum primum and septum secundum are pressed together at birth (Fig. 5.19). This abnormality is generally asymptomatic during infancy. However, the persistent increase in flow of blood into the right atrium can lead to hypertrophy of the right atrium, right

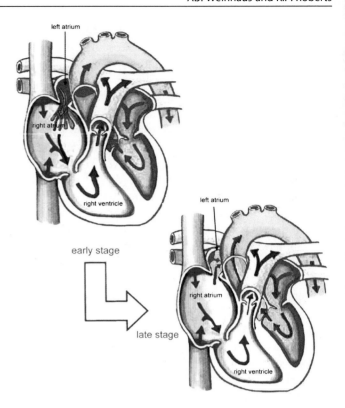

Fig. 5.19 Atrial septal defect (ASD). Incomplete formation of the septum secundum over the ostium secundum results in a persistent opening in the interatrial septum. After birth, the pressure in the left atrium is greater than the right, and there is modest left-to-right shunting of blood. However, the right atrium responds to continuous increases in volume. The result is increased pressure generated by the right atrium and a reverse in the flow from the right to the left atrium, further resulting in oxygen-poor blood in the aortic artery and symptoms of hypoxia. (Modified from Human Anatomy, 4th Edition (1995), K. M. Van De Graaff (ed.), Wm. C. Brown Communications, Inc., Dubuque, IA, p. 557. Reprinted by permission of The McGraw-Hill Companies.)

ventricle, and the pulmonary trunk. In some cases, during adulthood pulmonary hypertension develops, and the left-to-right converts to right-to-left shunt. Thus, increased pressure in the right atrium results in a right-to-left blood flow across the atrial septum. This causes oxygen-poor blood to mix with the oxygen-rich blood returning to the left atrium from the lungs. Oxygen-poor blood is then pumped out of the heart through the aortic artery and the symptoms of hypoxia ("low oxygen") result. Approximately 30% of normal hearts have a small patency with a valve-competent foramen ovale.

5.9 Other Fetal Remnants: Ventricular Atrial Septal Defect

The developmental formation of the interventricular septum is extremely complex. Simply, the septum forms as the growing walls of the right and left ventricles become more closely apposed to one another. The growth of the muscular septum commences at the inferior end and proceeds superiorly. Septation of the ventricles and formation of the ventricular outflow tracts (membranous interventricular septum) must occur in tight coordination. Ventricular septal defects can occur because of errors in this complex process. Failure of complete fusion of the membranous septum (from the aortic and pulmonary outflow tracts) and the muscular septum results in one type of ventricular septal defect (Fig. 5.20). Ventricular septal defects are the most common congenital heart defect.

Whatever the origin of a ventricular septal defect, the result is a massive left-to-right shunting of blood. This is associated with postnatal pulmonary hypertension and deficient closure of AV valves. This type of condition is often referred to, in lay terms, as "baby being born with a hole in the heart." Because of extreme hypoxia and pulmonary hypertension, there is usually immediate surgical repair of the defect. For additional information on such defects and the means for their repair, refer to Chapter 34.

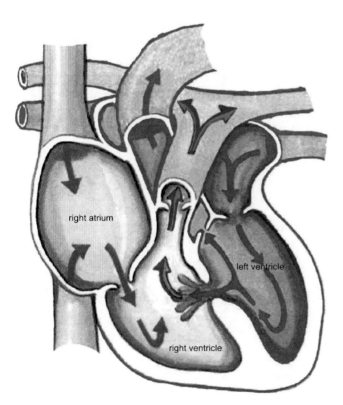

Fig. 5.20 Ventricular septal defect. Caused by abnormal development of the interventricular septum. This condition results in massive left-to-right shunting of blood. This is associated with pulmonary hypertension and deficient closure of atrioventricular valves after birth. Emergent surgical repair of this hole is indicated. (Figure modified from Human Anatomy, 4th Edition (1995), K. M. Van De Graaff (ed.), Wm. C. Brown Communications, Inc., Dubuque, IA, p. 557. Reprinted by permission of The McGraw-Hill Companies.)

5.10 Vasculature of the Heart

Although the heart is filled with blood, it provides very little nourishment and oxygen to the tissues of the heart. The walls of the heart are too thick to be supplied by diffusion alone. Instead, the tissues of the heart are supplied by a separate vascular supply committed only to the heart. The arterial supply to the heart arises from the base of the aorta as the right and left coronary arteries (running in the coronary sulcus). The venous drainage is via cardiac veins that return deoxygenated blood to the right atrium.

The coronary arteries arise from the ostia in the left and right sinuses of the aortic semilunar valve, course within the epicardium, and encircle the heart in the AV (coronary) and interventricular sulci (Fig. 5.21).

5.10.1 Right Coronary Artery

The right coronary artery emerges from the aorta into the AV groove. It descends through the groove, then curves posteriorly, and makes a bend at the crux of the heart and continues downward in the posterior interventricular sulcus. Within millimeters after emerging from the aorta, the right coronary artery gives off two branches (Figs. 5.21 and 5.22). The conus (arteriosus) artery runs to the conus arteriosus (right ventricular outflow tract), and the atrial branch to the right atrium. This atrial branch gives off the SA nodal artery (in 50–73% of hearts, according to

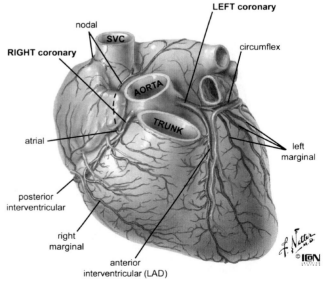

Fig. 5.21 Vascular supply to the heart. Arterial supply to the heart occurs via the right and left coronary arteries and their branches. Venous drainage occurs via cardiac veins

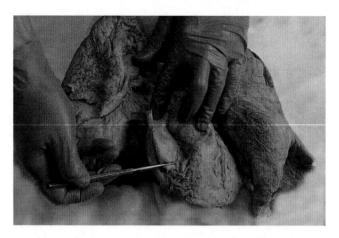

Fig. 5.22 Atrial branch of right coronary artery. This atrial branch gives off the sinoatrial (SA) nodal artery which runs along the anterior right atrium to the superior vena cava, encircles it in a clockwise, or sometimes counterclockwise, direction before reaching the SA node. The nodal artery can also pass intramurally through the right atrium to the SA node. The SA nodal artery supplies the SA node, Bachman's bundle, crista terminalis, and the left and right atrial free walls

most prominent of these is the right marginal branch which runs down the right margin of the heart supplying this part of the right ventricle. As the right coronary curves posteriorly and descends downward on the posterior surface of the heart, it gives off two to three branches. One is the posterior interventricular (posterior descending) artery that runs in the posterior interventricular sulcus. It is directed toward the apex of the heart to supply the posterior free wall of the right ventricle. In 85–90% of hearts, branches of this artery (posterior septal arteries) supply the posterior one-third of the interventricular septum (Fig. 5.23). The second artery is the AV nodal artery which branches from the right coronary artery at the crux of the heart and passes anteriorly along the base of the atrial septum to supply the AV node (in 50–60% of hearts), proximal parts of the bundles (branches) of His, and the parts of the posterior interventricular septum that surround the bundle branches. Another artery crosses the crux into the left AV groove to supply the diaphragmatic surface of the left ventricle and the posterior papillary muscle of the bicuspid valve. The right coronary artery also serves as an important collateral supply to the anterior side of the heart, left ventricle, and anterior two-thirds of the interventricular septum via the conus artery and communicating arteries in the interventricular septum (Fig. 5.23). Kugel's artery, which originates from either the right or left coronary artery, runs from anterior to posterior through the atrial septum. This artery serves as an important collateral connection from anterior arteries to the AV node and posterior arteries.

various reports), which runs along the anterior right atrium to the superior vena cava, encircling it in a clockwise or counterclockwise direction before reaching the SA node. The SA nodal artery supplies the SA node, Bachman's bundle, crista terminalis, and the left and right atrial free walls. The right coronary artery continues in the AV groove and gives off a variable number of branches to the right atrium and right ventricle. The

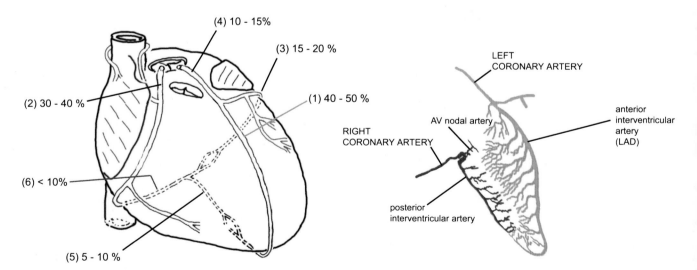

Fig. 5.23 Arterial supply to the interventricular septum. *Left*: Sites of coronary artery occlusion, in order of frequency and percentage of occlusions involving each artery. *Right*: The right coronary artery supplies the posterior one-third of the interventricular septum, and the left coronary supplies the anterior two-thirds. The artery to the atrioventricular node commonly branches off of the posterior interventricular artery. Occlusions occur most frequently in the anterior interventricular artery, which is the primary blood supply to the interventricular septum (and bundle branches within). AV = atrioventricular

5.10.2 Left Coronary Artery

The left coronary artery (left main coronary artery) emerges from the aorta through the ostia of the left aortic cusp within the sinus of Valsalva (Fig. 5.21). The plane of the semilunar valve is tilted so that the ostium of the left coronary artery is superior and posterior to the right coronary ostium. The left coronary artery travels from the aorta, and passes between the pulmonary trunk and the left atrial appendage. Under the appendage, the artery divides (and is thus a very short vessel) into the anterior interventricular (left anterior descending artery) and the left circumflex artery. The left coronary artery may be completely absent, i.e., the anterior interventricular and circumflex arteries arise independently from the left aortic sinus.

The anterior interventricular artery appears to be a direct continuation of the left coronary artery which descends into the anterior interventricular groove. Branches of this artery, anterior septal perforating arteries, enter the septal myocardium to supply the anterior two-thirds of the interventricular septum (in about 90% of hearts) (Fig. 5.23). The first branch, the first septal perforator, supplies a major portion of the AV conduction system. In about 80% of hearts, the second or third perforator is the longest and strongest of the septal arteries and is often called the *main septal artery*. This artery supplies the middle portion of the interventricular septum. This artery also sends a branch to the moderator band and the anterior papillary muscle of the tricuspid valve (right ventricle), which is reasonable considering that the moderator band is part of the septomarginal trabeculae of the interventricular septum. This artery is often called the *moderator artery*. Other branches of the anterior interventricular artery extend laterally through the epicardium to supply adjacent right and left ventricular free walls. The anterior interventricular artery also sends a branch to meet the conus artery from the right coronary to form an important collateral anastomosis called the *circle of Vieussens*, as well as branches to the anterior free wall of the left ventricle called *diagonal arteries*. These are numbered according to their sequence of origin as first, second, etc. diagonal arteries. The most distal continuation of the anterior interventricular artery curves around the apex and travels superiorly in the posterior interventricular sulcus to anastomose with the posterior descending from the right coronary artery. In summary, the anterior interventricular artery and its branches supply most of the interventricular septum—the anterior, lateral, and apical wall of the left ventricle; most of the right and left bundle branches; and the anterior papillary muscle of the bicuspid valve (left ventricle). It also provides collateral circulation to the anterior right ventricle, the posterior part of the interventricular septum, and the posterior descending artery.

The circumflex artery branches off of the left coronary artery and supplies most of the left atrium—the posterior and lateral free walls of the left ventricle and (with the anterior interventricular artery) the anterior papillary muscle of the bicuspid valve. The circumflex artery may give off a variable number of left marginal branches to supply the left ventricle. The terminal branch is usually the largest of these branches. More likely, the circumflex artery may continue through the AV sulcus to supply the posterior wall of the left ventricle and (with the right coronary artery) the posterior papillary muscle of the bicuspid valve. In 40–50% of hearts the circumflex artery supplies the artery to the SA node.

In 30–60% of hearts, the left coronary artery may give off one or more intermediate branches that originate *between* the anterior interventricular and circumflex arteries. These extend diagonally over the left ventricle toward the apex of the heart and are thus named diagonal or intermediate arteries.

The anterior interventricular artery is the most commonly occluded of the coronary arteries (Fig. 5.23). It is the major blood supply to the interventricular septum and the bundle branches of the conducting system. It is easy to see why coronary artery disease can lead to impairment or death (infarction) of the conducting system. The result is a "block" of impulse conduction between the atria and the ventricles known as "right/left bundle branch block." Furthermore, branches of the right coronary artery supply both the SA and AV node in at least 50% of hearts. An occlusion in this artery could result in necrosis of the SA or AV nodes, thus preventing or interrupting the conduction of electrical activity across the heart.

5.10.3 Cardiac Veins

The coronary arteries supply the heart with nutrients and oxygen. At the same time, waste products and carbon dioxide must be removed. An extensive network of intercommunicating veins provides venous drainage from the heart. The venous drainage of deoxygenated blood from the rest of the body is returned to the right atrium, as is the venous drainage of the heart. Venous drainage of the heart is accomplished through three separate systems: (1) the cardiac venous tributaries which converge to form the coronary sinus; (2) the anterior cardiac (anterior right ventricular) veins; and (3) the smallest cardiac (Thebesian) venous system (Fig. 5.24).

Fig. 5.24 Venous drainage of the heart. Three separate venous systems carry blood to the right atrium—the coronary sinus and it tributaries, the great, middle, and small cardiac veins; the anterior cardiac veins; and the smallest (Thebesian) cardiac veins

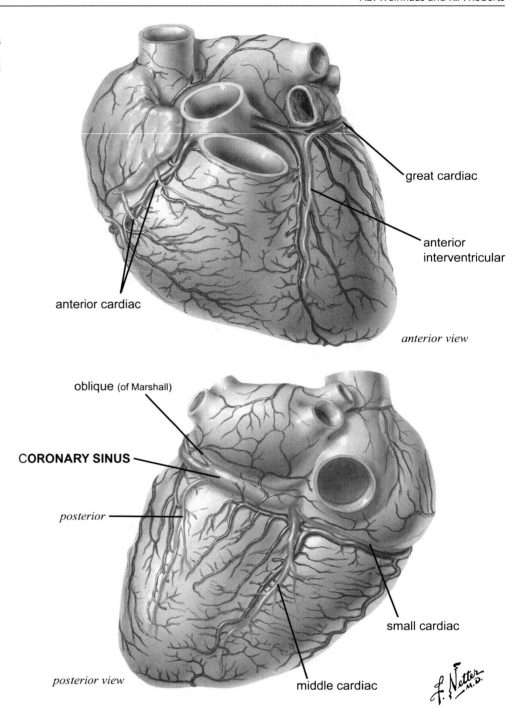

great cardiac

anterior interventricular

anterior cardiac

anterior view

oblique (of Marshall)

CORONARY SINUS

posterior

small cardiac

posterior view   middle cardiac

Most of the myocardium is drained by the cardiac veins that course parallel to the coronary arteries. These three large veins (the great, middle, and small cardiac veins) converge to form the coronary sinus.

On the anterior side of the heart, the anterior interventricular vein lies within the anterior interventricular sulcus and runs from inferior to superior beside the anterior interventricular artery (Figs. 5.24 and 5.25). At the base of the heart, near the bifurcation of the left coronary artery,

it turns and runs within the AV groove as the great cardiac vein around the left side of the heart to the posterior. In the AV groove on the posterior side of the heart, the great cardiac vein *becomes* the coronary sinus, which then empties into the right atrium. From the inside of the right atrium, it can be seen that the coronary sinus opens into the right atrium forming an opening or *os* that is located anteriorly and inferiorly to the orifice of the inferior vena cava. There is a valve (Thebesian valve) that

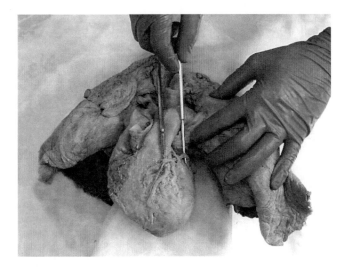

Fig. 5.25 The great cardiac vein. On the anterior side of the heart, the anterior interventricular vein lies within the anterior interventricular sulcus and runs from inferior to superior beside the anterior interventricular artery. At the base of the heart, it changes to the great cardiac vein as it runs within the atrioventricular groove around the left side of the heart to the posterior. In the atrioventricular groove on the posterior side of the heart, the great cardiac vein becomes the coronary sinus and empties into the right atrium

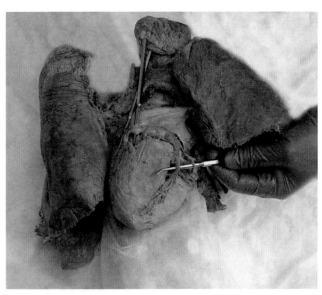

Fig. 5.26 The middle cardiac vein. The middle cardiac vein, located on the posterior surface of the heart, arises near the posterior aspect of the apex of the heart and runs from inferior to superior through the posterior interventricular sulcus before entering the coronary sinus. The middle cardiac vein is formed from venous confluence of tributaries that drain the posterior left and right ventricles and the interventricular septum

covers the opening of the coronary sinus to prevent backflow. The great cardiac vein is formed by the confluence of small venous tributaries from the left and right ventricles and anterior portion of the interventricular septum. As it ascends toward the coronary sinus, it receives small venous tributaries from the left atrium and left ventricle. It also receives a large left marginal vein, which runs parallel to the left marginal artery.

There are two structures that serve as the boundary between the termination of the great cardiac vein and the beginning of the coronary sinus. The first is the valve of Vieussens, which has the appearance of a typical venous valve and functions to prevent the backflow of blood from the coronary sinus into the great cardiac vein (Raymond Vieussens, French anatomist, 1641–1715). The second is the space between the entry points of the oblique vein of the left atrium (of Marshall) and the posterior (posterolateral) vein of the left ventricle (John Marshall, English anatomist, 1818–1891). The oblique vein of Marshall runs superior to inferior along the posterior side of the left atrium, providing venous drainage of the area. The posterior vein ascends to the coronary sinus from the inferior portion of the left ventricle and provides drainage of the area.

In addition to the great cardiac vein, the coronary sinus receives the posterior interventricular (or middle cardiac) vein (Figs. 5.24 and 5.26). Located on the posterior surface of the heart, it arises near the posterior aspect of the apex of the heart and runs from inferior to superior through the posterior interventricular sulcus. It then joins the coronary sinus within millimeters of the sinus entering into the right atrium. The middle cardiac vein is formed from venous confluence of tributaries that drain the posterior left and right ventricles and the interventricular septum.

The coronary sinus also receives the highly variable small cardiac vein. The small cardiac vein arises from the anterior/lateral/inferior portion of the right ventricle. It ascends and runs inferior to and roughly parallel with the marginal branch of the right coronary artery until it reaches the right AV sulcus. At this point, it turns and runs horizontally around to the posterior side of the heart and enters the coronary sinus with the middle cardiac vein. The small cardiac vein is extremely small or absent in 60% of hearts. In about 50% of hearts, the small cardiac vein enters the right atrium directly, and it infrequently drains into the middle cardiac vein.

Typically, about 85% of the venous drainage of the heart occurs through the great, middle, and small cardiac veins through the coronary sinus to the right atrium. This elaborate system of veins drains the left ventricle, some of the right ventricle, both atria, and the anterior portion of the interventricular septum.

The second system of venous drainage of the heart involves the variable and delicate anterior cardiac veins (Fig. 5.24 and 5.27). This system is distinguished from the other cardiac venous system because the anterior cardiac veins do not drain into the coronary sinus. The two to

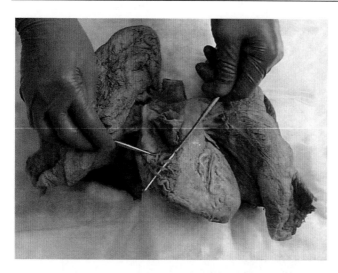

Fig. 5.27 Anterior cardiac veins. Two to four anterior cardiac veins originate and drain the anterior right ventricular wall. These veins travel superiorly to cross the right atrioventricular sulcus and enter into the right atrium. These veins are part of the smallest cardiac venous system which empties oxygen-poor blood directly into the right atrium without communication with the coronary sinus

four anterior cardiac veins originate and drain the anterior right ventricular wall, travel superiorly to cross the right AV sulcus, and enter the right atrium *directly*. The sulcus is usually packed with adipose tissue. Through this adipose tissue run the anterior cardiac veins, the right coronary artery, and a branch of the coronary artery, the right atrial or nodal artery. The anterior cardiac veins pass over the right coronary artery in close proximity and in a perpendicular angle. A right marginal vein (when present) runs parallel with the right marginal artery before entering the right atrium directly and is usually considered part of the anterior cardiac venous system.

The third system of venous drainage of the heart is the smallest cardiac venous system (Fig. 5.27). This system is composed of a multitude of small intramural ("within the walls") intramyocardial veins also called Thebesian veins (Adam C. Thebesius, German physician, 1686–1732). These are minute vessels that begin in the capillary beds of the myocardium and open directly into the chambers of the heart. Although called veins, they are valveless communications between myocardial capillaries and a chamber of the heart. Interestingly, ostia of Thebesian veins may be found in all chambers of the heart, but are most prevalent in the atrial and ventricular septa. They are more prevalent on the right side than the left. As much as 17% of myocardial drainage occurs through these smallest cardiac veins, with 49% through the cardiac veins and coronary sinus, and 24% through anterior cardiac veins.

5.10.4 Myocardial Bridges

The coronary arteries typically course upon the myocardium or under/within the epicardium of the heart. Frequently, a portion of an artery deviates from its usual subepicardial position to follow an intramyocardial (intramural) course, either by traveling a significant length within the myocardium or beneath an arrangement of muscular slips ("myocardial bridges"). Myocardial bridging is most common in the middle segment of the anterior interventricular artery [2]. The myocardial fibers that cover or "bridge over" the anterior interventricular artery are direct extensions of the myocardium of the conus arteriosus of the right ventricle and cross the artery in a perpendicular direction. Myocardial bridges over the right coronary and the circumflex arteries are much less common. When present, these bridges are extensions of the respective atrial myocardium [3]. The prevalence of myocardial bridges from various sources is reported to occur in 5.4–85.7% of hearts when measured from the cadaver [4–6], and 0.5–16% when measured from angiography in catheterization labs [4, 5, 7].

Coronary arteries have a tortuous pattern as they run across the heart. Interestingly, studies employing angiography followed by detailed micro-dissection show that a coronary artery with a typical tortuous shape takes on a perfectly straight pattern when it follows an intramyocardial course [8].

Angiography has also shown that myocardial bridges are associated with narrowing of the lumen of the coronary artery. The narrowing appears during systole and disappears during diastole [2]. The appearance of straight running or systolic narrowing patterns appears to be an important diagnostic technique during angiography to discover intramyocardial segments of coronary arteries [2].

Myocardial bridging is usually a benign condition. Although there is contrasting evidence, atherosclerosis is uncommon within a myocardial bridge [4]; bridging might provide some protection against plaque formation [2].

5.11 Autonomic Innervation of the Heart

The SA node produces a regular series of impulses and is called the "pacemaker" of the heart. The SA node spontaneously produces an impulse for contraction of the atrial myocardium, depolarizes the AV node, and sends an impulse through the bundle fibers to the ventricular myocardium. In addition to the pacemaker activity of the SA node, the heart is also under autonomic, or involuntary, control.

The autonomic nervous system is separated into the *sympathetic* and *parasympathetic* nervous systems. These two systems send neurons to the same target, but convey opposite effects. In emergency situations, sympathetic nerves travel to the heart and innervate the SA and AV nodes in order to increase the rate and force of contraction. In resting situations, parasympathetic nerves that innervate the SA and AV nodes to slow down the heart rate reduce the force of contraction and constrict the coronary arteries, thus saving energy.

Both the sympathetic and parasympathetic nerves are composed of a two-neuron pathway. These two neurons meet or synapse somewhere in the middle and form a structure called a *ganglion* ("swelling"). Neurons of the sympathetic nervous system emerge from the spinal cord. They emerge from all eight of the cervical segments, and the first five of the thoracic spinal cord segments. These neurons travel laterally just centimeters from the spinal cord before they synapse. All of the neurons to the heart are believed to synapse in only two places—the middle cervical ganglion and the cervicothoracic (fused inferior cervical/1st thoracic, or stellate "star-shaped") ganglion. Multitudes of fibers then emanate from these ganglia and run to the heart as sympathetic cardiac nerves.

Parasympathetic neurons emerge directly from the brain as part of the vagus nerve or cranial nerve X. The vagus nerve and its branches form the parasympathetic part of the cardiac nerves running toward the heart.

Sympathetic and parasympathetic cardiac nerves interconnect. In addition, nerves of the right and left side have connections. Altogether, this huge group of connections forms the cardiac plexuses. The dorsal cardiac plexus is located posterior to the arch of the aorta near the bifurcation of the trachea. The ventral plexus is located anterior to the aorta. Nerves from the cardiac plexuses extend to the atria and ventricles, SA node, AV node, coronary arteries, and the great vessels. It is generally believed that there is sympathetic and parasympathetic innervation of the myocardium that forms a network from the atria to the ventricles. For more details about the role of the autonomic nervous system in the physiological control of the heart, refer to Chapter 12.

References

1. Wenink ACG. The medial papillary complex. Br Heart J 1977;39:1012–8.
2. Kalaria VG, Koradia N, Breall JA. Myocardial bridge: A clinical review. Catheter Cardiovasc Interv 2002;57:552–6.
3. Garg S, Brodison A, Chauhan A. Occlusive systolic bridging of circumflex artery. Cathet Cardiovasc Diagn 2000;51:477–8.
4. Polacek P. Relation of myocardial bridge and loops on the coronary arteries to coronary occlusions. Am Heart J 1961;61:44–52.
5. Irvin RG. The angiographic prevalence of myocardial bridging. Chest 1982;81:198–202.
6. Noble J, Bourassa MG, Petitclerc R, Dyrda I. Myocardial bridging and milking effect of left anterior descending artery: Normal variant or obstruction. Am J Cardiol 1976;37:993–9.
7. Greenspan M, Iskandrin AS, Catherwood E, Kimbiris D, Bemis CE, Segal BL. Myocardial bridging of the left anterior descending artery: Evaluation using exercise thallium-201 myocardial scintigraphy. Cathet Cardiovasc Diagn 1980;6:173–80.
8. Lachman N, Satyapal KS, Vanker EA. Angiographic manifestation and anatomical presence of the intra-mural LAD: Surgical significance. Clin Anat 2002;15:426.

Supplementary Reference Texts and Suggested Reading

Berne RM, Levy MN, Koeppen BM, Stanton BA, eds. Physiology. 5th ed. St. Louis, MO: Mosby, 2004.

Garson A, et al., eds. The science and practice of pediatric cardiology. 2nd ed. Baltimore, MD: Williams and Wilkins, 1997.

Goss CM, ed. Anatomy of the human body: Gray's anatomy. Philadelphia, PA: Lea and Febiger, 1949.

Hurst JW, ed. Hurst's the heart. New York, NY: McGraw-Hill, 1990.

Kumar V, Cotran RS, Robbins SL, eds. Robbins basic pathology. 7th ed. Philadelphia, PA: Saunders, 2003.

Larson WJ, ed. Human embryology. 2nd ed. New York, NY: Churchill Livingstone, 1997.

Moore KL, Dalley AF, eds. Clinically oriented anatomy. 5th ed. Philadelphia, PA: Lippincott Williams and Williams, 2006.

Netter FH, ed. Atlas of human anatomy. 3rd ed. Teterboro, NJ: ICON Learning Systems, 2003.

Stedman TL, ed. Stedman's medical Dictionary. Baltimore, MD: Williams and Wilkins, 1972.

Chapter 6
Comparative Cardiac Anatomy

Alexander J. Hill and Paul A. Iaizzo

Abstract The need for appropriate animal models to conduct translational research is vital for advancements in the diagnosis and treatment of heart disease. The choice of animal model to be employed must be critically evaluated. In this chapter, we present the comparative cardiac anatomy of several of the commonly employed animal models (dog, pig, and sheep). A general comparison focuses on several specific anatomic features: the atria, the ventricles, the valves, the coronary system, lymphatics, and the conduction system. Finally, we present novel qualitative and quantitative data that we have obtained from perfusion fixed specimens of the most commonly used animal models.

Keywords Comparative anatomy · Human · Sheep · Dog · Pig · Heart · Cardiac

6.1 Historical Perspective of Anatomy and Animal Research

Anatomy is one of the oldest branches of medicine, with historical records dating back at least as far as the third century BC; animal research dates back equally as far. More specifically, Aristotle (384–322 BC) studied comparative animal anatomy and physiology, and Erasistratus of Ceos (304–258 BC) studied live animal anatomy and physiology [1]. Galen of Pergamum (129–199 AD) is probably the most notable early anatomist who used animals in his research in which he attempted to understand the normal structure and function of the body [2]. He continuously stressed the centrality of anatomy and made an attempt to dissect every day, as he felt it was critical to learning [3]. His most notable work was *De Anatomicis Administrationibus* (On Anatomical Procedures) which, when rediscovered in the sixteenth century, renewed interest in anatomy and scientific methods [2].

The Renaissance was a period of great scientific discovery and included important advances in our understanding of human and animal anatomy. Andreas Vesalius (1514–1564 AD) was arguably the greatest anatomist of the era [4]. To teach anatomy, he performed public nonhuman dissections at the University of Padua and is credited with creating the field of modern anatomy [2]. His immediate successors at Padua were Matteo Realdo Colombo (1510–1559 AD) and Gabriele Falloppio (1523–1562 AD). It was Colombo who, in great detail, described the pulmonary circulation and both the atrial and ventricular cavities; Falloppio is credited with the discovery of the Fallopian tubes among other things [4]. Animal research flourished during this period due to a number of popular ideas launched by both the Christian Church and one of the prominent scientific leaders at that time, Rene Descartes. The Church asserted that animals were under the dominion of man and, although worthy of respect, could be used to obtain information if it was for a "higher" purpose [2]. Descartes described humans and other animals as complex machines, with the human soul distinguishing man from all other animals. This beast–machine concept was important for early animal researchers because if animals had no souls, it was thought that they could not suffer pain. Interestingly, it was believed that the reactions of animals were responses of automata and not pain [2].

The concept of functional biomedical studies can probably be attributed to another great scientist and anatomist, William Harvey (1578–1657 AD). He is credited with one of the most outstanding achievements in science and medicine—a demonstration of the circulation of blood which was documented in his publication *Exercitatio Anatomica De Motu Cordis et Sanguinis in Animalibus* (*De Motu Cordis*) in 1628. Very importantly, his work ushered in a new era in science, where a hypothesis was

P.A. Iaizzo (✉)
University of Minnesota, Department of Surgery, B 172 Mayo, MMC 195, 420 Delaware St. SE, Minneapolis, MN 55455, USA
e-mail: iaizz001@umn.edu

P.A. Iaizzo (ed.), *Handbook of Cardiac Anatomy, Physiology, and Devices*, DOI 10.1007/978-1-60327-372-5_6,

formulated and then tested through experimentation [4]. Many great anatomists emerged during this period and made innumerable discoveries; many of these discoveries were named after the individuals who described them and include several researchers who studied cardiac anatomy such as the Eustachian valve (Bartolomeo Eustachio), the Thebesian valve and Thebesian veins (Thebesius), and the sinus of Valsava (Antonio Maria Valsava). It should be noted that during this time period, in addition to animal research, dissections on deceased human bodies were performed, but not to the degree that they are today. In fact, it is written that, in general, during the post-Renaissance era there was a serious lack of human bodies available for dissection. Oftentimes, bodies were obtained in clandestine manners such as by grave robbing or the bodies of executed criminals were provided for dissection. In spite of the lack of bodies, most structures in the human body, including microscopic ones, were described by various anatomists and surgeons between the fifteenth and early nineteenth centuries.

Early in the nineteenth century, the first organized opposition to animal research occurred. In 1876, the Cruelty to Animals Act was passed in Britain. It was followed in the United States by the Laboratory Animal Welfare Act of 1966, which was amended in 1970, 1976, and 1985. These two acts began a new era in how laboratory animals were treated and utilized in experimental medicine. Importantly, the necessity of animal research is still great and therefore animals continue to be used for a variety of purposes including cardiovascular device research.

6.2 Importance of Anatomy and Animal Research

Anatomy remains as quite possibly one of the most important branches of medicine. In order to diagnose and treat medical conditions, normal structure and function must be known, as it is the basis for defining what is abnormal. Furthermore, structure typically has a great impact on the function of an organ, such as with the heart. For instance, a stenotic aortic valve will usually cause functional impairment of the left ventricle and lead to further pathologic conditions (e.g., ventricular hypertrophy). Thus, knowledge of anatomy and pathology is fundamental in understanding not only how the body is organized but also how the body works and how disease processes can affect it.

Likewise, animal research has been fundamental for much of the progress made in medicine. Most, if not all, of what we know about the human body and biology, in general, has been initially made possible through animal research. A publication by the American Medical Association in 1989 listed medical advances emanating from animal research, including studies on AIDS, anesthesia, cardiovascular disease, diabetes, hepatitis, and Parkinson's disease, to name only a few [2]. Furthermore, it has been through animal research that nearly all advances in veterinary medicine have also been established.

Animal research is still fundamental in developing new therapies aimed at improving the quality of life for patients with cardiovascular disease. Specifically, early cardiac device prototype testing is commonly performed utilizing animal models, both with and without cardiovascular disease. More specifically, before any invasively used device (a Class III medical device) can be tested in humans, the Food and Drug Administration (FDA) requires that sufficient data be obtained from animal research indicating that the device functions in the desired and appropriate manner. Importantly, it is also critical to subsequently extrapolate that a given device will be safe when used in humans, that is, it will behave in humans in a manner similar to its determined function in the chosen animal models in which it was tested. More specifically, this extrapolation of animal testing data to the human condition requires that the animal model(s) chosen for testing possesses similar anatomy and physiology as that of humans (normal and/or diseased). Unfortunately, detailed information relating human cardiac anatomy to that of the most common large mammalian animal models has been relatively lacking.

The following historical example illustrates how such a lack of knowledge can have a dramatic effect on the outcomes of cardiovascular research. During the 1970s and 1980s, dogs were employed as the primary animal model in numerous studies to identify potential pharmacological therapies for reducing infarct size. However, a detailed understanding of the coronary arterial anatomy was lacking or overlooked at the time; subsequently, it was shown that dogs have a much more extensive coronary collateral circulation relative to humans (Fig. 6.1). Thus, even when major coronary arteries were occluded, reliable and consistent myocardial infarcts were difficult to create. This led to false claims about the efficacy of many drugs in reducing infarct size which, when subsequently tested in humans, usually did not produce the same results as those observed in the canine experiments [5]. Therefore, ischemia studies with human-sized hearts have shifted to alternative species, such as swine, which are considered to resemble the coronary collateral circulation of humans more precisely [6–9].

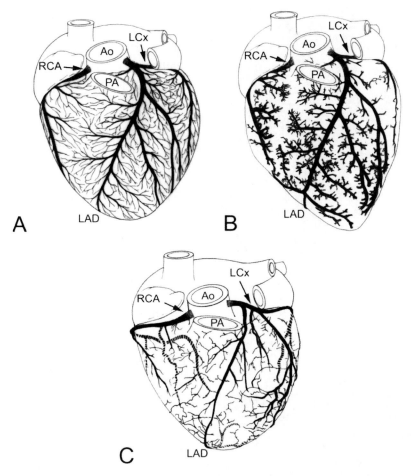

Fig. 6.1 Drawing of the coronary arterial circulation in the (**A**) dog, (**B**) pig, and (**C**) human. Notice the extensive network of coronary collateralization in the dog heart, including many arterial anastomoses. The normal pig and human hearts have significantly less collateralization; each area of myocardium is usually supplied by a single coronary artery. Ao = aorta; LAD = left anterior descending artery; LCx = left circumflex artery; PA = pulmonary artery; RCA = right coronary artery

6.3 Literature Review of Large Mammalian Comparative Cardiac Anatomy

In general, the hearts of large mammals share many similarities, and yet the sizes, shapes, and positions of the hearts in the thoracic cavity can vary considerably between species [10]. Typically, the heart is located in the lower ventral part of the mediastinum in large mammals [11]. Most quadruped mammals tend to have a less pronounced left-sided orientation and a more ventrally tilted long axis of the heart when compared to humans [11] (Fig. 6.2). Additionally, hearts of most quadruped mammals tend to be elongated and have a pointed apex, with the exception of: (1) dogs which tend to have an ovoid heart with a blunt apex [11]; (2) sheep which may have a somewhat blunt apex [12]; and (3) pigs which have a blunt apex that is oriented medially [12]. Comparatively, human hearts typically have a trapezoidal shape [13] with a blunt apex. However, the apices of normal dog, pig,

sheep, and human hearts are all formed entirely by the left ventricles [12–15] (Fig. 6.3).

It is important to note that differences exist in the heart weight to body weight ratios reported for large mammals. It is generally accepted that adult sheep and adult pigs have smaller heart weight to body weight ratios than those of adult dogs. More specifically, the adult dog may have as much as twice the heart weight to body weight ratio (6.95 g/kg, 7 g/kg) as pigs (2.89 g/kg, 2.5 g/kg) or sheep (3.13 g/kg, 3 g/kg) [16, 17], yet such findings will also likely be breed specific. The normal adult human heart weight to body weight ratio has been reported to be 5 g/kg which, on a comparative note, is similar to that of young pigs (25–30 kg animals) [7].

All large mammalian hearts are enclosed by the pericardium, which creates the pericardial cavity surrounding the heart. The pericardium is fixed to the great arteries at the base of the heart and is attached to the sternum and diaphragm in all mammals, although the degree of these

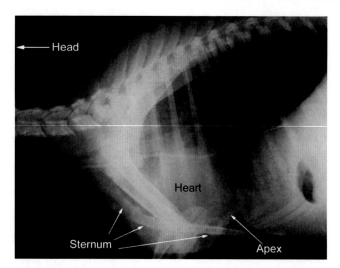

Fig. 6.2 Lateral radiograph of sheep thorax showing orientation of the heart while the animal is standing. The cranial direction is to the left and ventral to the bottom. The apex of the heart is more ventrally tilted (down toward the sternum) than is seen in humans, due to the posture of quadruped mammals. It should be noted, however, that this tilting is limited due to extensive attachments of the pericardium to the sternum and diaphragm

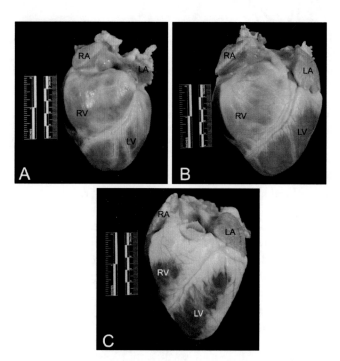

Fig. 6.3 The anterior aspect of the dog (**A**), pig (**B**), and sheep (**C**) hearts. The apex is formed entirely by the left ventricle in these hearts. Also notice the differences in overall morphology of the hearts. The dog heart is much more rounded than the pig and sheep hearts and has a blunt apex. The pig heart has more of a "valentine" shape with a somewhat blunt apex compared to the sheep heart. The sheep heart is much more conical in shape and has a much more pronounced apex than dog or pig hearts. Also noteworthy is the presence of significant amounts of epicardial fat on the sheep heart, compared with dog and pig hearts. LA = left atrium; LV = left ventricle; RA = right atrium; RV = right ventricle

attachments to the diaphragm varies between species [10, 11]. Specifically, the attachment to the central tendinous aponeurosis of the diaphragm is firm and broad in humans and pigs, the phrenopericardial ligament is the only pericardial attachment in dogs, and the caudal portion of the pericardium is attached via the strong sterno-pericadial ligament in sheep [10, 11].

The pericardium consists of three layers—the serous visceral pericardium (epicardium), the serous parietal pericardium, and the fibrous pericardium. The serous parietal pericardium lines the inner surface of the fibrous pericardium, and the serous visceral pericardium lines the outer surface of the heart. The pericardial cavity is found between the serous layers and contains the pericardial fluid. The pericardium is considered to serve many functions including: (1) preventing dilatation of the heart; (2) protecting the heart from infection and adhesions to surrounding tissues; (3) maintaining the heart in a fixed position in the thorax; and (4) regulating the interrelations between the stroke volumes of the two ventricles [18–20]. However, it should be noted that the pericardium is not essential for survival, since humans with congenital absence of the pericardium and pericardiectomized animals or humans can survive with minimal consequences for many years [18, 21].

Although the basic structure of the pericardium is the same, there are important differences between species [18, 19, 22]. For instance, pericardial wall thickness increases with increasing heart size [18]. Nevertheless, humans are the notable exception to this rule, having a much thicker pericardium than animals with similar heart sizes [18]. Specifically, the pericardium of the human heart varies in thickness between 1 and 3.5 mm [20], while the average thickness of the pericardiums of various animal species was found to be considerably thinner (sheep hearts, 0.32 ± 0.01 mm; pig hearts, 0.20 ± 0.01 mm; dog hearts, 0.19 ± 0.01 mm) [19]. Differences in the amount of pericardial fluid are considered to exist as well. Holt reported that most dogs have 0.5–2.5 ml of pericardial fluid, with some dogs having up to 15 ml, compared to 20–60 ml in adult human cadaver hearts [18]. For additional information on the pericardium, see Chapter 8.

The normally formed hearts of large mammals consist of four chambers—two thin-walled atria and two thicker walled ventricles. From both anatomical and functional perspectives, the heart is divided into separate right and left halves, with each half containing one atrium and one ventricle. In the fully developed heart with no associated pathologies, deoxygenated blood is contained in the right side of the heart and kept separate from oxygenated blood, which is in the left side of the heart. The normal path of blood flow is similar among all large mammals. Specifically, systemic deoxygenated blood returns to the right atrium via the caudal (inferior in humans) vena cava and the cranial (superior in humans) vena cava, subsequently passing into the right ventricle through the open tricuspid valve. At the same time, oxygenated blood returns from the lungs via the pulmonary veins to the left atrium and then through the open mitral valve to fill the left ventricle. After atrial contraction forces the last of the blood into the ventricles, ventricular contraction ejects blood through the major arteries arising from each ventricle, specifically the pulmonary trunk from the right ventricle and the aorta from the left ventricle. Via the pulmonary arteries, blood travels to the lungs to be oxygenated, whereas aortic blood travels through both the coronary arterial system (to feed the heart) and the systemic circulation (to oxygenate bodily tissue). For additional discussions of flow patterns and function see Chapters 1 and 18.

6.3.1 The Atria

The right and left atria of the adult mammalian heart are separated by the interatrial septum. They are located at what is termed "the base" of the heart. The base receives all of the great vessels and is generally oriented cranially or superiorly, although there are reported differences in orientation among species which are mostly dependent on the posture of the animal [13, 14, 23]. During fetal development, blood is able to pass from the right atrium to the left atrium, effectively bypassing the pulmonary circulation through a hole in the interatrial wall termed the "foramen ovale." The foramen ovale has a valve-like flap located on the left atrial side of the interatrial septum, which prevents backflow into the right atrium during left atrial contraction [24]. At the time of birth or soon thereafter, the foramen ovale closes and is marked in the adult heart by a slight depression on the right atrial side of the interatrial wall termed the "fossa ovalis" [14, 24, 25]; it should be noted that it can remain patent in some individuals. As compared to humans, the fossa ovalis is more posteriorly (caudally) positioned in dogs and sheep [11], but more deep-set and superior in the pig heart [13].

The sinus venosus, a common separate structure in nonmammalian hearts, is incorporated into the right atrium and is marked by the sinoatrial node in large mammals [24, 25]. According to Michaëlsson and Ho [11], all the mammals studied (including dogs, pigs, and sheep) have principally the same atrial architecture including the sinus venosus, crista terminalis, fossa ovalis, Eustachian valve (valve of the inferior vena cava), and Thebesian valve (valve of the coronary sinus). All large mammalian atria also have an ear-like flap called the auricle or appendage [13, 14, 25], although the size and shape of the auricles vary considerably between species [11, 13]. In general, the junction between the right atrium and the right appendage is wide, whereas the junction on the left side is much more narrow [13]. Multiple pectinate muscles are found in both the right and left atrial appendages and on the lateral wall of the right atrium [11, 13, 14] (Figs. 6.4 and 6.5). Commonly, there is one posterior (caudal or inferior) and one anterior (cranial or superior) vena cava, although in some mammals there are two anterior venae cavae [24] and the location of the ostia of the venae cavae entering into the atrium varies [11, 13]. Specifically, the ostia of the inferior and superior venae cavae enter at right (or nearly right) angles in large mammalian animal models, while entering the atrium nearly in line in humans [13]. Typically, the extent of the inferior vena cava between the heart and liver is long in domestic animals (>5 cm) and short in humans (1–3 cm) [11]. The coronary sinus ostium is normally located in the posterior wall of the right atrium, but its location can differ slightly between species. Interestingly, the number of pulmonary veins entering the left atrium also varies considerably between species; human hearts typically have four [13] or occasionally five [15], dog hearts have five or six [14], and pig hearts have two primary pulmonary veins [13]. In all large mammalian hearts, the atria are separated from the ventricles by a layer of fibrous tissue called the "cardiac skeleton," which serves as an important support for the valves as well as to electrically isolate the atrial myocardium from the ventricular myocardium [23].

6.3.2 The Ventricles

The left and right ventricles of the large mammals used for cardiovascular research essentially contain the same components which are also structurally very similar to those in humans, including an inlet (inflow) region, an apical region, and an outlet (outflow) region. The ventricles can be considered the major ejection/pumping chambers of the heart and, as expected, their walls are significantly more muscular in nature than those of the atria. It should also be noted that the left ventricular walls are notably more muscular than those of the right ventricle, due to the fact that the left ventricle must generate enough pressure to overcome the resistance of the systemic circulation, which is much greater than the resistance of the pulmonary circulation (normally more than four times greater). The walls of both ventricles near the apex have interanastomosing muscular ridges and columns termed the "trabeculae carneae" which serve to strengthen the walls and increase the force exerted during contraction

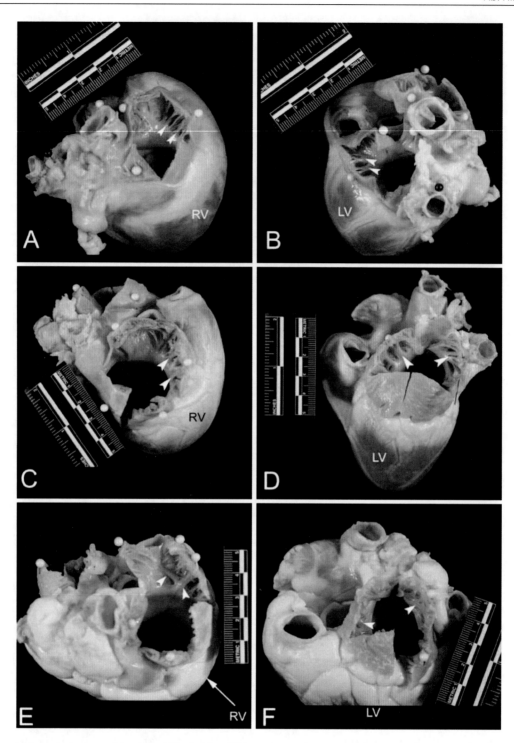

Fig. 6.4 The cranial (superior) aspect of dog (**A** and **B**), pig (**C** and **D**), and sheep (**E** and **F**) hearts. Images on the left of the figure (**A**, **C**, and **E**) show opened right atrial appendages, while images on the right (**B**, **D**, and **F**) show opened left atrial appendages. *White arrows* point to pectinate muscles that line the right and left atrial appendages. Notice that the right and left atrial appendages of the dog heart are tubular in nature. In contrast, the right and left atrial appendages of the pig and sheep hearts are more triangular in morphology. LV = left ventricle; RV = right ventricle

[11, 14, 24, 25]. However, large mammalian hearts reportedly do not have the same degree of trabeculations located in the ventricles as normal adult human hearts, and the trabeculations in animal hearts are commonly much coarser than those of human hearts [11, 13] (Figs. 6.6 and 6.7). Papillary muscles supporting the atrioventricular valves are found attached to the walls of the ventricles. Similar to human anatomy, in the majority of large mammalian

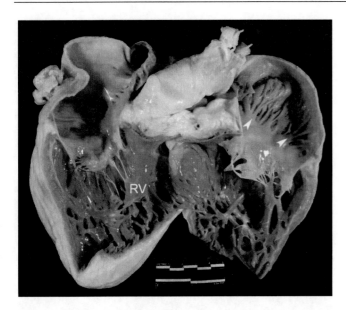

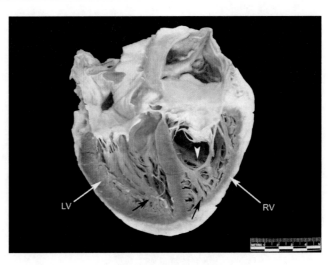

Fig. 6.7 Image of a human heart opened on the long axis to show both ventricular cavities. The left ventricle is on the *left* and the right ventricle on the *right*. *Black arrows* point to ventricular trabeculations, which are fine and numerous. The *white arrow* points to the moderator band, which is thick and muscular. It is different in size, shape, and location from the animal hearts shown in Fig. 6.6. LV = left ventricle; RV = right ventricle

Fig 6.5 A human heart opened on the inferior and superior aspects of the right ventricle, to show the anterior and posterior walls. *White arrows* point to pectinate muscles in the right atrial appendage on the anterior aspect. RV = right ventricle

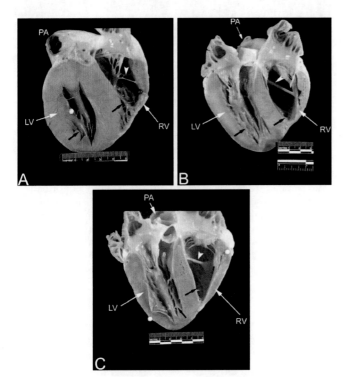

Fig. 6.6 Images showing dog (**A**), pig (**B**), and sheep (**C**) hearts that have been opened along the long axis to show both ventricular cavities. The anterior half of the heart is shown (left ventricle on the *left* and right ventricle on the *right*). *Black arrows* point to ventricular trabeculations which are large and coarse. *White arrows* point to the moderator band. Notice that a fibrous, branched moderator band extends from the anterior papillary muscle to the free wall in the canine heart. In contrast, a muscular, nonbranched moderator band extends from the septal wall to the anterior papillary muscle in pig and sheep hearts. Additionally, notice the presence of fibrous bands in the left ventricle. LV = left ventricle; PA = pulmonary artery; RV = right ventricle

animal hearts, the right ventricle has three papillary muscles and the left ventricle has two, although variations in individuals and species do occur [11]. Both ventricles typically have cross-chamber fibrous or muscular bands which usually contain Purkinje fibers. Within the right ventricle of most dogs, pigs, and ruminants, a prominent band termed the "moderator band" is typically present [11]. However, the origin and insertion of the band, as well as the composition of the band, differ notably between species. For example, in the pig heart, the band originates much higher on the septal wall compared to the analogous structure in the human heart [13], and the sheep heart has a similar moderator band as the pig heart (Figs. 6.6, 6.7, 6.8, and 6.9). In the dog heart, a branched or single muscular strand extends across the lumen from the septal wall near, or from the base of, the anterior papillary muscle [14] (Figs. 6.6, 6.7, 6.8, and 6.9). However, Truex and Warshaw reported that they [26] did not find any moderator bands in the dog hearts they examined (*n* = 12), but did observe them in all sheep hearts (*n* = 12) and all pig hearts (*n* = 12), compared to 56.8% of the human hearts they examined (*n* = 500). Furthermore, they described three subtypes of moderator bands: a free arching band, a partially free arching band, and a completely adherent band. Nevertheless, one must also consider the potential for breed differences in animals and ethnic variability in humans. It is interesting to note that while, in general, anatomical textbooks state there is no specific structure named the moderator band in the left ventricle, left ventricular bands similar to the moderator band of the right ventricle have been described in the literature. For example, Gerlis et al. found left ventricular bands

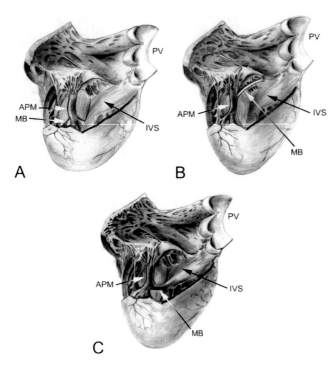

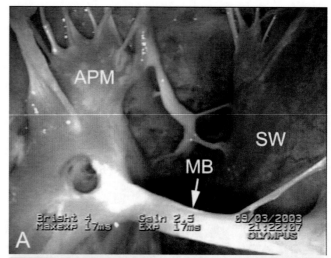

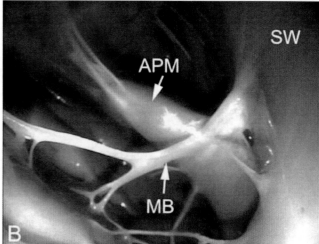

Fig. 6.8 Drawing of an opened right ventricular cavity in dog (**A**), pig and sheep (**B**), and human (**C**) hearts. The structure of the moderator band differs greatly between these hearts. In the dog heart, there is a branching fibrous band that runs from the anterior papillary muscle to the free wall of the right ventricle. In the human heart, the moderator band is typically located near the apex and is thick and muscular. In the pig and sheep hearts, the moderator band originates much higher on the interventricular septum and travels to the anterior papillary muscle. It is not as thick as in the human heart, but is still muscular in nature. Also, note that the anterior papillary muscle in the dog heart originates on the septal wall, as opposed to originating on the free wall of the human, pig, and sheep hearts. APM = anterior papillary muscle; IVS = interventricular septum; MB = moderator band; PV = pulmonary valve

Fig. 6.9 Images showing the moderator band in the right ventricle of an ovine heart (**A**) and canine heart (**B**). The moderator band in the sheep is muscular, originating on the septal wall and running to the anterior papillary muscle. In contrast, the moderator band in the canine heart appears fibrous. It originates on the septal wall, runs to the anterior papillary muscle, and continues to the free wall of the right ventricle. APM = anterior papillary muscle; MB = moderator band; SW = septal wall

in 48% of the hearts of children and in 52% of the adult human hearts studied [27] (Fig. 6.7). They also reported that left ventricular bands were highly prevalent in sheep, dog, and pig hearts [27] (Fig. 6.6).

6.3.3 The Cardiac Valves

Large mammalian hearts have four cardiac valves with principally similar structures and locations. Two atrioventricular valves are located between each atrium and ventricle on both the right and left sides of the heart, and two semilunar valves lie between the ventricles and the major arteries arising from their outflow tracts (the pulmonary artery and aorta). Chordae tendinae connect the fibrous leaflets of both atrioventricular valves to the papillary muscles in each ventricle and serve to keep the valves from prolapsing

into the atria during ventricular contraction, thereby preventing backflow of blood into the atria. The semilunar valves, the aortic and pulmonic, do not have attached chordae tendinae and close due to pressure gradients developed across them. See Chapter 31 for more details on valvular structures, functions, and defects.

The valve separating the right atrium from the right ventricle is termed the "tricuspid valve" because it has three major cusps—the anterosuperior (anterior), inferior (posterior), and septal cusps. Typically, there are also three associated papillary muscles in the right ventricle. Interestingly, the commissures between the anterosuperior leaflet and the inferior leaflets can be fused in dog hearts [14] giving the appearance of only two leaflets. Interindividual and interspecies variations in the number of papillary muscles have also been reported [11]. The valve separating the left atrium from the left ventricle is termed the "mitral or bicuspid valve" because it typically has two cusps, the anterior (aortic) and the posterior (mural). However, according to Netter [15], the human mitral valve actually can be considered to have four cusps, including the two major cusps listed above and two small commissural cusps or scallops; further publications on the mitral valve describe large variations in the number of scallops present in human hearts. In large mammalian hearts, two primary leaflets of the mitral valve are always present, but variations in the number of scallops exist and can be quite marked, giving one the impression of extra leaflets [11]. A fibrous continuity between the mitral valve and the aortic valve is present in humans and most large mammals, extending from the central fibrous body to the left fibrous trigone [11]. The length of this fibrous continuity, termed the "intervalvar septum or membranous septum," varies considerably in length in different animals, but notably is completely absent in sheep [28]. There are also differences in the fibrous ring supporting the mitral valve and in the composition of the leaflets of the mitral valve between species. For instance, according to Walmsley a segment of the ring at the base of the mural cusp is always present in the human heart, but is difficult to distinguish in certain breeds of dogs and is inconspicuous in the sheep heart [28].

Differences in aortic valve anatomy have also been reported in the literature. For example, Sands et al. compared aortic valves of human, pig, calf, and sheep hearts [29], and they reported that interspecies differences in leaflet shape exist, but that all species examined had fairly evenly spaced commissures. Additionally, they found that variations in leaflet thickness existed; in particular, sheep aortic valves were described as especially thin and fragile. They also noted that there was a substantially greater amount of myocardial tissue supporting the right and left coronary leaflet bases in the animal hearts relative to humans [29].

6.3.4 The Coronary System

Mammalian hearts have an intrinsic circulatory system that originates with two main coronary arteries [11] whose ostia are located directly behind the aortic valve cusps. Deoxygenated coronary blood flow returns to the right atrium via the coronary sinus into which the coronary veins drain, and also to the right atrium, the right and left ventricles [24, 30], and the left atrium [31, 32] by

Thebesian veins. According to Michaëlsson and Ho [11], differences in perfusion areas exist between large mammalian species as well as within species (e.g., between breeds); these differences have also been described in humans. Dogs and sheep typically have a left coronary type of supply, such that the majority of the myocardium is supplied via branches arising from the left coronary artery. In contrast, pigs typically have a balanced supply where the myocardium is supplied equally from both right and left coronary arteries [11]. Yet Crick et al. [13] reported that most of the pig hearts they examined (80%) possessed right coronary dominance. Additionally, Weaver et al. [33] found that the right coronary artery was dominant in 78% of the pigs they studied. Most human hearts (approximately 90%) also display right coronary arterial dominance [34].

Another important aspect of the coronary arterial circulation, one that is of great importance in myocardial ischemia research, is the presence or absence of significant collateralization of the coronary circulation. Normal human hearts tend to have sparse coronary collateral development, which is very similar to that seen in normal pig hearts [33]. In contrast, it is now widely known that extensive coronary collateral networks can be seen in normal dog hearts [5, 35–38]. Furthermore, Schaper et al. [39] found that the coronary collateral network of dogs was almost exclusively located at the epicardial surface, while that of pig hearts, when present, was located subendocardially. They were unable to detect a significant collateral network in the hearts of sheep (Fig. 6.1).

There are three major venous pathways that drain the heart—the coronary sinus, anterior cardiac veins, and Thebesian veins [32, 40]. Drainage from each of these venous systems is present in human hearts as well as in dog, pig, and sheep hearts [13, 14, 24, 32]. While the overall structure of the coronary venous system is similar across species, interindividual variations are common. Nevertheless, there is one notable difference in the coronary venous system between species that warrants mention, that is, the presence of the left azygous vein draining the left thoracic cavity directly into the coronary sinus; such a left azygous vein is typically present in both pig [13] and sheep hearts [11] (Fig. 6.10).

6.3.5 The Lymphatic System

In addition to an intrinsic circulatory system, large mammalian hearts have an inherent and substantial lymphatic system which serves the same general function of the lymphatic system in the rest of the body. More specifically, the mammalian lymphatic system has been described as

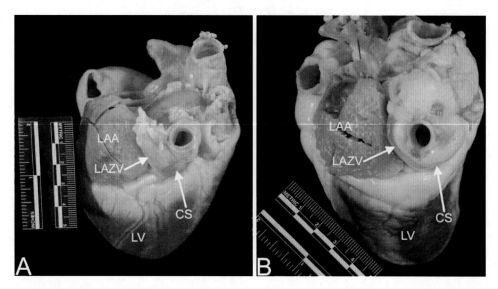

Fig. 6.10 Images showing the left azygous (hemiazygous) vein entering the coronary sinus in the pig (**A**) and sheep (**B**) hearts. The left azygous vein drains the thoracic cavity directly into the coronary sinus in these animals, rather than emptying into the superior vena cava via the azygous as seen in dog and human hearts. Notice that it travels between the left atrial appendage and the pulmonary veins; the oblique vein of Marshall (oblique vein of the left atrium) travels this path in human and dog hearts. CS = coronary sinus; LAA = left atrial appendage; LAZV = left azygous vein; LV = left ventricle

follows: hearts have subepicardial lymphatic capillaries that form continuous plexuses covering the whole of each ventricle [41]. Furthermore, the lymphatic channels are divided into five orders, with the first order draining the capillaries and joining to become the second order and so on, until the lymph is drained from the heart via one large collecting duct of the fifth order. In general, it has been described that dogs, pigs, and humans have extensive subepicardial and subendocardial networks with collecting channels directed toward large ducts in the atrioventricular sulcus that are continuous with the main cardiac lymph duct [42]. Furthermore, it was found that the lymphatic vessels of the normal heart are distributed in the same manner as the coronary arteries and follow them as two main trunks to the base of the heart [43].

6.3.6 The Conduction System

All large mammalian hearts have a very similar conduction system whose main components are the sinoatrial node, atrioventricular node, bundle of His, right and left main bundle branches, and Purkinje fibers. Yet interspecies variations are well recognized, especially with regard to the finer details of the arrangement of the transitional and compact components of the atrioventricular node [11]. In the mammalian heart, the sinoatrial node is the normal pacemaker [11, 24, 25] and is situated in roughly the same location in all hearts: high on the right atrial wall near the junction of the superior vena cava and the right atrium. Conduction spreads through the atria to the atrioventricular node (which interestingly is unique to both birds and mammals) [25], and then to the bundle of His, which is the normal conducting pathway from the atria to the ventricles, penetrating through the central fibrous body. Right and left main bundle branches emanate from the bundle of His and branch further into the Purkinje fibers which then rapidly spread conduction to the ventricles [11]. The atrioventricular node and bundle of His are typically located subendocardially in the right atrium within a region known as the "triangle of Koch," which is delineated by the coronary sinus ostium, the membranous septum, and the septal/posterior commissure of the tricuspid valve. The presence of the "os cordis" has been noted to be present in the sheep heart, but not in dog, pig, or human hearts. Specifically, it is a small, fully formed bone that lies deep in the atrial septum which, in turn, influences the location and course of the bundle of His in sheep hearts. Other known differences in the atrioventricular conduction system between human, pig, dog, and sheep hearts are illustrated in Table 6.1. For more details on the conduction system please see Chapter 11.

Table 6.1 Similarities and differences in the atrioventricular conduction system of dog, pig, sheep, and human hearts [44–47]

	Location of the AV node	AV node and His bundle junction	Length of the His bundle	Route of the His bundle
Human	Located at the base of the atrial septum, anterior to the coronary sinus, and just above the tricuspid valve	End of the AV node and the beginning of the His bundle are nearly impossible to distinguish	Total length of the unbranched portion is 2–3 mm. Penetrating bundle is 0.25–0.75 mm in length. Bundle bifurcates just after emerging from the central fibrous body	Bundle lies just beneath the membranous septum at the crest of the interventricular septum
Pig	Lies on the right side of the crest of the ventricular septum and is lower on the septum than in humans	No explicit information found	Penetrating bundle is very short in comparison to humans	Climbs to the right side of the summit of the ventricular septum, where it enters the central fibrous body. The bifurcation occurs more proximally than in humans
Dog	Same as in humans	Consists of internodal tracts of myocardial fibers	Penetrating bundle is 1–1.5 mm long, significantly longer than the human penetrating bundle	His bundle runs forward and downward through the fibrous base of the heart, just beneath the endocardium. There are at least three discrete His bundle branches of myocardium that join the atrial end of the AV node via a proximal His bundle branch
Sheep	Located at the base of the atrial septum, anterior to the coronary sinus, just above the tricuspid valve, and at the junction of the middle and posterior one-third of the os cordis	Junction is characterized by finger-like projections, where the two types of tissue overlap; size and staining qualities of the initial Purkinje cells of the His bundle make it easy to distinguish between the end of the AV node and the beginning of the His bundle	Portion of the bundle passing through the central fibrous body is ~1 mm. Bundle extends 4–6 mm beyond the central fibrous body before it bifurcates	Unbranched bundle must pass beneath the os cordis to reach the right side of the ventricular septum. His bundle then remains relatively deep within the confines of the ventricular myocardium. Branching occurs more anteriorly in sheep than in humans

AV = atrioventricular.

6.4 Qualitative and Quantitative Comparisons of Cardiac Anatomy in Commonly Used Large Mammalian Cardiovascular Research Models

The following section describes original research conducted at the University of Minnesota by the authors of this chapter.

6.4.1 Importance for Comparing the Anatomy of Various Animal Models

Selection of the proper experimental model for use in cardiovascular research depends on many factors including: (1) cost; (2) quality and quantity of data; (3) familiarity with the model; and/or (4) relevance to the human condition [48]. Typically, a balance as to the relative importance of these factors is determined when optimizing any experimental protocol. Yet one important parameter that is often overlooked in such a design is the comparative cardiac anatomy of the model in question relative to that of humans.

Even today, there is often considerable debate over which cardiovascular research model most closely resembles the human heart anatomically. Surprisingly, in spite of this debate, the comparative cardiac anatomy of such models as a specific topic is largely unexplored. Nevertheless, this question is especially important for biomedical device design and testing in which the goal is to test a product that directly interacts with specific anatomical structures. Furthermore, such comparisons often become even more complicated due to: (1) the relative orientation and/or position of each species' heart and (2) the various terminologies used to describe heart anatomy and position (attitudinally correct anatomy) which can vary between various animal models and in comparison to humans. In addition, one hopes to match the cardiac dimensions across species, but this can be further complicated by both gender and age. For example, a 6- to 7-month-old Yorkshire swine has a typical cardiac mass between 300 and 400 g, which is similar to that of the healthy adult human. Finally, genetic heritage influences expressed cardiac anatomy and specific descriptors are often missing in previous reports (i.e., specific breeds of animals studied).

Thus, the following studies were designed to elucidate the major similarities and differences between the hearts of several major large mammalian cardiovascular research models and then relate these findings to humans. Specifically, qualitative and quantitative techniques were employed on postmortem, formalin fixed porcine, ovine, canine, and human hearts.

6.4.2 Methods and Materials

For this study, we obtained fresh hearts of humans (*Homo sapiens*; man), pigs (*Sus domestica*; swine, porcine), dogs (*Canis lupus familiaris*; canine), and sheep (*Ovis aries*; ovine). Human hearts (*n* = 8) were obtained from the Anatomy Bequest Program at the University of Minnesota. All human hearts were previously unfixed and devoid of clinically diagnosed heart disease or defect. Swine (Yorkshire cross), canine (hound cross), and ovine (Polypay cross) (*n* = 10 each) hearts were obtained from either the Research Animal Resources at the University of Minnesota or the Physiological Research Laboratories at Medtronic, Inc.; these animals were used for prior research studies that did not alter their anatomy. In other words, in all cases, care was taken to ensure that hearts were only obtained from individuals and animals in which cardiac anatomy was not considered to be altered by disease processes or any prior experimental protocols.

6.4.2.1 Heart Preservation

To preserve the hearts and prepare them for comparative anatomical study, specimens were all similarly "pressure perfusion fixed." Briefly, this consisted of suspending each heart in a large container of 10% buffered formalin from cannulae tied into the following major vessels: the superior caval vein, the pulmonary trunk, the aorta, and one pulmonary vein. All remaining vessels were sealed, with the exception of small vents positioned both in the inferior caval vein and in one of the pulmonary veins. Formalin was gravity fed down the cannulae from a

reservoir chamber positioned 35–40 cm above the fluid level in the suspension chamber. This system generated a reproducible perfusion pressure between 45 and 50 mmHg. The hearts were allowed to fix under these conditions for a minimum of 24 h in order to allow for adequate penetration of fixative. This method of fixation was quite reproducible to ensure that the hearts maintained a similar anatomical configuration.

6.4.2.2 Qualitative Anatomical Assessment of Perfusion Fixed Hearts

Several observational assessments, similar to those conducted and previously described by Crick et al. [13], were completed on each heart. In addition to these assessments, a 6 mm endoscopic camera (Olympus Optical, Tokyo, Japan) was inserted into each chamber of each heart, with care taken not to distort any structure to be observed. This allowed for direct visualization of the internal chambers of the heart without dissection, hence allowing the anatomic structures to be examined in a more realistic state. Specific anatomical features assessed included:

- Overall shape of entire heart (conical, valentine, trapezoidal, elliptical, or rounded with blunt apex; Fig. 6.3)
- Overall shape and size of atria and free portions of the appendages (triangular, half-moon, or tubular)
- Ventricular formation of the apex (right, left, or both ventricles)
- Number of pulmonary veins (best estimates were made as some pulmonary veins were dissected close to the atrium)
- Presence or absence of noncardiac coronary sinus tributaries (left azygous vein)
- General shape of

  o Inferior caval vein ostiums
  o Superior caval vein ostiums
  o Pulmonic valves
  o Tricuspid valves
  o Aortic valves
  o Mitral valves
  o Coronary sinus ostiums

- Presence or absence of the valve of the coronary sinus ostium (Thebesian valve)
- Presence or absence of the moderator bands of the right ventricles (if present, the locations of attachment points were noted)
- Number of papillary muscles found in the right and left ventricles

- Degree of trabeculation of right and left ventricular endocardium (1–5; 1 = no trabeculations, 5 = highly trabeculated)
- Presence or absence of any left ventricular bands (i.e., similar structures to the moderator bands of the right ventricle).

6.4.2.3 Quantitative Anatomical Assessments of Perfusion Fixed Hearts

The following quantitative measurements were performed on each heart by employing a novel 3D technique. Briefly, a Microscribe® 3D digitizing arm (3DX, Immersion Corp., San Jose, CA), consisting of a touch probe with six degrees of freedom, was used to gather the 3D data points. First, each heart was suspended and stabilized within a rectangular metal frame via sutures placed into the aorta, the right and left lateral ventricular walls, and the apex. More specifically, the heart was suspended in the classic "valentine heart" position, with the apex pointing toward the bottom of the frame and base toward the top, for easy comparison between hearts. In all cases, attitudinally correct nomenclature was used to describe structures in a more meaningful manner (Figs. 6.11 and 6.12; see also Chapter 2). To allow for the generation of a consistent coordinate axis system, three small holes for touch probe placement were drilled into a right angle scribe that was affixed to a corner of the support structure. This setup allowed for a consistent reference frame for all subsequent digitizations; each heart was maintained within the same 3D space, allowing for precise measurement between all digitized locations.

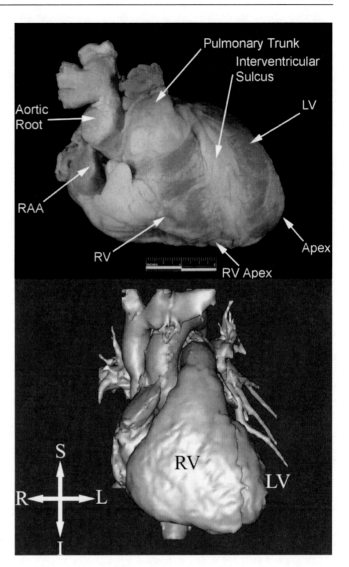

Fig. 6.12 Anterior surface of a fixed human heart and end-diastolic volumetric reconstruction of a human heart from magnetic resonance images. Note that the apex of the human heart is pointed to the left and slightly anteriorly. LV = left ventricle; RAA = free portion of right atrial appendage; RV = right ventricle

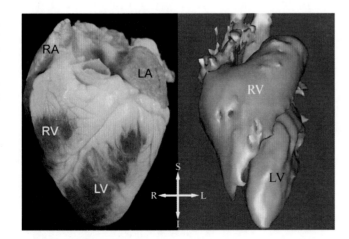

Fig. 6.11 Anterior surface of a fixed sheep heart and end-diastolic volumetric reconstruction of a sheep heart from magnetic resonance images. Note that the apex of the sheep heart is pointed inferiorly and slightly anteriorly. LA = left atrium; LV = left ventricle; RA = right atrium; RV = right ventricle

Furthermore, this overall setup and experimental design allowed for free movement of the 3DX probe as the reference frame could be regenerated following each movement, allowing for complete probe access to all desired aspects of the heart.

For probe initialization, the coordinate axes were set up using the acquisition software (Inscribe, Immersion Corp., San Jose, CA) on the right angle scribe by digitizing the location of the three holes that were set up as the origin, a point on the x-axis and a point on the y-axis; the software then automatically generated the z-axis. Prior to dissection, eight external locations were digitized in each heart (Table 6.2) such that comparisons of the major external dimensions could be performed (Table 6.3).

Then, small incisions were made in the right and left atrial appendages to allow for internal access in each heart. With the simultaneous use of endoscopic cameras, the touch probe was navigated to specific locations in each heart such that comparisons of valve dimensions, ventricular chamber dimensions, and those of the coronary sinus ostium could be subsequently calculated (Tables 6.2 and 6.3). It should be noted that all orientational terms are in relation to the reference frame, which closely mimics the orientation of the animal hearts in vivo. However, these terms do not necessarily describe the exact positions of the human hearts in vivo (terms in parenthesis below describe

Table 6.2 Digitized locations

External locations	Description
Base	Anterior (antero-superior) at the origin of the pulmonary trunk
	Posterior (postero-inferior) at the junction of the coronary sulcus and the interventricular sulcus
	Right lateral at the right atrial/right ventricular junction
	Left lateral at the left atrial/left ventricular junction
Apex	At the true apex of the heart (LV)
Coronary sinus	The entry of the coronary sinus into the right atrium on the posterior aspect of the heart and three evenly spaced points to the end of the coronary sinus, defined as the junction of the great cardiac vein and the oblique vein of the left atrium (Marshall)

Internal locations	Description
Tricuspid valve	Anterior (superior)
	Posterior (inferior)
	Septal (posterior)
	Lateral (anterior)
	Center—best approximation
Coronary sinus	Superior (postero-lateral)
	Inferior (antero-septal)
	Septal (inferior)
	Thebesian valve leading edge (when present)
	Center—best approximation
Pulmonic valve	Mid-point on anterior cusp
	Mid-point of right cusp
	Mid-point of left cusp
	Center—best approximation
RV apex	Deepest point in the RV apex
Mitral valve	Anterior (superior)
	Posterior (inferior)
	Spetal (posterior)
	Lateral (anterior)
	Center—best approximation
Aortic valve	Mid-point of right coronary cusp
	Mid-point of left coronary cusp
	Mid-point of noncoronary cusp
	Right coronary/left coronary commissure tip
	Right coronary/noncoronary commissure tip
	Left coronary/noncoronary commissure tip
	Center—best approximation
LV apex	Deepest point in the LV apex

Table 6.3 Calculated measurements

External measurments	Description
Base to apex length	Anterior (antero-superior) to apex
	Posterior (postero-inferior) to apex
	Right lateral to apex
	Left lateral to apex
Coronary sinus	Length of the coronary sinus

Internal measurements	Description
Coronary sinus ostium	Superior (postero-lateral) to inferior (antero-septal) diameter
	Lateral (inferior) to septal (superior) diameter
	Functional ostium—Thebesian valve to septal (superior) diameter
Tricuspid valve	Anterior (superior) to posterior (inferior) diameter
	Septal (posterior) to lateral (anterior) diameter
Right ventricular inflow	Anterior (superior) tricuspid valve to apex distance
	Posterior (inferior) tricuspid valve to apex distance
	Septal (posterior) tricuspid valve to apex distance
	Lateral (anterior) tricuspid valve to apex distance
	Center tricuspid valve to apex distance
Pulmonic valve	Sinotubular junction diameter
	Basal annular diameter
Right ventricular outflow	Mid-anterior cusp pulmonic valve to apex distance
	Mid-right cusp pulmonic valve to apex distance
	Mid-left cusp pulmonic valve to apex distance
	Center pulmonic valve to apex distance
Mitral valve	Anterior (superior) to posterior (inferior) diameter
	Septal (posterior) to lateral (anterior) diameter
Left ventricular inflow	Anterior (superior) mitral valve to apex distance
	Posterior (inferior) mitral valve to apex distance
	Septal (posterior) mitral valve to apex distance
	Lateral (anterior) mitral valve to apex distance
	Center mitral valve to apex distance
Aortic valve	Sinotubular junction diameter
	Basal annular diameter
Left ventricular outflow	Mid-right coronary cusp aortic value to apex distance
	Mid-left coronary cusp aortic value to apex distance
	Mid-noncoronary cusp aortic valve to apex distance
	Center aortic valve to apex distance

the attitudinally correct terms for describing the human hearts). It should be further noted that, in total, only three measurements from porcine heart number 1 needed to be removed due to improper coordinate axis regeneration. These were: (1) posterior base to whole heart apex; (2) aortic valve mid-left coronary cusp to left ventricular apex; and (3) aortic valve center to left ventricular apex.

All calculations were analyzed both as raw data and as normalized data (divided by the given heart weight). Statistical significance tests were performed using one-way ANOVA and Bonferroni post-analyses; significance was set at $\alpha = 0.05$. All values are presented as means $\pm$ standard deviation.

6.4.3 Results

The average heart weights were 367.3 ± 65.8 g for humans, 274.6 ± 50.4 g for pigs, 258.1 ± 36.2 g for dogs, and 353.1 ± 120.7 g for sheep. Human heart weights were significantly larger than dog heart weights ($p < 0.05$). The average age of the human donors was 63.8 ± 19.5 years. Although the exact age of the animals was not known, all porcine hearts were from younger rapidly growing animals (<1 year old); all canine (1–2 years old) and ovine hearts (1–3 years old) were from mature animals. Six of the human hearts were obtained from females and two were from males. All porcine and canine hearts were from male animals, while all ovine hearts were from female animals.

6.4.3.1 Qualitative Comparisons

The human hearts had the largest variation in overall shape compared to the animal hearts. Three human hearts were classified as having an elliptical shape, two were conical, two were rounded with a blunt apex, and one was valentine shaped. The overall defined shapes of the animal hearts were as follows: 6 ovine hearts were considered conical and 4 were valentine; 8 porcine hearts were valentine and 2 were trapezoidal; and all 10 canine hearts were elliptical. Nevertheless, the apexes of the hearts were formed entirely by the left ventricles in all animal hearts and in five of the eight human hearts. In the other three human hearts, the apexes were mostly left but were considered slightly shifted toward a "joint apex."

Generally, the free portions of the right atrial appendages of the human hearts were defined as either triangular (seven of eight) or tubular on the left (eight of eight). The size of the free portion of the appendages was variable in the human hearts with three having larger right appendages, three having larger left appendages, and two having similar sized appendages. The free portions of the right atrial appendages of the ovine hearts were in the shape of a half-moon (9 of 10) and typically characterized as triangular on the left (8 of 10). The free portions of the right atrial appendages were larger than the left in seven hearts and the same size as the left in the remaining three hearts. The free portions of the right atrial appendages of the porcine hearts were generally in the shape of a half-moon (9 of 10) and typically triangular on the left (6 of 10). The left atrial appendage was larger than the right in nine hearts and the same size in the remaining heart. In the canine hearts, the free portions of both atrial appendages were considered to be tubular in nine hearts and triangular in one heart. The free portions of the right atrial appendages were larger than the left in five hearts and the same size as the left in the other five hearts. The left azygous (hemiazygous) vein was present as a tributary to the coronary sinus in all ovine and porcine hearts examined; it was not present in any of the canine hearts or human hearts. Thebesian valves covering some aspect of the coronary sinus ostium were present in all human hearts, but absent in all animal hearts examined.

Moderator bands were present in the right ventricles of all hearts examined (Figs. 6.6, 6.7, 6.8, and 6.9). However, the origin and attachment of these bands, as well as their appearance, were varied among species. In the human hearts, the moderator band typically arose more apically on the septal wall and attached to the base of the anterior papillary muscle (APM). Interestingly, the band was a free arc in six of the hearts and a ridge in two hearts. In both sheep and pigs, the moderator bands presented as muscular structures that originated on or near the septal papillary muscle (SPM), inserted at the body or head of the APM, and were free arcs in all. In contrast, the moderator bands of the canine hearts presented as fibrous networks that originated on the APM or septal wall and inserted on the free walls of the right ventricles (usually at multiple sites). Similar to all pig and sheep hearts and 75% of the human hearts, the canine moderator band was a free arching structure across the ventricular cavity. There were left ventricular bands, similar to the moderator band (composed of or containing what are considered to be conduction fibers), identified in all but one porcine heart and one human heart.

All human, ovine, and porcine hearts had one well-defined APM in the right ventricle. In contrast, six canine hearts had two APMs and four hearts had a single APM. Nine ovine hearts had a single posterior papillary muscle (PPM) in the right ventricle and one heart had two PPMs. Six porcine hearts had a single PPM, three hearts had two PPMs, and one heart had three PPMs. Only one canine heart had a single PPM, five hearts had two PPMs, and four hearts had three PPMs. Three human hearts had a single PPM, one heart had two PPMs, and four hearts had three PPMs. Eight ovine hearts had a single SPM and two hearts had two SPMs. In contrast, four canine hearts had a single SPM and six hearts had three or more SPMs. Additionally, only two porcine hearts had a single SPM, four hearts had two SPMs, and four hearts had three or more SPMs. Three human hearts had a single SPM, three hearts had two SPMs, and two hearts had three SPMs. All hearts from all species had other small papillary muscles on the septal wall which were not fully formed and projected into the right ventricle, as well as chordae appearing to attach directly to the septal wall.

In the left ventricle, all animal hearts from all species had a single APM with varying numbers of heads. In contrast, five human hearts had a single APM, one heart had two APMs, and two hearts had three APMs. All porcine and canine hearts had a single PPM in the left ventricle, while eight ovine hearts had a single PPM and two hearts had two PPMs. Four human hearts had a single PPM in the left ventricle and four hearts had two PPMs.

Generally, the right ventricle and left ventricle apices of human hearts were far more trabeculated as compared to each species of animal hearts. In the right ventricle, the canine hearts were more trabeculated than those of porcine and ovine hearts. In contrast, the degree of trabeculation in the left ventricular apexes was similar across animal hearts. It was also noted that the epicardiums of the ovine hearts were typically covered in greater amounts of fatty tissue relative to the canine and porcine hearts.

The shapes of the ostiums of the superior vena cavae and the inferior vena cavae were circular in all hearts examined, with the exception of one human heart in which the inferior vena cava ostium was removed during heart removal. The shapes of the tricuspid valves and mitral valves ranged within species and included elliptical, circular, nearly circular, and half-moon. Similarly, the aortic and pulmonary valves were circular in all hearts examined. The coronary sinus ostiums were elliptical in the majority of hearts.

Due to cannulation of the hearts for perfusion and dissection of the pulmonary veins near the left atrium, the number of pulmonary veins could not be reliably determined in all hearts. Typically, major ostia were seen within

each heart, but bifurcation patterns were different within and between species. Oftentimes, the myocardium traveled deep into the "vein" which was defined by a major ostium, yet the veins could be bifurcated almost directly at the myocardial/venous tissue junction into two to four veins. The canine hearts were the only exception to this generalization, in which seven hearts had greater than five pulmonary veins (range five to eight).

6.4.3.2 Quantitative Comparisons

In general, calculated dimensions and heart weights were not well correlated, with the highest correlations found in ovine hearts. Therefore, statistical analyses were performed on both raw measurements and on those normalized to heart weight values. Statistically significant differences between the species were found for both raw and normalized data. Although some overlap of statistically significant differences existed between the raw and normalized values, oftentimes statistical significance was not conserved between the two methods. Therefore, only raw data is presented throughout the remaining portion of this chapter and in Tables 6.4 and 6.5, with statistically significant differences noted.

Externally, the average anterior (anterosuperior) base to apex distance was significantly longer in sheep hearts than canine hearts. The average base to apex distance on the posterior (posteroinferior) and left lateral aspects was significantly longer in the human hearts than swine, canine, and ovine hearts. The average right lateral base to apex distance was significantly longer in human hearts compared to swine and canine hearts, and the ovine hearts were also significantly longer than the swine hearts. The average external length of the coronary sinus was significantly longer in the human hearts compared to the swine, canine, and ovine hearts (Table 6.4).

Internally, the average superior (posterolateral) to inferior (anteroseptal) coronary sinus ostium diameter was significantly larger in human hearts compared to swine, canine, and ovine hearts. The average lateral (inferior) to septal (superior) diameter was significantly smaller in canine hearts compared to human, swine, and ovine

Table 6.4 External dimensions (mean ± std. dev)

Measurement	Human	Swine	Canine	Ovine	
Anterior (antero-superior) base to apex distance (mm)	98.7 ± 14.6	101.2 ± 6.8	93.5 ± 4.1	111.1 ± 16.8	ζ
Posterior (postero-inferior) base to apex distance (mm)	87.7 ± 12.4	65.6 ± 4.2	71.3 ± 2.9	72.6 ± 7.6	$\alpha\beta\theta$
Right lateral base to apex distance (mm)	106.4 ± 10.9	88.4 ± 4.8	94.3 ± 5.8	103.8 ± 12.7	$\alpha\beta\varepsilon$
Left lateral base to apex distance (mm)	99.7 ± 9.5	80.8 ± 5.3	78.6 ± 3.5	87.4 ± 10.2	$\alpha\beta\theta$
Coronary sinus length	46.5 ± 5.2	25.1 ± 2.7	29.8 ± 6.7	29.9 ± 8.6	$\alpha\beta\theta$

Significant differences are noted by the following symbols: α—human, swine; β—human, canine; θ—human, ovine; δ—swine, canine; ε—swine, ovine; ζ—canine, ovine.

Table 6.5 Internal dimensions (mean ± std. dev)

Measurement	Human	Swine	Canine	Ovine	
Coronary sinus ostium					
CS Os superior (postero-lateral) to inferior (antero-septal) diameter (mm)	12.3±4.2	7.7±1.4	5.0±1.0	8.1±3.2	αβθ
CS Os lateral (inferior) to septal (superior) diameter (mm)	15.7±2.4	16.4±2.9	9.8±2.2	18.3±5.0	βδζ
CS Os functional ostium—Thebesian valve to opposite edge diameter (mm)	8.1±2.9	NA	NA	NA	αθδζ
Tricuspid valve					
Tricuspid valve anterior (superior) to posterior (inferior) diameter (mm)	43.0±3.1	37.2±4.2	38.8±3.0	39.9±3.8	α
Tricuspid valve septal (posterior) to lateral (anterior) diameter	37.7±7.2	30.3±5.5	29.5±4.6	36.0±9.4	
RV inflow tract					
Tricuspid valve anterior (superior) to RV apex distance (mm)	86.9±12.9	72.0±4.7	65.3±4.1	66.1±15.9	αβθ
Tricuspid valve posterior (inferior) to RV apex distance (mm)	78.9±19.9	55.5±3.3	49.3±3.6	51.9±11.1	αβθ
Tricuspid valve septal (posterior) to RV apex distance (mm)	77.4±14.0	61.8±4.3	55.5±4.8	59.5±10.1	αβθ
Tricuspid valve lateral (anterior) to RV apex distance (mm)	83.7±21.0	61.6±4.9	55.7±3.8	58.7±16.7	αβθ
Tricuspid valve center to RV apex distance (mm)	73.1±19.2	51.8±2.7	45.7±4.5	50.4±9.8	αβθ
Pulmonic valve					
Pulmonic valve sinotubular junction diameter (mm)	28.1±3.8	18.7±1.6	18.3±3.3	22.8±5.7	αβθ
Pulmonic valve basal annular diameter (mm)	31.1±3.2	25.6±2.0	25.5±2.9	29.8±6.8	
RV outflow tract					
Pulmonic valve mid-anterior cusp to apex distance (mm)	86.9±14.7	93.3±6.2	84.8±5.0	90.4±16.0	
Pulmonic valve mid-right cusp to apex distance (mm)	93.9±15.0	85.4±5.9	76.7±4.1	82.4±21.1	
Pulmonic valve mid-left cusp to apex distance (mm)	87.9±13.6	79.0±4.7	69.4±4.3	79.2±9.7	β
Pulmonic valve center to apex distance (mm)	90.4±16.7	85.6±6.5	77.9±4.3	81.4±11.3	
Mitral Valve					
Mitral valve anterior (superior) to posterior (inferior) diameter (mm)	37.9±4.6	31.0±3.9	31.3±4.6	36.9±7.4	
Mitral valve septal (posterior) to lateral (anterior) diameter (mm)	32.5±5.6	23.7±2.7	22.0±4.9	25.8±6.3	αβθ
LV inflow tract					
Mitral valve anterior (superior) to LV apex distance (mm)	83.7±18.0	76.8±6.3	63.1±6.0	75.7±13.5	β
Mitral valve posterior (inferior) to LV apex distance (mm)	78.2±18.2	68.2±5.5	60.0±5.8	67.4±11.6	β
Mitral valve septal (posterior) to LV apex distance (mm)	80.7±15.7	70.6±6.1	65.2±5.8	70.2±13.4	β
Mitral valve lateral (anterior) to LV apex distance (mm)	77.4±17.3	72.1±5.3	59.4±4.8	72.1±13.2	β
Mitral valve center to LV apex distance (mm)	69.5±16.2	62.0±5.9	52.1±4.9	62.3±11.3	β
Aortic valve					
Aortic valve sinotubular junction diameter (mm)	26.4±3.0	21.4±2.3	16.8±2.7	20.4±3.8	αβθδ
Aortic valve basal annular diameter (mm)	30.0±2.6	25.1±3.2	23.2±4.1	28.9±5.4	βζ
LV outflow tract					
Aortic valve mid-right coronary cusp to LV apex distance (mm)	89.9±18.6	72.5±6.2	65.2±5.8	76.2±13.3	αβ
Aortic valve mid-left coronary cusp to LV apex distance (mm)	89.7±18.6	77.1±5.5	67.1±6.1	77.3±14.5	β
Aortic valve mid-noncoronary cusp to LV apex distance (mm)	92.7±20.1	73.8±6.2	67.1±7.1	73.0±11.9	αβθ
Aortic valve center to LV apex distance (mm)	90.8±18.3	75.9±5.8	63.7±6.6	75.2±12.8	βθ

Significant differences are noted by the following symbols: α—human, swine; β—human, canine; h–human, ovine; δ— swine, canine; ε—swine, ovine; ζ—canine, ovine.

hearts. As stated earlier, Thebesian valves were present in all human hearts. Due to this valve, the functional ostium of the coronary sinus (i.e., that which was not covered by a Thebesian valve) was reduced in the superior/inferior dimension in these hearts as the attachment of the valve was typically in the posterolateral/anteroseptal direction. When taking into account the Thebesian valve, the average diameter of the functional ostium of the human hearts was significantly smaller than that of the swine and ovine hearts (Table 6.5).

The average tricuspid valve diameters were all of similar size, with the exception of the anterior (superior) to posterior (inferior) dimension, which was significantly larger in human hearts than pig hearts. The average right ventricular inflow tract length was significantly longer in human hearts compared to the animal hearts in all dimensions analyzed. No significant differences were seen in the average lengths of the outflow tracts of the right ventricles, with the exception of the mid-left cusp to apex dimension, which was significantly shorter in canine hearts than human hearts. The average diameter of the sinotubular junction of the pulmonic trunk was significantly greater in the human hearts as compared to the animal hearts. No significant differences were observed in the average diameters of the basal annular ring of the pulmonic valve (Table 6.5).

No significant differences were observed in the average diameter of mitral valve in the anterior (superior) to posterior (inferior) dimension. However, the average diameter of the mitral valve in the septal (posterior) to lateral (anterior) dimension was significantly larger in the human hearts as compared to the animal hearts. The average dimensions of the inflow tracts of the left ventricle were significantly shorter in the canine hearts compared to human, swine, and ovine hearts in all dimensions analyzed. The average diameters of the left ventricular outflow tract were generally longer in the human hearts than the animal hearts. The average human dimensions were significantly longer than the swine and canine hearts in the mid-right cusp dimension, significantly longer than the canine hearts in the mid-left dimension, significantly longer than all hearts in the noncoronary dimension, and significantly longer than the canine and ovine hearts from the center of the aortic valve. The average diameter of the sinotubular junction of the aorta was significantly larger in the human hearts than all animal hearts. Additionally, the average diameter of the swine hearts was significantly longer than the canine hearts at this location. Finally, the average diameters of the basal annulus of the aortic valve were significantly larger in human and ovine hearts than canine hearts (Table 6.5).

6.4.4 Discussion and Consideration of Previous Studies on Comparative Anatomy

In the present study, we examined the gross morphology of the hearts of humans, pigs, dogs, and sheep and compared them both qualitatively and quantitatively. To the authors' knowledge, this is the first study specifically aimed at elucidating both qualitative and quantitative similarities and/or differences in the cardiac anatomy of these commonly employed species for cardiovascular research. These presented findings should be seen as a unique initial database on the overall shapes of hearts, appendages, and valves, the presence or absence of specific anatomical features, and quantitative dimensions, which were measured in nondissected pressure fixed, end-diastolic volume hearts. These comparisons demonstrate that important anatomic differences exist between hearts isolated from humans, pigs, dogs, and sheep. Hopefully, these results can be used by future investigators as an aid in making critical choices as to which animal model would be best for their specific biomedical/cardiovascular research.

A sizeable quantity of literature has been published on many qualitative aspects of large mammalian cardiac anatomy. However, much of this research is very general (i.e., all mammalian hearts have a right and left atrial appendage) [11, 13, 14, 25] or very specific (i.e., comparative cardiac anatomy of the cardiac foramen ovale) [49] and, importantly, most research is not done in a truly comparative fashion. Furthermore, much of this literature does not provide information useful for those specifically performing cardiovascular research with the hope of translating such results to relevant human research.

There are specific examples of anatomic structure that we studied in these comparative analyses that have been described somewhat differently in the previous literature. Crick et al. [13] reported that the shape of the porcine heart was valentine; we observed this shape in 8 of 10 hearts. They also reported a trapezoidal shape of the human hearts they examined. Greater variability was seen in the observed shape of our human hearts, with no general trend seen. The formation of the apex of the heart entirely by the left ventricle has also been previously reported for all animals examined in this study [12–14]; this is also the case for most of the human hearts in this study and is widely reported in literature and textbooks. The presence of a moderator band in the right ventricle in all hearts examined has also been previously noted [11, 13, 50]. However, Truex and Warshaw [26], while finding a moderator band in the right ventricle of all sheep and pigs studied, failed to find such a band in the canine hearts they examined and only found a band in 56.8% of human hearts. This discrepancy was likely due to definition and to the different morphology presented by the band in these animals. Interestingly, we observed left ventricular bands in nearly all of the hearts examined (7 human, 9 swine, 10 canine, and 10 ovine). Gerlis et al. [27] reported that they found left ventricular bands in 100% of ovine hearts ($n = 42$), 100% of canine hearts ($n = 12$), and 86% of porcine hearts they examined ($n = 36$), but only in 52% of adult hearts examined ($n = 50$). Joudinaud and colleagues cataloged the papillary muscles of the swine heart in 2006 [50], classifying them based on the leaflets they supported. They defined them as anteroposterior (APM in this study), anteroseptal (SPM in this study), and posteroseptal (PPM in this study). They found, on average, 1.08 anteroposterior papillary muscles, 2.42 posteroseptal papillary muscles, and 1.78 anteroseptal papillary muscles. These findings are similar to our observations of an average of 1 APMs 1.9 PPMs, and 2.1 SPMs, with a slightly different weighting toward more SPMs than PPMs in our study compared to their research. While a specific report on the number of papillary muscles in the ventricles of other hearts could not be found, it has been reported that human, canine, porcine, and ovine hearts typically have three papillary muscles (APM, PPM, and SPM) in the right ventricle and two (APM and PPM) in the left ventricle [11]. While our findings are similar for the left ventricle, we found a much greater variability in the number of papillary muscles in the right ventricle of all species examined, with some canine hearts having as many as six right ventricular papillary muscles.

Relative to recent interest in the development of access and closure devices for the atria or means for occluding the left atrial appendages in patients with atrial fibrillation, it should be noted that some of our qualitative findings were different from what has been previously reported. For example, Crick et al. [13] reported that the right atrial appendages of the swine hearts typically had a tubular shape, while we found that the right atrial appendages were shaped more like a half-moon. Also, they reported that the right and left atrial appendages of swine hearts were of similar size; we found that the left atrial appendages were larger in 90% of the hearts examined. This discrepancy could be related to the breed differences; Crick et al. did not provide the specific breed of the animals used in their study. Interestingly, they reported that the right atrial appendages of the human hearts were "appreciably" larger than the left, a finding which is similar to our findings in three of the eight hearts examined. It should be noted that we believe the authors of that study were referring to the free portion of the right appendage for comparison, as it is believed that the atrial appendage of the right atrium technically includes all pectinate portions of the atrium arising from the terminal crest [51]. However, the authors reference that the appendage on the right side consists of pectinate muscles and that these pectinate muscles "surround entirely the parietal margin of the vestibule of the tricuspid valve." If the definition is used to describe the right atrial appendage, one would find that only in rare cases (most likely pathological) would the left atrial appendage be larger than the right as the pectinate muscles of the left atrium are nearly always contained within the free portion.

As mentioned previously, there has been a lack of published information comparing canine, porcine, and ovine hearts quantitatively. Yet Lev, Rowlatt, and Rimoldi [52] eloquently described methods to study the congenitally malformed heart quantitatively in 2D in 1961, and followed with an excellent paper on the anatomy of the normal human child heart in 1963 [53]. These methods were applied to the swine heart in a publication by Eckner et al. [54]. More specifically, they measured the inflow and outflow tracts of right and left ventricle of the swine using methods as described by Lev et al. in 1961. From 27 porcine hearts weighing in the range of 200–300 g, they found the length of the right ventricular inflow tract to be 5.396 ± 0.386 cm, the length of the right ventricular outflow tract to be

8.550 ± 0.461 cm, the length of the left ventricular inflow tract to be 7.623 ± 0.348 cm, and the length of the left ventricular outflow tract to be 7.388 ± 0.391. In the present study, we found the length of the right ventricular inflow tract to be 5.55 ± 0.33 cm, the right ventricular outflow tract to be 7.9 ± 0.47 cm, the length of the left ventricular inflow tract to be 6.82 ± 0.55 cm, and the length of the left ventricular outflow tract to be 7.25 ± 0.62 cm. Overall, the measurements from the two studies are similar; however, the right ventricular outflow tract and left ventricular inflow tract were noticeably shorter in the hearts examined in this study compared to those of Eckner et al. It should be noted that the methods described by Lev et al. and used by Eckner et al. were slightly ambiguous regarding their definitions of the measurement end points. For instance, the right ventricular inflow tract measurement was described as "the length of the inflow tract of the right ventricle is measured from a point at the tricuspid annulus in the center of the posterior wall to the apex" [52]. Thus, depending on one's interpretation of the location of this point, significantly varied measurements could be obtained. In spite of this, the measurement locations in the present study were selected so that they were as close as possible to as those measured by Eckner et al. Similarly, another group of investigators, Alvarez et al. [55], applied similar assessment methods to the right ventricles of 75 porcine hearts. They found that the length of the right ventricular inflow tract was on average 5.881 ± 0.842 cm and the outflow tract was 8.437 ± 1.026 cm. Interestingly, the outflow tract length was again longer than that measured in the current study, while the inflow tract length was similar among all three studies. While the breed of swine used by Eckner et al. was not reported, Alvarez et al. used hearts obtained from the Europa breed. The hearts used in the present study were from Yorkshire cross animals; this variation in breed may explain the differences in measured dimensions.

In contrast to the lack of publications examining the gross dimensions of the hearts, there have been publications concerned with the dimensions of the cardiac valves, mostly focused on the aortic and mitral valves. The sheep is the most common model used in experimental models of mitral regurgitation and, due to this, there are numerous studies examining both the normal and pathological anatomy of the mitral valve (see also Chapter 25). Yet many of these studies do not provide comparable measurements. However, in 1997, Gorman et al. published a study of six sheep, demonstrating that the end-diastolic anterior–posterior dimension was 26.6 mm and the end-diastolic commissure–commissure dimension was 35.4 mm [56]. In 2002, Timek et al. reported, in a study of six sheep instrumented with radiopaque markers, that the end-diastolic anterior–posterior dimension of the mitral valve was 2.63 ± 0.32 cm and the end-diastolic commissure–commissure dimension was 3.59±0.43 cm [57]. While the nomenclature used between these studies and the data we presented is slightly different, these reported measurements are very similar overall: our measurements were 25.8±6.3 mm septal–lateral (anterior–posterior) and 36.9±7.4 mm anterior–posterior (superior–inferior or commissure–commissure). Tsakiris et al. reported that the average early diastolic anterior–posterior dimension of five canine hearts was 2.1±0.2 cm, similar to our findings of 22.0±4.9 mm [58]. Chandraratna and Aronow reported a mean maximal diastolic anterior–posterior diameter of 2.2±0.22 cm and end-systolic anterior–posterior diameter of 1.76±0.22 cm from 23 normal human subjects studied with echocardiography [59]. Nordblom and Bech-Hanssen reported a mean end-diastolic anterior–posterior dimension of 2.9±0.35, mean end-systolic anterior–posterior dimension of 3.3±0.32 cm, and mean end-diastolic commissure–commissure dimension of 3.7±0.43 cm in 38 normal human subjects [60]. These two publications show the wide variation of reported results in the literature; reporting on all of the mitral publications is beyond the scope of this paper. However, it should be noted that our results provided above were more similar to the publication by Nordblom than that of Chandraratna. Added considerations in comparing anatomic studies that one needs to keep in mind are that differing methodologies may slightly skew obtained data, or that newer methodologies may provide more accurate measurements. For example, this could be due to changes in the definition of the dimensions measured and also to higher resolution offered by newer ultrasound technology which provides important in vivo measurements.

Regarding the aortic valve, Sands et al. published the only available quantitative study examining the aortic valves of multiple hearts, including 10 swine, 9 ovine, 9 bovine, and 7 humans [29]. Interestingly, in their investigations, aortic valve diameters were measured via passing an obturator through fresh hearts until a snug fit was determined. They reported the average annulus diameters of 26.4±3.15 mm in human hearts, 26.6±1.84 mm in pig hearts, and 25.8±.29 mm in sheep hearts. It may be assumed that, by annulus, they were actually referring to the basal portion of the annulus. For the in vitro data on perfusion fixed hearts we provided above, larger average basal annular diameters in human hearts (30.0±2.6 mm) and in sheep hearts (28.9±5.4 mm) were observed, and slightly smaller average diameters in pig hearts (25.1±3.2 mm) were found. More recently, Lansac and colleagues published a sonometric study of eight ovine aortic valves and ascending aortas, in which they reported average basal annular diameters of 20.7±0.4 mm and commissure diameters of 14.1±0.2 mm, which are both smaller than our reported diameters [61]. Sim and colleagues published a comparison of 12 human and 12 swine aortic valves in which they

reported mean diameters of 2.55±0.13 cm for human hearts ($n = 12$) and 2.20±0.32 cm for swine hearts [62], both which are smaller than those observed in our studies. Interestingly, Swanson and Clark published a study of five normal human aortic valves in 1974, using silicone casts of aortic valves prepared at various pressures (0–120 mmHg) [63]. Regardless of the pressure used, on average, the basal annulus in their study was smaller than that observed in this study. Finally, in support of the fact that sheep are the most commonly used animal model for aortic valve studies, we found that the average basal annulus diameters were most similar between sheep and human hearts. However, we noted that the sinotubular junction diameters were significantly smaller in all animals studied as compared to the human hearts. This could have implications for selection of an animal model for newer technologies such as transcatheter-delivered aortic valves, as some technology engages the sinotubular junction for fixation of the device.

Publications on the valves on the right side of the heart are scarce, especially the pulmonic valve, and none were found with comparable measurements. The tricuspid valve has been quantitatively studied in sheep, canines, and humans, although similar to mitral valve studies, similar measurements to this study are not evident in many publications. Jouan and colleagues studied the tricuspid annulus of seven sheep and showed that during the cardiac cycle the minimum diameter (approximately perpendicular to the septum) changed from 17.8±1.9 mm to 21.2±2.0 mm and maximum diameter (approximately parallel to the septum) changed from 36.4±2.4 to 40.1±2.6 mm [64]. While this report does not specifically give orientational references for these numbers, the minimum diameter is described as perpendicular to the septum and therefore is much smaller than that observed in this study. The maximum diameter, however, is similar to the anterior–posterior (superior–inferior) diameter of this study. In 2007, Anwar and colleagues reported the average tricuspid annular diameter of 100 normal patients to be 4.0±0.7 cm [65]. Again, no orientational references are given to this diameter, but rather it appears to be the maximal diameter, which most likely correlates to the anterior–posterior (superior–inferior) diameter of this study with similar values observed.

The dimensions analyzed in perfusion fixed hearts we provided above can also be used to illustrate some differences in the gross morphology of the hearts examined. Interestingly, the average right ventricular inflow tract of the human hearts examined in this study was significantly longer than that of the other hearts examined, although the outflow tracts of the right ventricles were relatively the same length among all hearts. This has direct applicability to right ventricular apical pacemaker lead design, in which the designs intended ultimately for human hearts are studied in any of the animal species examined in this study—the lead length to reach the right ventricular apex from the tricuspid valve in the animal species is on average 1–2 cm shorter than in human hearts. The rest of the implant anatomy would also need to be considered for complete analysis. Another interesting finding was the significantly smaller diameter of the coronary sinus ostiums in canine hearts compared to the other hearts examined. Coupled with the external measured length of the coronary sinus, which was significantly longer in human hearts than other hearts, implications for animal model selection in biomedical device research become obvious. Similar to the right ventricular apical lead length mentioned above, coronary venous-delivered left ventricular pacing lead lengths may need to be shortened for animal work. Furthermore, when choosing an animal model to simulate coronary sinus access similar to humans with Thebesian valves, the canine model becomes an obvious choice due to the similarity in size. Maric et al. examined the diameter of the coronary sinus ostium in humans and dogs; they found the diameter to be 8.43 ± 2.6 mm in humans and 6.5 ± 1.31 mm in dogs [66]. Unfortunately, Maric does not mention which diameter was measured (i.e., superior/inferior or lateral/septal).

6.5 Summary

Cardiac research is an important field that will continue to thrive for many years to come. It is critical that the appropriate animal models are employed to perform well-designed translational research prior to human clinical trials. In this chapter, we presented a unique set of comparative information relative to cardiac anatomy of several large mammalian models commonly used for such laboratory testing: the pig, dog, and sheep. Important differences and similarities exist that may impact research results relative to either device testing or pharmacological therapeutic trials. The novel research data presented here from our laboratory were specifically designed to systematically compare the anatomical features of these animal models to humans, both qualitatively and quantitatively. The techniques employed were unique in that they allowed study of nondissected hearts, providing measurements from realistic geometric configurations. We observed that specific differences in the cardiac anatomy exist between the species, for hearts isolated and pressure perfusion fixed with similar weights, and that these differences may be useful in choosing an animal model for certain types of biomedical research. It is likely as CT and MRI methodologies continue to advance, more specific structural

comparisons can be better performed on functioning hearts, yet details about animal age, weight, health status, and/or breed will need to be well described in order to make such data sets of higher value.

References

1. Paul EF, Paul J. Why animal experimentation matters: The use of animals in medical research. New Brunswick, NJ: Social Philosophy and Policy Foundation: Transaction, 2001.
2. Monamy V. Animal experimentation: A guide to the issues. Cambridge, United Kingdom; New York, NY: Cambridge University Press, 2000.
3. Nutton V. Portraits of science. Logic, learning, and experimental medicine. Science 2002;295:800–1.
4. Persaud TVN. A history of anatomy: The post-Vesalian era. Springfield, IL: Charles C Thomas Publisher, 1997.
5. Hearse DJ. The elusive coypu: The importance of collateral flow and the search for an alternative to the dog. Cardiovasc Res 2000;45:215–9.
6. Christensen GC, Campeti FL. Anatomic and functional studies of the coronary circulation in the dog and pig. Am J Vet Res 1959;20:18–26.
7. Hughes HC. Swine in cardiovascular research. Lab Anim Sci 1986;36:348–50.
8. Kong Y, Chen JT, Zeft HJ, et al. Natural history of experimental coronary occlusion in pigs: A serial cineangiographic study. Am Heart J 1969;77:45–54.
9. Verdouw PD, van den Doel MA, de Zeeuw S, et al. Animal models in the study of myocardial ischaemia and ischaemic syndromes. Cardiovasc Res 1998;39:121–35.
10. Getty R. General heart and blood vessels. In: Getty R, ed. Sisson and Grossman's: The anatomy of the domestic animals. 5th ed. Philadelphia, PA: Saunders, 1975:164–75.
11. Michaëlsson M, Ho SY. Congenital heart malformations in mammals: An illustrated text. London, UK; River Edge, NJ: Imperial College Press, 2000.
12. Ghoshal NG. Ruminant, carnivore, porcine: Heart and arteries. In: Sisson S, Grossman JD, Getty R, eds. Sisson and Grossman's: The anatomy of the domestic animals. 5th ed. Philadelphia, PA: Saunders, 1975:960–1023, 1594–1651, 1306–42.
13. Crick SJ, Sheppard MN, Ho SY, et al. Anatomy of the pig heart: Comparisons with normal human cardiac structure. J Anat 1998;193:105–19.
14. Evans HE. The heart and arteries. In: Miller ME, Evans HE, eds. Miller's anatomy of the dog. 3rd ed. Philadelphia, PA: Saunders, 1993:586–602.
15. Netter FH, Ciba Pharmaceutical Company. Medical Education Division. Heart. West Caldwell, NJ: The Division, 1979.
16. Holt JP, Rhode EA, Kines H. Ventricular volumes and body weight in mammals. Am J Physiol 1968;215:704–15.
17. Lee JC, Taylor FN, Downing SE. A comparison of ventricular weights and geometry in newborn, young, and adult mammals. J Appl Physiol 1975;38:147–50.
18. Holt JP. The normal pericardium. Am J Cardiol 1970;26:455–65.
19. Naimark WA, Lee JM, Limeback H, et al. Correlation of structure and viscoelastic properties in the pericardia of four mammalian species. Am J Physiol 1992;263:H1095–106.
20. Spodick DH. The pericardium: A comprehensive textbook. New York, NY: M. Dekker, 1997.

21. Moore T, Shumacker HJ. Congenital and experimentally produced pericardial defects. Angiology 1953;4:1–11.

22. Elias H, Boyd L. Notes on the anatomy, embryology and histology of the pericardium. J New York Med Coll 1960;2:50–75.

23. Hurst JW. Atlas of the heart. New York, NY: McGraw-Hill: Gower Medical Pub, 1988.

24. Montagna W. Comparative anatomy. New York, NY: Wiley, 1959.

25. Kent GC, Carr RK. Comparative anatomy of the vertebrates. 9th ed. Boston, MA: McGraw Hill, 2001.

26. Truex RC, Warshaw LJ. The incidence and size of the moderator band in man and mammals. Anat Rec 1942;82:361–72.

27. Gerlis LM, Wright HM, Wilson N, et al. Left ventricular bands. A normal anatomical feature. Br Heart J 1984;52:641–7.

28. Walmsley R. Anatomy of human mitral valve in adult cadaver and comparative anatomy of the valve. Br Heart J 1978;40:351–66.

29. Sands MP, Rittenhouse EA, Mohri H, et al. An anatomical comparison of human pig, calf, and sheep aortic valves. Ann Thorac Surg 1969;8:407–14.

30. Ansari A. Anatomy and clinical significance of ventricular Thebesian veins. Clin Anat 2001;14:102–10.

31. Pina JAE, Correia M, O'Neill JG. Morphological study on the Thebesian veins of the right cavities of the heart in the dog. Acta Anat 1975;92:310–20.

32. Ruengsakulrach P, Buxton BF. Anatomic and hemodynamic considerations influencing the efficiency of retrograde cardioplegia. Ann Thorac Surg 2001;71:1389–95.

33. Weaver ME, Pantely GA, Bristow JD, et al. A quantitative study of the anatomy and distribution of coronary arteries in swine in comparison with other animals and man. Cardiovasc Res 1986;20:907–17.

34. Anderson RH, Becker AE. The heart: Structure in health and disease. London, UK; New York, NY: Gower Medical Pub, 1992.

35. Kloner RA, Ganote CE, Reimer KA, et al. Distribution of coronary arterial flow in acute myocardial ischemia. Arch Pathol 1975;99:86–94.

36. Koke JR, Bittar N. Functional role of collateral flow in the ischaemic dog heart. Cardiovasc Res 1978;12:309–15.

37. Redding VJ, Rees JR. Early changes in collateral flow following coronary artery ligation: The role of the sympathetic nervous system. Cardiovasc Res 1968;2:219–25.

38. Weisse AB, Kearney K, Narang RM, et al. Comparison of the coronary collateral circulation in dogs and baboons after coronary occlusion. Am Heart J 1976;92:193–200.

39. Schaper W, Flameng W, De Brabander M. Comparative aspects of coronary collateral circulation. Adv Exp Med Biol 1972;22:267–76.

40. Gregg D, Shipley R. Studies of the venous drainage of the heart. Am J Physiol 1947;151:13–25.

41. Patek PP. The morphology of the lymphatics of the mammalian heart. Am J Anat 1939;64:203–49.

42. Johnson RA, Blake TM. Lymphatics of the heart. Circulation 1966;33:137–42.

43. Symbas PN, Cooper T, Gantner GEJ, et al. Lymphatic drainage of the heart: Effect of experimental interruption of lymphatics. Surg Forum 1963;14:254–6.

44. Anderson RH, Becker AE, Brechenmacher C, et al. The human atrioventricular junctional area. A morphological study of the A-V node and bundle. Eur J Cardiol 1975;3:11–25.

45. Bharati S, Levine M, Huang SK, et al. The conduction system of the swine heart. Chest 1991;100:207–12.

46. Frink RJ, Merrick B. The sheep heart: Coronary and conduction system anatomy with special reference to the presence of an os cordis. Anat Rec 1974;179:189–200.

47. Ho SY, Kilpatrick L, Kanai T, et al. The architecture of the atrioventricular conduction axis in dog compared to man: Its significance to ablation of the atrioventricular nodal approaches. J Cardiovasc Electrophysiol 1995;6:26–39.

48. Hearse DJ, Sutherland FJ. Experimental models for the study of cardiovascular function and disease. Pharmacol Res 2000;41:597–603.

49. Macdonald AA, Johnstone M. Comparative anatomy of the cardiac foramen ovale in cats (Felidae), dogs (Canidae), bears (Ursidae) and hyaenas (Hyaenidae). J Anat 1995;186:235–43.

50. Joudinaud TM, Flecher EM, Duran CM. Functional terminology for the tricuspid valve. J Heart Valve Dis 2006;15:382–8.

51. Anderson RH, Cook AC. The structure and components of the atrial chambers. Europace 2007;9:vi3–9.

52. Lev M, Rowlatt UF, Rimoldi HJ. Pathologic methods for the study of the congenitally malformed heart. AMA Arch Pathol 1961;72:493–511.

53. Rowlatt UF, Rimoldi HJ, Lev M. The quantitative anatomy of the normal child's heart. Pediatr Clin N Am 1963;10:499–588.

54. Eckner FA, Brown BW, Overll E, et al. Alteration of the gross dimensions of the heart and its structures by formalin fixation. A quantitative study. Virchows Arch A Pathol Pathol Anat 1969;346:318–29.

55. Alvarez L, Rodriquez JE, Saucedo R, et al. Swine hearts: Quantitative anatomy of the right ventricle. Anat Histol Embryol 1995;24:25–7.

56. Gorman JH, III, Gorman RC, Jackson BM, et al. Distortions of the mitral valve in acute ischemic mitral regurgitation. Ann Thorac Surg 1997;64:1026–31.

57. Timek TA, Lai DT, Tibayan F, et al. Atrial contraction and mitral annular dynamics during acute left atrial and ventricular ischemia in sheep. Am J Physiol Heart Circ Physiol 2002;283:H1929–35.

58. Tsakiris AG, Padiyar R, Gordon DA, et al. Left atrial size and geometry in the intact dog. Am J Physiol 1977;232:H167–72.

59. Chandraratna PA, Aronow WS. Mitral valve ring in normal vs dilated left ventricle. Cross-sectional echocardiographic study. Chest 1981;79:151–4.

60. Nordblom P, Bech-Hanssen O. Reference values describing the normal mitral valve and the position of the papillary muscles. Echocardiography 2007;24:665–72.

61. Lansac E, Lim HS, Shomura Y, et al. A four-dimensional study of the aortic root dynamics. Eur J Cardiothorac Surg 2002;22:497–503.

62. Sim EK, Muskawad S, Lim CS, et al. Comparison of human and porcine aortic valves. Clin Anat 2003;16:193–6.

63. Swanson M, Clark RE. Dimensions and geometric relationships of the human aortic valve as a function of pressure. Circ Res 1974;35:871–82.

64. Jouan J, Pagel MR, Hiro ME, et al. Further information from a sonometric study of the normal tricuspid valve annulus in sheep: Geometric changes during the cardiac cycle. J Heart Valve Dis 2007;16:511–8.

65. Anwar AM, Geleijnse ML, Soliman OI, et al. Assessment of normal tricuspid valve anatomy in adults by real-time three-dimensional echocardiography. Int J Cardiovasc Imaging 2007;23:717–24.

66. Maric I, Bobinac D, Ostojic L, et al. Tributaries of the human and canine coronary sinus. Acta Anat (Basel) 1996;156:61–9.

Chapter 7
The Coronary Vascular System and Associated Medical Devices

Sara E. Anderson, Ryan Lahm, and Paul A. Iaizzo

Abstract Even as recent as several hundred years ago, the function of the coronary vascular system was largely unknown. Today, it is well established that the coronary system is a highly variable network of both arteries supplying and veins draining the myocardium of oxygenated and deoxygenated blood, respectively. Due to recent advances in technology, the coronary vascular system has been utilized as a therapeutic conduit in a variety of biomedical applications, e.g., cardiac resynchronization therapy. Additionally, symptomatic diseases such as coronary artery disease can be alleviated with stenting or coronary artery bypass grafts. It is well accepted that a comprehensive understanding of the geometric anatomical characteristics of the coronary system will allow for future medical devices to be engineered to successfully deliver novel therapies to a variety of cardiac patients.

Keywords Coronary arteries · Coronary veins · Venous valves · Stents · Transvenous pacing leads

7.1 Introduction

While anatomical studies of the heart began centuries ago, Herophilus (c. 335–c. 280 BC) was the first to observe and record differences between coronary arteries and veins, including the discovery that arteries were much thicker than veins and veins, in contrast to arteries, collapsed when emptied of blood [1]. More than 1,000 years later, in 1628 AD, William Harvey, court physician to King James I and King Charles I, published "On the motion of the heart and blood in animals," the first accurate description of the circulatory system [2].

Subsequently, in 1689, Scaramucci conjectured that the contraction of the heart displaced blood from deeper coronary vessels into coronary veins [3]. However, details of coronary blood flows were not well understood until the technology capable of measuring arterial and venous flows was more recently developed [3].

Today, it is known that the coronary system is comprised of arteries, arterioles, capillaries, and cardiac veins and venules. The coronary arteries originate with right and left main coronary arteries which exit the ascending aorta just above the aortic valve. These two branches subdivide and course over the surface of the heart (epicardium) as they traverse away from the aorta. These arteries arborize into progressively smaller branches that then progress inward to penetrate the epicardium and supply blood to the transmural myocardium. Coronary arteries eventually branch into arterioles; arterioles then branch into innumerable capillaries that deliver oxygenated blood to all of the heart's cells. Blood continues through the capillaries to begin the return back into the cardiac chambers through venules, and then coalesce into the coronary veins. It is the coronary veins that collect deoxygenated blood and return it to the right atrium through the coronary sinus, where it joins the systemic deoxygenated blood entering from the superior and inferior venae cavae. A corrosion cast of a human heart reveals the complexity and extensiveness of the coronary vascular system (Fig. 7.1).

Coronary blood flow is critical in supporting cardiac function. If disease states or acute events occur that obstruct coronary flow, consequences are commonly quite detrimental and/or fatal. For example, changes in electrocardiograms can be recorded within beats when there is inadequate blood flow delivered to a region of the heart. Whenever coronary blood flow falls below what is required to meet metabolic needs, the myocardium is considered ischemic; the pumping capability of the heart is impaired, and there are associated changes in electrical activity (e.g., increased risk of fibrillation). Prolonged ischemia can lead to myocardial infarction, commonly

S.E. Anderson (✉)
University of Minnesota, Departments of Biomedical Engineering and Surgery and Covidien, 5920 Longbow Dr., Boulder, CO 80301, USA
e-mail: sara.e.andersson1@gmail.com

P.A. Iaizzo (ed.), *Handbook of Cardiac Anatomy, Physiology, and Devices*, DOI 10.1007/978-1-60327-372-5_7,
© Springer Science+Business Media, LLC 2009

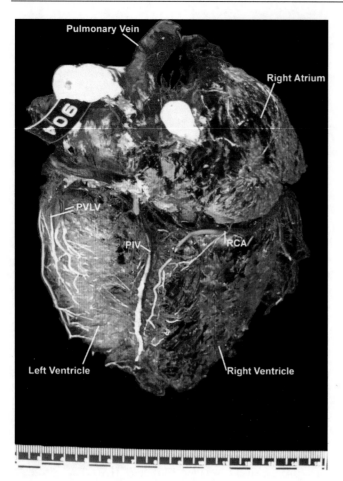

Fig. 7.1 *Red* and *blue* plastics were injected into the arterial and venous systems of this heart, respectively. The rest of the myocardial tissue was "corroded" away with digestive enzymes; thus only the extensive coronary system remains. The heart is viewed from the diaphragmatic surface. It is important to note that this heart represents one example of the coronary system. PIV = posterior interventricular vein; PVLV = posterior veins of the left ventricle; RCA = right coronary artery. Figure courtesy of Alexander Hill (Medtronic, Inc.)

called a heart attack, which can cause irreversible myocardial cell death. Coronary artery disease, which is associated with obstruction of arterial blood flow, is the most common type of heart disease and the leading cause of death in the United States in both males and females [4]. For more details on cardiac oxygen and nutrient delivery and its association with ischemia, refer to Chapter 19.

7.2 Coronary Arteries

7.2.1 Coronary Arteries: Anatomical Description

Oxygenated blood is pumped into the aorta from the left ventricle. Located just above the aortic valve are the ostia of the left and right coronary arteries in the left and right

sinuses of Valsalva, respectively (see Fig. 5.22). The left main coronary artery typically bifurcates into the left anterior descending and left circumflex branches shortly after exiting the aorta [4–6]. The left circumflex artery typically traverses under the left atrial appendage to the lateral wall of the left ventricle. Both the left anterior descending and left circumflex branches decrease in diameter along their lengths [4]. The left coronary artery and its branches supply the majority of oxygenated blood to ventricular myocardium and additionally to the left atrium, left atrial appendage, pulmonary artery, and aortic root [5, 6]. The right coronary artery courses along the right anterior atrioventricular groove below the right atrial appendage, along the epicardial surface adjacent to the tricuspid valve annulus. When the right coronary artery reaches the posterior surface of the heart, it becomes known as the posterior descending artery and runs toward the apex of the left ventricle. Note that the right coronary artery does not typically taper in diameter until it gives rise to the posterior descending artery [4]. In general, coronary arteries traverse the surface of the heart and are encased in varying amounts of epicardial fat. However, some arteries course into myocardium [4]. Numerous clinically relevant arterial branches arise from the right coronary artery, including the conus branch, artery to the sinus node, right superior septal artery, right atrial branches, preventricular branch, anterior ventricular branches, right marginal branch, right atrioventricular node branch, right posterior ventricular branches, posterior interventricular artery, and posterior septal branches. Notably, the right coronary artery branches supply the sinus and atrioventricular nodes; hence, blockage in these vessels can lead to conduction abnormalities. For a more detailed anatomical description of the coronary arteries, see Chapter 5.

7.2.2 Coronary Arteries: Disease

Coronary arterial functional anatomy changes throughout a person's life span; in the elderly, coronary arteries typically become more tortuous, their inner diameters expand, and more calcific deposits can be observed [7]. While these changes are common with aging, certain disease states can significantly increase flow restrictions to the point of causing detrimental damage and/or even death. More specifically, coronary artery disease is generally defined as the gradual narrowing of the lumen of the coronary arteries due to atherosclerosis. An example of an artery with calcifications is shown in Fig. 7.2. Atherosclerosis is a condition that involves thickening of the arterial walls via cholesterol and fat deposits that

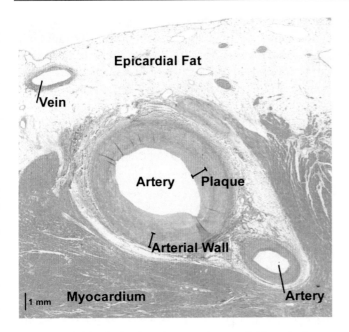

Fig. 7.2 This histologic view of an anterior arterial branch shows a layer of plaque that makes the interior lumen of the artery irregular. Additionally, this figure shows that this particular arterial branch was not completely encased by epicardial fat, but was partially surrounded by myocardium

build up along the endoluminal surface of the arteries. With severe disease, these plaques may become calcified, increase in size, and eventually cause significant stenosis; a stenotic vessel has an increased vascular resistance relative to that of healthy vessels. A steady decrease in arterial cross-sectional area can eventually lead to complete blockage of the artery. As a result, oxygen and nutrient supply to the myocardium decreases below the level of demand. As the disease progresses, the myocardium downstream from the occluded artery becomes ischemic. Eventually, myocardial infarction may occur if the coronary artery disease is not detected and treated in a timely manner. See Chapter 19 for additional description of cardiac ischemia.

Myocardial ischemia not only impairs the electrical and mechanical function of the heart, but also commonly results in intense, debilitating chest pain known as "angina pectoris." Yet, while at rest, anginal pain can often be absent in individuals with coronary artery disease (or in individuals with early disease stages), but induced during physical exertion or with emotional excitement. Such situations are associated with an increase in sympathetic tone that increases myocardial oxygen consumption (and subsequently ischemia) when blood flow cannot keep up with myocardial metabolic needs. To date, typical treatment for angina resulting from coronary artery disease includes initial pharmacological approaches, such as the administration of: (1) coronary vasodilator drugs (e.g., nitroglycerin); (2) nitrates to

reduce myocardial demand by dilating systemic veins and thus reducing preloads; or (3) β-blockers (e.g., propranolol).

7.3 Cardiac Capillaries

Capillaries are the smallest blood vessels in the human body and branch numerous times to ensure that every myocyte lies within a short distance (microns) of at least one of these branches. Via diffusion, nutrients and metabolic end products move between the capillary vessels and the surroundings of the myocytes through the interstitial fluid. Subsequent movement of these molecules into a cell is accomplished by both diffusion and mediated transport. Nevertheless, as with all organs, blood flow through the capillaries within the heart can be considered passive and occurs only because coronary arterial pressure is higher than venous pressure, which is the case in the heart during diastole. Although capillaries are a very important part of the coronary system, their current use for device therapies is relatively nonexistent due to their small diameters (i.e., size of a red blood cell).

7.4 Coronary Veins

Coronary venous flow occurs during diastole and systole, and the coronary venous system drains the myocardium of oxygen-depleted blood.

7.4.1 Coronary Veins: Anatomical Description

The cardiac venous system dominates the arterial system; there are at least twice as many veins as arteries in human myocardial tissue [8, 9]. In general, veins are considered as "low-resistance conduits" to the heart and can alter their capacity to maintain venous pressure [10]. The coronary sinus serves as the primary collector of cardiac venous blood [11–13] and is located in the posterior portion of the coronary sulcus on the diaphragmatic or posterior surface of the heart [6, 14–19]. A movie clip (MPG 7.1) from the Companion CD shows a representative coronary sinus. The coronary sinus empties directly into the right atrium near the conjunction of the posterior interventricular sulcus and the coronary sulcus (crux cordis area) [19–21], located between the inferior vena cava and tricuspid valve [6, 11, 14, 22, 23]. The atrial ostium can be partially covered by a Thebesian valve, although the anatomy of this valve is highly variable [11, 13–17, 19–29]. The coronary sinus receives drainage from most epicardial ventricular veins, including the oblique vein of the left atrium (and other left and right atrial veins), the great cardiac vein, the posterior vein of the left ventricle, the left marginal vein, and the posterior interventricular vein [6, 11, 14, 16, 18, 19, 21, 23–25, 30–33]. The great cardiac vein, the longest venous vessel of the heart, consists of two primary portions—the anterior interventricular vein and its continuation, the great cardiac vein (see Fig. 5.25) [19, 27, 31, 34]. As the great cardiac vein courses from the apex of the heart toward the base of the heart, it is commonly joined by numerous venous contributors from the interventricular septum, anterior aspects of both ventricles, and the apical region [6, 11, 16, 18, 19, 31, 35]. The anterior interventricular vein typically continues toward the base of the heart in the anterior interventricular groove until it reaches the left coronary sulcus, where it becomes the great cardiac vein [11, 16, 19, 20, 24, 31, 34]. As the great cardiac vein courses around the inferior atrioventricular sulcus, it is joined by venous drainage from the left atrium, including the vein of Marshall [16]. At this point, the left obtuse marginal vein and left inferior veins from the left ventricle are also considered to flow toward the great cardiac vein [16, 20]. As the great cardiac vein follows the left atrioventricular groove around the left side of the heart, the great cardiac vein is considered to be in close proximity to the anterolateral commissure of the mitral valve [15]. The great cardiac vein commonly continues until the left inferior portion of the coronary sulcus and finally merges with the coronary sinus [19, 20, 27, 34].

The amalgamation of the great cardiac vein and coronary sinus typically occurs about 15–20 mm inferior to the ostium of the left inferior pulmonary vein [31]. The valve of Vieussens, which covers the ostium of the great cardiac vein as it enters the coronary sinus, typically delineates the beginning of the coronary sinus [31, 36]. The junction of the great cardiac vein and coronary sinus can also be defined by the existence of the vein of Marshall [20]. The great cardiac vein typically enters the coronary sinus at an approximate angle of 180° [31, 36]. The left marginal vein courses the left side of the heart and drains the left ventricular myocardium [19, 31]; it is commonly located in an inferior position at an obtuse angle of the heart [33] and parallels the course of the left marginal branch of the left coronary artery [31]. The posterior vein of the left ventricle is typically a left ventricular venous branch that originates from the lateral and posterior aspects of the left ventricle and courses between the great cardiac vein and posterior interventricular vein [19, 24, 35, 36]. The posterior interventricular vein, commonly

referred to as the middle cardiac vein [19], is a major coronary vein that typically originates near the apex and usually ascends in or very near to the posterior interventricular sulcus [6, 16, 19, 24, 26, 35–37]. The small cardiac vein commonly drains the posterior and lateral wall of the right ventricle. A small vein in comparison to the previously mentioned veins, the small cardiac vein originates in the posterior part of the right coronary sulcus and courses the base of the right ventricle, paralleling the right coronary artery [19].

7.4.1.1 Coronary Veins: Valves

The role of venous valves, in general, is to prevent retrograde blood flow. Such valves in the heart are often present at the ostia to the coronary sinus [11, 13, 14, 16, 17, 19–29], the left marginal vein [27, 30], the posterior vein of the left ventricle [19], and the posterior interventricular vein [16, 19, 20, 38, 39]. A predominant valve can also be identified at the delineation between the coronary sinus and the great cardiac vein [20, 31, 36]. Venous valves within the major left ventricular veins have been observed to be comparable in number of valves per vein except in the left marginal vein, which has fewer valves per vein [40]. These valves are most prevalent at the ostia to smaller contributor veins [40]. An example of a valve covering a venous contributor ostia is shown in Fig. 7.3 and in MPG 7.2 in the Companion CD.

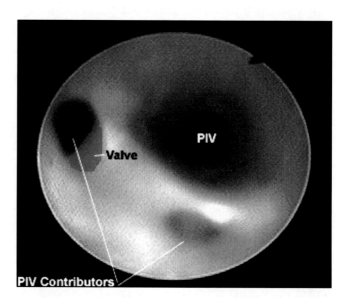

Fig. 7.3 View from the base of the heart toward the apex along the length of the posterior interventricular vein (PIV). Two venous contributors can be seen toward the bottom of the image. The ostia of the contributor to the upper left was partially covered by a venous valve (shown by *highlight*)

7.4.2 Coronary Veins: Disease

Cardiac veins are less likely to develop clinically significant disease states such as atherosclerosis. This is probably due to the inherently lower pressure within the venous portion of coronary circulation and the higher distensibility of the walls of the cardiac veins. When diseases such as heart failure induce myocardial remodeling, the venous system adapts to maintain both blood volume and venous pressure. However, it is generally accepted that the coronary venous system is not affected by atherosclerotic disease, and its "dense meshwork with numerous interconnections" allows blood to return to the heart via numerous pathways [41].

7.5 Microanatomy of Coronary Arteries and Veins

In general, vessels are composed of three layers, which vary in thickness depending on both vessel type and their relative size [42–44]. These layers are the tunica intima, tunica media, and tunica adventitia and can be seen in Fig. 7.4. The tunica intima is comprised of endothelium, subendothelial connective tissue, and an internal elastic lamina [5, 44]. The endothelium of vessels entering the heart is continuous with the heart's endothelium [42]. In veins, the tunica intima and tunica media are less distinct than in arteries, e.g., the venous tunica intima is difficult to distinguish at low power magnification [42]. Concentric layers of smooth muscle, along with collagenic and elastic fibers, make up the tunica media [42–44].

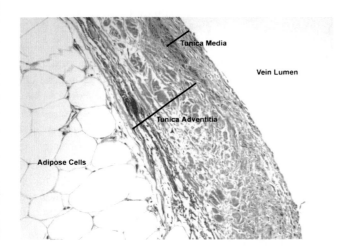

Fig. 7.4 View of coronary venous wall at 20 × magnification. To the left are adipose cells and the far right is the vein lumen. The layers of the tunica adventitia and tunica media comprising the venous wall can be seen. The tunica intima cannot be observed at this magnification

The tunica media for a vein is much smaller than for an artery of similar size, as can be seen in Fig. 7.5 [42, 44]. The tunica adventitia is composed of longitudinally arranged collagen fibers [42–44]. In contrast, the tunica adventitia is much larger in veins than in arteries [42].

7.6 Anastomoses and Collaterals

Connections between arteries that supply or veins that drain the same regions, known as "anastomoses," provide alternate routes for blood to reach (via arteries) or leave (via veins) the same cardiac region. While numerous anastomoses have been observed on the epicardial surface of the heart, even more are considered present within the myocardium [5]. During fetal development, anastomoses are somewhat prominent; after birth, these channels decrease in both size and functionality [5].

In the general population, anterior interventricular and posterior interventricular veins typically have the same origin and termination and follow the same course, while veins between the interventricular sulci are highly variable in number, size, course, and occurrence of anastomoses [19]. In addition, in general, coronary veins have a higher occurrence of anastomoses than coronary arteries [19], resulting in a highly interconnected venous network [6, 9, 41]. More specifically, the apical region of the heart will typically elicit the greatest density of venous anastomoses [45, 46].

Interestingly, in hearts with atherosclerotic damage, small anastomoses develop into larger, more efficient collaterals due to hypertrophic remodeling [5]. Such collaterals may help to protect against ischemia by continuing to allow blood to flow to a given region of the heart when an original arterial route becomes obstructed [21, 46]. Collaterals protect against hypoxia and ischemia by continuing to supply oxygenated blood to a specific region of myocardium [5]. While collaterals increase in size and number with age, whether this increase is related to atherosclerosis is unknown [47, 48]. Nevertheless, large and significant collaterals are often found near an infarcted area, which may indicate a slow remodeling process [21, 49]. However, in severe stages of coronary artery disease, even extensive collaterals will not allow certain regions of the myocardium to be adequately perfused. To treat coronary artery disease patients, either the arterial branch needs to be reopened by coronary angioplasty and/or stenting or a new pathway should be created via coronary artery bypass grafting. If such an obstruction is an acute event, collaterals will not have sufficient time to develop to adequately protect a given heart region from myocardial tissue damage.

Fig. 7.5 This figure shows the relative differences between coronary arteries and veins. To the left is a coronary vein, with a very thin venous wall. Both the tunica media and adventitia can be observed. The tunica intima cannot be observed at this magnification (10×). To the right, the coronary artery is significantly thicker in both the tunica media and adventitia layers. Epicardial fat encases both of these vessels

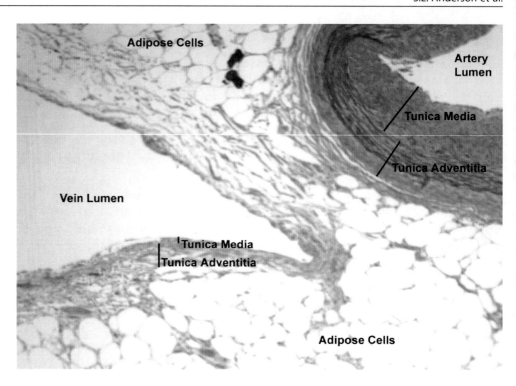

7.7 Assessment and Visualization of the Coronary System

Catheterization of the heart is an invasive but commonly employed procedure for visualization of the heart's coronary arteries, chambers, valves, and/or great vessels. It can also be used to: (1) measure pressures in the heart and blood vessels; (2) assess function, cardiac output, and diastolic properties of the left ventricle; (3) measure the flow of blood through the heart and coronary vessels; (4) determine the regional oxygen content of the blood (e.g., aortic and within the coronary sinus); (5) determine the status of the electrical conduction properties of the heart; and/or (6) assess septal or valvular defects.

Basic catheterization techniques involve inserting a long, flexible, radio-opaque catheter into a peripheral vein (for right heart catheterization) or a peripheral artery (for the left heart) under fluoroscopy (continuous x-ray observation). Commonly, during this invasive procedure, a radio-opaque contrast medium is injected into a cardiac vessel or chamber. The procedure may specifically be used to visualize the anatomical features of the coronary arteries, coronary veins, aorta, pulmonary blood vessels, and/or ventricles. Such investigations may provide pertinent clinical information about structural abnormalities in blood vessels that restrict flow (such as those caused by atherosclerotic plaque), abnormal ventricular blood volumes, inappropriate myocardial wall thicknesses, and/or altered wall motion. A sample venogram from an isolated heart preparation can be seen in MPG 7.3 in the Companion CD; the balloon catheter was

inserted into the coronary sinus to block off antegrade flow, and then contrast was injected retrograde such that the coronary venous tree was more easily observable.

To date, coronary angiography has been the primary visualization modality used clinically. However, multiple contrast injections can potentially be acutely deleterious to patients such as those with compromised cardiac output [50]. Left coronary angiography [50–52] or intracardiac ultrasound [50] can be employed to aid in locating the coronary sinus ostium for coronary venous system procedures. More recently, digital subtraction angiography has been observed to allow examination of venous occlusions and anatomical variants [53].

In the future, improving the quality of cardiac visualization will allow for better planning of implantation and, therefore, decreased patient risk [54]. For example, in coronary artery bypass surgery, planning where sutures should be fixed is essential to avoid suturing to a rigid calcified arterial wall [5]. Several visualization modalities have recently been used and developed to enhance visualization of the coronary system. For instance, prior to lead implantation, tissue Doppler imaging can be utilized to identify the target implant region for a transvenous pacing lead [55, 56]. Additionally, noncontact electrical mapping (see Chapter 29) could be used to identify electrically viable target regions [57].

Several other visualization methodologies are worth mentioning. First, electron beam computed tomographic angiography allows minimally invasive, detailed visualization of the coronary system [58]. Second, multislice computed tomography uses a 4D functional imaging computed tomography scanner to obtain structural and functional features. High-quality, virtual images show details such that transvenous lead implantation, for instance, can be planned to reduce procedure time and patient risk [54]. It is likely that future innovation in imagery technologies, including 4D intracardiac ultrasound, will further increase efficiency of assessing the presence of coronary plaques and stenoses, coronary sinus cannulation, and/or venous paths for subselection.

7.8 Medical Devices and the Coronary System

7.8.1 Devices and the Coronary Arteries

Intricate medical devices are required for performing interventional procedures with the coronary arteries. For example, percutaneous transluminal coronary angioplasty is a procedure during which a balloon catheter is introduced into the narrowed portion of the coronary artery lumen and inflated to reopen the artery to allow the return of normal blood flow. During this procedure, often a coronary stent is also placed such that restenosis of the artery is significantly delayed. A stent is a device comprised of wire mesh that provides scaffolding to support the wall of the artery and keep its lumen open and free from the buildup of plaque. A picture of a balloon angioplasty catheter and a coronary stent is shown in Fig. 7.6.

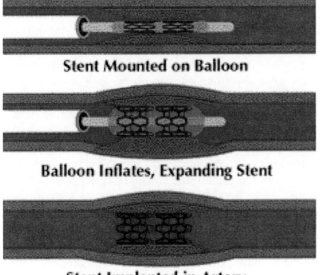

Stent Mounted on Balloon

Balloon Inflates, Expanding Stent

Stent Implanted in Artery

Fig. 7.6 An illustration of the stenting procedure. The balloon catheter with a collapsed stent mounted on it is placed in the artery at the location of narrowing. The balloon is inflated to open the artery and deploy the stent. Finally, the catheter is removed, and the stent is left behind

Balloon angioplasty and coronary stents have prevented numerous patients from having to undergo immediate coronary artery bypass graft surgery, which can be costly and painful. More recently, such stents have been produced with a variety of drug coatings in further attempts to minimize or eliminate the possibility of restenosis. The most common drug used to coat stents is siroliumus (also known as rapamycin). Drugs like sirolimus work by stopping cell growth; they also stop scar tissue from forming within arteries that have been opened. For more details, refer to Chapters 13 and 38.

While these drug-eluting stents have been a great improvement over angioplasty [59], it is generally considered that success rates could be further improved via new techniques. For example, the STAR (subintimal tracking and reentry) technique utilizes a small wire to dissect into the obstruction [60]. Additionally, several novel devices have recently been developed, e.g., radiofrequency signals can warn the user when the wire tip is too close to the vessel wall to prevent perforation, and can also be pulsed to facilitate passage through a coronary artery obstruction [61]. Another catheter design pulses the face of the obstruction to create a path into the obstruction [61]. Finally, the use of proteolytic enzymes has been proposed to digest parts of the obstruction to aid in mechanical passage of a guidewire [61].

7.8.2 Devices and the Coronary Veins

The coronary venous system has been utilized in a variety of ways to enhance cardiac therapies due to the venous system's "dense meshwork with numerous interconnections" and its relative immunity to atherosclerotic disease [41]. For example, local electrograms recorded from the coronary venous system can indicate various arrhythmias and potential ablation target sites for left-sided accessory pathways [13, 62, 63]. Additionally, defibrillation coils implanted within the coronary venous system and, in particular, the posterior interventricular or anterior interventricular veins can lower defibrillation thresholds significantly [64, 65]. The lower thresholds are likely attributable to more efficient transfer of the defibrillation current through the heart [64]. Furthermore, from the coronary venous system, the coronary flow reserve can be determined [13] and coronary perfusion during percutaneous transluminal angioplasty of coronary arteries can be monitored [66].

Because the coronary venous system is not prone to the effects of atherosclerotic disease, it is considered that it may also serve as an effective conduit for drug delivery or as a potential avenue for coronary artery bypass. For example, for decades, the distribution of cardioplegia through the coronary sinus has been proven to be safe and effective in myocardial protection, and even superior to the traditional method of antegrade cardioplegia, especially in patients with coronary artery disease [13, 67]. More recently, since restoration of coronary blood flow prior to an acute myocardial infarction can significantly reduce infarct size and improve myocardial function, the administration of recombinant tissue-type plasminogen through the coronary venous system was shown to result in both shorter recovery times and significant reduction in infarct size when compared to intravenous administration [68]. The coronary venous system also can be employed to deliver cell therapy directly to the myocardium as a potential treatment for heart failure [69]. In one case study, it was demonstrated that a catheter-based system allowed arterialization of a cardiac vein to bypass a totally occluded left anterior descending coronary artery [70].

In the past decade, the coronary venous system has also been used as a pacing lead implant site for biventricular pacing systems or primary left ventricular pacing. More specifically, cardiac resynchronization therapy (CRT) involves simultaneously pacing at least two ventricular sites in order to minimize the required time for total ventricular activation and thus improve cardiac synchrony in certain patients with heart failure eliciting ventricular dyssynchrony [71, 72]. Implantation of pacing leads via the coronary venous system is currently the most popular approach for left ventricular pacing and is accomplished by a transvenous approach [73]. For example, several studies have reported the beneficial results of pacing from the lateral or posterolateral region of the left ventricle [52, 73–76]; either the left marginal vein or posterior vein of the left ventricle are considered optimal implant sites [71, 77]. However, it should be noted that, to date, response rates to CRT are still suboptimal with a typical success rate of around two-thirds [78, 79]. An example of a pacing lead implant in the coronary venous system is shown in MPG 7.4 in the Companion CD. Transvenously placing the pacing lead is considered less invasive and allows for greater patient comfort [80]. For additional information on cardiac pacing, see Chapter 27.

7.8.3 Long-Term Effects of Devices Placed Within Coronary System

Bare metal stents were an improvement over angioplasty, and now it is accepted that drug-eluting stents are an improvement over bare metal stents with respect to patients requiring additional interventional procedures. However, it was recently noted that long-term survival rates of patients were not significantly different in one study comparing these groups [59]. Importantly, it is considered that the possibility of restenosis is perpetual, even with drug-eluting stents.

Only recently have devices been chronically implanted in the coronary venous system. Therefore, the long-term risks of chronically implanted pacing leads in the coronary venous system have not been thoroughly explored, but the potential exists for coronary sinus thrombosis, circumflex artery injury (due to its close proximity to the coronary sinus and great cardiac vein), and/or myocardial injury [52, 81–83].

Lead extraction from the coronary venous system, if required, can be particularly difficult due to thin venous walls [84], but can be necessary in the event of an infection, complication, phrenic nerve stimulation, high pacing threshold, and/or lead dislodgement [85]. To date, the risk of dissecting a vein wall and causing bleeding into the pericardial space remains unknown [84, 85]. Yet it has been suggested that lead designs with isodiametric profiles and reduced or near absent fixation tines may be associated with increased ease of lead extraction [85, 86].

7.9 Notable Engineering Parameters and Design Criteria Associated with the Coronary System

When designing and testing the devices used in the interventional procedures discussed in Section 7.8, a thorough understanding of the geometric parameters of the coronary system is considered as critical. The main purpose of the following text is to summarize, at a basic level, the important anatomical parameters that one needs to consider when designing interventional devices and/or associated delivery procedures related to the coronary system.

From an engineering perspective, the development of any medical device requires knowledge and application of several important parameters; this is especially true for coronary system devices due to the complexity and variations found in the human coronary system. As with any device placed in the human body, a solid understanding of the fundamental anatomical properties of the tissue with which the device interacts is vital to obtain acceptable results regarding: (1) delivery efficacy; (2) long-term device stability; and/or (3) overall performance. These results are important not only chronically, but also for initial device delivery. Although biological reactions to materials placed inside the human body must be understood to guarantee long-term stability and performance of medical devices, the following discussion focuses on the macroscopic physical properties of the coronary vessels.

To simplify the coronary system to its basic structure, each vessel branch can be defined in terms of a flexible cylinder or tube. A tube is a hollow cylindrical structure of a known but variable length, radius, and wall thickness. This means the coronary arterial and venous networks can be represented by a large number of interrelated tubes that supply blood to and receive blood from one another. The parameters described here are those that must be defined to understand fully the geometric and dynamic properties of this tube network so devices may be optimized to interact with them.

7.9.1 Diameter

The most basic parameter that must be known about arteries and veins is their diameter. However, both artery and vein diameters are not constant along their lengths [5, 87–89]. Typically, coronary arteries decrease in diameter along their length [87–89]. Thus, the left main and right coronary arteries generally have the largest diameters of the entire coronary arterial network; these diameters range from 1.5 to 5.5 mm for both vessels, with means of 4.0 and 3.2 mm, respectively [46, 90]. The more bifurcations an artery undergoes, the smaller its diameter will generally become. In the case of the coronary arteries, the vessels located at the very end of the network are the capillaries, which are typically on the order of 5–7 μm in diameter [91]. This diameter is approximately 600 times smaller than that of either the left main or right coronary arteries.

Conversely, veins increase in diameter as they move from their source to their termination. Thus, the largest diameter vessel in the coronary venous network is the coronary sinus, which serves as the primary collector of cardiac venous blood and has a diameter that ranges from 4.5 to 19 mm at its ostium; average diameters of the coronary sinus are 6–10 mm [22, 27, 92, 93]. The difference in diameter from one end of the venous system to the other is roughly a factor of 1,200. However, in diseased states such as heart failure, the ostium tends to increase in diameter [92]. The coronary sinus, although often reported as having a diameter, is usually elliptical (or ovular) in cross section [20, 33] and, therefore, has a major and minor axis dimension rather than a true diameter, as if it had a circular cross section. It is also important to recall that, because arteries and veins are made up of compliant tissue, their diameters change throughout the cardiac cycle because of pressure changes that occur during systole and diastole [94].

The design of coronary stents and balloon angioplasty catheters relies heavily on the diameter of the vessels in which they are meant to reside. If a stent or balloon is designed with too large a diameter, when it is deployed within the artery it may cause a wall strain so great that it could be damaging to the artery. On the other hand, if the design has a diameter that is too small, the device will be ineffective. In the case of the balloon catheter with a diameter that is too small, the lumen will not be opened up enough to cause any significant decrease in the degree of occlusion.

Another device that must be designed with vessel diameter in mind is the left ventricular pacing lead. Because such a lead is designed for placement in a posterolateral tributary of the coronary sinus, it must have a small enough diameter to fit inside the vein, yet have a large enough diameter to stay reliably in its intended location. If such criteria are not met, the leads may not be useful or safe.

7.9.2 Cross-Sectional Profile

Cross-sectional shape profile is another parameter that is closely related to vessel diameter. Cross-sectional shape profile is determined by the shape of the vessel that results after slicing it perpendicular to its centerline. In a hypothetical cylinder, this profile would be a perfect circle. When arteries are diseased and contain significant amounts of atherosclerotic plaque, their cross-sectional profiles can change from roughly circular to various different, and often quite complex, profiles, depending on the amount and orientation of the plaque. To date, coronary venous shape profiles have not been well documented, but they can be considered as noncircular, in general, because of the lower pressures within the vessel as well as the more easily deformable vessel walls in relation to the arteries. In Fig. 7.5, an example of the differences between arterial and venous cross-sectional profiles can be observed.

The design of two devices in particular should be considered in relation to the cross-sectional shape of the coronary vessels—coronary stents and angioplasty catheter balloons. Because coronary arteries are typically circular in cross section, stents are designed also to be circular in their cross section. If a similar device were ever needed for placement in the relatively healthy coronary venous network, a different design would probably be initially considered because the cross-sectional profile of a coronary vein, especially the coronary sinus, is generally noncircular. Angioplasty balloons have also been designed with the consideration that coronary arteries are typically circular in cross section. When inflated, the balloon generates a shape that has a uniform diameter in cross section, which may be consistent with what a healthy coronary artery looks like in cross section.

7.9.3 Ostial Anatomy

Understanding the anatomy of the ostia of each of the three most prominent vessels in the coronary system (right coronary artery, left main coronary artery, and coronary sinus) is especially important when interventional procedures require cannulation of the ostia to perform a specific procedure within the lumen of the vessel. This is true of nearly all procedures done on coronary vessels because they are typically aimed at the lumen of the vessel but, on occasion, one may want to block off or place a flow-through catheter in the ostium.

The ostia of the coronary arteries are generally open with no obstructions except when coronary plaques form; in this case, they can become partially or even fully occluded. When occlusion is not present at the ostial origin of the coronary arteries, there are generally no naturally occurring anatomical structures to impede entrance to the vessels.

The coronary sinus ostium, as discussed in Section 7.4, often has some form of Thebesian valve covering its opening into the right atrium [20, 33]. This valve can take many different forms and morphologies and can cover the coronary sinus ostium to varying degrees [13, 27, 32, 95–98]. When the Thebesian valve is significantly prominent in the manner in which it covers the coronary sinus ostium, cannulation can be much more difficult than in other cases [96, 97].

This consideration is important as it specifically applies to the implantation of pacing leads into the left ventricular coronary veins for CRT. In the process of delivering a lead to the coronary veins, coronary sinus cannulation is of paramount importance because it is currently considered the primary point of entry into the coronary venous network for pacemaker lead introduction for eventual pacing of the left ventricle. Additionally, venous valves are often present at the ostia and within the major left ventricular veins; an example can be seen in Fig. 7.3 [40, 99]. Coronary venous valves, such as the valve of Vieussens, could hinder or help advancement of guidewires, catheters, and pacing leads for a variety of cardiac interventional procedures, especially during subselection of venous branches where a large number of venous valves are observed [40]. To design the optimal catheter or lead delivery procedure, the presence of the Thebesian valve and other venous valves should be fully considered in addition to other anatomical features.

7.9.4 Vessel Length

Each tube that makes up a section of the coronary arterial or venous network is also a branch that arises from a parent vessel. Each of these vessel branches has starting and ending points. Typically, vessel lengths can be measured directly on a specimen after the heart has been extracted. With the advent of 3D medical imaging technologies such as magnetic resonance imaging and computerized tomographic angiography, coronary vessel lengths can be measured in vivo by reconstructing them in space [100–102]. The length of the coronary sinus is often defined from its ostium at the right atrium to the location of the valve of Vieussens or the point where the vein of Marshall intersects it. The length of the coronary sinus varies from 15 to 65 mm [20]. Although there are published data on incidence and qualitative morphology of the tributaries of the coronary sinus [14, 23], their length is generally not addressed.

Because coronary catheterization is both expensive and invasive, knowledge of coronary arterial lengths prior to implanting a stent, for example, can screen patients and lead to reduced procedure times. When percutaneous transluminal coronary angioplasty procedures are performed, it is critical that the physician know the exact location along the length of an artery the occlusion occurs and the relative distance needed from catheter entry to that site. These parameters are often measured using contrast angiography. When contrast is injected and fluoroscopic images are acquired, the location of the occluded arterial region can be quickly identified. An application for which coronary venous length is an important consideration is implantation of left ventricular leads in the posterolateral branches of the coronary sinus. Optimal lead designs should take into account the average length along the coronary sinus of the normal and/or diseased human heart where a candidate posterolateral branch enters. Prior knowledge of this parameter, either in a specific patient or across a population, might improve ease of implant and long-term efficacy of therapy. This information could also be useful in understanding the likelihood of a lead dislodging after initial implantation.

7.9.5 Tortuosity

Since the vessels in the coronary system course along a nonplanar epicardial surface, they are by nature tortuous. Thus, they have varying degrees of curvature along their lengths according to the topography of the epicardial surfaces on which they lie. If vessels were simply

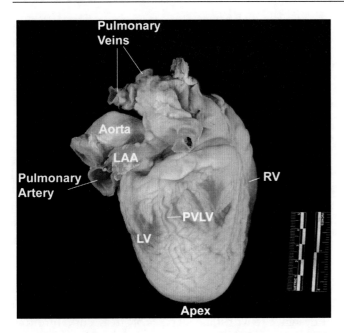

Fig. 7.7 Posterolateral view of a formalin fixed human heart. The posterior vein of the left ventricle (PVLV) has at least four significant curves as seen from this image. There is a modest amount of fat present on the surface of the heart. LAA=left atrial appendage; LV=left ventricle; RV=right ventricle

curvilinear entities such that they traversed in a single plane only, their tortuosities could be much more easily defined. But, in reality, the vessels of the coronary system are not curvilinear, rather, they are 3D curves that twist and turn in more than two dimensions. When the third dimension is added, the tortuosity becomes much more complex; both the curvature of each segment element and the direction of curve orientation must be defined. Figure 7.7 shows an example of a posterior vein of the left ventricle that is highly tortuous.

The levels of tortuosity encountered in the coronary vessels may significantly influence device delivery and chronic performance. When a device such as a catheter or lead must be passed through a tortuous anatomy such as that of the coronary vessels, the greater the curvature and change in curvature over the length of a vessel, the more difficult it will be to pass the device through it due to friction generated at locations where a device contacts tissue. For vessels that more closely resemble a straight line, these devices should pass through more easily.

7.9.6 Wall Thickness

All coronary vessel walls have thickness related to their function as discussed earlier in this chapter. When a device is placed into the coronary system, there is always

a danger of perforation. In general, perforation takes place when a device is inadvertently introduced into the vessel lumen with a level of force and angle of incidence to the vessel wall that causes the device to create a hole in the vessel wall. This situation, although not very common, is not only very dangerous but can be lethal if not dealt with appropriately. Perforation is more often fatal when it happens in arteries as opposed to veins for two reasons: (1) more blood is lost under high pressures in the arteries; and (2) loss of oxygenated blood to the body and the heart itself is more immediately detrimental than if deoxygenated blood were to exit the coronary veins.

Although it is clear that no device is meant to perforate the vessels of the coronary system, each should be developed with the worst-case scenario of perforation in mind, such that the devices will not be problematic for patients or physicians. It should be noted that the wall thickness of the larger coronary arteries, the thickest in the coronary system, is roughly 1 mm [103, 104]. To our knowledge, only one study has defined venous wall thicknesses [87]. In general, anterior and posterior interventricular vein wall thicknesses (0.11–0.17 mm) were significantly larger when compared with the left marginal vein and posterior vein of the left ventricle vein wall thicknesses (0.09–0.13 mm). Vein wall thicknesses in apical regions of all four major left ventricular veins were significantly smaller than those in basal regions; average vein wall thicknesses in apical regions ranged from 0.09 to 0.13 mm, in comparison to 0.11–0.17 mm in basal regions. Examples of relative wall thicknesses for arteries and veins can be seen in Fig. 7.5.

7.9.7 Relationship to Myocardium

The relationship between the coronary vessel and the myocardium is an important parameter to take into consideration when designing certain medical devices. Both coronary arteries and veins exhibit tortuosity on the surface of the heart and sometimes course into the myocardium (see Section 7.2). Additionally, the hearts of "most adults in Western countries contain varying physiological amounts of fat, found mainly in the subepicardial region" [105]. Epicardial fat can represent a significant cardiac component [106–111] and may comprise up to half of the heart's weight, particularly in obese patients that have hypertension and atherosclerotic coronary artery disease [109]. In general, large epicardial fatty deposits are in the atrioventricular sulci and surround the anterior and posterior descending coronary arteries [110–112]; coronary vessels often are displaced off the epicardial surface of the heart and are surrounded by epicardial fat. As can be seen in Figs. 7.4 and 7.5, adipose cells surround both epicardial arteries and veins.

The distance added by epicardial fat could significantly affect medical device efficacy, particularly for transvenous pacing leads. Pacing thresholds for leads implanted in coronary veins have previously been shown to be smaller at distal positions than at more proximal positions [3, 21, 113]. While increases in pacing thresholds toward the base of the heart could be due to larger vein circumferences, a larger amount of epicardial fat present at the base of the heart could also play a role. With increasing rates of obesity, particularly in the United States, epicardial fat must be taken into account when designing devices that depend on close proximity to myocardial tissue.

7.9.8 Branch Angle

As a vessel bifurcates, "daughter" branches are diverted in a different direction from the parent vessel. This creates a situation in which the smaller vessel has a certain branching angle in relation to the direction of the parent vessel. Branching angles can be measured by calculating the angle between the trajectory of the parent vessel and its daughter. An example of this idea is illustrated in Fig. 7.8. Using electron beam computed tomography, branching angles of coronary sinus tributaries are 117±25.3° for the posterior interventricular vein, 88.9±24.0° for the posterior vein of the left ventricle, 85.3±30.0° for the left marginal vein, and 19.2±54.1° for the anterior interventricular vein [114].

The branch angle of a daughter vessel is important since it applies, for example, directly to the situation in which a transvenous pacing lead enters a posterior or lateral branch of the coronary sinus. Thus, the only way to optimize the design of this type of lead and its delivery system, such that it can easily make the turn into a branching vessel, is to know the general severity of the branching angle. The more gradual the turn a lead has to take from a parent vessel to its daughter, the easier it is for an implanter to navigate in general.

7.9.9 Motion Characteristics

Since the vessels of the coronary system are attached directly to the epicardium, it follows that they are not stationary due to the motion of the heart. Along with the simple 3D displacement that occurs over time because of motion, there are other mechanical parameters that are dynamic, such as curvature, stress, and torsion. Each of these fundamental mechanical parameters can have significant effects on devices placed in the lumen of a deforming vessel. Devices such as stents and leads must be designed to withstand all types of stress, curvature, and torsion changes that patients are expected to experience over their lifetimes within an arterial or venous vessel lumen. Additional necessary considerations include: (1) the relative changes in both the 3D path of each vessel and changes in lumen diameter during a given cardiac cycle; and (2) the relative influences associated with alterations in contractility states (e.g., the effects of exercise increasing cardiac output four- to sixfold).

7.10 Summary

Several hundred years ago, the function of the coronary system was unknown. Now, the coronary system is commonly considered as a highly variable network of arteries and veins supplying and draining the myocardium of oxygenated and deoxygenated blood, respectively. Due to advances in technology, the coronary system has been

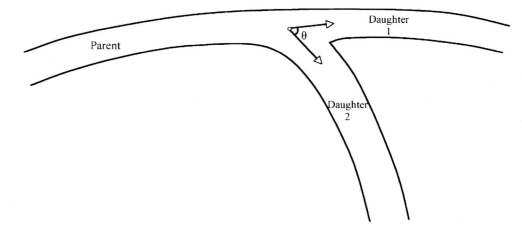

Fig. 7.8 Diagram of the branching angle between a parent vessel and its daughter. Angle θ represents the branching angle generated between the parent vessel and daughter 2

utilized in a variety of biomedical applications, including CRT. Additionally, symptomatic diseases such as coronary artery disease can be alleviated with stenting or coronary artery bypass grafts. An understanding of the structural and geometric anatomical characteristics of the coronary system will allow for future medical devices to be engineered to successfully deliver therapies to a variety of patients.

References

1. Harris CRS. The heart and the vascular system in ancient Greek medicine; from Alcmaeon to Galen. Oxford: Clarendon Press, 1973.
2. Phillips RE, Jr. The heart and circulatory system. Access Excellence at the National Health Museum. http://www.accessexcellence.org/AE/AEC/CC/heart_background.php. Access: 5/5/08.
3. Kajiya F, Kimura A, Hiramatsu O, Ogasawara Y, Tsujioka K. Coronary venous flow. In: Hirakawa S, Rothe CF, Shoukas AA, Tyberg JV, eds. Veins: Their functional role in the circulation. Tokyo: Springer-Verlag, 1993.
4. Alexander RW, Schlant RC, Fuster V, O'Rourke RA, Roberts R, Sonnenblick EH, eds. Hurst's the heart. New York, NY: McGraw-Hill, 1999.
5. von Ludinghausen M. The clinical anatomy of coronary arteries. Adv Anat Embryol Cell Biol 2003;167:III–VIII, 1–111.
6. Williams PL, Bannister LH, Berry MM, et al., eds. Gray's anatomy. London: Churchill Livingston, 1995.
7. Vlodaver Z, Edwards JE. Pathology of coronary atherosclerosis. Prog Cardiovasc Dis 1971;14:256–74.
8. Hutchins GM, Moore GW, Hatton EV. Arterial-venous relationships in the human left ventricular myocardium: Anatomic basis for countercurrent regulation of blood flow. Circulation 1986;74:1195–202.
9. Truex RC, Angulo AW. Comparative study of the arterial and venous systems of the ventricular myocardium with special reference to the coronary sinus. Anat Rec 1952;113:467–91.
10. Widmaier EP, Raff, H, Strang KT, eds. Vander, Sherman, & Luciano's human physiology: The mechanisms of body function. 9th ed. Boston: McGraw-Hill, 2004.
11. Giudici M, Winston S, Kappler J, et al. Mapping the coronary sinus and great cardiac vein. Pacing Clin Electrophysiol 2002; 25:414–9.
12. Hood WB, Jr. Regional venous drainage of the human heart. Br Heart J 1968;30:105–9.
13. Silver MA, Rowley NE. The functional anatomy of the human coronary sinus. Am Heart J 1988;115:1080–4.
14. Adatia I, Gittenberger-de Groot AC. Unroofed coronary sinus and coronary sinus orifice atresia: Implications for management of complex congenital heart disease. J Am Coll Cardiol 1995;25:948–53.
15. El-Maasarany S, Ferrett CG, Firth A, Sheppard M, Henein MY. The coronary sinus conduit function: Anatomical study (relationship to adjacent structures). Europace 2005; 7:475–81.
16. Ho SY, Sanchez-Quintana D, Becker AE. A review of the coronary venous system: A road less traveled. Heart Rhythm 2004;1:107–12.
17. Malhotra VK, Tewari SP, Tewari PS, Agarwal SK. Coronary sinus and its tributaries. Anat Anz 1980;148:331–2.
18. Ratajczyk-Pakalaska E. The coronary venous anatomy. In: Meerbaum S, ed. Myocardial perfusion, reperfusion, coronary venous retroperfusion. New York: Springer, 1990:51–92.
19. von Ludinghausen M. The venous drainage of the human myocardium. Adv Anat Embryol Cell Biol 2003;168:I–VIII, 1–104.
20. Singh JP, Houser S, Heist EK, Ruskin JN. The coronary venous anatomy: A segmental approach to aid cardiac resynchronization therapy. J Am Coll Cardiol 2005;46:68–74.
21. Vlodaver DP, Amplatz MH, Burchell MH, Edwards MB. Coronary heart disease, clinical, angiographic, and pathologic profiles. New York: Springer, 1976.
22. Maric I, Bobinac D, Ostojic L, Petkovic M, Dujmovic M. Tributaries of the human and canine coronary sinus. Acta Anat (Basel) 1996;156:61–9.
23. Roberts JT. Arteries, veins, and lymphatic vessels of the heart. In: Luisada AA, ed. Development and structure of the cardiovascular system. New York: McGraw-Hill, 1958:85–118.
24. Kawashima T, Sato K, Sato F, Sasaki H. An anatomical study of the human cardiac veins with special reference to the drainage of the great cardiac vein. Ann Anat 2003;185:535–42.
25. Maros TN, Racz L, Plugor S, Maros TG. Contributions to the morphology of the human coronary sinus. Anat Anz 1983;154:133–44.
26. McAlpine WA. Heart and coronary arteries: An anatomical atlas for clinical diagnosis, radiological investigation, and surgical treatment. Berlin; New York: Springer-Verlag, 1975.
27. Ortale JR, Gabriel EA, Iost C, Marquez CQ. The anatomy of the coronary sinus and its tributaries. Surg Radiol Anat 2001;23:15–21.
28. Sun Y, Arruda M, Otomo K, et al. Coronary sinus-ventricular accessory connections producing posteroseptal and left posterior accessory pathways: Incidence and electrophysiological identification. Circulation 2002;106:1362–7.
29. Von Ludinghausen M. Microanatomy of the human coronary sinus and its major tributaries. In: Meerbaum S, ed. Myocardial perfusion, reperfusion, coronary venous reperfusion. Darmstadt: Steinkopff Verlag, 1990:93–122.
30. Mochizuki S. Vv. cordis. In: Adachi B, ed. Das venensystem der Japaner. Kioto: Kenkyusha, 1933:41–64.
31. Pejkovic B, Bogdanovic D. The great cardiac vein. Surg Radiol Anat 1992;14:23–8.
32. Piffer CR, Piffer MI, Zorzetto NL. Anatomic data of the human coronary sinus. Anat Anz 1990;170:21–9.
33. Schaffler GJ, Groell R, Peichel KH, Rienmuller R. Imaging the coronary venous drainage system using electron-beam CT. Surg Radiol Anat 2000;22:35–9.
34. Bales GS. Great cardiac vein variations. Clin Anat 2004;17:436–43.
35. Gerber TC, Sheedy PF, Bell MR, et al. Evaluation of the coronary venous system using electron beam computed tomography. Int J Cardiovasc Imaging 2001;17:65–75.
36. Gilard M, Mansourati J, Etienne Y, et al. Angiographic anatomy of the coronary sinus and its tributaries. Pacing Clin Electrophysiol 1998;21:2280–4.
37. Schumacher B, Tebbenjohanns J, Pfeiffer D, Omran H, Jung W, Luderitz B. Prospective study of retrograde coronary venography in patients with posteroseptal and left-sided accessory atrioventricular pathways. Am Heart J 1995;130:1031–9.
38. Bergman RA, Thompson SA, Saadeh FA. Absence of the coronary sinus. Anat Anz 1988;166:9–12.
39. Parsonnet V. The anatomy of the veins of the human heart with special reference to normal anastomotic channels. J Med Soc N J 1953;50:446–52.
40. Anderson SE, Quill JL, Iaizzo PA. Venous valves within left ventricular coronary veins. J Interv Card Electrophysiol 2008 Nov; 23(2):95–9.
41. Mohl W. Basic considerations and techniques in coronary sinus interventions. In: Mohl W, ed. Coronary sinus interventions in cardiac surgery. Austin: R.G. Landes Company, 1994:1–10.

42. Histology of the Blood Vessels: http://www.courseweb/uottawa.ca/medicine-histology/English/Cardiovascular/HistologyBloodVessels.htm

43. Junqueira LC, Carneiro J, Kelley RO. Basic histology. Stamford, Connecticut: Appleton & Lange, 1998.

44. Kessel RG. Basic medical histology: The biology of cells, tissues, and organs. New York: Oxford University Press, 1998.

45. von Ludinghausen M. Clinical anatomy of cardiac veins, Vv. cardiacae. Surg Radiol Anat 1987;9:159–68.

46. Baroldi G, Mantero O, Scomazzoni G. The collaterals of the coronary arteries in normal and pathologic hearts. Circ Res 1956;4:223–9.

47. Kitzman DW, Edwards WD. Age-related changes in the anatomy of the normal human heart. J Gerontol 1990;45:M33–9.

48. Moberg A. Anatomical and functional aspects of extracardial anastomoses to the coronary arteries. Pathol Microbiol (Basel) 1967;30:689–94.

49. Waller BF, Schlant RC. Anatomy of the heart. In: Schlant RC, Alexander RW, eds. Hurst's the heart. 8th ed. New York: McGraw-Hill, 1994:59–112.

50. Leon AR. Cardiac resynchronization therapy devices: Patient management and follow-up strategies. Rev Cardiovasc Med 2003;4 Suppl 2:S38–46.

51. Macias A, Gavira JJ, Alegria E, Azcarate PM, Barba J, Garcia-Bolao I. Effect of the left ventricular pacing site on echocardiographic parameters of ventricular dyssynchrony in patients receiving cardiac resynchronization therapy. Rev Esp Cardiol 2004;57:138–45.

52. Walker S, Levy T, Rex S, Brant S, Paul V. Initial United Kingdom experience with the use of permanent, biventricular pacemakers: Implantation procedure and technical considerations. Europace 2000;2:233–9.

53. Oginosawa Y, Abe H, Nakashima Y. Prevalence of venous anatomic variants and occlusion among patients undergoing implantation of transvenous leads. Pacing Clin Electrophysiol 2005;28:425–8.

54. Coatrieux JL, Hernandez AI, Mabo P, Garreau M, Haigron P. Transvenous path finding in cardiac resynchronization therapy. Functional Imaging and Modeling of Heart, Proceedings, 2005:236–45.

55. Ansalone G, Giannantoni P, Ricci R, Trambaiolo P, Fedele F, Santini M. Doppler myocardial imaging to evaluate the effectiveness of pacing sites in patients receiving biventricular pacing. J Am Coll Cardiol 2002;39:489–99.

56. Cazeau S, Leclercq C, Lavergne T, et al. Effects of multisite biventricular pacing in patients with heart failure and intraventricular conduction delay. N Engl J Med 2001;344:873–80.

57. Lambiase PD, Rinaldi A, Hauck J, et al. Non-contact left ventricular endocardial mapping in cardiac resynchronisation therapy. Heart 2004;90:44–51.

58. Shinbane JS, Girsky MJ, Mao S, Budoff MJ. Thebesian valve imaging with electron beam CT angiography: Implications for resynchronization therapy. Pacing Clin Electrophysiol 2004;27:1566–7.

59. Prasad A, Rihal CS, Lennon RJ, Wiste HJ, Singh M, Holmes DR, Jr. Trends in outcomes after percutaneous coronary intervention for chronic total occlusions: A 25-year experience from the Mayo Clinic. J Am Coll Cardiol 2007;49:1611–8.

60. Colombo A, Mikhail GW, Michev I, et al. Treating chronic total occlusions using subintimal tracking and reentry: The STAR technique. Catheter Cardiovasc Interv 2005;64:407–11; discussion 412.

61. Weisz G, Moses JW. New percutaneous approaches for chronic total occlusion of coronary arteries. Expert Rev Cardiovasc Ther 2007;5:231–41.

62. Cappato R, Schluter M, Weiss C, Willems S, Meinertz T, Kuck KH. Mapping of the coronary sinus and great cardiac vein using a 2-French electrode catheter and a right femoral approach. J Cardiovasc Electrophysiol 1997;8:371–6.

63. Stellbrink C, Diem B, Schauerte P, Ziegert K, Hanrath P. Transcoronary venous radiofrequency catheter ablation of ventricular tachycardia. J Cardiovasc Electrophysiol 1997;8:916–21.

64. Dosdall DJ, Rothe DE, Brandon TA, Sweeney JD. Effect of rapid biphasic shock subpulse switching on ventricular defibrillation thresholds. J Cardiovasc Electrophysiol 2004;15:802–8.

65. Huang J, Walcott GP, Killingsworth CR, Smith WM, Kenknight BH, Ideker RE. Effect of electrode location in great cardiac vein on the ventricular defibrillation threshold. Pacing Clin Electrophysiol 2002;25:42–8.

66. Nitsch J. Continuous monitoring of coronary perfusion during percutaneous transluminal coronary angioplasty of the left anterior descending artery. J Intervent Cardiol 1989;2:205–10.

67. Gundry SR. A comparison of retrograde cardioplegia versus antegrade cardioplegia in the presence of coronary artery obstruction. 66th Annual Scientific Sessions of the American Heart Association. Dallas, TX, 1982.

68. Miyazaki A, Tadokoro H, Drury JK, Ryden L, Haendchen RV, Corday E. Retrograde coronary venous administration of recombinant tissue-type plasminogen activator: A unique and effective approach to coronary artery thrombolysis. J Am Coll Cardiol 1991;18:613–20.

69. Thompson CA, Nasseri BA, Makower J, et al. Percutaneous transvenous cellular cardiomyoplasty. A novel nonsurgical approach for myocardial cell transplantation. J Am Coll Cardiol 2003;41:1964–71.

70. Oesterle SN, Reifart N, Hauptmann E, Hayase M, Yeung AC. Percutaneous in situ coronary venous arterialization: Report of the first human catheter-based coronary artery bypass. Circulation 2001;103:2539–43.

71. Barold SS. What is cardiac resynchronization therapy? Am J Med 2001;111:224–32.

72. Casey C, Knight BP. Cardiac resynchronization pacing therapy. Cardiology 2004;101:72–8.

73. Daubert JC, Ritter P, Le Breton H, et al. Permanent left ventricular pacing with transvenous leads inserted into the coronary veins. Pacing Clin Electrophysiol 1998;21:239–45.

74. Gasparini M, Mantica M, Galimberti P, et al. Is the left ventricular lateral wall the best lead implantation site for cardiac resynchronization therapy? Pacing Clin Electrophysiol 2003;26:162–8.

75. Stevenson WG, Sweeney MO. Single site left ventricular pacing for cardiac resynchronization. Circulation 2004;109:1694–6.

76. Valls-Bertault V, Mansourati J, Gilard M, Etienne Y, Munier S, Blanc JJ. Adverse events with transvenous left ventricular pacing in patients with severe heart failure: Early experience from a single centre. Europace 2001;3:60–3.

77. Alonso C, Leclercq C, d'Allonnes FR, et al. Six year experience of transvenous left ventricular lead implantation for permanent biventricular pacing in patients with advanced heart failure: Technical aspects. Heart 2001;86:405–10.

78. Conti CR. Cardiac resynchronization therapy for chronic heart failure: Why does it not always work? Clin Cardiol 2006;29:335–6.

79. Yu CM, Wing-Hong Fung J, Zhang Q, Sanderson JE. Understanding nonresponders of cardiac resynchronization therapy—current and future perspectives. J Cardiovasc Electrophysiol 2005;16:1117–24.

80. Mair H, Sachweh J, Meuris B, et al. Surgical epicardial left ventricular lead versus coronary sinus lead placement in biventricular pacing. Eur J Cardiothorac Surg 2005;27:235–42.

81. Ellery SM, Paul VE. Complications of biventricular pacing. Eur Heart J Suppl 2004;6:D117–21.

82. Sack S, Heinzel F, Dagres N, et al. Stimulation of the left ventricle through the coronary sinus with a newly developed 'over the wire' lead system—early experiences with lead handling and positioning. Europace 2001;3:317–23.

83. Sharifi M, Sorkin R, Sharifi V, Lakier JB. Inadvertent malposition of a transvenous-inserted pacing lead in the left ventricular chamber. Am J Cardiol 1995;76:92–5.

84. Tacker WA, Vanvleet JF, Schoenlein WE, Janas W, Ayers GM, Byrd CL. Post-mortem changes after lead extraction from the ovine coronary sinus and great cardiac vein. Pacing Clin Electrophysiol 1998;21:296–8.

85. De Martino G, Orazi S, Bisignani G, et al. Safety and feasibility of coronary sinus left ventricular leads extraction: A preliminary report. J Interv Card Electrophysiol 2005;13:35–8.

86. Bulava A, Lukl J. Postmortem anatomy of the coronary sinus pacing lead. Pacing Clin Electrophysiol 2005;28:736–9.

87. Anderson SE, Hill AJ, Iaizzo PA. Microanatomy of human left ventricular coronary veins. Anat Rec 2009 Jan; 292(1):23–8.

88. Dodge JT, Jr., Brown BG, Bolson EL, Dodge HT. Lumen diameter of normal human coronary arteries. Influence of age, sex, anatomic variation, and left ventricular hypertrophy or dilation. Circulation 1992;86:232–46.

89. Zubaid M, Buller C, Mancini GB. Normal angiographic tapering of the coronary arteries. Can J Cardiol 2002;18:973–80.

90. Angelini P. Normal and anomalous coronary arteries: Definitions and classification. Am Heart J 1989;117:418–34.

91. Ono T, Shimohara Y, Okada K, Irino S. Scanning electron microscopic studies on microvascular architecture of human coronary vessels by corrosion casts: Normal and focal necrosis. Scand Electron Microsc 1986:263–70.

92. Hellerstein HK, Orbison JL. Anatomic variations of the orifice of the human coronary sinus. Circulation 1951;3:514–23.

93. Potkin BN, Roberts WC. Size of coronary sinus at necropsy in subjects without cardiac disease and in patients with various cardiac conditions. Am J Cardiol 1987;60:1418–21.

94. Ge J, Erbel R, Gerber T, et al. Intravascular ultrasound imaging of angiographically normal coronary arteries: A prospective study in vivo. Br Heart J 1994;71:572–8.

95. Felle P, Bannigan JG. Anatomy of the valve of the coronary sinus (Thebesian valve). Clin Anat 1994;7:10–2.

96. Hill AJ, Ahlberg SE, Wilkoff BL, Iaizzo PA. Dynamic obstruction to coronary sinus access: The Thebesian Valve. Heart Rhythm 2006;3:1240–1.

97. Hill AJ, Coles JA, Jr., Sigg DC, Laske TG, Iaizzo PA. Images of the human coronary sinus ostium obtained from isolated working hearts. Ann Thorac Surg 2003;76:2108.

98. Jatene M, Jatene F, Costa R, Romero S, Monteiro R, Jatene A. Anatomical study of the coronary sinus valve—Thebesius valve. Chest 1991;100 (Suppl):90S.

99. Anderson SE, Hill AJ, Iaizzo PA. Venous valves: Unseen obstructions to coronary access. J Interv Card Electrophysiol 2007;19:165–6.

100. Achenbach S, Kessler W, Moshage WE, et al. Visualization of the coronary arteries in three-dimensional reconstructions using respiratory gated magnetic resonance imaging. Coron Artery Dis 1997;8:441–8.

101. Achenbach S, Ulzheimer S, Baum U, et al. Noninvasive coronary angiography by retrospectively ECG-gated multislice spiral CT. Circulation 2000;102:2823–8.

102. Li D, Kaushikkar S, Haacke EM, et al. Coronary arteries: Three-dimensional MR imaging with retrospective respiratory gating. Radiology 1996;201:857–63.

103. Gradus-Pizlo I, Feigenbaum H. Imaging of the left anterior descending coronary artery by high-frequency transthoracic and epicardial echocardiography. Am J Cardiol 2002;90:28L–31L.

104. Kim WY, Stuber M, Bornert P, Kissinger KV, Manning WJ, Botnar RM. Three-dimensional black-blood cardiac magnetic resonance coronary vessel wall imaging detects positive arterial remodeling in patients with nonsignificant coronary artery disease. Circulation 2002;106:296–9.

105. Basso C, Thiene G. Adipositas cordis, fatty infiltration of the right ventricle, and arrhythmogenic right ventricular cardiomyopathy. Just a matter of fat? Cardiovasc Pathol 2005; 14:37–41.

106. Corradi D, Maestri R, Callegari S, et al. The ventricular epicardial fat is related to the myocardial mass in normal, ischemic and hypertrophic hearts. Cardiovasc Pathol 2004; 13:313–6.

107. Hangartner JR, Marley NJ, Whitehead A, Thomas AC, Davies MJ. The assessment of cardiac hypertrophy at autopsy. Histopathology 1985;9:1295–306.

108. Reiner L, Mazzoleni A, Rodriguez FL, Freudenthal RR. The weight of the human heart. I. Normal cases. AMA Arch Pathol 1959;68:58–73.

109. Shirani J, Berezowski K, Roberts WC. Quantitative measurement of normal and excessive (cor adiposum) subepicardial adipose tissue, its clinical significance, and its effect on electrocardiographic QRS voltage. Am J Cardiol 1995;76:414–8.

110. Shirani J, Roberts WC. Clinical, electrocardiographic and morphologic features of massive fatty deposits ("lipomatous hypertrophy") in the atrial septum. J Am Coll Cardiol 1993;22:226–38.

111. Sons HU, Hoffmann V. Epicardial fat cell size, fat distribution and fat infiltration of the right and left ventricle of the heart. Anat Anz 1986;161:355–73.

112. Rokey R, Mulvagh SL, Cheirif J, Mattox KL, Johnston DL. Lipomatous encasement and compression of the heart: Antemortem diagnosis by cardiac nuclear magnetic resonance imaging and catheterization. Am Heart J 1989;117:952–3.

113. Anderson SE, Iaizzo PA. Effect of pacing lead positions and venous microanatomy on pacing parameters. Submitted to Heart, February 2009.

114. Mao S, Shinbane JS, Girsky MJ, et al. Coronary venous imaging with electron beam computed tomographic angiography: Three-dimensional mapping and relationship with coronary arteries. Am Heart J 2005;150:315–22.

Chapter 8
The Pericardium

Eric S. Richardson, Alexander J. Hill, Nicholas D. Skadsberg, Michael Ujhelyi, Yong-Fu Xiao, and Paul A. Iaizzo

Abstract The pericardium is a unique structure that surrounds the heart and serves several important physiological roles; the removal of the pericardium, certain pericardial disorders, or the build-up of fluids within this space will ultimately alter hemodynamic performance. Recent therapeutic approaches have been directed to exploit the space that exists between the pericardium and the epicardial surface of the heart. New devices and techniques are being developed to access this space in a minimally invasive fashion. The pharmacokinetics of many drugs may be greatly enhanced if the drug is delivered into the pericardium. As more is learned about the pericardium, it may play a more significant role in cardiac therapies.

Keywords Pericardium · Pericardial fluid · Mechanical effects · Pericardial disorders · Comparative anatomy · Intrapericardial therapeutics

8.1 Introduction

The pericardium is a fibro-serous conical sac structure encasing the heart and roots of the great cardiac vessels. In humans, it is located within the mediastinal cavity posterior to the sternum and cartilage of the 3rd through 7th ribs of the left thorax and is separated from the anterior wall of the thorax. It is encompassed from the posterior resting against the bronchi, the esophagus, the descending thoracic aorta, and the posterior regions of the mediastinal surface of each lung. Laterally, the pericardium is covered by the pleurae and lies along the mediastinal surfaces of the lung. It can come into direct contact with the chest wall near the ventricular apical region, but this varies with the dimensions of the long axis of the heart or with various disease states. Under normal circumstances, the pericardium separates and isolates the heart from contact by the surrounding tissues, allowing freedom of cardiac movement within the confines of the pericardial space (Fig. 8.1).

8.2 Anatomy

In humans, the 1–3 mm thick fibrous pericardium is commonly described as a "flask-shaped bag." The neck of the pericardium (superior aspect) is closed by its extensions surrounding the great cardiac vessels, while the base is attached to the central tendon and to the muscular fibers of the left side of the diaphragm (Fig. 8.2). Much of the pericardium's diaphragmatic attachment consists of loose fibrous tissue that can be readily separated and/or isolated, but there is a small area over the central tendon where the diaphragm and the pericardium are completely fused.

Examination of the pericardium reveals that it is comprised of two interconnected structures, the serous pericardium and the fibrous pericardium. The serous pericardium is one continuous sac with a large in-fold that contains the heart (Fig. 8.3). An appropriate analogy would be a fist (representing the heart) pushed into the side of a deflated balloon (representing the serous pericardium), therefore enveloped by two individual layers of material. The interior surface of the pericardium is intimately connected to the surface of the heart and is known as the "visceral pericardium," or the "epicardium." The exterior surface of the serous pericardium is known as the "parietal pericardium" and is fused with the thick lining of the fibrous pericardium. The pericardial space, where the pericardial fluid resides, is bounded on either side by the parietal and visceral pericardium. To the naked eye, however, the visceral pericardium cannot be distinguished

E.S. Richardson (✉)
University of Minnesota, Departments of Biomedical Engineering and Surgery, B172 Mayo, MMC 195, 420 Delaware St. SE Minneapolis, MN 55455, USA
e-mail: richa483@umn.edu

P.A. Iaizzo (ed.), *Handbook of Cardiac Anatomy, Physiology, and Devices*, DOI 10.1007/978-1-60327-372-5_8,
© Springer Science+Business Media, LLC 2009

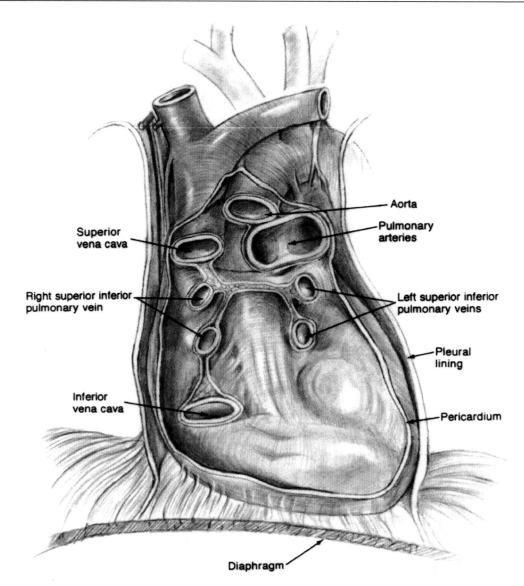

Fig. 8.1 Shown is the posterior view of the pericardial sac, with the anterior surface and heart cut away. One can see that the great vessels of the heart penetrate through the pericardium, which extends up these vessels for several centimeters

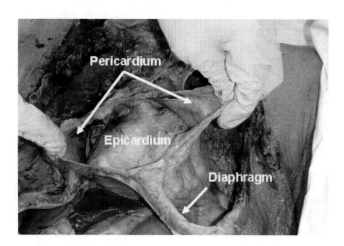

Fig. 8.2 The fibrous pericardium of a fresh human cadaver is opened to expose the epicardium of the heart. Note the attachment of the pericardium to the diaphragm

from the epicardial surface of the heart, and the parietal pericardium cannot be distinguished from the fibrous pericardium. For this reason, the general use of the term "pericardium" refers to the composite of the parietal and fibrous pericardium, which appears to be a single sac that surrounds the heart. Yet, more accurately, the pericardium should be described as three total layers, with fluid lining between two of them (Fig. 8.3).

The inferior vena cava enters the pericardium through the central tendon of the diaphragm where there exists a small area of fusion between the pericardium and the central tendon, but it receives no covering from this fibrous layer. Between the left pulmonary artery and subjacent pulmonary vein is a triangular fold of the serous pericardium known as the "ligament of the left vena cava" (vestigial fold of Marshall). It is formed by a serous layer over the remnant of the lower part of the left superior

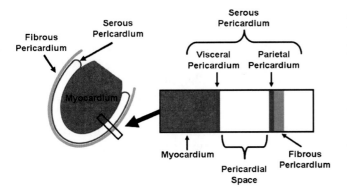

Fig. 8.3 On the *left*, a schematic diagram of the serous and fibrous pericardium is shown with respect to the heart. On the *right*, an expanded cross-section view shows the attachment of two layers of the serous pericardium (visceral and parietal) to the myocardium and fibrous pericardium, respectively

vena cava (duct of Cuvier) which regresses during fetal life, but remains as a fibrous band stretching from the highest left intercostal vein to the left atrium, where it aligns with a small vein known as the "vein of the left atrium" (oblique vein of Marshall), eventually opening into the coronary sinus. The pericardium is also attached to the posterior-sternal surface by superior and inferior sternopericardial ligaments that securely anchor the pericardium and also act to maintain the orientation of the heart inside the thorax.

As previously mentioned, the serous pericardium is a closed sac that lines the fibrous pericardium consisting of a visceral and a parietal portion. The visceral portion that covers the heart and great vessels is commonly referred to as the "epicardium" and is continuous with the parietal layer that lines the fibrous pericardium. The parietal portion covering the remaining vessels is arranged in the form of two tubes. The aorta and pulmonary artery are enclosed in one tube (the "arterial mesocardium"), while the superior and inferior venae cavae and the four pulmonary veins are enclosed in the second tube (the "venous mesocardium") (see JPG 8.1 in the Companion CD). There is an attachment to the parietal layer between the two branches, behind the left atrium, commonly referred to as the "oblique sinus." There is also a passage between the venous and arterial mesocardia (i.e., between the aorta and pulmonary artery in front and the atria behind) that is termed the "transverse sinus." The "superior sinus or superior aortic recess" extends upward along the right side of the ascending aorta to the origination point of the innominate artery. The superior sinus also joins the transverse sinus behind the aorta, and they are both continually fused until they reach the aortic root. For additional text describing this anatomy, also see Chapter 5.

The arteries of the pericardium are derived from the internal mammary and its musculophrenic branch, and

also from the descending thoracic aorta. The nerves innervating the pericardium are derived from the vagus and phrenic nerves, as well as the sympathetic trunks.

8.3 Physiology of the Normal Pericardium

8.3.1 Pericardial Fluid

In normal hearts, the pericardium should be considered as only a potential space. It contains 20–60 ml of pericardial fluid, most of which resides in the major pericardial sinuses and the atrioventricular grooves [1]. The fluid is an ultrafiltrate of plasma and therefore has many similarities to plasma in its electrolyte composition; pericardial fluid, however, contains about half the total protein concentration, one-third the triglyceride and cholesterol content, and one-fifth the amount of white blood cells [2]. A more complete comparison of plasma and pericardial fluid composition is shown in Table 8.1.

The details of the formation, clearance, and turnover of pericardial fluid have not yet been fully explained. Yet it is generally agreed that pericardial fluid is derived from plasma leakage from myocardial capillaries [3], and this filtrate is eventually drained by the lymphatic system. During situations of high pericardial fluid pressure, such as in cardiac tamponade, investigators have found that fluid may pass through the pericardium and enter the pleural space [4]. The turnover time of pericardial fluid in humans has not been established, but in sheep it is observed to be every 5.4 h [5].

As mentioned previously, pericardial fluid distribution is not uniform. The majority of the fluid, found in the major sinuses and grooves of the heart, makes up the pericardial reserve volume. Yet the fluid is considered to be well mixed due to the motion of the heart, and agents injected into the pericardial space quickly and evenly

Table 8.1 Normal plasma composition compared to the pericardial fluid composition of 30 patients undergoing cardiac surgery

	Normal plasma range	Pericardial fluid mean value	Mean fluid:serum ratio
Total protein (g/dl)	6.5–8.2	3.3	0.6
Albumin (g/dl)	3.6–5.5	2.4	0.7
Glucose (mg/dl)	70–110	133	1.0
Urea (mg/dl)	15–45	33	1.0
Calcium (mg/dl)	8.1–10.4	7.3	0.9
LDH (IU/l)	100–260	398	2.4
Creatinine (mg/dl)	0.8–1.2	0.9	0.9
Cholesterol (mg/dl)	130–240	43	0.3
Triglycerides (mg/dl)	50–170	34	0.3
White blood cells (K/μl)	4.0–10.8	1.4	0.2

Data are from Ben-horin [2].

Fig. 8.4 As pericardial fluid volume increases, the pericardial reserve volume is filled. Once the reserve volume is full, pressure within the pericardium rapidly rises and cardiac performance may be compromised. Adapted from Spodick [1]

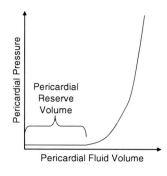

disperse throughout [5]. Yet, too much pericardial fluid, either due to disease or due to an intervention, may cause increased pericardial pressure and compromise cardiac performance, a syndrome called "cardiac tamponade." As shown in Fig. 8.4, the pericardial fluid volume acts as a buffer against increasing pressure; once these groves and sinuses have filled, however, the pressure quickly increases with additional fluid volume.

8.3.2 Mechanical Effects of the Pericardium

The degree to which the pericardium alters heart wall movement(s) varies depending on the ratio of cardiac to pericardial size, loading conditions, and the degree of active and passive filling. Closure of the pericardial sac following open-heart surgery has been proposed to: (1) avoid possible postoperative complications; (2) reduce the frequency of ventricular hypertrophy; and/or (3) facilitate future potential reoperations by reducing fibrosis [6]. Furthermore, reported differences in ventricular performance, dependent on the presence of the pericardium, have been observed following cardiac surgery [7, 8].

In general, the presence of a pericardium physically constrains the heart, often resulting in a depressive hemodynamic influence limiting cardiac output by restraining diastolic ventricular filling [9, 10] (see MPG 8.1 in the Companion CD). The physical constraint by the pericardium is translated into direct external mechanical forces that can also alter patterns in myocardial and systemic blood flow [10, 11]. Direct primary and indirect secondary effects are observed as additional forces through the chamber free walls. Because both the left and right side atria and the left and right side ventricles are bound by a common septum, geometrical changes from chamber interaction(s) are dynamic, depending on the different filling rates and ejection rates of each of the four chambers [12, 13]. Thus, it is important to note that chamber-to-chamber interactions through the interventricular

septum and by the pericardium further promote direct mechanical chamber interactions [14–16].

The effects of the pericardium on mechanical measures of cardiac performance are generally not evident until ventricular and atrial filling limitations are reached, changing geometrical and mechanical properties through factors such as maximum chamber volumes and elasticity. These effects become more evident as these pericardial limitations become extended [17, 18]. With the known force–length dependence of cardiac muscle, variation of chamber volumes through removal of the pericardium will, in turn, alter isometric tensions and therefore directly impact systolic ejection. On the other hand, in specific cases where the restrictive role of the pericardium greatly increases, such as during cardiac tamponade, an increased intrapericardial fluid volume may result in critical restriction by the pericardium that then reduces cardiac performance (Fig. 8.5) [19, 20].

It should also be noted that increases in intrathoracic pressure will also create an additional interaction between the ventricles, as well as between the heart and lungs in a closed chest. Thus, studying cardiac function in situ (with an opened chest) or in vitro allows for the elimination of these influences of intrathoracic pressures, thus allowing for more direct identification and quantification of pericardial influences on cardiac performance and ejection [21]. Furthermore, such isolation of these pericardial effects from diastolic filling is an important consideration since normal ventricular output is dependent on diastolic pressure, independent of the presence of the pericardium [22].

8.4 Pericardial Disorders: Congenital, Pathological, and Iatrogenic

Sir William Osler, considered as the father of modern medicine, referred to pericardial disease when he stated "probably no serious disease is so frequently overlooked by the practitioner" [23]. Many pericardial disorders are asymptomatic and often go unnoticed throughout the patient's life, but some may be fatal (Fig. 8.6). Pericardial disorders may be generally classified as congenital, pathological, or iatrogenic.

Congenital abnormalities of the pericardium are extremely rare. Partial absence of the pericardium may occur, usually exposing the left side of the heart. Complete absence of the pericardium is even less frequent [23]. Cysts may also form during development in, on, or around the pericardium. These usually are not clinically significant and need to be treated only if they become symptomatic [1]. A list of these major congenital abnormalities is found in Table 8.2.

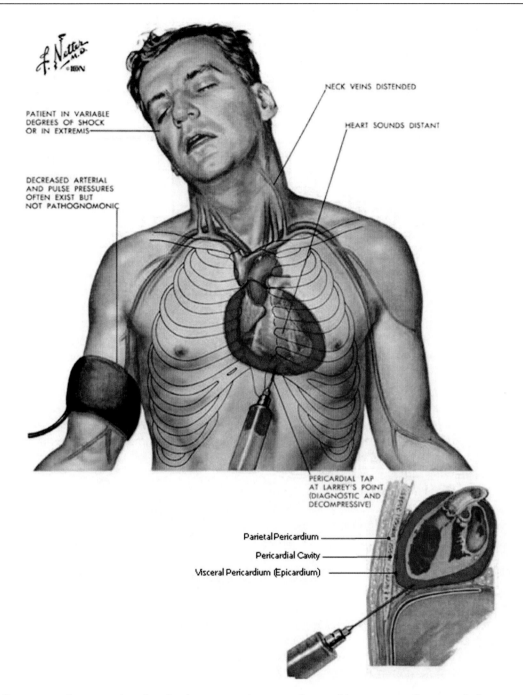

Fig. 8.5 Cardiac tamponade occurs when there is a large accumulation of fluid in the pericardium (*top*). During tamponade, hemodynamics may be seriously compromised. Distended neck veins, decreased blood pressure, various degrees of shock, and distant heart sounds may all be symptoms of tamponade. In most cases, tamponade is treated by pericardiocentesis, or drainage of the sac with a long hypodermic needle (*bottom*). Reproduced from Atlas of Human Anatomy 2003, with permission from ICON Learning Systems

During disease or injury, the pericardium responds with the production of fluid, fibrin, cells, or a combination of the three [23]. The amount of each depends on the type of disease or injury. Numerous forms of pericarditis can initiate an inflammatory response, including fibrinous pericarditis, fibrous pericarditis, infective pericarditis, and cholesterol pericarditis. Diseases unrelated to the pericardium may also trigger a pericardial response, such as a nearby neoplasm or even a myocardial infarction. After a transmural myocardial infarction, for example, patients almost always form adhesions between the necrotic area of the myocardium and the fibrous pericardium [23]. Pericardial effusions, or excess fluid in the pericardium, may occur with disease. Large volumes of lymph, chyle, or blood may accumulate in the pericardial sac. If the accumulation of fluid is significant, this may result in

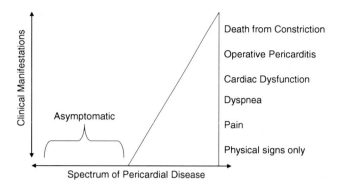

Fig. 8.6 Most pericardial diseases are discovered postmortem, implying that they were asymptomatic throughout the patient's life. Serious pericardial disease, however, may have many clinical manifestations, as shown in the figure. Adapted from Reddy [23]

impaired cardiac function, the condition noted above as cardiac tamponade that, if not treated, can be fatal. A list of several major pathologically induced pericardial disorders is also found in Table 8.2.

Finally, iatrogenic disorders often occur during the treatment of unrelated diseases. During cardiac surgery, the pericardium is often removed (partially or entirely) and, to date, is rarely repaired. There has been much debate as to whether closing the pericardium after surgery would be beneficial to the patient. Most surgeons believe that closing the pericardium may acutely compromise postoperative hemodynamics and increase the risk of tamponade. More recent research has shown that there are no clinical benefits, but there may be adverse effects resulting from closure of the pericardium after cardiac surgery [24]. Nevertheless, if the pericardium is left open, the exposed epicardium tends to become very fibrous, complicating future interventions. It should be noted that noncardiac surgical procedures performed near the heart may also induce trauma to the pericardium and cause an inflammatory response. Furthermore, even some nonsurgical interventions may damage the pericardium. For example, resuscitation from cardiac arrest (CPR) may cause a fibrous response. In some patients,

irradiation may create an effusion and subsequent tamponade [23]. The pericardium may also adversely react to a number of commonly prescribed drugs such as procainamide, penicillin, doxorubicin, anticoagulants, and/or antithrombotics [1]. The reader is again referred to Table 8.2 for a list of major iatrogenic pericardial disorders.

In general, pericardial disorders can be diagnosed using ECG, echocardiography, radiography, and/or auscultation. Pericardial fluid samples and pericardial tissue biopsies may also aid in complicated diagnoses. Typically, once diagnosed, pericardial disorders are often treatable with a number of drugs and/or interventions [25]. In situations of large pericardial effusions, pericardiocentesis is performed by draining the effusion with a hypodermic needle inserted near the xyphoid process (Fig. 8.5). This is usually done under guidance of echocardiography or fluoroscopy to prevent myocardial puncture, but in emergency situations (such as during acute cardiac tamponade), it may be done without guidance ("blindly"). Chronic effusions or other diseases may necessitate a partial or complete pericardiotomy. This is done by creating an opening into the mediastinum (called a pericardial window) to view and remove portions of the pericardium; visualization of the procedure can be enhanced by a laparoscope or thoracoscope. Balloon pericardiotomy is a more recently employed minimally invasive technique that uses a balloon to enlarge a small hole in the pericardium [3].

8.5 Comparative Anatomy of the Pericardium

The pericardium is fixed to the great arteries at the base of the heart and is attached to the sternum and diaphragm in all mammals, although the degree of these attachments to the diaphragm varies between and within species [26, 27]. Specifically, the attachment to the central tendinous aponeurosis of the diaphragm is firm and broad in humans and pigs, the phrenopericardial ligament is the only

Table 8.2 Major sources of pericardial disorders (congenital, pathological, or iatrogenic)

Congenital	Pathological	Iatrogenic
Primary	Idiopathic pericarditis	Surgical
Pericardial absence	Due to living agents—infectious, parasitic	Instrument trauma
Cysts	Vasculitis—connective tissue disease	Cardiac resuscitation
Teratoma	Immunopathies/hypersensitivity states	Iatrogenic pneumopericardium
Lymphangioma	Disease of contiguous structures	Drug reactions and complications
Diverticulom	Disorders of metabolism	Radiation
Pericardial bands	Trauma—indirect, direct	
Secondary	Neoplasms—primary, metastatic, multicentric	
Pericarditis due to maternal lupus	Uncertain pathogenesis	
Intrapericardial hernia of abdominal organs		

Adapted from Spodick [1].

attachment in dogs, and the caudal portion of the pericardium is attached via the strong sternopericardial ligament in sheep [26, 27] (see MPG 8.2 in the Companion CD).

Although the basic structure of the pericardium is the same, differences exist between various species with respect to both geometry and structure [28–30]. Generally, pericardial wall thickness usually increases with increasing heart and cavity size between the various species [28]. However, humans are a notable exception to this rule, having a much thicker pericardium than animals with similar heart sizes [28]. Specifically, the pericardium of human hearts varies in thickness between 1 and 3.5 mm [1], while the average pericardial thickness of various animal species was found to be considerably thinner (ovine hearts: 0.32 ± 0.01 mm, porcine hearts: 0.20 ± 0.01 mm, and canine hearts: 0.19 ± 0.01 mm) [29]. Differences in the relative volume of pericardial fluid also exist. Holt [28] reported that most dogs have between 0.5 and 2.5 ml of pericardial fluid (with some dogs having up to 15 ml) compared to 20–60 ml in adult human cadaver hearts. In the Visible Heart® lab, we have found that 70–80 kg swine have about 7–8 ml of pericardial fluid. In selecting an appropriate animal model for pericardial access procedures or intrapericardial therapeutics, the significant differences in pericardial thickness, pericardial fluid volume, and pericardial attachments between humans and various animal models must be considered.

8.6 Surgical Uses of the Pericardium

Due to the inherent mechanical properties of the fibrous pericardium, it has been used in various applications during surgery and has also been used in bioprosthetic heart valves. During cardiac surgery, fresh autografts, cryopreserved homografts, or glutaraldehyde fixed xenografts can be used as patches during reconstructive repairs in both congenital and acquired heart diseases. For example, in congenitally malformed hearts, pericardial patches are used during surgical repairs of the right ventricular outflow tracts and/or during repair of torn aortic leaflets, among other things. Pericardial patches have also been used in acquired diseases to repair the mitral and aortic valves as well as ventricular walls [31].

The use of pericardium in heart valves is a relatively recent development. The search for an alternative to mechanical valves has led people to investigate many types of bioprosthetic valves. These bioprostheses consist of homografts (preserved cadaveric valves), autografts (transplant of a patient's pulmonic valve to the aortic

position—the Ross procedure), and xenografts. Xenograft valves have included preserved porcine aortic tissue as well as preserved bovine pericardium. More specifically, glutaraldehyde fixed bovine or porcine pericardium has been used in the design of aortic and mitral bioprosthetic valves, which have realized wide clinical success. Such pericardium is prepared and fixed using specific processes (which typically vary slightly between manufacturers) and then cut to resemble a tri-leaflet semilunar valve and assembled into a stent with a sewing cuff.

8.7 Intrapericardial Therapeutics

8.7.1 Clinical Pericardial Access

Traditionally, pericardial access has been limited to patients with pericardial effusions. The effusion gives physicians a buffer between the fibrous pericardium and the epicardium during pericardiocentesis or creating a pericardial window, thus preventing damage to the myocardium and coronary vessels. Recently, there has been an interest in accessing the healthy pericardium for the delivery of various therapeutics. The challenge of accessing a healthy pericardium is to puncture and catheterize the pericardium with minimal risk to the heart. This is a difficult task considering the almost negligible layer of pericardial fluid in a healthy pericardial sac.

Several unique biomedical devices or tools have been (or are being) developed to aid in accessing pericardial space via use of novel catheter designs, e.g., allowing controlled myocardial penetration during fluoroscopic visualization. Specifically, a recently introduced technology has been developed that uses a sheathed needle with a suction tip designed for grasping the pericardium and accessing the pericardial space using a transthoracic approach while, at the same time, minimizing the risk of myocardial puncture; the PerDUCER® instrument (Comedicus, Inc., Columbia Heights, MN) is placed following subxiphoid access into the mediastinum under fluoroscopic guidance from the apparatus positioned onto the anterior outer surface of the pericardial sac (Fig. 8.7). Under manual suction, the sac is retracted and a needle is inserted, allowing for the placement of a guidewire into the space via the needle lumen. The needle is then removed and a standard delivery catheter is placed into position. The Philipps University of Marburg has also been developing a similar product called the Marburg Attacher (http://cardiorepair.com) that is currently undergoing clinical trials. Other percutaneous subxyphoid techniques have been proposed [32], but are not in current clinical use.

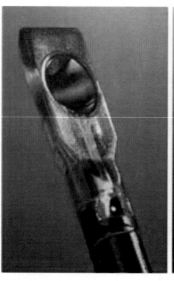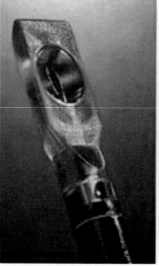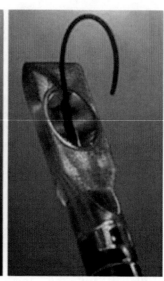

A novel transatrial technique has been recently developed by Verrier and colleagues [33] which has been very successful in animal studies. In this procedure, a guide catheter is introduced into the right atrium from the femoral vein, and a needle catheter is advanced through the guide catheter to pierce the right atrial appendage. A guidewire is then passed through the needle catheter into the pericardial space. A soft delivery catheter can be passed over the guidewire and can reside in pericardial space for long-term drug delivery or for fluid sampling. Recent studies in swine have shown that catheters left in the pericardial space over long periods of time can remain patent and cause minimal fibrosis and inflammatory response at the epicardium [34, 35].

The ability to access the pericardial space has created new opportunities to further understand the role of the pericardium under normal cardiac function and/or following cardiac disease(s). Despite the growing literature establishing the feasibility of intrapericardial therapeutics and diagnostics, the results of clinical trials employing pericardially delivered agents directed toward angiogenesis, restenosis, and/or other coronary and myocardial indications are currently lacking.

8.7.2 Potential Intrapericardial Therapies

With recent advances in minimally invasive cardiac surgical procedures, it is likely that instances and abilities in preserving the integrity of the pericardium during cardiac surgery will increase. The diminished ability of cardiac cells to regenerate under adverse loading conditions impairs the ability to regenerate lost myocardial function, making

procedures to reduce myocardial trauma of particular interest. In addition, access into the pericardial space provides a new route for numerous novel treatments and therapies that can be applied directly to the epicardial surface and/or the coronary arteries. For quite some time, nonsurgical intrapericardial therapy has been employed in patients with sufficient fluid in the pericardial space allowing a needle to be safely placed within the space [1]. This methodology has been used for patients with such clinical indications as, but not limited to, malignancies, recurrent effusions, uremic pericarditis, and connective tissue disease. As mentioned above, instrumenting the pericardium has been made possible by numerous techniques that allow for the study of intrapericardial therapeutics and diagnostics by clinicians and investigators alike. More specifically, the endoluminal delivery of various agents has been found to be clinically limited due to short residence time, highly variable deposited agent concentration, inconsistency in delivery concentrations, and relatively rapid washout of agents from the target vessel [36]. A desired example of targeted application includes infusion of concentrated nitric oxide donors, which could present undesirable effects if systemically delivered. Further, one is allowed increased site specificity and the delivery of label-specific therapeutic agents to target cells, receptors, and channels. A great deal of interest has been focused on delivery of angiogenic agents and various growth factors into the intrapericardial space [37–39]. In particular, research has concentrated on administration in patients with ischemic heart disease [40, 41]. Early results indicate several benefits associated with the delivery of angiogenic agents that include increased collateral vessel development, regional myocardial blood flow, myocardial function in the ischemic region, and myocardial vascularity.

In our lab, we have shown that intrapericardial delivery of omega-3 fatty acids can drastically reduce infarct size and lower the occurrence of ventricular arrhythmias. In a recent study [42], 23 swine were treated with either an infusion of omega-3 fatty acids or saline in the pericardial sac prior to occluding the left anterior descending artery. Prior to, during, and after the occlusion, hemodynamic and electrophysiological data were recorded. Upon sacrificing the animal, the heart was sectioned and stained to determine infarct size. We found that both infarct size and arrhythmia scores were reduced by half in animals treated with omega-3 fatty acids. Furthermore, the treatment had a minimal effect on hemodynamics, which is in contrast to the use of many anti-arrhythmic drugs. Current research is underway to determine if this therapy would be feasible in a clinical setting.

8.7.3 Pericardial Pharmacokinetics

As described previously, the pericardium in humans is generally believed to contain 20–60 ml of physiologic fluid (0.25±15 ml/kg) situated within the cavity space [43]. Yet dye studies suggest that pericardial fluid is not uniformly distributed over the myocardium, with the majority of pericardial fluid residing within the atrioventricular and interventricular grooves as well as the superior-transverse sinuses (in supine individuals). Although the pericardial fluid is not uniformly distributed, pharmacokinetic studies suggest that there is complete mixing of the fluid so that pericardial fluid content is spatially uniform [44–46]. Hence, sampling pericardial fluid content should not vary functionally by sampling location [45].

Tissue distribution and drug clearance clearly affect all drug response. Because specific pericardial pharmacokinetic data remain unknown for the majority of compounds, pericardial drug disposition must be gleaned from physical–chemical properties based on a few select studies. Pericardial fluid is cleared via lymphatics and epicardial vasculature, with the former being a very slow process [47]. In addition to these passive clearance mechanisms, the epicardial tissues contain metabolic enzymes that may clear compounds via a biotransformation process. This is likely to occur with certain labile peptides and small molecules such as nitric oxide. Unfortunately, there is very little known today about pericardial drug metabolism. In general, it is considered that whether or not a compound residing in the pericardial space is cleared via lymphatic drainage, passive diffusion, or biotransformation will depend on its molecular size, tissue affinity, water solubility, and enzymatic stability. Thus, compounds such as large proteins do not rapidly diffuse into the vascular space and are slowly cleared from the pericardial space perhaps via lymphatics unless, of course, they are biotransformed [45, 48]. Importantly, this yields a pericardial fluid clearance and residence time longer than the corresponding plasma half-life. For example, administering atrial naturetic peptide into the pericardial fluid space had a five-fold longer clearance and residence time within the pericardial fluid space, as compared to plasma clearance of an intravenous dose [48]. Similarly, small water-insoluble compounds may also have very prolonged pericardial fluid residual times.

One case report documented that the pericardial fluid half-life of 5-fluorouracil (sparingly soluble in water) was approximately 10-fold longer than plasma half-life (168 versus 16 min); it should be noted that the patient in this investigation had metastatic breast carcinoma with pericardial involvement [44]. The patient had received a relatively large pericardial 5-fluorouracil dose (200 mg) to manage recurrent pericardial effusion. This large dose, however, was associated with nearly undetectable plasma levels, indicating minimal spillover from pericardial fluid into the systemic circulation. While it was expected that 5-fluorouracil would have a longer pericardial residual time because it is water insoluble, it is unknown if these findings would occur in a healthy pericardial fluid space.

On the other hand, small water-soluble compounds have up to five- to eight-fold shorter pericardial fluid clearance and residence times as compared to plasma [46]. For example, procainamide is a water-soluble compound that has a pericardial fluid half-life ranging from 30 to 41±2.1 min as compared to the 180-min plasma half-life; it has been reported that the procainamide rapidly diffused out of the pericardial space with a terminal elimination half-life approximately five to seven times shorter than plasma [49]. However, procainamide spillover from pericardial fluid into plasma was considered not to produce measurable plasma concentrations because of the relatively low pericardial doses (0.5–2 mg/kg). Similarly, it is not surprising that the converse was also true, that intravenously administered procainamide rapidly diffused into the pericardial space, across a plasma to pericardial fluid concentration gradient, such that pericardial fluid procainamide concentrations were similar to plasma approximately 20–30 min following an intravenous injection. The likely explanation for these findings is that the vast ventricular epicardial blood supply served as a clearing system (pericardial administration) or a delivery system (intravenous administration) according to drug concentration diffusion gradient. Importantly, the diffusion of pericardial-administered procainamide into the vascular space will likely prevent drug accumulation in ventricular tissue and a global pharmacologic response.

In addition to pericardial drug residence and clearance times, the determination of distribution volume may be of considerable importance, particularly to achieve desired peak drug concentrations. There is a direct and inverse relationship between peak drug concentrations and drug distribution volumes, such that a low drug distribution volume achieves higher peak concentrations. Perhaps of clinical importance, with the very small pericardial fluid volume, it is likely that pericardial drug doses can be substantially reduced to achieve therapeutic concentrations. This was evident whereby sequential pericardial procainamide doses of 0.5, 1, and 2 mg/kg produced peak pericardial fluid concentrations that ranged from 250 to 900 μg/ml; these concentrations were nearly 1,000-fold greater than peak plasma concentrations of procainamide following the administration of a 2 mg/kg intravenous dose. In a follow-up study in which a single procainamide dose was employed, similar findings were documented; it was also reported that a pericardial fluid volume of distribution of 1.6 ± 0.16 ml/kg was observed, which is approximately 1,000-fold smaller than plasma procainamide volume of distribution of 2,000 ml/kg. While pericardial procainamide dosing produced very large pericardial fluid concentrations, procainamide could not be detected in the plasma given the very small doses. With such a powerful diffusion gradient, it is likely that pericardial procainamide delivery can achieve very high atrial tissue concentrations. Indirect evidence of tissue distribution is a procainamide distribution volume that is larger (40–50 ml) than the estimated pericardial fluid volume of 20–30 ml. Since the procainamide pericardial volume of distribution exceeded the expected pericardial volume, there was some tissue distribution. These pharmacodynamic data suggest that tissue distribution mainly occurs in the atrium, likely because the atrium is a very thin structure with a low blood supply. Thus, this tissue architecture is ideal for specialized therapeutic drug diffusion and therefore differs from that of the ventricle(s).

Unfortunately, most pericardial procainamide pharmacokinetic studies performed to date have not directly measured tissue concentrations following infusion. However, in one study which evaluated the pharmacodynamic effects of pericardial amiodarone delivery, the amiodarone tissue distribution was quantified at several myocardial locations [50]. Not surprisingly, it was reported that atrial and epicardial ventricular tissue had the highest amiodarone tissue concentration, while ventricular endocardial amiodarone tissue concentrations were approximately 10-fold lower. However, importantly, the amiodarone levels were likely still within a therapeutic range. This was supported by the fact that pericardial amiodarone delivery prolonged endocardial ventricular refractory periods by up to 13%, which was equivalent to epicardial ventricular refractory period measurements and the magnitude of atrial refractory period prolongation. The similar refractory response between epicardial and endocardial measurements, with very large differences in amiodarone tissue concentrations, indicates that amiodarone effects are maximal at low tissue concentrations. Unlike pericardial amiodarone administration, pericardial procainamide had no effect on endocardial ventricular refractory periods [46]. It is likely that such a beneficial ventricular tissue distribution does not occur with more water-soluble compounds such as procainamide. On the other hand, it is not surprising that amiodarone, when administered into the pericardial space, could penetrate ventricular tissue and affect global ventricular electrophysiology because it is highly lipophilic and has a huge tissue distribution including the intracellular space [50].

Lastly, perhaps it is possible to modify molecules to achieve an optimal pericardial fluid residence time and thus therapeutic outcomes (benefits). More specifically, for some agents, it may be desirable to have a short residence time. For example, pericardial drug delivery to cardiovert atrial fibrillation may require very high drug concentrations for only a brief duration, given the acute nature of the therapy. On the other hand, the ability to manage chronic conditions such as ischemic heart disease or heart failure may necessitate longer pericardial residual times. In this regard, Baek et al. recently showed that a derivitized nitric oxide donor molecule, diazeniumdiolate, with bovine serum albumin resulted in a five-fold increase in pericardial fluid clearance and residence time versus a small molecule nitric oxide donor (diethylenetriamine/NO) [51]. This group went on to show that it may be possible that a single pericardial dose of the nitric oxide donor could inhibit in-stent restenosis. Unlike patients with any type of effusion, the normal pericardium is a very thin layer, bringing it closer to the heart, and subsequently increasing the risk of harm to the patient.

8.8 Summary

The pericardium is a unique structure that surrounds the heart and serves several important physiological roles. The removal of the pericardium, certain pericardial disorders, and or the build-up of fluids within this space will ultimately alter hemodynamic performance. Recent therapeutic approaches have been directed to exploit the space that exists between the pericardium and the epicardial surface of the heart. New devices and techniques are being developed to access this space in a minimally invasive fashion. An important consideration when utilizing animal models to study such devices is that the pericardium in humans is much thicker, and there is more pericardial fluid than in commonly employed animal models. The pharmacokinetics of many drugs may be greatly enhanced if the drug is delivered into the pericardium. As more is learned about the pericardium, it may play a significant role in cardiac therapies.

References

1. Spodick DH, ed. The pericardium: A comprehensive textbook. New York, NY: Marcel Dekker, 1997.
2. Ben-horin S, Shinfeld A, Kachel E, Chetrit A, Livneh AR. The composition of the normal pericardial fluid and its implications for diagnosing pericardial effusions. Am J Med 2005;118:636–40.
3. Shabetai R. The pericardium. Boston, MA: Kluwer Academic Publishers, 2003.
4. Pegram BL, Bishop VS. An evaluation of the pericardial sac as a safety factor during tamponade. Cardiovasc Res 1975;9:715–21.
5. Boulanger B, Yuan Z, Flessner M, Hay J, Johnston, M. Pericardial fluid absorption into lymphatic vessels in sheep. Microvasc Res 1999;57:174–86.
6. Angelini GD, Fraser AG, Koning MM, et al. Adverse hemodynamic effects and echocardiographic consequences of pericardial closure soon after sternotomy and pericardiotomy. Circulation 1990;82:IV397–406.
7. Reich DL, Konstadt SN, Thys DM. The pericardium exerts constraint on the right ventricle during cardiac surgery. Acta Anaesthesiol Scand 1990;34:530–3.
8. Daughters GT, Frist WH, Alderman EL, Derby GC, Ingels NB, Jr., Miller DC. Effects of the pericardium on left ventricular diastolic filling and systolic performance early after cardiac operations. J Thorac Cardiovasc Surg 1992;104:1084–91.
9. Hammond HK, White FC, Bhargava V, Shabetai R. Heart size and maximal cardiac output are limited by the pericardium. Am J Physiol 1992;263:H1675–81.
10. Abel FL, Mihailescu LS, Lader AS, Starr RG. Effects of pericardial pressure on systemic and coronary hemodynamics in dogs. Am J Physiol 1995;268:H1593–605.
11. Allard JR, Gertz EW, Verrier ED, Bristow JD, Hoffman JI. Role of the pericardium in the regulation of myocardial blood flow and its distribution in the normal and acutely failing left ventricle of the dog. Cardiovasc Res 1983;17:595–603.
12. Beloucif S, Takata M, Shimada M, Robotham JL. Influence of pericardial constraint on atrioventricular interactions. Am J Physiol 1992;263:H125–34.
13. Calvin JE. Optimal right ventricular filling pressures and the role of pericardial constraint in right ventricular infarction in dogs. Circulation 1991;84:852–61.
14. Hess OM, Bhargava V, Ross J, Jr., Shabetai R. The role of the pericardium in interactions between the cardiac chambers. Am Heart J 1983;106:1377–83.
15. Janicki JS, Weber KT. The pericardium and ventricular interaction, distensibility, and function. Am J Physiol 1980;238:H494–503.
16. Shabetai R, Mangiardi L, Bhargava V, Ross J, Jr., Higgins CB. The pericardium and cardiac function. Prog Cardiovasc Dis 1979;22:107–34.
17. Belenkie I, Dani R, Smith ER, Tyberg JV. The importance of pericardial constraint in experimental pulmonary embolism and volume loading. Am Heart J 1992;123:733–42.
18. Watkins MW, LeWinter MM. Physiologic role of the normal pericardium. Ann Rev Med 1993;44:171–80.

19. Janicki JS. Influence of the pericardium and ventricular interdependence on left ventricular diastolic and systolic function in patients with heart failure. Circulation 1990;81:III15–20.
20. Netter FH, ed. Atlas of human anatomy. 3rd ed. Teterboro, NJ: ICON Learning Systems, 2003.
21. Weber KT, Janicki JS, Shroff S, Fishman AP. Contractile mechanics and interaction of the right and left ventricles. Am J Cardiol 1981;47:686–95.
22. Kingma I, Smiseth OA, Frais MA, Smith ER, Tyberg JV. Left ventricular external constraint: Relationship between pericardial, pleural and esophageal pressures during positive end-expiratory pressure and volume loading in dogs. Ann Biomed Eng 1987;15:331–46.
23. Reddy RS, Leon DF, Shaver JA, eds. Pericardial disease. New York, NY: Raven Press, 1982.
24. Bittar MN, Bernard JB, Khasati N, Richardson S. Should the pericardium be closed in patients undergoing cardiac surgery? Inter Cardiovasc Thorac Surg 2005;4:151–5.
25. Fowler N. The pericardium in health and disease. Mount Kisco, NY: Futura Publishing Company, Inc., 1985.
26. Getty R. General heart and blood vessels. In: Getty R, ed. Sisson and Grossman's the anatomy of the domestic animals. 5th ed. Philadelphia, PA: Saunders, 1975:164–75.
27. Michaëlsson M, Ho SY, eds. Congenital heart malformations in mammals: An illustrated text. River Edge, NJ: Imperial College Press, 2000.
28. Holt JP. The normal pericardium. Am J Cardiol 1970; 26:455–65.
29. Naimark WA, Lee JM, Limeback H, Cheung DT. Correlation of structure and viscoelastic properties in the pericardia of four mammalian species. Am J Physiol 1992;263:H1095–106.
30. Elias H, Boyd L. Notes on the anatomy, embryology and histology of the pericardium. J New York Med Coll 1960;2:50–75.
31. David TE. The use of pericardium in acquired heart disease: A review article. J Heart Valve Dis 1998;7:13–8.
32. Laham RJ, Simons M, Hung D. Subxyphoid access of the normal pericardium: A novel drug delivery technique. Catheter Cardiovasc Interv 1999;47:109–11.
33. Verrier RL, Waxman S, Lovett EG, Moreno R. Transatrial access to the normal pericardial space. Circulation 1998;98:2331–3.
34. Kolettis TM, Kazakos N, Katsouras CS, et al. Intrapericardial drug delivery: Pharmacologic properties and long-term safety in swine. Intern J Cardiol 2005;99:415–21.
35. Bartoli CR, Akiyama I, Godleski JJ, Verrier RL. Catheter Cardiovasc Interv 2007;70:221–7.
36. March KL. Methods of local gene delivery to vascular tissue. Semin Interv Cardiol 1996;1:215–23.
37. Laham RJ, Rezaee M, Post M, et al. Intrapericardial administration of basic fibroblast growth factor: Myocardial and tissue distribution and comparison with intracoronary and intravenous administration. Catheter Cardiovasc Interv 2003;58: 375–81.
38. Lazarous DF, Shou M, Stiber JA, et al. Pharmacodynamics of basic fibroblast growth factor: Route of administration determines myocardial and systemic distribution. Cardiovasc Res 1997;36:78–85.
39. Tio RA, Grandjean G, Suurmeijer AJ, et al. Thoracoscopic monitoring for pericardial application of local drug or gene therapy. Int J Cardiol 2002; 82:117–21.
40. Laham RJ, Hung D. Therapeutic myocardial angiogenesis using percutaneous intrapericardial drug delivery. Clin Cardiol 1999;22:I6–9.
41. Landau C, Jacobs AK, Haudenschild CC. Intrapericardial basic fibroblast growth factor induces myocardial angiogenesis in a rabbit model of chronic ischemia. Am Heart J 1995; 129:924–31.

42. Xiao YF, Sigg DC, Ujhelyi MR, Wilhelm JJ, Richardson ES, Iaizzo PA. Pericardial delivery of omega-3 fatty acid: A novel approach to reducing myocardial infarct sizes and arrhythmias. Am J Physiol Heart Circ Physiol 2008;294:H2212–8.

43. Choe YH, Im JG, Park JH, Han MC, Kim CW. The anatomy of the pericardial space: A study in cadavers and patients. AJR Am J Roentgenol 1987;149:693–7.

44. Lerner-Tung MB, Chang AY, Ong LS, Kreiser D. Pharmacokinetics of intrapericardial administration of 5-fluorouracil. Cancer Chemother Pharmacol 1997;40:318–20.

45. Stoll HP, Carlson K, Keefer LK, Hrabie JA, March KL. Pharmacokinetics and consistency of pericardial delivery directed to coronary arteries: Direct comparison with endoluminal delivery. Clin Cardiol 1999;22:I10–6.

46. Ujhelyi M, Hadsell K, Euler D, Mehra R. Intrapericardial therapeutics: A pharmacodynamic and pharmacokinetic comparison between pericardial and intravenous procainamide. J Cardiovasc Electrophysiol 2002;13:605–11.

47. Hollenberg M, Dougherty J. Lymph flow and 131-I-albumin resorption from pericardial effusions in man. Am J Cardiol 1969;24:514–22.

48. Szokodi I, Horkay F, Kiss P, et al. Characterization and stimuli for production of pericardial fluid atrial natriuretic peptide in dogs. Life Sci 1997;61:1349–59.

49. Nolan PE. Pharmacokinetics and pharmacodynamics of intravenous agents for ventricular arrhythmias. Pharmacotherapy 1997;17:65–75S; discussion 89–91S.

50. Ayers GM. Rho TH, Ben-David J, Besch HR, Jr., Zipes DP. Amiodarone instilled into the canine pericardial sac migrates transmurally to produce electrophysiologic effects and suppress atrial fibrillation. J Cardiovasc Electrophysiol 1996; 7:713–21.

51. Baek SH, Hrabie JA, Keefer LK, Hou D, Fineberg N, Rhoades R, March KL. Augmentation of intrapericardial nitric oxide level by a prolonged-release nitric oxide donor reduces luminal narrowing after porcine coronary angioplasty. Circulation 2002;105:2779–84.

Chapter 9
Congenital Defects of the Human Heart: Nomenclature and Anatomy

James D. St. Louis

Abstract There are numerous congenital defects of the human heart and many typically require medical intervention. The primary goal of this chapter is to briefly define such abnormalities and introduce the reader to the various classification schemes that have been used to describe their relative anatomic and functional features.

Keywords Septal defect · Aortopulmonary window defect · Coarctation of the aorta · Interrupted aortic arch · Tetralogy of Fallot · Atresia · Ebstein's anomaly · Transposition of the great vessels · Total anomalous pulmonary venous connection · Persistent truncus arteriosus

9.1 Introduction

Congenital defects of the human heart present a unique challenge in establishing an accurate and consistent nomenclature that is secondary to our somewhat incomplete understanding of their embryologic origin and vast complexity of varied anatomic presentation. In any attempt to describe a complex system, several lines of reasoning may evolve that foster not only controversy but also confusion. An adequate system to describe congenital lesions of the human heart is no exception. Nevertheless, several leading clinicians and investigators in this field can be credited with the primary elucidation of a system that attempts to organize and categorize these complex lesions.

Of importance, Richard Van Praagh presented a system based on the segmental anatomy of the developing heart [1, 2]. His generalized theory states that by understanding the anatomical position of the cardiac segments, the majority of cardiac defects may be accurately described. The three segments which Van Praagh described consist of the atria, the ventricle, and the great vessels. These segments may be described by delineating their relative positional relationships. The *visceroatrial situs* is defined as the relative position of the right and left atria to the sidedness of the abdominal (visceral) organs; the term situs means position or location. The *bulb ventricular loop* is described as the orientation of the right and left ventricles to the great vessels (pulmonary artery and aorta). These segments are referenced in sequence, with each being designated by a letter. The connection of the visceral venous vessels (the superior and inferior venae cavae) and the atrial body is termed the visceroatrial situs and is described by the following letters: S, *Situs Solitus*; I, *Situs Inversus*; and A, *Situs Ambiguous*. When the visceral situs is normal (*Situs Solitus*), the stomach and spleen lie to the left, the right lobe of the liver is larger than the left, and the appendix is right sided. In Situs Inversus, the position of the abdominal organs is reversed, with the stomach and spleen lying on the right and the dominant lobe of the liver to the left; the appendix and inferior vena cava are to the left, with the left lung being typically trilobed. Situs Ambiguous describes a group of anomalies in which the dominant characteristic is a lack of visceral sidedness. The abdominal organs may be positioned to the anatomic left or right, often with the liver lying in the midline. A unique characteristic of these individuals is the abnormal existence or a complete lack of a spleen. In general, polysplenic patients tend to have all atrial and pulmonary structures consistent with left-sided morphology, while asplenic patients tend to be right-sided dominant [3].

The orientation of the right or left ventricular mass is described by how the embryonic cardiac tube loops during its development. In this system, the terms "right" and "left" are used to refer to the specific morphology of the ventricular mass rather than their spatial arrangement. The anatomic right ventricle has a very trabeculated endocardium, while the left ventricular endocardium is smooth with finer trabeculation. The rightward (normal)

J.D. St. Louis (✉)
University of Minnesota, Departments of Surgery and Pediatrics, MMC 495, 420 Delaware St. SE, Minneapolis, MN 55455, USA
e-mail: stlou012@umn.edu

P.A. Iaizzo (ed.), *Handbook of Cardiac Anatomy, Physiology, and Devices*, DOI 10.1007/978-1-60327-372-5_9,
© Springer Science+Business Media, LLC 2009

orientation is given the term "D" for *D-loop*. This indicates that the morphologic right ventricle is oriented to the right and anterior to the morphologic left ventricle. If the cardiac tube undergoes looping in the leftward direction, the segment is given the reference letter "L" for *L-loop*. In this situation, the morphologic right ventricle lies posterior and to the left of the morphologic left ventricle. The final segmental orientation described by Van Praagh deals with the relationship of the great vessels and semilunar valves to the ventricles. The aorta is normally committed to the morphologic left ventricle, with the aortic valve located leftward and posterior to the pulmonary valve. This normal relationship is given the reference letter "S." When the great vessels are transposed, with the aortic valve being rightward and anterior to the pulmonary valve, the convention used is "D." With *D-transposed* great vessels, the aorta is committed to the morphologic right ventricle and the pulmonary artery and valve to the morphologic left ventricle. When the orientation of these great vessels and semilunar valves is normal, but the aorta is committed to the right ventricle and the pulmonary artery to the left ventricle, the term *L-transposed* great vessels is used.

Throughout this chapter, anatomic lesions of the heart will be described and organized based on this aforementioned physiologic derangement (Table 9.1). Furthermore, cyanotic lesions refer to cardiac defects that typically result in systemic arterial desaturation. Finally, shunts refer to an anomalous pathway of blood flow resulting from anatomic defects and their relative resultant downstream pressures.

9.2 Atrial Septal Defect

The classification of an *atrial septal defect* is based on the location in the interatrial septum (Table 9.2). A *patent foramen ovale* is considered a small interatrial communication that does not result from a defect in either the septum primum or the septum secundum. The lesion exists in the region of the foramen ovale and is the result of the failure of the septum primum to fuse with the septum secundum. A secundum-type atrial septal defect occurs when there is a deficiency in the septum primum (Fig. 9.1); this defect may be large or exist as multiple fenestrations in the septum primum. For additional details on fetal anatomy, see Chapter 3.

An atrial septal defect in the region of the sinus venosus, usually superiorly near the junction of the superior vena cava and atrium, is classified as a *venosus-type atrial septal defect*. These defects are commonly associated with partial anomalous pulmonary venous return [4]. A coronary sinus atrial septal defect or unroofed coronary sinus defect results from a deficiency in all or part of the wall separating the left atrium from the coronary sinus. When this deficiency is complete, the coronary sinus is absent and

Table 9. 1 Anatomic lesions of the heart based on physiologic derangement

Acyanotic
- Left-to-right shunts
  - ☐ Atrial septal defect
  - ☐ Ventricular septal defect
  - ☐ Atrioventricular septal defect
  - ☐ Aortopulmonary window
- Left-sided obstructive lesions
  - ☐ Aortic coarctation
  - ☐ Congenital aortic stenosis
  - ☐ Interrupted aortic arch

Cyanotic
- Right-to-left shunts
  - ☐ Tetralogy of Fallot
  - ☐ Pulmonary stenosis
  - ☐ Pulmonary atresia
    - ♦ With intact ventricular septum
    - ♦ With ventricular septal defect
  - ☐ Tricuspid atresia
  - ☐ Ebstein's anomaly
- Complex mixing defects
  - ☐ Transposition of the great vessels
  - ☐ Total anomalous pulmonary venous connection
  - ☐ Truncus arteriosus
  - ☐ Hypoplastic left heart syndrome

Table 9.2 Classification of atrial septal defects
- Secundum type
- Venosus type
- Coronary sinus type

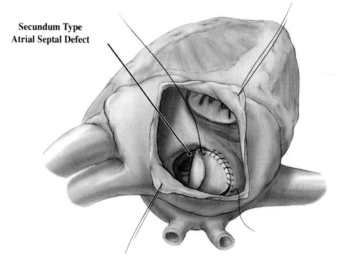

Secundum Type
Atrial Septal Defect

Fig. 9.1 Secundum-type atrial septal defect seen via an incision in the right atrial appendage

communication exists in the posteroinferior region of the atrial septum. The presence of a left superior vena cava is often associated with this type of defect which enters the upper corner of the left atrium [5].

9.3 Ventricular Septal Defect

A *ventricular septal defect* (VSD) is generally defined as a deficiency in the interventricular septum. Importantly, VSDs make up approximately 20% of all congenital heart defects that are identified and require surgical corrections. Because of the numerous anatomic descriptions that one can find in the literature relative to the ventricular septum, an adequate and accepted classification of the defect has remained elusive.

Here we consider that the ventricular septum may be divided into four anatomic regions based on the anterior and posterior extension of the *Septomarginal Trabecularis* (Fig. 9.2) [6]. The clinical management of specific types of

Table 9.3 Classification of ventricular septal defects

Type 1	Subarterial
	Supracristal
	Conal
	Infundibular
Type 2	Perimembranous
	Paramembranous
	Conoventricular
Type 3	Inlet
	Atrioventricular canal type
Type 4	Muscular
	• Anterior
	• Midventricular
	• Posterior
	• Apical

VSDs is based on these anatomic regions (Table 9.3) [7]. Defects that exist in (or within proximity of) the membranous portion of the septum are termed *perimembranous* or *paramembranous VSDs* (Fig. 9.3). Defects that exist in the infundibular region, i.e., superior to the anterior portion of the Septomarginal Trabecularis, are termed *supracristal VSDs*. It should be noted that other terms that have been used to describe such defects include *subarterial, conal,* or *infundibular VSDs*. The third type of VSD is located posterior to the posterior arm of the Septomarginal Trabecularis and involves the inlet of the right ventricular septum immediately inferior to the atrioventricular valve apparatus. These defects have been described as *inlet* or *atrioventricular canal*-type VSDs. The final type of VSD is one that exists in a portion of the trabecular (muscular) septum. These defects are termed *muscular VSDs* and can be further described based on their relative position in the muscular

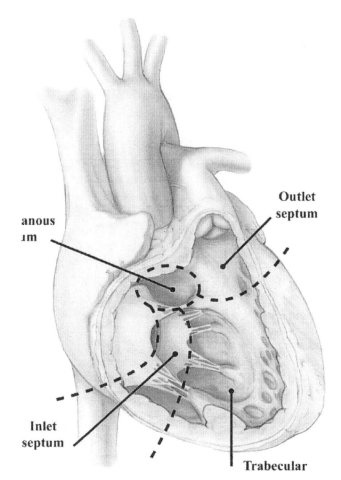

anous
ım

Outlet
septum

Inlet
septum

Trabecular

Fig. 9.2 Ventricular septum visualized through the right ventricular free wall. Note the three regions, including the inlet region supporting the tricuspid valve, the trabeculated muscular septum, and the outlet septum forming the pulmonary annulus

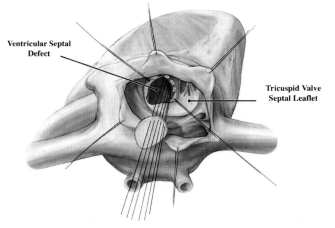

Ventricular Septal
Defect

Tricuspid Valve
Septal Leaflet

Fig. 9.3 A perimembranous ventricular septal defect seen through the tricuspid valve. The septal leaflet of the tricuspid valve is retracted superiorly. Sutures are placed into the right side of the septum to avoid creating heart block

septum. Furthermore, such defects can be completely surrounded by muscle and removed from all conduction tissue; yet, they may also exist as multiple coalescing holes termed *Swiss cheese* defect [8].

9.4 Atrioventricular Septal Defect

Atrioventricular septal defects, also referred to as *endocardial cushion defects* or *atrioventricular canal defects*, are typically characterized by a common atrioventricular junction [9]. Such defects are primarily due to the absence of the membranous atrioventricular septum with concomitant deficiencies in the overlying regions of the atrial and ventricular musculatures [10]. In general, atrioventricular septal defects may be placed into three separate categories based on the relative complexity of underlying anatomy: (1) partial AV canal defects; (2) transitional AV canal defects; and (3) complete AV canal defects.

A partial (incomplete) AV canal defect has an ostium primum atrial septal defect and a cleft in the anterior leaflet of the left atrioventricular valve. The important characteristic of this defect is that there are generally two distinct atrioventricular valves with separate annuli. A complete AV canal defect, representing the opposite extreme in this spectrum of anomalies, consists of a defect in the atrial and ventricular septum and is also associated with a single atrioventricular annulus with a varying number of remaining leaflets. More specifically, two dominate leaflets, the superior (anterior) and inferior (posterior), form the basis by which complete AV canal defects are generally classified. Finally, transitional AV canals have two distinct atrioventricular annuli with septal defects at both the atrial and ventricular levels [11].

9.5 Aortopulmonary Window Defect

The separation of the great vessels occurs when two opposing tissue cushions form on the right superior and left inferior portions of the common arterial trunk. Failure of these tissue cushions to properly develop will result in an *aortopulmonary defect* (Fig. 9.4) [12]. Previously, Mori and coworkers classified aortopulmonary defects into three types, based on their relative location [13]. Type I defects are the most common, and exist just above the atrioventricular valves. Type II aortopulmonary window defects are located in the most distal aspect of the ascending aorta, and thus surgical repairs are more complicated. Finally, Type III defects involve the majority of the ascending aortic pulmonary union.

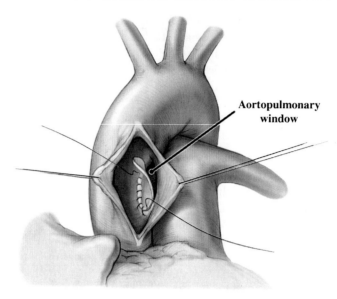

Fig. 9.4 An aortopulmonary window is created by a deficiency in the separation of the truncus. This defect is visualized through an incision in the ascending aorta

9.6 Coarctation of the Aorta

Coarctation of the aorta can be defined as varying degrees of obstruction to blood flow through the descending aorta. It should be noted that early attempts to classify these lesions as either infantile or adult have fostered confusion and debate [14]. Hence, these and other terms, such as pre- and post-ductal, should be considered as anatomically incorrect as they provide little value in planning the subsequent surgical correction. In the early 1990s, Amato and colleagues proposed a classification system based on the degree of aortic hypoplasia and existence of associated cardiac lesions (Table 9.4) [15]. In this scheme, Type I lesions are defined to involve narrowing of the segment of aorta adjacent to the insertion of the ductus arteriosus (Fig. 9.5); Type II defects involve the primary site of narrowing (Type I) in association with hypoplasia of the segment of the aorta between the left subclavian artery and the ductus arteriosus (*isthmus hypoplasia*); and Type III is the most severe form of coarctation, in which there is severe hypoplasia in a large portion of the aortic arch. In these later cases, the

Table 9.4 Coarctation of the aorta

Type I	Primary coarctation
Type II	Coarctation with isthmus hypoplasia
Type III	Coarctation with tubular hypoplasia of the distal arch
	• Coarctation associated with ventricular septal defects
	• Coarctation associated with other major cardiac defects

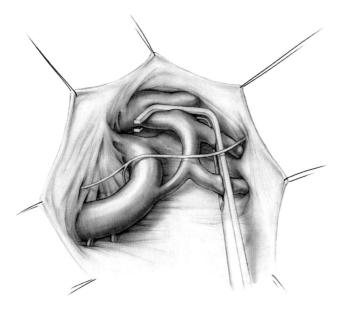

Fig. 9.5 Coarctation of the newborn is often associated with severe hypoplasia of the transverse aortic arch. A proximal vascular clamp has been placed in preparation for coarctation resection. Notice the recurrent laryngeal nerve rapping around the ductus arteriosus

hypoplasia most often involves the segment of aorta between the left carotid artery and left subclavian artery.

9.7 Interrupted Aortic Arch

Interruption of the aortic arch involves complete loss of continuity between the ascending and descending aorta. Blood flow to the lower body is provided by a patent ductus arteriosus. In patients with an *interrupted aortic arch* (IAA) this defect is often associated with a large, posteriorly oriented ventricular septal defect. Back in the late 1950s, Celoria and Pattern [16] devised a classification system that continues to have both anatomic and surgical significance (Fig. 9.6). In this scheme, a Type "A"

interruption occurs when there is lack of continuity between the left subclavian artery and the descending aorta. In Type "B" interruptions, the defects occur between the left carotid artery and the left subclavian artery. In general, Type "C" is the rarest form and such defects occur between the innominate and the left carotid arteries.

9.8 Tetralogy of Fallot

Tetralogy of Fallot is described as a tetrad of malformations consisting of: (1) pulmonary artery stenosis; (2) a ventricular septal defect; (3) hypertrophy of the right ventricular outflow tract; and (4) an overriding of the aortic valve to the right (Fig. 9.7). Nevertheless, this

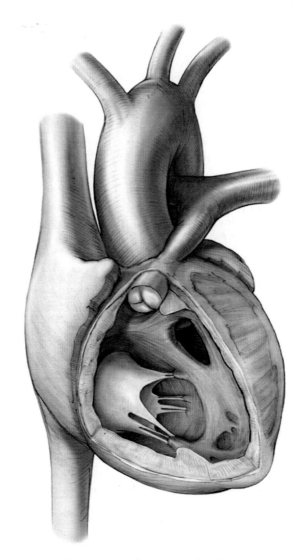

Fig. 9.7 Four components of Tetralogy of Fallot include pulmonary annular hypoplasia, a malaligned ventricular septal defect, right ventricular hypertrophy, and an overriding aortic annulus. The defect is viewed by removal of the right ventricular free wall

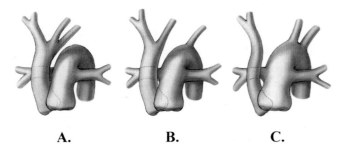

A.   **B.**   **C.**

Fig. 9.6 Classification scheme for interrupted aortic arch. Type A occurs when all the arch vessels originate proximal to the interruption. Type B occurs when the left subclavian artery originates distal to the discontinuous segment. Type C occurs when the left carotid originated distal to the discontinuous segment

constellation of defects can all be accounted for by hypoplasia of the subpulmonary infundibulum, and therefore should not be considered as a separate anomaly [17]. It should be noted that although an elaborate classification system has not evolved for this lesion, confusion with the terminology to describe the variants of tetralogy has persisted.

9.9 Pulmonary Atresia with Ventricular Septal Defect

Intense debate exists regarding the proper distinction between Tetralogy of Fallot with or without pulmonary atresia. For example, there are groups who believe that Tetralogy of Fallot with pulmonary atresia should be clinically grouped with all Tetralogy of Fallot patients. Still others feel that this defect should be a subgroup under the heading of pulmonary atresia with ventricular septal defect. Nevertheless, the surgical considerations and outcomes, however classified, are similar. It is of interest to note that, in an attempt to address these issues, Tchervenkov and Roy proposed a unifying classification system that is based on the anatomy and morphology of the pulmonary circulation [18]. As such, they place these defects into the category of pulmonary atresia with ventricular septal defect (PA-VSD). More specifically, in Type "A" PA-VSD, there are continuous pulmonary arteries with pulmonary blood flow being supplied by the ductus arteriosus; multiple aortopulmonary collateral arteries (MAPCA) are absent. It was further proposed that Type "B" includes those patients who have continuous pulmonary arteries in the presence of MAPCAs. Finally, Type "C" consists of no or discontinuous pulmonary arteries and multiple aortopulmonary collaterals.

9.10 Tricuspid Atresia

Tricuspid atresia involves complete absence of the right atrioventricular connection. The rudimentary right ventricular body lacks an inlet portion, while the size of the trabecular and outlet portion is typically determined by the size of the VSD and the nature of the ventriculoarterial connection. The most common valve morphology is a muscular atresia in which no tricuspid valvular tissue is found, but there is a dimple in the muscular floor of the right atrium [19]. Various described anatomic subtypes of tricuspid atresia are based on the morphology and orientation of the great vessels and have undergone several revisions over the last century [20, 21]. The most commonly employed classification system is divided into three types

Table 9.5 Tricuspid atresia

Normally related great vessels
- Type I (a) Pulmonary atresia
- Type I (b) Pulmonary hypoplasia, small VSD
- Type I (c) No pulmonary hypoplasia, large VSD

D-transposed great vessels
- Type II (a) Pulmonary atresia
- Type II (b) Pulmonary or subpulmonary stenosis
- Type II (c) Large pulmonary artery

L-transposed great vessels
- Type III (a) Pulmonary or subpulmonary stenosis
- Type III (b) Subaortic stenosis

based on the orientation of the great vessels: Type I, with normally related great vessels; Type II, in which the great vessels are transposed; and Type III, consisting of congenital corrected transposition of the great vessels (Table 9.5). It should be noted that each of these groups may be further subdivided based on the degree of obstruction to pulmonary blood flow. For example, subtype "a" consists of atretic pulmonary arteries, subtype "b" has either pulmonary stenosis or hypoplasia, and subtype "c" is made up of those individuals with no obstruction to pulmonary blood flow.

9.11 Ebstein's Anomaly

Ebstein's anomaly is characterized by structural defects within both the tricuspid valve and the right ventricle. Most commonly, the annulus of the tricuspid valve is displaced downward with a deformed and tethered anterior leaflet, and the right ventricle is dilated, with the atrialized portion cephalad to the tricuspid annulus being very thin [22]. In 1988, Carpentier and colleagues attempted to classify Ebstein's anomaly based on the relative volume of the right ventricle [23]. More specifically, these authors proposed four subtypes: Type A, the volume of the right ventricle is adequate; Type B, there is a large atrialized component of the right ventricle, but the anterior leaflet moves freely; Type C, the anterior leaflet is severely restrictive in its movement and may cause significant obstruction of the right ventricular outflow tract; and Type D in which there is almost complete atrialization of the ventricle, with the exception of a small infundibular component.

9.12 Transposition of the Great Vessels

Transposition of the great vessels is characterized by a reversal in the anatomic relationship of the great vessels with respect to the ventricles. In "D"-transposition of the great vessels, the pulmonary artery arises leftward and posterior to the aorta; these defects are physiologically uncorrected. The pulmonary artery is committed to the left ventricle, while the aorta arises from the right ventricle. "L"-transposition of the great vessels is synonymous with anatomically corrected transposition; the aortic valve is anterior and to the left of the pulmonary valve. In such cases, the aortic valve is connected to the left-sided morphologic right ventricle and the right ventricle receives oxygenated blood from the left ventricle. Long-term issues arise from the fact that the morphologic right ventricle is functioning as a systemic pump, with eventual failure being documented in several studies.

9.13 Total Anomalous Pulmonary Venous Connection

In *total anomalous pulmonary venous connection*, all of the pulmonary veins connect to the right atrium through one of several venous tributaries, i.e., none of the veins connect to the left atrium. The clinical classification systems for this defect have undergone several revisions; to date, the system set forth by Darling and associates has been widely accepted for use by the congenital cardiovascular community [24]. In general, this classification system is based on the origin of the anomalously draining veins: Type I, the anomalous connection is at a supracardiac level, either to a left superior vena cava or to the brachiocephalic vein; Type II, the connection is directly to the heart, either the coronary sinus or right atrium; Type III, anomalous veins originate from below the diaphragm, usually from the sinus venosus; and Type IV, consisting of a combination of two or more of the other types.

9.14 Persistent Truncus Arteriosus

Persistent truncus arteriosus, in general, consists of a single arterial vessel that arises from a common semilunar valve and overrides a larger VSD. The truncal artery supplies blood to the aorta, lungs, and coronary arteries [25]. Persistent truncus arteriosus results from failure of the truncal ridges and aortopulmonary septum to develop and divide into the aorta and pulmonary trunk. In 1949, Collett and Edwards described truncus arteriosus based on the origin of the pulmonary artery from the truncal artery [26]. Like many other congenital defects, several subtypes have been subsequently defined. Type I consists of an arterial trunk that originates from the common semilunar valve with its immediate bifurcation into a pulmonary artery and ascending aorta (Fig. 9.8). Type II

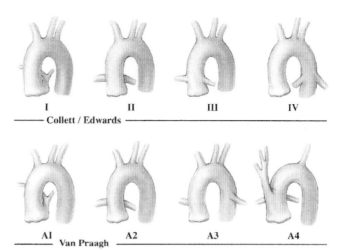

Fig. 9.8 Classification of truncus arteriosus

refers to a separate origin of the left and right pulmonary arteries from the posterior wall of the truncal artery. Type III describes similar anatomy as Type II, but with the right and left pulmonary arteries each originating further apart. In Type IV, often referred to as *pseudotruncus*, there is an absence of the main pulmonary artery, with the lungs receiving blood supply via pulmonary collaterals. It should be noted that, today, most would agree this entity should not be described as a truncal defect, but rather as a form of pulmonary atresia with VSD.

References

1. Van Praagh R. Terminology of congenital heart disease: Glossary and commentary. Circulation 1977;56:139.
2. Van Praagh R, Vlad P. Dextrocardia, mesocardia, and levocardia: The segmental approach in congenital Heart disease. In: Keith JD, Rowe RD, Vlad P, eds. Heart disease in infancy and childhood. 3rd ed. New York, NY: Macmillan, 1978.
3. Seo JW, Brown NA, Ho SY, Anderson RH. Abnormal laterality and congenital cardiac anomalies. Relations of visceral and cardiac morphologies in the mouse. Circulation 1992;86:642–50.
4. Anderson RH. Sinus kenosis interfacial communication and sinus node problems. Am J Cardiol 1987;59:724.
5. Shunmacker HB, King H, Waldhausen JA. The persistent left superior vena cava. Surgical implications, with special reference to caval drainage into the left atrium. Ann Surg 1967;165:797.
6. Wilcox BR, Cook AC, Anderson RH. Abnormal segmental connections. In: Wilcox, BR, Cook AC, Anderson RH, eds. Surgical anatomy of the heart. 3rd ed. United Kingdom: Cambridge University Press, 2005:157–70.
7. Van Praagh R, Geva AT, Kreutzer J. Ventricular septal defects: How shall we describe, name and classify them? J Am Coll Cardiol 1989;14:1298–9.
8. Mace L, Dervanian P, Le Bret E, et al. "Swiss cheese" septal defects: Surgical closure using a single patch with intermediate fixings. Ann Thorac Surg 1999;67:1754–8.
9. Becker AE, Anderson RH. Atrioventricular septal defects: What's in a name? J Thorac Cardiovasc Surg 1982;83:461–9.

10. Wilcox BR, Cook AC, Anderson RH. Abnormal segmental connections. In: Wilcox, BR, Cook AC, Anderson RH, eds. Surgical anatomy of the heart. 3rd ed. United Kingdom: Cambridge University Press, 2005:141–57.

11. Penkoske PA, Neches WH, Anderson RH, Zuberbuhler JR. Further observations on the morphology of atrioventricular septal defects. J Thorac Cardiovasc Surg 1985;90:611–22.

12. Kutsche LM, Van Mierop LHS. Anatomy and pathogenesis of aortopulmonary septal defects. Am J Cardiol 1987;59:442.

13. Mori K, Ando M, Takao A. Distal type of aortopulmonary window: Report of 4 cases. Br Heart J 1978;40:681–9.

14. Bonnet LM. Congenital stenosis of the aorta. REV Med Paris 1903;104:227–30.

15. Amato JJ, Galdier RJ, Cotroneo JV. Role of extended aortoplasty related to the definition of coarctation of the aorta. AM Thorac Surg 1991;52:615–20.

16. Celoria GC, Pattern RP. Congenital absence of the aortic arch. Am Heart J 1959;58:407–20.

17. Van Praagh R, Van Praagh S, Nebesar R, Muster A, Sachehida N, Paul M. Tetralogy of Fallot: Underdevelopment of the pulmonary infundibulum and its sequelae. Am J Cardiol 1970;26:25–33.

18. Tchervenkov C, Roy N. Congenital heart surgery nomenclature and database project: Pulmonary atresia-ventricular septal defect. Ann Thorac Surg 2000;69:S97–105.

19. Wilcox BR, Cook AC, Anderson RH. Abnormal segmental connections. In: Wilcox, BR, Cook AC, Anderson RH, eds. Surgical anatomy of the heart. 3rd ed. United Kingdom: Cambridge University Press, 2005:229–36.

20. Edwards WS, Burchell HB. Congenital tricuspid atresia: A classification. Med Clin North Am 1949;33:1117–96.

21. Kuhne M. Ulber zwei salle congenitally amnesia des ostium venosum dextnmA. Jahrbuch fur kinderheikunde und physicks erziehung 1906;63:235.

22. Anderson KR, Zuberbuhler JR, Anderson RH. Morphologic spectrum of Ebstein's anomaly of the heart: A review. Mayo Clin Proc 1979;54:174–80.

23. Carpentier A, Chauvaud S, Mace L. A new reconstructive operation for Ebstein's anomaly of the tricuspid valve. J Thorac Cardiovasc Surg 1988;96:92–101.

24. Darling RC, Rothney WB, Craig JM. Total pulmonary venous drainage into the right side of the heart: Report of 17 autopsied cases not associated with other major cardiovascular anomalies. Lab Invest 1957;6:44–64.

25. Anderson R, Thiene G. Categorization and description of hearts with a common arterial trunk. Eur J Cardiothorac Surg 1989;3:481–7.

26. Collett RW, Edwards JE. Persistent trances arterioles: A classification according to anatomic types. Surg Clin North Am 1949;29:1245.

Part III
Physiology and Assessment

Chapter 10
Cellular Myocytes

Vincent A. Barnett

Abstract The function of the heart as a pump is ultimately dependent on the coordinated contractions of its chambers to move blood throughout the body. These contractions are produced by cardiac myocytes, the muscle cells of the heart. Understanding of the structure and function of these cells on an individual level provides insights into adaptations of the heart due to normal as well as pathophysiological changes over the course of a lifetime.

Keywords Actin · Action potential · Adenosine triphosphate (ATP) · Gap junctions · Intercalated disk · Membrane potential · Myofibril · Myosin · Sarcomere · Sarcoplasmic reticulum · Tropomyosin · Troponin · Transverse tubules

10.1 General Cellular Morphology

All human cells can be thought of as biological machines that are surrounded by a membrane bilayer (plasma membrane). The average thickness or diameter of a non-muscle cell is approximately 10–20 μm. The encapsulating membrane is primarily composed of a bilayer of phospholipids, bipolar molecules with hydrophilic head groups, and hydrophobic lipid tails (Fig. 10.1). In addition, the plasma membrane is studded with receptors (Fig. 10.1) for various biochemical signaling molecules (hormones, neurotransmitters, etc.). Also resident in the plasma membrane are a number of ion-specific pumps and channels which function to regulate the internal environment of the cell (endoplasm). The interior of each cell contains enzymes and organelles that are specialized to support a wide array of biological functions. Key organelles include the nucleus (which contains the genetic blueprint for cellular function), mitochondria (which converts various energy sources to adenosine triphosphate (ATP), the endoplasmic reticulum, and the Golgi apparatus (which supports protein synthesis).

10.2 Cardiac Muscle Cell Morphology

Muscle cells are similar in that they contain these common organelles, but distinct in that they also include an elaborate protein scaffold that is anchored to the cell membrane (Fig. 10.2). Force generation by proteins within the matrix leads to the contraction of the cells and pumping of blood by the heart. Mammalian cardiac cells are roughly cylindrical, but may also include short branch-like projections. Diameters of the cells are in the range of 10–20 μm and lengths are on the order of 50–100 μm. Force is produced primarily along the long axis of the cell. Most of the internal volume of myocytes is devoted to a cytoskeletal lattice of contractile proteins whose liquid crystalline order gives rise to a striated appearance under the microscope (Figs. 10.2 and 10.3). As with other cell types, the membrane bilayer contains a collection of ion channels and ion pumps and receptor proteins. In addition, the membranes of cardiac muscle cells contain proteins designed to connect cardiac myocytes to one another as both mechanical and electrical partners.

10.3 Cardiac Cell Membranes

The surface (or plasma) membranes of cardiac cells are punctuated by openings of membrane-lined channels, the *transverse tubules* (or T-tubules), that pass envagenated

V.A. Barnett (✉)
University of Minnesota, Department of Integrative Biology
and Physiology, 6-125 Jackson Hall, 321 Church St.
SE Minneapolis, MN 55455, USA
e-mail: barne014@umn.edu

Fig. 10.1 A typical mammalian cell. The intracellular environment is separated from the extracellular environment by a lipid bilayer membrane (see area encircled in figure). Each cell contains a nucleus containing chromosomes and a collection of organelles to support biosynthetic and other "housekeeping" tasks. Shown here are the endoplasmic reticulum, ribosomes, mitochondria, Golgi apparatus, lysosomes, various ion channels, and biochemical receptors

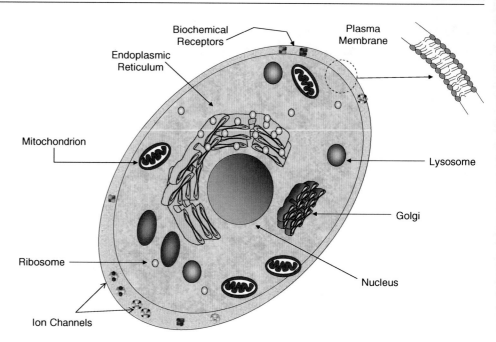

through the cell and are filled with extracellular fluid (Fig. 10.4). As they pass through the cell, the T-tubule network encircles internal contractile structures known as myofibrils. Abutting the T-tubules, in the sarcoplasm (cytoplasm) of the myocytes, is the sarcoplasmic (endoplasmic) reticulum, a cytosolic organelle that is specialized to store calcium. The T-tubules provide a pathway for conduction of action potentials through the entire thickness of a cardiac myocyte. Their close association with the sarcoplasmic reticulum helps to couple cardiac action potentials to the release of calcium from internal stores.

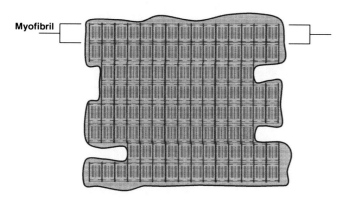

Fig. 10.2 A typical cardiac cell. The intracellular space is largely filled with contractile structures called myofibrils. The nucleus and other organelles that support cellular function are present, but are often crowded to the periphery by the contractile apparatus

10.4 Intercalated Disks

A structure referred to as the *intercalated disk* forms strong mechanical links between myocytes (Fig. 10.5). The intercalated disk structures are formed by the association of membrane-bound proteins on the surfaces of the neighboring cells. The protein components of these membrane plaques include N-cadherin, desmin, vinculin, α- and β-catenin, desmoplakin-1, desmocollin-2, and plakoglobin-2 [1, 2]. The tight cell-to-cell coupling of the intercalated discs contributes structural integrity to branches of myocardial cells. The connection of the cardiac myocytes in this manner facilitates some lateral shifting and the interdigitation of the cells. However, longitudinal shifting of cardiac myocytes relative to one another is practically impossible (Fig. 10.5). Importantly, it is the structural integrity of the intercalated disks between individual cells that allows force to be transmitted across the myocardium.

10.5 Gap Junctions

Gap junctions form electrical connections between cardiac cells [3]. Membrane proteins known as connexins form six-membered rings called connexons on the sarcolemma (surface) of cardiac cells (Fig. 10.6A). The connexons on the surface of one cell dock with connexons on the surface of a neighboring cell, forming a gap junction (Fig. 10.6B).

Fig. 10.3 A cross-section of cardiac tissue showing two cells separated by a blood vessel containing red blood cells. The repeating sarcomeric structure of the myofibrils and the names of the sarcomeric landmarks are highlighted on the *left* of the figure. On the *right* of the figure the legend points out the membrane specializations of the cell. These include the intercalated disks, gap junctions, the transverse tubules that punctuate the sarcolemma (plasma membrane), and the sarcoplasmic reticulum. Also shown are mitochondria compacted into a limited space because of the abundance of the myofibrils

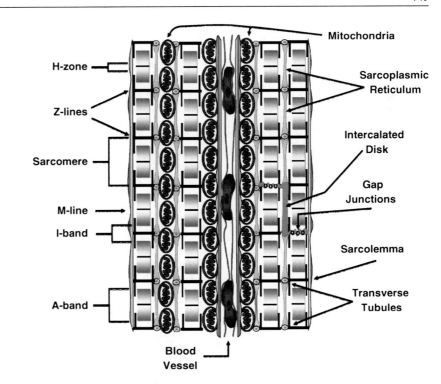

When gap junctions are open, they provide direct communication between the sarcoplasmic spaces of adjoining cells, creating a functional syncytium or network of synchronized cells. This connectivity allows activation signals to be passed from cell to cell in cardiac tissue. Electrical communication, provided by the gap junctions, facilitates the seemingly simultaneous, coordinated contractions of cardiac muscle. For more details on movement of electrical signals through heart tissue, the reader is referred to Chapter 11.

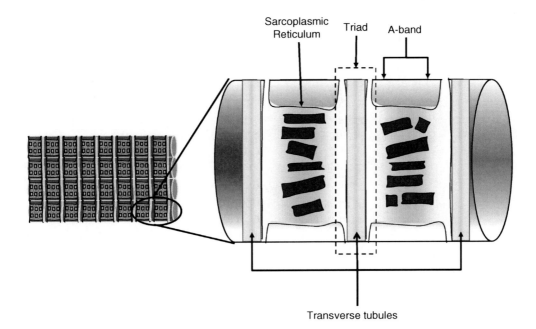

Fig. 10.4 A section of a cardiac cell showing the relationship of the sarcoplasmic reticulum and the transverse tubules (T-tubules). The sarcoplasmic reticulum surrounds each myofibril and lays adjacent to the T-tubules as they pass through a cardiac cell. The junction of the T-tubule with the adjacent sarcoplasmic reticulum is referred to as the *triad*. This close proximity allows the action potentials that pass through the T-tubular system to influence calcium release from the sarcoplasmic reticulum

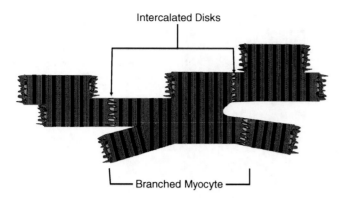

Intercalated Disks

Branched Myocyte

Fig. 10.5 A collection of interconnected cardiac muscle cells showing their characteristic branched structure. At the interface of adjoining cells there is an interconnection of membrane-bound proteins known as the intercalated disk. This structure mechanically couples the cardiac cells so that the forces generated by each cell are communicated through the vessels of the heart

A.

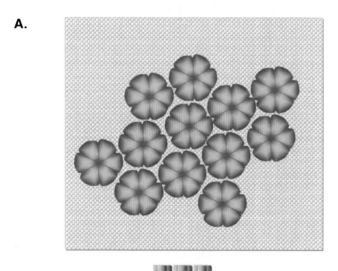

B.

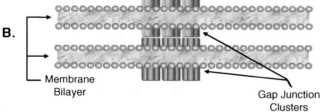

Membrane Bilayer

Gap Junction Clusters

Fig. 10.6 (**A**) Overhead representation of a plaque of connexons on a cardiac membrane. Six connexins form each pore structure (connexons) on the membrane surface which cluster in the intercalated disk regions at cell–cell interfaces. (**B**) Side view of the interface between two cells showing the docking of connexons to form a gap junction between adjacent cells

10.6 Myofibrillar Structure

The arrangement of the contractile proteins in cardiac muscle cells is similar to that found in skeletal muscle. The contractile subunits known as myofibrils run parallel to one another along the long axis of the cell (Fig. 10.2). Myofibrils fill most of the cytoplasmic space of each cardiac myocyte, with the remainder of the cell occupied by the normal intracellular machinery (Fig. 10.3). Each myofibril is composed of smaller contractile units called sarcomeres, the smallest functional unit in muscle (Figs. 10.3 and 10.7). It is the arrangement of contractile proteins into the sarcomeres that gives cardiac and skeletal muscle their characteristic striated appearance under microscopic examination. At regular intervals along each myofibril, a transverse matrix of the proteins α-actinin and actin forms boundaries known as *Z-disks* (or Z-lines; Fig. 10.7). A sarcomere is defined as the arrangement of contractile proteins that resides between two consecutive Z-disks along a myofibril. Actin filaments anchored on each face of a Z-disk extend for 1 μm toward the center of adjacent sarcomeres (thin filaments). Thick filaments of the protein myosin sit in the center of each sarcomere and extend toward the Z-disks at the ends of the sarcomere (thick filament length ~1.6 μm). The thick filaments are connected at their centers by a protein matrix referred to as the M-line (or M-disk). The region of the sarcomere in which the myosin filaments reside is known as the "A-band" (Figs. 10.3 and 10.7). The area between A-bands is known as the *I-band*; each I-band is bisected by a Z-line and is traversed by the actin thin filaments (Figs. 10.3 and 10.7).

10.7 Thin Filament

As noted above, the principle structural component of the thin filaments is a double-stranded filament of the globular protein actin (Fig. 10.7). The thin filaments also incorporate the regulatory proteins tropomyosin (Tm) and troponin (Tn). Tropomyosin is a double-stranded α-helical coiled-coil protein that spans seven actin monomers (~35 nm). Troponin is a globular protein complex with three subunits: TnC, a calcium-binding subunit; TnI, a subunit which facilitates inhibition of muscle contraction; and TnT, a subunit that connects the troponin complex to tropomyosin and actin. Tropomyosin molecules are aligned end to end around the helical coil of the thin filament with one Tn complex attached to each Tm molecule. In relaxed muscle, the track traced by tropomyosin as it binds to actin on the thin filament impedes the binding of the myosin heads to actin-binding sites [4]. However, upon muscle activation and the subsequent increase in myoplasmic calcium concentrations, free calcium binds to TnC inducing a conformational change of the entire troponin complex that is transmitted to tropomyosin. Tm then shifts its position on the actin thin filament revealing the site on actin required for strong myosin binding. Myosin can then bind to the thin

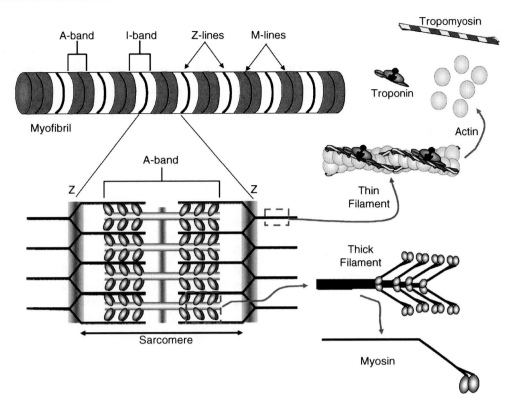

Fig. 10.7 Myofibrils are constructed of repeating sarcomeres within cardiac muscle cells. Each sarcomere is defined as the structures bounded on each end by Z-disks (Z-lines). Thin filaments of the protein actin are attached to the Z-line and reach toward the center of each sarcomere. Two regulatory proteins are found on the double-stranded actin thin filaments—tropomyosin and troponin. Tropomyosin is a double-stranded a-helical protein dimer that binds across seven actin monomers on the thin filament obscuring a binding site for myosin. Troponin is a three-subunit globular protein that binds one per tropomyosin. Thick filaments of the protein myosin are found in the center of the sarcomere. The area that contains the thick filaments is also known as the A-band. The myosin molecules are asymmetrically shaped with a coiled-coil "tail" and two globular "head" domains. The head domains bind to actin to form crossbridges between the filaments and generate contractile force

filament in a manner conducive to force production. This association of a tropomyosin–troponin complex over seven actin monomers represents a de facto regulatory subunit along the thin filament. The overlap of Tm molecules creates a mechanism for the communication of the activation signal along the thin filament making the initiation of force generation via this mechanism highly cooperative [4].

This thin filament-based mechanism for the regulation of contraction is also used for the control of skeletal muscle. In contrast, the activation of smooth muscle, the muscle of the vascular system, gut, and airways is also calcium dependent. However in smooth muscle troponin is absent. The rise in calcium concentration is sensed by the cytosolic protein calmodulin and activation occurs via a different thick filament-based mechanism.

10.8 Thick Filament

Myosin is the molecular motor protein responsible for force production and movement of muscle cells. The protein is asymmetrically shaped with a long alpha-helical

"tail" and two globular "head" domains (Fig. 10.7). The tails associate in an anti-parallel manner to form the backbone of the thick filament. This results in a bipolar structure that has a bare zone in the center and the globular "head" domains of the myosin molecules projecting from each end. These head domains contain an actin-binding site and an ATP hydrolysis site. As will be discussed later, the cyclic interaction of these head domains to the actin thin filaments forming crossbridges provides the underlying mechanism for myocyte contraction.

10.9 Energy Metabolism

ATP production in cardiac muscle is primarily accomplished via oxidative phosphorylation. Oxidative phosphorylation is a multistep enzymatic process that extracts energy primarily from glucose and other energy-rich compounds and converts it to ATP. The energy extraction and ATP production occur in the mitochondria found in the cytoplasmic space of cardiac myocytes.

Intracellular concentrations of ATP hover in the 4–5 mM range, with additional energy stored in creatine phosphate which acts as a backup to the ATP supply. Creatine phosphate (~20 mM) can be used to regenerate ATP in a one-step enzymatic process catalyzed by the enzyme creatine kinase. There is an absolute requirement for oxygen in the ATP production mechanism and it is the reason that blood flow to the heart is so critical. The amount of ATP and creatine phosphate normally present is insufficient to power the contractile activities and other uses of ATP in heart cells for more than a few beats. For a more detailed description see Chapter 19.

10.10 Force Production: The Crossbridge Cycle

During diastole, myosin crossbridges bind ATP and hydrolyze it, but cannot use the energy released during hydrolysis to produce force (Fig. 10.8) because of the inhibition of tropomyosin and troponin on the thin filament. The hydrolytic event (Fig. 10.8, Step 1) induces a conformational change in myosin that allows it to hold on to the products of ATP hydrolysis (inorganic phosphate (Pi) and adenosine diphosphate (ADP)). It also retains most of the energy released during the hydrolysis of the high-energy phosphate bond of ATP. During systole, calcium from the extracellular milieu and the sarcoplasmic reticulum floods the cytoplasm, raising the intracellular concentration of calcium rises from micromolar to millimolar levels (Fig. 10.10). The binding of calcium to troponin removes the inhibition of the Tm–Tn complex on the thin filament. The energized myosin crossbridges can then bind to actin to the thin filament (Fig. 10.8, Step 2). This association with actin catalyzes the release of Pi and ADP, and a concomitant force-generating conformational change of the myosin head occurs while it is bound to actin (Fig. 10.8, Step 3). The conformational change pulls the thin filament past the thick filament. At the end of the force-generating transition, myosin can rebind ATP (Fig. 10.8, Step 4) which reduces the affinity of the crossbridge for actin and causes crossbridge detachment. The subsequent hydrolysis of the myosin-bound ATP, in turn, reenergizes the crossbridge and prepares it for the next force-generating cycle. The cycle continues as long as the calcium concentration is high enough to keep the Tm–Tn complexes from blocking the myosin-binding sites.

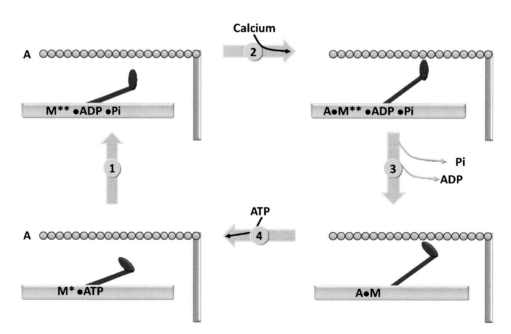

Fig. 10.8 Crossbridge cycle. Step 1: Myosin (M) binds ATP on its globular head domain and hydrolyzes it to ADP and phosphate (Pi); the energized myosin crossbridge (M**ADP-Pi) then waits for activation of the actin (A) thin filament. Step 2: After activation, the energized crossbridge binds to the actin thin filament. Step 3: The association with actin triggers the rapid release of ATP hydrolysis products ADP and Pi from the crossbridge; the release of ADP and Pi is coupled to a conformational change of the crossbridge domain which produces force, pulling the actin thin filament relative to the thick filament. Step 4: ATP binds to the crossbridge as it completes its powerstroke causing the dissociation of myosin and actin; this forms the M*ATP state as the conformation of myosin changes again. The crossbridge cycle continues as long as the intracellular calcium concentration is high. At rest the system sits with myosin in an equilibrium between the M*ATP state and the M**ADP-Pi state

10.11 Length–Tension Relationship

The myofibrils of a cardiac myocyte are tethered to the membranes and intercalated disks at each end of the cell via connective protein linkages. Cell length is a dynamic variable with shortening of a cardiac cell occurring with each systolic contraction and stretch of the cell occurring during each diastole as the chambers refill with blood. This means that the myofibrils and sarcomeres also shorten and lengthen during the cardiac cycle. It is important then to realize that there is a direct connection between the overlap of the thick and thin filaments and the resultant force output developed by cardiac muscle cells.

It is therefore fairly straightforward to see that when the majority of crossbridges are capable of binding to actin and thus inducing force, the cell will produce its maximum force. Sarcomere length is simply the distance from one Z-line to the next Z-line along a myofibril. In general, when the sarcomere length is approximately $2\,\mu m$, nearly all of the myosin crossbridge domains can bind to the thin filaments and maximal isometric force can be elicited (Fig. 10.9). It is also relatively straightforward to see that if the myocyte is stretched, potential force decreases because of the decrease in overlap of the thick and thin filaments; this is because of the reduced potential for possible crossbridge formations (Fig. 10.9). If the myocyte is shortened from the full overlap position and then activated, the subsequent force generation also decreases but for a different reason. We have already stated that the arrangement of the thick and thin

filaments in the sarcomere is semi-crystalline. When the cells become overshortened, several types of filament misalignment are possible such as: (1) the thick filaments can run into the Z-disks and become disordered; or (2) the thin filaments can cross the M-line and interact with each other or with myosin crossbridges from the other half-sarcomere. This disorder and/or interference that may occur in an overly shortened sarcomere are the cause for the decrease in myocyte tension. From the graph of the length–tension relationship (Fig. 10.9), you will notice a peak representing the noncompressed full overlap position. Shortening or lengthening the myocyte from this set point will decrease resultant muscle tension. In a normal cardiac cycle, the cell shortens during systole and has its length reset by stretching of the vessel wall during diastole. Since adjustment of the cell length changes the amount of force (or pressure) that can be generated, it is sometimes referred to as the preload of the cell.

10.11.1 Practical Applications of the Length–Tension Relationship

In general, the length of cardiac cells or myocytes is controlled in vivo through their shortening during systole and their being stretched during diastole (Fig. 10.9). That the set point of the length–tension relationship can be tuned in this manner is, in part, the mechanical underpinning for Starling's Law of the Heart (e.g., stroke volume increases as cardiac filling increases). Furthermore, if cardiac filling

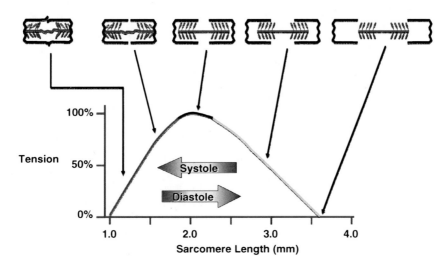

Fig. 10.9 Length–tension relationship. Mechanical coupling between the myofibrils and the membrane are such that a stretch or contraction of the cell alters the overlap of the thin and thick filaments of each sarcomere. At a sarcomere length of near $2.1\,\mu m$, there is complete overlap of the thick and thin filaments; if the length is unchanged, the cells have their maximal force production potential. At sarcomere lengths less than $\sim 1.8\,\mu m$, the filaments become compressed in the sarcomere and interfere with one another, reducing the force that can be produced. As the sarcomere length is increased from the region that produces maximal force, the overlap of the crossbridge domains of the thick filament and the thin filament decreases with a near linear decline in force-generating potential

adjusts the sarcomere length to a point closer to the plateau of the length–tension relationship (Fig. 10.9), this length change produces an alignment of the contractile proteins that can then result in greater force production during the next systolic period. It then also follows that the increased force, which can occur during the isovolumic (isometric) phase of systole, will result in a greater stroke volume. However, in hypertrophic cardiomyopathies, filling pressures are less likely to stretch the myocytes and reset the length of the cells. In contrast, in dilated myopathies, myocytes may be overstretched during diastole, reducing the pressure-building capacity of ventricular muscle.

10.12 Force and Velocity

The velocity of muscle cell shortening depends on the load that it works against. In cardiac muscle the load for the left ventricle is the systemic blood pressure and it is referred to as the *afterload*. Importantly, as afterload increases the velocity of myocyte shortening decreases. This relationship can impact ejection fraction as the ventricles are less effective in expelling blood against high systemic pressures.

10.13 Cardiac Cell Action Potentials

The electrical activity of cardiac muscle cells is fundamental to normal function and takes advantage of the properties of the cell membrane to selectively pass charged species from inside to outside and vice versa. Most cells build a charge gradient through the action of ion pumps and ion selective channels. The charge difference across a membrane creates an electrical potential known as the resting membrane potential of the cell. In the resting state, the interior of the cell carries a negative charge relative to the exterior interstitial environment. The energy related through the discharging of this potential is commonly coupled with cellular functions. In excitable cells, transient changes in the electrical potential (action potentials) are used to either communicate or do work. Importantly, in the myocyte, action potentials required to initiate the process known as *excitation contraction coupling*.

The extracellular fluid has an ionic composition similar to that of blood serum. The total intracellular concentration of calcium is higher, but much of it is bound to proteins or sequestered in organelles (mitochondria, sarcoplasmic reticulum). Hence, free myoplasmic concentrations are very low and are in the micromolar range (Table 10.1).

Table 10.1 Major ionic species contributing to the resting potential of cardiac muscle cells

Ion	Inside (mM)	Outside (mM)	Ratio of inside/outside	E_{ion}* (mV)
Sodium	15	145	9.7	+60
Potassium	150	4	0.027	−94
Chloride	5	120	24	−83
Calcium	10^{-7}	2	2×10^4	+129

*E_{ion} is the equilibrium potential calculated from the Nernst equation.

ATP-dependent ion pumps, ion-specific channel proteins, and ion exchange proteins are all required to maintain the difference in ion concentrations. This separation of charged species across a resistive barrier (in this case, the cell membrane) generates the electrical potential (E_{ion}) mentioned above. For individual ions, the value of this potential can be calculated using the Nernst equation:

$$E_{ion} = -\frac{RT}{zF} \ln \frac{[\text{outside}]}{[\text{inside}]}$$

where R is the gas constant, T is the temperature (K), z is the valence of the ion (charge and magnitude), and F is the Faraday constant.

In Table 10.1, the concentrations of the ions (inside and outside) that play a role in the resting membrane potential of cardiac muscle cells are shown with their respective calculated equilibrium potentials. The measured membrane potential of a cardiac muscle cell is in the range of −90 mV, suggesting that it is primarily determined by either the chloride or potassium distribution. However, measurements of ion movements have shown that chloride is distributed passively across the cell membrane (because of its negative charge, it follows positive ion movement) and can therefore be ignored in such a calculation; this leaves potassium as the dominant ion species in determining the resting potential of the cardiac myocyte.

The membrane potentials of living cells depend not just on the potassium distribution, but also on several parameters including the concentrations of the other major ion species on both sides of the membrane as well as their relative permeabilities. To determine the overall membrane potential (E_m), a modified Goldman–Hodgkin–Katz equation [5] is used to take into account the equilibrium potentials for individual ions and the permeability (conductance) of the membrane for each species such that

$$E_m = \frac{g_{Na}}{g_{tot}} E_{Na} + \frac{g_K}{g_{tot}} E_K + \frac{g_{Ca}}{g_{tot}} E_{Ca}$$

where g_{Na} is the membrane conductance for sodium (Na), g_K is the membrane conductance for potassium (K), g_{Ca} is the membrane conductance for calcium (Ca), g_{tot} is the total membrane conductance, E_{Na} is the equilibrium potential for sodium, E_K is the equilibrium potential for potassium, and E_{Ca} is the equilibrium potential for calcium. Evaluation of the Goldman–Hodgkin–Katz equation using the values in Table 10.1 and the conductance values for sodium, potassium, and calcium results in a membrane potential of –90 mV.

As noted above, cells can have a variety of ion selective channels in their membranes. The term gating refers to the trigger required for opening such a channel. More specifically, voltage-gated ion channels respond to changes in the local membrane potential of the cell, and ligand-gated ion channels respond to specific circulating biochemical factors; spontaneously active ion channels have a random frequency of opening and closing, whereas leak channels seem to be constitutively open though at a low level. In addition to classification based on their control mechanisms, channels are also classified by their ion selectivity and/or the direction of ion passage that such a channel facilitates.

Cardiac action potentials occur because of transient changes in the cellular permeability to Na^+, Ca^{2+}, and K^+. An initial electrical depolarization (threshold is $\sim$40 mV above the resting potential) causes the transient opening of voltage-dependent Na-channels (Figs. 10.10 and 10.12). This brief increase in sodium permeability further depolarizes the cell and drives the membrane potential toward the sodium equilibrium potential (Table 10.1; Figs. 10.10 and 10.12). The larger magnitude depolarization activates voltage-gated Ca- and K-channels. The subsequent opening of the voltage-gated L-type (long opening duration) calcium channels allows calcium to enter the myocyte and sustains the depolarized state. The opening of the voltage-gated K-channels allows potassium efflux from the cell and thus drives the membrane potential back toward the potassium equilibrium potential (more negative) (Fig. 10.11). The timing of these changes depends on the isoforms of the Ca- and K-channel proteins present in each cell, with sinoatrial and atrioventricular action potentials lasting $\sim$150 ms, ventricular muscle $\sim$250 ms,

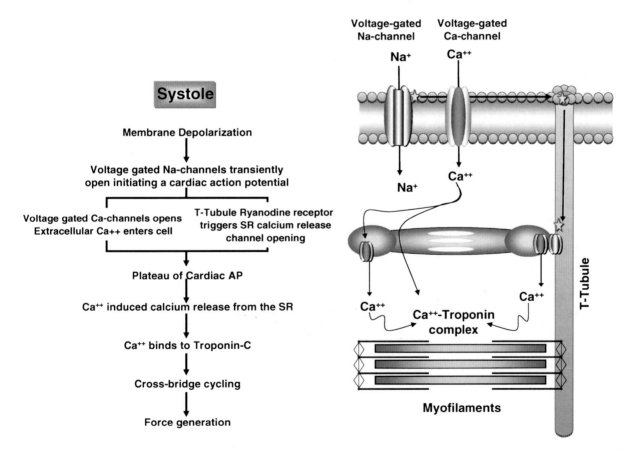

Fig. 10.10 Excitation contraction coupling. In systole, an electrically depolarizing signal triggers the transient opening of voltage-gated Na-channels; the influx of positively charged Na ions further depolarizes the cell. This further depolarization causes the opening of L-type Ca-channels (long duration opening) and calcium enters the cell. This also causes ryanodine receptors in the T-tubules to trigger the release of calcium from Ca-channels in the sarcoplasmic reticulum. This initiates the plateau of the cardiac action potential. The rise in intracellular calcium concentration triggers additional calcium release from the sarcoplasmic reticulum via Ca-channels. The calcium binds to troponin on the thin filaments, inducing the movement of tropomyosin. Crossbridge cycling begins generating tension in the cardiac myocytes

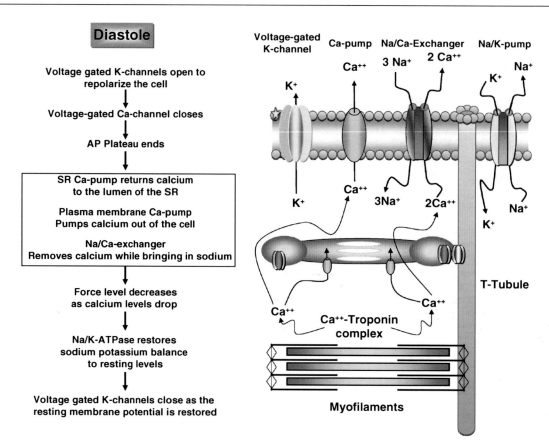

Fig. 10.11 Relaxation of cardiac muscle cells. The depolarization eventually opens voltage-gated K-channels. K flows out of the cell and, as the sarcolemmal Ca-channels close, the cell begins to repolarize. Calcium is pumped out of the cytoplasm by ATP-driven pump proteins on the sarcoplasmic reticulum and sarcolemma. Calcium is also expelled from the cell via the Na/Ca-exchange protein. To combat the rise in intracellular Na that this causes, the Na/K-ATPase pumps K into the cell and Na out, helping to restore the resting potential and the ionic environment that existed before the cell was activated

and Purkinje fingers ~300 ms (also see Chapter 11). The primary difference between these cell types is often the duration of the plateau phase (phase 2) which is primarily a response to Ca-channels (Figs. 10.12 and 10.13).

The various phases of the cardiac action potential are associated with changes in the flow of ionic currents across the cell membrane. Atrial and ventricular cardiac muscle cells have an extremely rapid initial transition from the resting membrane potential to depolarization (*phase 0*). In phase 0, the Na-channels open and there is a large-amplitude, short-duration inward Na-current (Fig. 10.13). As the sodium channels begin to close, *phase 1* is defined as a small initial repolarization. The opening of the L-type calcium channels causes a calcium influx and is balanced by the potassium efflux via the now open K-channels. This balance results in the electrically positive plateau (*phase 2*) of the cardiac action potential profile. As the Ca-channels close, the flux of ions through the K-channels begins to dominate the membrane potential and repolarization of the cells begins (*phase 3*). *Phase 4* is the restoration of the resting membrane potential and

the closing of the K-channels. From the initiation of the action potential through approximately half of the repolarization, the cell is considered refractory, meaning that it could not respond to a new depolarization signal.

10.14 Pacemaker Cells

The sinoatrial and atrioventricular nodal cells have what is considered to be unstable resting potentials; a gradual rise in resting potential crosses the threshold for opening of T-type (transiently open) calcium channels. The movement of calcium into the cells (phase 0) initiates depolarization. No initial repolarization or plateau occurs, so phases 1 and 2 are said to be absent. Repolarization (phase 3) is accomplished through the opening of voltage-gated K-channels. Once the cell is repolarized (phase 4), leak channels (often attributed to slow Na-channels) contribute to instability of the resting potential and a gradual rise to the threshold value of the T-type Ca-channels (Fig. 10.12).

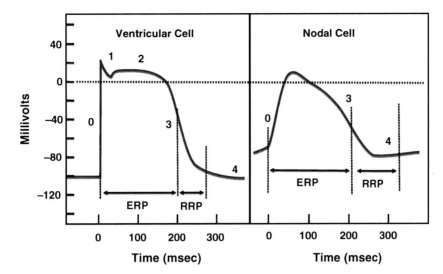

Fig. 10.12 Action potential profiles for ventricular and nodal cardiac cells. *Ventricular cell*: Before activation, the cell's membrane potential is negative (phase 0—*upstroke*). A small depolarizing event triggers the opening of voltage-gated Na-channels (phase 1—*initial repolarization*). As the Na-channels close, there is a small recovery in polarization; the voltage-gated Ca- and K-channels open followed by a *plateau* (phase 2) in the membrane potential. In phase 3—*repolarization,* as the Ca-channels close, the K-channels remain open and the membrane potential grows more negative eventually returning to *resting membrane potential* level (phase 4) where the K-channels also close. From phase 0 through the middle of phase 3 is the effectively refractory period (ERP), meaning that another depolarization would not trigger the opening of the Na-channels. The remainder of phase 3 is the relative refractory period (RRP); a new depolarizing signal would cause some of the Na-channels to reopen. *Nodal cell*: Pacemaker cells have a different electrical signature to their action potentials. The cells spontaneously rise to the threshold of T-type Ca-channels whose opening is the cause of phase 0 upstroke that is not as rapid as that of the ventricular cells. There is no phase 1 or 2 as in ventricular cells. The opening of voltage-gated K-channels causes repolarization—phase 3, ultimately reaching an unstable resting potential minimum from which the cells repeat the cycle. The spontaneous rise of the membrane potential has been attributed to leaky Na-channels. The refractory periods of nodal cells reflect the potential for opening the T-type Ca- channels

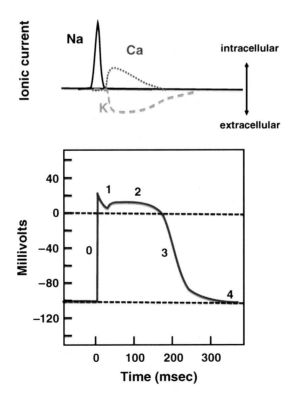

Fig. 10.13 Ionic currents corresponding to the phases of the ventricular action potential. The inward current associated with the opening of the voltage-gated Na-channels is responsible for phase 0 of the cardiac action potential. The closing of the Na-channels is reflected in the initial repolarization of phase 1. The depolarization of the cell by the Na-current triggers the opening of the voltage-gated Ca-channels and the voltage-gated K-channels whose ionic currents are in balance during phase 2, the plateau. The closing of the Ca-channels while the K-channels are still passing an outward current causes the repolarization (phase 3) and return to the resting membrane potential (phase 4)

The sinoatrial node is a specialized collection of cardiac myocytes in the right atrium. These cells have unstable resting potentials that lead to spontaneous depolarizations of this cell cluster with a relatively rapid and regular repeat (i.e., more rapid than all other myocytes). Cardiac activation is governed by the principle of overdrive suppression. This principle states that the myocytes with the most rapid frequency of depolarization control the overall rhythm of the heart. Furthermore, the action potential of the sinoatrial node is referred to as a "slow response" because the upstroke of the depolarization is slower than that of the non-nodal cardiac cells that provide the contractile force during atrial or ventricular contraction. However, the rapid repeat of this depolarization gives the sinoatrial node overall control of the heart rate. For additional details on this process see the next chapter.

References

1. Colaco CALS, Evans WH. A biochemical dissection of the cardiac intercalated disk: Isolation of subcellular fractions containing fascia adherentes and gap junctions. J Cell Sci 1981;52:313–25.
2. Kaplan SR, Gard JJ, Protonotarios N, et al. Remodeling of myocyte gap junctions in arrhythmogenic right ventricular cardiomyopathy due to a deletion in plakoglobin (Naxos disease). Heart Rhythm 2004;1:3–11.
3. Beauchamp P, Yamada KA, Baertschi AJ, et al. Relative contributions of connexins 40 and 43 to atrial impulse propagation in synthetic strands of neonatal and fetal murine cardiomyocytes. Circ Res 2006;99:1216–24.
4. Boussouf SE, Geeves MA. Tropomyosin and troponin cooperativity on the thin filament. Adv Exp Med Biol 2007;592:99–109.
5. Sperelakis N. Origin of the cardiac resting potential. In: Berne RM, Sperelakis N, Geiger SR, eds. The handbook of physiology Section 2, The cardiovascular system Section 1. American Physiological Society, 1979:187–267.

Other Resources

Berne RM, Levy MN, eds. Cardiovascular physiology. 7th ed. St. Louis: Mosby, 1979. Chapter 2, Electrical activity of the heart, pp. 7–54; Chapter 3, The cardiac pump, pp. 55–82.

Berne RM, Levy MN, eds. Physiology. 4th ed. St. Louis: Mosby, 1998. Chapter 23, The cardiac pump, pp. 360–78.

Costanzo LS. Physiology. Philadelphia: Saunders, 1998. Chapter 4, Cardiovascular physiology, pp. 99–162.

Germann W, Stanfield C, eds. Principles of human physiology. San Francisco: Benjamin Cummings, 2002. Chapter 12, The cardiovascular system: Cardiac function, pp. 369–402.

Mohrman DE, Heller LJ, eds. Cardiovascular physiology. 5th ed. New York: McGraw-Hill, 2003. Chapter 2, Characteristics of cardiac muscle cells, pp. 19–46.

Rhoades RA, Tanner GA, eds. Medical physiology. Boston: Little, Brown, 1995. Chapter 10, Cardiac muscle, pp. 193–206.

Vander A, Sherman J, Luciano D. Human physiology: The mechanisms of body function. 8th ed. Boston: McGraw-Hill, 2001. Chapter 14, Section C: The heart, pp. 387–406.

Chapter 11
The Cardiac Conduction System

Timothy G. Laske, Maneesh Shrivastav, and Paul A. Iaizzo

Abstract The intrinsic conduction system of the heart is comprised of several specialized subpopulations of cells that either spontaneously generate electrical activity (pacemaker cells) or preferentially conduct this activity throughout the chambers in a coordinated fashion. This chapter will discuss the details of this known anatomy as well as put such discoveries into a historical context. The cardiac action potential underlies signaling within the heart and the various populations of myocytes will elicit signature waveforms. The recording or active sensing of these potentials is important in both research and clinical arenas. This chapter aims to provide a basic understanding of the cardiac conduction system to provide the reader with a foundation for future research and reading on this topic. The information in this chapter is not comprehensive and should not be used to make decisions relating to patient care.

Keywords Cardiac conduction · Sinoatrial node · Depolarization · Atrioventricular node · Electrophysiology · Cardiac action potential · Gap junction

11.1 Introduction

Orderly contractions of the atria and ventricles are regulated by the transmission of electrical impulses that pass through an intricate network of modified cardiac muscle cells, "the cardiac conduction system." These cells are interposed within the contractile myocardium. This intrinsic conduction system is comprised of several specialized subpopulations of cells that spontaneously generate electrical activity (pacemaker cells) and/or preferentially conduct this activity throughout the heart. Following an initiating activation (or depolarization) within the

myocardium, this electrical excitation spreads throughout the heart in a rapid and highly coordinated fashion. This system of cells also functionally controls the timing of the transfer of activity between the atrial and ventricular chambers. Interestingly, a common global architecture is present in mammals, but significant interspecies differences exist at the histologic level [1, 2] (see also Chapter 6).

Discoveries relating to this intrinsic conduction system within the heart are relatively recent relative to cardiac function and anatomy. Johannes E. von Purkinje first described the ventricular conduction system in 1845 and Gaskell, an electrophysiologist, coined the phrase "heart block" in 1882. Importantly, Gaskell also related the presence of a slow ventricular rate to disassociation with the atria [3]. The discovery of the mammalian sinoatrial node was published by Sir Arthur Keith and Martin Flack in 1907 in the *Journal of Anatomy and Physiology*. Nevertheless, novel findings relating to the functionality of this node are still being made today [4].

The elucidation of the bundle of His is attributed to its namesake, Wilhelm His Jr. [5], who described the presence in the heart of a conduction pathway from the atrioventricular node through the cardiac skeleton that eventually connected to the ventricles. Tawara later verified the existence of the bundle of His in 1906 [6]. Due to the difficulty in distinguishing the atrioventricular nodal tissue from the surrounding tissue, he defined the beginning of the bundle of His as the point at which these specialized atrioventricular nodal cells enter the central fibrous body (which delineates the atria from the ventricles). Tawara is also credited with being the first to clearly identify the specialized conduction tissues (modified myocytes) that span from the atrial septum to the ventricular apex, including the right and left bundle branches and Purkinje fibers.

Walter Karl Koch (1880–1962) was a distinguished German surgeon who discovered a triangular-shaped area in the right atrium of the heart that marks the atrioventricular node (known today as *Koch's triangle*). Among Koch's notable research findings was his hypothesis that the last

T.G. Laske (✉)
University of Minnesota, Department of Surgery, and Medtronic, Inc., 8200 Coral Sea St. NE, MVS84, Mounds view, MN 55112, USA
e-mail: tim.g.laske@medtronic.com

part of the heart to lose activity when the whole organ died was the pacemaker region (*ultimum moriens*). Koch localized this last region of the heart to lose function through his detailed anatomical and histological studies of the hearts of animals and stillborn human fetuses. He postulated that the cardiac region near the opening of the wall of the coronary sinus was the true pacemaker of the heart [7, 8]; the atrioventricular node will elicit an escape rhythm when the sinoatrial node in the right atrium fails (see below).

Early discoveries by distinguished researchers such as Koch, Tawara, and Aschoff have been immortalized in medical terminology (Koch's triangle, Tawara's node, and Aschoff's nodule). As history demonstrates, a thorough understanding of the anatomy and function of the cardiac conduction system is important for those designing cardiovascular devices and procedures. More specifically, surgical interventions (heart valve replacement repair, repair of septal defects, coronary bypass grafting, congenital heart repair, etc.) are commonly associated with temporary or permanent heart block due to trauma or damage of the conduction system and/or disruption of its blood supply [9–13]. Hence, if one is designing corrective procedures and/or devices to be used, she/he needs to consider ways to avoid damage to cellular structures of the conduction system. For example, advances in surgical techniques for the repair of ventricular septal defects have reduced the incidence of complete atrioventricular block from 16% in the 1950s to less than 1% currently [14, 15]. Additionally, many rhythm control devices such as pacemakers and defibrillators aim to return the patient to a normal rhythm and contraction sequence [16–24]. More recent research is even investigating repair/replacement of the intrinsic conduction system using gene therapies [25].

A final example illustrating why an understanding of the heart's conduction system is critical to the design of devices and procedures is the therapeutic use of cardiac ablation. These methodologies purposely modify the heart to: (1) destroy portions of the conduction system (e.g., atrioventricular nodal ablation in patients with permanent atrial fibrillation); (2) eliminate aberrant pathways (e.g., accessory pathway ablation in Wolff–Parkinson–White syndrome); and/or (3) destroy inappropriate substrate behavior (e.g., ablation of ectopic foci or reentrant pathways in ventricular tachycardias, Cox's Maze ablation for atrial fibrillation, etc.) [26–29].

11.2 Overview of Cardiac Conduction

The "sinoatrial node" is located in the right atrium in the healthy heart and serves as the natural pacemaker (Fig. 11.1). These pacemaker cells manifest spontaneous depolarizations and are thus responsible for generating

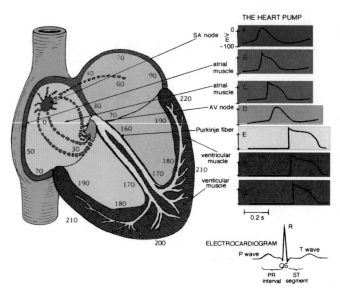

Fig. 11.1 The conduction system of the heart. Normal excitation originates in the sinoatrial node, then propagates through both atria (internodal tracts shown as *dashed lines*). The atrial depolarization spreads to the atrioventricular node, passes through the bundle of His (not labeled), and then to the Purkinje fibers which make up the left and right bundle branches; subsequently all ventricular muscle becomes activated. AV = atrioventricular; SA = sinoatrial

the normal cardiac rhythm; such a rhythm can also be described as intrinsic or automatic. Importantly, the frequency of this earliest depolarization is modulated by both sympathetic and parasympathetic efferent innervation. In addition, the nodal rate can also be modulated by local changes within perfusion and/or the chemical environment (neurohormonal, nutritional, oxygenation, etc.). Although the atrial rhythms normally emanate from the sinoatrial node, variations in the initiation site of atrial depolarization have been documented outside of the histological nodal tissues, particularly when high atrial rates are elicited [30–33].

One of the most conspicuous features of sinoatrial nodal cells is that they possess poorly developed contractile apparati (a common feature to all of the myocytes specialized for conduction), comprising only about 50% of the intracellular volume [34]. In general, although it cannot be seen grossly, the location of the sinoatrial node is on the "roof" of the right atrium at the approximate junctions of the superior vena cava, the right atrial appendage, and the sulcus terminalis. In the adult human, the node is approximately 1 mm below the epicardium, 10–20 mm long, and up to 5 mm thick [35]. For more details on cardiac anatomy, refer to Chapters 5 and 6.

After initial sinoatrial nodal excitation, depolarization spreads throughout the atria. The exact mechanisms involved in the spread of impulses (excitation) from the sinoatrial node across the atria are somewhat controversial [36]. However, it is generally accepted that: (1) the spread of depolarizations from nodal cells can go directly to adjacent myocardial cells; and (2) preferentially ordered myofibril pathways allow this excitation to rapidly traverse the right atrium to both the left atrium and the atrioventricular node. It is believed that there are three preferential anatomic conduction pathways from the sinoatrial node to the atrioventricular node (known as the node of Tawara) [37]. In general, these can be considered as the shortest electrical routes between the nodes. They are microscopically identifiable structures, appearing to be preferentially oriented fibers that provide a direct node-to-node pathway. In some hearts, pale staining Purkinje-like fibers have also been reported in these regions (tracts are shown as dashed lines in Fig. 11.1; also see JPG 11.1 on the Companion CD). More specifically, the anterior tract is described as extending from the anterior part of the sinoatrial node, bifurcating into the so-called Bachman's bundle (delivering impulses to the left atrium) and a second tract that descends along the interatrial septum which connects to the anterior part of the atrioventricular node. The middle (or Wenckebach's pathway) extends from the superior part of the sinoatrial node, runs posteriorly to the superior vena cava, then descends within the atrial septum, and may join the anterior bundle as it enters the atrioventricular node. The third pathway is described as being posterior (Thorel's) which, in general, is considered to extend from the inferior part of the sinoatrial node, passing through the crista terminalis and the Eustachian valve past the coronary sinus to enter the posterior portion of the atrioventricular node. In addition to excitation along these preferential conduction pathways, general excitation spreads from cell to cell throughout the entire atrial myocardium via the specialized connections between cells, "the gap junctions," which exist between all myocardial cell types (see below).

Toward the end of atrial depolarization, the excitatory signal reaches the atrioventricular node. This excitation reaches these cells via the aforementioned atrial routes, with the final excitation of the atrioventricular node generally described as occurring via the slow or fast pathways. The slow and fast pathways are functionally, and usually anatomically, distinct routes to the atrioventricular node. The slow pathway generally crosses the isthmus between the coronary sinus and the tricuspid annulus and has a longer conduction time, but a shorter effective refractory period than the fast pathway. The fast pathway is commonly a superior route, emanating from the interatrial septum, and has a faster conduction rate but, in turn, a longer effective refractory period. Normal conduction during sinus rhythm occurs along the fast pathway, but higher heart rates and/or premature beats are often conducted through the slow pathway, since the fast pathway may be refractory at these rates.

Recent advances in the optical mapping of the human atrioventricular junction further elucidate the dual pathway electrophysiology [38]. More specifically, the dual characteristics of this function have been revealed using an S1–S2 pacing protocol; in this procedure, a stimulus (S1) of constant duration and amplitude is applied followed by a second stimulus (S2) of varying duration and amplitude. The S1–S2 interval is iteratively reduced until conduction block in the fast pathway occurs due to the long refractory period [38].

Though the primary function of the atrioventricular node may seem simple, that is to relay conduction between the atria and ventricles, its structure is very complex. As a means to describe these complexities, mathematical arrays and finite element analysis models have been constructed to elucidate the underlying structure–function relationship of the node [39]. Figure 11.2 shows a 3D reconstruction of the region using a model of the heart stained with the voltage sensitive dye di-4-ANEPPS. The reconstruction includes histology and immunolabeling of marker proteins to identify various tissue types. Figure 11.3 shows the nodal reconstruction of a normal human heart as well as one from a patient who had an implanted left ventricular assist device. For movies of these reconstructions, see AVI 11.2, AVI 11.3, and AVI 11.4 on the Companion CD.

In general, the atrioventricular node is located in the so-called "floor" of the right atrium, over the muscular part of the interventricular septum, and inferior to the membranous septum. Following atrioventricular nodal excitation, the slow pathway conducts impulses to the "His bundle," indicated by a longer interval between atrial and His activation (note that the bundle of His has also been referred to as the "common bundle"). As mentioned above, the anatomical region in which the His bundle and the atrioventricular node both reside has been termed the "triangle of Koch." The triangle is bordered by the coronary sinus, the tricuspid valve annulus along the septal leaflet, and the tendon of Todaro.

After leaving the bundle of His, the normal wave of cardiac depolarization spreads to both the left and right bundle branches; these pathways carry depolarization to the left and right ventricles, respectively. Finally, the signal broadly travels through the remainder of the Purkinje fibers and ventricular myocardial depolarization spreads (see MPG 11.5 on the Companion CD).

In addition to the normal path of ventricular excitation, direct connections to the ventricular myocardium from the atrioventricular node and the penetrating portion of the bundle of His have been described in humans [40]. Yet, the function and prevalence of these connections, termed "Mahaim fibers," is poorly understood. An

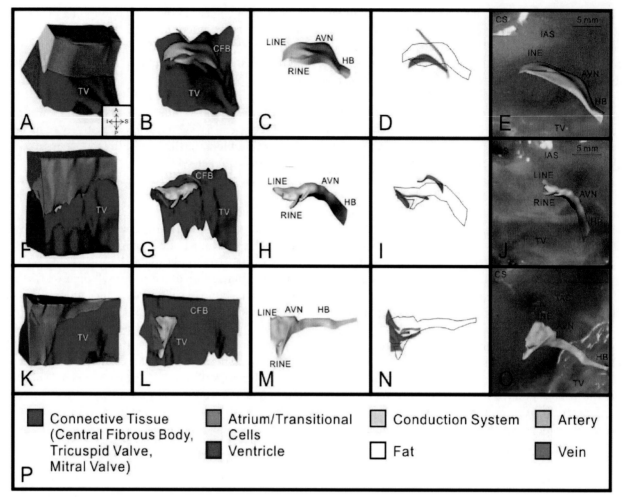

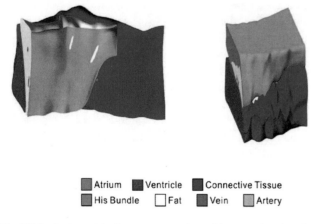

Fig. 11.3 Atrioventricular reconstruction with normal and pathologic human hearts. The normal human heart (*left*) and the heart of a left ventricular assist device patient (*right*) show different proportions of tissue type in the nodal region

additional aberrant pathway existing between the atria and ventricles has been termed the "bundle of Kent" (the clinical manifestation of ventricular tachycardias due to the presence of this pathway is termed "Wolff–Parkinson–White syndrome"). Therapeutically, this accessory pathway is commonly ablated.

Alternate representations of the cardiac conduction system are shown in Figs. 11.4 and 11.5, with details of the ventricular portion of the conduction system shown in Fig. 11.6. More specifically, the left bundle branch splits into fascicles as it travels down the left side of the ventricular septum just below the endocardium (these can be visualized with proper staining). Its fascicles extend for a distance of 5–15 mm, fanning out over the left ventricle. Importantly, typically about midway to the apex of the left ventricle, the left bundle separates into two major

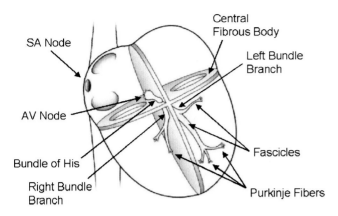

Fig. 11.4 The conduction system of the heart. Normal excitation originates in the sinoatrial node then propagates through both atria. The atrial depolarization spreads to the atrioventricular node and passes through the bundle of His to the bundle branches/Purkinje fibers. AV = atrioventricular; SA = sinoatrial

divisions, the anterior and posterior branches (or fascicles). These divisions extend to the base of the two papillary muscles and the adjacent myocardium. In contrast, the right bundle branch continues inferiorly, as if it were a continuation of the bundle of His, traveling along the right side of the muscular interventricular septum. This bundle branch runs proximally just deep to the endocardium, and its course runs slightly inferior to the septal

papillary muscle of the tricuspid valve before dividing into fibers that spread throughout the right ventricle. The complex network of conducting fibers that extends from either the right or left bundle branches is composed of the rapid conduction cells known as "Purkinje fibers." The Purkinje fibers in both the right and left ventricles act as preferential conduction pathways to provide rapid activation and coordinate the excitation pattern within the various regions of the ventricular myocardium. As described by Tawara, these fibers travel within the trabeculations of the right and left ventricles, as well as to within the myocardium. Due to the tremendous variability in the degree and morphology of the trabeculations existing both within and between species, it is likely that variations in the left ventricular conduction patterns also exist. It should be noted that one of the most easily recognized conduction pathways commonly found in mammalian hearts is the moderator band, which contains Purkinje fibers from the right bundle branch (see also Chapter 6).

Three criteria for considering a myocardial cell as a "specialized conduction cell" were first proposed by Aschoff [41] and Monckeberg [42] in 1910, which include: (1) the ability to histologically identify discrete features; (2) the ability to track cells from section to section; and (3) these cells are insulated by fibrous sheaths from the

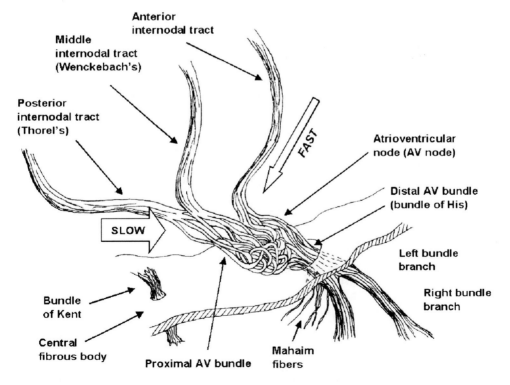

Fig. 11.5 Details of the atrioventricular nodal region. The so-called slow and fast conduction pathways are indicated by the *arrows*. To improve clarity in the visualization of the conduction anatomy, the fascicles of the atrioventricular node are not drawn to scale (their size was increased to allow the reader to visualize the tortuosity of the conduction pathway) and the central fibrous body has been thinned. AV = atrioventricular

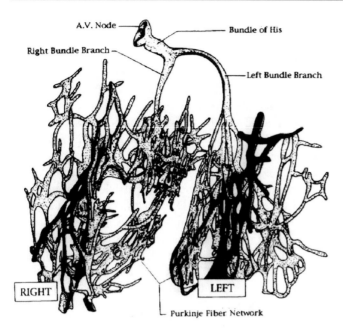

Fig. 11.6 The ventricular conduction system. The Purkinje network has a high interspecies and intraspecies variation, which likely results in variability in excitation and contractile patterns within the ventricles. This variability is evident in the dramatic differences seen in the degree and morphology of the cardiac trabeculations (which typically contain these fibers). Modified from DeHann DL, Circulation 1961;24:458

nonspecialized contractile myocardium. It is noteworthy that only the cells within the bundle of His, the left and right bundle branches, and the Purkinje fibers satisfy all three criteria. No structure within the atria meets all three criteria, including Bachman's bundle, the sinoatrial node, and the atrioventricular node (which are all uninsulated tissues).

11.3 Cardiac Rate Control

Under normal physiologic conditions, the dominant pacemaker of the heart is the sinoatrial node which, in adults, fires at rates between 60 and 100 beats/min, faster than any other cardiac region. In an individual at rest, modulation by the parasympathetic nervous system dominates which slows the sinoatrial nodal rate to about 75 action potentials per minute (or beats per minute when contractions are elicited).

In addition to the cells of the sinoatrial node, other specialized conduction system cells are capable of developing spontaneous diastolic depolarization, specifically those found in the specialized fibers in the atrioventricular junction and His–Purkinje system. Rhythms generated by impulse formation within these cells range from 25 to 55 beats/min in the human heart (Fig. 11.7). These lower rate rhythms are commonly referred to as "ventricular escape rhythms," and are important for patient survival, since they maintain some degree of cardiac output in situations when the sinoatrial and/or atrioventricular nodes are nonfunctional or are functioning inappropriately. Note that the various populations of pacemaker myocytes (i.e., in the sinoatrial and atrioventricular nodes) elicit

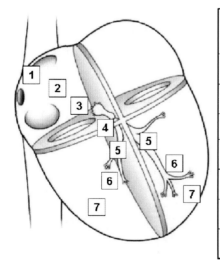

Normal Activation Sequence	Structure	Conduction velocity (m/sec)	Pacemaker rate (beats/min)
1	SA node	< 0.01	60 – 100
2	Atrial myocardium	1.0 – 1.2	None
3	AV node	0.02 – 0.05	40 – 55
4	Bundle of His	1.2 – 2.0	25 – 40
5	Bundle branches	2.0 – 4.0	25 – 40
6	Purkinje network	2.0 – 4.0	25 – 40
7	Ventricular myocardium	0.3 – 1.0	None

Fig. 11.7 Conduction velocities and intrinsic pacemaker rates of various structures within the cardiac conduction pathway. The structures are listed in the order of activation during a normal cardiac contraction, beginning with the sinoatrial node. Note that the intrinsic pacemaker rate is slower in structures further along the activation pathway. For example, the atrioventricular nodal rate is

slower than the sinoatrial nodal rate. This prevents the atrioventricular node from generating a spontaneous rhythm under normal conditions, since it remains refractory at rates <55 beats/min. If the sinoatrial node becomes inactive, the atrioventricular nodal rate will then determine the ventricular rate. Tabulation adapted from Katz AM, ed. Physiology of the heart. 3rd ed. 2001

so-called slow-type action potentials (slow response action potential; see below).

In addition to the normal sources of cardiac rhythms, myocardial tissue can also exhibit abnormal self-excitability; such a site is also called an "ectopic pacemaker" or "ectopic focus." This pacemaker may operate only occasionally, producing extra beats, or it may induce a new cardiac rhythm for some period of time. Potentiators of ectopic activity include caffeine, nicotine, electrolyte imbalances, hypoxia, and/or toxic reactions to drugs such as digitalis. For more detail on rate control of the heart, refer to Chapter 12.

11.4 Cardiac Action Potentials

Although cardiac myocytes branch and interconnect with each other (mechanically via the intercalated disk and electrically via the gap junctions; see below), under normal conditions the heart should be thought to form two separate functional networks—the atria and the ventricles. The atrial and ventricular tissues are separated by the fibrous skeleton of the heart (the central fibrous body). This skeleton is comprised of dense connective tissue rings that surround the valves of the heart, fuse with one another, and merge with the interventricular septum. The skeleton can be thought to: (1) form the foundation to which the valves attach; (2) prevent overstretching of the valves; (3) serve as a point of insertion for cardiac muscle bundles; and (4) act as an electrical insulator that prevents the direct spread of action potential from the atria to the ventricles. See also Chapter 5 for further details on the cardiac skeleton.

A healthy myocardial cell has a resting membrane potential of approximately –90 mV. The resting potential is described by the Goldman–Hodgkin–Katz equation, which takes into account the permeabilities ("Ps") as well as the intracellular and extracellular concentrations of ions [X], where X is the ion:

$$V_m = (2.3 R^* T/F)^* \log_{10} \frac{P_K[K]_o + P_{Na}[Na]_o + P_{Cl}[Cl]_i + \cdots}{P_K[K]_i + P_{Na}[Na]_i + P_{Cl}[Cl]_o + \cdots}$$

In the cardiac myocyte, the membrane potential is dominated by the K^+ equilibrium potential. An action potential is initiated when this resting potential becomes shifted toward a more positive value of approximately –60 to –70 mV (Fig. 11.8). At this threshold potential, the cell's voltage-gated Na^+ channels open and begin a cascade of events involving other ion channels. In artificial electrical stimulation, this shift of the resting potential and subsequent depolarization is produced by the excitation delivered through the pacing system. The typical ion

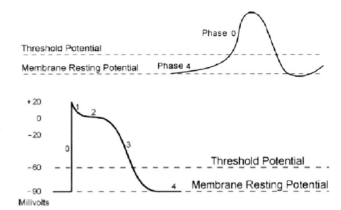

Fig. 11.8 Typical cardiac action potentials (slow on top and fast below). The resting membrane potential, threshold potential, and the phases of depolarization (0–4) are shown

Table 11.1 Ion concentrations for mammalian myocytes

Ion	Intracellular concentration (mM)	Extracellular concentration (mM)
Sodium (Na)	5–34	140
Potassium (K)	104–180	5.4
Chloride (Cl)	4.2	117
Calcium (Ca)		3

Adapted from Katz AM, ed. Physiology of the heart. 3rd ed. 2001.

concentrations for a mammalian cardiac myocyte are summarized in Table 11.1 and graphically depicted in Fig. 11.9.

When a myocyte is brought to the threshold potential, normally via a neighboring cell, voltage-gated fast Na^+ channels actively open (activation gates); the permeability of the sarcolemma (plasma membrane) to sodium ions ($P_{Na}+$) dramatically increases. Because the cytosol is electrically more negative than extracellular fluid, and the Na^+ concentration is higher in the extracellular fluid, Na^+ rapidly crosses the cell membrane. Importantly, within a few milliseconds, these fast Na^+ channels automatically inactivate (inactivation gates) and P_{Na}^+ decreases.

The membrane depolarization due to the activation of the Na^+ induces the opening of the voltage-gated slow Ca^{2+} channels located within both the sarcolemma and sarcoplasmic reticulum (internal storage site for Ca^{2+}) membranes. Thus, there is an increase in the permeability of Ca^{2+} (P_{Ca}^{2+}), which allows the concentration to dramatically increase intracellularly (Fig. 11.10). At the same time, the membrane permeability to K^+ ions decreases due to closing of K^+ channels. For approximately 200–250 ms, the membrane potential stays close to 0 mV, as a small outflow of K^+ just balances the inflow of Ca^{2+}. After this fairly long delay, voltage-gated K^+ channels open and active repolarization is initiated. The opening

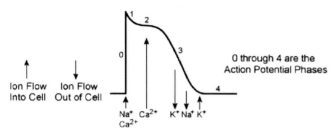

Fig. 11.9 A cardiac cell at rest. The intracellular space is dominated by potassium ions, while the extracellular space has a higher concentration of sodium and calcium ions

PHASES OF ACTION POTENTIAL AND ION FLOW

Fig. 11.10 Ion flow during the phases of a cardiac action potential

of these K^+ channels (increased membrane permeability) allows for K^+ to diffuse out of the cell due to its concentration gradient. At the same time, Ca^{2+} channels begin to close, and net charge movement is dominated by the outward flux of the positively charged K^+, restoring the negative resting membrane potential to approximately –90 mV (Figs. 11.10 and 11.11).

As mentioned above, not all action potentials that are elicited in the cardiac myocardium have the same time courses; slow and fast response cells have differing shaped action potentials with different electrical properties in each phase. Recall that the pacemaker cells (slow response type) have the ability to spontaneously depolarize until they reach threshold and thus elicit action potentials. Action potentials from such cells are also characterized by a slower initial depolarization phase, a lower amplitude overshoot, a shorter and less stable plateau phase, and repolarization to an unstable, slowly depolarizing resting potential (Fig. 11.12). In the pacemaker cells, at least three mechanisms are thought to underlie the slow depolarization that occurs during phase 4 (diastolic

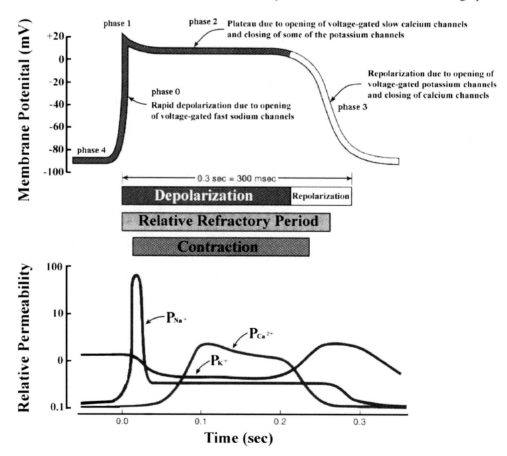

Fig. 11.11 A typical action potential of a ventricular myocyte and the underlying ion currents. The resting membrane potential is approximately –90 mV (phase 4). The rapid depolarization is primarily due to the voltage-gated Na^+ current (phase 0), which results in a relatively sharp peak (phase 1) and transitions into the plateau

(phase 2) until repolarization (phase 3). Also indicated are the refractory period and timing of the ventricular contraction. Modified from Tortora GJ, Grabowski SR, eds. Principles of anatomy and physiology. 9th ed. 2000

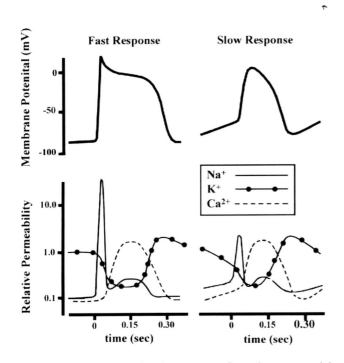

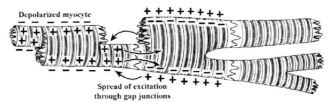

Fig. 11.13 Shown are several cardiac myocytes in different states of excitation. The depolarization that occurred in the cell on the left causes depolarization of the adjacent cell through cell-to-cell conduction via the gap junctions (nexus). Eventually all adjoining cells will depolarize. An action potential initiated in any of these cells will be conducted from cell to cell in either direction

Fig. 11.12 The comparative time courses of membrane potentials and ion permeabilities that would typically occur in a fast response (*left*, e.g., ventricular myocyte) and a slow response cell (*right*, e.g., a nodal myocyte). Modified from Mohrman DE, Heller LJ, eds. Cardiovascular physiology. 5th ed. 2003

interval): (1) a progressive decrease in P_K+; (2) a slight increase in $P_{Na}+$; and (3) an increase in P_{Ca}^{2+}.

11.5 Gap Junctions (Cell-to-Cell Conduction)

In the heart, cardiac muscle cells (myocytes) are connected end to end by structures known as "intercalated disks." These are irregular transverse thickenings of the sarcolemma, within which there are "desmosomes" that hold the cells together and to which the myofibrils are attached. Adjacent to the intercalated disks are the gap junctions, which allow action potentials to directly spread from one myocyte to the next. More specifically, the disks join the cells together by both mechanical attachment and by protein channels. The firm mechanical connections are created between the adjacent cell membranes by proteins called adherins in the aforementioned structures, the desmosomes. The electrical connections (low resistance pathways, gap junctions) between the myocytes are via the channels formed by the protein connexin. These channels allow ion movements between cells (Fig. 11.13).

As noted above, not all cells elicit the same types of action potentials, even though excitation is propagated from cell to cell via their interconnections (gap junctions).

The action potentials elicited in the sinoatrial nodal cells are of the slow response type and those in the remainder of the atria have a more rapid depolarization rate (Fig. 11.14). Although a significant temporal displacement in the action potentials elicited by the myocytes of the two nodes (sinoatrial and atrioventricular) occurs, the action potential morphologies are similar.

It takes approximately 30 ms for excitation to spread between the sinoatrial and atrioventricular nodes, and atrial activation occurs over a period of approximately 70–90 ms (Fig. 11.14). The speed at which an action potential propagates through a region of cardiac tissue is called the "conduction velocity" (Fig. 11.7). The conduction velocity varies considerably in the heart and is directly dependent on the diameter of a given myocyte. For example, action potential conduction is greatly slowed as it passes through the atrioventricular node. This is due to the small diameter of these nodal cells, the tortuosity of the cellular pathway [2], and the slow rate of rise of their elicited action potentials. This delay is important to allow adequate time for ventricular filling.

Action potentials in the Purkinje fibers are of the fast response type (Fig. 11.14), i.e., rapid depolarization rates that, in part, are due to their large diameters. This feature allows the Purkinje system to transfer depolarization to the majority of cells in the ventricular myocardium nearly in unison. Because of the high conduction velocities in these cells which span the myocardium, there is a minimal delay in the cell's time of onset. It is important to note that the ventricular cells that are last to depolarize have shorter duration action potentials (shorter Ca^{2+} current), and thus are the first to repolarize. The ventricular myocardium repolarizes within the time period represented by the T-wave in the electrocardiogram.

11.6 The Atrioventricular Node and Bundle of His: Specific Features

The atrioventricular node and the bundle of His play critical roles in the maintenance and control of ventricular rhythms. As mentioned previously, the atrioventricular

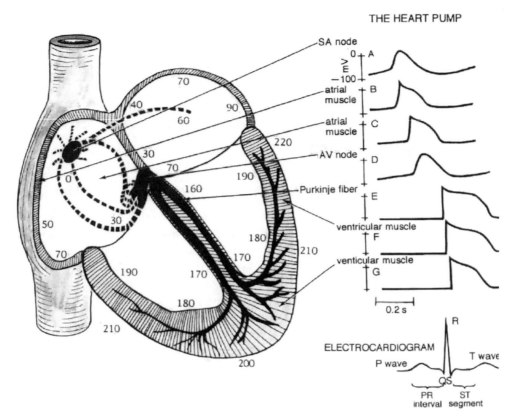

Fig. 11.14 Shown are the predominant conduction pathways in the heart and the relative time, in milliseconds, that cells in these various regions become activated following an initial depolarization within the sinoatrial node. To the right are typical action potential waveforms that would be recorded from myocytes in these specific locations. The sinoatrial and atrioventricular nodal cells have similar shaped action potentials. The nonpacemaker atrial cells elicit action potentials that have shapes somewhat between the slow response (nodal) and fast response cells (e.g., ventricular myocytes). The ventricular cells elicit fast response type action potentials; however, their durations vary in length. Due to the rapid excitation within the Purkinje fiber system, the initiation of depolarization of the ventricular myocytes occurs within 30–40 ms and is recorded as the QRS complex in the electrocardiogram

node is composed of heterogeneous gap junctions with electrical communication via the protein connexin. Specifically, there are four connexin proteins identified to date: Cx43, Cx40, Cx45, and Cx30.2/31.9. Cx43 and Cx40 are associated with the fast conduction pathway, whereas Cx45 and Cx30.2/31.9 are generally expressed in the slow conduction pathway [43]. The expression of these proteins is also species dependent; it should be noted that one study found that, in the human atrioventricular junction, Cx43, Cx40, and Cx45 are expressed [44].

Additionally, both structures are frequently accessed during cardiac catheterization procedures: (1) as anatomic landmarks; (2) to allow insight into atrial–ventricular conduction behaviors; and/or (3) to ablate these structures or the surrounding tissues to terminate aberrant behaviors (e.g., reentrant tachycardias) or to prevent atrioventricular conduction in patients with chronic atrial fibrillation. Today, there is a strong interest by the medical device designer to understand the details of the structural and functional properties of the atrioventricular node and the bundle of His to develop new therapies and/or to avoid inducing complications.

The myocytes located within the region of the atrioventricular node and the bundle of His have many unique characteristics. Specifically, both the atrioventricular node and His bundle are comprised primarily of "spiraled" myofibers that are then combined to form many collagen-encased fascicles. These fascicles are generally arranged in a parallel fashion in the proximal atrioventricular bundle (PAVB, the region of the atrioventricular node transitioning from the atrium into the body of the nodal tissues) and the distal atrioventricular bundle (DAVB, the penetrating portion of the bundle of His), and are interwoven within the atrioventricular node itself (the tortuosity of the cellular pathway within the atrioventricular node likely is a major contributor to the conduction delay in this region). In general, the myocytes of the His are larger than those of the PAVB and the atrioventricular node, and the perinuclear regions of these myocytes are filled with glycogen. These cells uniquely utilize anaerobic metabolism instead of the normal aerobic metabolism used by the more abundant contractile myocardium. His myocytes have longer intercalated disks and, although all of the nodal tissues have thin end processes, they are less numerous in this region. His myocytes are innervated, but to a lesser extent than those in the atrioventricular node. Unlike the sinoatrial and atrioventricular nodes, the His bundle has no large blood vessels that supply it specifically. Table 11.2 is a summary of the histological characteristics of the His in comparison to the other nodal tissues.

It should be noted that the bundle of His can receive inputs from both the atrioventricular node and from transitional cells in the atrial septum. In general, the His bundle is located adjacent to the annulus of the tricuspid valve, distal to the atrioventricular node, and slightly proximal to the right bundle branch and left bundle branch. The functional origin may be ill defined, but as described above, it is typically considered to anatomically begin at the point where the atrioventricular nodal tissue enters the central fibrous body. The bundle of His is described as having three regions—the penetrating bundle, nonbranching bundle, and branching bundle. The penetrating bundle is the region that enters the central fibrous body. At this point, the His fascicles are insulated but are surrounded by atrial tissue (superiorly and anteriorly), the ventricular septum (inferiorly), and the central fibrous body (posteriorly). Thus, the exact point where the atrioventricular nodal tissues end and the bundle begins is difficult to define, since it occurs over a transitional region. The penetrating bundle has been described as oval in shape and was found to be 1–1.5 mm long in young canines and 0.25–0.75 mm long in neonates [1]. The nonbranching bundle passes through the central fibrous

Table 11.2 Summary of the histological characteristics of the nodal and perinodal tissues in canines

Feature	Atrioventricular bundle (DAVB, His bundle)	Atrioventricular node (AVN)	Proximal atrioventricular bundle (PAVB)
Nucleus	Clear perinuclear zone filled with glycogen	Clear perinuclear zone filled with glycogen	Clear perinuclear zone filled with glycogen
Metabolism	Anaerobic	Anaerobic	Anaerobic
Myofiber size	Largest	Mid	Smallest
Myofibers in fascicles	Yes	Yes	Yes
Primary fascicles encased in collagen	Yes	Yes	Yes
Secondary fascicles present	Yes	Yes	Yes
Secondary fascicles encased in collagen	Yes	Yes	Yes
Fascicular arrangement	Parallel	Interwoven ("massive whorl")	Parallel
Myofiber arrangement within fascicles	Least spiraling	Spiraled	Most spiraling
Cross-striations	Delicate	Delicate	Delicate
End processes present on the myocytes	Yes. Short and delicate	Yes. Most numerous. Extend from proximal parallel myofibers to central whorled fibers	Yes
Intercalated disks	Broad	Form short stacks	Broadest
Fat vacuoles	Little or none	Little or none	Yes
Vascularization	No large vessels	No large vessels	Large vessels present
Innervation	Tendrils (sympathetic). No packets or fascicles of nerve endings present	Fascicles of boutons, tendrils (sympathetic), and varicosities (parasympathetic) present	Fascicles of boutons, tendrils (sympathetic), and varicosities (parasympathetic) present. Sheaves of nerve endings extend along the length of the myofibers

Compiled from Racker and Kadish [2].

body and is surrounded on all sides by the central fibrous body. In this cardiac region, the His bundle still has atrial tissue superior and anterior to it, the ventricular septum inferior to it, and now the aortic and mitral valves posterior to it. The branching bundle is described to begin as the His exits the central fibrous body. At this point, it is inferior to the membranous septum and superior to the ventricular septum. The bundle is also at its closest proximity to both the right and left ventricular chambers at this point. After leaving the central fibrous body, the bundle then bifurcates into the bundle branches; the right bundle branch passes into the myocardium of the interventricular septum and the left bundle branch travels subendocardially along the septum in the left ventricle (as noted above). Figures 11.15 and 11.16 show canine histological sections of the bundle of His as they exit the central fibrous body (the branching bundle).

Electrophysiologic studies of the bundle of His have most commonly been performed using catheters with polished electrodes and a short interelectrode spacing (i.e., those with diameters of 2 mm). Due to the small amplitude of the His potential, special high pass filtering must be used (>30 Hz). This high pass setting must be used in order to separate the His signal from the low-frequency shift in the isopotential line between the atrial depolarization and the atrial repolarization/ventricular depolarization. His potentials can commonly be mapped by deploying an electrode in one of three ways: (1) endocardially in the right atrium at a point on the tricuspid annulus near the membranous septum; (2) epicardially at the base of the aorta near the right atrial appendage; or (3) intra-arterially within the noncoronary cusp of the aortic valve [16–18, 20, 45].

Today, His potentials are commonly mapped to provide a landmark for ablation of the atrioventricular node as well as to assess A-to-V conduction timing. In addition to direct electrical mapping, much can be learned about the general anatomical and functional properties of the cell lying within the bundle via attempts to directly stimulate it. For example, direct stimulation of the His produces normal ventricular activation due to the initiation of depolarization into the intrinsic conduction pathway [16, 17, 19]. Thus, if one frequently experiences failed attempts to selectively stimulate the His bundle, she/he may assume pathological changes [20].

The His bundle has historically been thought to act only as a conduit for transferring depolarization. Ventricular escape rhythms have been known to emanate from the His, but it was thought to be, in general, a relatively simple structure. To the contrary, recent evidence indicates that at least two general sources serve as inputs to the His, and that it functions as at least two functionally distinct conduits. Using alternans (alternate beat variation in the direction, amplitude, and duration of any component of the EKG), the duality of its electrophysiology was recently demonstrated in isolated preparations from the region of the triangle of Koch in rabbit hearts [45].

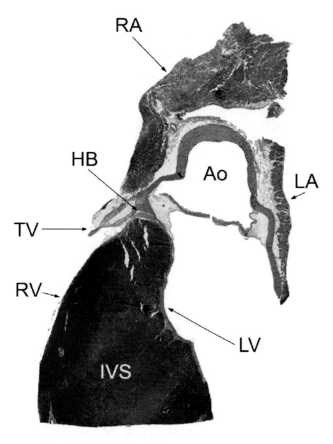

Fig. 11.15 Histologic section through the bundle of His in a canine heart. The section was prepared using a modified Masson's trichrome stain (collagen/nuclei stains *blue*, muscle/keratin/cytoplasm stains *red*). Ao = aorta; HB = His bundle; IVS = interventricular septum; LA = left atrium; LV = left ventricular endocardium; RA = right atrium endocardium; RV = right ventricle endocardium; TV = tricuspid valve

11.7 Comparative Anatomy

All large mammalian hearts are considered to have a very similar conduction system whose main components are the sinoatrial node, the atrioventricular node, the bundle of His, right and left main bundle branches, and Purkinje fibers. Yet, interspecies variations are well recognized [1, 46–48]. For a summary of the major differences in the atrioventricular conduction systems between human, pig, dog, and sheep hearts, refer to Chapter 6.

Fig. 11.16 Histologic section through the bundle of His in a canine heart. The region enlarged is noted by the *dashed lines* in the original histologic section. Both sections were prepared using a modified Masson's trichrome stain (collagen/nuclei stain *blue*, muscle/keratin/cytoplasm stain *red*). Ao = aorta; CFB = central fibrous body (provides structure and isolates the atrial from the ventricular tissues); HB = His bundle; IVS = interventricular septum; LA = left atrium; LV = left ventricular endocardium; RA = right atrium endocardium; RV = right ventricle endocardium; TV = tricuspid valve

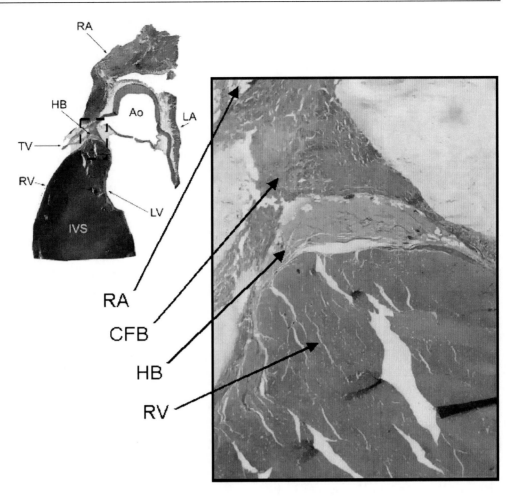

More specifically, Bharati et al. made a comparison of the electrophysiologic properties of the swine and human hearts (Table 11.3) [46]. In addition to significant differences in atrial (HRA–LRA) and A–V conduction times (much shorter in the swine), the authors also found significantly more autonomic innervation within the atrioventricular node and penetrating bundle of the swine heart (thought to be both adrenergic and cholinergic). They concluded that this indicates a more important neurogenic component to the swine conduction system, relative to the human heart. Due to this difference, they cautioned using swine as a model for assessing cardiac arrhythmias. Although the neurogenic differences between the human and swine are significant in vivo, isolation of such hearts results in denervation of the conduction system and thus reduces or eliminates the relevance of this finding.

The canine is another commonly used model in biomedical device research. Information on A-to-V timing in canines was published by Karpawich et al. [18]. They placed tripolar electrodes on the right atrial epicardium near the noncoronary cusp of the aorta of canines; the resulting timing recorded was extracted from the paper and is tabulated in Table 11.4.

Table 11.3 Comparison of swine to human electrophysiology

Parameter	Swine: average ± std dev (range)	Normal human
Heart rate (beats/min)	132 ± 32 (91–167)	60–100
PR interval (ms)	94 ± 27 (50–120)	3–5 year old: 110–150 5–9 year old: 120–160
QT interval (ms)	256 ± 69 (150–340)	HR = 150: 210–280 HR = 100: 260–350
HRA–LRA (ms)	10 ± 0 (10)	2–5 year old: 6–38 6–10 year old: 0–41
LRA–H (ms)	63 ± 2 (60–65)	2–5 year old: 45–101 6–10 year old: 40–124
H–V (ms)	25 ± 7 (20–35)	2–5 year old: 27–59 6–10 year old: 28–52

Adapted from Bharati et al. [46].
H = His; HR = heart rate; HRA = high right atrium; LRA = low right atrium; V = ventricle.

Table 11.4 Tabulation of activation timing

	P-wave to R-wave interval (ms)	Atrial activation to His bundle electrogram (ms)	His bundle electrogram to ventricular activation (ms)
Mean	92.1	77.5	29
Std dev	18.4	11.5	8.9
Max	120	100	50
Min	70	60	20

Data compiled from Karpawich et al. [15].

11.8 The Recording of Action Potentials and/or the Spread of Excitation Through the Myocardium

Action potential waveforms can be actively monitored from the epicardial, endocardial, or transmural surfaces of the heart. Several methods exist for the acquisition of such signals. Such methods include the use of: (1) glass micropipette electrodes; (2) metal electrodes of various designs; (3) multielectrode arrays; (4) optical mapping; or (5) contact or noncontact endocardial mapping. When contact or noncontact endocardial mapping technologies are employed, they measure the intracardiac electrograms (endocardial, see also Chapter 29) rather than those from the epicardial surface or globally from the whole myocardium, as in a standard 12-lead ECG. It should be noted that for many ablative arrhythmia therapies, it is the measurement of intracardiac electrograms within a given cardiac chamber that is more common than the recordings from the epicardium (see Chapter 26) [49]. Furthermore, algorithms employed by implantable devices typically use the intercardiac (transmural) electrogram (EGM) signal when detecting an arrhythmia; it is

common to use active fixation leads with distal electrodes screwed into the myocardium [50].

Typically, glass micropipettes are produced from small diameter capillary tubing and then employed for intracellular recordings. These glass tubes are heated (with a burner or heating element) and then, under tension, elongated (stretched) to produce a constriction that eventually breaks. Currently, this process is typically facilitated by a commercially available micropipette puller which reproducibly creates electrodes with tips of about 0.1 μm with resistances of 10–40 MΩ. The pipette is then filled with an electrolyte such as 3 M KCl. A silver, platinum, or stainless steel wire is then positioned inside the pipette until it is in contact with the electrolytic solution [51]. The user must be careful while manipulating the fragile electrode tip, especially when recording directly from a beating, moving cell. The ultimate goal with this recording approach is to impale the microelectrode through the cell membrane, so that the tip is into the myoplasm of a single cell while not inducing major damage to the cell; the membrane seals around the tip and the cell does not become depolarized.

There are various designs for metal recording electrodes which can be employed to monitor action potential waveforms extracellularly. One of the most common methods is to use a needle with two closely spaced embedded conductors. Yet, the relative spacing between the active and reference conductors can be manipulated to control the sensing area [52]. Another method is to use an internal conductor needle with the cannula of the needle as the reference electrode. In such cases, the internal conducting wire is electrically isolated from the cannula. In a monopolar configuration, the needle is a single shaft, and the reference is taken from the subject ground. Each of these designs can have needle tip diameters as small as 0.30 mm.

Various types of electrode designs and typical signals that can be recorded with each are shown in Fig. 11.17.

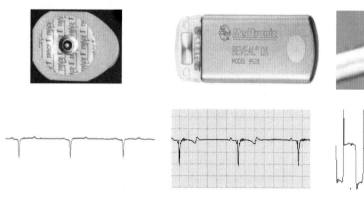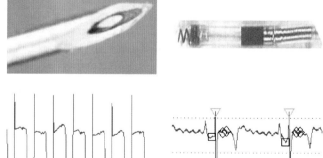

Fig. 11.17 Representative cardiac signals. The *leftmost signal* is from a standard Ag/AgCl surface electrode. The *second signal* was collected subcutaneously with a Medtronic Reveal® Dx insertable cardiac monitor. The *third signal* was collected from a concentric bipolar needle electrode with 0.3 mm spacing between conductors. The *last endocardial signal* was obtained with a Medtronic 5076 screw-in electrode in the right ventricle; this electrogram has key fiducial points marked

Note that the morphology of a recorded signal will typically depend on: (1) the configuration of the electrode employed (monopolar or bipolar); (2) the relative surface area that the electrode will monitor; (3) the anatomical placement (atrium or ventricle); and/or (4) the site-specific myocardial wall recording location (endocardial, epicardial, or transmural). Multiple ECG patches, for example, are used to cover a larger surface area on the skin and thus detect potential changes from a large transmural field, whereas a bipolar concentric needle placed epicardially records from a focal population of cells. In other words, the surface electrodes will provide a signal representative of a major portion of the whole heart, while the small bipolar needle electrode provides a much more localized signal.

For comparison, modern pacemaker lead diameters range from 4 to 10 French (Fr; 1 Fr is one-third millimeter). Additionally, catheters used for noncontact cardiac mapping of endocardial activation and repolarization processes are typically 9 Fr.

As noted above, active and passive pacing leads can be used to detect action potential waveforms, commonly used today in either unipolar or bipolar configurations (i.e., with those leads that have both a distal tip electrode and a distal ring electrode). Such leads can be used for either sensing or pacing. Note that their relative dimensions will ultimately dictate the size of the field from which they are sensing electrical potentials. As with any active fixation lead or metal electrode which is engaged into the myocardium, an initial injury potential can be associated with its placement [53]. It should also be noted that the current trend in the pacing lead industry is to continually decrease the diameter of both the body and tip dimensions (i.e., 2 Fr leads are currently in development and clinical trials).

One can consider that an extension of the single electrode approach is the multielectrode array. As the name implies, such systems consist of an array of equally spaced electrodes supported by a base. Conducting wires are attached to the electrodes on the array. Depending on the design, one or more of the electrodes on the array can serve as the reference electrode, while the others become the active electrodes. These arrays allow for the mapping of electrical potentials within a given region of the heart [54]. The designer or eventual user must determine the appropriate electrode spacing for a given application, while also considering the relative electrode configurations, the employed sampling rates, and/or the density of electrodes necessary to elucidate the nature of the desired local events to monitor.

Catheter-based cardiac mapping systems are primarily used to understand the underlying mechanisms of arrhythmias. In principle, electroanatomical mapping systems use low magnetic fields to reconstruct 3D maps and electrical activation sequences of the chamber of interest. Briefly, in sequential mapping systems, mapping catheters with radiofrequency capability are placed into the heart chamber with fluoroscopic guidance. Low magnetic fields are generated by pads located under the patient's bed. The sensor tip of the catheter attains data in order to compute information regarding magnetic field amplitude, frequency, and phase to reconstruct a spatial 3D position. After chamber reconstruction, sequential recording of electrical activation is recorded by dragging the catheter along the endocardial wall. The intercardiac electrogram is measured and typically the activation time is superimposed on the reconstructed 3D chamber, resembling a contour map. The reconstruction process can be conducted in real time, however, the process is time consuming since it is a sequential process. Hence, one can gain insights on the relative spread of excitation through a given chamber or portions of the conduction system.

Contact mapping can also be conducted with basket catheters that typically contain 32–64 nickel or titanium electrodes that are 1–2 mm long and 1 mm in diameter with interelectrode distances from 3 to 10 mm. The endocardial surface is mapped as the basket's splines, making contact with the chamber wall. This technique has limitations, however, since a catheter that is too small or too large will result in poor-quality electrogram recordings. The technique is also susceptible to movement artifacts from the continuously beating heart [55, 56]. Nevertheless, one can track relative electrical activities through the heart with such methodologies.

A more recent advancement in 3D chamber mapping is noncontact mapping technology. One such product is the EnSite® system by Endocardial Solutions (St. Jude Medical, St. Paul, MN). This system includes catheter 64 laser-etched unipolar electrodes that lie within the chamber; using such systems, one can track, on a beat-to-beat basis, the activation and repolarization patterns in a given chamber (see Chapter 29 for more details on these systems). It is the continued development of such cardiac mapping systems that helps physicians localize sites for catheter ablation for the treatment of complex cardiac arrhythmias such as tachycardia or atrial fibrillation [55, 57].

11.9 Future Research

Although much is already known, a great deal of supposition and controversy remains related to our understanding of the cardiac conduction system. Specifically, characterization of the anatomy and electrophysiology of the atrioventricular nodal region and the bundle of His continues to be an area of great scientific interest and debate [58–60]. For example, current clinical interest in the atrioventricular node and His bundle has focused research on their potential stimulation to ultimately improve hemodynamics in patients requiring pacing [16–21] and their use in treating atrioventricular nodal reentrant tachycardias [1, 2, 54, 61]. In addition to these applied research investigations, there is a need for additional basic scientific investigations to improve our understanding of the fundamental physiology of the heart's conduction system and the mechanisms of cardiac activation in normal and diseased tissues; the findings from these studies will provide a better foundation for future therapies.

11.10 Summary

This chapter reviewed the basic architecture and function of the cardiac conduction system in order to provide the reader with a working knowledge and vocabulary related to this topic. While a great deal of literature exists regarding the cardiac conduction system, numerous questions remain related to the detailed histological anatomy and cellular physiology of these specialized conduction tissues and how they become modified in disease states. Future findings associated with the function and anatomy of the cardiac conduction system will likely lead to improvements in therapeutic approaches and medical devices.

Acknowledgments Medtronic Training and Education and Gorinka Shrivastav for graphical support; Rebecca Rose, DVM, Louanne Cheever, and Alexander Hill, PhD of Medtronic for the histological sectioning and staining; Anthony Weinhaus, PhD for additional details on atrial anatomy; Igor Efimov, PhD from Washington University in St. Louis, MO for 3D images of the human atrioventricular node.

References

1. Ho SY, Kilpatrick L, Kanai T, et al. The architecture of the atrioventricular conduction axis in dog compared to man—Its significance to ablation of the atrioventricular nodal approaches. J Cardiovasc Electrophysiol 1995;6:26–39.
2. Racker DK, Kadish AH. Proximal atrioventricular bundle, atrioventricular node, and distal atrioventricular bundle are distinct anatomic structures with unique histological characteristics and innervation. Circulation 2000;101:1049–59.
3. Furman S. A brief history of cardiac stimulation and electrophysiology—The past fifty years and the next century. NASPE Keynote Address, 1995.
4. Boyett D, Dobrzynski H. The sinoatrial node is still setting the pace 100 years after its discovery. Circ Res 2007;100:1543–5.
5. His W, Jr. Die Tatigkeit des embryonalen herzens und deren bedcutung fur die lehre von der herzbewegung beim erwachsenen. Artbeiten aus der Medizinischen Klinik zu Leipzig, 1893;1:14–49.
6. Tawara S. Das Reizleitungssystem des Saugetierherzens: Eine anatomisch-histologische Studie uber das Atrioventrikularbundel und die Purkinjeschen Faden. Jena, Germany: Gustav Fischer, 1906: 9–70, 114–56.
7. Conti AA, Giaccardi M, Yen Ho S, Padeletti L. Koch and the "ultimum moriens" theory—The last part to die of the heart. J Interv Card Electrophysiol 2006;15:69–70.
8. Koch WK. Der funktionelle bau des menschlichen herzen. Berlin and Vienna: Urban und Schwarzenberg, 1922.
9. Sorensen ER, Manna D, McCourt K. Use of epicardial pacing wires after coronary artery bypass surgery. Heart Lung 1994; 23:487–92.
10. Villain E, Ouarda F, Beyler C, Sidi D, Abid F. Predictive factors for late complete atrioventricular block after surgical treatment for congenital cardiopathy. [Article in French.] Arch Mal Coeur Vaiss 2003;96:495–8.
11. Bae EJ, Lee JY, Noh CI, Kim WH, Kim YJ. Sinus node dysfunction after fontan modifications—Influence of surgical method. Int J Cardiol 2003;88:285–91.
12. Hussain A, Malik A, Jalal A, Rehman M. Abnormalities of conduction after total correction of Fallot's Tetralogy: A prospective study. J Pak Med Assoc 2002;52:77–82.
13. Bruckheimer E, Berul CI, Kopf GS, et al. Late recovery of surgically-induced atrioventricular block in patients with congenital heart disease. J Interv Card Electrophysiol 2002;6:191–5.
14. Ghosh PK, Singh H, Bidwai PS. Complete A–V block and phrenic paralysis complicating surgical closure of ventricular septal defect—A case report. Indian Heart J 1989;41:335–7.
15. Hill SL, Berul CI, Patel HT, Rhodes J, Supran SE, Cao QL, Hijazi ZM. Early ECG abnormalities associated with transcatheter closure of atrial septal defects using the Amplatzer Septal Occluder. J Interv Card Electrophysiol 2000;4:469–74.
16. Deshmukh P, Casavant DA, Romanyshyn M, Anderson K. Permanent direct His-bundle pacing: A novel approach to cardiac pacing in patients with normal His-Purkinje activation. Circulation 2000;101:869–77.
17. Karpawich P, Gates J, Stokes K. Septal His-Purkinje ventricular pacing in canines: A new endocardial electrode approach. PACE 1992;15:2011–5.
18. Karpawich PP, Gillette PC, Lewis RM, Zinner A, McNamera DG. Chronic epicardial His bundle recordings in awake nonsedated dogs: A new method. Am Heart J 1983;105:16–21.
19. Scheinman MM, Saxon LA. Long-term His-bundle pacing and cardiac function. Circulation 2000;101:836–7.
20. Williams DO, Sherlag BJ, Hope RR, El-Sherif N, Lazzara R, Samet P. Selective versus non-selective His bundle pacing. Cardiovasc Res 1976;10:91–100.
21. Karpawich PP, Rabah R, Haas JE. Altered cardiac histology following apical right ventricular pacing in patients with congenital atrioventricular block. PACE 1999;22:1372–7.
22. de Cock CC, Giudici MC, Twisk JW. Comparison of the haemodynamic effects of right ventricular outflow-tract pacing with right ventricular apex pacing: A quantitative review. Europace 2003;5:275–8.
23. Cleland JG, Daubert JC, Erdmann E, et al. CARE-HF study Steering Committee and Investigators. The CARE-HF study (CArdiac REsynchronisation in Heart Failure study): Rationale, design and end-points. Eur J Heart Fail 2001;3:481–9.
24. Leclercq C, Daubert JC. Cardiac resynchronization therapy is an important advance in the management of congestive heart failure. J Cardiovasc Electrophysiol 2003;14:S27–9.
25. Miake J, Marban H, Nuss B. Biological pacemaker created by gene transfer. Nature 2002;419:132–3.

26. Nattel S, Khairy P, Roy D, et al. New approaches to atrial fibrillation management: A critical review of a rapidly evolving field. Drugs 2002;62:2377–97.

27. Takahashi Y, Yoshito I, Takahashi A, et al. Ablation and Pacing Therapy Working Group. AV nodal ablation and pacemaker implantation improves hemodynamic function in atrial fibrillation. Pacing Clin Electrophysiol 2003;26:1212–7.

28. Bernat R, Pfeiffer D. Long-term Rand learning curve for radio frequency ablation of accessory pathways. Coll Antropol 2003;27:83–91.

29. Gaita F, Riccardi R, Gallotti R. Surgical approaches to atrial fibrillation. Card Electrophysiol Rev 2002;6:401–5.

30. Betts TR, Roberts PR, Ho SY, Morgan JM. High density mapping of shifts in the site of earliest depolarization during sinus rhythm and sinus tachycardia. PACE 2003;26:874–82.

31. Boineau JB, Schuessler RB, Hackel DB, et al. Widespread distribution and rate differentiation of the atrial pacemaker complex. Am J Physiol 1980;239:H406–15.

32. Boineau JB, Schuessler RB, Mooney CR. Multicentric origin of the atrial depolarization wave: The pacemaker complex. Relation to the dynamics of atrial conduction, P-wave changes and heart rate control. Circulation 1978;58:1036–48.

33. Lee RJ, Kalman JM, Fitzpatrick AP, et al. Radiofrequency catheter modification of the sinus node for 'inappropriate' sinus tachycardia. Circulation 1995;92:2919–28.

34. Tranum-Jensen J. The fine structure of the atrial and atrioventricular (AV) junctional specialized tissues of the rabbit heart. In: Wellens HJJ, Lie KI, Janse MJ, eds. The conduction system of the heart: Structure, function, and clinical implications. Philadelphia, PA: Lea & Febiger, 1976:55–81.

35. Waller BF, Gering LE, Branyas NA, Slack JD. Anatomy, histology, and pathology of the cardiac conduction system: Part I. Clin Cardiol 1993;16:249–52.

36. Boyett MR, Honjo H, Kodama I, et al. The sinoatrial node: Cell size does matter. Circ Res 2007;101:e81–2.

37. Garson AJ, Bricker JT, Fisher DJ, Neish SR, eds. The science and practice of pediatric cardiology. Volume I. Baltimore, MD: Williams & Williams, 1998:141–3.

38. Hucker WJ, Fedorov VV, Foyil KV, Moazami N, Efimov IR. Optical mapping of the human atrioventricular junction. Circulation 2008;117:1474–7.

39. Li JL, Greener ID, Inada S, et al. Computer three-dimensional reconstruction of the atrioventricular node. Circ Res 2008; 102:975–85.

40. Becker AE, Anderson RH. The morphology of the human atrioventricular junctional area. In: Wellens HJJ, Lie KI, Janse MJ, eds. The conduction system of the heart: Structure, function, and clinical implications. Philadelphia, PA: Lea & Febiger, 1976:263–86.

41. Aschoff L. Referat uber die herzstorungen in ihren bezeihungen zu den spezifischen muskelsystem des herzens. Verh Dtsch Ges Pathol 1910;14:3–35.

42. Monckeberg JG. Beitrage zur normalen und pathologischen anatomie des herzens. Verh Dtsch Ges Pathol 1910;14: 64–71.

43. Hucker WJ, McCain ML Laughner JI, Iaizzo PA, Efimov IR. Connexin 43 expression delineates two discrete pathways in the human atrioventricular junction. Anat Rec (Hoboken) 2008; 291:204–15.

44. Davis LM, Rodefeld ME, Green K, Beyer EC, Saffitz JE. Gap junction protein phenotypes of the human heart and conduction system. J Cardiovasc Electrophysiol 1995;6:813–22

45. Zhang Y, Bharati S, Mowrey KA, Shaowei Z, Tchou PJ, Mazgalev TN. His electrogram alternans reveal dual-wavefront inputs into and longitudinal dissociation within the bundle of His. Circulation 2001;104:832–8.

46. Bharati S, Levine M, Huang SK, et al. The conduction system of the swine heart. Chest 1991;100:207–12.

47. Anderson RH, Becker AE, Brechenmacher C, Davies MJ, Rossi L. The human atrioventricular junctional area. A morphological study of the A–V node and bundle. Eur J Cardiol 1975;3:11–25.

48. Frink RJ, Merrick B. The sheep heart: Coronary and conduction system anatomy with special reference to the presence of an os cordis. Anat Rec 1974;179:189–200.

49. El-Sherif N, Lekieffre J. Practical management of cardiac arrhythmias. Armonk, NY: Futura Publishing Co., 1997:xv, 348.

50. Shrivastav M, Iaizzo P. Discrimination of ischemia and normal sinus rhythm for cardiac signals using a modified k means clustering algorithm. Conf Proc IEEE Eng Med Biol Soc 2007;3856–9.

51. Webster JG. Bioinstrumentation. Hoboken, NJ: John Wiley & Sons,2004:xiv, 383.

52. Shrivastav M. Methods of ambulatory detection and treatment of cardiac arrhythmias using implantable cardioverter-defibrillators. Biomed Instrum Technol 1999;33:505–21.

53. Webster JG, ed. Design of cardiac pacemakers. Piscataway, NJ: IEEE Press, 1995.

54. Sahakian AV, Peterson MS, Shkurovich S, et al. A simultaneous multichannel monophasic action potential electrode array for in vivo epicardial repolarization mapping. IEEE Trans Biomed Eng 2001;48:345–53.

55. Shenasa M, Borggrefe M, Breithardt G, eds. Cardiac mapping. 2nd ed. New York, NY: Futura, 2003:xxiii, 784.

56. Shrivastav M, Iaizzo PA. In vivo cardiac monophasic action potential recording using electromyogram needles. Proceedings of the IEEE Biomedical Circuits and Systems Conference. London, United Kingdom, 2006.

57. Schilling RJ, Kadish AH, Peters NS, Goldberger J, Davies DW. Endocardial mapping of atrial fibrillation in the human right atrium using a non-contact catheter. Eur Heart J 2000;21: 550–64.

58. Becker AE, Anderson RH. Proximal atrioventricular bundle, atrioventricular node, and distal atrioventricular bundle are distinct anatomic structures with unique histological characteristics and innervation—Response. Circulation 2001;103:e30–1.

59. Bharati S. Anatomy of the atrioventricular conduction system—Response. Circulation 2001;103:e63–4.

60. Magalev TN, Ho SY, Anderson RH. Special report: Anatomic-electrophysiological correlations concerning the pathways for atrioventricular conduction. Circulation 2001;103:2660–7.

61. Kucera JP, Rudy Y. Mechanistic insights into very slow conduction in branching cardiac tissue—A model study. Circulation Res 2001;89:799–806.

Additional Reference Texts

Mohrman DE, Heller LJ, eds. Cardiovascular physiology. 5th ed. New York, NY: Langer Medical Books/McGraw-Hill, 2003.

Wellens HJJ, Lie KI, Janse MJ, eds. The conduction system of the heart: Structure, function, and clinical implications. Philadelphia, PA: Lea & Febiger, 1976.

Alexander RW, Schlant RC, Fuster V, eds. Hurst's: The heart: Arteries and veins. 9th ed. New York, NY: McGraw-Hill, 1998.

Katz AM, ed. Physiology of the heart. 3rd ed. Philadelphia, PA: Lippincott, Williams, and Wilkins, 2001.

Tortora GJ, Grabowski SR, eds. Principles of anatomy and physiology. 9th ed. New York, NY: John Wiley & Sons, Inc., 2000.

Chapter 12
Autonomic Nervous System

Kevin Fitzgerald, Robert F. Wilson, and Paul A. Iaizzo

Abstract The autonomic nervous system and the role it plays in governing the behavior of the cardiovascular system is immense in both its complexity and importance to life. The antagonistic nature of the parasympathetic and sympathetic branches of this system allows rapid and essential changes in cardiac parameters such as heart rate, contractility, and stroke volume in order to deliver metabolites and nutrients to tissues and organs that need them at any given time. Increased sympathetic outflow relative to normal resting conditions most often causes an excitatory response in physiologic parameters (such as heart rate and/or smooth muscle contraction), whereas parasympathetic stimulation usually results in calming adjustments (decreased contractility and/or vasodilatation). It is important to note that both branches exhibit influences that do not rigidly fit into these general guidelines.

Keywords Sympathetic anatomy · Parasympathetic anatomy · Baroreceptors · Homeostasis · Hypothalamic control · Effector pathways · Heart rate · Stroke volume · Contractility · Arteriolar pressure · Cardiac denervation

column, but are classified by fundamental differences. Anatomically, the origin of the sympathetic (thoracolumbar) division of the central nervous system lies between the first thoracic (T1) and the second or third lumbar sections (L2 or L3). In contrast, the exiting fibers of the parasympathetic division (craniosacral) originate from both the medulla oblongata and the sacral portion of the spinal cord (S2–S4). The primary neurotransmitter released during depolarization is another means of characterizing the two branches of the autonomic nervous system. In the sympathetic division, norepinephrine is the principal postsynaptic neurotransmitter, whereas acetylcholine is the chief transmitter found throughout the parasympathetic division. The primary physiological response induced by each respective neurotransmitter is also a useful way to categorize the divisions of the autonomic nervous system. Such classifications are important considerations when investigating the autonomic nervous system regulation and function of the heart.

12.1 Introduction

The autonomic nervous system coordinates involuntary control of the viscera and other tissues throughout the body, with the exception of skeletal muscle. This branch of the central nervous system, organized into parasympathetic and sympathetic divisions, integrates efferent and afferent fibers that regulate the activities of the majority of organs, glands, and smooth musculature found in the body. The presynaptic cell bodies of these neurons comprising both categories originate in the gray matter of the spinal

12.2 Sympathetic Anatomy

Cell bodies of presynaptic sympathetic efferent neurons are found in the paired lateral horns of the spinal cord, an area identifiable between the T1 and the L2 or L3 vertebrae. The axons of these cells exit the interior of the spinal cord through ventral rootlets, which coalesce to form the larger ventral roots and eventually become ventral rami. Sympathetic fibers almost immediately divert into white rami communicantes (Fig. 12.1) branching from these spinal nerves, which connect them to paired columns of sympathetic ganglia located on either side of the spinal cord called the "sympathetic trunks." Vertebrae from T1 to S5 have corresponding pairs of ganglia, each of which

K. Fitzgerald (✉)
Medtronic, Inc., 1129 Jasmine St., Denver, CO 80220, USA
e-mail: kevin.fitzgerald@medtronic.com

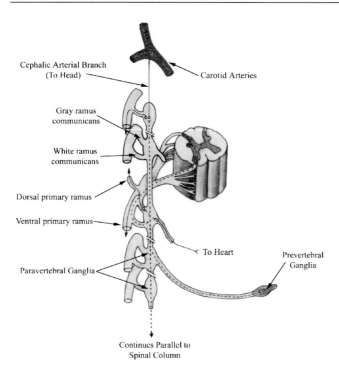

Cephalic Arterial Branch
(To Head)

Carotid Arteries

Gray ramus
communicans

White ramus
communicans

Dorsal primary ramus

Ventral primary ramus

To Heart

Prevertebral
Ganglia

Paravertebral Ganglia

Continues Parallel to
Spinal Column

Fig. 12.1 Pathways of sympathetic motor fibers. The three potential paths of travel taken by presynaptic sympathetic motor fibers are shown. Preganglionic fibers traveling to the heart and other areas of the thoracic cavity synapse either immediately upon reaching the sympathetic trunk or traverse to other levels to synapse. Complete passage through the paired trunks also occurs with prevertebral ganglia. Modified from Moore and Dalley [1]

are interconnected with both ascending and descending nerve fibers, forming the complex column-like structures.

Preganglionic sympathetic neurons synapse within the ganglia of the sympathetic trunk. The 10–20 nm separation distance [1] between presynaptic and postsynaptic cells is called the synaptic cleft, where neurotransmitter is released from synaptic vesicles. Acetylcholine is the neurotransmitter released from preganglionic neurons in both the sympathetic and the parasympathetic branches of the autonomic nervous system (Fig. 12.2). This compound binds to receptors on postsynaptic cell bodies, causing localized depolarizations of cell membranes, which may subsequently initiate action potentials that propagate down the axons of postsynaptic cells. In the sympathetic nervous system, norepinephrine is the primary postsynaptic neurotransmitter released. Such junctions can also be activated by epinephrine, and both can often be found with cotransmitters such as dopamine [2] and/or histamine [3]. Both norepinephrine and epinephrine play important roles during sympathetic stimulation of the heart, as will be discussed in later portions of this chapter.

Three primary paths of travel are commonly identified for presynaptic (also referred to as "preganglionic") nerve fibers upon reaching the sympathetic trunk. A preganglionic fiber can immediately synapse on the cell body of a postganglionic fiber at the level of the trunk upon which the fiber entered. Preganglionic fibers can also follow a route that traverses through the sympathetic trunk, either ascending or descending to synapse within a higher or lower level ganglion. A third but less common path of travel for presynaptic neurons involves passing through the sympathetic trunk completely, then synapsing within a prevertebral ganglion in close proximity to the viscera innervated. In general, presynaptic fibers traveling to the head, neck, thoracic cavity, and limbs will follow one of the first two courses. Innervation of organs and glands located in the abdominopelvic cavity follow the third path through prevertebral ganglia (Fig. 12.1).

A variation of the second path discussed above occurs primarily with innervation of sweat glands, hair follicles, and peripheral arteries. Presynaptic nerves that arrive at the paired sympathetic ganglion as discussed previously traverse through the white rami communicantes. Instead of immediately continuing to peripheral regions of the body after synapsing, the postsynaptic neurons next travel through gray (unmyelinated) rami (Fig. 12.1) and exit along large bundles of nerve fibers called "primary rami." From the primary rami, smaller nerve branches bifurcate and act to control the vasculature (vasodilatation and vasoconstriction), hair follicle stimulation, and sweating. If the nerves are destined for the head, their cell bodies are located in the superior cervical ganglion and their axons follow the path of the carotid arteries to their respective destinations; the muscles of the eye are also innervated by this collection of sympathetic neurons.

Nerve fibers traveling from the central nervous system to a destination elsewhere in the body are termed efferent. Afferent nerves carry information from various locations in the body to the central nervous system. Frequently, these respective paths of travel occur in parallel but the flow of excitation is in the opposite direction, and thus their fibers are bunched closely together to form larger nerve branches. The main nerve branches controlling the sympathetic behavior of the heart and lungs are the cardiopulmonary splanchnic nerves, which consist of both efferent and afferent fibers. Efferent nerves navigate a route originating from the ganglia in the upper cervical region (superior, middle, and inferior cervical ganglia) and the upper thoracic (T1–T5) levels of the sympathetic trunk. The inferior, middle, and superior cardiac nerves, in turn, originate from corresponding cervical ganglia and approach the base of the heart before splitting into smaller nerves and distributing themselves throughout much of the myocardium and vasculature. The cardiac

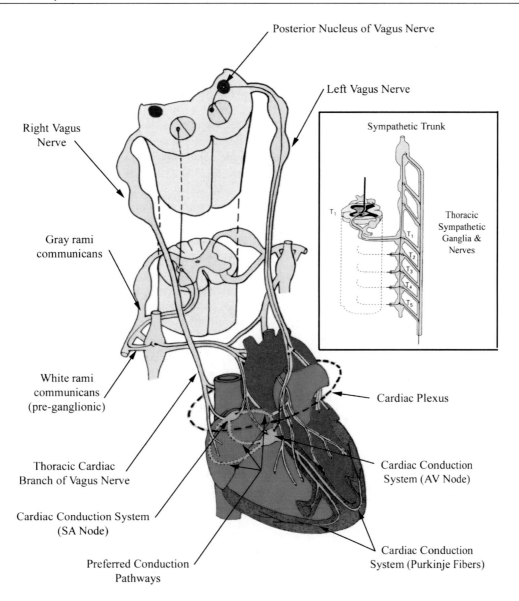

Fig. 12.2 Autonomic innervation of the heart. Vagal innervation of the right atrium can be observed. The area where many axons congregate just prior to innervation of the heart is depicted as the cardiac plexus. Sympathetic fibers branching from an arbitrary vertebral level of the paired sympathetic trunks are also illustrated. AV, atrioventricular; SA, sinoatrial. Modified from Martini [4]

plexus can be considered as groupings of the nerve bundles destined to and originating from the heart, which is depicted in Fig. 12.2; they are extremely difficult to visualize with the naked eye.

Incoming postsynaptic sympathetic neurons which innervate the human heart are highly concentrated around and near the aortic arch. Some of this innervation occurs throughout the aortic arch itself, as well as at the base of the ascending portion of the vessel. Many branches from these nerves continue down the aorta or under the arch to the pulmonary trunk, where they again diverge and track with the pulmonary arteries. Still more

neuronal bifurcations have been identified which extend to reach other areas of the heart, including both the atria and the right and left ventricles. Sympathetic innervation of both the sinoatrial and the atrioventricular nodes is important for control of heart rate, but has not been distinguished in greater concentration at these areas relative to elsewhere in the atria [5, 6]. Many nerves have been identified epicardially, often following the path of the coronary arteries and veins [5, 7]. In general, sympathetic innervation is more highly concentrated in the ventricles than in the atria [8]. Within the ventricles, a higher distribution is observed toward the base of the heart as opposed to the apex, with nerves in the epicardium at a slightly greater concentration than in the endocardium. This latter tendency is also evident in the atria [8].

12.3 Adrenal Medulla

The sympathetic nervous system also controls the hormonal secretions of the paired suprarenal (adrenal) glands in the abdomen, which are components of the endocrine system. Specifically, preganglionic fibers, with their cell bodies located in the lower thoracic (T10–T12) segments of the spinal cord, travel to the adrenal medulla by means of the abdominopelvic splanchnic nerves. It is in the medulla, or central portions of the suprarenal glands, that norepinephrine and epinephrine are released into the bloodstream [1]. The release of these catecholamines into the blood is considered a postsynaptic response initiated from this type of sympathetic activation. Specifically, the cortex surrounding the medulla portions of the adrenal glands is responsible for producing multiple steroid hormones. As blood drains from the highly vascularized cortex to the medulla, the aforementioned hormones can be used to convert norepinephrine to epinephrine. The respective mechanisms of action for these two similarly structured catecholamines will be discussed later.

12.4 Parasympathetic Anatomy

The parasympathetic (craniosacral) nervous system branches from four paired cranial nerves and the lower sacral segment of the spinal cord (S2–S4). The vagus nerve (cranial nerve X) is the main effector pathway for cardiac functions that are controlled by input from the parasympathetic branch of the autonomic nervous system (Fig. 12.2). Efferent fibers of the vagus nerves originate in the medulla oblongata and weave through the neck alongside the carotid arteries to the thoracic and abdominopelvic cavities, bifurcating many times along the way to innervate an assortment of organs including the heart. More specifically, the efferent fibers of the cranial parasympathetic branch communicate with blood vessels of the head and other viscera; the sacral portion of the spinal cord innervates viscera of the lower abdominopelvic cavity like the urinary bladder and colon, as well as their respective blood vessels.

Unlike the short sympathetic preganglionic fibers, the parasympathetic division of the autonomic nervous system generally has very long preganglionic fibers and short postsynaptic fibers. Hence, the parasympathetic ganglia

are often located very proximal to, or actually within, the target organ. As discussed previously, acetylcholine is this branch of the autonomic nervous system and is the primary neurotransmitter at both preganglionic and postganglionic junctions.

Within the heart, the majority of the parasympathetic ganglia are located near the sinoatrial node and within the conduction tissue surrounding the atrioventricular node [5]. Consequently, the right and left vagus nerves envelope a large and overlapping portion of the atria, where short postsynaptic fibers from both branches act on the conduction centers of the heart (Fig. 12.2). However, the endings of the right vagus primarily innervate the sinoatrial nodal region, while a great number of projections from the left are typically observed at the atrioventricular node [5]. In fact, high concentrations of vagal innervation situated within a localized region of epicardial fat near the atrioventricular node have been described for the human heart, and it is hypothesized that nerves located within this "pad" have little effect on behavior of the sinoatrial node [9]. Thus, it is likely that each region is controlled independently of the other. Parasympathetic junctions are also observed in the ventricles, but only at one-half to one-sixth as frequently as sympathetic innervation [8]. Nevertheless, nerves of the parasympathetic division of the autonomic nervous system outnumber those of the sympathetic division in the atria by some 30–60% [8]. Interestingly, while sympathetic innervation has been described to occur at approximately an equal distribution between the endocardial and the epicardial surfaces of the heart, vagal nerve endings are reportedly located at almost twice the density (1.7–1) transmurally (within the myocardium) when compared with their epicardial distribution [8].

12.5 Baroreceptors

The autonomic nervous system plays a vital role in the overall regulation of blood pressure throughout the body. Specialized receptors sensitive to changes in arterial diameter are located at various strategic locations within the upper thoracic cavity and neck; these nerve clusters are commonly known as "arterial baroreceptors." Substantial groupings of such baroreceptors can be found at the arch of the aorta and on the internal carotid arteries (just distal to where the common carotid bifurcates). This focal density of carotid baroreceptors is also termed the "carotid sinus." The majority of such receptors are located at areas within these arteries where the walls decrease in thickness, enabling pressure changes to be somewhat magnified at these locations (Fig. 12.3). Under even minimal pressure

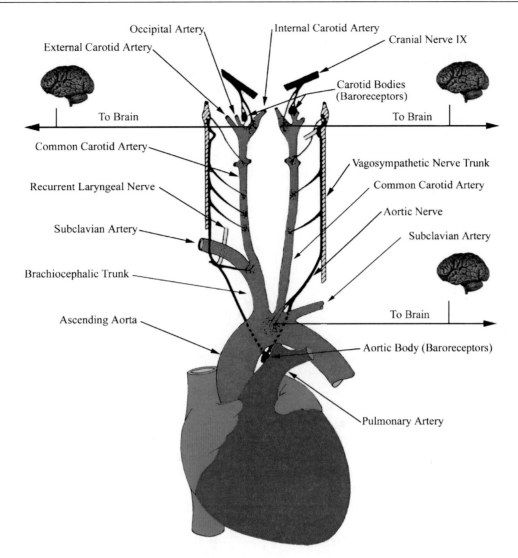

Fig. 12.3 Arterial baroreceptors. Receptors located at the bifurcations of the carotid arteries and aortic arch convey information to the brain and vasculature to help regulate pressure fluctuations. Modified from Mountcastle [10]

increases, these large arteries will elicit detectable wall dilatations. In contrast, under decreased pressure, their internal diameters will decline, also resulting in changes of the firing frequencies of these receptors. The axons of these afferent neurons travel from baroreceptors along parasympathetic corridors to the medullary cardiovascular center in the brainstem. Under increases in the mean pressure detected by these arterial baroreceptors, efferent sympathetic stimulation will decrease, which is accompanied by an increase in parasympathetic outflow to the heart. This neural activity is intended to return the mean pressure to a normal state. The opposite autonomic response would commence if the mean arterial pressure at the baroreceptor locations decreased. The synergistic functioning briefly noted here between both divisions of the autonomic nervous system will be discussed in much

greater detail in the following sections. It should be noted that the direct application of pressure to an individual's neck at the site of the carotid sinus can induce a reflex decrease in blood pressure, even to the point of causing unconsciousness, i.e., the so-called "sleeper hold."

12.6 Homeostasis

The tendency to maintain the internal environment of the body at a relatively constant level is known as "homeostasis." The heart itself exerts perhaps the greatest control influences on countless parameters involving the circulation of blood throughout the body. The heart communicates with the central nervous system via both branches of the autonomic nervous system. Both the sympathetic and the parasympathetic divisions work together in synergistic control of antagonistic influences in order to prevent potentially harmful fluctuations in many vital bodily functions. While it is obvious that significant changes do occur, an array of physiologic responses involving the heart (homeostatic control mechanisms) mediated by the autonomic nervous system quickly reverses these changes to return within the reasonable ranges required to maintain overall health. In general, homeostatic control functions are the underlying determinants of the relative parasympathetic and sympathetic activation.

12.7 Hypothalamic Control

The autonomic control of the heart is greatly influenced by the activity within the portion of the brain known as the "hypothalamus." Afferent fibers from the brainstem (medulla oblongata) and spinal cord convey information via the autonomic afferent system to the hypothalamic nuclei within the central nervous system [11], whereas impulses that leave the hypothalamus travel along efferent fibers to the various sympathetic and parasympathetic ganglia as noted above. Most parasympathetic response signals have been determined to originate from the anterior portions of the hypothalamus, while sympathetic activity stems primarily from the posterior portions [6, 11]. Direct electrical stimulation of specific sites within the hypothalamus can initiate preprogrammed simultaneous patterned changes in heart rate, blood pressure, and peripheral resistance [5].

As noted above, afferent axons from the aortic and carotid baroreceptors principally travel to the medullary cardiovascular centers, with neural pathways continuing onward to hypothalamus [6]. It should be noted that temperature regulation of the body is also centered within the hypothalamus. Thus, during exposure to cold, the hypothalamus initiates appropriate autonomic responses to maintain body temperature, like vasoconstriction and shivering. The contraction of the peripheral vasculature motivates a redistribution of blood flow to vital organs like the heart and brain, in order to maintain their suitable function [2]. The shiver reflex induced by the hypothalamus increases heat production which, in turn, causes additional adjustments in blood flow and cardiac activity. The opposite outcome occurs during exposure to high degrees of heat, such that sweating is initiated via postganglionic sympathetic neurons, and vasodilation of the vasculature supplying the skin is amplified. The regulation of bodily processes is an important responsibility of the hypothalamus, and it performs such tasks via the autonomic

pathways, hence regulating countless systems within the body simultaneously. Keeping this relative state of constancy throughout the body regardless of extreme changes that may occur externally is referred to as "homeostasis;" in nearly all cases, there are direct effects on cardiac performance.

In addition to the influence the hypothalamus has on autonomic pathways, emotional and hormonal changes are controlled in this region of the brain in order to promote homeostasis. The pituitary gland function is also mediated by the hypothalamus, initiating or suppressing hormonal release from this important part of the endocrine system to the rest of the body. Some of these hormones act as cotransmitters in the presence of acetylcholine or norepinephrine during synapses eliciting parasympathetic or sympathetic activity [2], dopamine being one example.

12.8 Effector Pathways to the Heart

Within the myocardium, parasympathetic nerve fibers release acetylcholine upon stimulation. Cardiac cells contain muscarinic receptors embedded within their lipid bilayer, which can activate G-proteins found in their cytoplasm upon binding with acetylcholine. Activation occurs when a bound GDP (guanosine diphosphate) molecule is replaced by a GTP (guanosine triphosphate) structure. Subsequently, this response allows the altered protein to bind with potassium channels in the membrane and causes them to open, thus increasing potassium permeability (Fig. 12.4). As a result, heart rate will generally decrease due to an efflux of potassium ions (K^+) from cardiac cells, since the cellular membrane becomes more polarized as the potential moves closer to the K^+ equilibrium potential of -90 mV [6]. This hyperpolarization makes the spontaneous generation of action potentials more difficult, and thus slows the rate of firing of the sinoatrial node. Activated G-proteins will remain in such a state until GTP is hydrolyzed to form inactive GDP [2, 12].

The type of regulatory control in the case described above involves the direct opening of K^+ channels via G-proteins within a cardiac muscle cell. It should also be noted that indirect opening of potassium channels may also occur after acetylcholine binds to the muscarinic receptors. Furthermore, activated G-proteins may also cause some increase in the production of arachidonic acid, which acts as a secondary messenger that can result in increased K^+ permeability due to cleavage of membrane lipids [12].

Modulation of G-proteins is also an important aspect of the underlying sympathetic effects on cardiac behavior. Sympathetic fibers release norepinephrine at postsynaptic terminals of cardiac muscle cells, and receptors located

Fig. 12.4 The effect of acetylcholine on cardiac muscle cells. Potassium channels within a cellular membrane are opened as a result of binding an activated G-protein. Acetylcholine released by parasympathetic neurons activates these G-proteins by binding with muscarinic receptors within the membrane. The effect of norepinephrine on cardiac muscle cells is propagated in a similar manner, with differences as described in the text. GTP, guanosine triphosphate

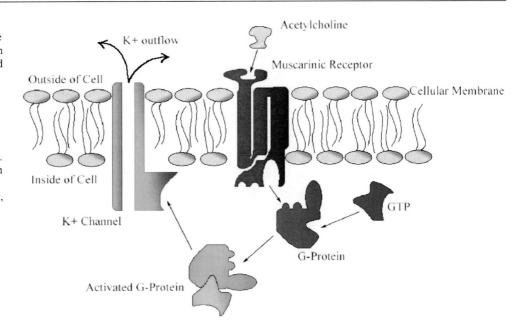

within the cellular membrane bind with the norepinephrine to stimulate β_1 adrenergic receptors. Next, G-proteins replace GDP at their binding sites with GTP upon activation by the excited β_1 receptors, causing an increase in the production of cyclic AMP within the cardiac myocytes. The increased cAMP levels cause molecules of protein kinase A to phosphorylate large numbers of calcium channels within the cellular membrane. This addition of a phosphate group not only causes Ca^{2+} channels to remain open longer but also allows for a greater number of channels to open, thus contributing to the influx of calcium ions into each cell upon activation [6]. In other words, the threshold for depolarization will be more easily attained due to the greater number of available calcium channels, thus allowing greater calcium incursion during activation and resulting in higher contraction strength.

An advantage of the mechanisms of action involving G-proteins is that autonomic modulation can be sustained without constant nerve fiber stimulation. That is, a burst of synaptic activity causing the release of either acetylcholine or norepinephrine can initiate the respective processes described above. For more details on cardiac receptors and intracellular signaling, refer to Chapter 13.

12.9 Specific Sympathetic and Parasympathetic Cardiac Controls

12.9.1 Heart Rate

The rate at which a normal adult heart completes cardiac cycles during rest is approximately 70 beats/min [6]. The heart rate is maintained at this relatively constant value via a continuous firing (activation) of the vagus nerve, called "basal (or vagal) tone." The heart rate will increase when vagal tone is overcome by increased activity of sympathetic nerves to the heart, which releases norepinephrine and causes a rise in the sinoatrial nodal depolarization rate (Fig. 12.5). A rate increase of this nature is referred to as a "positive chronotropic effect." As stated above, the fundamental cause of this increase in heart rate is due to an increase in activated calcium channels in myocardial cell membranes, increasing the speed at which depolarization occurs. This increased sympathetic outflow can be initiated by a large array of internal and external stimuli, including but not limited to exercise, an

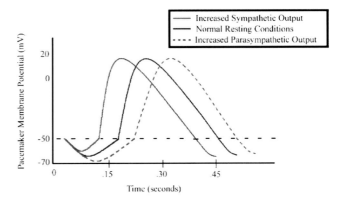

Fig. 12.5 The effects of changes in sympathetic and parasympathetic outflows to the heart. The heart will increase its rate of contraction during increased sympathetic neural stimulation. This time is required for the cardiac pacemaker cells to reach threshold decreases. In contrast, increased parasympathetic outflow will decrease the heart rate and increase the time to threshold

increase in body temperature, trauma, and/or stress. Additionally, a concurrent release of epinephrine from the adrenal medulla can further amplify these same effects on myocardial ion channels, although to elicit a significant rise in heart rate, the amount of the hormone liberated must be fairly substantial [6].

Parasympathetic discharge, in part, increases potassium ion permeability in cardiac myocytes, thus increasing the threshold for depolarization to occur spontaneously particularly within the sinoatrial node; as a result, the heart rate declines (Fig. 12.5). This autonomic neural input predominates during sleep and other sedentary states, eliciting an increase in cardiac cycle time and therefore enabling the heart to expend less energy [2]. In addition to decreasing the slope of the pacemaker potential, parasympathetic stimulation may also induce a so-called pacemaker shift [5]; true pacemaker cells can become more inhibited than the latent pacemakers, thus shifting the initiation of spontaneous depolarization from the true pacemakers to the latent ones [5].

Conduction velocity is the measure of the spread of action potentials through the heart. Parasympathetic stimulation above normal tonic activity slows this conduction velocity, and this response is termed "negative dromotropic." It follows that an increase in conduction velocity, which commonly accompanies sympathetic stimulation, has a "positive dromotropic" effect. The atrioventricular node is the location within the heart where conduction speed variation is most notable. The reader is referred to Chapter 11.

The control mechanisms of heart rate are also, in part, dependent on gender [13]. For example, women have been shown to exhibit higher frequency parasympathetic input (using spectral analysis procedures) than men of similar age, possibly indicating a more dominant control of heart rate via vagal stimulation than their male counterparts [13].

12.9.2 Stroke Volume and Contractility

Like heart rate, the amount of blood ejected from the ventricles during systole is greater when the heart is modulated by an increased sympathetic input (Fig. 12.6). The underlying mechanism for this increased stroke volume is enhanced cardiac myocyte contractility, and the magnitude of this response is strongly affected by preload and afterload conditions, as predicted by the Frank–Starling law [6]. Such an increase in contractility is characterized as a "positive inotropic" effect. By and large, myocytes increase in length in proportion to their preload, and since they become more elongated, they also have the capability to shorten over this

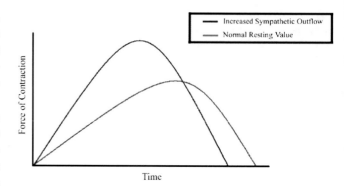

Fig. 12.6 Effect of increased sympathetic stimulation on contractility (see text for details)

greater distance. This increased amount of shortening leads to an enhanced strength of contraction of the heart (see also Chapter 10). As described previously, sympathetic excitation facilitates a larger and more rapid Ca^{2+} influx into cardiac cells, which further augments the degree of overall contraction during systole [12].

Combined with a larger preload, the increased contractility due to calcium ion influx will raise the stroke volume of the heart (Fig. 12.7). Likewise, the ejection fraction of blood from a given chamber of the heart also elevates accordingly [2]. However, stroke volume is also dependent on afterload created by the relative diameter of the peripheral arteries and will not increase as significantly under sympathetic stimulation if the afterload is elevated due to vasoconstriction. As expected from the often antagonistic nature of the autonomic nervous system, parasympathetic stimulation decreases contractility. However, the relative decrease in contractility is much less significant than the increase in this parameter that sympathetic input provides [2].

An important concept to note involves simultaneous increases in heart rate and stroke volume. Since cardiac output is the product of these two quantities, its overall value commonly increases with sympathetic stimulation.

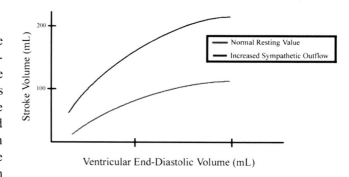

Fig. 12.7 Effect of increased sympathetic stimulation on stroke volume (see text for details)

Conversely, cardiac output normally decreases with a higher rate of parasympathetic input. This is common when the body is in a sedentary state, hence tissue oxygen and metabolite requirements are not as high.

The time necessary for the heart to fully contract and relax decreases under sympathetic stimulation, due primarily to the larger proportion of the cardiac cycle that is made available for filling. While an increase in heart rate makes the total duration of the cardiac cycle shorter [2], the corresponding rise in contractility causes the muscular contractions to commence more rapidly and with greater force than under resting conditions. This translates to a decrease in the amount of time necessary for contraction of the heart during a complete cardiac cycle. Thus, the heart is relaxed for a greater portion of the cycle, enabling enhanced filling of the chambers to provide a greater volume of blood ejected for each contraction.

12.9.3 Baroreceptor Pressure Regulation

Arterial pressure, or afterload, is regulated in the short-term by baroreceptors in the walls of the aorta and carotid arteries. In particular, baroreceptors sense both the magnitude and the rate of stretch of arterial walls due to pressure fluctuations within the vessels [6]. The afferent fibers projecting from the baroreceptors convey this information concerning pressure shifts to the autonomic nervous system which, in turn, responds by either increasing or decreasing sympathetic and/or parasympathetic drive. A basal tonic activity can be identified from the receptors, which progresses to the higher cardiovascular

centers. The frequency of impulses can be observed to increase or decrease in response to these pressure changes. Decreased arterial dilatation causes sympathetic nerves to increase their discharge rate and escalate the release of norepinephrine, thus increasing heart rate, stroke volume, and peripheral resistance [2]. The baroreceptor reflex functions as a negative feedback system [6], such that a decrease in arterial stretch will induce an increased sympathetic discharge, accordingly raising cardiac output (Fig. 12.8). This, in turn, will increase blood delivered to the vessels containing baroreceptors, increase pressure, and decrease the tonic activity of the receptors. Homeostatic control of arterial pressure is thus administered, since the decreased baroreceptor discharge rate will cause a lowered degree of sympathetic activity and revert the cardiac output back toward its basal value. In other words, the response of the baroreceptors ultimately removes the stimulus causing the initial response [6]. Carotid artery massage is sometimes suggested in an attempt to decrease overall sympathetic tone in the body, e.g., an individual eliciting an arrhythmia due to stress can sometimes convert back to a normal sinus rhythm by such a maneuver.

Importantly, long-term pressure regulation is not accomplished via baroreceptor input, due to their adaptive nature (accommodation). That is, if pressure in the aorta and carotid arteries remains elevated for sustained periods, the tonic firing rates will eventually return toward resting values regardless of whether or not the pressures remain elevated. Long-term regulation of pressure involves numerous complex hormonal mechanisms, which are extensively influenced by the hypothalamic and medullary cardiovascular centers.

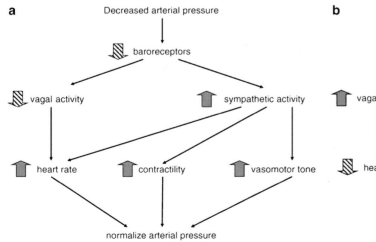

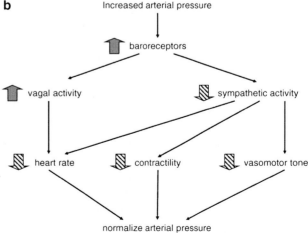

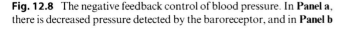

Fig. 12.8 The negative feedback control of blood pressure. In **Panel a**, there is decreased pressure detected by the baroreceptor, and in **Panel b**

there is an elevated pressure. The relative responses that occur in order to maintain an overall normal systemic pressure are indicated

12.9.4 Arteriolar Pressure Regulation

Because the heart is responsible for delivery of blood to every part of the body, homeostatic control often involves changing the amount of blood provided by the circulatory system to a given tissue, organ, or organ system. For example, the gastrointestinal system normally receives approximately 20% of the blood pumped by the heart during each cardiac cycle. However, during times of intense stress or exertion, the blood provided to this area may drastically decrease, while the proportion of blood provided to the heart and skeletal muscles may increase notably. Such changes in blood supply are commonly mediated by changes in resistance of the peripheral vasculature (see also Fig. 1.7 in Chapter 1).

At rest, the smooth muscle cells in the walls of arterioles throughout the body remain slightly contracted due to a combination of influences from the central nervous system, hormonal distribution within the vasculature, and/or localized organ effects. The relative degree of contraction within the arterioles is referred to as their basal tone. The stretching of the arterioles due to pulsatile blood pressure is thought to be the cause of the constant state of stress within such vessels [6]. Arterioles innervated by sympathetic fibers possess an increased contractile tone, termed the "neurogenic tone," due to the sustained activation of these fibers. Control of the vascular peripheral resistance is achieved by varying the firing frequency within these sympathetic fibers. More specifically, postganglionic fibers release the neurotransmitter norepinephrine, which binds to alpha (α_1) adrenergic receptors within the smooth muscle cells in arteriolar walls. Thus, an increase in the firing activity of these neurons produces an increase in norepinephrine levels which, in turn, binds with more α_1 receptors and causes an overall decrease in the diameters of arterioles. In contrast, a lowering of the basal tonic activity causes vasodilation, since less neurotransmitter is available for binding, causing the smooth muscle cells to relax.

The relative firing rates of arteriolar sympathetic neurons innervating a given tissue are also modulated by the need for blood elsewhere in the body. For example, if a hemorrhage occurs in the abdomen which results in significant bleeding, sympathetic activity to that area will increase, causing less blood to flow to these damaged tissues in an attempt to preserve adequate levels of flow to the heart and brain. It should be noted that other regulators exist for the control of vasomotion and the tonic activity of the sympathetic system. Local increases in extracellular cation concentrations, acetylcholine levels, and even norepinephrine itself can act to prevent extreme vasoconstriction. Adrenergic receptors that are pharmacologically different from those in smooth muscle

cells [6] have been identified on postganglionic sympathetic neurons themselves and are given an α_2 designation. These receptors bind with the neurotransmitter and inhibit its release if the amount previously liberated is excessive (negative feedback).

Blood flow through the coronary arterioles is primarily regulated by local metabolic controls that are highly coupled with oxygen consumption. That is, subtle increases in oxygen consumption by the heart will result in an increase in blood flow through the coronaries. Elevated sympathetic activity of the systemic vasculature typically induces a subsequent decrease in the diameter of the peripheral arteries. However, upon sympathetic excitation, vasodilatation predominates in the coronary arterioles instead of vasoconstriction, since oxygen consumption is raised significantly by concurrently inducing higher heart rates and levels of contractility. The factors motivating metabolic regulation therefore outweigh the vasoconstrictive effects of sympathetic innervation of the coronaries.

Blood flow to skeletal muscle is controlled in a similar manner to that of the coronary arteries, in that local metabolic factors play a vital role in regulating vessel resistance. While increased sympathetic activity may decrease the blood flow to a resting skeletal muscle by a factor of four [6], a muscle undergoing exercise (and thus in the presence of elevated sympathetic activity) can elicit an increase in blood flow almost 20 times that of normal resting values [6]. However, this muscle response must occur in conjunction with a drastic decrease in the blood flow to other tissues or organs, such as those of the abdominal cavity or nonexercising muscles. This course of action allows the total peripheral resistance to remain at a functional level. Homeostatic control during exercise also exists at the skin. In order to cool the body from the increased metabolic heat production, sweat glands become active and blood flow increases significantly over the normal resting value in order to dissipate excess body heat. The active vasodilatation is the result of metabolic activity overcoming the increased sympathetic outflow to skin arterioles.

During the digestion of food, increased sympathetic activity predominates at the vasculature of skeletal muscles and increases blood flow to the stomach and intestines. Parasympathetic discharge to the heart increases, while the sympathetic stimulus declines, lowering the heart rate. This concentration of blood to the abdominal organs facilitates the movement of nutrients to areas of the body in need and is a good example of how both branches of the autonomic nervous system work together to sustain a level of balance throughout the entire body.

The suprarenal glands can also contribute to vasomotion. Since norepinephrine is released directly into the bloodstream from these endocrine glands, arteriolar constriction in the systemic organs can result. The "fight or flight" response in humans elicited under stressful or exciting circumstances originates from the hypothalamus via hormones that travel to the pituitary gland and later the adrenal cortex, where the agent cortisol is released into the bloodstream and adrenal medulla. It is in the medulla that cortisol activates the enzyme necessary to convert norepinephrine to epinephrine, which is released into the bloodstream to amplify increased sympathetic activity [2, 3]. Blood flow to the skin and other internal organs (like the stomach and intestines) is greatly decreased by increasing sympathetic (and decreasing parasympathetic) tonic activity, while flow to skeletal muscles and the heart increases considerably. This process can be thought of as simply delivering blood to the areas of the body most in need to deal with the demanding circumstances. The direct release of these agents into the bloodstream allows for their rapid circulation, which helps contract arterioles along with conventional sympathetic outflow. The "adrenaline rush" one experiences during periods of great tension or exhilaration comes from the adrenal glands.

Regulation of the veins and venules in the body is carried out by many of the same mechanisms as that for arterioles. While veins have smooth muscle in their walls complete with α_1 receptors that respond to norepinephrine, their basal tonic activity is much lower than that observed in arterioles. Thus, venules at rest can be considered to be in a more dilated state. The wall thickness of veins is also significantly less than that found in arteries, which enables the consequences of physical effects to be more prominent in veins. That is, the overall blood volume associated with veins can be greatly affected by compressive forces. For example, in skeletal muscle, the degree of muscle contraction around the vessel can push large amounts of blood back toward the heart, which enables quicker filling within the right atrium and enables sustained physical activity. If skeletal muscles surrounding veins are relaxed, the venous system can act as a blood reservoir (see also Fig. 1.3 in Chapter 1).

Vasculature of skeletal muscles and the liver can have a unique effect on homeostasis via noninnervated β_2 receptors located in arteriolar walls. Increased blood levels of epinephrine can activate these receptors which, along with G-proteins [6, 12], act to catalyze an intracellular chemical reaction resulting in decreased cytoplasmic levels of Ca^{2+} and a hyperpolarization of the cellular membrane. This decreases the contractile machinery sensitivity to Ca^{2+}, causing vasodilatation [6]. Vasodilatation in the presence of epinephrine is in contrast to the decrease in vessel diameter caused by the chemically similar compound norepinephrine. The β_2 receptors are more sensitive to epinephrine than the α_1 receptors [6]. Thus, a small elevation in the concentration of epinephrine in the bloodstream (e.g.,

provided by the adrenal medulla) can cause vasodilatation. However, if the level of catecholamine increases, the more numerous α_1 receptors will be activated and cause vasoconstriction. It is important to note that there is no neural input to β_2 receptors, and norepinephrine therefore has no effect on their activation.

It can be seen that the parasympathetic and sympathetic effects of the heart and vasculature often elicit opposite physiologic responses, yet work in conjunction to synergistically maintain homeostasis.

12.10 Cardiac Denervation

Denervation can be divided into two categories—preganglionic and postganglionic. Preganglionic denervation can be caused primarily by disease or injury of the vasomotor centers in the brain or spinal cord above T10; it leaves intact the postganglionic nerve fiber and many reflexes that occur at the ganglionic level. Preganglionic denervation results not only in loss of centrally mediated cardiac reflexes but also leads to abnormalities in the control of peripheral vascular tone and inability to control blood pressure with changes in body position. Shy–Drager syndrome is a classic example of preganglionic denervation affecting the cardiovascular system [14].

Postganglionic denervation of the heart occurs as the result of several neurodegenerative processes, after certain types of cardiac surgery and/or after cardiac transplantation. Loss of the postganglionic nerve cell body results in Wallerian degeneration of the distal nerve, with loss of axonal integrity and neurotransmitters. Loss of neurotransmitters at the neural junction with the distal target (e.g., cardiac conduction tissue or cardiac myocytes) leads to an increase in neurotransmitter receptor number and density. This, combined with a loss of neurotransmitter metabolism by the degenerated neuron, makes both the cardiac conduction system and the muscle hypersensitive to circulating catecholamines (the so-called denervation hypersensitivity).

Cardiac transplantation is the most complete form of cardiac denervation, resulting in loss of both sympathetic and parasympathetic innervation, with subsequent Wallerian degeneration of the intracardiac nerve fibers [15]. Diabetes is the most common cause of denervation in the general non-transplant population [16]. More specifically, a diabetic neuropathy can result in loss of both sympathetic and parasympathetic efferent and afferent pathways. As with other neurodegenerative diseases, neuronal loss is typically patchy and permanent. Other diseases leading to cardiac denervation include infiltrative diseases such as amyloidosis.

12.10.1 Effects of Denervation on Basal Cardiac Function

Loss of tonic parasympathetic vagal inhibition of sinus node depolarization causes a rise in basal heart rate and loss of heart rate fluctuation with respiration. The resting heart rate of heart transplant patients typically is 95–100 beats/min. A number of reflexes that are mediated primarily through the vagal nerves are absent, including carotid sinus slowing of heart rate, the pulmonary inflation reflex, and the Bezold–Jarisch reflex.

In contrast, resting inotropic state of the cardiac muscle and myocardial blood flow are normal after denervation; basal ventricular function is changed minimally by denervation. Measures of systolic contraction (such as dP/dt, ejection fraction, and cardiac output) are usually preserved. Preservation of pump function after denervation may be related, in part, to an upregulation of beta catecholamine receptors on myocytes and the conduction system, leading to an amplification of the response to bloodborne catecholamines [17].

Coronary blood flow is unchanged at rest and increases normally with exercise. Coronary flow reserve (a measure of maximal coronary blood flow) is normal, although in animals the response to ischemia is blunted [18, 19].

Afferent sensation to pain (e.g., from ischemia), chemoreceptor stimulation (e.g., from ischemia, hyperosmolar contrast media), and stretch receptor stimulation (e.g., from pressure overload) are all initially absent. This aspect of denervation is important because coronary occlusion due to transplant-related coronary arteriorpathy is common and the absence of anginal pain removes an important warning symptom.

12.10.2 Effects of Denervation on Exercise Hemodynamics

Cardiac denervation results in a blunting of the chronotropic response to exercise. With exercise, heart rate rises due to an increase in plasma catecholamines (released primarily from the adrenal glands) rather than from direct sympathetic stimulation of the sinus node. The heart rate increase is delayed; heart rate peaks well after cessation of exertion and remains elevated until the circulating catecholamines can be metabolized (Fig. 12.9).

Exercise or stress also results in a delayed increase in inotropic state, similar to the changes in chronotropic response. Unlike resting ventricular function, peak inotropic state and ejection fraction are typically reduced.

12.10.3 Reinnervation

Sympathetic neural reinnervation of the heart occurs in nearly all animals undergoing auto-transplantation and in most patients undergoing orthotropic transplantation. Reinnervation typically occurs over both the aortic and the atrial suture lines (left more than right), extending from the base of the heart to the apex. The rate of reinnervation is slow (years), and in humans it is patchy and incomplete. The anterior wall typically reinnervates earlier and more densely than the rest of the left ventricle [20]. The sinus node reinnervates to some degree in over 75–80% of the patients.

Reinnervation results in partial normalization of the chronotropic and inotropic response to exercise [21, 22]. Reinnervated patients exercise longer and have higher

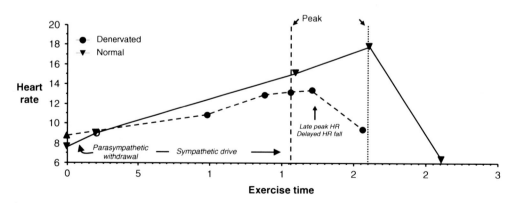

Fig. 12.9 The heart rate response to treadmill exercise is shown for normally innervated subjects (*solid line*) and patients with cardiac denervation after heart transplantation (*dashed line*). The denervated patients have higher resting heart rates, but heart rates rise more slowly with exercise because the increase in heart rate is dependent primarily on circulating catecholamines. After cessation of exercise, heart rates in the denervated patients continue to rise briefly and then fall slowly as circulating catecholamines are metabolized

maximal oxygen consumptions. Additionally, cardiac pain sensation (i.e., angina) can return, although the regional nature of reinnervation results in reduced or patchy sensation to ischemia in most transplant recipients [23]. Parasympathetic reinnervation has been reported in a small number of transplant recipients; it is accompanied by return of respiratory-mediated fluctuation in heart rate and carotid sinus slowing of heart rate.

It should be noted that in some transplant patients, the native sinus node is left intact, yet due to the suture line, these individuals require pacing therapy. There are known causes in which the activity in natively innervated nodes is sensed by a pacing system which then rate adjusts the ventricular pacing accordingly; hence, a more functional control of heart rate is maintained relative to the intrinsic activity within the autonomic nervous system.

12.11 Summary

The autonomic nervous system and the role it plays in governing the behavior of the cardiovascular system is immense in both its complexity and importance to life. The antagonistic nature of the parasympathetic and sympathetic branches of this system allows rapid and essential changes in cardiac parameters such as heart rate, contractility, and stroke volume in order to deliver metabolites and nutrients to tissues and organs that need them at any given time. Increased sympathetic outflow relative to normal resting conditions most often causes an excitatory response in physiologic parameters (such as heart rate and/or smooth muscle contraction), whereas parasympathetic stimulation usually results in calming adjustments (decreased contractility and/or vasodilatation). It is important to note that both branches exhibit influences that do not rigidly fit into these general guidelines.

References

1. Moore KL, Dalley AF II, eds. Clinically oriented anatomy. 4th ed. Philadelphia, PA: Lippincott Williams & Wilkins, 1999.
2. Vander A, Sherman J, Luciano D, eds. Human physiology. 8th ed. Boston, MA: McGraw Hill, 2001.
3. Hansen JT, Koeppen BM, eds. Netter's atlas of human physiology. 1st ed. Teterboro, NJ: Icon Learning Systems LLC, 2002.
4. Martini, FH, ed. Fundamentals of anatomy and physiology. 5th ed. New York, NY: Benjamin Cummings, 2001.
5. Berne RM, Levy MN, eds. Cardiovascular physiology. 3rd ed. St. Louis, MO: C.V. Mosby Company, 1977.
6. Mohrman DE, Heller LJ, eds. Cardiovascular physiology. 5th ed. New York, NY: Lange Medical Books/McGraw Hill, 2003.
7. Netter FH, ed. Atlas of human anatomy. 2nd ed. East Hanover, NJ: Novartis, 1998.
8. Kawano H, Okada R, Yano K. Histological study on the distribution of autonomic nerves in the human heart. Heart & Vessels 2003;18:32–9.
9. Quan K, Lee JH, Van Hare G, Biblo L, Mackall J, Carlson M. Identification and characterization of atrioventricular parasympathetic innervation in humans. J Cardiovasc Electrophysiol 2002;13:735–9.
10. Mountcastle VB, ed. Medical physiology. 14th ed. St. Louis, MO: C.V. Mosby Company, 1980.
11. Nolte J, ed. The human brain: An introduction to its functional anatomy. 5th ed. St. Louis, MO: Mosby, 2002.
12. Matthews GG, ed. Cellular physiology of nerve and muscle. 3rd ed. Malden, MA: Blackwell Science, Inc., 1998.
13. Evans JM, Ziegler MG, Patwardhan AR, et al. Gender differences in autonomic cardiovascular regulation: Spectral, hormonal and hemodynamic indexes. J Appl Physiol 2001;91:2611–8.
14. Ziegler MG, Lake CR, Kopin IJ. Sympathetic nervous system defect in primary orthostatic hypotension. N Engl J Med 1977;296:293.
15. Williams VL, Cooper T, Hanlon CR. Neural responses following autotransplantation of the canine heart. Circulation 1963;27:713.
16. Watkins PJ, MacKay JD. Cardiac denervation in diabetic neuropathy. Ann Intern Med 1980;92:304–7.
17. Vatner DE, Lavallee M, Amano J, Finizola A, Homcy CJ, Vatner SF. Mechanisms of supersensitivity to sympathomimetic amines in the chronically denervated heart of the conscious dog. Circ Res 1985;57:55–64.
18. Lavallee M, Amano J, Vatner SF, Manders WT, Randall WC, Thomas JX. Adverse effects of chronic denervation in conscious dogs with myocardial ischemia. Circ Res 1985;57:383–92.
19. McGinn AL, Wilson RF, Olivari MT, Homans DC, White CW. Coronary vasodilator reserve after human orthotopic cardiac transplantation. Circulation 1988;78:1200–9.
20. Schwaiger M, Hutchins GD, Kalff V, et al. Evidence for regional catecholamine uptake and storage sites in the transplanted human heart by positron emission tomography. J Clin Invest 1991;87:1681–90.
21. Wilson RF, Johnson TH, Haidet GC, Kubo SH, Mianuelli M. Sympathetic reinnervation of the sinus node and exercise hemodynamics after cardiac transplantation. Circulation 2000;101:2727–33.
22. Bengel FM, Ueberfuhr P, Schlepel N, Reichart B, Schwaiger M. Effect of sympathetic reinnervation on cardiac performance after heart transplantation. N Engl J Med 2001;345:731–8.
23. Stark RP, McGinn AL, Wilson RF. Chest pain in cardiac transplant recipients: Evidence for sensory reinnervation after cardiac transplantation. N Engl J Med 1991;324:1791–4.

Chapter 13
Cardiac and Vascular Receptors and Signal Transduction

Daniel C. Sigg and Ayala Hezi-Yamit

Abstract Cellular physiological functions are regulated via signaling mechanisms in essentially any cell type of any organ. While myocardial cells are unique in that they are interconnected to each other via gap junctions and thus act as an electrical syncytium, there is nevertheless an enormous number of important cellular receptors that allow individual cells to receive and respond to various signals. Inflammation plays a very important role in cardiovascular disease. For example, device-based interventions such as coronary stenting may activate inflammation via a series of complex signaling processes. Importantly, inflammation pathways also play a central role in the elicitation of atherosclerosis, myocardial infarction, and/or heart failure. It is the general aim of this chapter to review the role and signaling mechanisms of selected physiologically and pathophysiologically important cardiac and vascular receptors with emphasis on G-protein-coupled receptors (e.g., beta-adrenergic receptors), non-G-protein-coupled receptor systems, such as guanylyl cyclase-related receptors (e.g., receptors for nitric oxide), and finally, to discuss the importance and complexity of inflammation in the pathobiology of coronary artery disease and stenting.

Keywords Cardiovascular cell receptors · Intracellular function · Signal transduction · Receptor coupling · G-protein receptor · Beta-adrenergic receptor · Alpha-adrenergic receptor · Muscarinic receptor · Receptor cross-talk

13.1 Introduction

Cellular physiological functions are regulated via signaling mechanisms in essentially any cell type of any organ. While myocardial cells are somewhat unique in that they are interconnected to each other with gap junctions and act as an electrical syncytium, there is nevertheless an enormous number of important cellular receptors that allow the cells to receive and respond to various signals. Many of these receptors are located on the cellular membrane. It would be elusive and clearly beyond the scope of this review to discuss all the receptors of all the cell types in the cardiovascular system. Our understanding of molecular cardiovascular biology is continuously growing. Therefore, it is the general aim of this chapter to focus on selected physiologically and pathophysiologically important cardiac and vascular receptors. Nevertheless, many of the principles and mechanisms discussed in the following pages, using certain receptor subtypes as examples, are applicable to related receptor systems and should make it easier to study and understand a "new" receptor signaling system. Furthermore, a thorough review of the normal function of these receptors is important and very helpful in understanding the altered function of the same receptor systems and associated signaling mechanisms in disease states. For example, it will be reviewed how a β-receptor antagonist (beta-blocker, a drug that is known to depress cardiac contractility) may be beneficial in the treatment of heart failure, a state of depressed cardiac function. This chapter will also largely focus on the large and important family of G-protein-coupled receptors, with particular emphasis on the β-adrenergic receptor (β-AR) signaling system; this system has important functions in both normal cardiac physiology and cardiac disease. Other important G-protein-coupled receptors will be reviewed, such as α-adrenergic receptors and muscarinic receptors. Non-G-protein receptor systems, such as tyrosine–kinase-linked receptors and guanylate cyclase-related receptors, will be briefly discussed.

D.C. Sigg (✉)
1485 Hoyt Ave W, Saint Paul, MN 55108
e-mail: siggx001@umn.edu

Finally, we want to provide an overview of the basic biology of coronary stenting. Our goal is to depict the biological cascade that is triggered by coronary angioplasty and stenting, as well as the complexity of subsequent biological responses, and to explain how these responses are modulated by drug-eluting stents.

13.2 Definition

Cell receptors allow extracellular substances to bind for regulation of intracellular function or metabolism, typically without having to enter the cell. A number of types of cellular receptors can initiate a signal that ultimately modulates cellular function. Most of the "classic" receptors are cell-surface receptors, spanning the whole cell membrane and thereby allowing mediation of signals from the extracellular site to the intracellular site. The largest, and possibly most important, group is the family of G-protein-coupled receptors. An attempt to classify cardiovascular receptors either by location or by receptor type is provided in Table 13.1.

13.3 G-Protein-Coupled Receptor (Seven-Transmembrane-Spanning Receptors) and Signal Transduction

13.3.1 Overview

G-protein-coupled receptors are functionally closely related to ion channels. The G-protein-coupled receptors are part of a growing gene family being identified that binds agonists such as adenosine, catecholamines, acetylcholine, odorants, angiotensin, histamine, opioids, and many others.

Table 13.1 Classification of cardiovascular receptors

By location	By receptor types
Cardiac receptors	G-protein-coupled
• Myocardial	receptors
• Conduction system	Tyrosine–kinase-
• Other	linked receptors
	Guanylate-cyclase-
	linked receptors
Vascular receptors	Other receptors
• Endothelial	(low-sensitivity
• Vascular smooth muscle	lipoprotein receptor;
• Other	nicotin acetylcholine
	receptor;
	peptidergic)

13.3.2 Receptor Structure

Interestingly, there are several structural similarities between ion channels and G-protein-coupled receptors. Both are integral membrane proteins with seven-transmembrane domains, which form bundles with a central pocket. In G-proteins, the pockets are the binding sites for the receptor ligands, and they are typically located on the extracellular site of the protein; the N-terminal tail is located extracellularly as are three extracellular loops. Three loops connecting the transmembrane domains and the C-terminal domain are located intracellularly (Figs. 13.1 and 13.2). The exact functions of the extracellular loops remain largely unknown. It is considered that the transmembrane domains are involved in receptor binding. The intracellular loops, particularly loop III and the C-terminal tail, are important for receptor coupling to the associated G-protein. Finally, both loop III and C-terminal tail are important for regulation of receptor function and contain phosphorylation and other posttranslational modification sites.

13.3.3 Receptor Coupling

The G-protein receptors interact intimately with G-proteins. G-proteins are complexes consisting of three subunits—α, β, and χ. There are different classes of G-proteins and attempts have been made to classify them as subtypes. For example, common α subunits include: (1) α_s (stimulatory) which activates adenyl cyclase; (2) α_i (inhibitory) which inhibits adenylyl cyclase; (3) α_0 which modulates calcium channels and phospholipase C; and (4) α_z which activates phospholipase C. In general, each α subunit contains a region that interacts with the receptor, a site that binds GTP (guanosine triphosphate) and a site interacting with the effector system.

13.3.4 Receptor Function and Regulation

The traditional concepts of G-protein-coupled receptor function are best illustrated in Fig. 13.1. First, an agonist binds to a receptor molecule, and then the seven-transmembrane-spanning receptor molecule interacts with a specific G-protein; this, in turn, modulates a specific effector. Examples of typical agonists, receptors, G-proteins, and effectors are provided in Fig. 13.1. While this illustration provides a general

Fig. 13.1 G-protein receptor-coupled signaling. The ubiquitous seven-transmembrane receptor systems are composed of a receptor, a heterotrimeric G-protein, and an effector system. The complexity of this system can be appreciated by the number of receptor types and subtypes, G-protein subtypes, and different effector systems

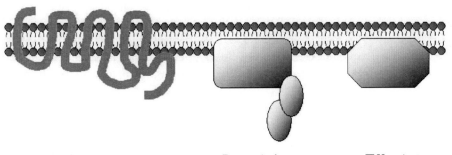

Receptor	G protein	Effector
Adrenergic	15 α-subunits	Adenylyl cyclase
Dopaminergic	6 β-subunits	Phospholipases A2, C
Opioid	12 χ-subunits	cGMP PDE
Lipids		K⁺ channels
Glycoprotein hormones		Ca⁺⁺ channels
Sensory		

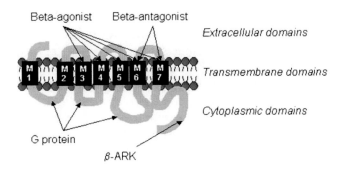

Fig. 13.2 The molecular schematic structure of a β-adrenergic receptor. Note the three main domains—extracellular, transmembrane, and cytoplasmic. The transmembrane domains are important for ligand binding. The transmembrane domain, M3-7, is important in agonist binding, whereas the domains M6 and M7 are involved in antagonist binding (β-receptor blockers). The cytoplasmic domains contain important binding sites for interactions with G-proteins, as well as various kinases such as β-AR kinase (β-ARK)

13.4 Beta-Adrenergic Receptors (β-ARs)

13.4.1 Classification of β-Adrenergic Receptors

Table 13.2 summarizes the general features of β-AR subtypes identified to date; note that there are three subtypes [1]. While all of the subtypes can be found in the heart, the predominant subtype in the vasculature is the β-2 AR. Importantly, norepinephrine and epinephrine are the endogenous agonists (catecholamines) which bind specifically to all three β-AR subtypes.

Pharmacologically, β-1 and β-2 receptors are characterized by an equal affinity for both the exogenous

summary of the individual components needed for proper G-protein-coupled receptor function, a more thorough understanding of the G-protein receptor-mediated signaling, as well as its regulation, is best accomplished by the more specific example of the well-characterized beta-adrenergic receptor (β-AR) system. Therefore, we will start our discussion with these physiologically, pathophysiologically, and clinically highly relevant seven-transmembrane spanning β-ARs.

Table 13.2 Beta-adrenergic receptor subtypes: G-proteins, tissue distributions, effectors, and signals

Receptor	β-1	β-2	β-3
Primary G-protein	Gs	Gs/Gi	Gs/Gi
Tissue distribution	Heart	Vessels, heart, lung, kidney	Adipose, heart
Primary effector in heart tissue	Adenylyl cyclase, L-type calcium channel	Adenylyl cyclase, L-type calcium channel	Adenylyl cyclase
Signals	cAMP/PKA	cAMP/PKA, MAPK	cAMP/ PKA

cAMP = cyclic adenosine 3′,5′-monophosphate (cyclic AMP); Gi = inhibitory G-protein; Gs = stimulatory G-protein; MAPK = mitogen-activated protein kinase; PKA = protein kinase A.

agonists isoproterenol and epinephrine, while norepinephrine (the neurotransmitter of the sympathetic nervous system) has a 10- to 30-fold greater affinity for the β-1 AR subtype. Also, β-1 ARs are more closely located to synaptic nerve termini than β-2 ARs, thereby being exposed and activated by higher concentrations of released norepinephrine.

13.4.2 β-AR Activation and Cardiovascular Function

Cardiac β-ARs are probably one of the most important (and most widely studied) types of receptor systems. Activation of β-ARs regulates important cardiovascular functions and is integral to the body's "flight or fight" response. For example, during exercise, heart rate and contractility both increase, cardiac conduction accelerates, and cardiac relaxation (which is an active process requiring adenosine triphosphate [ATP]) is enhanced. Moreover, vascular relaxation (vasodilation) of many vascular beds can be observed during exercise (e.g., in skeletal muscles). All these effects are at least partially a direct consequence of β-AR activation and involve key elements of G-protein receptor signaling: (1) receptor binding; (2) G-protein activation; and (3) activation of an effector system. Importantly, most of these specific physiological cardiac effects are mediated via activation of β-1 AR, while the vascular effects are mediated through the β-2 receptor subtype. However, heart muscle also contains β-2 receptors (as well as β-3 receptors). Nevertheless, the β-1 receptor subtype is the predominant cardiac isoform in healthy humans. More specifically, while there is a substantial population of β-2 receptors in the atria, only around 20–30% of the total β-AR population is β-2 ARs in the left ventricle [2]. Not only is the activation of β-ARs and their associated signaling transduction key in understanding the physiology of the cardiovascular system, but it has been recognized over the past decades that β-AR activations also play key roles in cardiac disease processes such as heart failure [3]. For example, an apparent paradox exists, namely that β-adrenergic blockers (β-receptor antagonists) are beneficial in patients with heart failure; this will be discussed in more detail later in this chapter.

13.4.2.1 Effects of β-receptor Activation on the Heart

β-receptor activation on the heart regulates cardiac function on a beat-to-beat basis. Specifically, β-AR stimulation causes: (1) increases in heart rates (a positive "chronotropic" effect); (2) increases in contractility (a positive "inotropic" effect); (3) enhancements in cardiac relaxation (a positive "lusitropic" effect); and/or (4) increases in conduction velocities (a positive "dromotropic" effect). The molecular mechanisms leading to each of these specific effects will be discussed. For further details, the reader is referred to the textbook by Opie [4]. Other important effects on cardiac myocytes that should be noted include those due to enhanced metabolism; the most significant effects on dilation in the coronary vasculature are mediated via metabolic waste products (CO_2, etc.). Also see Chapter 19 for a detailed discussion of energy metabolism and feedback mechanisms.

13.4.2.2 Positive Chronotropic Effect

When activated, β-ARs located on the cells that make up the sinoatrial node increase the firing rate of the sinoatrial node. While the mechanisms of these effects are not fully understood, they are known to involve activation of G-proteins and formation of cyclic adenosine monophosphate (cAMP) called a "second messenger." Cyclic AMP can then bind to ion channels which are, in part, responsible for the diastolic (phase 4) depolarization of sinoatrial nodal cells. These ion channels, referred to as hyperpolarization-activated cyclic nucleotide-gated channels, have several unique properties, as they: (1) activate during hyperpolarization (more negative membrane potentials); (2) are responsive to cAMP; (3) are conductive for both Na^+ and K^+ ions; and (4) can be blocked by caesium. Cyclic AMP binding to the intracellular domain of these ion channels shifts their activation curves to more positive potentials, which increases the rates of "spontaneous" depolarization of sinoatrial nodal cells, and ultimately their firing rates. The chronotropic effects can also be mediated via norepinephrine released from sympathetic nerve endings in the sinoatrial node and/or from circulating catecholamines (epinephrine and norepinephrine). From an integrative physiology standpoint, increasing heart rates are an adaptive response to an increased demand of oxygen and cardiac output in the periphery. Accelerating the heart rate will, in turn, increase cardiac output if stroke volume remains constant (cardiac output = heart rate x stroke volume).

13.4.2.3 Positive Inotropic Effects

As mentioned before, cardiac output needs to increase during exercise. One way to accomplish this is by increasing the heart rate; another is to increase stroke volume, e.g., by increasing cardiac filling (or increasing the preload). This can be accomplished by increasing the venous tone of the great veins that will increase filling of the heart chambers. It should be noted that this is an effect that is also mediated by adrenergic receptors but, in this particular case, by α-ARs causing venoconstriction (secondary to increased calcium influx). Such an increased preload then induces increased filling (and stretching) of the myocardial chambers, and via the "Frank-Starling" mechanism, stroke volume becomes augmented. However, stroke volume can also be efficiently improved by increasing the contractile force of the heart muscle at a given constant muscle length (i.e., independent of fiber length); this is called a positive inotropic effect and is mediated by activation of β-ARs, both β-1 AR and β-2 AR. The detailed molecular mechanisms involve the following processes (Fig. 13.3):

1. β-agonist binds to either β-1 or β-2 receptor.
2. GTP binds to the stimulatory α-subunit of the G-protein (Gαs) and activates it.
3. The G-subunits dissociate (the α-subunit dissociates from the β-subunit and χ-subunit).
4. The α-subunit (containing GTP) stimulates an effector protein called adenylyl cyclase (AC).
5. Cyclic 3'-5' cAMP is formed and GTP is hydrolyzed to GDP (guanosine diphosphate) plus Pi (the α-subunit/GTP is a GTPase).
6. The α-subunit/GDP binds to the β- and χ-subunits, and the initial (inactive) resting state reforms.

13.4.2.4 The Second Messenger Concept

Cyclic adenosine monophosphate is one of the key effector molecules in many of the signaling processes involving β-ARs (but also in many other biologic receptor systems). This molecule is commonly referred to as a "second messenger" and is one of many such molecules identified that are involved in cellular signal transduction. Another highly relevant second messenger is cyclic guanosine monophosphate (cGMP); cGMP is typically formed in vascular cells after binding nitric oxide, but can also be formed in cardiac and other cells after binding natriuretic peptides. As the name implies, these molecules trigger additional signaling mechanisms. Importantly, cAMP is present in all cardiac myocytes; it is rapidly turned over, and there is a constant dynamic balance between cAMP generation and breakdown via phosphodieasterases (enzymes which break down cAMP). While cAMP can increase in response to β-adrenergic activation, there are other pharmacologically active agents that can lead to increased cAMP levels via alternate mechanisms. For examples, glucagon is known to stimulate AC via a non-

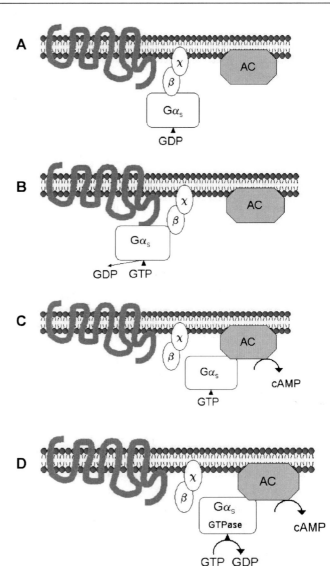

Fig. 13.3 G-protein receptor activation and coupling with adenylyl cyclase (AC) during β-adrenergic receptor activation. **Panel A**: The receptor is inactive; GDP (guanosine diphosphate) is bound to α-subunit of stimulatory G-protein. **Panel B**: The agonist binds to receptor which leads to receptor G-protein interaction; GTP (guanosine triphosphate) binds to stimulatory G-proteins (α-subunit, Gαs). **Panel C**: The G-subunits dissociate and Gαs stimulates adenylate cyclase, with subsequent formation of cAMP (cyclic adenosine monophosphate). **Panel D**: Gαs GTPase becomes active, GDP reforms, and the activation cycle ends

β-AR mechanism; forsokolin stimulates AC directly; phosphodieasterase inhibitors such as milrinone, amrinone, and others inhibit the breakdown of cAMP resulting in increased cAMP levels. The exact mechanism of how formation of cAMP leads to increased cardiac contractility in cardiac myocytes will be further discussed below.

It is known that cAMP enhances the activity of protein kinase A. Once activated, protein kinase A causes the subsequent phosphorylating of numerous proteins including voltage-dependent sarcolemmal calcium channels, phospholamban (located in the sarcoplasmic reticulum), troponin I, and troponin C. The primary effect of phosphorylating the calcium channels and phospholamban is that this will increase calcium influx during a cardiac activation cycle and also increase calcium uptake by the sacroplasmic reticulum. Working in concert, these effects will ultimately result in increased calcium transients during cardiac excitation–contraction coupling. Further, these increased intracellular calcium transients will result in increased ATP splitting by the myosin ATPase, which then increases the rate of development of contractile force (and also increases deinhibition of actin and myosin by the interaction of calcium with troponin C), ultimately causing an increase in total cardiac force development. If this stimulation is maintained, this effect or response often becomes attenuated over time. Also, cAMP levels may decrease, for example, due to activation of calmodulin which activates cAMP breakdown via phosphodieasterase activation and also via activation of β-AR kinase (β-ARK activation and downregulation).

It is important to recognize that the response to β-AR stimulation cannot simply be explained by overall increased tissue levels of cAMP. It has been speculated that cAMP may be compartmentalized in the heart, with a specific compartment available to increase contractility [5]. In addition, it has been shown that both β-2 ARs and β-1 ARs, which both mediate positive inotropic responses, do so largely independent of cAMP generation. This latter response may, in some cases, be one of the myopathic mechanisms in chronic heart failure by resulting in increased systolic and diastolic calcium levels [6]. The complexity of the β-AR stimulatory G-protein adenylyl cyclase signaling system can be further illustrated by the fact that there are about 20 identified Gα-subtypes, about five β-subtypes, and about 11 χ-subtypes, in addition to about nine isoforms of AC [7]. In cardiac tissue, isoforms V and VI of AC are considered to predominate. It should also be noted that specific anchoring proteins enable the juxtaposition of protein kinase A with its specific target proteins (A-kinase-anchoring proteins), which may account for the resulting compartmentalization (and complexity) of responses.

13.4.2.5 Positive Lusitropic Effects

Phospholamban can be activated by protein kinase A (via cAMP) or by increased calcium levels subsequent to voltage-gated calcium channel activation (secondary to protein kinase A phosphorylation). This typical phosphorylation of phospholamban leads to increased activity

of this enzyme, which then results in enhanced calcium removal from the cytosol back into the sarcoplasmic reticulum. It is known that the activation of troponin I, via protein kinase A, increases the rate of cross-bridge detachment and thus relaxation. Importantly, both of these responses will increase the rate of relaxation, an active process to remove calcium from the cytosol. A basic summary of the mechanisms of β-adrenergic increase in cardiac contractility and relaxation is provided in Fig. 13.4.

13.4.2.6 Dromotropic Effects

Activation of the voltage-gated (L-type) calcium channels in the atrioventricular node may enhance conduction in these nodal cells, as well as those of the Purkinje fibers.

13.4.2.7 Metabolic Effects

In general, the metabolic effects mediated via the β-AR system include: (1) increases in glycogen formation (via increased glycogenolysis as well as decreased formation of glycogen); (2) the stimulation of lipolysis; and/or (3) increases in ATP production (via glycolysis/citrate cycle). Some of these metabolic effects may be mediated

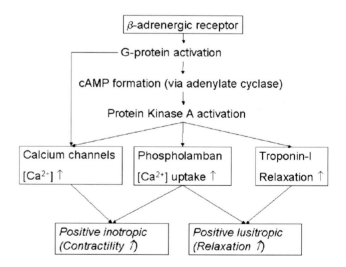

Fig. 13.4 The major intracellular signaling mechanisms involved in the regulation of cardiac contractility and relaxation following β-adrenergic receptor activation. It should be noted that there is also the possibility that L-type voltage-dependent calcium channels can be activated via a direct effect of a stimulatory G-protein (Gαs) subsequent to β-adrenergic receptor (both β-1 and β-2 adrenergic receptors) activations. This overall signaling pathway is cAMP-independent. The resulting increased systolic and diastolic calcium fluxes are considered to become a potentially myopathic mechanism in chronic heart failure

via the β-3 AR (e.g., control of lipolysis). The β-3 AR is also considered to have some regulatory function in cardiac (and vascular) contractility (e.g., negative inotropic effects) [8].

13.4.2.8 Effects of β-Receptor Activation in the Vasculature

The main physiological function of β-AR activation in the vasculature is induced relaxation (vasodilation), which is induced via a reduction of cytosolic calcium levels in the smooth muscle cells (SMCs) composing these vessels, with relaxation having the greatest importance in arterioles. These relaxation responses are mediated via the β-2 AR subtype and are antagonized by α-AR activation (α-1 receptor subtype). The effects of α-receptor signal transduction will be discussed further below.

13.4.3 β-AR Regulation

To best understand β-AR regulation, it is useful to review the molecular structure of this receptor. Basically, the receptor is composed of three types of domains: (1) the extracellular domain; (2) the transmembrane domains which are involved in the agonist and antagonist binding (ligand binding); and (3) the intracellular or cytoplasmic domains which are important for G-protein interactions and interactions with kinases such as β-ARK (β-adrenergic receptor kinase) (Fig. 13.2).

13.4.3.1 β-Adrenergic Receptor Desensitization and Downregulation

Receptor "downregulation" can be defined as a reduced presence in functional numbers of receptors in the cell membrane. Downregulation can result from internalization (and destruction in lysosomes), decreased rates of receptor degradation (nonlysosomal), and/or decreased synthesis. "Desensitization" is typically defined as receptor refractoriness, a "state of decreased activity following continued stimulation." Yet, it should be noted that one cannot always identify a clear distinction between these two definitions in the literature. For example, the β-receptor can become desensitized during isoproterenol stimulation (a classic pharmacological β-adrenergic agonist). In contrast, during continuous β-AR stimulation, the enzyme β-ARK increases its activity; β-ARK phosphorylates the cytoplasmic domain sites of the β-AR

(Fig. 13.2) and is able to uncouple the receptor from the Gαs (stimulatory G-protein). This response acts as a block of the signal and activation of adenylyl cyclase is decreased; in other words, adenylyl cyclase is uncoupled from the β-AR. Resensitization occurs once the receptor has been dephosphorylated; this mechanism is called "agonist-specific desensitization." In contrast, "nonagonist-specific" desensitization can occur via second messenger cAMP (and also via diacylglycerol which activates protein kinase A and C) which phosphorylates the G-protein-coupled receptors.

Specific examples of "physical" downregulation include internalization of receptors during continuous prolonged β-AR stimulation, which can be induced either pharmacologically (such as in an intensive care unit setting) or which is observed in heart failure (increased sympathetic tone and circulating catecholamines). This latter response may be a protective mechanism to minimize calcium overload of the cardiac myocytes secondary to β-adrenergic stimulation. Additional clinical examples of receptor regulation include "hypersensitivity" to β-AR agonists after propranolol (a β-AR blocker) withdrawal following long-term use. This enhanced sensitivity is considered to be due to receptor externalization. Another example is drug tolerance to dobutamine (or other β-AR agonists); the molecular mechanisms underlying this clinical phenomenon may be desensitization.

While agonist-specific and -unspecific desensitization can be viewed as one of the classical concepts of receptor regulation, G-protein receptor kinases, such as β-ARK and associated proteins (β-arrestins), seem to function by other mechanisms. For example, β-arrestins are considered to interact with a G-protein-coupled receptor and thus inhibit further G-protein coupling after the receptor has been phosphorylated by β-ARK. While this more traditional role is now well established, β-arrestins have also been shown to be involved in receptor internalization as well as complex additional signaling mechanisms (e.g., mitogen-activated protein kinase pathways) [9, 10]. Internalization (also known as "sequestration" or "endocytosis") is generally considered to serve various other functions including: (1) receptor resensitization (dephosphorylation) and recycling; and/or (2) altering signaling processes. Typically, the mechanisms of internalization involve the classical described clathrin-coated pit processes (caveolae) and also non-coated pit mechanisms. Another interesting role of β-arrestins is in ubiquitination; this is a means by which proteins are marked for subsequent degradation. For example, β-arrestin ubiquitination is important for β-1 AR internalization, while receptor ubiquitination is necessary for lysosomal targeting and degradation of the receptors [11]. The gene regulation of the β-AR has been reviewed nicely elsewhere [7].

13.4.4 The Association Between β-ARs and Cardiac Disease

The function of the β-AR-signaling pathway is not only of great importance in the normal regulation of physiological cardiac vascular function, but has critical, although different, roles in the development of chronic heart failure. In general, heart failure is a syndrome defined by an inability of the heart to pump adequate amounts of blood to the body organs. The normal physiological response to an inadequate blood (oxygen) supply is to increase the cardiac output (and thereby oxygen delivery) via activation of the adrenergic nervous system (sympathetic nervous system); this response is characterized by an increase in circulating catecholamines. While this sympathetic response would intuitively be seen as beneficial, and indeed is also initially adaptive, in reality, the sustained β-AR activation and increased norepinephrine tissue levels [12] are considered to be associated with "negative biological effects." Therefore, a sustained β-AR response in the cardiac patient may be, in fact, considered both maladaptive and inappropriate. Consistent with this notion, adrenergic drive is increased in all chronically failing human hearts with systolic dysfunction, as well as in all animal models of hemodynamic overload. Thus, adrenergic drive can also be considered as a "servo-control" mechanism to maintain cardiac performance at an acceptable level [7]. For example, the proportion of β-1 to β-2 adrenergic subreceptor population in normal human ventricles shifts from 70:30 in diseased human ventricles to about 50:50 in normal human ventricles [13]. Also on the molecular level, both receptor subtypes are typically desensitized, due to uncoupling of the receptors from their signaling pathways associated with both increased β-AR phosphorylation and upregulation of the inhibitory G-protein, Gi.

To illustrate the maladaptive β-AR signaling response, it is important to consider that β-adrenergic agonists, given to patients with chronic heart failure, may actually increase mortality. In contrast, the administration of β-blockers has been shown to improve survival; β-AR blockers are currently (2003) one of the cornerstones of medical/drug therapy for patients with chronic heart failure.

In certain patients with cardiac failure, there is a situation where increased adrenergic drive is required to maintain the circulatory needs of their bodies; the more the heart is activated adrenergically, the more profound are the effects of desensitization which, in turn, activates the adrenergic system even more, ultimately causing myocardial tissue damage. Based on the studies in which β-AR blocking agents were administered, it is generally believed that the β-AR system is central in this vicious pathological cycle (or positive feedback loop), which is commonly characterized by progressive remodeling and myocardial dysfunction.

13.4.4.1 Beta-Adrenergic Signaling and Heart Failure

One of the hallmarks of chronic heart failure is adrenergic overdrive leading to β-AR downregulation and desensitization. In particular, β-1 ARs have been shown to be downregulated selectively, while the β-2 ARs are relatively increased so that, as mentioned above, the population of β-1 to β-2 shifts from 75/25 to about 50/50. The marked uncoupling of the β-AR receptors from the G-proteins is due to increased levels of β-ARK1, as well as an increased inhibitory G-protein (Gi) [14]. This, in turn, results in not only attenuated β-AR signaling but also activation of additional pathways involved in ventricular remodeling (see below).

The shift of the β-1/β-2 AR subpopulation to an increased number of β-2 receptors is only one of the phenomena associated with chronic heart failure. More specifically, β-2 ARs couple to a number of signaling pathways, including a potential coupling to an inhibitory G-protein (Gαi). Also, β-2 ARs may modulate several G-protein independent pathways, including inhibition of sodium–hydrogen exchanges as well as a non-protein kinase A-dependent interaction with L-type calcium channels [15, 16]. There are other G-protein-independent pathways in which the β-2 ARs have been implicated, such as those associated with phosphatidylinositol kinase, phospholipase C/protein kinase C, and/or arachidonic acid signaling. And while many details of these pathways remain poorly understood, it is becoming more clear that some of these pathways play important roles in the molecular pathobiology of heart failure.

One of the widely recognized mechanisms of β-AR desensitization is agonist-dependent β-ARK-mediated phosphorylation of the β-AR itself. Moreover, the beta-gamma subunits of the G-proteins can act as signaling molecules themselves, with the potential of activating many downstream targets of pathways such as adenylyl cyclases, PLC, PLA2, PI3K, K$^+$ channels, and/or Src-Ras-Raf-MEK-MAPK (mitogen-activated protein kinase) [7].

The potentially toxic effects of long-term β-1 AR receptor activation are also illustrated by the fact that selective β-1 AR agonist or receptor overexpression leads to increased cardiac "apoptosis" or programmed cell death [17–19]. The mechanisms by which such apoptosis is activated have been attributed, in part, to initial activation of calcineurin via increased intracellular calcium through L-type calcium channels [20]. Additionally, direct toxic effects of catecholamines on the myocytes have been described as a result of direct β-AR activation [12]. Other effects of chronic β-AR signaling include production of cytotoxicity via calcium overload, increased free radical formation, as well as stimulation of pathologic hypertrophy [7]. For example, the marked uncoupling

Table 13.3 β-adrenergic receptor signaling pathways in heart failure

Molecule	Change
β1-AR	$\downarrow$, uncoupled
β2-AR	NC, uncoupled
β-ARK1	$\uparrow$
β-arrestin 1 and 2	NC
Galpha1	$\uparrow$

Modified from Rockman et al. [1].
AR = adrenergic receptor; ARK = adrenergic receptor kinase.

of β-1 and β-2 receptors from their physiological signaling pathways not only results in attenuation of the β-AR signaling, but also allows for the coupling of the receptors with other possible myopathic signaling pathways involved in ventricular remodeling (e.g., MAPK and PI(3)K cascades). As alluded to earlier, β-receptor antagonists may be a beneficial therapy in the chronic heart failure patient. Specifically, the β-1-specific β-AR-blocking drug metoprolol produces reverse remodeling similar to a combined α-β blocker carvedilol, suggesting that β-1 AR receptor signaling is an important determinant of pathologic hypertrophy in human heart failure [21].

Lastly, genetic heterogeneity in expression of the β-AR in the general population has been identified which may be associated with disease susceptibility. For example, a substitution of threonine to isoleucine at amino acid 164 in the β-2 AR has been linked with reduced survival and exercise tolerance in patients with heart failure [22, 23].

A summary of the known changes in β-AR signaling is provided in Table 13.3. Lastly, it should be mentioned that investigations using transgenic animal models have greatly helped to elucidate some of the important disease mechanisms associated with adrenergic receptor reception pathways; they have also served as tools in identifying and testing novel or evolving therapeutic targets for the treatment of heart failure [1].

13.5 Alpha-Adrenergic Receptors (α-AR)

13.5.1 Physiology

Two major α-AR subtypes have been identified—α-1 and α-2. The α-1 type receptors have been described to be present in the heart, as well as in the vessels and smooth muscle. The primary response to their activation in cardiac cells is phospholipase C-β which leads to an increase in diacylglycerol, inositol triphosphate (InsP$_3$), and also activates both protein kinase C and MAPKs. Physiological receptor agonists include norepinephrine and epinephrine, and a Gq protein is the primary associated G-protein [24]. In general, the primary physiological importance of α-1

receptors is far greater in the vasculature, leading to calcium influx and vasoconstriction via the second messenger InsP$_3$. In cardiac muscle cells, α-1 receptors have been shown to induce a positive inotropic effect; like β receptors, this response is also associated with formation of InsP$_3$ [25]. Alpha-2 receptors have been identified on coronary vessels, as well as in the central nervous system (presynaptic); they reduce the activity of AC (and protein kinase A) via an inhibitory G-protein.

In summary, the primary physiological role of α-1 receptors is for the vasculature regulation of tone via vasoconstriction, which is secondary to calcium influx into the SMCs of the circulatory arterioles.

13.5.2 Role in Disease States

In general, in heart failure patients, the α-1 AR system will elicit an increase in receptor density and is also characterized by changes in inotropic responses [26]. In addition, α-1 AR activation has been shown to promote cardiomyocyte hypertrophy via activation of hypertrophic MAPK pathways.

13.6 Role of Adrenergic and Other Receptors in Myocardial Hypertrophy

Prolonged or repeated increased workloads on the heart lead to cardiac hypertrophy. Hypertrophy is typically characterized by increased contractile protein content (and muscle mass), myofilament reorganization, and reexpression of embryonic markers. As discussed earlier, myocyte cell growth by G-protein-coupled receptors may involve not only ras and MAPK pathways but also other signaling pathways (e.g., calcineurin, PI3K, and phosphotidylinositol-3-OH). Abnormal β-AR function with elicited hypertrophy is also characteristic; in particular, elevated myocardial levels of β-ARK1 can be detected [27]. As mentioned above, α-1 receptor signaling also may be very important in the development of cardiac hypertrophy. Specifically, Gq-coupled receptors, such as angiotensin, α-1 AR, and endothelin, can all activate hypertrophic MAPK pathways [28, 29]. To summarize, the cardiac hypertrophic response may not be compensatory to reduce wall stress, but rather maladaptive and thus increase mortality. In particular, signaling pathways involving elevated catecholamine levels (norepinephrine and epinephrine) and activated Gq-coupled receptors seem to promote hypertrophic responses. Thus, targeting these specific signaling pathways may be a novel therapeutic approach for the potential treatment of "maladaptive" cardiac hypertrophy, and ultimately heart failure. For further details on this topic, the reader is referred to the review by Rockman et al. [1].

13.7 Muscarinic Receptors

13.7.1 Physiology

The muscarinic receptor system in the heart is also an associated G-protein-coupled receptor system, one fairly similar to the β-AR. The main cardiac receptor subtype (M2 receptor) is a cholinergic receptor, and thus mediates primary "parasympathetic" (syn. nervus vagus, cholinergic, acetylcholine mediated) nervous system responses. For more details, refer to Chapter 12. Its general function is to simultaneously balance and antagonize the sympathetic effects of β-AR activation, with its most pronounced effects on the controls of the sinoatrial (heart rate, chronotropic effect) and atrioventricular nodes (conduction, dromotropic effect). There exist very few muscarinic M2 receptors in the ventricles, so activated negative inotropic (contractility) effects subsequent to M2 receptor activation are very small. The primary control signal mediated via the vagus nerve is that which leads to a local release of acetylcholine in the sinoatrial and atrioventricular nodes. Acetylcholine then binds to the M2 receptor, activates an inhibitory G-protein (Gαi), and essentially decreases the activity of adenylyl cyclase, which directly leads to opening of K$^+$ channels. Thus, in the sinoatrial node, vagal stimulation tends to a flattening of the diastolic depolarization,

which then induces a slowing of heart rate (bradycardia, negative chronotropic effect) possibly via the effects of reduced cAMP availability on I$_f$ current (hyperpolarization activated cyclic nucleotide gated channel), but also via activation of a potassium outward current which in concert decrease the spontaneous firing rate of the sinoatrial node. In the atrioventricular nodal tissue, vagal stimulation also activates an inhibitory G-protein, which typically causes a slowing conduction velocity via a decreased calcium influx through L-type calcium channels. Clinically, the effects of vagal stimulation on the atrioventricular node are detected as increased atrioventricular nodal conduction times (e.g., prolonged PR interval).

The M3 muscarinic subtype is primarily found in vascular SMCs. Its activation leads to contraction of vascular smooth muscles via a Gq/11-PLC-InsP3-mediated calcium influx (as well as diacylglycerol/phospholipase C/protein kinase, cAMP elevation).

13.8 Other G-Protein-Coupled Cardiovascular Receptors

There is a variety of other G-protein-coupled cardiovascular receptor systems which have important roles in cardiac physiology and pathophysiology. Yet, it is beyond the scope of this chapter to review all these systems in detail; however, for some degree of comprehensiveness, a current list of considered important G-protein-coupled receptor systems and their respective functions is provided in Table 13.4.

Table 13.4 Other cardiovascular G-protein-coupled receptor systems

Family	Type	Cardiovascular function	G-protein	Signaling
Adenosine	A1	Bradycardia	Gi/o	AC inhibition, K$^+$ opening
	A2A	Vasodilation	Gs/G15	AC, PLC-β
	A2B	Vascular smooth muscle relaxation	Gq/11	PLC/AC-mediated calcium activation
	A3	A1 modulation	Gi3	AC inhibition, PLC, InsP3-mediated calcium increase
Angiotensin	AT1	Vascular smooth muscle contraction; cell proliferation; cell hypertrophy; antinatriuresis	Gq/11	PLC/PKC-mediated calcium elevation
	AT2	Vasodilatation; apoptosis; growth inhibition; natriuresis; nitric oxide production	Gia2/Gia3	MAPK activation, K$^+$ opening, PTPase activation leading to T-type calcium channel closure
Endothelin	ETA	Vasoconstriction	Gq/11	PLC/InsP3, cAMP
	ETB	Vasodilatation/vasoconstriction (ETB2)	Gi; Gq/11	cAMP inhibition, PLC/InsP3 calcium increase
Opioid	OP1 (delta), OP3 (mu)	Central cardiovascular regulation (OP1, 3); cardioprotection (OP1)	Gialpha1/3; Go	IK conductance activation; reduction in neuronal Ica, AC inhibition, PKC and KATP channel activation (cardioprotection)

AC = adenylyl cyclase; cAMP = cyclic adenosine monophosphate; MAPK = mitogen-activated protein kinase; PKC = phospholipase C/protein kinase.

13.9 Receptor Cross-Talk

"Cross-talk" between receptors refers to a biological phenomenon whereby interactive regulatory (or modulatory) messages are sent from one receptor to another. Many of the aforementioned receptor pathways are engaged in some degree of cross-talk, which is commonly via second messengers and/or protein kinases which, in turn, modulate G-protein-mediated messages. While the current understanding of receptor cross-talk is far from being complete, it is clear that receptor cross-talk is integral for sustaining a coherent function of the cardiovascular system and has implications in both normal physiology and elicited cardiac disease states.

The following is an example of one such cardiovascular cross-talk interaction and its relevance to the pharmacological treatment of disease. As reviewed previously, heart failure, in general, is characterized by dysfunction of the β-AR receptor system (downregulation of β-1 receptors, uncoupling of β-AR and AC), but also the renin–angiotensin system (downregulation of AT1 receptors); distinct signaling pathways have been identified which then characterizes both β-AR (e.g., via Gs and AC) and AT1 receptor signaling (e.g., via Gq/11 and PLCβ). In a recent study, it was shown that selective blockade of β-AR-inhibited angiotensin-induced contractility, while selective blockade of AT1 receptors reduced catecholamine-induced reduction in heart rate [30]. These unusual transinhibitory effects were considered to be caused by underlying G-protein receptor uncoupling. Furthermore, direct interactions of these receptor systems were demonstrated in vivo, and it is speculated that such interactions may have a profound role in determining the ultimate responses to drugs designed to block a given receptor subtype (e.g., β-AR blockers, AT1-receptor blockers). Note that cardiovascular receptor cross-talk has been extensively reviewed by Dzimiri [31].

universal signaling molecule present in all tissues, and its role is important not only in normal physiology but also in disease processes. Physiologically, nitric oxide is produced by several isoforms of the enzyme nitric oxide synthase (NOS). To date, three isoforms have been described to function within the cardiovascular system—eNOS, iNOS, and nNOS. Nitric oxide is a small, lipid-soluble, gas molecule that readily crosses cell membranes. Inside the cell, it typically binds to a receptor, the soluble (cytoplasmatic) guanylyl cyclase (GC, an enzyme which converts GTP to cyclic 3'-5' GMP). Cyclic GMP is the second messenger in this signaling cascade and, in the cardiovascular system, can activate two major effector systems—cGMP-regulated phosphodiesterases and cGMP-dependent protein kinases (cGKs).

In the vascular SMCs, nitric oxide inhibits vascular smooth muscle constriction (causes vasodilation) via inhibition of cytoplasmic calcium release. However, the underlying mechanisms for the important vasodilatatory effect of nitric oxide are complicated, and minimally involve a cGMP-dependent protein kinase (cGKI); these pathways have been reviewed in detail elsewhere [32]. Nitric oxide has also been shown to reduce vascular smooth muscle proliferation (clinically important in in-stent restenosis) and migration. It is well established that nitric oxide release may reduce platelet adhesion and activation, as well as vascular inflammation [33]. Importantly, nitric oxide insufficiency is considered to be an important factor in endothelial dysfunction, leading to the increased susceptibility for arterial thrombosis formation [34].

Nevertheless, the relevance of nitric oxide signaling is not limited to vascular biology or pathobiology; it has been demonstrated that nitric oxide has an important pathophysiological role in heart failure as well, i.e., in the modulation of cardiac function, cardiovascular protection, and/or in the regulation of apoptosis [35–37].

13.10 Guanylate-Cyclase-Linked Receptors

13.10.1 Soluble Guanylyl Cyclase (Receptor for Nitric Oxide)

Although structurally different, the general principles of receptor signaling as discussed for the β-AR apply also for nitric oxide/guanylyl cyclase signaling. Specifically, the agonist nitric oxide is considered as a

13.10.2 Membrane Guanylyl Cyclase A (Receptors for Natriuretic Peptides)

To date, at least seven membrane bound enzymes synthesizing cyclic GMP (cGMP) have been identified. All seven of these membrane guanylyl cyclases (GCs) have a common structure (Fig. 13.5). For the purpose of this discussion, guanylyl cyclase-A has the greatest importance relative to the heart, and thus will be discussed in detail.

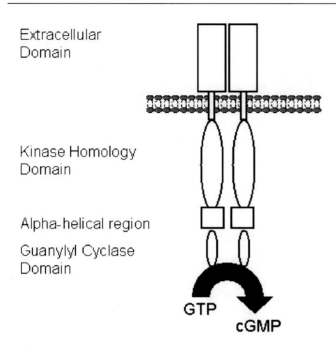

Extracellular
Domain

Kinase Homology
Domain

Alpha-helical region

Guanylyl Cyclase
Domain

GTP

cGMP

Fig. 13.5 Basic topology of membrane GC-A receptor. The membrane GC (guanylyl cyclase) form homodimers or higher order structures (modified from Kuhn [38]). cGMP = cyclic guanosine monophosphate; GTP = guanosine triphosphate

ANP/BNP are around 2–5 min. Interestingly, although both ANP and BNP bind to the same receptors, it has been shown that targeted genetic disruption of ANP or BNP in mice induces a unique phenotype; ANP-deficient mice show arterial hypertension, hypertrophy, and cardiac death. In contrast, the BNP-deficient mice phenotype is characterized by mostly cardiac fibrosis. More specifically, BNP has a lower affinity to GC-A than ANP and may act mostly as a local paracrine (antifibrotic) factor. Also, under physiological conditions, the ANP levels are much higher than BNP levels in the circulating blood, and the potency for induced vasorelaxation is also less for BNP vs. ANP [38].

Nevertheless, the cardiovascular effects of ANP-GC-A are complex, but can generally be summarized as inducing hypovolemic and hypotensive effects, which are induced via hormonal, renal, vascular, central nervous system, and/or other mechanisms. The most important hypotensive effects also involve associated decreased sympathetic activity and complex renal responses which subsequently lead to increased diuresis [38].

13.10.3 Physiology

Currently, three natriuretic peptides have been identified—ANP, BNP, and CNP. Both ANP and BNP bind to GC-A and are released in the heart; they are considered as cardiac hormones. In general, CNP is mainly produced by the vascular endothelium and may be a regulator of vascular tone and cell growth through GC-B activation. This receptor consists of an extracellular domain, a kinase homology domain, an α-helical amphipathic region (hinge region), and a C-terminal guanylyl cyclase (catalytic) domain (Fig. 13.5). This receptor is considered to exist in dimers (two molecules coupled together).

The major effects of GC-A are via the formation of, and the activation by, cGMP. Since, in general, the agonists are circulating hormones (peptides), a variety of organ systems can be affected simultaneously following ANP/BNP release. ANP is mainly produced in the atrium, while BNP is produced primarily in the ventricles. The primary triggering factors for ANP/BNP release are wall stretch and/or pressure increases, but their release may also involve neurohumoral factors (glucocorticoids, catecholamines, angiotensin II, etc.). The primary effect of ANP/BNP release is modulation of blood pressure/volume; the half-lives of

13.10.4 Role in Cardiac Disease

During chronic hemodynamic overload, ANP and, to an even greater level, BNP expression in the cardiac ventricles is significantly increased. This response may not only be for the maintenance of both arterial blood pressure and volume homeostasis, but also as local antihypertrophic (ANP) and antifibrotic (BNP) factors. While ANP/BNP levels are increased in patients with cardiac hypertrophy and/or heart failure, the GC-A-mediated effects of these peptides are diminished. Mechanisms for these responses may be postreceptor defects such as dephosphorylation of GC-A, sequestration of natriuretic peptides by a clearance receptor, altered transcriptional regulation at the gene level, and/or others [31]. However, to date, the processes regulating GC-A activity (and desensitization) are largely unknown. Yet, synthetic BNP (nesiritide) and ANP (anaritide) have been shown to be highly beneficial as an acute treatment of heart failure. Hence, it is conceivable that the thorough understanding of the mechanisms for chronic desensitization, as well as regulation of GC-A receptor signaling, might be important for the development of novel therapeutic approaches for various forms of cardiac disease.

13.11 Vascular Response to Drug-Eluting Stents: Inflammation, Neointimal Formation, and Endothelial Function

13.11.1 The History of Angioplasty/Stenting

Percutaneous transluminal coronary angioplasty (PTCA) was introduced in 1977 as a novel device-based therapy for occlusive coronary artery disease and has been quickly accepted due to its established benefits [39, 40]. Basically, this technology enabled the physician to advance a balloon catheter to an occluded coronary artery via a minimally invasive image-guided catheter procedure. After identification of the culprit lesion, the physician would advance the catheters to that site and, using wire and catheter technology, inflate the balloon catheter to reopen the narrowed vessel and thus restore critically reduced blood flow. While this technique revolutionized the treatment of coronary artery disease, it was not without problems. Balloon angioplasty may, in itself, result in vessel injury, initiating negative vessel remodeling and neointimal proliferation, thus leading to a high incidence (30–50%) of restenosis [38]. The introduction of bare metal stents in 1994 changed the face of interventional cardiology. Bare metal stents clearly demonstrated superiority over balloon angioplasty alone due to prevention of the elastic recoil and the negative remodeling effects [41–44]; nevertheless, neointimal proliferation continued to be a significant problem. In fact, bare metal stenting created a new disease—in-stent restenosis (ISR). The prevalence of ISR increased proportionally with use of stent implantation [45]. This was particularly true in patients with complex lesion subsets, such as diabetes, bifurcated lesions, long diffuse lesions, and/or in small vessels in which the restenosis rate remained as high as 30–60% [46, 47]. Drug-eluting stents (DESs) were introduced in 2003 to prevent or minimize ISR; they combined the mechanical benefits of bare metal stents with the controlled elution of a pharmacological agent that aimed to suppress neointimal proliferation [40, 48, 49]. Most DESs employed today consist of a metallic stent and a polymeric coating that controls a release of anti-proliferative drugs [50]. Currently, about 6 million people worldwide have been treated with DESs [51]. Drug-eluting stents have dramatically transformed the landscape of interventional cardiology, demonstrating substantial reduction in angiographic and clinical restenosis [52]. However, despite reduced restenosis rates, the frequency of in-stent thrombosis has not statistically decreased with DESs compared with bare metal stents [53, 54]. Stent thrombosis after percutaneous coronary intervention is an uncommon and potentially catastrophic event that might manifest as myocardial infarction and sudden death. Furthermore, recent data raise questions regarding the increased risk of late stent thrombosis; these events occur up to 3 years after implantation, and association with late stent thrombosis is often a more complex lesion in a higher-risk patient [55, 56]. There is still widespread controversy regarding the actual risks associated with DESs, as it relates to high morbidity and mortality [57].

13.11.2 The Vascular Biology of Restenosis

13.11.2.1 Overview

Restenosis can be defined as the arterial wall's healing response to mechanical injury, which results in neointimal hyperplasia and vessel wall remodeling [58, 59]. The cellular and molecular events and temporal sequence of events leading to restenosis have been described in animal models [60, 61] and include: (1) platelet aggregation; (2) inflammatory cell infiltration with release of inflammatory and growth factors; (3) medial SMC modulation and proliferation; and/or (4) proteoglycan deposition and extracellular matrix remodeling.

Interestingly, specific elastic wall remodeling is virtually absent after stent procedures, as observed by studies using volumetric intravascular ultrasound. Concerning ISR, the current paradigm is that injury, deendothelialization, and crush of the plaque due to stent deployment lead to immediate platelet activation and fibrin deposition [62]. The activated platelets, in turn, recruit circulating leukocytes from the blood stream to the injury site via surface expression of adhesion molecules, such as P-selectin. The leukocytes then bind tightly to the surface through these leukocyte integrin Mac-1 (CD11b/CD18) molecules. Driven by the chemical gradients of chemokines released from SMCs and resident macrophages, activated leukocytes then migrate into the tissue, and this is where they, in turn, release additional chemokines and growth factors. The growth factors that are subsequently released from platelets, leukocytes, and SMCs are believed to stimulate the migration of SMCs from the media into the neointima. The resultant neointima consists of SMCs, extracellular matrix, and macrophages recruited over several weeks. Cellular division takes place in this phase, which appears to be essential for the subsequent development of restenosis [62]. Subsequently, the artery enters the next phase of cell driven remodeling involving both extracellular matrix protein degradation and resynthesis. Accompanying this period is a shift to fewer cellular elements and greater production of extracellular matrix protein, which is composed of various collagen subtypes and proteoglycans and constitutes the major component of the mature restenotic plaque. It should be noted that in the balloon-angioplastied artery, subsequent reorganization of the extracellular matrix protein (e.g., replacing hydrated molecules by collagen) may lead to shrinkage of the entire artery and thus negative remodeling [63]. In the stented artery, this phase has a reduced clinical impact because of negative remodeling, although constituents of extracellular matrix protein such as hyaluronan, fibronectin, osteopontim, and vitornectin also facilitate SMC migration [64]. In both balloon-angioplastied and stented arteries, reendothelialization of at least part of the injured vessel surface may occur. Continuous endothelial coverage, provided that the endothelium is properly functional, endows the stented vessel with a hemocompatable, antithrombotic, and anti-inflammatory lining [65]. Refer to Table 13.5 for a summary of the pathobiological events associated with coronary angioplasty and stenting.

Biology of Smooth Muscle Cells

In a normal vessel uninterrupted by turbulent flow, inflammation, or vascular disease, the SMCs are quiescent and thus elicit low levels of proliferative activity. In contrast, in response to mechanical injury following percutaneous coronary intervention and stenting, a biological cascade will be triggered that prompts SMCs to progress into an activated state [59]. More specifically, activated SMCs exhibit several phenotypic changes including switches in their differentiation phenotype (de-differentiation), migrations, proliferations, and/or increased protein syntheses [66]. In general, differentiated SMCs are spindle-shaped, show contractile properties, and exhibit low frequency of proliferation, whereas de-differentiated SMCs are rhomboid-shaped and show a high degree of protein synthesis, proliferation, and migratory activity (66). Platelet-derived growth factor-BB, produced by activated platelets, can modulate SMCs to evoke de-differentiation phenotypes and has been shown to induce a suppression of the SMC marker genes such as SM α-actin, SM-myosin heavy chain, and SM22α [67, 68].

The source of heterogeneous SMC populations that contributes to this vascular remodeling after vascular interventions is controversial and has been extensively studied by many researchers using various preclinical models. It is speculated that some of the potential sources of heterogeneous SMC are: (1) adventitia [69, 70]; (2) in situ differentiation and expansion; and/or (3) distant sources such as the bone marrow [71].

Several signaling pathways have been described to be involved in SMC phenotype switching from differentiated to de-differentiated SMCs. The most prominent pathway is the MAPK–MEKK1/2-extracellular signal-regulated kinase (ERK)1/2 pathway. The transposition of MAPK

Table 13.5 Pathobiology of coronary angioplasty and stenting

PCI/Stenting-related biology (post-PCI/ stenting)	Effector cells (molecules)	Target cells	Therapeutically relevant agents
Endothelial denudation (min)	Endothelial cells	Smooth muscle cells Platelets	Nitric oxide inducers
Plaque rapture (min-days)	Macrophages (tissue factor, inflammatory cytokines)	Platelets	TF antagonists, Platelets activation inhibitors, PAR1 and PAR4 (platelets-activated receptors) antagonists
Acute thrombosis (min-days)	Platelets (adhesion molecules)	Leukocytes/ Monocytes Neutrophils/T cells	Platelets activation inhibitors
Acute inflammation (h-days)	Monocytes (growth factors and inflammatory mediators) Smooth muscle cells	Monocytes Smooth muscle cells Platelets	Anti-inflammatory agents
Neointimal formation	Smooth muscle cells Endothelial cells	Smooth muscle cells Endothelial cells	Inhibitors of cell cycle and proliferation, Multiple MOA that modulate smooth muscle cell phenotype
Healing/ reendothelialization (days-weeks)	Endothelial progenitor cells Platelets (SDF alpha, adhesion molecules, extracellular matrix)	Endothelial cells	Inducers of endothelial growth/function, cell- and gene-based therapy aimed at healing
Late stent thrombosis (30 days to years)	Endothelial cells Platelets Monocytes/Macrophages	NA	

PAR1 = protease-activated receptor 1; PCI = percutaneous coronary intervention; TF = tissue factor.

to the nucleus inhibits transcription of genes associated with the contractile phenotype and stimulates expression of genes associated with growth. The MAPK/ERK cascade is a well-known signal transduction pathway which governs migration, proliferation, survival, and apoptosis responses in SMC and various other cell types. MAPK/ERK is also considered to regulate the induction of growth factor secretion [72, 73]. Upstream of the MAPK/ERK is a pertinent protein-tyrosine kinase receptor that is activated by a growth factor, resulting in receptor phosphorylation and binding of adaptor proteins such as Grb2 and Shc to the activated receptor. Adaptor protein binding leads to ras activation of the GTP-binding protein family, by the mammalian son-of-sevenless (mSOS; guanine nucleotide exchange factor), activating Raf MAPKK/MEK and the downstream molecules, p44 MAPK/p42 MAPK (ERK1/2). Next, phosphorylated MAPK enters the nucleus to form a complex with the transcriptional factors Elk-1 and Sap1 (an Ets family member), inducing transcription by binding to the SRE promoter of genes such as c-fos. This mechanism is thought to be critical in the regulation of gene expression for proliferation, migration, differentiation, and phenotypic switching [74–76].

It should be noted that Kawai and Owens recently reviewed several pathways that may be involved in SMC phenotype modulation. Some of these pathways include Krüppel-like factor 4, phosphorylated Elk-1, HERP1, FOXO4, YY1, FHL2, and several homeobox proteins [67, 77, 78].

Extracellular Matrix Accumulation

Irrespective of the origin of SMCs in vascular lesions, their interactions with the extracellular matrix are fundamental to initiate a proliferative response and to direct their migration [79]. These interactions are dependent upon specific cell-surface integrins and can trigger intracellular signaling and cell cycle entry and also facilitate cell cycle progression induced by mitogens. In addition, extracellular matrix interactions may also control the availability and activity of growth factors such as heparin-binding mitogens which, in turn, can be sequestered by heparan sulfate containing extracellular matrix components, and thus regulate SMC proliferation [79]. Extracellular matrix remodeling is the net result of the balance of matrix production and degradation; extracellular matrix synthesis is generally regulated primarily by the matrix metalloproteinases, whereas extracellular matrix degradation is regulated by matrix metalloproteinase inhibitors such as the tissue inhibitor of metalloproteinase. Conversely, both the production and the

degradation of the extracellular matrix following vascular injury are required for SMC migration, proliferation, and thus the formation of the neointima [80]. Various mitogens, such as platelet-derived growth factor, angiotensin II, and TGF-β, have the ability to control extracellular matrix stability; this occurs primarily by changing the extracellular matrix components synthesized and secreted by SMCs [81].

SMC Cell Cycle and Proliferation

The factors that stimulate SMC proliferation might include growth factors, inflammatory cytokines, coagulation, and prothrombotic factors. These factors are produced by SMCs and endothelial cells as a result of either vascular wall injury or by activation of platelets, leukocytes, monocytes, neutrophils, or macrophages. The resultant mitogenic stimuli that these factors provide will then converge into a final common signaling pathway regulating the cell cycle [82].

When quiescent SMCs enter more proliferative states, they first transit from the G0 to the G1 phase of the cell cycle and then enter the S phase in order to ultimately undergo replication [83]. Cell cycle progression is under the control of cyclins and cyclin-dependent kinases (CDKs), which phosphorylate the retinoblastoma gene product (pRB) [84, 85]. pRB phosphorylation represents the critical checkpoint of the phase transition and increased pRB phosphorylation correlates with the induction of SMC proliferation in injured vessels; high levels of phosphorylated pRB are required for the development of intimal hyperplasia following PTCA and stenting [86] (Fig. 13.6). Upon pRB phosphorylation, sequestered E2F transcription factors are released to induce the transcription of genes involved in the regulation of S phase DNA synthesis. Through CDK-inhibitors such as p27 (KIP1), the activity of cyclin/CDK complexes in quiescent SMCs is inhibited, providing an additional layer of regulation. In response to mitogens, p27 undergoes ubiquitination and degradation through the proteasome pathway allowing CDK/cyclin complexes to phosphorylate pRB [87–89].

Drugs for DESs

The Limus Drugs: Rapamycin (sirolimus) was the first DES drug that was clinically shown to reduce or inhibit restenosis [90]. Rapamycin is a natural macrocyclic lactone that is structurally related to the immunosuppressive agents, tacrolimus, and cyclosporine A. Yet, the mechanism of action of Rapamycin differs significantly from

Fig. 13.6 Schematic representation of the smooth muscle cell (SMC) cycle. (**A**) The retinoblastoma gene product (RB) and the CDK-inhibitor, p27, are the key regulators of the quiescent SMC cell cycle. (**B**) Initiation of a proliferative cell cycle in SMC, in response to mitogens, is controlled via the phosphorylation of Rb (pRb) by cyclins and cyclin-dependent kinases (CDKs), and by the removal of p27 through ubiquitination and degradation. The removal of the cell cycle inhibition allows the transcription factor E2F to induce activation of genes that are required for cell growth and proliferation

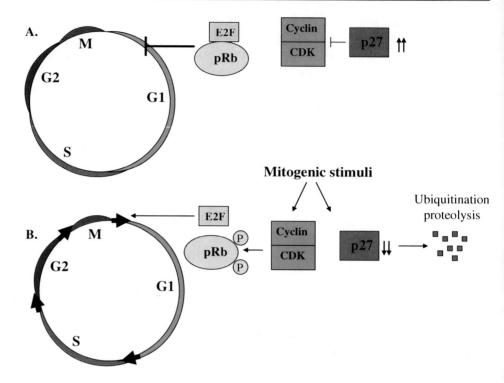

these later agents, as it does not inhibit calcineurin and the subsequent T-cell activation pathway [91]. Rapamycin is a highly specific inhibitor of a multifunctional serine–threonine kinase, also known as the mammalian target of Rapamycin. In essence, Rapamycin gains function by binding to the immunophilin FK506-binding protein 12 (FKBP12) and the resultant complex inhibits the activity of the mammalian target of Rapamycin. To date, the mammalian target of Rapamycin is known to have two main functions: (1) activation of p70S6 kinase; and (2) activation of the eukaryotic initiation factor 4E-BP1 (Fig. 13.7). The activation of p70S6 kinase leads to phosphorylation of 40S ribosomal protein that is phosphorylated on multiple sites after mitogen stimuli. These modifications are believed to favor the recruitment of the 40S subunit into actively translating polysomes, resulting in protein synthesis and mRNA translation. Furthermore, p70S6 kinase leads to an increase in the expression of proliferating nuclear antigen, thereby promoting DNA replication. Rapamycin blocks the activation of these downstream signaling elements, which results in G1 cell cycle arrest in various cells, including T and B cells, as well as non-immune cells such as fibroblasts, endothelial cells, and SMCs [92]. Rapamycin is also thought to prevent cyclin-dependent kinase (cdk) activation by the induction of its inhibitor, p27, which inhibits pRb phosphorylation and thus accelerates the turnover of cyclin D1; this leads to a deficiency of active cdk4/cyclin D1 complexes, all of which potentially contribute to the prominent inhibitory effects of Rapamycin at the G(1)/S phase transition.

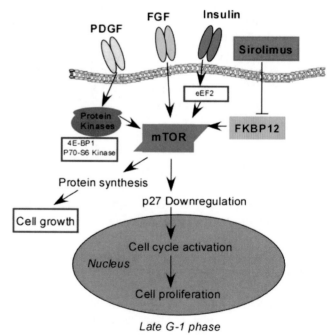

Fig. 13.7 Schematic representation of the mTOR signaling pathway and the mechanism of action of Sirolimus (Rapamycin). Sirolimus forms a complex with FKBP 12 which modulates downstream signaling events. mTOR = mammalian target of Rapamycin

The fact that Rapamycin can block the cell cycle progression of SMCs and inhibit their proliferation was the primary finding that led to its incorporation into DESs [93]. Subsequently, Rapamycin has been demonstrated to successfully control arterial renarrowing after percutaneous intervention and to abolish restenosis [94]. Currently, there are additional potent analogs of Rapamycin which have been incorporated into DESs, including Zotarolimus and Everolimus, that exhibit similar mechanisms of action (i.e., the inhibition of mammalian target of Rapamycin). Importantly, they have shown initial clinical efficacy in controlling ISR [90].

Paclitaxel: Paclitaxel is a microtubule-stabilizing agent belonging to the chemical class of taxanes, obtained originally from the yew tree. Paclitaxel promotes the assembly of microtubules from tubulin dimers and stabilizes microtubules by preventing depolymerization. This stability results in the inhibition of the normal dynamic reorganization of the microtubule network that is essential for vital interphase and mitotic cellular functions. Furthermore, Paclitaxel induces abnormal arrays or "bundles" of microtubules throughout the cell cycle and multiple asters of microtubules during mitosis. Paclitaxel has also demonstrated potent antitumor activity and thus is an approved drug for the treatment of various types of cancers [95]. Paclitaxel inhibits both the migration and the proliferation of SMCs. More recently, Paclitaxel-eluting stents were shown to efficiently prevent angiographic and clinical restenosis [96].

Other Potential Drug Targets for DESs: Many candidate molecules that regulate vascular SMC growth have been studied in preclinical models using a variety of pharmacological and gene therapy approaches [97]. Results have suggested important roles in this process for: (1) the renin–angiotensin system; (2) catecholamines; (3) ET-1; (4) natriuretic peptides; (5) thrombin; (6) platelet-derived growth factor; (7) TGF and other activins [98, 99]; (8) fibroblast growth factor; and (9) other stimuli including oxidative stress nitric oxide and the estrogen receptor [97, 100, 101].

Endothelial Cells

The healthy vascular endothelium is primarily a continuous single cell lining of the cardiovascular system that forms a critical interface between the blood and its components on one side and the tissues and organs on the other. Endothelial integrity is essential for maintaining vascular homeostasis [102]. Yet, the endothelium can also be considered as heterogenous and has many synthetic and metabolic functions, i.e., it can synthesize several powerful vasodilators including nitric oxide, prostacyclin, and endothelium-derived relaxing factors which, in turn, control vascular tone. It also acts as a non-thrombogenic, non-inflammatory and selective permeable barrier. Importantly, endothelial-derived nitric oxide participates in the control of vascular healing by attenuating vascular

inflammation and inhibiting SMC proliferation and migration [103]. Endothelial cells can also promote healing by close interaction with the extracellular matrix and with adjacent cells including pericytes and SMCs within the vessel wall [104]. In response to injury such as angioplasty or stenting, vascular endothelium has the ability to respond by modulating its microenvironment, e.g., activated endothelial cells can rapidly alter the interrelated processes of coagulation, fibrinolysis, growth, and inflammation by secreting prothrombotic molecules such as Willebrand factor and surface expression of adhesion molecules such as P-selectin. In addition, activated endothelial cells can induce plasminogen activator (tPA) that, in turn, inhibits clot lysis. The endothelium also loses its vasodilating ability, rendering the underlying vascular smooth muscle susceptible to the effects of vasoconstrictive and growth-promoting stimuli [105–107].

Importantly, endothelial denudation during PTCA has been postulated to be a fundamental incident contributing to development of restenosis. In addition, endothelial dysfunction has been associated with poor outcomes of coronary revascularization [108]. The term "endothelial dysfunction" most commonly refers to impairment of endothelium-dependent vasodilation and implies presence of widespread abnormalities in endothelial integrity and homeostasis.

In recent years, endothelial function and regeneration have been the focus of multiple preclinical and clinical studies aimed at establishing the mechanisms of action linking incomplete endothelial regeneration, as well as dysfunctional endothelium, with increased risk of vascular disease, including the increased risk for restenosis and late stent thrombosis [109]. Based on the established links, diverse strategies are currently being pursued to promote healing through restoration of proper endothelial growth and function. These strategies include: (1) pharmacological modulation strategies to increase eNOS and nitric oxide production; (2) tissue engineering, gene and stem cell therapies, and procedural modifications (i.e., direct stenting); (3) vessel reconstruction with autologous endothelial cell/fibrin matrix; and (4) the use of estrogen-loaded stents and stents designed to capture progenitor endothelial cells [110, 111].

Effect of Shear Stress on Endothelial Cells and the Link to Restenosis

Biomechanical forces such as fluid shear stresses can activate the endothelium to stimulate the production of an array of biological mediators. Some of these mediators act by altering gene regulation and are analogous to endothelial activation by inflammatory cytokines

[45, 112]. The endothelial cell is capable of responding not only to the magnitude of the applied forces but also to their temporal and spatial fluctuations (e.g., steady versus pulsatile flow, uniform laminar, disturbed laminar, or turbulent flow regions). In turn, this suggests the existence of primary flow sensors (receptors) that are coupled via distinct signaling pathways to nuclear events [113]. Endothelial cells have the capacity to discriminate among specific biomechanical forces and translate these input stimuli into distinctive phenotypes [114].

Endothelial cells subjected to weak shear stress exhibit increased proliferation, while strong shear stresses are associated with increased nitric oxide production and inhibition of endothelial cell proliferation [115]. In addition, in vitro modeling studies [116] have demonstrated focal areas within stents that have low shear stress values and may provide a milieu for endothelial cell activation and vascular proliferation. In vivo, coronary stent implantation can change the three-dimensional geometry and shear stress distribution of the vessel [117].

13.11.2.2 The Role of Inflammation in Restenosis

Based on experimental and clinical data, the important role of inflammation in vascular healing and ISR has been suggested and its importance increasingly emphasized [118, 119]. Endothelial injury, platelet and leukocyte interactions, and subcellular inflammatory mediators are pivotal in the development of the inflammatory response following PTCA and stenting.

The modulation of vascular repair by inflammatory cells is achieved via multiple mechanisms: (1) generation of injurious reactive oxygen intermediates; (2) release of growth and chemotactic factors; and (3) production of enzymes (e.g., matrix metalloproteinases, cathepsin S) capable of degrading extracellular constituents and thereby facilitating cell migration [120].

Leukocytes Recruitment

In animal models in which a stent is deployed to produce deep vessel wall trauma, it has been shown that a brisk early inflammatory response can be induced with abundant surface-adherent neutrophils and monocytes [121]. Days and weeks later, macrophages accumulate within the developing neointima and are observed clustering around stent struts. The number of vessel wall monocytes/macrophages is positively correlated with the neointimal area, suggesting a possible causal role for monocyte activity in restenosis [122]. The mechanisms that govern leukocytes recruitment and infiltration into these tissues

following stent deployment are comprised of multistep adhesive and signaling events. More specifically, the initial adhesion tethering and rolling of leukocytes to the activated platelets at the site of stent deployment is mediated by the platelet adhesion molecule, P-selectin, which then accelerates fibrin formation and deposition. P-selectin also mediates the adherence of platelets to neutrophils via specific interaction with its endogenous ligand, P-selectin glycoprotein-1 (PSGL-1) [122]. Following initial rolling, the leukocytes adhere more firmly through the direct interaction of the surface integrin, Mac-1 (CD11b/ CD18) [123], with the platelet receptors, such as GP Ib, and through cross-linking with fibrinogen to the GP IIb/IIIa receptor. Migration of leukocytes across the platelet-fibrin layer and diapedesis into the tissue is then driven by the chemical gradients of the chemokines produced by inflammatory cells, by inflammation deranged SMCs, and by the resident macrophages [124]. Finally, Mac-1 integrin also functions to amplify the inflammatory response by inducing neutrophil activation, upregulating the expression of cell adhesion molecules, and generating signals that promote integrin activation and chemokine synthesis.

Chemokines and Proinflammatory Cytokines

"Chemokines" are a group of chemoattractant cytokines produced by a number of somatic cells, including endothelial cells, SMCs, and leukocytes. Chemokines elicit a chemotactic stimulus to the adherent leukocytes, directing their migration into the intima [125]. Recent research has identified several candidate chemoattractant molecules responsible for leukocytes transmigration to areas of vascular injury, including monocyte chemoattractant protein (MCP-1) and proinflammatory cytokines such as TNF alpha and interleukins (IL)-1 beta [126, 127]. In addition, T cells encounter signals that cause them to elaborate inflammatory cytokines such as γ-interferon and lymphotoxin (tumor necrosis factor [TNF]-β) that, in turn, can stimulate macrophages as well as vascular endothelial cells and SMCs. These leukocytes, as well as resident vascular wall cells, will secrete cytokines and growth factors (such as platelet-derived growth factor, basic fibroblast growth factor, and epidermal growth factor) that will promote the migration and proliferation of SMCs [45].

MCP-1: MCP-1 belongs to the subfamily of C–C chemokines-beta and is considered responsible for the direct migration of monocytes into the intima at sites of lesion formation [120]. In addition to promoting the transmigration of circulating monocytes into tissues, MCP-1 exerts various other effects on monocytes including superoxide anion induction, cytokine production, and adhesion molecule expression. Inflammatory cytokines or peptide growth factors induce MCP-1 expression in endothelial cells or vascular SMCs. Since elevated levels of MCP-1 have been demonstrated in myocardial infarction, heart failure, and after angioplasty, this chemokine is considered as a probable key factor in initiating the inflammatory process and maintaining the proliferative response to vascular injury restenosis [128, 129]. Furthermore, following stent placement, MCP-1 levels in plasma increase after several days and are more likely to be elevated at follow-up 6 months later in patients who have restenosis.

M-CSF: In addition to MCP-1, macrophage colony-stimulating factor (M-CSF) contributes to the differentiation of the blood monocyte into the macrophage foam cell. Inflammatory mediators such as M-CSF augment expression of macrophage scavenger receptors, leading to the formation of lipid-laden macrophages. M-CSF promotes the replication of macrophages within the intima as well [130]. Moreover, elevated plasma levels of M-CSF were demonstrated in patients with restenosis after PTCA compared to patients without restenosis. Positive correlation was also observed with regard to elevated plasma levels of M-CSF and the extent of lumen loss by restenosis [131].

IL-1beta: Interleukin-1beta (IL-1beta) is the prototypical inflammatory cytokine and is believed to be a critical early mediator of inflammation [132]. Patients with coronary artery disease have markedly elevated levels of IL-1, with its levels being particularly elevated in unstable disease. IL-1beta is capable of inducing smooth muscle activation and leukocyte recruitment in restenosis and atherosclerosis. Recent experimental data reveal that various components of the IL-1 signaling pathway, namely IL-1beta cytokine, IL-1 receptor antagonist (IL-1ra), and IL-1 receptors (IL-1RI and IL-1RII), exhibit differential but concomitant expression patterns following stenting [131] and likely play distinct roles in neointima formation. In addition, local release of IL-1beta cytokine occurs shortly after coronary stent placement, including DESs, which is possibly related to plaque rupture and/or endothelium trauma following the stenting procedure [133].

TNF$_\alpha$: Tumor necrosis factor alpha (TNF-alpha) is a multifunctional cytokine which is considered to play a key role in inflammation and immunity, as well as in apoptosis and cell survival [134]. TNF$_\alpha$ that is secreted from endothelial muscle cells, SMCs, and macrophages has been associated with coronary atheroma. It enhances monocyte recruitment into developing atherosclerotic lesions and is considered as a potential link between obesity and atherosclerosis. TNF$_\alpha$ was also shown to act locally at sites of tissue injury induced by vessel wall damage and

may exert critical influence on the development of restenosis after percutaneous coronary intervention [135].

Systemic Markers of Inflammation and ISR

After balloon angioplasty and/or stenting procedures, there are several systemic markers of inflammation that appear to be predictive of restenosis. These markers are upregulated, transiently or sustained, following stent implantation and are also associated with an increased risk of clinical and angiographic restenosis. They include the C-reactive protein, the most common biomarker for inflammation and coronary disease. Formerly considered solely as a biomarker for inflammation, C-reactive protein is now viewed as a prominent component of the vascular inflammatory process [136]. It can activate the complement pathway, induce the secretion of inflammatory and procoagulant cytokines such as interleukin-6 and endothelin-1, and decrease the expression of endothelial nitric oxide synthase in endothelial cells. In addition, the C-reactive protein activates macrophages to express cytokine and tissue factors [137]. Several studies have indicated a positive association between elevated plasma levels of the C-reactive protein and stent restenosis [138].

Other markers of inflammation and coronary disease encompass key components of innate immunity, vascular injury, and disruption of the atherosclerotic plaque. These include elevated numbers of circulating leukocytes and monocytes in peripheral blood [139, 140], as well as increased levels of the integrin MAC-1 which marks their activation and adhesion [123]. Furthermore, levels of the proinflammatory and proatherothrombotic cytokines, IL-6, and soluble CD40L (sCD40L), each located in the culprit coronary arteries (measured in blood taken from the coronary artery ostium), have been found to increase early after coronary stenting and are associated with risk of restenosis of the revasculized coronary artery [141, 142]. Interleukin-6 is the principal procoagulant cytokine expressed by various cells, including macrophages, T cells, endothelial cells, and SMCs. It triggers an increase in plasma concentrations of fibrinogen, plasminogen activator inhibitor type 1, and the C-reactive protein [143]. Similarly, elevated levels of IL-6 are also associated with increased risk of future myocardial infarction in healthy men [144]. Furthermore, sCD40L was described to be released from activated platelets and interacts with CD40L expressed on vascular cells initiating inflammatory and proatherothrombotic cascade [145]. Importantly, elevated plasma levels of sCD40L can be used to identify patients with acute coronary syndromes at heightened risk of death and recurrent myocardial infarction, independent of other predictive variables [146].

The Cross-Talk Between Inflammation and Thrombosis

Importantly, plaque rupture, whether spontaneous or as a result of stenting, then promotes the activation of an inflammatory response. In turn, one of the primary consequences of increased proinflammatory cytokines in the vasculature is the elevated procoagulant state and an increase in thrombosis [147]. Proinflammatory cytokines such as IL-1β IL-6, MCP-1, and TNFαd α will then increase the expression of a number of other specific proteins that serve to regulate coagulation. Foremost among these is the induction of "tissue factor" expression by endothelial cells, underlying SMCs, and monocytes [147]. Tissue factor (coagulation factor III or CD142) is a 46-kDa transmembrane glycoprotein that serves as one of the primary initiators of blood coagulation [148]. In this biochemical cascade, cell-anchored tissue factor interacts with soluble factor VIIa (FVIIa) to induce factor Xa (FXa) activation, leading to cleavage of prothrombin to thrombin, the proteolytically active protease. Thrombin, in turn, is responsible for conversion of plasma fibrinogen to fibrin, which envelopes and stabilizes developing thrombi (blood clots). Thrombin also cleaves and activates the platelet receptor protease-activated receptor 1 (also known as the thrombin receptor), which induces platelet aggregation and thrombus growth [149]. Activated platelets will release the contents of granules,

which further promotes platelet recruitment, adhesion, aggregation, and activation. In addition to initiating coagulation, interaction of tissue factor with the adhesion molecule, P-selectin, has been demonstrated to accelerate the rate and extent of fibrin formation and deposition. P-selectin is expressed on activated platelets and endothelium and serves as the receptor for the endogenous ligand, P-selectin glycoprotein-1 (PSGL-1), expressed on various leukocytic cell types. In addition to mediating transient interactions between endothelial cells and leukocytes, P-selectin has been reported to mediate adherence of platelets to monocytes and neutrophils via specific interaction with PSGL-1. Finally, P-selectin is rapidly cleaved off the surface of the platelet membrane and appears in the circulation as a soluble form, which has been reported to be elevated in patients with acute coronary syndromes including unstable angina and non-Q-wave myocardial infarction [147].

The Molecular Signaling Leading to Inflammation Due to Vascular Interventions

Inflammatory responses to vascular interventions are governed by the activation of signaling cascades central to inflammation and vascular disease and facilitated via thrombotic signaling (Fig. 13.8). These combine the

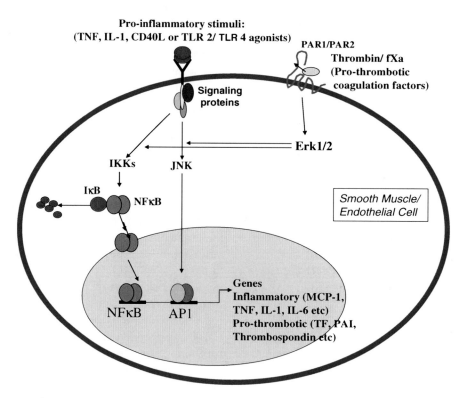

Fig. 13.8 Schematic representation of the cross-talk between inflammatory and thrombotic signaling pathways, including the activation of the AP-1 and the NF-kB transcription factors

classic, well-studied signal transduction pathways, triggered by the proinflammatory cytokines, such as TNF-α, IL-1β, and CD40L, with other signaling pathways which were recently elucidated, including toll-like receptor-2 (TLR-2) and toll-like receptor-4 (TLR-4). It should be noted that metabolic abnormalities such as high LDL, high glucose, and insulin resistance that are prevalent in diabetic and atherosclerotic patients undergoing PTCA can specifically impair or trigger undesired signaling pathways which will further accelerate inflammation, coagulation, and/or thrombosis. These include impaired IGF-1 signaling, impaired PPAR signaling, and the activation of TLR-4 signaling [150–154].

TNF-α Signaling: The interaction of TNF-α **d** α with TNF receptor 1 and receptor 2 (TNFR-1, TNFR-2) activates several signal transduction pathways, leading to the diverse functions of TNF-α **d** α. It has been recently shown that in the arterial wall, TNFR1 mediates this signaling that will contribute to the pathogenesis of atherosclerosis; this response includes enhancing arterial wall chemokine and adhesion molecule expression, as well as by augmenting medial SMC proliferation and migration [155]. The signaling molecules of TNFR-1 (collectively called the TNFR-1 signalosom) have been elucidated quite well, even though the regulation of the signaling still remains unclear. TNFR-1 signalosom consists of signaling proteins that mutual cross-talk will trigger the activation of nuclear factor kappa B (NFκB) [156]. In addition, the TNFR-1 signalosom mediates the activation of the mitogen-activated protein kinases (MAPKs), including the MEK1 and MEK2 and their substrates extracellular-regulated kinases 1 and 2 (ERK1 and ERK2, ERK1/2) pathway, and also the p38-MAPK and c-Jun N-terminal kinase (JNK) stress kinase pathways [155].

CD40-CD40L Signaling: Ligation of CD40 in circulating cells or in the vessel wall may promote mononuclear cell recruitment, participate in the weakening of the plaque, and contribute to thrombosis and neointimal formation [157]. CD40 belongs to the TNF receptor (TNFR) superfamily that also includes TNFR-1 and TNFR-2. CD40 has been shown to express in vascular cells, endothelial cells, and SMCs, and in additional cells implicated in vascular disease, such as monocytes and macrophages. These cells commonly express the receptor constitutively in vitro and show basal expression in non-diseased tissue. Stimulation with inflammatory cytokines enhances expression of CD40 in vitro [158, 159]. CD40 ligand (recently renamed CD154) is a member of the TNF gene superfamily that also includes TNF-α **d** α. Numerous cell types can express CD40L, particularly those implicated in atherogenesis, namely endothelial cells, SMCs, macrophages, and platelets. The precise signaling

mechanism by which the interaction between CD40L and its receptor CD40 mediates inflammatory secretion is not yet fully understood. The cytoplasmic region of CD40 consists of two major signaling domains that through the association with binding proteins termed TNFR-associated factors (TRAFs) can trigger the activation of NFκB, MAPKs, ERK1/2, p38MAPK, and JNK [160, 161]. It is notable that this signaling activation, resulting from CD40 ligation, appears to be cell specific and differs significantly within certain cell types and at various stages of activation and differentiation [161]. For example, within endothelial cells, CD40 ligation-induced activation of NFκB, interferon regulatory factor-1 (IRF-1), JNK and p38-MAPK signaling pathways, and CD40-mediated signaling events in SMCs include tyrosine phosphorylation as well as the activation of NFκB. In monocytes, ligation of CD40 triggers activation of MEK1/2–ERK1/2, as well as the JNK pathway.

IL-1β Signaling: Increased levels of IL-1 enhance vascular adhesion, vascular permeability, macrophage activation, endothelial cell and SMC proliferation, and protease-induced plaque rupture—all key steps in the progression of vascular disease [162]. IL-1 activity is mediated by the formation of a complex involving the type 1 receptor, IL-1R [163]. This receptor is a member of a larger related family, most of which are involved in the mechanisms of host defense. IL-1R was the first receptor discovered in this superfamily and the IL-1-mediated signaling pathway serves as a prototype for the other family members. This large superfamily is collectively called toll/interleukin1 receptor (TIR) and encompasses the Ig domain family (IL-1 receptors, IL-18 receptors, and IL-1R-like receptors), the leucine-rich domain family (the toll-like receptors and similar receptors), and a series of TIR domain-containing intracellular adapter molecules. IL-1R mediates a complex pathway involving a cascade of kinases organized by multiple adapter molecules into signaling complexes, leading to activation of the transcription factors NFκB, p38-MAPK (activating the transcription factor ATF), and JNK pathways (activating the transcription complex AP-1, activator protein 1) [164].

Remarkably IL-1 and TNF-mediated signaling pathways also share several biological properties, particularly the inflammatory molecules they trigger (secretion of inflammatory cytokines and expression of surface adhesion molecules) and the downstream signaling activation such as NFκB and MAPKs, p38, and JNK pathways. The prominent difference is that TNF receptor signaling induces programmed cell death, whereas IL-1 receptor signaling does not.

Initiation of IL-1R activation requires the assistance of the receptor accessory protein (IL-1RAcP) after which the death domain (containing protein MyD88) is recruited to the activated receptor complex. MyD88 functions as an adaptor to recruit the serine–threonine IL-1 receptor-associated kinase IRAK to the receptor through its death domain. IRAK then leaves the receptor complex and interacts with TRAF6, another adaptor signaling molecule that is required for the activation of NFκB. To date, the TRAF family of adaptor proteins (a total of six) has been elucidated in several signaling pathways that lead to NFκB activation, such as TNF and CD40L. Finally, different TRAFs have been found to be used by the various NFκB-dependent pathways [165, 166].

Toll-like Receptors and Vascular Pathogenesis: Members of the TLR subfamily (TLR1-9) will identify alarm indications incoming from microbial pathogens or the host itself and then, in response, mediate the initiation of the innate immunity [164]. Toll-like receptor ligation induces expression of a wide variety of genes such as genes encoding proteins involved in cytokine production (TLR4 in particular), leukocyte recruitment, and phagocytosis that all contribute to the inflammatory response. Toll-like receptors can form dimeric receptor complexes consisting of two different TLRs or homodimers in the case of TLR4. Recently, the expression of TLRs (TLR1, TLR2, and TLR4) was described in human atherosclerotic plaques [167, 168], and a significant amount of evidence is beginning to accumulate indicating that the TLRs are important in cardiovascular pathologies. Toll-like receptor expression has been shown to be elicited by both arterial and myocardial cells. The importance of TLR4 as well as TLR2 was recently considered to be verified through mouse knock-out studies [169]. Among other data, it was demonstrated that the endothelium-dependent dilation in response to acetylcholine in vessels from TLR4(−/−) mice was greatly reduced, thus illustrating a novel role for TLR4 also in the homeostatic control of a functional endothelium [170]. In addition, TLR2 (−/−) mice exhibited marked suppression of neointimal hyperplasia. In addition, endogenous TLR-2 seems to play significant role in inflammatory responses and ROS production after vascular injury. In addition, flow-dependent regulation of TLR2 was demonstrated in endothelial cells, both in vitro and in vivo; expression of endothelial TLR2 is induced under disturbed flow, but not laminar flow, which may explain how a TLR2 could be involved in atherogenesis with regional specificity of lesion development [171]. Similarly, human studies on polymorphisms also point to a role of TLR4 in neointima formation and atherosclerosis.

More specifically, TLRs are type I transmembrane receptors with extracellular leucine repeats and a carboxy terminal intracellular tail containing a conserved region called TIR homology domain. The TIR domain is indispensable for signal transduction since it serves as a scaffold for a series of protein–protein interactions which result in the activation of a unique signaling module consisting of the adaptor protein myeloid differentiation factor 88 (MyD88), interleukin-1 receptor-associated kinase (IRAK) family members, and Tollip, which is used exclusively by TIR family members. Subsequently, several central signaling pathways are activated in parallel, the activation of NFκB being the most prominent event of the inflammatory response.

The extracellular domains of these receptors are involved in ligand binding, but are also necessary for dimerization; various ligands have been identified through in vitro systems or knock-out mouse models. Most of these ligands can be classified as pathogen-associated molecular pattern molecules which are highly conserved. However, recent evidence suggests that TLR4 and TLR2 also respond to endogenous factors produced by stress or cell damaging, like heat shock proteins, extracellular matrix components of fibronectin and hyaluronan, as well as disturbed shear flow [164, 172].

NFκB: Among the various signal transduction pathways that are triggered by vascular inflammation, the activation of the transcription factor NFκB is considered today as the most prominent one. TNF-α, CD40L, IL-1β, and TLR vascular receptors use parallel proximal signaling components that distally converge into the activation of the transcriptional factor NFκB (Fig. 13.8). Once NFκB is fully activated, it participates in the regulation of various target genes in different vascular and immune cells to exert its biological functions. NFκB controls the expression of many inflammatory cytokines, chemokines, immune receptors, and cell-surface adhesion molecules.

NFκB is also a collective term for a family of proteins that exist either as heterodimers or as homodimers. In unstimulated cells, NFκB is sequestered in the cytoplasm because of its association with a member of the IκB family of inhibitory proteins [173]. IκB makes multiple contacts with NFκB, and these interactions mask the nuclear localization sequence of NFκB and can interfere with sequences important for DNA binding [174]. Inflammatory stimulation leads to the phosphorylation of IκBs by IκB kinases, which then targets the IκB for proteosomal degradation [175]. After IκB degradation, liberated NFκB translocates to the nucleus and triggers the transcription of its target genes. More recently, a second level of regulation of NFκB was demonstrated that relies on the phosphorylation of members of the second group of NFκB proteins (p65/RelA, RelB, and c-Rel), resulting in the activation of transcriptional activity of NFκB [176].

13.11.2.3 Late Stent Thrombosis

Although rare, stent thrombosis remains a severe complication after stent implantation owing to its associated high morbidity and mortality. Following stent implantation, patients are typically treated with antiplatelet agents such as clopidogrel and/or aspirin. Defined by the time of occurrence, thrombosis after stenting can be acute (<24 hours), subacute (<30 days), late (>30 days), or very late (>12 months) [55]. Recent data have associated the use of DESs with late and very late thrombosism, i.e., up to 3 years after implantation and predominantly after discontinuation of the antiplatelet therapy. Notable is a recent meta-analysis on 14 contemporary clinical trials that compared DESs (Paclitaxel or sirolimus) with bare metal stents; the authors concluded that even though the overall incidence of late stent thrombosis (more than 1 year after coronary revascularization) was low (~0.5%), DESs appeared to increase the risk for late stent thrombosis [177]. However, this remains a topic of lively debate, as some data from large registries and meta-analyses of randomized trials have indicated a higher risk for DES thrombosis, whereas others suggest an absence of such a risk.

The factors that are associated with an increased risk of late stent thrombosis include: (1) the procedure itself (such as stent malapposition); (2) the patient and his/her general health; and (3) specifics of lesion characteristics (such as small vessels) [55, 178]. In addition, the drugs that are released from current DESs exert their biological effects through inhibition of the cell cycle, aimed at preventing vascular SMC proliferation. Nevertheless, a combination of drug-induced inhibition of proliferation of endothelial cells, with denudation of endothelial cell layer caused by PTCA and stenting may, in fact, impair the reendothelialization and compromise arterial healing [179]. In addition, current DES drugs, such as sirolimus and Paclitaxel, have been reported to induce tissue factor expression [180], which results in a prothrombogenic environment and might ultimately increase the risk of late thrombosis. For example, it has been reported previously that the non-erodable polymers of the Cypher and Taxus stents provoke chronic eosinophilic infiltration of the arterial wall, suggestive of hypersensitivity reactions in a small number of cases [181].

In general, overwhelming evidence suggests a pivotal role of inflammation in restenosis following stent placement. Inflammation plays a role during initial stent placement through progression of restenosis, and most likely critically influences the pathobiology of stent-based thrombosis. It is unclear whether the striking similarity in the pathophysiology markers of atherosclerosis, restenosis, and the risk of cardiac events is due to underlying common pathology or due to a more direct, causal etiology.

13.12 Summary

Cellular physiological functions are regulated via signaling mechanisms in essentially any cell type of any organ. While myocardial cells are unique in that they are interconnected to each other with gap junctions and act as an electrical syncytium, there is nevertheless an enormous number of important cellular receptors that allows the cells to receive and respond to various signals. Inflammation plays a very important role in cardiovascular disease. For example, device-based interventions such as coronary stenting may activate inflammation via a series of complex signaling processes, but importantly, inflammation plays also a central role in atherosclerosis, myocardial infarction, and heart failure. It was the general aim of this chapter to review the role and signaling mechanisms of selected physiologically and pathophysiologically important cardiac and vascular receptors with emphasis on G-protein-coupled receptors (e.g., beta-adrenergic receptors), non-G-protein-coupled receptor systems, such as guanylyl cyclase-related receptors (e.g., receptors for nitric oxide), and finally, to discuss the importance and complexity of inflammation in the pathobiology of coronary artery disease and stenting.

13.13 List of Abbreviations

AC	adenylyl cyclase
ATP	adenosine triphosphate
β-AR	beta-adrenergic receptor
β-ARK	beta-adrenergic receptor kinase
cAMP	cyclic adenosine monophosphate
cGMP	cyclic guanosine monophosphate
CDK	cyclin-dependent kinase
DES	drug-eluting stents
ERK	extracellular signal-regulated kinase
GC	guanylyl cyclase
GDP	guanosine diphosphate
GTP	guanosine triphosphate
IRAK	interleukin-1 receptor associated kinase
ISR	in-stent restenosis
JNK	Jun N-terminal kinase
MAPK	mitogen-activated protein kinase
NOS	nitric oxide synthase
pRB	retinoblastoma gene product
PTCA	percutaneous transluminal coronary angioplasty
SMC	smooth muscle cell
TIR	toll/interleukin1 receptor
TLR	toll-like receptor
TNF	tumor necrosis factor
TNFR	tumor necrosis factor receptor
TRAF	TNFR-associated factors

References

1. Rockman HA, Koch WJ, Lefkowitz RJ. Seven-transmembrane-spanning receptors and heart function. Nature 2002;415:206–12.

2. del Monte F, Kaufmann AJ, Poole-Wilson PA, et al. Coexistence of functioning beta-1 and beta-2 adrenoreceptors in single myocytes from human ventricle. Circulation 1993;88:854–63.

3. Bristow MR, Hershberger RE, Port JD, et al. Beta-adrenergic pathways in non-failing and failing human ventricular myocardium. Circulation 1990;82:112–25.

4. Opie L. Receptors and signal transduction. In:Opie L, ed. The heart: Physiology, from cell to circulation. 3rd ed. Philadelphia, PA: Lippincott Williams & Wilkins, 1998:173–207.

5. Hohl CM, Li Q. Compartmentation of camp in adult canine ventricular myocytes. Relation to single cell free calcium transients. Circ Res 1991;69:1369–79.

6. Lader AS, Xiao YF, Ishikawa Y, et al. Cardiac gsalpha overexpression enhances L-type calcium channels through an adenylyl cyclase independent pathway. Proc Natl Acad Sci USA 1998;95:9669–74.

7. Port JD, Bristow MR. Altered beta-adrenergic receptor gene regulation and signaling in chronic heart failure. J Mol Cell Cardiol 2001;33:887–905.

8. Gauthier C, Langin D, Balligand JL. Beta3-adrenoceptors in the cardiovascular system. Trends Pharmacol Sci 2000;21:426–31.

9. Laporte SA, Oakley RH, Holt JA, Barak LS, Caron MG. The interaction of beta-arrestin with the AP-2 adaptor is required for the clustering of beta-2 adrenergic recedptor into clathrin coated pits. J Biol Chem 2000;275:23120–6.

10. Luttrell LM, Ferguson SS, Daakay Y, et al. Beta-arrestin-dependent formation of beta-2 adrenergic receptor-Src protein kinase complexes. Science 1999;283:655–61.

11. Shenoy SK, McDonald PH, Kohout TA, Lefkowitz RJ. Regulation of receptor fate by ubiquitination of activated beta-2 adrenergic receptor and beta-arrestin. Science 2001;294:1574–77.

12. Mann D, Kent R, Parsons B, Cooper IVG. Adrenergic effects on the biology of the adult mammalian cardiocyte. Circulation 1992;85:790–804.

13. Bristow MR, Ginsburg R, Umans V, et al. Beta 1 and beta 2-adrenergic receptor subpopulations in nonfailing and failing human ventricular myocardium: Coupling of both receptor subtypes to muscle contraction and selective beta 1-receptor down-regulation in heart failure. Circ Res 1986;59:297–309.

14. Ungerer M, Parruti G, Böhn M, et al. Expression of beta-arrestins and beta-adrnergic receptor kinases in the failing human heart. Circ Res 1994;74:206–13.

15. Steinberg SF. The molecular basis for distinct beta-AR subtype action in cardiomyocytes. Circ Res 1999;85:1101–11.

16. Lader AS, Xiao YF, Ishikawa Y, et al. Cardiac gsalpha overexpression enhances L-type calcium channels through an adenylyl cyclase independent pathway. Proc Natl Acad Sci USA 1998;95:9669–74.

17. Communal C, Singh K, Sawyer DB, Colucci WS. Opposing effects of beta-1 and beta-2 adrenergic receptor on cardiac myocyte apoptosis: Role of a pertussis toxin sensitive G protein. Circulation 1999;100:2210–2.

18. Zaugg M, Xu W, Lucchinetti E, Shafiq SA, Jamali NZ, Siddiqui MA. Beta-adrenergic receptor subtypes differentially affect apoptosis in adult rat ventricular myocytes. Circulation 2000;102:344–50.

19. Bisognano JD, Weinberger HD, Bohlmeyer TJ, et al. Myocardial-directed overexpression of the human beta-1-adrenergic receptor in transgenic mice. J Mol Cell Cardiol 2000;32:817–30.

20. Saito S, Hiroi Y, Zou Y, et al. Beta-adrenergic pathway induces apoptosis through calcineurin activation in cardiac myocytes. J Biol Chem 2000;275:34528–33.

21. Lowes BD, Gill EA, Abraham WT, et al. Effects of carvedilol on left ventricular mass, chamber geometry, and mitral regurgitation in chronic heart failure. Am J Cardiol 1999;83:1201–5.

22. Liggett SB, Wagoner LE, Craft LL, et al. The Ile164 Beta-2 AR polymorphism adversely affects the outcome of congestive heart failure. J Clin Invest 1998;102:1534–9.

23. Wagoner LE, Craft LL, Singh B, et al. Polymorphisms of the beta-2 AR determine exercise capacity in patients with heart failure. Circ Res 2000;86:834–40.

24. Graham RM, Perez DM, Hwa J, Piascik MT. Alpha-AR subtypes. Molecular structure, function and signaling. Circ Res 1996;78:737–49.

25. Otani H, Otani H, Das DK. Alpha-1 adrenoreceptor mediated phosphoinisotidie breakdown and inotropic response in rate left ventricular papillary muscles. Circ Res 1988;62:8–17.

26. Hwang KC, Grady CD, Sweet WE, Moravec CS. Alpha-1 adrenergic receptor coupling with Gh in the failing human heart. Circulation 1996;94:718–26.

27. Choi DJ, Koch WJ, Hunter JJ, Rockman HA. Mechanism of beta-adrenergic receptor desensitization in cardiac hypertrophy is increased beta-ARK. J Biol Chem 1997;272:17223–9.

28. Knowlton KU, Michael MC, Itani, et al. The alpha1A-adrenergic receptor subtype mediates biochemical, molecular, and morphologic features of cultured myocardial cell hypertrophy. J Biol Chem 1993;268:15374–80.

29. Sugden PH. Signaling in myocardial hypertrophy: Life after calcineurin? Circ Res 1999;84:633–46.

30. Barki-Harrington L, Luttrell LM, Rockman HA. Dual inhibition of beta-adrenergic and angiotensin II receptors by a single antagonist. Circulation 2003;108:1611–8.

31. Dzimiri N. Receptor crosstalk: Implications for cardiovascular function, disease and therapy. Eur J Biochem 2002;269:4713–30.

32. Münzel T, Feil R, Mülsch A, Lohmann SM, Hofmann F, Walter U. Physiology and pathophysiology of vascular signaling controlled by cyclic guanosine 3',5'-cyclic monophosphate-dependent protein kinase. Circulation 2003;108:2172–83.

33. von der Leyen HE, Dzau VJ. Therapeutic potential of nitric oxide synthase gene manipulation. Circulation 2001;103:2760–5.

34. Loscalzo J. Nitric oxide insufficiency, platelet activation, and arterial thrombosis. Circ Res 2001;88:756–62.

35. Champion HC, Skaf MW, Hare JM. Role of nitric oxide in the pathophysiology of heart failure. Heart Fail Rev 2003;8:35–46.

36. Jugdutt BI. Nitric oxide and cardiovascular protection. Heart Fail Rev 2003;8:29–34.

37. Young-Myeong K, Bombeck CA, Billiar TR. Nitric oxide as a bifunctional regulator of apoptosis. Circ Res 1999;84:253–6.

38. Kuhn M. Structure, regulation, and function of mammalian membrane guanylyl cyclase receptors, with a focus on guanylyl cyclase A. Circ Res 2003;93:700–9.

39. Nobuyoshi M, Kimura T, Nosaka H, et al. Restenosis after successful percutaneous transluminal coronary angioplasty: Serial angiographic follow-up of 229 patients. J Am Coll Cardiol 1988;12:616–23.

40. Kipshidze NN, Tsapenko ML, Leon MB, Stone GW, Moses JW. Update on drug-eluting coronary stents. Expert Rev Cardiovasc Ther 2005;3:953–68.

41. van den Brand MJ, Rensing BJ, Morel MA, et al. The effect of completeness of revascularization on event-free survival at one year in the ARTS trial. J Am Coll Cardiol 2002;39:559–64.

42. Topol EJ, Serruys PW. Frontiers in interventional cardiology. Circulation 1998;98:1802–20.

43. Serruys PW, Foley DP, Suttorp MJ. A randomized comparison of the value of additional stenting after optimal balloon angioplasty for long coronary lesions: Final results of the additional value of NIR stents for treatment of long coronary lesions (ADVANCE) study. J Am Coll Cardiol 2002;39:393–9.

44. Fischman DL, Leon MB, Baim DS, et al. A randomized comparison of coronary-stent placement and balloon angioplasty in the treatment of coronary artery disease. Stent Restenosis Study Investigators. N Engl J Med 1994;331:496–501.

45. Scott NA. Restenosis following implantation of bare metal coronary stents: Pathophysiology and pathways involved in the vascular response to injury. Adv Drug Deliv Rev 2006;58:358–76.

46. Faries PL, Rohan DI, Takahara H. Human vascular smooth muscle cells of diabetic origin exhibit increased proliferation, adhesion, and migration. J Vasc Surg 2001;33:601–7.

47. El-Omar MM, Dangas G, Iakovou I, Mehran R. Update on in-stent restenosis. Curr Interv Cardiol Rep 2001;3:296–305.

48. Hill RA, Boland A, Dickson R, et al. Drug-eluting stents: A systematic review and economic evaluation. Health Technol Assess 2007;11:iii, xi-221.

49. Htay T, Liu MW. Drug-eluting stent: A review and update. Vasc Health Risk Manag 2005;1:263–76.

50. Steffel J, Tanner FC. Biological effects of drug-eluting stents in the coronary circulation. Herz 2007;32:268–73.

51. Mackman N. Triggers, targets and treatments for thrombosis. Nature 2008;451:914–8.

52. Kaul S, Shah PK, Diamond GA. As time goes by: Current status and future directions in the controversy over stenting. J Am Coll Cardiol 2007;50:128–37.

53. Bavry AA, Kumbhani DJ, Helton TJ, Bhatt DL. Risk of thrombosis with the use of sirolimus-eluting stents for percutaneous coronary intervention (from registry and clinical trial data). Am J Cardiol 2005;95:1469–72.

54. Moreno R, Fernández C, Hernández R, et al. Drug-eluting stent thrombosis: Results from a pooled analysis including 10 randomized studies. J Am Coll Cardiol 2005;45:954–9.

55. Luscher TF, Steffel J, Eberli FR, et al. Drug-eluting stent and coronary thrombosis: Biological mechanisms and clinical implications. Circulation 2007;115:1051–8.

56. Legrand V. Therapy insight: Diabetes and drug-eluting stents. Nat Clin Pract Cardiovasc Med 2007;4:143–50.

57. Kawaguchi R, Angiolillo DJ, Futamatsu H, Suzuki N, Bass TA, Costa MA. Stent thrombosis in the era of drug-eluting stents. Minerva Cardioangiol 2007;55:199–211.

58. Forrester JS, Fishbein M, Helfant R, Fagin J. A paradigm for restenosis based on cell biology: Clues for the development of new preventive therapies. J Am Coll Cardiol 1991;17:758–69.

59. Costa MA, Simon DI. Molecular basis of restenosis and drug-eluting stents. Circulation 2005;111:2257–73.

60. Libby P. Atherosclerosis: Disease biology affecting the coronary vasculature. Am J Cardiol 2006;98:3–9Q.

61. Casscells W, Engler D, Willerson JT. Mechanisms of restenosis. Tex Heart Inst J 1994;21:68–77.

62. Welt FG, Rogers C. Inflammation and restenosis in the stent era. Arterioscler Thromb Vasc Biol 2002;22:1769–76.

63. Mintz GS, Popma JJ, Hong MK, et al. Intravascular ultrasound findings after excimer laser coronary angioplasty. Cathet Cardiovasc Diagn 1996;37:113–8.

64. Lundmark K, Tran PK, Kinsella MG, Clowes AW, Wight TN, Hedin U. Perlecan inhibits SMC adhesion to fibronectin: Role of heparan sulfate. J Cell Physiol 2001;188:67–74.

65. Lerman A. Restenosis: Another "dysfunction" of the endothelium. Circulation 2005;111:8–10.

66. Muto A, Fitzgerald TN, Pimiento JM, et al. Smooth muscle cell signal transduction: Implications of vascular biology for vascular surgeons. J Vasc Surg 2007;45:A15–24.

67. Owens GK, Kumar MS, Wamhoff BR. Molecular regulation of vascular smooth muscle cell differentiation in development and disease. Physiol Rev 2004;84:767–801.

68. Li X, et al. Suppression of smooth-muscle alpha-actin expression by platelet-derived growth factor in vascular smooth-muscle cells involves Ras and cytosolic phospholipase A2. Biochem J 1997;327:709–16.

69. Zalewski A, Shi Y, Johnson AG. Diverse origin of intimal cells: Smooth muscle cells, myofibroblasts, fibroblasts, and beyond? Circ Res 2002;91:652–5.

70. Powell DW, Mifflin RC, Valentich JD, Crowe SE, Saada JI, West AB. Myofibroblasts. I. Paracrine cells important in health and disease. Am J Physiol 1999;277:C1–9.

71. Yokote K, Take A, Nakaseko C, et al. Bone marrow-derived vascular cells in response to injury. J Atheroscler Thromb 2003;10:205–10.

72. Bornfeldt KE, Krebs EG. Crosstalk between protein kinase A and growth factor receptor signaling pathways in arterial smooth muscle. Cell Signal 1999;11:465–77.

73. Seger R, Krebs EG. The MAPK signaling cascade. Faseb J 1995;9:726–35.

74. Asada H. Paszkowiak J, Teso D, et al. Sustained orbital shear stress stimulates smooth muscle cell proliferation via the extracellular signal-regulated protein kinase 1/2 pathway. J Vasc Surg 2005;42:772–80.

75. Nishida E, Gotoh Y. The MAP kinase cascade is essential for diverse signal transduction pathways. Trends Biochem Sci 1993;18:128–31.

76. Marshall CJ. Specificity of receptor tyrosine kinase signaling: Transient versus sustained extracellular signal-regulated kinase activation. Cell 1995;80:179–85.

77. Liu Y, McDonald OG, Shang Y, Hoofnagle MH, Owens GK. Kruppel-like factor 4 abrogates myocardin-induced activation of smooth muscle gene expression. J Biol Chem 2005;280:9719–27.

78. McDonald OG, Warnhoff BR, Hoofnagle MH, Owens GK. Control of SRF binding to CArG box chromatin regulates smooth muscle gene expression in vivo. J Clin Invest 2006;116:36–48.

79. Hedin U, Roy J, Tran PK. Control of smooth muscle cell proliferation in vascular disease. Curr Opin Lipidol 2004;15:559–65.

80. Geng YJ, Libby P. Progression of atheroma: A struggle between death and procreation. Arterioscler Thromb Vasc Biol 2002;22:1370–80.

81. Raines EW. The extracellular matrix can regulate vascular cell migration, proliferation, and survival: Relationships to vascular disease. Int J Exp Pathol 2000;81:173–82.

82. Dzau VJ, Braun-Dullaeus RC, Sedding DG. Vascular proliferation and atherosclerosis: New perspectives and therapeutic strategies. Nat Med 2002;8:1249–56.

83. Walworth NC. Cell-cycle checkpoint kinases: Checking in on the cell cycle. Curr Opin Cell Biol 2000;12:697–704.

84. Weinberg RA. E2F and cell proliferation: A world turned upside down. Cell 1996;85:457–9.

85. Harbour JW, Dean DC. Rb function in cell-cycle regulation and apoptosis. Nat Cell Biol 2000;2:E65–7.

86. Tanner FC, Boehm M, Akyürek LM, et al. Differential effects of the cyclin-dependent kinase inhibitors p27(Kip1), p21(Cip1), and p16(Ink4) on vascular smooth muscle cell proliferation. Circulation 2000;101:2022–5.

87. Gizard F, Bruemmer D. Transcriptional control of vascular smooth muscle cell proliferation by peroxisome proliferator-

activated receptor-gamma: Therapeutic implications for cardiovascular diseases. PPAR Res 2008;2008:429123.

88. Sherr CJ, Roberts JM. CDK inhibitors: Positive and negative regulators of G1-phase progression. Genes Dev 1999;13: 1501–12.

89. Braun-Dullaeus RC, Mann MJ, Dzau VJ. Cell cycle progression: New therapeutic target for vascular proliferative disease. Circulation 1998;98:82–9.

90. Quizhpe AR, Feres F, de Ribamar Costa J Jr., et al. Drug-eluting stents vs bare metal stents for the treatment of large coronary vessels. Am Heart J 2007;154:373–8.

91. Neuhaus P, Klupp J, Langrehr JM. mTOR inhibitors: An overview. Liver Transpl 2001;7:473–84.

92. Sehgal SN. Sirolimus: Its discovery, biological properties, and mechanism of action. Transplant Proc 2003;35:7–14S.

93. Ruygrok PN, Muller DW, Serruys PW. Rapamycin in cardiovascular medicine. Intern Med J 2003;33:103–9.

94. Abizaid A. Sirolimus-eluting coronary stents: A review. Vasc Health Risk Manag 2007;3:191–201.

95. Larkin JM, Kaye SB. Epothilones in the treatment of cancer. Expert Opin Investig Drugs 2006;15:691–702.

96. Sheiban I, Moretti C, Oliaro E, et al. Evolving standard in the treatment of coronary artery disease. Drug-eluting stents. Minerva Cardioangiol 2003;51:485–92.

97. Kukreja N, Onuma Y, Daemen J, Serruys PW. The future of drug-eluting stents. Pharmacol Res 2008;57:171–80.

98. Okamoto S, Inden M, Setsuda M, Konishi T, Nakano T. Effects of trapidil (triazolopyrimidine), a platelet-derived growth factor antagonist, in preventing restenosis after percutaneous transluminal coronary angioplasty. Am Heart J 1992;123:1439–44.

99. Powell JS, Clozel JP, Müller RK, et al. Inhibitors of angiotensin-converting enzyme prevent myointimal proliferation after vascular injury. Science 1989;245:186–8.

100. Garas SM, Huber P, Scott NA. Overview of therapies for prevention of restenosis after coronary interventions. Pharmacol Ther 2001;92:165–78.

101. Reidy MA, Fingerle J, Lindner V. Factors controlling the development of arterial lesions after injury. Circulation 1992;86:III43–6.

102. Meredith IT, Anderson TJ, Uehata A, Yeung AC, Selwyn AP, Ganz P. Role of endothelium in ischemic coronary syndromes. Am J Cardiol 1993;72:27–31C; discussion 31–32C.

103. Versari D, Lerman LO, Lerman A. The importance of reendothelialization after arterial injury. Curr Pharm Des 2007;13:1811–24.

104. Rao RM, Yang L, Garcia-Cardena G, Luscinskas FW. Endothelial-dependent mechanisms of leukocyte recruitment to the vascular wall. Circ Res 2007;101:234–47.

105. Berk BC. Vascular smooth muscle growth: Autocrine growth mechanisms. Physiol Rev 2001;81:999–1030.

106. Langille BL, O'Donnell F. Reductions in arterial diameter produced by chronic decreases in blood flow are endothelium-dependent. Science 1986;231:405–7.

107. Datta YH, Ewenstein BM. Regulated secretion in endothelial cells: Biology and clinical implications. Thromb Haemost 2001;86:1148–55.

108. Celermajer DS. Endothelial dysfunction: Does it matter? Is it reversible? J Am Coll Cardiol 1997;30:325–33.

109. Leopold JA, Loscalzo J. Clinical importance of understanding vascular biology. Cardiol Rev 2000;8:115–23.

110. Tanguay JF. Vascular healing after stenting: The role of 17-beta-estradiol in improving re-endothelialization and reducing restenosis. Can J Cardiol 2005;21:1025–30.

111. Adams B. Xiao Q, Xu Q. Stem cell therapy for vascular disease. Trends Cardiovasc Med 2007;17:246–51.

112. Sprague EA, Luo J, Palmaz JC. Endothelial cell migration onto metal stent surfaces under static and flow conditions. J Long Term Eff Med Implants 2000;10:97–110.

113. Davies PF. Flow-mediated endothelial mechanotransduction. Physiol Rev 1995;75:519–60.

114. Garcia-Cardena G, Comander J, Anderson KR, Blackman BR, Gimbrone MA Jr. Biomechanical activation of vascular endothelium as a determinant of its functional phenotype. Proc Natl Acad Sci USA 2001;98:4478–85.

115. Lin K, Hsu PP, Chen BP, et al. Molecular mechanism of endothelial growth arrest by laminar shear stress. Proc Natl Acad Sci USA 2000;97:9385–9.

116. Levesque MJ, Nerem RM, Sprague EA. Vascular endothelial cell proliferation in culture and the influence of flow. Biomaterials 1990;11:702–7.

117. LaDisa JF Jr., Guler I, Olson LE, et al. Three-dimensional computational fluid dynamics modeling of alterations in coronary wall shear stress produced by stent implantation. Ann Biomed Eng 2003;31:972–80.

118. Colombo A, Sangiorgi G. The monocyte: The key in the lock to reduce stent hyperplasia? J Am Coll Cardiol 2004;43:24–6.

119. Farb A, Sangiorgi G, Carter AJ, et al. Pathology of acute and chronic coronary stenting in humans. Circulation 1999;99:44–52.

120. Welt FG, Tso C. Edellman ER, et al., Leukocyte recruitment and expression of chemokines following different forms of vascular injury. Vasc Med 2003;8:1–7.

121. Tanaka H, Sukhova GK, Swnason SJ, et al. Sustained activation of vascular cells and leukocytes in the rabbit aorta after balloon injury. Circulation 1993;88:1788–803.

122. Rogers C, Welt FG, Karnovsky MJ, Edelman ER. Monocyte recruitment and neointimal hyperplasia in rabbits. Coupled inhibitory effects of heparin. Arterioscler Thromb Vasc Biol 1996;16:1312–8.

123. Rogers C, Edelman ER, Simon DI. A mAb to the beta2-leukocyte integrin Mac-1 (CD11b/CD18) reduces intimal thickening after angioplasty or stent implantation in rabbits. Proc Natl Acad Sci USA 1998;95:10134–9.

124. McEver RP, Cummings RD. Role of PSGL-1 binding to selectins in leukocyte recruitment. J Clin Invest 1997;100:S97–103.

125. Weber C. Platelets and chemokines in atherosclerosis: Partners in crime. Circ Res 2005;96:612–6.

126. Kitamoto S, Egashira K. Anti-monocyte chemoattractant protein-1 gene therapy for cardiovascular diseases. Expert Rev Cardiovasc Ther 2003;1:393–400.

127. Wainwright CL, Miller AM, Wadsworth RM. Inflammation as a key event in the development of neointima following vascular balloon injury. Clin Exp Pharmacol Physiol 2001;28:891–5.

128. Cipollone F, Marini M, Fazia M. Elevated circulating levels of monocyte chemoattractant protein-1 in patients with restenosis after coronary angioplasty. Arterioscler Thromb Vasc Biol 2001;21:327–34.

129. Oshima S, Ogawa H, Hokimoto S, et al., Plasma monocyte chemoattractant protein-1 antigen levels and the risk of restenosis after coronary stent implantation. Jpn Circ J 2001;65:261–4.

130. Bursill CA, Channon KM, Greaves DR. The role of chemokines in atherosclerosis: Recent evidence from experimental models and population genetics. Curr Opin Lipidol 2004;15:145–9.

131. Tashiro H, Shimokawa H, Sadamatsu K, Aoki T, Yamamoto K. Role of cytokines in the pathogenesis of restenosis after percutaneous transluminal coronary angioplasty. Coron Artery Dis 2001;12:107–13.

132. Arend WP, Guthridge CJ. Biological role of interleukin 1 receptor antagonist isoforms. Ann Rheum Dis 2000;59:i60–4.

133. Sardella G, Mariani P, D'Alessandro M, et al. Early elevation of interleukin-1beta and interleukin-6 levels after bare or drug-eluting stent implantation in patients with stable angina. Thromb Res 2006;117:659–64.

134. Odrowaz-Sypniewska G. Markers of pro-inflammatory and pro-thrombotic state in the diagnosis of metabolic syndrome. Adv Med Sci 2007;52:246–50.

135. Monraats PS, Pires NM, Schepers A, et al. Tumor necrosis factor-alpha plays an important role in restenosis development. Faseb J 2005;19:1998–2004.

136. Kawamoto R, Hatakeyama K, Imamura T, et al. Relation of C-reactive protein to restenosis after coronary stent implantation and to restenosis after coronary atherectomy. Am J Cardiol 2004;94:104–7.

137. Mazer SP, Rabbani LE. Evidence for C-reactive protein's role in (CRP) vascular disease: Atherothrombosis, immuno-regulation and CRP. J Thromb Thrombolysis 2004;17:95–105.

138. Gaspardone A, Versaci F, Tomai F, et al. C-Reactive protein, clinical outcome, and restenosis rates after implantation of different drug-eluting stents. Am J Cardiol 2006;97:1311–6.

139. Moreno PR, Bernardi VH, López-Cuéllar J, et al. Macrophage infiltration predicts restenosis after coronary intervention in patients with unstable angina. Circulation 1996;94:3098–102.

140. Stakos DA, Kotsianidis I, Tziakas DN, et al. Leukocyte activation after coronary stenting in patients during the subacute phase of a previous ST-elevation myocardial infarction. Coron Artery Dis 2007;18:105–10.

141. Funayama H, Ishikawa SE, Kubo N, Yasu T, Saito M, Kawakami M. Close association of regional interleukin-6 levels in the infarct-related culprit coronary artery with restenosis in acute myocardial infarction. Circ J 2006;70:426–9.

142. Cipollone F, Ferri C, Desideri G, et al. Preprocedural level of soluble CD40L is predictive of enhanced inflammatory response and restenosis after coronary angioplasty. Circulation 2003;108:2776–82.

143. Lin ZQ, Kondo T, Ishida Y, Takayasu T, Mukaida N. Essential involvement of IL-6 in the skin wound-healing process as evidenced by delayed wound healing in IL-6-deficient mice. J Leukoc Biol 2003;73:713–21.

144. Becker RC. Complicated myocardial infarction. Crit Pathw Cardiol 2003;2:125–52.

145. Vishnevetsky D, Kiyanista VA, Gandhi PJ. CD40 ligand: A novel target in the fight against cardiovascular disease. Ann Pharmacother 2004;38:1500–8.

146. Yan JC, Ding S, Liang Y, et al. Relationship between upregulation of CD40 system and restenosis in patients after percutaneous coronary intervention. Acta Pharmacol Sin 2007;28:339–43.

147. Shebuski RJ, Kilgore KS. Role of inflammatory mediators in thrombogenesis. J Pharmacol Exp Ther 2002;300:729–35.

148. Giesen PL, Fyfe BS, Fallon JT, et al. Intimal tissue factor activity is released from the arterial wall after injury. Thromb Haemost 2000;83:622–8.

149. Martorell L, Martinez-Gonzalez J, Rodriguez C, Gentile M, Calvayrac O, Badimon L. Thrombin and protease-activated receptors (PARs) in atherothrombosis. Thromb Haemost 2008;99;305–15.

150. Hideshima T, Rodar K, Chauhan D, Anderson KC. Cytokines and signal transduction. Best Pract Res Clin Haematol 2005;18:509–24.

151. Barish GD, Atkins AR, Downes M, et al. PPARdelta regulates multiple proinflammatory pathways to suppress atherosclerosis. Proc Natl Acad Sci USA 2008;105:4271–6.

152. Baron AD. Insulin resistance and vascular function. J Diabetes Complications 2002;16:92–102.

153. Kim F, Pham M, Luttrell I, et al. Toll-like receptor-4 mediates vascular inflammation and insulin resistance in diet-induced obesity. Circ Res 2007;100:1589–96.

154. Nilsson J, Nilsson LM, Chen YM, Molkentin JD, Erlinge D, Gomez MF. High glucose activates nuclear factor of activated T cells in native vascular smooth muscle. Arterioscler Thromb Vasc Biol 2006;26:794–800.

155. Zhang L, Peppel K, Sivashanmugam P, et al. Expression of tumor necrosis factor receptor-1 in arterial wall cells promotes atherosclerosis. Arterioscler Thromb Vasc Biol 2007;27:1087–94.

156. Heyninck K, Beyaert R. Crosstalk between NF-kappaB-activating and apoptosis-inducing proteins of the TNF-receptor complex. Mol Cell Biol Res Commun 2001;4:259–65.

157. Schonbeck U, Libby P. CD40 signaling and plaque instability. Circ Res 2001;89:1092–103.

158. Vanichakarn P, Blair P, Wu C, Freedman JE, Chakrabarti S. Neutrophil CD40 enhances platelet-mediated inflammation. Thromb Res 2008;Feb 18 [Epub ahead of print].

159. Lutgens E, Lievens D, Beckers L, Donners M, Daemen M. CD40 and its ligand in atherosclerosis. Trends Cardiovasc Med 2007;17:118–23.

160. Chakrabarti S, Blair P, Freedman JE. CD40-40L signaling in vascular inflammation. J Biol Chem 2007;282:18307–17.

161. Zirlik A, Bavendiek U, Libby P, et al. TRAF-1, –2, –3, –5, and –6 are induced in atherosclerotic plaques and differentially mediate proinflammatory functions of CD40L in endothelial cells. Arterioscler Thromb Vasc Biol 2007;27:1101–7.

162. Hoge M, Amar S. Role of interleukin-1 in bacterial atherogenesis. Drugs Today (Barc) 2006;42:683–8.

163. Fogal B, Hewett SJ. Interleukin-1beta: A bridge between inflammation and excitotoxicity? J Neurochem 2008;Mar 19 [Epub ahead of print].

164. Li X, Qin J. Modulation of Toll-interleukin 1 receptor mediated signaling. J Mol Med 2005;83:258–66.

165. Boraschi D, Tagliabue A. The interleukin-1 receptor family. Vitam Horm 2006;74:229–54.

166. Gottipati S, Rao NL, Fung-Leung WP. IRAK1: A critical signaling mediator of innate immunity. Cell Signal 2008;20:269–76.

167. Mullaly SC, Kubes P. Toll gates and traffic arteries: From endothelial TLR2 to atherosclerosis. Circ Res 2004;95:657–9.

168. Schoneveld AH, Oude Nijhuis MM, van Middelaar B, Laman JD, de Kleijn DP, Pasterkamp G. Toll-like receptor 2 stimulation induces intimal hyperplasia and atherosclerotic lesion development. Cardiovasc Res 2005;66:162–9.

169. Shishido T, Nozaki N, Takahashi H, et al. Central role of endogenous Toll-like receptor-2 activation in regulating inflammation, reactive oxygen species production, and subsequent neointimal formation after vascular injury. Biochem Biophys Res Commun 2006;345:1446–53.

170. Harrington LS, Belcher E, Moreno L, Carrier MJ, Mitchell JA. Homeostatic role of Toll-like receptor 4 in the endothelium and heart. J Cardiovasc Pharmacol Ther 2007;12:322–6.

171. de Kleijn MJ, Wilmink HW, Bots ML, et al. Hormone replacement therapy and endothelial function. Results of a randomized controlled trial in healthy postmenopausal women. Atherosclerosis 2001;159:357–65.

172. Martin MU, Wesche H. Summary and comparison of the signaling mechanisms of the Toll/interleukin-1 receptor family. Biochim Biophys Acta 2002;1592:265–80.

173. Karin M, Ben-Neriah Y. Phosphorylation meets ubiquitination: The control of NF-[kappa]B activity. Annu Rev Immunol 2000;18:621–63.

174. Chen FE, Huang DB, Chen YQ, Ghosh G. Crystal structure of p50/p65 heterodimer of transcription factor NF-kappaB bound to DNA. Nature 1998;391:410–3.

175. Li ZW, Chu W, Hu Y, et al. The IKKbeta subunit of IkappaB kinase (IKK) is essential for nuclear factor kappaB activation and prevention of apoptosis. J Exp Med 1999;189:1839–45.

176. Li X, Stark GR. NFkappaB-dependent signaling pathways. Exp Hematol 2002;30:285–96.

177. Bavry AA, Kumbhani DJ, Helton TJ, Borek PP, Mood GR, Bhatt DL. Late thrombosis of drug-eluting stents: A meta-analysis of randomized clinical trials. Am J Med 2006;119:1056–61.

178. Iakovou I, Schmidt T, Bonizzoni E, et al. Incidence, predictors, and outcome of thrombosis after successful implantation of drug-eluting stents. JAMA 2005;293:2126–30.

179. Waters RE, Kandzari DE, Phillips HR, Crawford LE, Sketch MH Jr. Late thrombosis following treatment of in-stent restenosis with drug-eluting stents after discontinuation of antiplatelet therapy. Catheter Cardiovasc Interv 2005;65:520–4.

180. Eisenreich A, Celebi O, Goldin-Lang P, Schultheiss HP, Rauch U. Upregulation of tissue factor expression and thrombogenic activity in human aortic smooth muscle cells by irradiation, rapamycin and paclitaxel. Int Immunopharmacol 2008;8:307–11.

181. Nakazawa G, Finn AV, Virmani R. Vascular pathology of drug-eluting stents. Herz 2007;32:274–80.

Chapter 14
Reversible and Irreversible Damage of the Myocardium: New Ischemic Syndromes, Ischemia/Reperfusion Injury, and Cardioprotection

James A. Coles, Daniel C. Sigg, and Paul A. Iaizzo

Abstract Ischemia and reperfusion injuries can lead to major compromises in cardiac function. While the intent of many of the past cardioprotective therapies was to protect the myocardium from ischemic necrosis, it may be that reperfusion injury following ischemia may occur despite such preventative attempts. There are continued efforts to identify improvements in myocardial protective strategies, and their ultimate goals are to minimize the risk of cellular injuries to all types of patients undergoing cardiovascular therapies, treatments, or surgeries. The goal of this chapter is to provide the reader with a general review of the physiology and pathophysiology of "myocardial ischemia."

Keywords Myocardial ischemia · Reperfusion injury · Cardioprotection · Myocardial stunning · Hibernating myocardium · Maimed myocardium · Ischemic preconditioning · Silent ischemia

14.1 Introduction

In the past, it was thought that a lack of blood flow to the heart resulted in irreversible myocardial damage and necrosis (infarction). However, recent evidence has suggested that there are several identifiable clinical scenarios that present between these basic definitions of "ischemia" and "infarction," and actually the heart may recover a variable degree of preischemic function, even when eliciting some degree of necrosis. Furthermore, with recent technological advances involving intentional cardiac arrest during cardiac surgery and noninvasive cardiac angioplasty (opening) of occluded coronary arteries, the phenomenon of reperfusion injury has also presented as a sometimes debilitating clinical syndrome. This chapter will explore these described ischemic syndromes and present an up-to-date overview of several methods to protect the heart from these conditions (cardioprotection).

14.2 Basic Cardiac Metabolism

The average healthy human heart weighs between 300 and 350 g and is approximately 0.5% of the total body mass, yet the oxygen demand of the heart accounts for 7% of the resting body oxygen consumption and, consequently, 5% of the cardiac output. The normal myocardial oxygen consumption (MVO_2) is approximately 8 ml O_2/100 g/min, yet this varies widely between normal, diseased, and exercising states. The MVO_2 is primarily dependent on coronary blood flow (CBF) and the removal of oxygen from the coronary blood arterial (CaO_2) minus venous (coronary sinus, CSO_2) contents, such that

$$MVO_2 = CBFx(CaO_2 - CSO_2).$$

Secondary determinants influencing MVO_2 include the relative heart rate, myocardial stroke work, afterload, and/or the inotropic state of the myocardium.

Importantly, associated with cardiac surgery, MVO_2 can vary extensively, with the greatest MVO_2 occurring immediately after bypass; replenishing energy stores requires a high oxygen demand (i.e., repaying oxygen debt). In contrast, cardiac arrest combined with myocardial hypothermia dramatically reduces MVO_2 (Fig. 14.1). It should be noted that hypothermic and normothermic modes of cardiac arrest differ in their degrees of MVO_2 reduction. However, in all cases, the arrested heart still elicits an oxygen demand, hence, there will always be some degree of imbalance between oxygen demand and delivery, with ischemia resulting.

J.A. Coles (✉)
Medtronic, Inc., 8200 Coral Sea St, MNV 41, Mounds View, MN 55112, USA
e-mail: james.coles@medtronic.com

P.A. Iaizzo (ed.), *Handbook of Cardiac Anatomy, Physiology, and Devices*, DOI 10.1007/978-1-60327-372-5_14,
© Springer Science+Business Media, LLC 2009

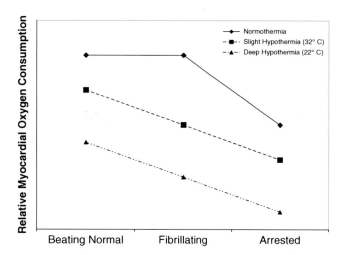

Fig. 14.1 Influence of temperature on myocardial metabolism. While it is expected that hypothermia decreases myocardial oxygen consumption in the beating and fibrillating heart, there also exists a significant difference between the normothermic and hypothermic arrested heart. This indicates that the heart still has a measurable oxygen demand while arrested. Also notable is the difference in myocardial oxygen consumption between the fibrillating and arrested heart at either temperature

14.3 Myocardial Ischemia

The basic definition of "myocardial ischemia" is a greater myocardial tissue oxygen demand than supply. During short-term ischemic episodes, the heart's defense mechanism seeks to remedy this imbalance by downregulating myocardial contractile function and, concomitantly, increasing the rate of glycolysis (anaerobic energy production). Consequently, sarcolemmal glucose transport increases, and intracellular acidosis resulting from a build-up of the glycolytic breakdown products causes further inhibition of the contractile apparatus. Even though energy production continues in the absence of oxygen, the glycolytic pathway is an inefficient means for producing ATP. As an ischemic episode becomes more severe or prolonged, the heart becomes unable to produce enough energy via glycolysis and cellular necrosis ensues. For example, 10 min of ischemia generally results in about 50% depletion of ATP; after approximately 30 min of normothermic ischemia without significant collateral blood flow, irreversible damage or necrosis occurs [1]. Anatomically, the most vulnerable layer of the heart is the subendocardium; due to the higher systolic wall stress in this layer compared to the mid and epicardial layers, there exists a relatively greater metabolic demand. For additional discussion on myocardial energetics, see Chapters 13 and 19.

14.4 New Ischemic Syndromes

In the past, it was generally believed that extending the period of myocardial ischemia would, in turn, lead to irreversible damage of the myocardial or infarcted (necrotic) tissue. However, more recently, between the clinical conditions of transient ischemia (angina pectoris) and myocardial infarction, five additional ischemic syndromes have been described (Figs. 14.2 and 14.3) [2, 3]. The *stunned myocardium* is characterized by postischemic impairment of myocardial function, but it is considered acute and completely reversible. The *hibernating myocardium* is also characterized by depressed myocardial function of variable duration, primarily caused by impaired oxygen delivery through an occluded vessel and, importantly, recovery of function occurs upon reflow to the ischemic region. Note that the hibernating myocardium is similar to the stunned myocardium, with the main difference being that reperfusion is not the cause of myocardial hibernation, as is the case with myocardial stunning. On the other hand, hibernation can be considered as a state of chronic stunning, yet the exact mechanism of hibernation remains largely unknown [4]. The *maimed myocardium* is considered the most severe of such syndromes and is characterized by irreversible myocardial damage that follows ischemia and reperfusion, and in which there is a delayed recovery to only partial preischemic function. *Ischemic preconditioning* is the condition where multiple brief ischemic episodes (<5 min) followed by reperfusion subsequently enhances the myocardial tolerances to a longer (<45 min) ischemic event (Figs. 14.3 and 14.4). Finally, patients with ECG changes of ischemia and contractile failure who lack chest pain may be experiencing *silent ischemia*. It has been proposed that these patients are either less sensitive to painful stimuli or the ischemia is somewhat milder [3].

14.4.1 Myocardial Stunning

There are two general theories for explaining the pathomechanism underlying myocardial stunning, and they are generally not considered to be mutually exclusive. Episodes of ischemia are caused by: (1) the formation of free radical reactive species; and/or (2) alterations in intracellular calcium [5]. Furthermore, in such cases, intracellular acidosis occurring during ischemia can potentially generate intracellular calcium oscillations and calcium overload upon reperfusion via activation of the sarcolemmal Na^+/H^+ exchanger (Fig. 14.4) [6].

Experimental studies have shown that the calcium sensitivity of the contractile apparatus is decreased in the

Fig. 14.2 Consequences of myocardial ischemia. The stunned myocardium usually results from a transient coronary occlusion followed by prompt reperfusion, however, it may also occur following prolonged ischemia in the preconditioned heart. Preconditioning lessens the infarct area following a sustained coronary occlusion but only the area is reperfused; however, the relationship between preconditioning and the maimed myocardium is unknown. Modified from Boden et al. [15]

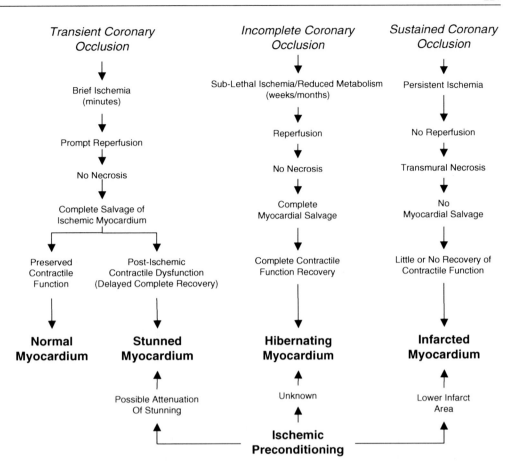

stunned myocardium, thereby resulting in lower maximal force generation even at higher than normal transient calcium levels [7, 8]. Furthermore, decreased myofilament sensitivity to calcium is considered primarily responsible for systolic dysfunction; for example, the stunned myocardium is still responsive to inotropic stimulation. Of additional interest is the finding that Troponin I (cTnI) degradation products were discovered in the human myocardium during aortic cross-clamping with bypass and that serum levels of cTnI increased during reperfusion, peaking approximately 24 h following cross-clamp removal [9]. This preliminary evidence further suggests that cTnI degradation products may potentially be utilized as biomarkers for stunning.

During the early stage of stunning, it is considered beneficial to prevent calcium oscillations and thus attenuate significant injury caused by reperfusion. This has been accomplished experimentally by utilizing Ca^{2+} antagonists, inorganic blockers, ryanodine, low-calcium reperfusion buffers, and/or Na^+/H^+ exchange blockers [10]. Conversely, when contractility is suppressed, as in the late stage of stunning, therapies should include those that increase the amplitude of intracellular calcium transients, inducing inotropic responses. Included in this subset of therapeutics are high-calcium buffers, Ca^{2+} agonists,

catecholamines, and/or phosphodiesterase inhibitors. Importantly, many of these therapies are specific to the stage or degree of stunning, and hence the timing of their use is critical so as not to become a detrimental therapy. For instance, hypocalcemia during and following cardiopulmonary bypass is a common occurrence mainly attributed to the utilization of priming fluids, citrated blood, and large doses of heparin during bypass [11]. Normally, hypocalcemia is successfully corrected with the administration of calcium chloride; however, calcium levels may return to preoperative levels prior to removal from cardiopulmonary bypass without supplemental calcium [12]. Therefore, the risk of stunning and myocardial damage may actually be increased with generalized calcium chloride administration. Note that, to date, there exists a lack of specific therapeutic guidelines for calcium administration during and following bypass.

14.4.2 Hibernating Myocardium

As previously discussed, myocardial stunning and hibernation are related in that a depressed state of contractility exists and, yet importantly, there is the potential to

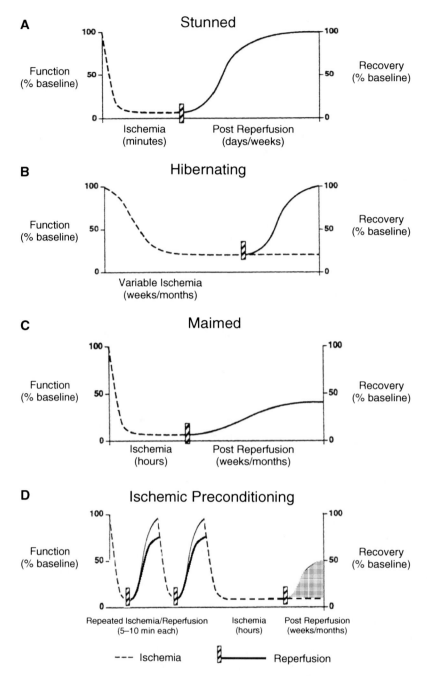

Fig. 14.3 New ischemic syndromes. New ischemic syndromes that do not fall within the realm of classic acute reversible and irreversible myocardial ischemia. (**A**) The stunned myocardium is characterized by a decrease in function following an ischemic event in which there is a complete absence of necrosis from ischemia or reperfusion and a complete functional recovery hours to days later. (**B**) The hibernating myocardium is characterized by chronic depressed myocardial function due to sublethal ischemia lasting for weeks to months, and revascularization may result in complete recovery of function. (**C**) The maimed myocardium has permanent damage resulting from a prolonged ischemic episode and has some functional recovery that does not return to preischemic levels. (**D**) Ischemic preconditioning exists when short ischemic episodes followed by reperfusion confer myocardial protection during a subsequent prolonged ischemic event. However, two areas of uncertainty exist in the preconditioning phenomenon: (1) functional recovery following the preceding short ischemic events may not return to preischemic levels and (2) while it is known that ischemic preconditioning lessens infarct size, it is uncertain whether long-term functional recovery following the prolonged ischemic episode is significantly improved (via decreased myocardial stunning). Only delayed ischemic preconditioning has been shown to attenuate myocardial stunning. Modified from Boden et al. [15]

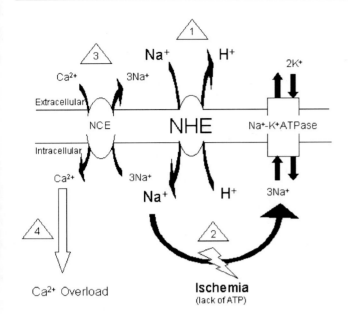

Fig. 14.4 Reperfusion injury via the Na^+–H^+ exchanger. Reperfusion injury-induced calcium overload can be explained, in part, by activation of the Na^+–H^+ exchanger (NHE). (1) Intracellular acidosis from a prior ischemic episode activates the NHE upon reperfusion, thereby decreasing intracellular acidosis and increasing Na^+ influx. (2) Intracellular sodium is primarily removed from the cell via the Na^+–K^+ ATPase during normal myocardial function. However, after ischemia (i.e., during the early stages of reperfusion), the lack of abundance of ATP does not allow for normal operation of the pump and intracellular $Na+$ increase. (3) Consequently, the Na^+–Ca^{2+} exchanger (NCE), which normally operates by extruding Ca^{2+} from the cytoplasm, is the primary mechanism for intracellular Na^+ removal operating in a reverse mode. (4) Intracellular Ca^{2+} overload results from NCE activation possibly causing arrhythmias, stunning, and necrosis

reversibly return the dysfunctional myocardium back to normal. However, it must again be restated that while stunning can be attributed to the reperfusion following a brief bout of ischemia, the hibernating myocardium is a chronic hypocontractile state due to a decreased oxygen supply and thus may only recover full function with revascularization. Additionally, many of the underlying mechanisms of stunning are considered directly related to the detrimental effects of reperfusion injury (to be discussed later) [13]. While there is a general absence of necrosis with myocardial hibernation, morphological changes to the myocardial architecture, such as loss of myofibrils and increased interstitial fibrosis, may occur if this state persists [14].

14.4.3 Maimed Myocardium

The maimed myocardium closely resembles that of a heart with a classic myocardial infarction in that ischemia-induced necrosis leads to loss of contractile

performance. In these cases, unlike in myocardial stunning, the duration of ischemia is long enough to result in necrosis. However, importantly there can be partial recovery of function to this ischemic region following timely reperfusion [15]. An example of the maimed myocardium syndrome would be a patient that exhibits an incomplete recovery of myocardial function following drug-induced or mechanical (angioplasty) reperfusion of an occluded coronary artery and then subsequently demonstrates regions of viable myocardium in the original ischemic area.

14.4.4 Ischemic Preconditioning

Ischemic preconditioning is a biological phenomenon whereby brief ischemic episodes followed by adequate reperfusion protect tissue from a subsequent "prolonged ischemic event" [16]. In the myocardium, ischemic preconditioning has been shown to be potentially infarct limiting [16] as well as antiarrhythmic [17], although the latter of these effects has been disputed. It is also well established that endogenous opioid receptor activation participates in myocardial ischemic preconditioning [18] and that preischemic administration of synthetic opioid agonists can mimic the benefits of ischemic preconditioning [19]. While ischemic and opioid preconditioning have both been convincingly shown to delay cell death in various experimental animal models, the clinical applicability of these therapies in humans may be limited to situations where the ischemic event can be anticipated (e.g., on- or off-bypass cardiac surgery, percutaneous transluminal coronary angioplasty, or stenting procedures) [20]. For a more comprehensive review of ischemic and opioid preconditioning, see articles by Yellon and Downey [ischemic preconditioning, 21] and Gross [opioid preconditioning, 22].

14.4.5 Silent Ischemia

"Silent ischemia" refers to single or multiple asymptomatic episodes of transient ischemia. In some cases, silent ischemia can occur in the week(s) following an acute myocardial infarction in patients with a history of coronary artery disease. In other scenarios, seemingly normal healthy individuals may experience episodes of silent ischemia that go relatively unnoticed. Detection of silent ischemia primarily relies on electrocardiographic monitoring, either in the form of 24-h Holtor monitoring (ambulatory) or exercise- and/or stress-induced assessment. In both cases, ischemia is typically detected by asymptomatic ST-segment elevations in an EKG tracing [23]; see also Chapter 17. Silent ischemia is postulated to be related to a lack of oxygen supply rather than an increase in oxygen demand, however, controversy remains regarding the mechanism whereby silent ischemia can proceed unnoticed.

14.4.6 How Can the Heart Be Protected from Ischemia?

As shown in Fig. 14.1, there are several means of decreasing myocardial oxygen demand when the oxygen supply is compromised. These include hypothermia, pharmacologically decreasing the heart rate, and/or controlled cardiac arrest. Additionally, as mentioned above, ischemic or pharmacological preconditioning of the heart are other ways to protect the heart from an ischemic episode and, hence, induce cardioprotection. However, these therapies require anticipation of the ischemic event, such that treatment can be administered prior to or early during the ischemia. In situations where anticipation of ischemia is not possible, for example in acute myocardial infarction, interventions which reestablish blood flow and oxygen to the ischemic zone (reperfusion) are the primary therapies. Nevertheless, it should be noted that dietary supplements such as omega-3 fatty acids have been considered as a potential means for prevention [24, 25]

14.5 Reperfusion Injury

While immediate restoration of blood flow and oxygen to ischemic tissue is ultimately a beneficial and important therapy, it should be noted that additional myocardial damage can occur upon myocardial reperfusion itself. In what has been termed the "oxygen paradox," the resupply of oxygen to a hypoxic cell simultaneously activates two intracellular processes of particular interest—the membrane-bound calcium pumps and the contractile apparatus. Resumption of contractile activity in the presence of oscillating and increasing intracellular Ca^{2+} levels can force the heart into a state of hypercontracture and thus cause intracellular edema. Collectively, these etiologies may ultimately result in membrane disruption and even cell death.

Reperfusion injury can present in (or is associated with) one or more of the following pathologies: (1) reperfusion arrhythmias; (2) microvascular damage and no-reflow; (3) accelerated cell death; (4) myocardial stunning; and/or (5) post-pump syndrome in procedures requiring cardiopulmonary bypass (Fig. 14.5). Reperfusion injury may cause immediate myocardial necrosis in severely damaged

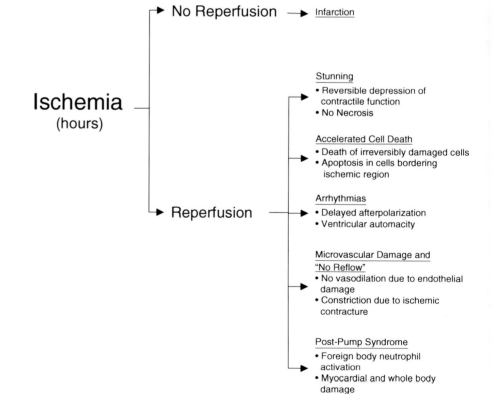

Fig. 14.5 Aspects of reperfusion injury. While reperfusion is still the most beneficial therapy for ischemia, any combination of stunning, accelerated cell death, arrhythmias, microvascular damage, or post-pump syndrome could occur, thus leading to postischemic dysfunction or necrosis

cells and delayed necrosis in cells adjacent to the ischemic region; conversely, complete recovery of myocardial function may occur despite an ischemic episode. Of importance, necrosis occurring during the ischemic episode must be differentiated from that which may occur following reperfusion, especially when discussing clinical therapies targeted at attenuating reperfusion injury.

Assessment of reperfusion injury following ischemia is often difficult, especially in the postsurgical patient. Yet, the determination of reperfusion injury and the relative extent of injury can be indirectly accomplished by hemodynamic monitoring (pressures, cardiac outputs, echocardiography) and examination of blood levels of cardiac enzymes (CK-MB, Troponin-I, LDH, and AST). Ideally, left ventricular end-diastolic pressure–volume measurements would provide functional and quantitative information relative to the degree of reperfusion injury; however, such data are difficult and rarely feasible to obtain clinically. However, with recent advances in echocardiography, relative changes in cardiac function and regional wall motion can be assessed in such patients (see Chapter 20). Furthermore, improvements in cardiac magnetic resonance imaging have allowed for the functional mapping of ischemic myocardial zones (see Chapter 22).

Myocardial viability can be fairly easily assessed with inotropic stimulation as the postischemic stunned (or the potentially reversibly injured) myocardium will both display an increased heart rate and contractility, while the irreversibly injured (necrotic) myocardium exhibits little to no response to the inotrope (e.g., by dopamine stress echocardiography). Note that, by definition, myocardial stunning is reversible; therefore, within days, a depressed cardiac function that is due to stunning should recover (Figs. 14.2 and 14.3). This phenomenon is commonly observed clinically when patients following coronary artery bypass grafting require 24–48 h of inotropic support.

14.5.1 Aspects of Reperfusion Injury

14.5.1.1 Myocardial Stunning

As previously discussed, the presence of intracellular oxygen free radicals and increased intracellular calcium during reperfusion leads to a reversible hypocontractile state of variability, yet this is relatively brief in duration.

14.5.1.2 Accelerated Cell Death

Typically, accelerated cell death upon reperfusion refers to cells that have been irreversibly damaged during the prior ischemic episode and are destined to die despite reperfusion. However, irreversible damage is not a prerequisite for cell death; upon reperfusion, detrimental ischemia-induced intracellular alterations may also occur in viable cells. More specifically, during reperfusion, the development of increased sarcolemmal permeability due to ischemia allows for the uncontrolled influx of calcium resulting in hypercontracture, decreased energy production, and/or cell death. Additionally, it should be noted that there is the paradoxical finding that apoptosis-related cell death in postischemic viable myocardium is reduced by early reperfusion and is accelerated in irreversibly ischemic-damaged cells [26].

14.5.1.3 Arrhythmias

Similar to myocardial stunning, increased episodes of arrhythmia upon reperfusion may be due, in part, to the presence of free radicals during ischemia and/or intracellular calcium oscillations at reflow. The restoration of flow enables the cell to resynthesize ATP. This abundance of energy and increased intracellular calcium at reperfusion may lead to excess cycling which, in turn, may cause delayed after-depolarizations and ventricular automaticity [27]. Interestingly, a bell-shaped relationship has been described between duration of ischemia and severity of reperfusion arrhythmias, with the peak occurring with reperfusion after 5–20 min of ischemia [3]. This is presumably due to the finding that, in severe ischemic episodes, the production of ATP during reperfusion is limited due to increased cellular necrosis, and consequently energy-dependent calcium oscillations are reduced [28].

The timing and speed of reperfusion are also considered to influence the occurrence and severity of induced arrhythmias. It has been speculated that sudden reperfusion is associated with a higher incidence of arrhythmias compared to a gradual reperfusion. Whether this phenomenon occurs in humans is controversial, as a study comparing revascularization of patients diagnosed with acute myocardial infarction, with either thrombolysis (a relatively slow reperfusion) or percutaneous transluminal coronary angioplasty (rapid reperfusion), revealed no differences in the occurrence of arrhythmias upon reperfusion [29]. In a recent study from our laboratory, the pericardial administration of omega-3 fatty acids as a preconditioning agent significantly reduced elicited arrhythmias during induced ischemia (coronary artery clamping) and also somewhat during subsequent reperfusion [25].

14.5.1.4 Microvascular Damage and "No-Reflow"

The "no-reflow" phenomenon is defined to occur when an attempt to reperfuse an ischemic area, by removing an occlusion regionally or reestablishing coronary flow globally, does not result in reflow to the area at risk. In fact, a recent study in patients diagnosed with acute myocardial infarction and treated with thrombolytic therapy revealed that approximately one-third of this study group showed impaired regional coronary flow 5 days after treatment [30]. There are two proposed mechanisms to explain this immediate or delayed "no-reflow:" (1) endothelial damage due to free radicals causes edema development and inhibits the release of vasodilatory agents into the coronary circulation; and/or (2) ischemic contracture of the myocardium mechanically constricts flow through the coronary system [3]. Additionally, activated neutrophils reintroduced upon reperfusion can adhere to damaged endothelium and, in severe cases, cause platelet aggregation and thus restenosis [31]. It is important to note that, in some cases, cardioplegia-induced global myocardial ischemia itself can cause regional no-flow, and regional infarctions will develop as a consequence of this phenomenon.

14.5.1.5 Post-pump Syndrome

When blood comes in contact with foreign nontissue surfaces, such as during cardiopulmonary bypass, a circulatory inflammatory response may be triggered. A large number of cells are typically activated during such a foreign body response, including monocytes, macrophages, endothelial cells, T cells, and, eventually, neutrophils. In a process collectively referred to as "neutrophil trafficking," these cells accumulate and adhere to the damaged endothelial layer [3]. They then migrate into the vascular interstitial space, the latter of which results in liberation of free radicals and leukotrienes [3]. This phenomenon may promote not only postsurgical myocardial damage, but also widespread systemic damage and/or even multiorgan dysfunction [32]. For example, it has been reported that cases of cerebral edema can develop after cardiopulmonary bypass which is considered to be mediated by bypass-related inflammation and endothelial cell activation [33]. For an additional discussion on the syndrome, see also Chapter 30.

14.6 Examples of Current Pharmacological Cardioprotective Therapies

Listed below are current examples of pharmacological therapies targeted at protecting the myocardium from damage due to ischemia and reperfusion injury. As noted above, our laboratory has recently investigated the pericardial delivery of omega-3 fatty acids, and we have observed significantly reduced infarct sizes in a swine model of ischemia/reperfusion injury by 50% [25].

14.6.1 Na+/H+ Exchange (NHE) Blockers

While activation of the exchanger in response to acidosis is a feedback mechanism that enables the myocardial cell to maintain a fairly stable pH range, NHE activation may not always be beneficial. During ischemia, there is often a build-up of metabolic products due to the anaerobic breakdown of ATP; the production of lactate and high CO_2 levels drive the intracellular pH below a tolerable level. However, a comparable decrease in the extracellular pH occurs during low-flow and no-flow ischemia and, importantly, NHE activity is inhibited. When blood flow is reestablished to the ischemic region, this inhibition is removed, and both the NHE and the $Na–HCO_3^-$ symport are simultaneously activated in an attempt to rapidly restore the internal pH [34]. With the normalization of intracellular pH via NHE, there is an associated increase in internal Na^+. Under normal conditions, cells primarily extrude Na^+ via the $Na^+–K^+$ ATPase; however, due to depleted energy reserves of such hearts, the postischemic cell relies on the $Na^+–Ca^{2+}$ exchanger for Na^+ normalization. Importantly, this results in increased intracellular Ca^{2+} levels which, as mentioned previously, significantly contribute to the pathology of reperfusion injury (Fig. 14.4).

In experimental animals, various NHE inhibitors have been shown to be beneficial when administered prior to either ischemia or reperfusion. Specifically, cariporide (NHE-1 specific) has been reported to reduce postischemic edema, arrhythmias, apoptosis, infarct size, contracture, enzyme efflux, and hypertrophy while also preventing free radical damage, preserving ATP, and enhancing myocardial preservation following prolonged storage [35–42]. Notably, in the GUARDIAN (GUARd During Ischemia Against Necrosis) clinical trial, cariporide pretreatment prior to coronary artery bypass grafting resulted in a 25% reduction in mortality or myocardial infarction following surgery [43]. Further supporting its use during routine cardiac surgery, Myers et al. found that hypothermia potentiated the benefits of cariporide, specifically when cariporide was administered during reperfusion [44]. However, in a follow-up clinical trial (the ESCAMI trial) where eniporide (another NHE-1 inhibitor) was administered upon reperfusion to patients undergoing percutaneous transluminal coronary angioplasty or thrombolysis for acute myocardial infarction, eniporide failed to show any significant reduction in either infarct size or occurrence of clinical events following treatment [45]. Furthermore, cariporide administration during reperfusion following global hypothermic ischemia failed to show any beneficial hemodynamic effects relative to control hearts (unpublished data from our laboratory). Nevertheless, while the use of NHE blockers is still considered experimental, their future use in cardiac surgery and ischemia/reperfusion remains promising. Interestingly, the prospect of using NHE blockers as a combined therapy with other cardioprotective therapies, such as ischemic preconditioning, is being addressed and initial results have suggested that the combined therapies produce additive benefit [46].

14.6.2 Antioxidants

Antioxidants are speculated to attenuate or prevent reperfusion injury by acting as: (1) free radical scavengers; (2) inhibitors of free radical generation; (3) metal chelators thereby removing the free radical generating catalyst; (4) promoters of endogenous antioxidant production; and/or (5) specific inhibitors of apoptosis via the upregulation of *Bcl-2* (a gene involved in the apoptosis signaling pathway) [47]. However, experimental animal models and human clinical trials have provided conflicting results as to the therapeutic benefits of antioxidants to attenuate reperfusion injury. Interestingly, many typical thiol-containing drugs commonly used for treating both coronary artery disease and heart failure have also been shown to exhibit antioxidant-like effects within the myocardium; these include β-adrenergic antagonists propanolol [48], metoprolol [49], and carvedilol [50], as well as angiotensin-converting enzyme inhibitors, iron chelating agents, and Ca^{2+} channel blockers [51]. Nevertheless, our laboratory is currently investigating the focal delivery of such agents into the pericardial space as a potential means to allow for higher therapeutic concentrations, but with lower systemic effects.

14.6.3 Calcium-Channel Antagonists

Experimentally, the administration of calcium-channel antagonists is believed to help preserve myocardial function and metabolism in case studies of normothermic ischemia, crystalloid cardioplegia, or blood cardioplegia [1]. More specifically, their use was reported to prevent ATP hydrolysis and calcium influx during ischemia and improve cardioplegia delivery by coronary vasodilation. However, the potential use of calcium-channel blockers for myocardial protection is considered to be limited due to their negative inotropic and dromotropic effects, which could be problematic in patients with preoperative poor ventricular function. Hence, further studies are needed to determine the potential utility of newer calcium-channel antagonists such as amlodipine and felodipine, agents which may elicit fewer side effects in very ill patients. Nevertheless, calcium-channel antagonists are typically administered in patients with normal preoperative function who are at risk for postoperative hypertension, tachycardia, coronary spasm, or ischemia [1].

14.6.4 Glucose–Insulin–Potassium

Perioperative depletion of myocardial glycogen stores has been correlated with a higher incidence of arrhythmias, low output syndrome, and/or infarction itself [51]. In one study, Iyengar et al. preoperatively dosed patients with a glucose–insulin–potassium solution and a bolus of exogenous glucose; subsequently, the researchers observed zero incidences of perioperative ischemic complications, compared to a 44% occurrence in patients not receiving the solutions [51]. This beneficial effect was attributed to increased preoperative glycogen stores, enhanced perioperative aerobic metabolism, and reduced free fatty acid circulation in the hypoxic hearts, all of which are mediated by glucose and insulin. Nevertheless, future studies are needed to validate such a therapy.

14.6.5 Growth Factors

The administration of growth factors for cardioprotection has been conducted in attempts to minimize or prevent apoptosis, which is known to occur in addition to necrosis during (prolonged) myocardial ischemia and reperfusion. In general, it is thought that reperfusion injury accelerates apoptosis in viable postischemic cells, adding to the overall necrosis [52]. More specifically, a link was described between apoptosis and reperfusion in humans following acute myocardial infarctions where apoptosis was significant in cells within and bordering the infarcted region [53]. Similarly, experimental animal studies have provided evidence of the infarct-reducing benefits of several growth factor proteins when given during ischemia and/or during reperfusion, including transforming growth factor-β1 (TGF-β1) [54], insulin [55], insulin-like growth factor (IGF-1) [56], fibroblast growth factor (FGF-1) [57], and cardiotrophin-1 (CT-1) [58].

14.6.6 Glutamate/Aspartate

The specific amino acids, glutamate and aspartate, when added to the cardiopulmonary bypass circuit, have been shown to reduce lipid peroxidation and preserve myocardial function following tissue reoxygenation [59]. Similarly, the addition of these amino acids to cardioplegia has yielded similar positive results [60]. While most of the benefits were attributed to the ability of the amino acids to anaerobically produce ATP via substrate phosphorylation, subsequent evidence has further linked their benefits to inhibition of free radical production and better retention of endogenous antioxidants [59].

14.6.7 Nitric Oxide (NO)

In addition to being a potent vasodilator, nitric oxide has also been shown to: (1) reduce platelet aggregation; (2) reduce neutrophil adherence; and (3) act as a free radical scavenger. Nitric oxide is primarily synthesized from the amino acid L-arginine by nitric oxide synthase. It is thought that l-arginine levels decline during ischemia leading to lower nitric oxide production, and thus a greater injury potential [1]. Furthermore, the addition of nitric oxide donors to cardioplegia solutions has been shown to beneficially increase ischemic nitric oxide levels [61]. Nevertheless, there are conflicting opinions regarding the benefits of nitric oxide due to its negative inotropic effects, hence future investigations are required.

14.7 Conclusions

The intent of this chapter was to outline the principles of ischemia and reperfusion injury and introduce the reader to the concept of cardioprotection. While the intent of many of the past cardioprotective therapies was to protect the myocardium from ischemic necrosis, it may be that reperfusion injury following ischemia in the forms of stunning, arrhythmias, and/or additional cellular necrosis may occur despite such cardioprotective efforts. Therefore, as a new era in the operating room and catheterization laboratories has evolved which allows for surgery on very ill patients, it is imperative that current myocardial protective strategies again be rigorously enhanced to account for the potential increased risks of ischemia and reperfusion injuries in such populations.

References

1. Edmunds LH, ed. Cardiac surgery in the adult. New York, NY: McGraw-Hill, 1997:295–318.
2. Yellon DM, Rahimtoola SH, Opie LH, et al. New ischemic syndromes: Beyond angina and infarction. New York, NY/Philadelphia, PA: Lippincott-Raven Publishers, 1997:10–20, 106–14.
3. Opie LH. The heart: Physiology, from cell to circulation. Philadelphia, PA: Lippincott-Raven, 1998:515–89.
4. Shen YT, Vatner SF. Mechanism of impaired myocardial function during progressive coronary stenosis in conscious pigs. Hibernation versus stunning? Circ Res 1995;76:479–88.
5. Bolli R, Marban E. Molecular and cellular mechanisms of myocardial stunning. Physiol Rev 1999;79:609–34.
6. Karmazyn M, Moffat MP. Role of Na+/H+ exchange in cardiac physiology and pathophysiology: Mediation of myocardial reperfusion injury by the pH paradox. Cardiovasc Res 1993;27:915–24.
7. Miller WP, McDonald KS, Moss RL. Onset of reduced Ca2+ sensitivity of tension during stunning in porcine myocardium. J Mol Cell Cardiol 1996;28:689–97.
8. Kusuoka H, Koretsune Y, Chacko VP, et al. Excitation-contraction coupling in postischemic myocardium. Does failure of activator Ca2+ transients underlie stunning? Circ Res 1990;66:1268–76.
9. McDonough JL, Labugger R, Pickett W, et al. Cardiac troponin I is modified in the myocardium of bypass patients. Circulation 2001;103:58–64.
10. Opie LH, du Toit EF. Postischemic stunning: The two-phase model for the role of calcium as pathogen. J Cardiovasc Pharmacol 1992;20:S1–4.
11. Aguilera IM, Vaughan RS. Calcium and the anaesthetist. Anaesthesia 2000;55:779–90.
12. Robertie PG, Butterworth JF, Royster RL, et al. Normal parathyroid hormone responses to hypocalcemia during cardiopulmonary bypass. Anesthesiology 1991;75:43–8.
13. Bolli R, Patel BS, Jeroudi MO, et al. Demonstration of free radical generation in "stunned" myocardium of intact dogs with the use of the spin trap alpha-phenyl N-tert-butyl nitrone. J Clin Invest 1988;82:476–85.
14. Heusch G, Schulz R. Myocardial hibernation. Ital Heart J 2002;3:282–4.
15. Boden WE, Brooks WW, Conrad CH, et al. Incomplete, delayed functional recovery late after reperfusion following acute myocardial infarction: "Maimed myocardium". Am Heart J 1995;130:922–32.
16. Murry CE, Jennings RB, Reimer KA. Preconditioning with ischemia: A delay of lethal cell injury in ischemic myocardium. Circulation 1986;74:1124–36.
17. Lawson CS, Coltart DJ, Hearse DJ. "Dose"-dependency and temporal characteristics of protection by ischaemic preconditioning against ischaemia-induced arrhythmias in rat hearts. J Mol Cell Cardiol 1993;25:1391–402.
18. Schultz JE, Rose E, Yao Z, et al. Evidence for involvement of opioid receptors in ischemic preconditioning in rat hearts. Am J Physiol 1995;268:H2157–61.
19. Coles JA, Jr., Sigg DC, Iaizzo PA. Role of kappa-opioid receptor activation in pharmacological preconditioning in swine. Am J Physiol Heart Circ Physiol 2003;284:2091–9.
20. Sigg DC, Coles JA, Jr., Gallagher WJ, et al. Opioid cardioprotection: Myocardial function and energy metabolism. Ann Thorac Surg 2001;72:1576–82.
21. Yellon DM, Downey JM. Preconditioning the myocardium: From cellular physiology to clinical cardiology. Physiol Rev 2003;83:1113–51.

22. Gross GJ. Role of opioids in acute and delayed preconditioning. J Mol Cell Cardiol 2003;35:709–18.

23. Cohn PF, Fox KM. Silent myocardial ischemia. Circulation 2003;108:1263–77.

24. Leaf A, Kang JX, Xiao YF. Fish oil fatty acids as cardiovascular drugs. Curr Vasc Pharmacol 2008;6:1–12. Review.

25. Xiao YF, Sigg DC, Ujhelyi MR, Wilhelm JJ, Richardson ES, Iaizzo PA. Pericardial delivery of Omega-3 fatty acid: A novel approach to reduce myocardial infarct sizes and arrhythmias. Am J Phyisol Heart Circ Physiol 2008;294:H2212–8

26. Fliss H, Gattinger D. Apoptosis in ischemic and reperfused rat myocardium. Circ Res 1996;79:949–56.

27. Opie LH, Coetzee WA. Role of calcium ions in reperfusion arrhythmias: Relevance to pharmacologic intervention. Cardiovasc Drugs Ther 1988;2:623–36.

28. Manning AS, Hearse DJ. Reperfusion-induced arrhythmias: Mechanisms and prevention. J Mol Cell Cardiol 1984;16:497–518.

29. Wehrens XH, Doevendans PA, Ophuis TJ, et al. A comparison of electrocardiographic changes during reperfusion of acute myocardial infarction by thrombolysis or percutaneous transluminal coronary angioplasty. Am Heart J 2000;139:430–6.

30. Maes A, Van de Werf F, Nuyts J, et al. Impaired myocardial tissue perfusion early after successful thrombolysis. Impact on myocardial flow, metabolism, and function at late follow-up. Circulation 1995;92:2072–8.

31. Forde RC, Fitzgerald DJ. Reactive oxygen species and platelet activation in reperfusion injury. Circulation 1997;95:787–9.

32. Menasche P, Peynet J, Haeffner-Cavaillon N, et al. Influence of temperature on neutrophil trafficking during clinical cardiopulmonary bypass. Circulation 1995;92:II334–40.

33. Anderson RE, Li TQ, Hindmarsh T, et al. Increased extracellular brain water after coronary artery bypass grafting is avoided by off-pump surgery. J Cardiothorac Vasc Anesth 1999;13:698–702.

34. Karmazyn M. The myocardial sodium–hydrogen exchanger (NHE) and its role in mediating ischemic and reperfusion injury. Keio J Med 1998;47:65–72.

35. Inserte J, Garcia-Dorado D, Ruiz-Meana M, et al. The role of the $Na+–H+$ exchange occurring during hypoxia in the genesis of reoxygenation-induced myocardial oedema. J Mol Cell Cardiol 1997;29:1167–75.

36. Garcia-Dorado D, Gonzalez MA, Barrabes JA, et al. Prevention of ischemic rigor contracture during coronary occlusion by inhibition of Na(+)–H(+) exchange. Cardiovasc Res 1997;35:80–9.

37. Klein HH, Bohle RM, Pich S, et al. Time delay of cell death by $Na+/H+$ exchange inhibition in regionally ischemic, reperfused porcine hearts. J Cardiovasc Pharmacol 1997;30:235–40.

38. Shipolini AR, Yokoyama H, Galinanes M, et al. $Na+/H+$ exchanger activity does not contribute to protection by ischemic preconditioning in the isolated rat heart. Circulation 1997;96:3617–25.

39. Yoshida H, Karmazyn M. Na(+)/H(+) exchange inhibition attenuates hypertrophy and heart failure in 1-wk postinfarction rat myocardium. Am J Physiol Heart Circ Physiol 2000;278:H300–4.

40. Myers ML, Farhangkhoee P, Karmazyn M. Hydrogen peroxide induced impairment of post-ischemic ventricular function is prevented by the sodium–hydrogen exchange inhibitor HOE 642 (cariporide). Cardiovasc Res 1998;40:290–6.

41. Mathur S, Karmazyn M. Interaction between anesthetics and the sodium–hydrogen exchange inhibitor HOE 642 (cariporide) in ischemic and reperfused rat hearts. Anesthesiology 1997;87:1460–9.

42. Hartmann M, Decking UK. Blocking Na(+)–H(+) exchange by cariporide reduces Na(+)-overload in ischemia and is cardioprotective. J Mol Cell Cardiol 1999;31:1985–95.

43. Theroux P, Chaitman BR, Danchin N, et al. Inhibition of the sodium–hydrogen exchanger with cariporide to prevent myocardial infarction in high-risk ischemic situations. Main results of the GUARDIAN trial. Guard during ischemia against necrosis (GUARDIAN) Investigators. Circulation 2000;102:3032–8.

44. Myers ML, Karmazyn M. Improved cardiac function after prolonged hypothermic ischemia with the $Na+/H+$ exchange inhibitor HOE 694. Ann Thorac Surg 1996;61:1400–6.

45. Zeymer U, Suryapranata H, Monassier JP, et al. The $Na+/H+$ exchange inhibitor eniporide as an adjunct to early reperfusion therapy for acute myocardial infarction. J Am Coll Cardiol 2001;38:1644–50.

46. Bugge E, Yterhus K. Inhibition of sodium–hydrogen exchange reduces infarct size in the isolated rat heart-A protective additive to ischaemic preconditioning. Cardiovasc Res 1995;29:269–74.

47. Dhalla NS, Elmoselhi AB, Hata T, et al. Status of myocardial antioxidants in ischemia-reperfusion injury. Cardiovasc Res 2000;47:446–56.

48. Khaper N, Rigatto C, Seneviratne C, et al. Chronic treatment with propranolol induces antioxidant changes and protects against ischemia-reperfusion injury. J Mol Cell Cardiol 1997;29:3335–44.

49. Kalaycioglu S, Sinci V, Imren Y, et al. Metoprolol prevents ischemia-reperfusion injury by reducing lipid peroxidation. Jpn Circ J 1999;63:718–21.

50. Feuerstein GZ, Yue TL, Cheng HY, et al. Myocardial protection by the novel vasodilating beta-blocker, carvedilol: Potential relevance of anti-oxidant activity. J Hypertens 1993;11:S41–8.

51. Iyengar SR, Charrette EJ, Iyengar CK, et al. Myocardial glycogen in prevention of perioperative ischemic injury of the heart: A preliminary report. Can J Surg 1976;19:246–51.

52. Yellon DM, Baxter GF. Reperfusion injury revisited: Is there a role for growth factor signaling in limiting lethal reperfusion injury? Trends Cardiovasc Med 1999;9:245–9.

53. Saraste A, Pulkki K, Kallajoki M, et al. Apoptosis in human acute myocardial infarction. Circulation 1997;95:320–3.

54. Baxter GFM., Brar BK, Latchman DS, Yellon DM. Infarct-limiting action of transforming growth factor beta-1 in isolated rat heart is abolished. Circulation 1998;100:1–9.

55. Baines CP, Wang L, Cohen MV, et al. Myocardial protection by insulin is dependent on phospatidylinositol 3-kinase but not protein kinase C or KATP channels in the isolated rabbit heart. Basic Res Cardiol 1999;94:188–98.

56. Buerke M, Murohara T, Skurk C, et al. Cardioprotective effect of insulin-like growth factor I in myocardial ischemia followed by reperfusion. Proc Natl Acad Sci USA 1995;92:8031–5.

57. Cuevas P, Carceller F, Martinez-Coso V, et al. Cardioprotection from ischemia by fibroblast growth factor: Role of inducible nitric oxide synthase. Eur J Med Res 1999;4:517–24.

58. Stephanou A, Brar B, Heads R, et al. Cardiotrophin-1 induces heat shock protein accumulation in cultured cardiac cells and protects them from stressful stimuli. J Mol Cell Cardiol 1998;30:849–55.

59. Morita K, Ihnken K, Buckberg GD, et al. Studies of hypoxemic/reoxygenation injury without aortic clamping. VIII. Counteraction of oxidant damage by exogenous glutamate and aspartate. J Thorac Cardiovasc Surg 1995;110:1228–34.

60. Drinkwater DC Jr., Cushen CK, Laks H, et al. The use of combined antegrade-retrograde infusion of blood cardioplegic solution in pediatric patients undergoing heart operations. J Thorac Cardiovasc Surg 1992;104:1349–55.

61. Nakanishi K, Zhao ZQ, Vinten-Johansen J, et al. Blood cardioplegia enhanced with nitric oxide donor SPM-5185 counteracts postischemic endothelial and ventricular dysfunction. J Thorac Cardiovasc Surg 1995;109:1146–54.

Chapter 15
The Effects of Anesthetic Agents on Cardiac Function

Jason S. Johnson and Michael K. Loushin

Abstract With the aging population and an increase in health problems such as obesity, diabetes, and coronary artery disease, the perioperative management and induction of general anesthesia in such patients, while providing cardiovascular stability, continues to offer both challenges and new developments in this field. These developments include new anesthesia medications, medical equipment and/or surgical technology, and anesthetic and surgical techniques. The goal of this chapter is to familiarize the reader with commonly employed clinical methodologies and anesthetics, with particular attention to the potential influences on the cardiovascular system.

Keywords Anesthesia · Inhalational anesthetics · Intravenous anesthetics · Anesthesia induction · Cardiac function · Hemodynamics · Cardioprotection · Myocardial preconditioning

15.1 Introduction

Anesthesia is considered necessary for many types of surgeries and procedures. In general, anesthesia may provide analgesia, amnesia, hypnosis, and/or muscle relaxation. The depth of anesthesia varies from minimal sedation to general anesthesia (Table 15.1). Importantly, medications used for general anesthesia can cause significant alterations in hemodynamics, especially during induction of anesthesia. Yet, understanding of anesthetic impact on cardiovascular physiology can allow induction and maintenance of anesthesia with minimal alterations from normal cardiovascular function. Both inhalational and intravenous anesthetics can affect cardiovascular

performance; this includes effects on cardiac output, heart rate, systemic vascular resistance, the cardiac conduction system, myocardial contractility, coronary blood flow, and/or blood pressure. The choice of inhalational and intravenous anesthetics is typically associated with the patient's underlying cardiovascular status such as heart failure, cardiac disease, and/or hypovolemia.

15.2 Anesthesia Induction Sequence

A focused patient history and physical is necessary prior to anesthesia to determine the most appropriate anesthetic for that individual. All patients undergoing elective surgery should be nil per os (NPO) of solid foods for at least six hours prior to an anesthetic; this is to minimize the risk of gastric regurgitation and thus aspiration of stomach contents into the lungs during the induction of anesthesia. Past history of any complications or reactions to anesthetics must also be considered. For example, patients with a history of porphyria should not receive a porphyria-inducing agent such as barbiturates or diazepam. Patients with a family history of malignant hyperthermia are at risk of eliciting an episode of malignant hyperthermia when a triggering agent such as succinylcholine or a volatile anesthetic is administered. Therefore, the need for laboratory studies is guided by the preexisting medical condition of each individual patient.

A typical general anesthesia induction sequence for an adult is as follows. After establishing intravenous access and placement of standard American Society of Anesthesiologist (ASA) [1] monitors, a patient is preoxygenated with 100% oxygen. An induction dose of an intravenous medication such as propofol and a muscle relaxant is administered to facilitate smooth induction of anesthesia (JPG 15.1). Once the patient is rendered unconscious and anesthetized, direct laryngoscopy is

M.K. Loushin (✉)
University of Minnesota, Department of Anesthesiology,
MMC 294, 420 Delaware Street SE, Minneapolis, MN 55455, USA
e-mail: loush001@umn.edu

P.A. Iaizzo (ed.), *Handbook of Cardiac Anatomy, Physiology, and Devices*, DOI 10.1007/978-1-60327-372-5_15,
© Springer Science+Business Media, LLC 2009

Table 15.1 Continuum of depth of sedation definition of general anesthesia and levels of sedation/analgesia

	Minimal sedation (anxiolysis)	Moderate sedation/analgesia ("conscious sedation")	Deep sedation/analgesia	General anesthesia
Responsiveness	Normal response to verbal stimulation	Purposeful response to verbal or tactile stimulation	Purposeful response following repeated or painful stimulation	Unarousable even with painful stimulus
Airway	Unaffected	No intervention required	Intervention may be required	Intervention often required
Spontaneous ventilation	Unaffected	Adequate	May be inadequate	Frequently inadequate
Cardiovascular function	Unaffected	Usually maintained	Usually maintained	May be impaired

ASA Standards, Guidelines and Statements [1].

performed and the trachea is intubated with an endotracheal tube. After confirmation of endotracheal intubation by auscultation of lungs and confirmation of end-tidal carbon dioxide, the patient is placed on an anesthesia ventilator and ventilated with a combination of anesthetic gases, oxygen, and/or air (JPG 15.2). Note, if a total intravenous anesthetic technique (such as propofol and opioid infusion) is chosen, anesthetic gases are not administered. A total intravenous anesthetic technique may be chosen in patients who have reactions to volatile anesthetics such as patients with malignant hyperthermia. The cardiovascular depressant effects of most anesthetics typically become evident during and immediately following induction. Maintaining cardiovascular stability requires: (1) careful titration of medications; (2) knowledge of clinical and basic science in physiology and pharmacology; and (3) diligent monitoring of vital signs (JPG 15.3)

For the induction of general anesthesia in children, one often utilizes a mask induction technique. Since placement of an intravenous catheter preinduction may be traumatic to the child or difficult due to noncooperation, mask induction with halothane, sevoflurane, and/or nitrous oxide is frequently employed; note that in current clinical practice, halothane is rarely used in the United States. After placement of ASA monitors, a high concentration of an inhalational anesthetic such as sevoflurane along with oxygen is administered via a face mask. After the patient becomes unconscious, a peripheral intravenous catheter is placed and a similar general anesthesia and airway management sequence subsequently follows.

It is important to note that direct laryngoscopy and endotracheal intubation can often stimulate the upper and lower airways which, in turn, may cause significant changes in blood pressures and heart rate if airway responses are not blunted. Commonly, titration of anesthetics and opioids are administered to blunt these airways and associated sympathetic responses.

15.3 Inhalational Anesthetics

Commonly used inhalational anesthetics include nitrous oxide, isoflurane, desflurane, and sevoflurane (Fig. 15.1). Each of these inhalational anesthetics has a specific minimum alveolar concentration (MAC) at which general anesthesia is induced (Table 15.2). MAC is defined as the minimum alveolar concentration of an inhaled anesthetic required to prevent movement in 50% of patients in response to a painful stimulus such as a surgical incision. It is important to note that infants and children have a higher MAC requirement than adults, while pregnant women and elderly patients have lower MAC requirements. MAC is additive, that is, 0.5 MAC of nitrous oxide and 0.5 MAC of isoflurane result in 1 MAC total anesthesia. More specifically, the brain anesthetic partial

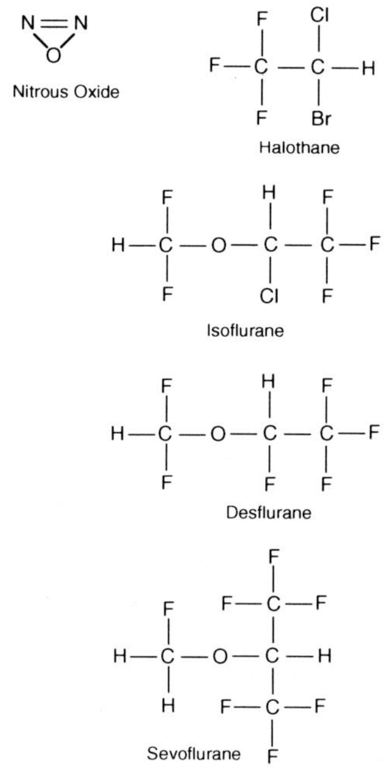

Fig. 15.1 Chemical structure of commonly administered inhalational anesthetics

Table 15.2 Minimal alveolar concentration (MAC) of inhalational anesthetics

Agent	MAC % (% of 1 atmosphere)	Vapor pressure (at 20°C)
Desflurane	6.0	680
Halothane	0.75	243
Isoflurane	1.2	240
Sevoflurane	2.0	160
Nitrous oxide	105	
Xenon	70	

pressure is dependent upon factors such as inspired (F_I) and alveolar (F_A) concentration of anesthetic gas. Brain (F_B) concentration of anesthetic is dependent upon F_A and F_I:

$$F_I \leftrightarrow F_A \leftrightarrow F_B$$

In general, anesthetic uptake is determined by blood solubility, cardiac output, and difference between alveolar to venous partial pressure [2]. The greater the uptake of anesthetic gas into blood, the slower the rate of induction. Inhalational anesthetics with lower blood:gas solubility (i.e., desflurane and sevoflurane) will cause faster induction and emergence from general anesthesia; higher concentrations of these agents are needed for the MAC requirement.

15.3.1 Blood Pressure and Systemic Vascular Resistance

All volatile anesthetics such as isoflurane, desflurane, sevoflurane, and halothane cause dose-dependent effects on cardiovascular function. For example, these agents cause a dose-dependent decrease in mean arterial blood pressure [3–6]. The relative decrease in mean arterial blood pressure is considered due to decreases in systemic vascular resistance, myocardial contractility, sympathetic output, or a combination of the above. In particular, isoflurane, desflurane, and sevoflurane cause greater decreases in systemic vascular resistances when compared to halothane (Table 15.3). Further, increasing doses of

halothane result in small changes in system vascular resistance [7], and decreases in mean arterial pressure with halothane administration are associated with decreases in cardiac output. In general, volatile anesthetics decrease systemic vascular resistance by causing peripheral vasodilation and thus increasing blood flow to cutaneous and skeletal muscle tissues [3]. It should be noted that nitrous oxide causes minimal alteration of systemic vascular resistance when administered alone. Typically, an initial drop in blood pressure following induction of anesthesia is associated with a decrease in systemic vascular resistance and preload. Low blood pressure can be increased by administration of intravenous fluids, placing the patient in a Trendelenburg position, and/or by giving peripheral vasoconstrictors such as phenylephrine or ephedrine.

15.3.2 Cardiac Conduction System and Heart Rate

Baroreceptors located near the aortic root, carotid arteries, and other sites detect changes in arterial blood pressure and affect cardiovascular function. A typical baroreceptor reflex from the carotid artery includes the afferent (cranial nerve IX) and efferent (cranial nerve X) nerves. An increase in arterial blood pressure is detected by the baroreceptor, causing reflex decrease in the heart rate. A decrease in arterial blood pressure then causes a reflex tachycardia to maintain cardiac output and organ perfusion. Importantly, volatile anesthetics will cause dose-dependent decreases in baroreceptor reflex activities [8]; hence, hemodynamic compensatory responses are attenuated by volatile anesthetics [9, 10]. It is common that alterations in hemodynamics due to volatile anesthetics may require administration of other pressor medications to offset the attenuation of these normal physiologic protective functions.

Volatile anesthetics may also cause specific cardiac dysrhythmias. Specifically, volatile anesthetics have been reported to both slow the rate of sinoatrial node discharge and increase ventricular and His bundle conduction times

Table 15.3 Cardiovascular effects of inhalational anesthetics

	Heart rate	Blood pressure	Systemic vascular resistance	Cardiac output	Sensitize to epinephrine	Coronary dilation
Desflurane	+	−	− −	0/−	0/+	+
Halothane	0	− −	0/−	−	+++	+
Isoflurane	+	− −	− −	−	0/+	++
Sevoflurane	0	− −	−	0/−	0/+	0
Nitrous oxide	+	0	0	0	0	0

[11], which may increase the development of nodal rhythms. Further, volatile anesthetics may increase ventricular automaticity by altering potassium and calcium ion channels [11]. It has been reported that halothane increases the incidence of ventricular dysrhythmias, especially when coadministered with epinephrine; in contrast, the coadministration of epinephrine with isoflurane, desflurane, or sevoflurane has noted minimal effects on increasing the incidence of ventricular dysrhythmias [12–14]. Furthermore, halothane may blunt the reflex increases in heart rates which typically accompany decreases in blood pressure; it may also slow conduction from the sinoatrial node, resulting in junctional ventricular rhythms. Sevoflurane and desflurane are also known to partially blunt sympathetic baroreflex sensitivity. Importantly, isoflurane is well known to cause significant decreases in systemic vascular resistance, and thus blood pressure. Yet, the baroreceptor response remains partially intact and thus cardiac output is maintained relatively stable with isoflurane by associated increases in heart rate.

In patient populations such as young children and the elderly, it is not uncommon to see decreases in heart rate following induction of anesthesia. An anticholinergic agent such as atropine or glycopyrrolate is frequently administered to prevent and/or treat such bradycardia.

15.3.3 Coronary Blood Flow

In general, volatile anesthetics cause a dose-dependent coronary vasodilation, i.e., with isoflurane having a greater effect than halothane [15, 16]. Increasing the concentration of isoflurane increases coronary blood flow, and this also has the potential to cause "coronary steal" syndrome [17, 18]. Coronary steal is caused by vasodilation of healthy coronary arteries and shunting of blood from myocardium at risk for ischemia to areas not at risk. More specifically, in coronary artery disease, cardiac areas at risk for myocardial ischemia have coronary arteries that are already maximally vasodilated. Desflurane and sevoflurane have not been associated with coronary steal syndrome [19, 20]. Nevertheless, the exact clinical significance of coronary steal in humans remains somewhat unresolved.

15.3.4 Contractility and Cardiac Output

Volatile anesthetics depress myocardial contractility by inducing alterations of calcium ion flux [21]. The mechanism of negative inotropic effects of volatile anesthetics include decreased free Ca^{2+}, decreased Ca^{2+} release

from sarcoplasmic reticulum, and/or altered contractile protein response to Ca^{2+} [21, 22]. Halothane diminishes myocardial contractility more than isoflurane, desflurane, and nitrous oxide below 1 MAC. Isoflurane and sevoflurane cause minimal change in contractility and thus allow for better maintained systemic cardiac output [22]. Due to better cardiovascular stability following either isoflurane or sevoflurane administration compared to halothane, the former agents are utilized frequently in patients with congenital heart defects and/or depressed myocardial function.

Due to the simultaneous stimulation of the sympathetic nervous system, the myocardial depressant effects of nitrous oxide are usually not evident in healthy individuals. Yet, in a compromised and failing myocardium, its depressant effects on contractility become much more evident. More specifically, nitrous oxide has been associated with sympathomimetic effects, as it: (1) increases plasma catecholamines; (2) causes mydriasis; and (3) induces vasoconstriction of systemic and pulmonary circulations [23]. When nitrous oxide is administered with opioids such as fentanyl, the sympathomimetic effects are minimized or abolished. Therefore, the combined administration of nitrous oxide and opioids may result in a significant decrease in mean arterial pressure and cardiac output.

The abrupt increase in a patient's desflurane concentration has been associated with a significant increase in sympathetic output, resulting in increased heart rate and mean arterial pressure. A proposed mechanism for this sympathetic stimulation is that it is due to airway and lung irritation with a high concentration of desflurane [24]. A smaller increase in sympathetic output is commonly associated with isoflurane administration, whereas sevoflurane, due to lack of airway irritation with its administration, is not associated with a significant increase in sympathetic output, even with a very rapid increase in concentration. Due to sevoflurane favorable airway properties, it is used frequently for inhalational induction of anesthesia in children; high concentrations of sevoflurane (4–8%) are needed for rapid mask induction and are well tolerated in children.

15.3.5 Pulmonary Blood Flow

Volatile anesthetics are potent bronchodilators and, in some cases, they have been used for the treatment of status asthmaticus. In general, it is considered that volatile anesthetics may cause a mild decrease in pulmonary vascular resistance, whereas nitrous oxide can cause a significant increase in pulmonary vascular resistance. Thus, the administration of nitrous oxide in patients with preexisting pulmonary artery hypertension may exacerbate the strain on the right heart by increasing pulmonary vascular resistance. This elevated pulmonary vascular resistance may also result in right-to-left intracardiac shunting in susceptible patients (i.e., ventriculoseptal defect). In general, volatile anesthetics also diminish the degree of hypoxic pulmonary vasoconstriction, which may result in hypoxia. It is important that in patients with congenital heart defects (i.e., intracardiac shunts, single ventricle, transposition of great arteries, Tetralogy of Fallot), the properties of select volatile anesthetics may be critical to offer better cardiovascular stability.

15.3.6 Cardioprotection/Preconditioning

The potential for myocardial preconditioning with volatile anesthetics has been extensively studied. Importantly, halogenated volatile anesthetics have been shown to provide cardioprotection against injury associated with ischemia and reperfusion [25–28]. The mechanism of cardioprotection seems to be similar to ischemic preconditioning first described by Murray et al. [29], and thus likely ultimately involves the mitochondrial potassium (K_{ATP}) channels [30].

15.3.7 Future Inhalational Anesthetics

Xenon was first used as an anesthetic gas in humans by Cullen and Gross in 1951 [31]. Xenon, an inert gas, has many properties that make it an ideal anesthetic gas; it has very low toxicity and is nonexplosive and nonflammable. The MAC of xenon is approximately 70%. Its very low blood to gas solubility partition coefficient (0.115) provides fast onset and emergence from anesthesia [32]. Recently, preliminary clinical studies with xenon have shown minimal adverse effects on the cardiovascular system and general hemodynamic parameters [32–34]. More specifically, xenon has been shown to induce minimal effects on alterations in heart rate, coronary blood flow, left ventricular pressure, and atrioventricular conduction time [35]. However, factors that may limit the use of xenon as an anesthetic gas are its cost and required unique delivery system; xenon must be extracted from the atmosphere and this process is expensive. Nevertheless, special breathing and delivery systems are in development.

It should be specifically noted that all volatile anesthetics trigger malignant hyperthermia in susceptible patients. Malignant hyperthermia is an inherited pharmacogenetic disorder that affects skeletal muscle and is characterized by a hypermetabolic response when exposed to a triggering agent such as volatile anesthetics and succinylcholine.

Disregulation of the ryanodine receptor, the calcium release channel of sarcoplasmic reticulum, is typically involved in this unregulated release of calcium from this storage site. Signs and symptoms of malignant hyperthermia include sympathetic hyperactivity, elevated carbon dioxide production, muscle rigidity, hyperthermia, metabolic acidosis, dysrhythmias, and hyperkalemia. Treatment of malignant hyperthermia requires removal of the triggering agent, intravenous administration of dantrolene, and management of the associated symptoms. For more details on malignant hyperthermia, see http://www.mhaus.org/.

15.4 Intravenous Anesthetics

15.4.1 Barbiturates

In general, barbiturates cause central nervous system inhibition (depression) by enhancing the effects of g-aminobutyric acid (GABA) [36]. Barbiturates bind to the GABA receptor complexes which, in turn, increase chloride channel activities, causing subsequent inhibition of the central nervous system. The GABA receptor complex has binding affinities for GABA, barbiturates, benzodiazepines, propofol, and/or alcohol [23].

Thiopental (3–5 mg/kg) and methohexital (1.5–2 mg/kg) are common barbiturates used for induction of general anesthesia (Fig. 15.2). After intravenous injection of thiopental or methohexital, anesthesia is induced rapidly, within seconds. Yet, the duration of induced anesthesia after a single bolus dose of intravenous barbiturate is short (approximately 5 min) due to rapid redistribution from the brain to other tissues such as muscle and adipose. Importantly, intraarterial injection of thiopental can result in severe vasospasm which may lead to thrombosis, tissue injury, and/or even gangrene. If intraarterial injections do occur, counteractive measures such as sympathetic nerve blocks or administration of papaverine, phenoxybenzamine, or lidocaine may be initiated to decrease induced arterial vasospasm.

The administration of barbiturates is typically associated with decreases in mean arterial pressure which result from both induced vasodilation and decreased myocardial contractility (Table 15.4). Barbiturates have

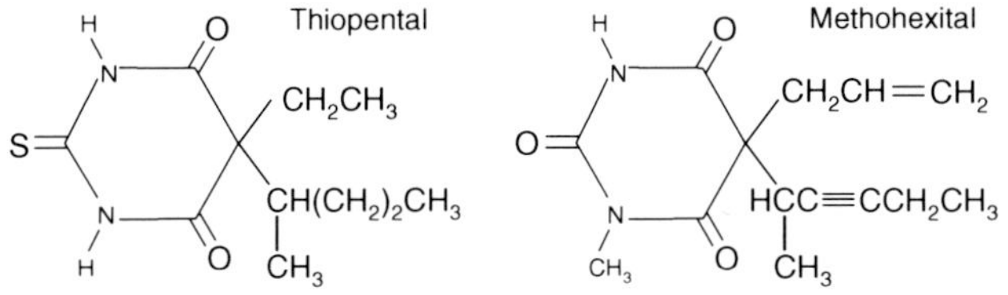

Fig. 15.2 Chemical structure of thiopental and methohexital

Table 15.4 Cardiovascular effects of intravenous anesthetics

	Heart rate	Blood pressure	Systemic vascular resistance	Cardiac output
Thiopental	+	−	−	+
Ketamine	++	++	+	++
Propofol	0/−	− −	− −	−
Etomidate	0	0/−	0	0
Fentanyl	0/−	0	0	0
Morphine	0/−	0/−	0/−	0
Midazolam	0	0	0	0
Methohexital	++	−	−	0/−
Meperidine	++	0/−	0/−	0/+

also been shown to cause dose-related myocardial depression, which is not as pronounced as that associated with volatile anesthetics. Yet, barbiturates may cause a small depression of the carotid and aortic baroreceptors, and therefore, an induced decrease in mean arterial pressure leading to reflex tachycardia. If intravenous barbiturates are administered slowly, relative hemodynamic stability can be maintained [37], especially in patients with normal intravascular volume status. In contrast, a rapid infusion of barbiturates, especially in hypovolemic patients, may result in significant hypotension. Subsequently, typical increases in heart rate upon barbiturate administration are not present if the baroreceptor reflex is not intact, as in heart transplant patients or in isolated heart preparations. Importantly, barbiturates do not generally sensitize the myocardium to the potential arrhythmic effects of administered catecholamines.

15.4.2 Benzodiazepines

Benzodiazepines are considered to produce central nervous system depression by binding to the GABA receptor complex and ultimately increasing chloride channel activities. Benzodiazepines, such as midazolam and diazepam, are often administered as adjuncts to anesthesia for sedation, amnesia, and anxiolysis. Benzodiazepines themselves do not have analgesic properties. Yet, they possess anticonvulsant properties and hence can be utilized in acute management of seizures. Interestingly, the acute administration of benzodiazepines is not associated with significant changes in hemodynamic parameters; blood pressure, heart rate, and systemic vascular resistance are fairly well maintained. However, systemic vascular resistance decreases in a dose-related fashion [38], but a typical dose required for sedation and anxiolysis in adults (1–2 mg intravenous) usually is not associated with any significant hemodynamic alteration.

More specifically, induction of anesthesia with midazolam (0.2–0.3 mg/kg intravenous) is associated with a decrease in systemic vascular resistance, but with minimal effects on cardiac output. Typically, the baroreceptor reflex remains intact and thus a relative decrease in mean arterial pressure will result in a responsive increase in heart rate. It has been reported that diazepam elicits even fewer cardiovascular effects than midazolam; a typical dose required for sedation and anxiolysis in adults usually is not associated with any significant hemodynamic alterations. At most, diazepam administration may cause a minimal change in blood pressure and systemic vascular resistance. Therefore, coadministration of diazepam and nitrous oxide is not associated with significant decreases in cardiovascular function [39]; thus, it is employed in patients where such concerns may be justified.

15.4.3 Opioids

Opioids are analgesics that are commonly administered as adjuncts to anesthesia. Opioids currently used in clinical practice include fentanyl, morphine, meperidine, alfentanil, sufentanil, and remifentanil (Table 15.5). All opioids exert their effect by interacting with opioid receptors (mu_1, mu_2, kappa, or delta; see Table 15.6); they are used as adjuncts to help blunt sympathetic responses to noxious stimuli. Overall, the clinical use of opioids causes minimal changes in cardiac output and blood pressure, yet opioids may generally cause bradycardia due to an increase in vagal tone. Typically at very high doses, opioids may have the following effects on hemodynamics: inhibition of autonomic nervous system, direct myocardial depression, and/or histamine release. More specifically, one *in vitro* study of human atrial myocardium found that fentanyl, remifentanil, and sufentanil did not modify inotropic effects, while alfentanil caused negative inotropy by affecting calcium regulation [40]. Yet, it has also been reported that opioids such as fentanyl may depress rat myocardial contractility by affecting calcium regulation [41]. Finally, it is considered that morphine may cause a decrease in mean arterial pressure by causing

Table 15.5 Opioid agonists commonly used in clinical practice

	Heart rate	Blood pressure	System vascular resistance	Contractility	Histamine
Meperidine	++	−	−	+/−	++
Morphine	0/−	−	−	−	++
Fentanyl	0/−	0	0	0	0
Alfentanil	−	0/−	−	0/−	0
Sufentanil	−	0/−	0/−	0/−	0
Remifentanil	−	0	0	0	0

Table 15.6 Opioid and opioid receptors

Drug	Mu receptor	Delta receptor	Kappa receptor
Morphine	+++	+?	+
Fentanyl	+++	?	
Sufentanil	+++	+	+
Buprenorphine	+		− −
Naloxone	− − −	−	− −
Naltrexone	− − −	−	− − −
Nalbuphine	− −		++
DPDPE		++	
DADLE	+	+++	+?
NorBNI	−	−	− − −
DSLET	+	++	
Naltrindole	−	− − −	−

Modified from Goodman and Gilman's The pharmacological basis of therapeutics. 10th ed. (Hardman JG, Limbird LE, eds). New York, NY: McGraw-Hill, 2001.

histamine release and bradycardia. It should be noted that high doses of an intravenous opioid such as fentanyl can cause chest wall rigidity, making manual ventilation of nonparalyzed patient difficult.

15.4.4 Ketamine

Ketamine is a phencyclidine derivative (Fig. 15.3) that causes intense analgesia and dissociative anesthesia. Patients who receive ketamine can obtain a cataleptic state with open eyes and/or ocular nystagmus. The typical routes for ketamine administration include intravenous (1–2 mg/kg), intramuscular (3–6 mg/kg), or oral (5–6 mg/kg). In general, ketamine's effects on the central nervous system are considered due to interactions with multiple receptors including N-methyl-D-asparate (NMDA), monoaminergic, opioid, and/or muscarinic. Due to interactions with pain receptors, ketamine possesses intense analgesic properties.

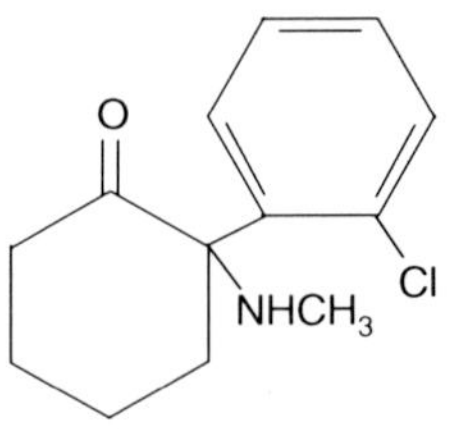

Potential side effects of ketamine administration include the stimulation of the central sympathetic nervous system and thus an increase in circulating epinephrine and norepinephrine. In patients where maintenance of myocardial contractility and systemic vascular resistance is vital (i.e., hypovolemia, trauma, and shock), ketamine may better stimulate the cardiovascular system to maintain cardiac output and blood pressure. More specifically, ketamine causes an increase in heart rate, blood pressure, cardiac output, and myocardial oxygen consumption. Due to stimulation of cardiovascular function, ketamine may not be appropriate in patients with aortic stenosis, coronary artery disease, and/or hypertrophic left ventricle. It should be noted that pulmonary artery pressure may also increase following administration of ketamine. Another important side effect attributed to ketamine administration is its bronchodilating effects; thus, patients with, or at risk for, bronchospasm may benefit from ketamine induction. In contrast, in patients with depleted catecholamine stores, ketamine may cause a serious depression of myocardial function [42]. In other words, the maintenance or elevation of cardiovascular function may not be seen following administration of ketamine in patients with depleted catecholamine stores such as those with sepsis. Furthermore, ketamine may also increase cerebral perfusion and intracranial pressures, and thus should be used carefully in patients with neurovascular disease.

15.4.5 Propofol

Propofol (1% solution) is a 2,6-diisopropylphenol (Fig. 15.4) that is typically administered intravenously for sedation and/or induction of anesthesia. Importantly, intravenous injections of propofol (1.5–2 mg/kg) are associated with rapid loss of consciousness (30–60 s); hence, this has obvious clinical advantages. Furthermore, a general anesthesia maintenance infusion of propofol is typically achieved with 100–200 mcg/kg/min intravenous.

Fig. 15.3 Chemical structure of ketamine

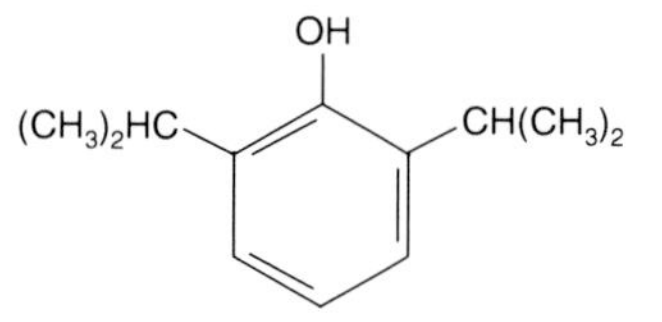

Fig. 15.4 Chemical structure of propofol

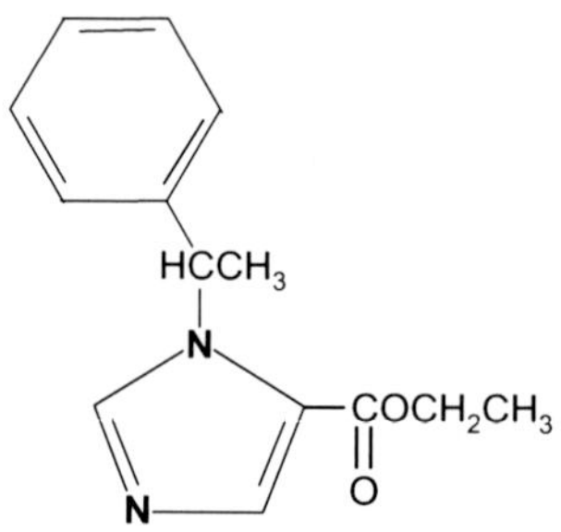

Fig. 15.5 Chemical structure of etomidate

Additional advantages of propofol include clear awakening, small cumulative effects, and/or decreased incidence of nausea and vomiting.

Propofol is considered to also interact with GABA receptors and activate them in a similar fashion as barbiturates. Likewise, activation of GABA receptors by propofol increases the conductance of chloride channels, resulting in inhibition of postsynaptic neurons.

Of clinical significance, the administration of propofol commonly causes a decrease in both systemic vascular resistance and cardiac contractility, hence resulting in decreased cardiac output and blood pressure. This reduction in systemic vascular resistance (and vasodilation) is considered due to decreased sympathetic vasoconstrictor activation of vascular smooth muscle [43]. The inhibition of sympathetic tone by propofol is reported to be greater than inhibition of parasympathetic activity; in some patients, this may result in significant bradycardia and even asystole [44–46]. The induced decrease in cardiac contractility is likely due to decreases in calcium uptake into the sarcoplasmic reticulum; decreased reuptake of calcium results in less calcium available for the next activation sequence [47].

Importantly, it should again be noted that in patients with decreased left ventricular function, the administration of propofol may result in severe hypotension and suppressed myocardial contractility. Therefore, the careful titration of propofol and adequate intravascular hydration are important in these types of patients.

15.4.6 Etomidate

Etomidate (Fig. 15.5) is an imidazole compound which is water soluble at lower pH and lipid soluble at physiologic pH. Rapid loss of consciousness is accomplished after intravenous injection of etomidate (0.2–0.4 mg/kg). It is important to recognize that etomidate lacks analgesic properties and does not blunt sympathetic responses to direct laryngoscopy and endotracheal intubation.

Generally, etomidate provides cardiovascular and pulmonary stability; typical induction doses of etomidate result in minimal changes in heart rate and cardiac output. Myocardial contractility is well maintained at doses needed

to induce general anesthesia [23] and is considered to produce less myocardial depression when compared to thiopental [48]. Etomidate does not induce significant histamine release, but it does depress adrenocortical function by inhibiting the conversion of cholesterol to cortisol [49]. Specifically, a single induction dose of etomidate can cause adrenal suppression for 5–8 h [50], and a continuous infusion of etomidate will cause further adrenocortical suppression. Typically, there is minimal clinical effect to adrenal suppression following a single induction dose of etomidate.

15.4.7 Nondepolarizing Muscle Relaxants

In general, the majority of nondepolarizing muscle relaxants have minimal effects on cardiovascular and hemodynamic stability. Yet, when induced, nondepolarizing muscle relaxants are believed to elicit cardiovascular effects by stimulating the release of histamine and affecting muscarinic and nicotinic receptors (Table 15.7). For example, pancuronium may cause vagal blockade (antimuscarinic effect) at the sinoatrial node, resulting in elevation of heart rate. The administration of pancuronium is also associated with activation of the sympathetic nervous system [51, 52]. Large doses of atracurium and mivacurium are associated with histamine release which may result in tachycardia and hypotension; such patients may display facial flushing as a result of histamine release. Interestingly, cisatracurium (a stereoisomer of atracurium) is not associated with clinically significant histamine

Table 15.7 Nondepolarizing muscle relaxants

	Histamine release	Vagal blockade
Atracurium	+	0
Cisatracurium	0	0
Mivacurium	+	0
Pancuronium	0	++
Rocuronium	0	0/+
Vecuronium	0	0
Tubocurarine	+++	0
Succinylcholine	0	−−

release. Finally, it is of interest to note that vecuronium and rocuronium are agents that are considered totally devoid of significant cardiovascular effects at clinical doses.

15.4.8 Depolarizing Muscle Relaxant

Succinylcholine is a depolarizing muscle relaxant; it has a similar structure to and mimics acetylcholine by binding to nicotinic cholinergic receptors. The duration of action of succinylcholine is short (min) and is broken down by the abundant pseudocholinesterase enzyme in the plasma. Importantly, the administration of succinylcholine may be associated with cardiac dysrhythmias (i.e., junctional rhythm and sinus bradycardia) by its muscarinic activity at the sinoatrial node. Administration of succinylcholine is associated with hyperkalemia in susceptible patients such as those with malignant hyperthermia, muscular dystrophy, spinal cord injury, and/or burn injury. More specifically, in boys with Duchenne muscular dystrophy, the administration of succinylcholine has been linked to episodes of sudden cardiac death.

15.4.9 Acupuncture

Acupuncture involves stimulation of specific anatomical locations on the skin to alter energy flow patterns throughout the body. The skin can be stimulated by manual or electrical stimulation, or the more typical placement of small metallic needles. Acupuncture has been used in China for thousands of years and, more recently, there has been a surge of interest in these nontraditional methodologies in the United States. Acupuncture has been utilized for treatment and prevention of multiple health conditions such as chronic pain, nausea and vomiting, obesity, substance abuse, and/or asthma. Stress responses and cardiovascular effects of pain have reportedly been attenuated by nonpharmacologic techniques such as acupuncture; it modulates the body's pain system, increases the release of endogenous opioids [53], and decreases postoperative pain [54]. In one study of a feline cardiovascular model, the utilization of electroacupuncture induced improvements in regional cardiac wall motion activity during myocardial ischemia [55]. Furthermore, it was reported that acupressure applied to females undergoing elective cesarean section with spinal anesthesia displayed a reduction in nausea and vomiting [56].

The potential advantages of acupuncture for the treatment of medical conditions continue to be investigated. Interestingly, with initial studies indicating some promising benefits of acupuncture for treatment of multiple medical conditions, the National Institutes of Health Consensus Conference has recommended that acupuncture be included in comprehensive management and may be useful as an adjunct treatment or an acceptable alternative [57]. Finally, limitations in the validation of acupuncture may stem from difficulty creating appropriate randomized, blinded, placebo-controlled clinical studies.

15.4.10 Anesthesia and Temperature Regulation

General and regional anesthesia is often associated with disregulation of body temperature and decreases in core body temperature. During the first hour of anesthesia, it is common for core body temperature to decrease by $0.5–1°C$. Most of the body heat lost during anesthesia is via convection and radiation, with some losses due to conduction and evaporation. Principally, anesthetics cause the core body heat to redistribute to the periphery, resulting in a drop in core body temperature [58]. In general, one can consider that, under anesthesia, patients become poikilotherms (minimal ability to thermoregulate). Therefore, multiple modalities to maintain normothermia during surgery have been developed, including forced air warming devices, fluid warmers, ventilator humidifiers, water mattresses and vests, radiant lamps, and warm blankets. Other modalities for warming patients include altering ambient room temperatures and/or the temperatures of irrigation solutions.

Importantly, postoperative hypothermia may be associated with: (1) delayed awakening from general anesthesia; (2) slowed drug metabolism; (3) coagulopathy; (4) vasoconstriction and poor tissue perfusion; (5) increases in blood viscosity; and/or (6) induced shivering. Postoperative shiver may be detrimental in patients with coronary artery disease, as shivering increases oxygen consumption and tachycardia. Currently, meperidine is clinically approved for treatment of excessive shivering in postoperative situations.

15.4.11 Myocardial Preconditioning with Inhalational and Intravenous Anesthetics

Since the initial report by Murray et al. [29] on ischemic preconditioning of dog myocardium, there has been great interest in myocardial preconditioning with pharmacologic agents. This includes myocardial preconditioning with volatile anesthetics such as desflurane [59], isoflurane [60, 61], and sevoflurane [62] as well as intravenous opioid agonists [63, 64]. Pharmacologic preconditioning is not just limited to cardiac tissue; other tissues such as lung, brain, and skeletal muscle [65] may benefit from preconditioning. In summary, preconditioning with anesthetics may offer life-extending benefits in cardiac, vascular, and/or organ transplantation surgical patients. For more details on this topic, see Chapter 14.

15.4.12 Heart Transplant

With the increasing numbers of individuals surviving heart transplants, the anesthetic management of the patient after a heart transplant procedure requires special considerations. A transplanted heart is initially totally denervated and usually elicits a higher basal heart rate (90–110 beats/min); direct autonomic nervous system effects are absent. Thus, agents such as atropine and glycopyrrolate will not cause an increase in heart rate. Vagal stimulation maneuvers such as carotid massage and oculocardiac reflex are also absent. However, acetylcholinesterase inhibitors such as neostigmine have been associated with severe bradycardia. If bradycardia develops, administration of direct acting cardiac agents such as isoproterenol or epinephrine may be required. The transplanted heart continues to respond to circulating catecholamines, and thus maintenance of cardiac output is aided by increased stroke volume (Frank–Starling relationship); maintaining adequate preload is considered essential in heart transplant patients postoperatively.

15.5 Summary

With the aging population and an increase in health problems such as obesity, diabetes, and coronary artery disease, the perioperative management and induction of general anesthesia in such patients, while providing cardiovascular stability, continues to offer both challenges and new developments in this field. These developments include new anesthesia medications, medical equipment and/or surgical technology, and anesthetic and surgical techniques. Nevertheless, with our growing understanding of inhalational and intravenous anesthetics, the maintenance of stable, physiologic cardiovascular function is common clinical practice today.

References

1. ASA Standards, Guidelines and Statements. American Society of Anesthesiologists. October 2001.
2. Eger EI II. Uptake of inhaled anesthetics: The alveolar to impaired anesthetic difference. In: Eger EI II, ed. Anesthetic uptake and action. Baltimore, MD: Williams & Wilkins, 1974:77.
3. Stevens W, Cromwell T, Halsey M, et al. The cardiovascular effects of a new inhalation anesthetic, Forane, in human volunteers at constant arterial carbon dioxide tension. Anesthesiology 1971;35:8–16.
4. Eger EI II, Smith N, Stoelting R. Cardiovascular effects of halothane in man. Anesthesiology 1970;32:396–409.
5. Weiskopf R, Cahalan M, Eger EI II, et al. Cardiovascular actions of desflurane in normocarbic volunteers. Anesth Analg 1991;73:143–56.
6. Holaday D, Smith F. Clinical characteristics and biotransformation of sevoflurane in healthy human volunteers. Anesthesiology 1981;54:100–6.
7. Pavlin EG, Su JY. Cardiopulmonary pharmacology. In: Miller RD, ed. Anesthesia Philadelphia, PA: Churchill Livingstone, 1994:145.
8. Muzi M, Ebert TJ. A comparison of baroreflex sensitivity during isoflurane and desflurane anesthesia in humans. Anesthesiology 1995;82:919–25.
9. Duke PC, Townes D, Wade JG. Halothane depresses baroreflex control of heart rate in man. Anesthesiology 1977;46:184–7.
10. Korly KJ, Ebert TJ, Vucins E, et al. Baroreceptor reflex control of heart rate during isoflurane anesthesia in humans. Anesthesiology 1984;60:173–9.
11. Atlee JL, Bosnjak ZJ. Mechanisms for cardiac dysrhythmias during anesthesia. Anesthesiology 1990;72:347–74.
12. Navarro R, Weiskopf RB, Moore MA, et al. Humans anesthetized with sevoflurane or isoflurane have similar arrhythmic response to epinephrine. Anesthesiology 1994;80:545–9.
13. Moore MA, Weiskopf RB, Eger EI, et al. Arrhythmogenic doses of epinephrine are similar during desflurane or isoflurane anesthesia in humans. Anesthesiology 1994;79:943–7.
14. Johnston PR, Eger EI, Wilson C. A comparative interaction of epinephrine with enflurane, isoflurane, and halothane in man. Anesth Analg 1976;55:709–12.
15. Crystal GJ, Khoury E, Gurevicius J, Salem MR. Direct effects of halothane on coronary blood flow, myocardial oxygen consumption, and myocardial segmental shortening in in situ canine hearts. Anesth Analg 1995;80:256–62.
16. Crystal GJ, Salem MR. Isoflurane causes vasodilation in the coronary circulation. Anesthesiology 2003;98:1030.
17. Priebe H, Foex P. Isoflurane causes regional myocardial dysfunction in dogs with critical coronary artery stenoses. Anesthesiology 1987;66:293–300.
18. Cason BA, Verrier ED, London MJ, et al. Effects of isoflurane and halothane on coronary vascular resistance and collateral myocardial blood flow: Their capacity to induce coronary steal. Anesthesiology 1987;67:665–75.
19. Kersten JR, Brayer AP, Pagel PS, et al. Perfusion of ischemic myocardium during anesthesia with sevoflurane. Anesthesiology 1994;81:995–1004.
20. Eger E. New inhaled anesthetics. Anesthesiology 1994;80:906–22.
21. Pavlin EG, Su JY. Cardiopulmonary pharmacology. In: Miller RD, ed. Anesthesia. Philadelphia, PA: Churchill Livingstone, 1994:148.
22. Rivenes SM, Lewin MB, Stayer SA, et al. Cardiovascular effects of sevoflurane, isoflurane, halothane, and fentanyl-midazolam in children with congenital heart disease. Anesthesiology 2001;94:223–9.
23. Stoelting RK, ed. Pharmacology and physiology in anesthetic practice. 3rd ed. Philadelphia, PA: Lippincott Williams & Wilkins, 1999.
24. Muzi M, Ebert TJ, Hope WG, et al. Site(s) mediating sympathetic activation with desflurane. Anesthesiology 1996;85:737–47.
25. Warltier DC, Wathiqui MH, Kampine JP, et al. Recovery of contractile function of stunned myocardium in chronically

instrumented dogs is enhanced by halothane or isoflurane. Anesthesiology 1988;69:552–65.

26. Marijic J, Stowe DF, Turner LA, et al. Differential protective effects of halothane and isoflurane against hypoxic and reoxygenation injury in the isolated guinea pig heart. Anesthesiology 1990;73:976–83.

27. Novalija E, Fujita S, Kampine JP, et al. Sevoflurane mimics ischemic preconditioning effects on coronary flow and nitric oxide release in isolated hearts. Anesthesiology 1999;91:701–12.

28. Conzen PF, Fischer S, Detter C, et al. Sevoflurane provides greater protection of myocardium than propofol in patients undergoing off-pump coronary artery bypass surgery. Anesthesiology 2003;99:826–33.

29. Murray CE, Jennings RB, Reimer KA. Preconditioning with ischemia: A delay of lethal cell injury in ischemic myocardium. Circulation 1986;74:1124–36.

30. Zaugg M, Lucchinetti E, Spahn DR, et al. Volatile anesthetics mimic cardiac preconditioning by priming the activation of mitochondrial K_{ATP} channels via multiple signaling pathways. Anesthesiology 2002;97:4–14.

31. Cullen SC, Gross EG. The anesthetic properties of xenon in animals and human beings with additional observation on krypton. Science 1951;1113:580–2.

32. Rossaint R, Reyle-Hahn R, Schulte J, et al. Multicenter randomized comparison of the efficacy and safety of xenon and isoflurane in patients undergoing elective surgery. Anesthesiology 2003;98:6–13.

33. Lachmann B, Armbruster S, Schairer W, et al. Safety and efficacy of xenon in routine use as an inhalational anesthetic. Lancet 1990;335:1413–5.

34. Luttrop HH, Romner B, Perhag L, et al. Left ventricular performance and cerebral hemodynamics during xenon anesthesia: A transesophageal echocardiography and transcranial Doppler sonography study. Anesthesia 1993;48:1045–9.

35. Stowe DF, Rehmert GC, Wai-Meng K, et al. Xenon does not alter cardiac function or major cation currents in isolated guinea pig hearts of myocytes. Anesthesiology 2000;92:516–22.

36. Franks NP, Lieb WR. Molecular and cellular mechanisms of general anaesthesia. Nature 1994;367:607–14.

37. Seltzer JL, Gerson JI, Allen FB. Comparison of the cardiovascular effects of bolus vs. incremental administration of thiopentone. Br J Anaesth 1980;52:527–9.

38. Sunzel M, Paalzow L, Berggren L, et al. Respiratory and cardiovascular effects in relation to plasma levels of midazolam and diazepam. Br J Clin Pharmacol 1988;25:561–9.

39. McCammon RL, Hilgenberg JC, Stoelting RK. Hemodynamic effects of diazepam-nitrous oxide in patients with coronary artery disease. Anesth Analg 1980;59:438–41.

40. Hanouz, J, Yvon A, Guesne G, et al. The in vitro effects of remifentanil, sufentanil, fentanyl, and alfentanil on isolated human right atria. Anesth Analg 2001;93:543–9.

41. Kanaya N, Kahary DR, Murray PA, Damron DS. Differential effects of fentanyl and morphine on intracellular calcium transients and contraction in rate ventricular myocytes. Anesthesiology 1998;89:1532–42.

42. Waxman K, Shoemaker WC, Lippmann M. Cardiovascular effects of anesthetic induction with ketamine. Anesth Analg 1980;58:355–8.

43. Robinson JF, Ebert TJ, O'Brien TJ, et al. Mechanisms whereby propofol mediates peripheral vasodilation in humans. Sympathoinhibition or direct vascular relaxation? Anesthesiology 1997;86:64–72.

44. Bray RJ. Fatal myocardial failure associated with a propofol infusion in a child. Anaesthesia 1995;50:94.

45. Tramer MR, Moore RA, McQuay HJ. Propofol and bradycardia: Causation, frequency and severity. Br J Anasth 1997;78:642–51.

46. James MFM, Reyneke CJ, Whiffler K. Heart block following propofol: A case report. Br J Anaesth 1989;62:213–5.

47. Sprun J, Lgletree-Hughes ML, McConnell BK, et al. The effects of propofol on the contractility of failing and nonfailing human heart muscles. Anesth Analg 2001;93:550–9.

48. Kissin I, Motomura S, Aultman DF, et al. Inotropic and anesthetic potencies of etomidate and thiopental in dogs. Anesth Analg 1983;62:961–5.

49. Fragen RJ, Shanks CA, Molteni A, et al. Effects of etomidate on hormonal responses to surgical stress. Anesthesiology 1984;61:652–6.

50. Wagner RL, White PF, Kan PB, et al. Inhibition of adrenal steroidogenesis by anesthetic etomidate. N Engl J Med 1984;310:1415–21.

51. Ivankovich AD, Miletich DJ, Albrecht RF, et al. The effect of pancuronium on myocardial contraction and catecholamine metabolism. J Pharm Pharmacol 1975;27:837–41.

52. Domenech JS, Garcia RC, Sastain JMR, et al. Pancuronium bromide: An indirect sympathomimetic agent. Br J Anaesth 1976;48:1143–8.

53. Han JS. Physiologic and neurochemical basis of acupuncture analgesia. In: Cheng TO, ed. The international textbook of cardiology. New York, NY: Pergamon, 1986:1124–6.

54. Felhendler DPT, Lisander B. Pressure on acupoints decreases postoperative pain. Clin J Pain 1996;12:326–9.

55. Li P, Pitsillides KF, Rendig SV, et al. Reversal of reflex-induced myocardial ischemia by median nerve stimulation: A feline model of electroacupuncture. Circulation 1998;97:1186–94.

56. Stein DJ, Birnbach DJ, Danzer BI, et al. Acupressure versus intravenous metoclopramide to prevent nausea and vomiting during spinal anesthesia for cesarean section. Anesth Analg 1997;84:342–5.

57. Acupuncture. NIH Consensus Conference. JAMA 1998;280:1518–24.

58. Sessler DI. Mild perioperative hypothermia. N Engl J Med 1997;336:1630–7.

59. Hanouz J, Yvon A, Massetti M, et al. Mechanisms of desflurane-induced preconditioning in isolated human right atria in vitro. Anesthesiology 2002;97:33–41.

60. Kersten JR, Schmeling TJ, Hettrick DA, et al. Mechanism of myocardial protection by isoflurane: Role of adenosine triphosphate-regulated potassium (KATP) channels. Anesthesiology 1996;85:794–807.

61. Belhomme D, Peynet J, Louzy M, et al. Evidence for preconditioning by isoflurane in coronary artery bypass graft surgery. Circulation 1999;100:II340–4.

62. De Hert S, ten Broeck P, Mertens E, et al. Sevoflurane but not propofol preserves myocardial function in coronary surgery patients. Anesthesiology 2002;97:42–9.

63. Sigg DC, Coles JA Jr, Gallagher WJ, Oeltgen PR, Iaizzo PA. Opioid preconditioning: Myocardial function and energy metabolism. Ann Thorac Surg 2001;72:1576–82.

64. Sigg DC, Coles JA Jr, Oeltgen PR, Iaizzo PA. Role of delta-opioid receptors in infarct size reduction in swine. Am J Physiol Heart Circ Physiol 2002;282:H1953–60.

65. Hong J, Sigg DC, Upson K, Iaizzo PA. Role of ∂-opioid receptors in preventing ischemic damage of isolated porcine skeletal muscle. Biophys J 2002;82:610a (Abstract 2982).

Chapter 16
Blood Pressure, Heart Tones, and Diagnoses

George Bojanov

Abstract The primary purpose of this chapter is to familiarize the reader with the basic concepts of blood pressure, heart tones, and some common diagnoses. It remains the general consensus that even the most sophisticated electronic monitors cannot fully reduce the need for sound clinical skills like proper patient inspection, palpation, percussion, and auscultation. Furthermore, it is important to reinforce the need for a deep understanding of basic physiological principles when interpreting physical examination findings. Invasive and noninvasive methods for assessing blood pressure are discussed in addition to new technologies.

Keywords Blood pressure measurement · Palpation · Doppler effect · Auscultation · Oscillometry · Plethysmography · Arterial tonometry · Arterial cannulation · Heart tones

16.1 Blood Pressure

Fundamental to providing comprehensive care to patients is the ability to obtain an accurate medical history and carefully perform a physical examination. The optimal selection of further tests, treatments, and use of subspecialists depends on well-developed history and physical examination skills. Key elements of a normal physical include obtaining a blood pressure reading and auscultation of the heart, both providing important information about the patient's hemodynamics and aiding in diagnosing anatomical and physiological pathology.

Naive ideas about circulation and blood pressure date as far back as ancient Greece. It took until the 18th century before the first official report describing an attempt to measure blood pressure was written, when Stephen Hales published a monograph on "haemastatics" in 1733. He conducted a series of experiments involving invasive cannulation of arteries in horses for the resultant direct blood pressure measurement. Unfortunately, his methods were not applicable for humans. During the subsequent two centuries, there were many contributions to the science of blood pressure control and its assessment. One of the greatest of these contributions was a publication in Gazetta Medica di Torino in 1896, called "A New Sphygmomanometer" by Dr. Riva-Rocci; this publication is still recognized as the single most important advancement in the field of practical noninvasive methods for blood pressure estimation.

In 1916, French physician Rene Laennec invented the first stethoscope, which was constructed from stacked paper rolled into a solid cylinder. Prior to his invention, physicians around the world would place an ear directly over the patient's chest to hear the heart and/or lung sounds. After Dr. Laennec's initial success, several new models were produced, primarily made of wood; this stethoscope was called a "monaural stethoscope." The "binaural stethoscope" was invented in 1829 by a doctor from Dublin and later gained widespread acceptance. In the 1960s, the Camman binaural stethoscope was considered the standard because of its superior auscultation capabilities.

It is essential for health care professionals and bioengineers to understand how blood pressure and heart tones are obtained, the advantages and disadvantages of the different methods used to obtain them, and how to interpret the gathered information.

16.1.1 Physiology of Blood Pressure

Blood pressure is the force applied on arterial walls as the heart pumps blood through the circulatory system. The rhythmic contractions of the left ventricle result in cyclic

G. Bojanov (✉)
University of Minnesota, Department of Anesthesiology,
MMC 294, 420 Delaware St. SE, Minneapolis, MN 55455, USA
e-mail: boja0003@umn.edu

P.A. Iaizzo (ed.), *Handbook of Cardiac Anatomy, Physiology, and Devices*, DOI 10.1007/978-1-60327-372-5_16,
© Springer Science+Business Media, LLC 2009

changes in the arterial blood pressure. During ventricular systole, the heart pumps blood into the circulatory system, and the pressure within the arteries reaches its highest level—a point known as "systolic blood pressure." During diastole, the pressure within the arterial system falls to its lowest level, a point called "diastolic blood pressure."

"Mean blood pressure," often used clinically, represents the time-weighted average of the arterial pressures recorded during one cardiac cycle. The alternating systolic and diastolic pressures create outward and inward movements of the arterial walls, perceived as arterial pulsation or arterial pulse. "Pulse pressure" is another clinical term and represents the difference between the systolic and diastolic blood pressures.

It is accepted convention that blood pressure is measured in millimeters of mercury (mmHg). A normal systolic blood pressure is less than 140 mmHg, and a normal diastolic blood pressure is less than 90 mmHg. Blood pressure higher than normal signifies "hypertension," and one lower than normal is called "hypotension." Normal mean arterial pressure is between 60 and 90 mmHg. The mean arterial pressure has significance in that it will drive tissue perfusion and can be measured directly using an automated blood pressure cuff or calculated using the following formulas:

$$MAP = DBP + PP/3 \text{ or } MAP = [SBP + (2 \times DBP)]/3$$

where $PP = SBP–DBP$, MAP = mean arterial pressure, DBP = diastolic blood pressure, PP = pulse pressure, and SBP = systolic blood pressure.

Blood flow throughout the circulatory system follows pressure gradients. By the time blood reaches the right atrium, representing the end point of the venous system, pressure will decrease to approx 0 mmHg. The two major determinants of the arterial blood pressure are: (1) cardiac output, representing the volume of blood pumped by the heart per minute; and (2) systemic vascular resistance, which is the impediment to blood flow created by the vascular bed. Cardiac output depends on a complexity of numerous factors including preload, contractility, afterload, heart rate, and/or rhythm. Systemic vascular resistance is equally complex and controlled by many additional factors including vasomotor tone of arterioles, terminal arterioles, and/or precapillary sphincters. Blood pressure as a function of the cardiac output and systemic vascular resistance can be expressed with the following abstract formula:

$$BP = CO \times SVR$$

where BP = blood pressure, CO = cardiac output, and SVR = systemic vascular resistance.

Blood pressure decreases by 3–5 mmHg in arteries 3 mm in diameter, and then reaches approximately 85 mmHg when entering arterioles; this accounts for approx 50% of the resistance of the entire systemic circulation. Blood pressure is further reduced to around 30–40 mmHg at the point of entry into capillaries, and then becomes approximately 10 mmHg at the venous end of the capillaries.

The speed of the advancing pressure wave during each cardiac cycle far exceeds the actual blood flow velocity. In the aorta, the pressure wave speed may be 15 times faster than the flow of blood. In an end artery, the pressure wave velocity may be as much as 100 times the speed of the forward blood flow.

As the pressure wave moves peripherally through the arterial tree, wave reflection, refraction, and interference distort the pressure waveform, causing an exaggeration of systolic and pulse pressures. This enhancement of the peripheral pulse pressure causes the systolic blood pressure in the radial artery to be 20–30% higher than the aortic systolic blood pressure and the diastolic blood pressure to be approx 10–15% lower than the aortic diastolic blood pressure. Nevertheless, the mean blood pressure in the radial artery will closely correspond to the mean aortic arterial pressure.

16.1.2 Methods of Measuring Blood Pressure

Arterial blood pressure can be measured both noninvasively and invasively, as described in the following sections.

16.1.2.1 Noninvasive Methods

Palpation

Palpation is a relatively simple and easy method for assessing systolic blood pressure. For example, a blood pressure cuff containing an inflatable bladder is applied to the arm and inflated until the arterial pulse felt distal to the cuff disappears. Pressure in the cuff is then released at a speed of approx 3 mmHg per heartbeat until an arterial pulse is felt again. The pressure at which the arterial pulsation can be detected is the systolic blood pressure; diastolic blood pressure and mean arterial pressure cannot be readily estimated using this method. Furthermore, the systolic blood pressure measured using the palpation method is typically an underestimation of the true arterial systolic blood pressure, i.e., because of insensitivity of the sense of touch and the relative delay between blood flow below the cuff and the appearance of arterial pulsations distal to the cuff.

Doppler Method

The Doppler method for blood pressure measurement is a modification of the palpation method described above. It uses a sensor Doppler probe to determine blood flow distal to the blood pressure cuff. The "Doppler effect" represents a shift in the frequency of a sound wave when a transmitted sound is reflected back from a moving object. Such a sound wave shift (e.g., caused by blood movement in an artery) is detected by a Doppler monitor and presented as a specific swishing sound. The pressure in the cuff, at which a blood flow is detected by the Doppler probe, is the systolic arterial blood pressure. Doppler-assisted blood pressure measurement is more accurate and less subjective in estimating systolic blood pressure, compared to the palpation method. Using Doppler for blood pressure assessment is quite useful for patients in shock and patients in low-flow states, as well as obese and pediatric (very young) patients. Disadvantages of the Doppler method include: (1) an inability to detect the diastolic blood pressure; (2) a necessity for sound-conducting gel between the skin and the probe (air is a poor conductor of ultrasound); (3) the likelihood of a poor signal if the probe is not applied directly over an artery; and/or (4) the potential for motion and electro-cautery artifacts.

Auscultation (Riva-Rocci Method)

The auscultation method uses a blood pressure cuff placed around an extremity (usually an upper extremity) and a stethoscope placed above a major artery just distal to the blood pressure cuff (e.g., the brachial artery if using the cuff on the upper extremity). Inflation of the blood pressure cuff above the patient's systolic blood pressure flattens the artery and stops blood flow distal to the cuff. As the pressure in the cuff is released, the artery becomes only partially compressed, which creates conditions for turbulent blood flow within the artery and produces the so-called "Korotkoff" sounds, named after the individual who first described them. Korotkoff sounds are caused by the vibrations created when blood flow in the partially flattened artery transforms from laminar into turbulent, and this state persists as long as there is a turbulent flow within the vessel. Systolic blood pressure is determined as the pressure of the inflated cuff at which Korotkoff sounds are first detected. Diastolic blood pressure is determined as the cuff pressure at which Korotkoff sounds become muffled or disappear.

Sometimes, in patients with chronic hypertension, there can be an auscultatory gap that represents disappearance of the normal Korotkoff sounds in a wide pressure range between the systolic and diastolic blood pressures. This condition will lead to inaccurately low blood pressure assessment. Korotkoff sounds can also be difficult to detect in patients who are in shock or in those with marked peripheral vasoconstriction. The use of microphones and electronic sound amplification can greatly increase the sensitivity of this method. Yet, considerations for systematic errors include motion artifact and electrocautery interference.

Oscillometry

Oscillometry is a noted method for blood pressure measurement which employs an automated blood pressure cuff. Arterial pulsations cause pressure oscillations in a cuff placed over an extremity. These oscillations are at their maximum when the cuff pressure equals the mean arterial pressure, and decrease significantly when the cuff pressure is above the systolic blood pressure or below the diastolic blood pressure. Advantages of this approach include the ease and reliability of use; some of the potential technical problems include motion artifacts, electrocautery interference, and inability to measure accurate blood pressure when patients experience arrhythmias.

When selecting a blood pressure cuff for noninvasive blood pressure measurement, it is important to select the cuff in accordance with the patient's size. Blood pressure cuffs for adult and pediatric patients come in variable sizes. An appropriate size means that the cuff's bladder length is at least 80% and the cuff width is at least 40% of the patient's arm circumference. If the cuff is too small, it will need to be inflated to a greater pressure to completely occlude the arterial blood flow, and the resultant measured pressure will be falsely elevated. On the other hand, if the cuff is too large, the pressure inside the cuff needed for complete occlusion of the arterial blood flow will be less, and the measured pressure will be falsely low.

Blood pressure is most commonly taken while the patient is seated with the arm resting on a table and slightly bent, which will typically position the patient's arm at the level of his/her heart. This same principle should be applied if the patient is in a supine position; the blood pressure cuff should be level with the patient's heart. If the location of the blood pressure cuff during blood pressure measurement is above or below the patient's heart level, measured blood pressure will be either falsely lower or higher than the actual pressure. This difference can be represented as the height of a column of water interposed between the level of the blood pressure cuff and the level of the patient's heart. To convert centimeters of water (cm H_2O) to millimeters of mercury, the measured height of the water column should be multiplied by a conversion factor of 0.74 (1 cm $H_2O = 0.74$ mmHg).

All of the aforementioned methods for assessing blood pressure do so indirectly by registering blood flow below a blood pressure cuff. Other noninvasive methods include plethysmography and arterial tonometry.

Plethysmography

The plethysmographic method for blood pressure assessment employs the fact that arterial pulsations cause a transient increase in the blood volume of an extremity, and thus in the volume of the whole extremity. A finger plethysmograph determines the minimum pressure needed by a finger cuff to maintain constant finger blood volume. A light-emitting diode and a photoelectric cell are used to detect changes in the relative finger volume; this information is, in turn, used to rapidly adjust the cuff pressure. Data can be displayed as a beat-to-beat tracing. Thus, in healthy patients, the blood pressure measured on a finger will correspond to the aortic blood pressure. Importantly, this relationship does not hold true for patients with low peripheral perfusion, such as those with peripheral artery disease, hypothermia, or patients in low-flow states.

Arterial Tonometry

Tonometry devices can determine beat-to-beat arterial blood pressure by adjusting the pressure required to partially flatten a superficial artery located between a tonometer and a bony surface (e.g., radial artery). These devices commonly consist of an electronic unit and a pressure-sensing head. The system includes an adjustable air chamber and an array of independent pressure sensors that, when placed directly over the artery, assess intraluminal arterial pressure. The resultant pressure record resembles an invasive arterial blood pressure waveform. Yet, limitations to this method include motion artifacts and the need for frequent calibration.

16.1.2.2 Invasive Methods of Blood Pressure Measurement

Indications

Indications for using direct blood pressure monitoring (arterial cannulation) include consistent hemodynamic instability, intraoperative monitoring in selected patients, and use of vasoactive drugs like dopamine, epinephrine, norepinephrine, and the like.

Cannulation Sites

Arteries most often selected for direct cannulation are the radial, ulnar, brachial, femoral, dorsalis pedis, or the axillary. Cannulation of an artery should be avoided if there is: (1) a considered lack of appropriate collateral circulation; (2) a skin infection on or near the site of cannulation; and/or (3) a known preexisting vascular deficiency (e.g., Raynaud's disease). The radial artery is the most often selected artery for invasive blood pressure monitoring because of easy access, superficial location, and good collateral flow to the region it supplies.

Techniques

The two frequently utilized techniques for arterial cannulation are: (1) a catheter over a needle; and (2) the "Seldinger's" technique. When using the catheter over a needle technique, the operator enters a selected artery with a needle over which a catheter has been placed. After free blood flow through the needle, the catheter is advanced over the needle and into the artery, after which the needle is withdrawn. The catheter is then connected to a pressure-transducing system. When using the Seldinger's technique, the operator first enters the artery with a needle. After confirmation of free blood flow through the needle, the operator places a steel wire into the artery and withdraws the needle. A plastic catheter is then advanced into the artery over the wire, then the wire is removed and the catheter is connected to a transducer system. Both methods require sterile techniques and skilled operators.

Considerations

Arterial cannulation provides beat-to-beat numerical information and thus tracings of appropriately monitored waveforms of arterial blood pressure, which is considered a "gold standard" in blood pressure monitoring. Invasive arterial pressure monitoring systems include a catheter (20 gauge catheter for adults), tubing, a transducer, and an electronic monitor for signal amplification, filtering, and analysis. Such pressure transducers are commonly based on the strain gauge principle—stretching a wire of silicone crystal changes its electrical resistance. The catheter, the connective tubing, and the transducer are prefilled with saline, and the use of a pressure bag provides continuous saline flush of the system at a typical rate of 3–5 mL/h. These systems should also allow for intermittent flush boluses.

Quality of information gathered using invasive blood pressure monitoring depends on the dynamic characteristics of the whole system. The complex waveform obtained from the arterial pulse can be expressed as a summation of simple sine and cosine waves using Fourier analysis. Most invasive blood pressure monitoring systems are designed to have natural frequencies of approximately 16–24 Hz, slightly exceeding the frequency of the arterial pulse waveform in order to reproduce it correctly. This natural frequency is described as that at which the system oscillates when disturbed. Another property of the catheter–tubing–transducer system is its dumping coefficient, characterizing how quickly oscillations in the system will spontaneously decay.

Both the natural frequency and the dumping coefficient are primarily determined by the employed length, size, and compliance of the catheter and tubing, as well as by presence of any air bubbles or blood clots that may be trapped in the tubing. This chapter is not intended to go into details about how to determine and change the system characteristics but, briefly, underdumping the system will exaggerate artifacts. For example, a catheter whip can result in a significant overestimation of the systolic blood pressure. Likewise, overdumping will blunt the response of the catheter–tubing–transducer system and lead to an underestimation of the systolic blood pressure. In addition, systems with low natural frequencies will show amplifications of the pressure curves, thus causing overestimation of the systolic blood pressure. Diastolic blood pressure will also be affected by altering the above-mentioned factors, but to a lesser degree. Note that system response characteristics can be optimized by using short, low-compliance tubing and by avoiding air trapping by using a flushing system.

When an invasive blood pressure system is connected to a patient, it should be zero referenced and calibrated. Zero referencing is performed by placing the transducer at the level of the midaxillary line, which corresponds to the level of the patient's heart when the patient is supine. The system is then opened to air, closed to the patient, and adjusted to a 0 mmHg baseline. Note that for proper zero referencing, it is not necessary for the transducer to be at the level of the patient's heart as long as the stopcock, which is opened to air during zero referencing, is at that level. The system is then directed to record from the patient and thus is ready for use.

System calibration is a separate procedure and involves connecting the invasive blood pressure system to a mercury manometer, closing the system to the patient, and pressurizing it to certain predetermined pressures. The gain of the monitor amplifier is then adjusted until displayed pressure equals the pressure in the mercury manometer. Recommendations are to perform zero referencing at least once on every clinical shift and this type of calibration at least once daily. It should be noted that some of the more contemporary transducer designs rarely require external calibration.

When connected to a patient, today's invasive blood pressure monitoring systems provide digital readings of systolic, diastolic, and mean blood pressures and pressure waveforms. Watching the trend of a waveform and its shape can provide other important information as well. More specifically, the top of the waveform represents the systolic blood pressure, and the bottom is the diastolic blood pressure. The dicrotic notch is caused by the closure of the aortic valve and backsplash of blood against the closed valve. The rate of the upstroke of the arterial blood pressure wave depends on the myocardial contractility, whereas the rate of the downstroke is affected by the systemic vascular resistance. Exaggerated variation in the size of the waves with respiration suggests hypovolemia. Thus, the trained eye can gain insight about a patient's cardiovascular status by evaluating aspects of this signal. Integrating the area under the waveform can be used for calculating the mean arterial pressure.

Complications

Potential complications associated with arterial cannulation include bleeding, hematoma, infection, thrombosis, ischemia distal to the cannulation site, vasospasm, embolization with air bubbles or blood clots, nerve damage, pseudoaneurysm formation, atheroma, and/or inadvertent intraarterial drug injection.

16.1.3 Diagnoses

16.1.3.1 Pulsus Paradoxus

Normally, the arterial and venous blood pressures fluctuate throughout the respiratory cycle, decreasing with inspiration and rising with expiration. Yet, this fluctuation in the blood pressure under normal conditions is less than 10 mmHg. Inspiration increases venous return, therefore increasing the right heart output transiently, according to the Frank–Starling law. As the blood is sequestered in the pulmonary circulation during inspiration, the left heart output is reduced and is expressed as a lower systolic blood pressure. The right ventricle contracts more vigorously and mechanically bulges the interventricular septum toward the left ventricle, reducing its size and accounting for even lower systolic blood pressure. Pulsus paradoxus is defined as an inspiratory decrease of systolic blood pressure by more than 10 mmHg.

Certain conditions drastically reduce the transmural or distending (filling) pressure of the heart and interfere with the diastolic filling of the ventricles. In such cases, there is typically an exaggeration of the inspiratory fall in the systolic blood pressure, which results from reduced left ventricular stroke volume and the transmission of the negative intrathoracic pressure to the aorta. Common causes for such reduction include pericardial effusion, adhesive pericarditis, cardiac tamponade, pulmonary emphysema, severe asthma, paramediastinal effusion, endocardial fibrosis, myocardial amyloidosis, scleroderma, mitral stenosis with right heart failure, tricuspid stenosis, hypovolemia, and/or pulmonary embolism. Associated clinical signs include a palpable decrease in pulse with inspiration and decrease in the inspiratory systolic blood pressure of more than 10 mmHg compared to the expiratory pressure. On clinical examination, one can detect extra beats on cardiac auscultation during inspiration, when compared to a peripheral pulse.

16.1.3.2 Pulsus Alternans

Pulsus alternans is an alternating weak and strong peripheral pulse, caused by alternating weak and strong heart contractions. A weak contraction will decrease the ejection fraction, hence increasing the end-diastolic volume (the volume of blood remaining in the ventricle after a weak heart contraction). As a result, in the next cardiac cycle, the heart will be stretched more; then, according to the Frank–Starling mechanism, this will generate higher pressures and a stronger perceived pulse. Pulsus alternans may be found in patients with severe heart failure, various degrees of heart block, and/or arrhythmias. Pulsus alternans is characterized by a regular rhythm and must be distinguished from pulsus bigeminus, which is an irregular heart rate (see below).

16.1.3.3 Bigeminal Pulse

A bigeminal pulse is caused by occurrences of premature contractions (usually ventricular) after every other heartbeat, resulting in an alternation in the relative pulse strength. Bigeminal pulse can often be confused with pulsus alternans. However, in contrast to the latter, in which the rhythm is regular, in pulsus bigeminus the weak beat always follows a shorter pulse interval; thus there is an arrhythmia.

16.1.3.4 Pulse Deficit

Pulse deficit is the inability to detect some arterial pulsations when the heart beats, as can be observed in patients with atrial fibrillation, in states of shock, or with premature ventricular complexes. The easiest way to detect pulse deficit is to place a finger over an artery while monitoring the QRS complexes on an electrocardiogram monitor. A QRS complex without a detected corresponding pulse represents a pulse deficit. In the presence of atrioventricular dissociation, when atrial activity is irregularly transmitted to the ventricles, the strength of the peripheral arterial pulse depends on the relative timing of the atrial and ventricular contractions. In a patient with rapid heartbeats, the presence of such variations suggests ventricular tachycardia. With an equally rapid rate, an absence of variation of pulse strength suggests a supraventricular mechanism. See Chapters 11 and 26 for an additional description of arrhythmias.

16.1.3.5 Wide Pulse Pressure

Wide pulse pressure, often called "water hammer pulse," is observed in cases of severe aortic regurgitation and consists of an abrupt upstroke (percussion wave) followed by a rapid collapse later in systole with no dicrotic notch.

16.1.3.6 Pulsus Parvus et Tardus

The phenomenon of pulsus parvus (small) et tardus (late) is observed in cases of aortic stenosis and is caused by reduction in stroke volume and prolonged ejection phase, producing reductions and delays in the volume increments inside the aorta. "Tardus" refers to delayed or prolonged early systolic acceleration; "parvus" refers to diminished amplitude and rounding of the systolic peak.

16.1.3.7 Bisferiens Pulse

A bisferiens (biphasic) pulse is characterized by two systolic peaks—the percussion and tidal waves—separated by a distinct midsystolic dip. The peaks are often equal, or one may be larger. Bisferiens pulse occurs in conditions in which a large stroke volume is ejected rapidly from the left ventricle and is observed most commonly in patients with either pure aortic regurgitation or with a combination of aortic regurgitation and stenosis. A bisferiens pulse can also be elicited by patients with hypertrophic obstructive cardiomyopathy. In these patients, the initial prominent percussion wave is associated with rapid ejection of blood into the aorta during early systole, followed by a rapid decline as the obstruction becomes prominent in midsystole followed by a tidal wave. Very rarely, bisferiens pulse occurs in individuals with a normal heart.

16.1.3.8 Dicrotic Pulse

Not to be confused with a bisferiens pulse, in which both peaks occur in systole, the dicrotic pulse is characterized by a second peak positioned in diastole immediately after the second heart sound. The normally small wave that follows aortic valve closure (dicrotic notch) is exaggerated and measures more than 50% of the pulse pressure on direct pressure recordings. A dicrotic pulse usually occurs in conditions such as cardiac tamponade, severe heart failure, and hypovolemic shock, in which a low stroke volume is ejected into a soft elastic aorta. Rarely, a dicrotic pulse can be noted in healthy adolescents or young adults.

16.2 Heart Tones

16.2.1 Physiology and Normal Heart Sounds

The primary heart tones are caused by vibrations created by pressure differentials during closure of the heart valves. Normal valve opening is relatively slow and makes little or no audible sounds. In general, heart tones are brief and characterized by varying intensity (loudness), frequency (pitch), and quality (timbre). To understand heart tones better, let us briefly review the physiology of the cardiac cycle. The electric impulse for cardiac contraction starts from the sinus node, located in the right atrium, thus causing the right atrium to contract first. Contraction of the ventricles begins with the left ventricle, resulting in mitral valve closure slightly before closure of the tricuspid valve. Ejection, on the other hand, starts in the right ventricle, because the right ventricular ejection normally occurs at a much lower pressure than the left ventricular ejection. Yet, ejection ends first in the left ventricle, causing the aortic valve to close slightly before the pulmonic valve.

The first heart sound (S1) arises from closure of the mitral valve (M1), and shortly thereafter by closure of the tricuspid valve (T1). The initial component of the first heart sound (M1) is most prominent at the cardiac apex. The second component (T1), when detected, normally presents at the left lower sternal border; it is less commonly heard at the apex and is seldom heard at the base. When the first heart sound noticeably splits, like in Ebstein's anomaly (often associated with delayed right ventricular activation), its first component is normally louder.

As mentioned previously, the intensity of heart sounds will increase with increases in pressure gradients across a particular valve. With an increasing pressure gradient, the blood velocity and the resultant force causing valve closure will increase, producing louder and more easily detectable sounds. Another factor affecting the intensity of the sound produced by an atrioventricular valve is the valvular position at the onset of systole. Note that when ventricular contraction occurs against a wide open valve, the leaflets will achieve higher velocity and thus the heart sound will be louder compared to a sound produced by a valve with partially closed leaflets at the beginning of systole.

The second heart sound (S2) is caused by closure of the aortic and the pulmonic valves. Normally the first component of this second heart sound is caused by the aortic valve closure (A2), followed shortly thereafter by the pulmonic valve closure (P2).

The physiological third heart sound (S3) (Fig. 16.1) occurs shortly after A2, and is a low-pitched vibration caused by rapid ventricular filling during diastole. Physiologic S3 sounds can commonly be heard in children, adolescents, and young adults. When detected after 30 years of age, S3 is referred to as "ventricular gallop" and is considered a sign of possible pathology. In most of the S3 ventricular gallop cases, there is diastolic dysfunction associated with ventricular failure. Normal third heart sounds sometimes persist beyond age 40 years and are more commonly found in women.

The physiological fourth heart sound (S4) (Fig. 16.2) is typically soft and low-pitched, and is best heard in late diastole just before S1. S4 is generated by rapid ventricular filling during atrial systole, causing vibrations of the left ventricular wall and the mitral apparatus. Normally, S4 is primarily heard in infants, small children, and adults over the age of 50 years. A loud S4, which can be

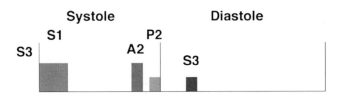

Fig. 16.1 Third heart sound (see text for details). A2 = aortic valve closure; P2 = pulmonic valve closure; S1 = first heart sound; S3 = third heart sound

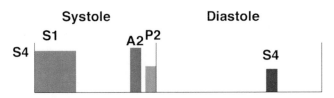

Fig. 16.2 Fourth heart sound (see text for details). A2 = aortic valve closure; P2 = pulmonic valve closure; S1 = first heart sound; S4 = fourth heart sound

associated with shock, is considered as a pathological sign and is referred to as an "S4 gallop."

16.2.2 Auscultatory Areas

Heart sounds generated by different valves are best heard over certain auscultatory areas, which bear the valve names but do not specifically correspond to the anatomical locations of the valves.

The aortic auscultation area is located over the second intercostal space at the right sternal border (Fig. 16.3). The pulmonic auscultation area is located in the second intercostal space at the left sternal border. The mitral auscultation area is just over the heart's apex, located in the fifth intercostal space, left of the sternum; this area is also called a left ventricular or apical area. The tricuspid auscultation area is located at the left lower sternal border. For patients with a left thoracic heart position (normal situs), auscultation should begin at the cardiac apex and continue with the left lower sternal border (following the inflow), and then the session should proceed interspace after interspace, up the left sternal border, up to the left myocardial base, and then move to the right base (outflow). This type of examination permits clinicians to think physiologically, i.e., following the inflow–outflow direction of the blood flow.

To most easily distinguish between the first and second heart sounds, one should take into account that there is a longer pause between S2 and S1 than between S1 and S2, caused by the fact that systole is shorter than diastole. S1 is also of longer duration and lower pitch, compared to the shorter duration and higher pitch of S2. In general, S1 is best heard at the heart's apex, and S2 is best auscultated over the aortic and pulmonic areas.

The normal heart sounds represent normally occurring phenomena in a normal heart, whereas cardiac pathologies can change the intensity and/or the timing of the occurrence of the sounds and/or even create new ones, often called "murmurs."

16.2.3 Abnormal Heart Sounds

Conditions that accentuate S1 sounds include mitral stenosis (most often), left-to-right shunts, hyperkinetic circulatory states, accelerated atrioventricular conduction, and/or tricuspid stenosis. A diminished S1 can be caused by mitral and tricuspid stenosis, moderate or severe aortic regurgitation, slow atrioventricular conduction, and/or hypocontractility states. A diminished S1 sound can also be observed in patients with thick chest walls, such as in individuals with excessively developed body musculature, obese patients, or in patients with emphysema.

Variability in the S1 sound can be observed in states causing variation in the velocity of atrioventricular valve closure, such as ventricular tachycardia, atrioventricular block, ventricular pacemakers, atrial fibrillation, and so on. An accentuated S2 is commonly detected in patients with: (1) diastolic or systolic hypertension; (2) aortic coarctation; (3) aortic dilation; (4) atherosclerosis of the aorta; and/or (5) pulmonary hypertension which is characterized by a loud pulmonary component of the second heart sound. A diminished S2 sound is detected most often in aortic valvular stenosis, pulmonic stenosis, and/or pulmonary emphysema.

Some degree of the splitting of the S2 sound can be normally heard during inspiration. Yet, abnormal or persistent S2 splitting is associated with: (1) delayed activation of the right ventricle; (2) prolonged right ventricular ejection time relative to left ventricular ejection time, like in pulmonic stenosis, mitral regurgitation, or ventricular septal defect; or (3) increased impedance of the pulmonary vasculature, as in massive pulmonary embolism or pulmonary hypertension. Persistent S2 splitting may also be observed in cases in which the aortic and pulmonic components of the second heart sound remain audible during both inspiration and expiration. This type of persistent splitting is often caused by a delay in the pulmonary component, such as that occurring in complete right bundle branch block, but it can also be caused by an early

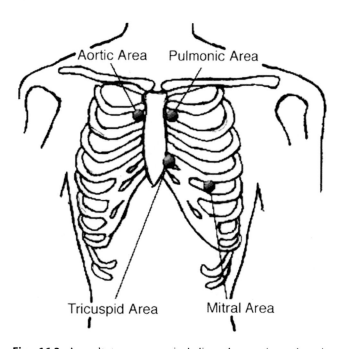

Fig. 16.3 Auscultatory areas, including the aortic, pulmonic, mitral, and tricuspid auscultation areas

timing of the aortic component often associated with mitral insufficiency. Changes in the duration of the split interval (greater with inspiration, lesser with exhalation) in the presence of both components define the split as persistent and not fixed.

Fixed splitting of S2 is commonly found in patients with atrial septal defect, severe pulmonic stenosis, or right ventricular failure. S2 fixed splitting is characterized by wide and persistent intervals between the aortic and pulmonary components, remaining unchanged during the respiratory cycle.

"Paradoxical splitting" refers to a reversed sequence of the semilunar valve (aortic and pulmonic) closures, with the pulmonary component (P2) preceding the aortic component (A2). Paradoxical splitting of S2 is caused by a delay in the A2, varying with the inspiratory cycle and can be caused by: (1) a complete left bundle branch block; (2) premature right ventricle contractions; (3) ventricular tachycardia; (4) severe aortic stenosis; (5) left ventricular outflow obstruction; (6) hypertrophic cardiomyopathy; (7) coronary artery disease; (8) myocarditis; and/or (9) congestive cardiomyopathy.

Normally, blood flow in the heart is laminar and does not produce vibrations. "Murmurs" are created whenever there is a pathology causing increased turbulent flow, often associated with abnormal shunts, obstructions, or even the reversing of flow. In other words, turbulent flow within the heart creates vibrations that can be heard as murmurs. The various murmurs are described both on the basis of appearance in relation to the cardiac cycle and on the basis of changes in features such as intensity (loudness), frequency (pitch), configuration (shape), quality, duration, and/or direction of radiation. For example, intensity or loudness can be graded from 1 to 6. Based on time of existence relative to the cardiac cycle, murmurs are classified as systolic, diastolic, or continuous. Depending on their life cycle during systole or diastole, they are further subclassified into early, mid, and late systolic or diastolic murmurs such that:

- Early systolic murmur begins with S1 and ends before the midsystole.
- Midsystolic murmur starts after S1 and ends before S2.
- Late systolic murmur begins in the middle of systole and ends at S2.
- Holosystolic murmur starts with S1 and continues for the duration of the whole systole.
- Early diastolic murmur begins with S2.
- Middiastolic murmur begins after S2.
- Late diastolic murmur begins just before S1.
- Continuous murmur continues during both systole and diastole.

Based on changes in intensity, murmurs are commonly described as: (1) crescendo, increasing in intensity; (2) decrescendo, decreasing in intensity; (3) crescendo–decrescendo, when the intensity of the murmur first increases and then decreases; or (4) plateau, the intensity of the murmur remains constant.

16.2.4 Dynamic Auscultation

The term dynamic auscultation refers to a technique of adjusting circulatory dynamics by means of respiration or various other planned physiological or pharmacological maneuvers and then determining their effects on the dynamics of the heart sounds and murmurs. Commonly altered variables that can affect sound and murmurs include: (1) changes in venous return affecting cardiac preload; (2) changes in systemic vascular resistance; (3) changes in contractility; (4) changes in heart rate or rhythm; and/or (5) maneuvers affecting pressure gradients within the heart. To date, diagnostic maneuvers frequently used for altering heart sounds include inspiration, expiration, exercise level, or body position (e.g., recumbent position, left semilateral position, standing up, sitting up, or leaning forward).

In general, spontaneous inspiration causes decreased intrathoracic pressure, increased venous return, increased right ventricular preload, and decreased pulmonary vascular resistance. Thus, modifying inspiration is used to increase the intensity of S3 and S4 gallops, tricuspid and pulmonic stenosis or regurgitation murmurs, or mitral and tricuspid clicks. Inspiration also causes some degree of splitting of S2, caused by prolonged right ventricular ejection. In contrast, expiration causes just the opposite— decreased venous return (preload) and decreased right-sided flow. Note that sounds and murmurs originating on the left side of the heart tend to be accentuated during expiration.

In addition, changes in a patient's positioning can affect heart sound intensity; this is caused by relative changes of ventricular preload, ventricular size, and movement of the heart closer to or farther from the chest wall. A recumbent position typically accentuates murmurs of mitral and tricuspid stenosis. Similarly, a left semilateral position accentuates left-sided S3 and S4, mitral opening snap, and mitral regurgitation murmurs. Standing will affect general hemodynamics by pooling blood in the lower extremities and decreasing heart filling pressure and ventricular size. Thus, standing up is clinically used to accentuate mitral and tricuspid clicks. Sitting up accentuates tricuspid valve opening snap, and sitting up and leaning forward are the best maneuvers for enhancing murmurs due to aortic and pulmonic regurgitation or aortic stenosis. Exercise causes increases in heart rate, shortens diastole, elevates left atrial pressure, and shortens the time for closure of the heart valves. Hence, physiological changes during exercise increase amplitudes of S1, S2, S3, S4, mitral opening snap, existing mitral regurgitation or stenosis, and/or patent ductus arteriosus murmur.

Two other pathological sounds, heard when auscultating the heart, are "clicks" and "opening snaps." Clicks are caused by the rapid movements of valvular structures. Systolic clicks are referred to as ejection or nonejection clicks, depending on their timing relative to systole. Ejection clicks, occurring early in systole, commonly indicate semilunar valve anomalies and, in rare conditions, great vessel lesions. Nonejection clicks are heard in mid to late systole and represent mitral (more often) or tricuspid valve prolapse. In contrast, a tricuspid valve opening snap is often heard when there is tricuspid valve stenosis and in conditions associated with increased blood flow across the tricuspid valve (e.g., presence of large atrial septal defect). Similarly, a mitral valve opening snap is caused by elevated left atrial pressure, resulting in rapid valve opening to the point of maximum excursion. Mitral valve opening snap is often associated with mitral stenosis and less often with ventricular septal defect, second or third degree atrioventricular block, patent ductus arteriosus, and hyperthyroidism. The mitral valve opening snap is similar in quality to normal heart sound and is often clinically confused with a splitting of S2.

16.2.5 Specific Murmurs

The murmur caused by aortic stenosis (Fig. 16.4) is characterized as a holosystolic crescendo–decrescendo murmur which is best heard at the aortic auscultation area. The high-velocity jet within the aortic root results in radiation of the murmur upward, to the right second intercostal space, and further into the neck. Although the murmur in the second right intercostal space is harsh, noisy, and impure, the murmur heard when auscultating over the left apical area can be pure and often

considered musical. The harsh "basal murmur" is believed to be caused by vibrations created when high-velocity blood jet is ejected through the aortic root. The musical second component of the aortic stenosis murmur originates from periodic high-frequency vibrations of the fibrocalcific aortic cusps and can be quite loud and heard even from a distance without an auditory aid. Murmurs of aortic stenoses are accentuated by expiration, sitting up, and/or leaning forward. The high-frequency apical midsystolic murmur of aortic stenosis should be distinguished from the high-frequency apical murmur of mitral regurgitation, a distinction that may be difficult or even impossible to detect, especially if the aortic component of the second heart sound is soft or absent. In such patients, echocardiography will likely be required to determine the relative cardiac pathophysiology; see Chapter 20 for more information on echocardiographic methods.

A murmur caused by pulmonary valve stenosis is a characteristic midsystolic murmur originating in the right side of the heart and best auscultated over the pulmonic auscultation area. This murmur begins after the first heart sound, rises to a peak in crescendo, and then decreases in slow decrescendo, finishing before a delayed or soft pulmonary component of the second heart sound. In general, the length and the profile of this murmur depend on the severity of the pulmonary valve obstruction.

The murmur caused by aortic insufficiency (Fig. 16.5) is an early decrescendo diastolic murmur originating in the left side of the heart and best heard over the aortic and pulmonic auscultation areas. This murmur begins with the aortic component of the second heart sound (S2). The intensity and configuration of such a murmur tend to reflect the volumes and rates of regurgitant flows. Radiation of this murmur to the right sternal border can signify aortic root dilation, often associated with Marfan's syndrome. In chronic aortic regurgitation, the aortic diastolic pressure always significantly exceeds the left ventricular diastolic pressure, so the decrescendo is subtle and yet the murmur is well heard throughout diastole. The diastolic murmur of acute severe aortic regurgitation differs from the chronic aortic regurgitation murmur primarily in that

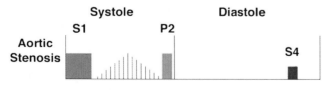

Fig. 16.4 Aortic stenosis murmur caused by stenotic aortic valve. Normally a holosystolic crescendo–decrescendo murmur is best heard at the aortic auscultatory area. P2 = pulmonic valve closure; S1 = first heart sound; S4 = fourth heart sound

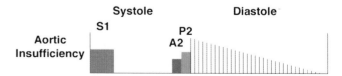

Fig. 16.5 Aortic insufficiency murmur. Early decrescendo diastolic murmur originating in the left side of the heart and best heard over the aortic and pulmonic auscultation areas. A2 = aortic valve closure; P2 = pulmonic valve closure; S1 = first heart sound

the diastolic murmur is relatively short. The short duration of the acute severe aortic regurgitation murmur is due to the fact that aortic diastolic pressure rapidly equilibrates with the rapidly rising diastolic pressure in the nondilated left ventricle. The aortic insufficiency murmur is accentuated during expiration, sitting up, or leaning forward.

A pulmonary regurgitation murmur is an early diastolic murmur originating from the right side of the heart. In this case, the second heart sound is often split with the murmur proceeding from its latter part; it is loud because of relatively high transvalvular pressure. The high pulmonary diastolic pressure generates high-velocity regurgitant flow resulting in a high-frequency blowing murmur that may last throughout diastole. Because of the persistent and significant difference between the pulmonary arterial and right ventricular diastolic pressures, the amplitude of this murmur is relatively uniform throughout most of the diastole.

Mitral stenosis murmur (Fig. 16.6) is caused by a stenotic mitral valve and is decrescendo–crescendo holodiastolic by nature. It is heard best at the mitral auscultation area and is typically accentuated both by exercise and assuming a recumbent position. Mitral stenosis murmur that lasts up to the first heart sound, even after long cardiac cycle, indicates that the stenosis is severe enough to generate a persistent gradient even at the end of long diastole.

The murmur caused by tricuspid stenosis is relatively middiastolic in origin and differs from the mitral stenosis middiastolic murmur in two important aspects: (1) the loudness of the tricuspid stenosis murmur increases with inspiration; and (2) to best hear this murmur, one auscultates over a relatively localized area along the left lower sternal border. Detectable inspiratory increases in loudness occur because of augmentation of the right ventricular volume, decreases in right ventricular diastolic pressure, and increases of the gradient and flow across the stenotic tricuspid valve. This murmur is best detected over the left lower sternal border, as it originates within the

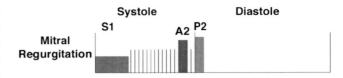

Fig. 16.7 Caused by an insufficiency of the mitral valve, the mitral regurgitation murmur is a systolic murmur best heard over the mitral auscultation area. A2 = aortic valve closure; P2 = pulmonic valve closure; S1 = first heart sound

inflow portion of the right ventricle and is then transmitted to the overlying chest wall.

Mitral regurgitation murmur (Fig. 16.7) is considered to be caused by an insufficiency of the mitral valve, and is a systolic murmur best heard at the mitral auscultation area; it is accentuated by exercise and left semilateral position. Acute severe mitral regurgitation is often accompanied by an early systolic murmur or holosystolic murmur that has a decrescendo pattern, which diminishes or ends before the second heart sound. The physiological mechanism responsible for this early systolic decrescendo murmur is acute severe regurgitation into a relatively normal size left atrium with limited distensibility. In such patients, the regurgitant flow is typically maximal early in systole and reaches minimum by late systole.

Another early systolic murmur is the "tricuspid regurgitation murmur" (Fig. 16.8), which is often associated with infective "endocarditis." The mechanisms responsible for the timing and configuration of this murmur are analogous to those described for mitral regurgitation. It is also a systolic murmur best heard over the tricuspid area and accentuated by inspiration.

The typical murmur associated with an atrial septal defect (Fig. 16.9) is also a systolic murmur which is caused by increased blood flow through the pulmonary valve, and thus is best heard over the pulmonic auscultation area. Most often, the atrial septal defect involves the fossa ovalis, which is midseptal in location, and is of the ostium secundum type (see Chapters 3 and 9 for more details). This type of defect is a true deficiency of the atrial septum and should not be confused with a patent foramen ovale. The magnitude of the left-to-right shunt through an atrial septal defect depends on the size of the defect and also the relative

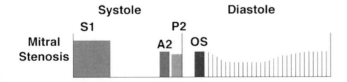

Fig. 16.6 Mitral stenosis murmur. Decrescendo–crescendo holodiastolic murmur, caused by a stenotic mitral valve. Best heard at the mitral auscultation area, this murmur is accentuated by exercise and by assuming a recumbent position. A2 = aortic valve closure; OS = opening snap; P2 = pulmonic valve closure; S1 = first heart sound

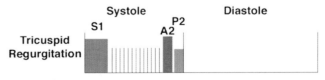

Fig. 16.8 The tricuspid regurgitation murmur is a systolic murmur best heard over the tricuspid area and is accentuated by inspiration. A2 = aortic valve closure; P2 = pulmonic valve closure; S1 = first heart sound

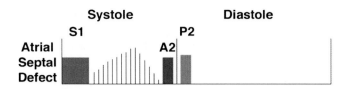

Fig. 16.9 The murmur associated with atrial septal defect is systolic and caused by increased blood flows through the pulmonic valve. Atrial sepal defect murmur is best heard over the pulmonic auscultation area. A2 = aortic valve closure; P2 = pulmonic valve closure; S1 = first heart sound

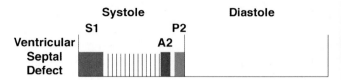

Fig. 16.11 Murmur associated with ventricular septal defect is systolic, caused by blood flow from the left to the right ventricle (or the right to the left ventricle in Eisenmenger's syndrome). A2 = aortic valve closure; P2 = pulmonic valve closure; S1 = first heart sound

compliance of the ventricles, as well as the relative resistance in both the pulmonary and systemic circulations. The increased pulmonary valve flow causes a delay (splitting) of the pulmonic component of the second heart sound.

The murmur associated with a patent ductus arteriosus (Fig. 16.10) is caused by an abnormal continuous turbulent flow through a patent ductus connecting the aorta with the main pulmonary artery. It is also considered a continuous "machinery murmur," heard in both systole and diastole, because aortic pressure is higher than the pressure in the pulmonary artery throughout the cardiac cycle. Other associated clinical findings in patients with patent ductus arteriosus include bounding peripheral pulses, wide pulse pressure, an infraclavicular and interscapular systolic murmur, precordial hyperactivity, hepatomegaly, bradycardia, episodes of apnea, and/or respiratory insufficiency.

The resultant murmur associated with a ventricular septal defect (Fig. 16.11) is systolic, with its intensity depending on the relative size of the defect. This ventricular sepal defect murmur is caused by abnormal blood flow from the left to the right ventricle or from the right to the left ventricle, as in Eisenmenger's syndrome. This latter syndrome is the reversing of the left-to-right shunt in patients with atrial septal defect, ventricular septal defect, or patent ductus arteriosus, all caused by increased pulmonary and right-sided pressures, secondary to increased pulmonary blood flow. This murmur is best heard over the mitral auscultation area located over the myocardial apex. Septal defects are commonly treated, sometimes noninvasively, thus eliminating these murmurs. See Chapter 34 for more details.

16.3 Recent Developments

The clinical application of cardiac auscultation has remained the same for centuries until recently, when some companies took auscultation to a whole new level by developing portable electronic stethoscopes. The central idea behind the electronic stethoscope is that human hearing is imperfect (or changes in its ability, i.e., aging) and can only detect a small fraction of the vast frequency range produced by the human heart. Therefore, recording the whole sound spectrum would provide novel information and thus increase our ability to diagnose pathology. More specifically, using electronic auscultation, heart sounds can be recorded for storage, later direct or remote playback or processing, such as e-mail, digital amplification, filtering for noise reduction, or electronic manipulation for accentuating particular sounds or noise. Today, electronic stethoscopes can easily record a phonocardiogram, providing visual sound representation, and can be viewed equally well by everyone thus eliminating errors associated with different hearing levels and/or clinical skills.

Currently several companies involved with digital stethoscope production include 3M Littmann, American Diagnostics Corp, Cardionics, Thinklabs, Welch Allyn, Doctors Research Group, and Andromed. Products from these companies typically employ proprietary technology and software, and therefore offer different filtering capabilities, presentation of information, size, weight, and/or ease of use.

It should be noted that an important part of each electronic stethoscope is the signal processing. There are several signal processing techniques employed, each providing slight advantages or disadvantages in obtaining different parts of the sound spectrum. Currently Fourier transform, short time Fourier transform, wavelet transform, and discrete wavelet transform are the incorporated sound processing techniques used in digital stethoscopes. Nevertheless, the main limitation of digital stethoscopy is the somewhat subjective nature of sound interpretation. Despite the superior quality of heart tones and murmurs, sounds obtained with digital stethoscopes have to be interpreted by physicians just like sounds obtained with acoustic stethoscopes. One way to deal with this

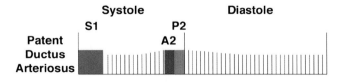

Fig. 16.10 Commonly associated with patent ductus arteriosus, this murmur is caused by a turbulent continuous flow through the ductus connecting the aorta with the main pulmonary artery. A2 = aortic valve closure; P2 = pulmonic valve closure; S1 = first heart sound

limitation is to run the digitally obtained and processed sound through an implemented algorithm to identify key parameters and yield relative diagnoses. In the near future, promising technology for achieving this diagnostic approach may be through the use of the artificial neural network, so that input data can be compared against learned data. The potential advantage of using an artificial neural network is that the network is adaptive and able to learn based on information fed to the system during a learning phase. For example, Zargis Medical recently developed Cardioscan, which is the first computer-aided medical device able to analyze heart sounds and identify suspected murmurs. Interestingly, Zargis has partnered with 3M Littmann and claims that using Cardioscan can reduce unnecessary referrals by 41%.

16.4 Summary

It remains the general consensus that even the most sophisticated electronic monitors cannot fully reduce the need for sound clinical skills like proper patient inspection, palpation, percussion, and auscultation. Furthermore, it is important to reinforce the need for a deep understanding of basic physiological principles when interpreting physical examination findings. In general, the application of technology in this area is viewed as helpful and can speed up decision making, but the knowledge of basic physiology and technology limitations can help us utilize these advancements to their maximum.

The primary purpose of this chapter was to familiarize the reader with the basic concepts of blood pressure, heart tones, and some common diagnoses. Many descriptions of the general scientific and clinical principles used in the chapter are simplified for clarity, along with their described underlying physiology and pathology; by no means is this chapter a complete review of the presented topics. There are many medical books dedicated to each topic alone and readers are strongly encouraged to further research sources and review in-depth information of interest.

General References and Suggested Reading

Faulconer A, Keys TE, eds. Foundations of anesthesiology, Vols. I and II. Park Ridge, IL: The Wood Library–Museum of Anesthesiology, 1993.

McVicker JT. Blood pressure measurement—does anyone do it right?: An assessment of the reliability of equipment in use and the measurement techniques of clinicians. J Fam Plann Reprod Health Care 2001;27:163–4.

O'Brien E, Pickering T, Asmar R, et al. Working group on blood pressure monitoring of the European Society of Hypertension, international protocol for validation of blood pressure measuring devices in adults. Blood Press Monit 2002;7:3–17.

Miller RD, Cucchiara RF, eds. Anesthesia. 4th ed, Vols. I and II. New York, NY: Churchill Livingstone, 1994.

Barash RG, Cullen BF, Stoelting RK, eds. Clinical anesthesia. 4th ed. Philadelphia, PA: Lippincott Williams & Wilkins, 2001.

Stoelting RK. Pharmacology and physiology in anesthetic practice. 3rd ed. Philadelphia, PA: Lippincott–Raven, 1999.

Kaplan JA, Reich DL, Konstadt SN, eds. Cardiac anesthesia. 4th ed. Philadelphia, PA: W.B. Saunders, 1999.

Braunwald E, ed. Heart disease: A textbook of cardiovascular medicine. 5th ed. Philadelphia, PA: W.B. Saunders, 1997.

Mohrman DE, Heller LJ, eds. Cardiovascular physiology. 4th ed. New York, NY: McGraw-Hill, 1997.

Chapter 17
Basic ECG Theory, 12-Lead Recordings and Their Interpretation

Anthony Dupre, Sarah Vieau and Paul A. Iaizzo

Abstract The recorded electrocardiogram (ECG) remains as one of the most vital monitors of a patient's cardiovascular status and is used today in nearly every clinical setting. This chapter discusses the ECG as a measure of how the electrical activity of the heart changes over time, as action potentials within each myocyte propagate throughout the heart during each cardiac cycle. By utilizing the resultant electrical field present in the body, electrodes can be placed around the heart to measure potential differences as the heart depolarizes and repolarizes. Furthermore, various techniques for obtaining ECG data are presented.

Electrocardiography has progressed rapidly since it was first employed back in the early 1900s. New instruments that are smaller and more sophisticated as well as innovative analysis techniques are continually being developed. The trend has been toward developing smaller, easier-to-use devices that can gather and remotely send a wealth of information to use for patient diagnosis and treatment.

Keywords Electrocardiogram · ECG waveform · 12-Lead ECG · ECG placement · ECG recording devices · Holter monitor · Loop recorder

17.1 The Electrocardiogram

An "electrocardiogram" (ECG) is a measure of how the electrical activity of the heart changes over time, as action potentials within each myocyte propagate throughout the heart as a whole during each cardiac cycle. In other words, the ECG is not a direct measure of the cellular depolarization and repolarization, but rather the recording of the cumulative signals produced by populations of cells eliciting changes in their membrane potentials at a given point in time. The ECG provides specific waveforms of electrical differences when the atria and ventricles depolarize and repolarize.

The human body can be considered, for the purposes of an ECG, as a large volume conductor. It is filled with tissues surrounded by a conductive medium in which the heart is suspended. During the cardiac cycle, the heart contracts in response to action potentials moving along the chambers of the heart. As this normally occurs, one part of the cardiac tissue is depolarized and another part is at rest, or polarized. This results in a charge separation, or dipole, which is illustrated in Fig. 17.1. The moving dipole causes current flow in the surrounding body fluids between the ends of the heart, resulting in fluctuating electric fields throughout the body. This is much like the electric field that would result, for example, if a common battery was suspended in a saltwater solution (an electrically conductive medium). The opposite poles of the battery would cause current flow in the surrounding fluid, creating an electric field that could be detected by electrodes placed in the solution. A similar electrical field around the heart can be detected using electrodes attached to the skin. The intensity of the voltage detected depends on the orientation of the electrodes with respect to that of the dipole ends. The amplitude of the signal is proportional to the mass of the tissue involved in creating that dipole at any given time. Typically, one employs electrodes on the surface of the skin to detect the voltage of this electrical field, which gives rise to the "electrocardiogram."

It is important to note that, because the surface ECG is measured on the skin, any potential differences within the body will have an effect on the resultant electrical fields that are being detected. This is why it is important for diagnostic purposes that, while recording an ECG, patients should remain as still as possible. Movements from skeletal muscle activation (electromyograms, EMGs) will contribute to the changes in voltages detected using electrodes on the surface of the body. A "resting

S. Vieau (✉)
Medtronic, Inc., 11386 Riverview Rd., Hanover, MN 55341, USA
e-mail: sarah.a.vieau@medtronic.com

P.A. Iaizzo (ed.), *Handbook of Cardiac Anatomy, Physiology, and Devices*, DOI 10.1007/978-1-60327-372-5_17,

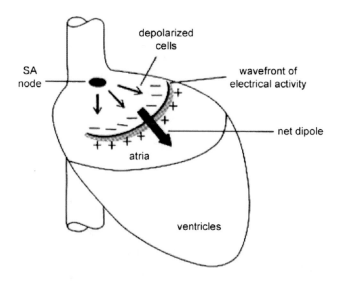

Fig. 17.1 After conduction begins at the sinoatrial node, cells in the atria begin to depolarize. This creates an electrical wavefront that moves down toward the ventricles, with polarized cells at the front, followed by depolarized cells behind. The separation of charge results in a dipole across the heart (with the large *black arrow* showing its direction). Modified from Mohrman and Heller (2003). SA = sinoatrial

ECG" is recorded when the monitored patient is essentially motionless; this type of ECG signal is discussed in the majority of this chapter.

17.2 ECG Devices

The invention of electrocardiography has had an immeasurable impact on the field of cardiology. It has provided insights into the structure and function of both healthy and diseased hearts. ECG has evolved into a powerful diagnostic tool for heart disease including the detection of arrhythmias, myocardial infarction, and hypertrophy, among others. The use of ECG has become a standard of care in cardiology, and new advances using this technology are continually being made.

17.3 History of the ECG

The discovery of intrinsic electrical activity of the heart can be traced back to as early as the 1840s. In 1842, the Italian physicist Carlo Matteucci first reported that an electrical current accompanies each heartbeat. Soon after, the German physiologist Emil DuBois-Reymond described the first action potential that accompanies muscle contraction. Rudolph von Koelliker and Heinrich

Miller recorded the first cardiac action potential using a galvanometer in 1856. Subsequently, the invention of the capillary electrometer in the early 1870s by Gabriel Lippmann led to the first recording of a human electrocardiogram by Augustus D. Waller.

The capillary electrometer is a thin glass tube containing a column of mercury that sits above sulfuric acid. With varying electrical potentials, the mercury meniscus moves and this can be observed through a microscope. Using this capillary electrometer, Waller was the first to show that the electrical activity precedes the mechanical contraction of the heart. He was also the first to show that the electrical activity of the heart can be seen by applying electrodes to both hands, or to one hand and one foot. Waller's work was the first description of "limb leads." Interestingly, Waller would often publicly demonstrate his experiments with his dog Jimmy who would stand in jars of saline during the recording of the ECG.

A major breakthrough in cardiac electrocardiography came with the invention of the string galvanometer by Willem Einthoven in 1901. He reported the first electrocardiogram using his string galvanometer the following year. Einthoven's string galvanometer consisted of a massive electromagnet with a thin silver-coated string stretched across it; electric currents that passed through the string would cause it to move from side to side in the magnetic field generated by the electromagnet. The oscillations in the string would provide information regarding the strength and direction of the electrical current. The deflections of the string were then magnified using a projecting microscope and were recorded on a moving photographic plate (Fig. 17.2). Years earlier, utilizing recordings from a capillary electrometer, Einthoven was also the first to label the deflections of the heart's electrical activity as P, Q, R, S, and T.

In 1912, Einthoven made another major contribution to the field of cardiac electrophysiology by deriving a mathematical relationship between the direction and the size of the deflections recorded by the three limb leads. This hypothesis became known as Einthoven's Triangle. The standard three limb leads were used for three decades before Frank Wilson described unipolar leads and the precordial lead configuration. The 12-lead ECG configuration used today consists of the standard limb leads of Einthoven and the precordial and unipolar limb leads based on Wilson's work (see the following discussion for details on these recordings).

Following Einthoven's invention of the string galvanometer, electrocardiography quickly became a research tool for both physiologists and cardiologists. Much of the current knowledge involving arrhythmias was developed using ECG. In 1906, Einthoven published the first results of ECG tracings of atrial fibrillation, atrial flutter,

Fig. 17.2 Willem Einthoven's string galvanometer consisted of a massive electromagnet with a thin silver-coated string stretched across it. Electric currents passing through the string caused it to move from side to side in the magnetic field generated by the electromagnet. The oscillations in the string provided information on the strength and direction of the electrical current. The deflections of the string were then magnified using a projecting microscope and recorded on a moving photographic plate. Reprinted with permission from NASPE-Heart Rhythm Society History Project

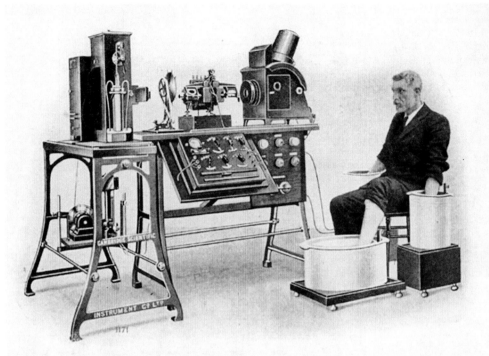

PHOTOGRAPH OF A COMPLETE ELECTROCARDIOGRAPH, SHOWING THE MANNER IN WHICH THE ELECTRODES ARE ATTACHED TO THE PATIENT, IN THIS CASE THE HANDS AND ONE FOOT BEING IMMERSED IN JARS OF SALT SOLUTION

ventricular premature contractions, ventricular bigeminy, atrial enlargement, and induced heart block in a dog. Einthoven was awarded the Nobel Prize for his work and inventions in 1924.

Thomas Lewis was one of the pioneering cardiologists who utilized the capabilities of the ECG to further scientific knowledge of arrhythmias. His findings were summarized in his books *The Mechanism of the Heart Beat* and *Clinical Disorders of the Heart Beat* published in 1911 and 1912, respectively. He also published over 100 research papers describing his work. Lewis was also the first to use the following terms: sinoatrial node, pacemaker, premature contractions, paroxysmal tachycardia, and atrial fibrillation.

Myocardial infarction and angina pectoris were also extensively studied with ECG using the string galvanometer device. Numerous clinical investigators also studied the changes within the ECG signal that were associated with the onset of myocardial infarction in both animals and humans. By the 1930s, the characteristic features of the ECG for the diagnostic indications of myocardial infarction had been identified, and later on, the connection between angina pectoris and coronary occlusion was made. While studying electrocardiographic changes accompanying angina pectoris, Francis Wood and Charles Wolferth performed the first use of the exercise electrocardiographic stress test. Their use of exercise for ECG

analyses stemmed from the observation that many of their patients experienced angina only during physical exertion. This technique was not routinely used, however, since it was thought to be very dangerous. Nevertheless, with these advances in protocols and technologies, the ECG emerged as a common diagnostic tool for physicians.

ECG equipment has come a long way since Einthoven's string galvanometer. The Cambridge Scientific Instrument Company in London was the first to manufacture this instrument back in 1905. It was massive, weighing in at 600 pounds. A telephone cable was used to transmit the electrical signals from a hospital over a mile away to Einthoven's laboratory. A few years later, Max Edelman of Cambridge Scientific Instrument Company manufactured a smaller version of the instrument (Fig. 17.3). However, it was not until the 1920s that bedside machines became available. A few years later, a "portable" version was manufactured in which the instrument was contained in two wooden cases, each weighing close to 50 pounds. In 1935, the Sanborn Company manufactured an even smaller version of the unit that weighed only about 25 pounds.

The use of ECG in a nonclinical setting became possible in 1949 with Norman Jeff Holter's invention of the Holter monitor. The first version of this instrument was a 75-pound backpack that could continuously record the ECG and transmit these signals via radio. Subsequent

Fig. 17.3 A diagram of Cambridge Scientific Instrument Company's smaller version of the string galvanometer. Reprinted with permission from NASPE-Heart Rhythm Society History Project

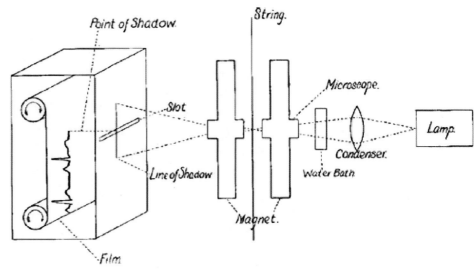

Diagrammatic representation of the electrocardiograph.

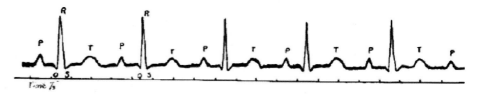

A diagrammatic electrocardiogram of a normal rhythm. The auricular impulse is shown by the upright curve *P*, and the ventricular impulse by the complicated curve or "complex" *QRST*, the beginning and end of which mark the beginning and end of systole.

versions of such systems have been dramatically reduced in size, and now a digital recording of the signal is used. Today, miniaturized systems (Fig. 17.4) allow patients to

be monitored over longer periods of time (usually 24 h) to help diagnose any problems with rhythm or ischemic heart disease.

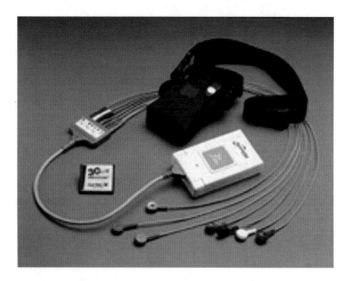

Fig. 17.4 A version of the Holter monitor that is used currently. The one seen here is manufactured by Medical Solutions, Inc. (Maple Grove, MN)

17.4 The ECG Waveform

As an ECG is recorded, a signal of voltage versus time is produced, which is normally displayed in millivolts (mV) versus seconds. A typical Lead II ECG waveform is shown in Fig. 17.5. For this recording, the negative electrode was placed on the right wrist and the positive electrode placed on the left ankle, a standard Lead II ECG. As such, one can observe a series of peaks and waves that correspond to ventricular or atrial depolarization and repolarization, with each segment of the signal representing a different event within the cardiac cycle.

The cardiac cycle begins with the firing of the sinoatrial node in the right atrium. This firing is not detected by the ECG because the sinoatrial node is not composed of an adequately large quantity of cells to

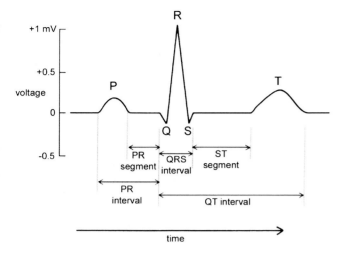

Fig. 17.5 A typical ECG waveform for one cardiac cycle, measured from the Lead II position. The P-wave denotes atrial depolarization, the QRS ventricular depolarization, and the T-wave denotes ventricular repolarization. The events on the waveform occur on a scale of hundreds of milliseconds. Modified from Mohrman and Heller (2003)

create an electrical potential with an amplitude high enough to be recorded with distal electrodes. The depolarization of the sinoatrial node is conducted rapidly throughout both the right and the left atria, giving rise to the P-wave. This represents the depolarization of both atria and the onset of atrial contraction; the P-wave is normally around 80–100 milliseconds (ms) in duration. As the P-wave ends, the atria are thus depolarized and this relates to the initiation of contraction. The signal then returns to baseline while action potentials (not large enough to be detected) spread through the atrioventricular node and bundle of His. Then, roughly 200 ms after the beginning of the P-wave, the right and left ventricles begin to depolarize resulting in the recordable QRS complex, which is approximately 100 ms in duration. The first negative deflection (if present) is the Q-wave, the large positive deflection is the R-wave, and if there is a negative deflection after the R-wave, it is called the S-wave. As the QRS complex ends, the ventricles are completely depolarized and are beginning contraction. Importantly, the exact shape of the QRS complex depends on the placement of electrodes from which the signals are recorded.

Simultaneous with the QRS complex, atrial contraction has ended and the atria are repolarizing. However, the effect of this global atrial repolarization is sufficiently masked by the much larger amount of tissue involved in ventricular depolarization, and is thus not normally detected in the ECG. Toward the end of ventricular contraction, the ECG signal returns

to baseline. The ventricles then repolarize after contraction, giving rise to the T-wave. The T-wave is normally the last detected potential in the cardiac cycle, thus it is followed by the P-wave of the next cycle, repeating the process.

It is clear that the QRS complex has a much higher and shorter duration peak than either the P- or T-waves. This is due to the fact that ventricular depolarization simultaneously occurs over a greater mass of cardiac tissue (i.e., a greater number of myocytes depolarizing at nearly the same time) and the fact that ventricular depolarization is much more synchronized than either atrial depolarization or ventricular repolarization. For additional details relative to the types of action potential that occur in various regions of the heart, the reader is referred to Chapter 11. It is important to note that deflections in the ECG waveform represent the changes only in electrical activity and have different time courses of generalized cardiac contractions or relaxations that take place on a slightly longer timescale. Figure 17.6 details certain points on the ECG waveform and how they relate to other events in the heart during the cardiac cycle.

Lastly, the ECG waveform in some individuals may show a potential referred to as the U-wave. Its presence is not fully understood, but is considered by some to be caused by late repolarization of the Purkinje system. If detected, the U-wave will be toward the end of the T-wave and has the same polarity (positive deflection). However, it has a much shorter amplitude and usually ascends more rapidly than it descends (which is the opposite of the T-wave).

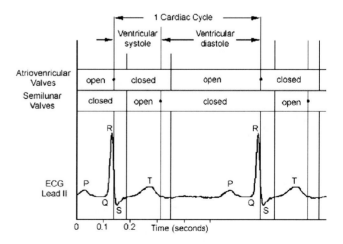

Fig. 17.6 A typical Lead II ECG waveform is compared to the timing of atrioventricular and semilunar valve activity, along with which segments of the cardiac cycle the ventricles are in systole/diastole. ECG = electrocardiogram

17.5 Measuring the ECG

The ECG is typically measured from electrodes placed on the surface of the skin; this can be done by placing a pair of electrodes directly on the skin and then monitoring the potential difference between them, as these signals are transmitted throughout the body. The detected waveform features depend not only on the amount of cardiac tissue involved but also on the orientation of the electrodes with respect to the major dipoles in the heart. Recall that the ECG waveform will look different when measured from different electrode positions, and typically an ECG is obtained using a number of different electrode locations (e.g., limb leads or precordial) or configurations (unipolar, bipolar, modified bipolar), which have been standardized by universal application of certain conventions.

17.5.1 Bipolar Limb Leads

Today, the three most commonly employed lead positions are referred to as Leads I, II, and III. Imagine the torso of the body as an equilateral triangle as illustrated in Fig. 17.7. This forms what is known as "Einthoven's Triangle" (named after the Dutch scientist who first described it). Electrodes are placed at each of the vertices of the triangle, and a single ECG trace (either Lead I, II, or III) is measured along the corresponding side of the triangle using the electrodes at each end. Because each lead uses one electrode on either side of the heart, Leads I, II, and III are also referred to as the bipolar leads. The

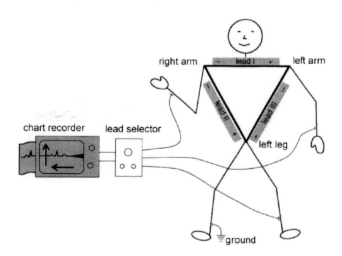

Fig. 17.7 The limb leads are attached to the corners of Einthoven's Triangle on the body. Each lead uses two of these locations for a positive and negative lead. The "+" and "−" signs indicate the orientation of the polarity conventions. Modified from Mohrman and Heller (2003)

positive and negative signs shown in Fig. 17.7 indicate the polarity of each lead measurement and are notably considered as the universal convention. The vertices of the triangle can be considered to be at the wrists and left ankle for electrode placement, as well as the shoulders and lower torso.

As an example, if the Lead II ECG trace shows an upward deflection, it would mean that the voltage measured at the left leg (or bottom apex of the triangle) is more positive than the voltage measured at the right arm (or upper right apex of the triangle). One time point where this happens is during the P-wave. Imagine the orientation of the heart as shown in Fig. 17.8, with the action potential propagation across the atria creating a dipole pointed downward and to the left side of the body. This can be represented as an arrow (Fig. 17.8) showing the magnitude and direction of the dipole in the heart. This dipole would, overall, create a more positive voltage reading at the left ankle electrode than at the right wrist electrode, thus eliciting the positive deflection of the P-wave on the Lead II ECG.

Now, imagine how that same action potential propagation would appear on the other lead placements, Leads I and III, if placed at the center of Einthoven's Triangle (Fig. 17.8, right side). One can think of each of these lead placements as viewing the electrical dipole from three different directions—Lead I from the top, Lead II from the lower right side of the body, and Lead III from the lower left side—all looking at the heart along the frontal plane. In this example, the atrial depolarization creates a dipole that gives a positive deflection for all three leads, because the arrow's projection onto each lead (in other words, measuring the cardiac dipole from each lead) results in the positive end of the dipole pointed more toward the positive end of the lead than toward the negative end. This is why atrial depolarization (P-wave) always appears as a *positive deflection*, but a different wave *magnitude*, for Leads I, II, and III. Ventricular depolarization, however, is a bit more complicated and results in various directions of the Q- and S-wave potentials depending on which lead trace is being utilized for recording.

17.5.2 Electrical Axis of the Heart

The direction and magnitude of the overall dipole of the heart at any instant is also known as the heart's "electrical axis," which is a vector originating in the center of Einthoven's Triangle such that the direction of the dipole is typically assessed in degrees. The convention for this is to use a horizontal line across the top of Einthoven's Triangle as 0° and move clockwise downward (pivoting

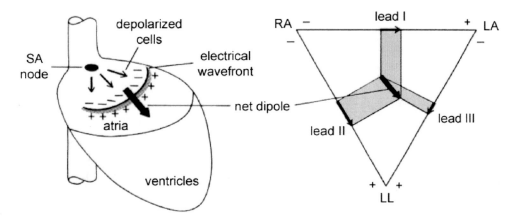

Fig. 17.8 The net dipole occurring in the heart at any one point in time is detected by each lead (I, II, and III) in a different way, due to the different orientations of each lead set relative to the dipole in the heart. In this example, the projection of the dipole on all three leads is positive (the *arrow* is pointing toward the positive end of the lead), which gives a positive deflection on the ECG during the P-wave.

Furthermore, Lead II detects a larger amplitude signal than Lead III does from the same net dipole (i.e., the net dipole projects a *larger arrow* on the Lead II side of the *triangle* than on the Lead III side). Figure from Mohrman and Heller (2003). LA = left arm; LL = left leg; RA = right arm; SA = sinoatrial

on the negative end of Lead I) as the positive direction. The electrical axis changes direction throughout the cardiac cycle as different parts of the heart depolarize and repolarize in different directions. The top row of panels in Fig. 17.9 shows the dipole spreading across the heart during a typical cardiac cycle, beginning with atrial depolarization. The bottom row shows the corresponding deflections on each ECG lead (I, II, and III). Note that, at certain points, the electrical axis of the heart may give opposite deflections on the different ECG leads.

As can be observed in Fig. 17.9, depolarization begins at the sinoatrial node in the right atrium, forming the P-wave. The atria depolarize downward and to the left, toward the ventricles, followed by a slight delay at the atrioventricular node before the ventricles depolarize. The initial depolarization in the ventricles normally occurs on the left side of the septum, creating a dipole pointed slightly down and to the right. This gives a negative deflection of the Q-wave for Leads I and II, however it is positive in Lead III. Depolarization then continues to spread down the ventricles toward the apex, which is when the most tissue mass is depolarizing at the same time, with the same orientation. This gives the large positive deflection of the R-wave for all three leads. Ventricular depolarization then continues to spread through the cardiac wall and finally finishes in the left ventricular wall. This results in a positive deflection for Leads I and II; however, Lead III shows a lower R-wave amplitude along with a negative S-wave deflection. After a sustained depolarized period (the S–T segment), the ventricles then repolarize. However, this occurs in the opposite anatomical direction of depolarization. The arrow in Fig. 17.9 represents the electrical axis of the heart (or the dipole) and

does not necessarily show the direction in which the repolarization wave is moving. Thus, even though the wave is moving from epicardium to endocardium, the dipole (and therefore the electrical axis) remains in the same orientation as during depolarization. Therefore, the T-wave is also a positive deflection on Leads I and II and negative (if present) on Lead III. The ventricles are then repolarized returning the signal to its baseline potential.

During the cardiac cycle, the electrical axis of the heart is always changing in both magnitude and direction. The average of all instantaneous electrical axis vectors gives rise to the "mean electrical axis" of the heart. Most commonly, it is taken as the average dipole direction during the QRS complex, being that this is the highest and most synchronized signal of the overall ECG waveform. Typically, to find the mean electrical axis, area calculations from under the QRS complexes from at least two leads are needed. However, it is easier and more commonly determined by an estimate using the deflection (positive or negative) and height of the R-wave. Figure 17.10 shows a simple example of using Leads I and II to find the electrical axis of the heart. It should be noted that, in the normal human heart, the electrical axis of the heart corresponds to the anatomical orientation of the heart (from base to apex). Also see Chapter 2 for more details on the heart orientation.

17.5.3 The 12-Lead ECG

Leads I, II, and III are the bipolar limb leads that have been discussed thus far. There are three other leads that use the limb electrodes, called the "unipolar limb leads."

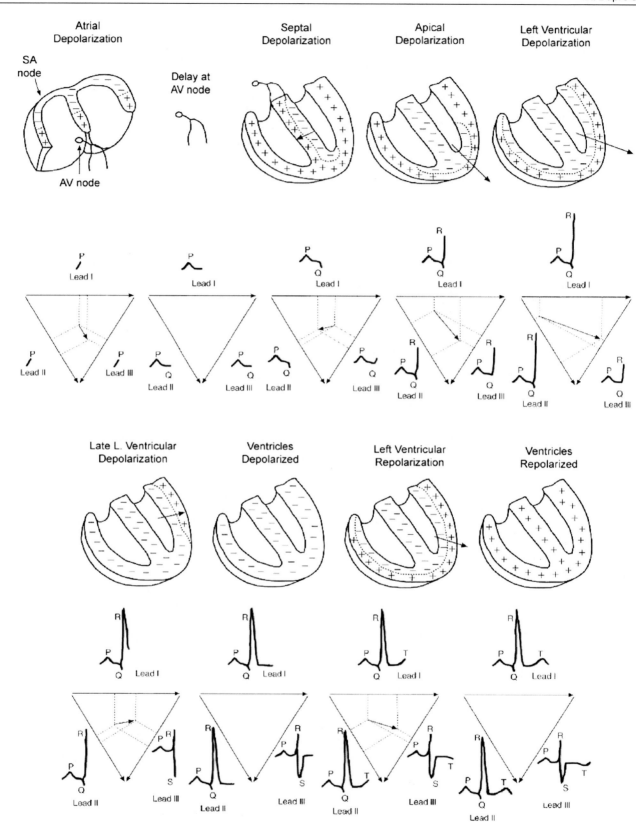

Fig. 17.9 The net dipole of the heart (indicated by the *arrow*) as it progresses through one cardiac cycle, beginning with firing of the sinoatrial node and finishing with the complete repolarization of the ventricular walls. The *bottom row* of panels displays how the net dipole is detected by each of the three bipolar limb Leads I, II, and III. Note the change in direction and magnitude of the dipole during one complete cardiac cycle. Modified from Johnson (2003)

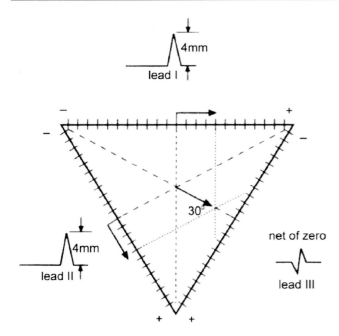

Fig. 17.10 The amplitudes of the Lead I and II R-waves are plotted along the corresponding leg of Einthoven's Triangle starting at the midpoint and drawn with a length equal to the height of the R-wave (units used to measure the amplitude can be arbitrary, since the direction, not the magnitude, of the axis is important). The direction of the plot is toward the positive end of the lead if the R-wave has a positive deflection and negative if it has a negative deflection. Perpendiculars from each point are then drawn into the triangle and meet at a point. A *line* drawn from the center of the *triangle* to this point gives the angle of the mean electrical axis. Since the normal activation sequence in the heart generally goes down and left, this is also the direction of the mean electrical axis in most people. The normal range is anywhere from 0° to +90°. Modified from Johnson (2003)

Each of these leads uses an electrode pair that consists of one limb electrode and a "neutral reference lead" that is created by hooking up the other two limb locations to the negative lead of the ECG amplifier. In other words, each lead has its positive end at the corresponding limb lead and runs toward the heart where its "negative" end is located, directly between the other two limb leads. These are referred to as the "augmented unipolar limb leads." The voltage recorded between the left-arm limb lead and the neutral reference lead is called Lead aVL; similarly, the right-arm limb lead is aVR, and the left-leg lead is aVF (Fig. 17.11).

The remaining 6 of the 12 lead recordings are the chest leads. These leads are also unipolar; however, they uniquely measure electrical activity in the traverse plane instead of the frontal plane. Similar to the unipolar limb leads, a neutral reference lead is "created," but this time using all three limb leads connected to the negative ECG lead, which basically puts it in the center of the chest. The six positive, or "exploring," electrodes are placed as shown in Fig. 17.12 (around the chest) and are labeled V1 through V6 (V designates voltage). These chest leads are also known as the "precordial" leads. Figure 17.12A shows a simple cross-section (looking superior to inferior) of the chest, depicting the relative position of each electrode in the traverse plane. Figure 17.12A also shows a typical waveform obtained from each of these leads. In summary, three bipolar limb leads, three unipolar limb leads, and six chest leads make up the 12-lead ECG.

The 12-lead ECG is widely used to evaluate cardiac electrical activity since it provides multiple "views" of how

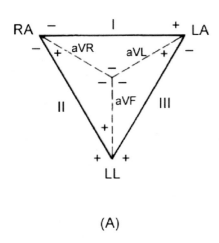

(A)

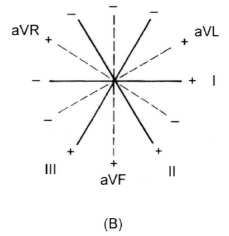

(B)

Fig. 17.11 (A) The augmented leads are shown on Einthoven's Triangle along with the other three frontal plane leads (I, II, and III). (B) A hex-axial reference system for all six limb leads is shown, with *solid* and *dashed lines* representing the bipolar and unipolar leads, respectively. Modified from Mohrman and Heller (2003).

aVF = voltage recorded between left-leg lead and neutral reference lead; aVL = voltage recorded between left-arm limb lead and neutral reference lead; aVR = voltage recorded between right-arm limb lead and neutral reference lead; LA = left arm; LL = left leg; RA = right arm

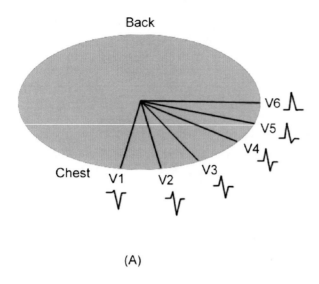

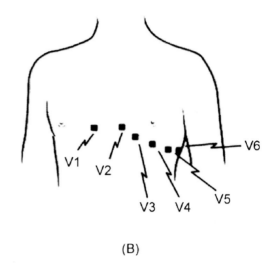

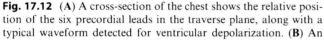

(A)   (B)

Fig. 17.12 (**A**) A cross-section of the chest shows the relative position of the six precordial leads in the traverse plane, along with a typical waveform detected for ventricular depolarization. (**B**) An anterior view of the chest shows common placement of each precordial lead, V1 through V6

electrical conduction moves through the heart. It can be used to help determine the location of many cardiac abnormalities including: (1) conduction disturbances (such as bundle branch block); (2) myocardial infarction or ischemia; (3) atrial or ventricular hypertrophy; or (4) electrolyte disturbances and drug effects.

17.6 Some Basic Interpretation of the ECG Trace

Analyses of the ECG waveforms and mean electrical axes are quite useful in the clinical setting. The ECG is considered to be one of the most important monitors of a patient's cardiovascular status and can be used for measurements as basic as heart rate. Most monitoring devices used today include automated systems that detect changes in durations between subsequent QRS complexes.

Of clinical importance in the ECG waveform are several parameters (regions), which include: the P–R interval, the QRS interval, the S–T segment, and the Q–T interval (Fig. 17.5). The P–R interval is measured from the beginning of the P-wave to the beginning of the QRS complex and is normally 120–200 ms long. This is a measure of the time it takes for an impulse to travel from sinoatrial excitation through the atria and atrioventricular node to the general onset of ventricular depolarization. The QRS interval measures how long the process of overall ventricular depolarization takes and is normally 60–100 ms. The S–T segment is the period of time when the ventricles are completely depolarized and is

contracting and is measured from the S-wave to the beginning of the T-wave. The Q–T interval is measured from the beginning of the QRS complex to the end of the T-wave; this is the time segment from when the ventricles begin their depolarization to the time when they have repolarized to their resting potentials and is normally about 400 ms in duration.

Determination of the P–R intervals provides useful information as to whether a patient may be eliciting some degree of heart block. Elongated P–R intervals (longer than ~200 ms) serve as a good indication that conduction through the atrioventricular node is slowed to some degree (first-degree heart block). Conduction in the atrioventricular node may even intermittently fail, which would elicit a P-wave without a subsequent QRS complex before the next P-wave (second-degree heart block). An ECG trace showing P-waves and QRS complexes beating independently of each other indicates that the atrioventricular node has ceased to transmit impulses at all (third-degree heart block). For information on atrioventricular blocks, see Chapter 11 or 27.

A wide QRS complex (greater than 100 ms) can indicate conduction blocks or delays in the bundle branches or Purkinje fibers that run through the ventricle. Delays or alterations in the conduction pathway through the ventricles can impact ventricular contraction and possibly cause dysynchrony between the right and left ventricles. This, in turn, will negatively impact cardiac function and hemodynamics.

Prolonged Q–T intervals (which are usually not more than 40% of the cardiac cycle length) are normally an indication of delayed repolarization of the cardiomyocytes, possibly caused by irregular opening or closing of sodium or potassium channels. A long Q–T interval may indicate that a patient is at risk of developing a ventricular tachyarrhythmia (see Chapter 27 for more details).

Another very clinically important interval is the S–T segment. Depression of the S–T segment (below the baseline) can indicate a regional ventricular ischemia. S–T segment elevations or depressions can also be used as an indication of many other abnormalities, including myocardial infarction, coronary artery disease, and/or pericarditis. For patients with established coronary artery disease, it is important to compare current ECG recordings to historical ones to establish if any new regions of ischemia or infarction exist.

Estimation of the electrical axis is also a helpful diagnostic measure. In the case of left ventricular hypertrophy, the left side of the heart is enlarged with greater tissue mass. This could cause the dipole during ventricular contraction to shift to the left. Much more can be said about specific interpretations of the intervals and segments that make up the ECG waveform. For more details on changes in ECG patterns associated with various clinical situations, the reader is referred to Chapters 11 and 26.

17.7 Lead Placement in the Clinical Setting

In a clinical setting, all 12 leads may not be displayed at the same time and, most often, not all leads are being measured simultaneously. A common setup used is a five-wire system consisting of two arm leads, which are actually placed on the shoulder areas, two leg leads placed low where the legs join the torso, and one chest lead. This arrangement allows one to display any of the limb leads (I, II, III, aVR, aVL, and aVF) and one of the precordial leads, depending on where the chest electrode is placed. Figure 17.13 shows the positioning of these five electrodes on the patient's body.

It should be noted that the exact anatomical placement of the leads is very important to obtain accurate ECG traces for clinical evaluations; moving an electrode even slightly away from its correct position could cause dramatically different traces and possibly lead to misdiagnosis. A slight exception to this rule is the limb leads, which do not necessarily need to be placed at the distal portion of the limb as described earlier. However, the limb leads need to be, for the most part, equidistant from each other relative to the heart for determination of the electrical axis to be accurate.

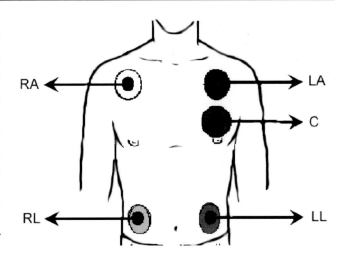

Fig. 17.13 Placement of the common five-wire ECG electrode system leads on the shoulders, chest, and torso. The chest electrode is placed according to the desired precordial lead position. C = chest; LA = left arm; LL = left leg; RA = right arm; RL = right leg

17.8 Computer Analyses

The use of computers for the analysis of ECG began in the 1960s. In 1961, Hubert Pipberger described the first computer analysis of ECG signals, an analysis that recognized basic abnormal activity. Computer-assisted ECG analyses were introduced into the general clinical setting in the 1970s. The use of computers, microcomputers, and microelectronic circuits has had a huge impact on electrocardiography. The size of the equipment has been drastically reduced to pocket size or even smaller for some applications. This has allowed broader deployment of continuous monitoring of patients over much longer time periods, which has greatly helped in the diagnosis of patients with infrequent symptoms (paroxysmal).

Computer programs can also provide summaries of information recorded from the ECG, including heart rates, multiple types of arrhythmias, and specific variations in QRS, ST, QT, or T patterns. Additionally, there are several computer analysis techniques that have been developed to further identify patients with cardiac dysfunction and previous myocardial infarctions that may be at risk for sudden death, e.g., signal-averaged ECG, microvolt T-wave alternans, and heart rate variability. Signal-averaged electrocardiography is a technique that uses computer analysis to identify late potentials appearing at the end of the QRS complex. Additionally, these late potentials have been associated with an increased risk of ventricular arrhythmias. Microvolt T-wave alternans is another method that may be used to identify patients at risk of ventricular arrhythmias. This technique measures the presence of small changes in T-wave amplitude that occur on an alternating beat-to-beat basis. Similarly, heart rate variability analysis measures subtle variations in ventricular rate to assess autonomic status (modulation of heart rate due to the influence of the autonomic nervous system). It is noteworthy that patients with low heart rate variability following a myocardial infarction may be at higher risk for sudden death. Studies have shown that these techniques have high negative predictive value and they have been proposed as screening techniques but, to date, they are not yet widely used in the clinical setting due, in part, to their relatively low positive predictive value.

17.9 Long-Term ECG Recording Devices

Currently, there are four general types of devices that are utilized in the collection of long-term electrocardiographic recordings: continuous recorders, event recorders, real-time monitoring systems, and implantable recorders.

Continuous recorders, like the Holter monitor described above, are attached to the surface of the body and continuously record signals for a predetermined duration (usually 24–48 h). Most such systems record from at least three different ECG leads. When using this method, patients must also record their daily activities and the time of the onset of symptoms (e.g., were they beginning to exercise?).

Event recorders are another type of instrument used for ECG collection. There are two basic types of event recorders—a postevent and a preevent recorder. Typically, a postevent recorder is worn continuously and is activated by the patient to store a recording when symptoms appear. Another type of postevent recorder, a miniature solid-state recorder, records the rhythm when symptoms appear by placing the unit on the precordium. Today, these devices can be as small as a credit card. Preevent, or loop recorders, are similar to postevent recorders, but a memory loop is used to enable the recording of information several minutes before and after the onset of symptoms. Examples of loop recorders are shown in Figs. 17.14 and 17.15.

The third type of ECG instrument that is used is a real-time monitoring system. With this type of instrument, the data are not recorded within the device, but it is transmitted trans-telephonically to a distal recording station. Such instruments are commonly used for monitoring of patients that have a potentially dangerous condition, so that the technician can quickly identify the rhythm abnormality and make arrangements for proper management of the condition.

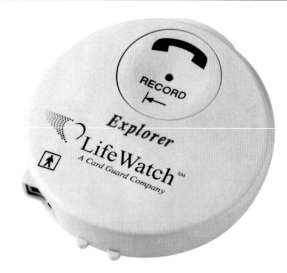

Fig. 17.14 A loop recorder with pacemaker and detection capabilities is shown. This model is manufactured by LifeWatch, Inc. (Rosemont, IL)

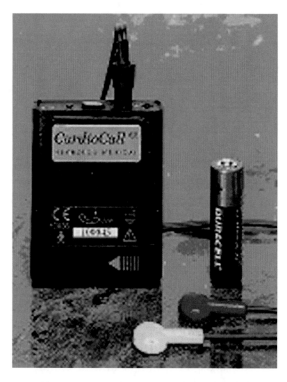

Fig. 17.15 The picture shows a loop recorder that is small enough to fit in your hand, measuring 55 mm across and weighing 79 g

Finally, implantable recorders are miniaturized loop recording devices that can be implanted subcutaneously. One of these devices, the Reveal™, is shown in Fig. 17.16 (Medtronic, Inc., Minneapolis, MN). For example, this device is used for patients that elicit infrequent symptoms (hence they remain undiagnosed) and for those in whom

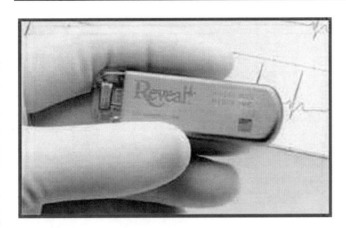

Fig. 17.16 The Reveal™, an implantable ECG loop recorder, is manufactured by Medtronic, Inc. (Minneapolis, MN)

external recorders are considered impractical. An implantable loop recorder can be programmed to automatically store data when fast or slow heart rhythms are detected. Additionally, the patient can also self-trigger the device to store data when symptoms are felt. The latest implantable loop recorders can be placed for up to 3 years and can also be used as a diagnostic tool to help manage the medical treatment of arrhythmias.

17.10 Summary

As cardiomyocytes depolarize and propagate action potentials throughout the heart, an electrical dipole is created. By utilizing the resultant electrical field present in the body, electrodes can be placed around the heart to measure potential differences as the heart depolarizes and repolarizes. This measurement gives rise to the ECG, normally consisting of the P-wave for atrial depolarization, the QRS complex for ventricular depolarization, and the T-wave for ventricular repolarization.

To date, there are 12 standard lead positions, which are clinically employed to detect the ECG. Most commonly, a five-wire system is used clinically and can be used for the three bipolar limb leads (which make up Einthoven's Triangle), the three unipolar limb leads, and one precordial (chest) lead at a time. At least two lead traces are needed to calculate the heart's electrical axis, which gives the general direction of the heart's dipole at any given instant. The heart's mean electrical axis is then the average dipole direction during the cardiac cycle (or more commonly, during ventricular depolarization).

The recorded ECG remains as one of the most vital monitors of a patient's cardiovascular status and is used today in nearly every clinical setting. Electrocardiography has come a long way since it was first employed back in the early 1900s. New instruments that are smaller and more sophisticated as well as innovative analysis techniques are continually being developed. ECG has also been used in combination with other implantable devices such as pacemakers and defibrillators. The trend has been toward developing smaller, easier-to-use devices that can gather and remotely send a wealth of information for use in patient diagnosis and treatment.

General References and Suggested Reading

Alexander RW, Schlant RC, Fuster V, eds. Hurst's: The heart, arteries and veins. 9th ed. New York, NY: McGraw-Hill, 1998.

Bloomfield D, Steinman RC, Namerow PB, et al. Microvolt T-wave alternans distinguishes between patients likely and patients not likely to benefit from implanted cardiac defibrillator therapy: A solution to the Multicenter Automatic Defibrillator Implantation Trial (MADIT) II Conundrum. Circulation 2004;110:1885–9.

Burchell HB. A centennial note on Waller and the first human electrocardiogram. Am J Cardiol 1987;59:979–83.

Drew BJ. Bedside electrocardiogram monitoring. AACN Clin Issues 1993;4:25–33.

Fye BW. A history of the origin, evolution, and impact of electrocardiography. Am J Cardiol 1994;73:937–49.

Garcia TB, Holtz NE. 12-Lead ECG: The art of interpretation. Sudbury, MA: Jones and Bartlett Publishers, 2001.

Hurst JW. Naming of the waves in the ECG, with a brief account of their genesis. Circulation 1998;98:1937–42.

Jacobson C. Optimum bedside cardiac monitoring. Prog Cardiovasc Nurs 2000;15:134–7.

Johnson LR, ed. Essential medical physiology. 3rd ed. San Diego, CA: Elsevier Academic Press, 2003.

Katz A, Liberty IF, Porath A, Ovsyshcher I, Prystowsky EN. A simple bedside test of 1-minute heart rate variability during deep breathing as a prognostic index after myocardial infarction. Am Heart J 1999;138:32–8.

Kossmann CE. Unipolar electrocardiography of Wilson: A half century later. Am Heart J 1985;110:901–4.

Krikler DM. Historical aspects of electrocardiography. Cardiol Clin 1987;5:349–55.

Mohrman DE, Heller LJ, eds. Cardiovascular physiology. 5th ed. New York, NY: McGraw-Hill, 2003.

Rautaharju PM. A hundred years of progress in electrocardiography: Early contributions from Waller to Wilson. Can J Cardiol 1987;3:362–74.

Scher AM. Studies of the electrical activity of the ventricles and the origin of the QRS complex. Acta Cardiol 1995;50:429–65.

Wellens HJJ. The electrocardiogram 80 years after Einthoven. J Am Coll Cardiol 1986;3:484–91.

Chapter 18
Mechanical Aspects of Cardiac Performance

Michael K. Loushin, Jason L. Quill, and Paul A. Iaizzo

Abstract Monitoring of hemodynamic and mechanical parameters of the heart are reviewed. Clinical methodologies are discussed along with tools used in a research setting. Specifically, these include: arterial blood pressure, central venous pressure, pulmonary artery pressure, mixed venous oxygen saturation, cardiac output, pressure–volume loops, flow monitoring, and Frank–Starling curves. These parameters are monitored using technology such as pressure transducers, Swan–Ganz catheters, thermodilution, sonomicrometry crystals, conductance catheters, ultrasound transducers, and loop recorders.

Keywords Cardiac pressure–volume loops · Blood pressure monitoring · Central venous pressue monitoring · Pulmonary artery pressure monitoring · Cardiac output · Cardiac index monitoring · Mixed venous saturation monitoring · Flow monitoring · Implantable monitoring

18.1 Introduction

This chapter is a review of commonly utilized monitoring techniques which are employed to assess the function of the general cardiovascular system. Specifically, means to assess arterial blood pressure, central venous pressure, pulmonary artery pressure, mixed venous oxygen saturation, cardiac output, pressure–volume loops, and Frank–Starling curves are described. Basic physiological principals underlying cardiac function are also briefly discussed.

Under normal physiologic conditions, the human heart functions as two separate pumps functioning in series; the right heart pumps blood through the pulmonary circulation and the left heart pumps blood through the systemic circulation. Each contraction of the heart and subsequent ejection of blood creates pressures, which can be monitored clinically to assess the function of the heart and its work against resistance. In general, the mechanical function of the heart is described by the changes in pressures, volumes, and flows that occur within each phase of the cardiac cycle, which is one complete sequence of myocardial contractions and relaxations.

18.2 Cardiac Cycle

The normal electrical and mechanical events of a single cardiac cycle of the left heart are correlated in Fig. 18.1. The mechanical events of the left ventricular pressure–volume curve are displayed in Fig. 18.2. During a single cardiac cycle, the atria and ventricles do not beat simultaneously; the atrial contraction occurs prior to ventricular contraction. This timing delay allows for proper filling of all four chambers of the heart. Recall that the left and right heart pumps function in series, but contract simultaneously. The diastolic phase of the cardiac cycle begins with the opening of the tricuspid and mitral valves (atrioventricular valves). These valves open when the pressures in the ventricles fall below those in the atria. This can be observed in Fig. 18.1 for the left heart, in which the mitral valve opens when the left ventricular pressure falls below the left atrial pressure. At this moment, passive filling of the ventricle begins. In other words, blood that has accumulated in the atria behind the closed atrioventricular valves passes rapidly into the ventricles, and this causes an initial drop in the atrial pressures. Later, pressures in all four chambers rise together as the atria and ventricles continue to passively fill in unison with blood returning to the heart through the veins (pulmonary veins to the left atrium, and the superior and inferior venae cavae to the right atrium).

J.L. Quill, (✉)
University of Minnesota, Department of Biomedical Engineering and Surgery, B172 Mayo, MMC 195, 420 Delaware St. SE, Minneapolis, MN 55455, USA
e-mail: quill010@umn.edu

P.A. Iaizzo (ed.), *Handbook of Cardiac Anatomy, Physiology, and Devices*, DOI 10.1007/978-1-60327-372-5_18,

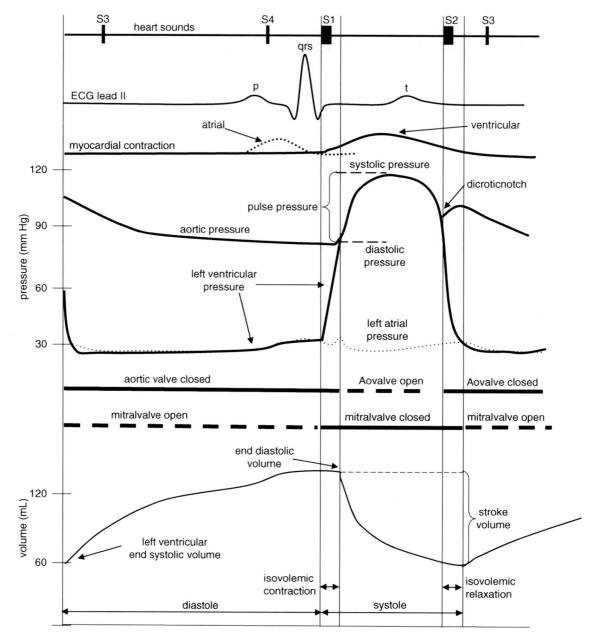

Fig. 18.1 Electrical and mechanical events of a single cardiac cycle within the left heart (see text for details)

Contractions of the atria are initiated near the end of ventricular diastole, which is initiated by depolarization of the atrial myocardial cells (sinoatrial node). Atrial depolarization is elicited at the P wave of the electrocardiogram (Fig. 18.1, ECG lead II). The excitation and subsequent development of tension and shortening of atrial cells cause atrial pressures to rise. Active atrial contraction forces additional volumes of blood into the ventricles (often referred to as "atrial kick"). The atrial kick can contribute a significant volume of blood toward ventricular preload (approximately 20%). At normal heart rates, the atrial contractions are considered essential for adequate ventricular filling. As heart rates increase, atrial filling becomes

increasingly important for ventricular filling because the time interval between contractions for passive filling becomes progressively shorter. Atrial fibrillation and/or asynchronized atrial–ventricular contractions can result in minimal contribution to preload, via the lack of a functional atrial contraction. Throughout diastole, atrial and ventricular pressures are nearly identical due to the open atrioventricular values which offer little or no resistance to blood flow. It should also be noted that contraction and movement of blood out of the atrial appendage (auricle) can be an additional source for increased blood volume.

Ventricular systole begins when the excitation passes from the right atrium through the atrioventricular node

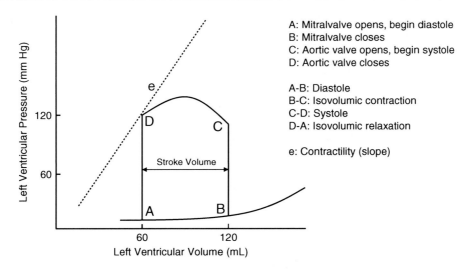

Fig. 18.2 Pressure–volume diagram of a single cardiac cycle (see text for details)

and through the remainder of the conduction system (His bundle and left and right bundle branches) to cause ventricular myocardial activation. This depolarization of ventricular cells underlies the QRS complex within the ECG (Fig. 18.1). As the ventricular cells contract, intraventricular pressures increase above those in the atria, and the atrioventricular valves abruptly close. Closure of the atrioventricular valves results in the first heart sound, S1 (Fig. 18.1). As pressures in the ventricles continue to rise together in a normally functioning heart, they eventually reach a critical threshold pressure at which the semilunar valves (pulmonary valve and aortic valve) open. The mechanical events of a single cardiac cycle and its pressure–volume relationship are displayed in Fig. 18.2. The normal time period between semilunar valve closures and atrioventricular valve openings is referred to as the "isovolumic contraction phase." During this interval, the ventricles can be considered as closed chambers. Ventricular wall tension is greatest just prior to opening of the semilunar valves. Ventricular ejection begins when the semilunar valves open. In early left heart ejection, blood enters the aorta rapidly and causes the pressure within it to rise. Importantly, pressure builds simultaneously in both the left ventricle and the aorta as the ventricular myocardium continues to contract. This period is often referred to as the "rapid ejection phase." A similar phenomenon occurs in the right heart; however, the pressures developed and those required to open the pulmonary valve are considerably lower.

Pressures in the ventricles and outflow vessels (the aorta and pulmonary arteries) ultimately reach maximum peak systolic pressures. Under normal physiologic conditions, the contractile forces in the ventricles diminish after achieving peak systolic pressures. Throughout ejection,

there are minimal pressure gradients across the semilunar valves due to their normally large annular diameters. Eventually the ventricular myocardium elicits minimal contraction to a point where intraventricular pressures fall below those in the outflow vessels. This fall in pressures causes the semilunar valves to close rapidly and is associated with the second heart sound, S2 (Fig. 18.1). A quick reversal in both aortic and pulmonary artery pressures is observed at this point, due to back pressure filling the semilunar valve leaflets. The back pressure on the valves causes the "incisura" or "dicrotic notch," which can be detected by local pressure recording (e.g., with a locally placed Millar catheter). After complete closure of these valves, the intraventricular pressure falls rapidly and the ventricular myocardium relaxes. For a brief period, all four cardiac valves are closed, which is commonly referred to as the "isovolumetric relaxation phase." Eventually, intraventricular pressure falls below the rising atrial pressures, the atrioventricular valve opens, and a new cardiac cycle is initiated.

18.3 Cardiac Pressure–Volume Curves

Ventricular function can be analyzed and graphically displayed with a pressure–volume diagram. Both systolic and diastolic pressure–volume relationships during a single cardiac cycle are displayed in Fig. 18.2. Pressure–volume assessment of myocardial function on intact myocardium involves multiple factors such as preload, afterload, heart rate, and contractility. The area inside the pressure–volume loop is an estimate of the myocardial energy (work = pressure × volume) utilized for each stroke volume (stroke volume = end-diastolic volume – end-systolic volume). The shape of the normal pressure–volume loop changes with alterations in myocardial compliance, contractility, and valvular and myocardial disease.

Pressure–volume loops are displayed by plotting ventricular pressure (y axis) against ventricular volume (x axis) during a single cardiac cycle (Fig. 18.2). Points and segments along the pressure–volume loop correlate with specific mechanical events of the ventricle. The width of the pressure–volume loop is the stroke volume. Myocardial contractility is represented by the slope of the end-systolic pressure–volume relationship; this relationship defines the maximal pressure generated over time with a given myocardial contractility state. Contractility is proportional to change in pressure over time (dP/dt). The passive ventricular filling during diastole is defined by the end-diastolic pressure–volume relationship, and ventricular compliance is inversely proportional to the slope of the end-diastolic pressure–volume relationship. The effect of heart rate on the pressure–volume relationship cannot be assessed with a single pressure–volume loop. Instead, multiple pressure–volume loops must be obtained to assess effects of heart rate on the pressure–volume loop. By altering variables such as afterload, contractility, and/or preload, the mechanical events and pressure–volume relationship are displayed.

The pressure–volume diagram shows events of a single cardiac cycle (Fig. 18.2):

A: mitral valve opens, begin diastole;
B: mitral valve closes, end diastole;
C: aortic valve opens, begin systole;
D: aortic valve closes, end systole;
A–B: diastole, ventricular filling;
B–C: isovolumic contraction;
C–D: systole, ventricular ejection;
D–A: isovolumic relaxation;
e: contractility (slope).

18.3.1 Preload

Preload is determined by the end-diastolic ventricular volume; it results from passive and active emptying of the atrium into the ventricle. Factors that affect this relationship, such as mitral stenosis and/or ventricular hypertrophy, will affect preload. The Frank–Starling curve also defines the relationship between preload and stroke volume; as end-diastolic volume increases, the stroke volume increases until the end-diastolic volume gets too excessive to allow proper ventricular contraction

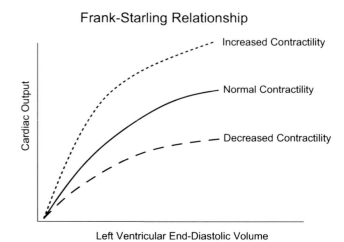

Fig. 18.3 The "Frank–Starling relationship." As the end-diastolic volume increases, the cardiac output also increases. Excessive preload may eventually result in decreased cardiac output

(Fig. 18.3). A pressure–volume loop is an alternative way to display the relationship between preload and stroke volume (Fig. 18.4); preload is the volume of blood in the ventricle at the end of diastole (point B in Fig. 18.4). An increase in preload is displayed by a right shift of the end-diastolic volume curve (A–B* in Fig. 18.4). In a normally functioning ventricle, an increase in preload while maintaining normal contractility and afterload results in increased stroke volume (SV* in Fig. 18.4). Excessive preload will not continue to result in increased stroke volume; excessive overdistention of the ventricle may result in heart failure (Fig. 18.5).

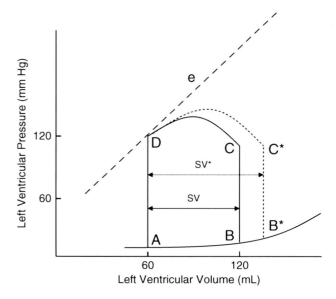

Fig. 18.4 Effect of acutely increased preload on the pressure–volume loop. Increasing preload while maintaining normal afterload and contractility results in increased stroke volume (SV*). e – contractility line; SV = stroke volume

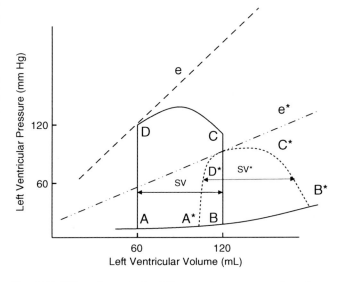

Fig. 18.5 Effect of ventricular failure on the pressure–volume loop. In heart failure, the myocardium compensates its inability to contract by increasing preload in an attempt to maintain stroke volume. Excessive preload eventually leads to worsening of heart failure. e and e* = contractility lines; SV = stroke volume

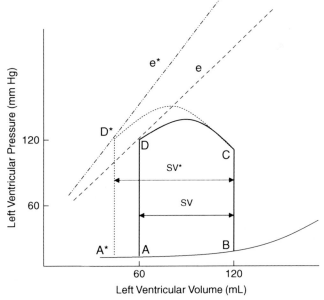

Fig. 18.6 Effects of acutely increasing contractility on the pressure–volume loop. Increasing contractility while maintaining normal preload and afterload results in increased stroke volume (SV*). Note the increased slope of the contractility line (e*). The area of loop D* is larger, indicating greater myocardial work per stroke volume. e and e* = contractility lines; SV = stroke volume

18.3.2 Contractility

Contractility is the relative ability of the myocardium to pump blood without changes in preload or afterload; it is influenced by intracellular calcium concentrations, the autonomic nervous system, humoral changes, and/or pharmacologic agents. A sudden increase in contractility with unchanged preload and afterload will result in increased stroke volume by ejecting more volume out of the ventricle (Fig. 18.6). The aortic valve opens at the same pressure and the ventricle ejects blood forward. Increased myocardial contractility forces more blood out of the ventricle during systole, which is displayed by a lower end-systolic volume. Note the change in SV* (Fig. 18.6) with increased contractility; the end-systolic volume is lower due to increased contractility resulting in increased stroke volume. With increased myocardial contractility and unchanged preload, the resulting pressure–volume loop shifts to the left, maintaining normal stroke volume. An increase in contractility is graphically displayed by the increase in the slope of line e* in Fig. 18.6. During ejection, the myocardium contracts from C to D* (Fig. 18.6). During conditions of lower end-diastolic volume, a normal stroke volume may be maintained by increasing contractility. Inotropes such as dopamine and epinephrine will increase contractility, which assists in maintaining adequate stroke volume during low contractility states such as heart failure and/or cardiogenic shock.

In heart failure, the myocardium has decreased capacity to pump blood and maintain normal cardiac output.

Heart failure may be acute (e.g., acute myocardial infarction, acute cardiogenic shock, or fluid overload) or it may be chronic (e.g., chronic congestive heart failure). In progressive heart failure, the myocardium often compensates its inability to contract by increasing preload and decreasing afterload in an attempt to maintain stroke volume (Fig. 18.5).

The increase in preload moves the myocardium up the Frank–Starling curve such that, by increasing end-diastolic volume, normal stroke volume may be maintained. The increase in preload and worsening heart failure eventually leads to ventricular dilatation and venous congestion. During heart failure, sympathetic tone increases as levels of circulating norepinephrine and epinephrine attempt to maintain normal cardiac output by increasing contractility and heart rate. The body's compensatory mechanism for heart failure may eventually become counterproductive and thus even worsen the situation.

18.3.3 Afterload

Afterload is another vital factor relative to stroke volume and therefore blood pressure. Afterload is most often equated with ventricular wall tension, which is also considered as the pressure the ventricle must overcome to eject a volume of blood past the aortic valve. In most normal clinical situations, afterload is assumed to be proportional to systemic vascular resistance. Wall tension is greatest at the moment just before opening of the aortic valve and can be described by LaPlace's law:

$$\text{Circumferential stress} = Pr/2H$$

where circumferential stress = wall tension, P = intraventricular pressure, r = ventricular radius, and H = wall thickness.

An increase in afterload requires ventricular pressure to increase during isovolumic contraction before the aortic valve opens (Fig. 18.7). Due to the increase in afterload, the ability of the ventricle to eject blood is decreased. This results in decreased stroke volume (SV* in Fig. 18.7A) and increased end-systolic volume (B* in Fig. 18.7B). If afterload remains increased, the myocardium establishes a new steady state that is shifted to the right and stroke volume is restored. A patient with severe aortic stenosis will likely elicit a pressure–volume loop as in Fig. 18.7. The myocardium usually compensates by increasing contractility to maintain adequate stroke volume. Thus, patients with hemodynamically significant aortic stenosis often develop left ventricular hypertrophy.

Afterload may be inversely related to cardiac output. In a dysfunctional myocardium, such as congestive heart failure, stroke volume decreases with increases in afterload. Importantly, increase in afterload also requires the myocardium to expend more energy to eject blood during systole.

18.3.4 Sonomicrometry Crystals

A common method for obtaining pressure–volume loops, and the changes observed by varying preload, afterload, or contractility, is to use sonomicrometry crystals for volume measurements in combination with a pressure-sensing catheter placed in the left ventricle. Sonomicrometry consists of piezoelectric crystals that transmit ultrasound signals through tissue to other crystals, where the signal is received; a distance measurement between two given crystals can be determined based upon the travel time of the ultrasound signal and the fiber orientation of the tissue. The piezoelectric (sonomicrometry) crystals function omnidirectionally and act as both receiver and transmitter with as many as 32 peers (in most commonly available systems). Complex, moving 3D geometries can then be modeled using techniques like sonomicrometry array localization. A sonomicrometry crystal can be seen in Fig. 18.8, where it is held in preparation for insertion through the epicardium.

Placement of four sonomicrometry crystals transmurally within the left ventricle, as well as the resulting pressure–volume loops, can be viewed on the Companion CD (WMV 18.1 and WMV 18.2). The method shown in the

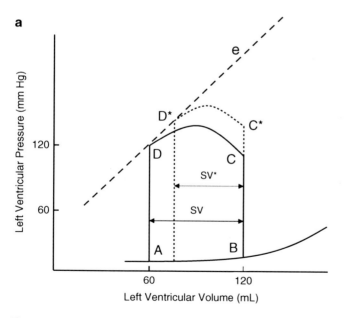

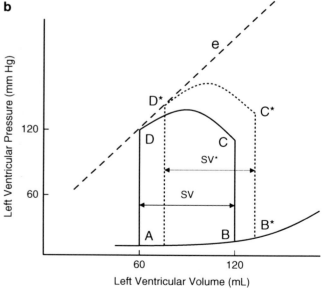

Fig. 18.7 (A) Effects of acutely increasing afterload on the pressure–volume loop. An increase in afterload while maintaining normal contractility and preload results in decreased stroke volume (SV*). A higher pressure is also required before the aortic valve opens (C*). (B) Restoration of stroke volume after increasing afterload. An increase in afterload while maintaining normal contractility and preload results in decreased stroke volume (SV*). A higher pressure is also required before the aortic valve opens (C*). e = contractility line; SV = stroke volume

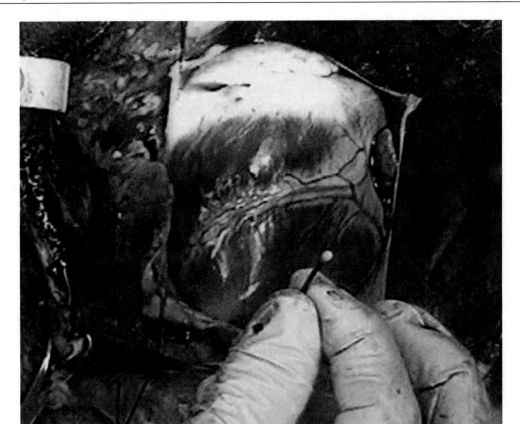

Fig. 18.8 A common sonomicrometry crystal placement. The crystal is shown prior to transmural implantation in a swine heart

supplemental video places four sonomicrometry crystals: one on the anterior surface, the second on the posterior surface, a third crystal at the base of the left ventricle (superior), and a final crystal at the left ventricular apex (inferior). The placement of the crystals in this pattern creates two distance measurements (anterior–posterior and base–apex) that are measured continuously through the cardiac cycle. By assuming that the left ventricle is the shape of an ellipsoid, changes in volume can be continuously estimated.

Traditionally, sonomicrometry has been used to determine cardiac function relative to large research animals (dogs, pigs, sheep, etc.). Both in vivo and in vitro studies can be performed which elucidate global cardiac function under a variety of conditions. Understanding the velocity of ultrasound through tissue is critical to acquiring accurate dimensions in a sonomicrometry system. The velocity of ultrasound is affected by a variety of factors including muscle fiber direction and composition, as well as the contractile state. In most biological tissues, the velocity of sound is approximately 1540 m/s.

A sonomicrometry system can use as few as 2 transducers, but typically employs between 6 and 32 transducers. Transducers are the piezoelectric crystals which are attached to electronics consisting of a pulse generator

and a receiver. Distance is measured by energizing the transmitter with a train of high-voltage spikes or square waves (both less than a microsecond in duration) to produce ultrasound. This excites the piezoelectric crystal to begin oscillating at its resonant frequency. This vibratory energy propagates through the medium and eventually comes in contact with piezoelectric crystals acting as receivers. These crystals begin vibrating and generate signals on the order of 1 mV. The piezoelectric signals are amplified and the distances between pairs of crystals are calculated. By monitoring the difference in time from transmission to reception of such signals, and knowing the speed of sound through the particular medium, the intercrystal distances can be calculated. With current systems, these computations take less than 1 ms.

In addition to sonomicrometry crystals being used in the manner described, several other types of studies have found sonomicrometry measurements to be helpful. Regional studies have been performed that focus on specific areas of the heart, investigating regional timing and left ventricular shortening [1]. The advent of 3D sonomicrometry, or "sonomicrometry array localization," has made possible the detailed study of discrete anatomical points throughout the cardiac cycle [2, 3]. A volume of data now exist describing the motion of valves, papillary muscles, ventricles, and atria. Another application involves tracking mobile components through the heart such as cardiac catheters [4]. We believe that these applications of sonomicrometry are important enough to be described in detail below.

In sonomicrometry array localization, the 3D position of each crystal is calculated from multiple intertransducer distances. This is done using a statistical technique called "multidimensional scaling;" such assessment gives the experimenter the ability to take the scalar sonomicrometer measurements and generate 3D geometry. Multidimensional scaling generates 3D coordinates for each crystal from a group of chord lengths in the array. By starting with an initial coordinate estimate and applying the Pythagorean theorem, a matrix of estimated distances is generated which corresponds to the actual measured distances. Using an iterative approach, multidimensional scaling then optimizes the value for the distance calculation by minimizing what is called the "stress function." If the distances measured between crystals are exact (no measurement error), then one solution with zero stress exists, which represents the intercrystal distances exactly. As measurement error increases, a zero solution to the stress function becomes impossible and the iterations begin seeking a minimum value. The globally minimum stress point defines the optimum 3D configuration. A similar style is used to generate an estimate of the error associated with each distance. The result of this analysis is a 3D moving model with an average error of approximately 2 mm. The advent and description of the feasibility assessment of this technique is described in detail by Ratcliffe et al. [2] and Gorman et al. [3]. The first reported application of this technology described the 3D modeling of the ovine left ventricle and mitral valve. The study involved a 16-transducer array in which 3 transducers were sutured to the chest wall and the remaining 13 were placed both epicardially and endocardially on the ventricular wall, the papillary muscles, and the mitral valve. The three crystals attached to the chest wall provided a fixed coordinate system from which whole body motion could be differentiated from cardiac motion. This study produced 3D depictions of the shape of the mitral annulus throughout the cardiac cycle, as well as quantitative images of ventricular torsion. Such applications open up many possibilities relative to chronic studies focusing on ventricular remodeling following traumas like myocardial infarction.

Another interesting application of sonomicrometry, available due to the development of sonomicrometry array localization, is the cardiac catheter tracking described by Meyer et al. [4]. The system involved placing seven sonomicrometric crystals in the epicardium of an ovine heart and tracking the position of a catheter with anywhere from one to five attached crystals. In this system, average distance errors on the order of 1.0 mm were demonstrated. The clinically relevant end point for this tool would be to replace the epicardial transceivers with transceivers mounted in catheters and deployed endocardially in a minimally invasive manner.

18.3.5 Conductance Catheter

Conductance catheters offer an alternative method for obtaining pressure–volume loops. In this method, a catheter is typically equipped with eight electrodes and a pressure lumen. The conductance catheter is placed retrograde across the aortic valve, so that the first electrode is positioned in the left ventricular apex and the eighth electrode is positioned across the aortic valve (Fig. 18.9). The pressure lumen is located within the left ventricle, usually at the distal tip of the conductance catheter.

The outermost electrodes of the conductance catheter produce an electric field, with the remaining electrodes

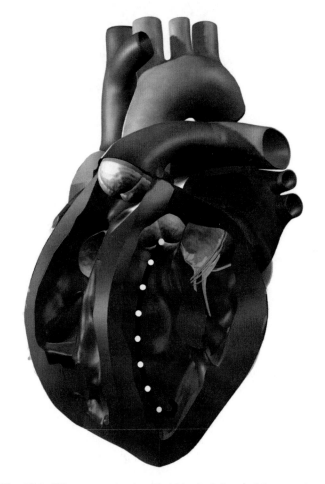

Fig. 18.9 When properly placed within the left ventricle, a conductance catheter spans from the apex to the aortic valve. The outermost electrodes (*yellow*) produce an electric field, and the inner electrodes (*white*) measure voltage differences that are related to volume changes within the chamber. A pressure sensor is typically incorporated into the distal tip of the catheter

sensing differentials in voltage potential. The use of conductance to measure volume arises from the fact that blood is a good conductor relative to the surrounding myocardium (160 vs. 400 Ω cm) [5]. When the ventricle is in diastole and filled with blood, the conductivity of the chamber will be much higher than during systole. The volume of the heart chamber is then analyzed as a series of conductive cylinders stacked upon each other, with a height predetermined as the distance between the electrodes. A change in the cross-sectional area of one of these cylinders is synonymous with a decrease in blood volume and a change in resistance, which is measured by the sensing electrodes.

The left ventricular volume can then be calculated as a voltage varying with time ($V(t)$), based upon the distance between the electrodes (L), the specific conductivity of blood (σ), the sum of the conductances that vary with time ($G(t)$), a dimensionless constant (α), and a correction term (C) [6]:

$$V(t) = \frac{L^2}{\alpha\sigma} G(t) - C$$

The conductance catheter was developed in the early 1980s by Baan et al. [6]. This method has shown reliable left ventricular segmental volumes when compared to cine CT scans [7] and sonomicrometry crystals. Additionally, the conductance methods could be optimally suited for right ventricular pressure–volume curves [8]. Sonomicrometry methods and angiography require the assumption of an ellipsoid shape for left ventricular measurements; the complex geometric shape of the right ventricle makes these methods ill-suited for volume measurements on the right side of the heart.

Both sonomicrometry crystals and conductance catheters are proven techniques for the measurement of left ventricular and aortic root volumes [9]. These technologies are applicable to many different study designs, yet care should be taken to choose the best method based upon the needs of the study. For studies involving complex geometric shapes, a conductance catheter may be the easiest method to obtain absolute volume changes, but a technique such as sonomicrometry array localization may be advantageous if the relative motion of geometric components is of interest.

18.4 Blood Pressure Monitoring

The cardiovascular system is most commonly assessed by monitoring arterial blood pressure. Blood pressure is proportional to the product of cardiac output and systemic vascular resistance:

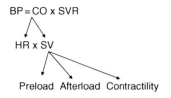

Fig. 18.10 Blood pressure monitoring which is proportional to the product of cardiac output and systemic vascular resistance. BP = blood pressure; CO = cardiac output; HR = heart rate; SV = stroke volume; SVR = systemic vascular resistance

$$BP = CO \times SVR$$
$$CO = HR \times SV$$
$$MAP = 1/3SBP + 2/3DBP$$

where BP = blood pressure, CO = cardiac output, SVR = systemic vascular resistance, HR = heart rate, SV = stroke volume, MAP = mean arterial pressure, SBP = systolic blood pressure, and DBP = diastolic blood pressure. Stroke volume is dependent upon preload, afterload, and contractility (Fig. 18.10).

Blood pressure can be defined to consist of three components: systolic blood pressure, mean arterial pressure, and diastolic blood pressure. Systolic blood pressure is the peak pressure during ventricular systole, mean arterial pressure is a crucial determinant for adequate perfusion of other major organs, and diastolic blood pressure is the main determinant for myocardial perfusion. Recall that the majority of coronary blood flow occurs during diastole.

Commonly, arterial blood pressure monitoring involves two primary techniques—noninvasive (indirect) and invasive (direct) methods. The decision to utilize either blood pressure monitoring method depends on multiple factors such as: (1) the patient's cardiovascular stability or instability; (2) the perceived need for frequent arterial blood samples; (3) the relative frequency of blood pressure recordings; and/or (4) the type of major surgery or trauma the patient will undergo. One of the advantages of an invasive blood pressure monitor is that it provides continuous, beat-to-beat blood pressures (JPG 18.1). Typically, direct arterial blood pressure monitoring is considered to be required when a cardiopulmonary bypass machine is utilized during cardiac surgery. Since there is no pulsatile flow during such surgery, the noninvasive methods to monitor blood pressure cannot be employed.

18.4.1 Noninvasive Arterial Blood Pressure Monitoring

Noninvasive blood pressure assessment is the most utilized and simplest technique to monitor arterial blood pressure. This technique utilizes a blood pressure cuff and the principle of pulsatile flow. A blood pressure cuff is applied to a limb such as forearm or leg and is inflated to a pressure greater than systolic blood pressure, which stops blood flow distal to the inflated cuff. As the pressure in the cuff is gradually decreased, blood flow through the artery is restored. The change in arterial pressure and flow creates oscillations which can be detected by auscultation of Korotkoff sounds and oscillometric methods. For accurate blood pressure measurement, the width of the cuff should be approximately one-third the circumference of the limb. A small, improperly sized cuff will overestimate systolic blood pressure, while a large cuff will underestimate the pressure. The rate of cuff deflation should be slow enough to hear Korotkoff sounds or detect oscillations. Noninvasive blood pressure monitors do not work if there is no pulsatile flow.

The automated method of noninvasive blood pressure monitoring is the "oscillometric" technique. Most oscillometric blood pressure monitors have oscillotonometers and a microprocessor. The blood pressure cuff is inflated until no oscillation is detected. As the cuff pressure is decreased, flow in the distal blood vessel is restored and amplitude of oscillations increases. A large increase in arterial wave oscillation amplitude is recorded as systolic blood pressure, the peak oscillation as mean arterial pressure, and the sudden decrease in amplitude as diastolic blood pressure (Fig. 18.11). Due to the sensitivity of the monitoring system, the mean arterial pressure is usually the most accurate and reproducible. For more details on such monitoring, refer to Chapter 16.

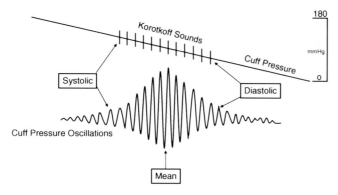

Fig. 18.11 An example of noninvasive blood pressure monitoring. As blood flow is restored with release of the blood pressure cuff, the arterial wave oscillations increase. The increase in oscillation amplitudes is associated with systolic blood pressure and presence of Korotkoff sounds. The peak of oscillations is associated with mean arterial pressure. Return of oscillations to baseline is diastolic blood pressure and end of Korotkoff sounds

18.4.2 Invasive Arterial Blood Pressure Monitoring

Continuous blood pressure monitoring is best accomplished by direct intraarterial blood pressure monitoring. Direct pressure monitoring allows for continuous beat-to-beat monitoring of arterial pressure, and the recorded arterial waveform provides temporal information relative to cardiovascular function. Direct pressure monitoring is often employed in clinical settings such as: (1) during major trauma and vascular surgery; (2) in patients with sepsis; and (3) during cardiopulmonary bypass where there is no pulsatile flow. Further, patients with significant cardiopulmonary disease (i.e., those in an intensive care unit) may require invasive arterial blood pressure monitoring (Table 18.1).

As noted above, besides providing blood pressure information, the arterial waveform also presents information about cardiovascular function. For example, the upstroke of an arterial waveform correlates with myocardial contractility (dP/dT), while the downstroke gives information relative to peripheral vascular resistance. The position of the dicrotic notch gives insights as to the systemic vascular resistance; a low dicrotic notch position on the arterial waveform may infer low vascular resistance, while a high dicrotic notch usually relates to higher systemic vascular resistance. Furthermore, by integrating the area under the curve of the arterial waveform, the stroke volume may also be estimated.

Direct arterial blood pressure monitoring typically involves cannulation of a peripheral artery and transducing the pressure (JPGs 18.2 and 18.3). An indwelling arterial catheter is connected to pressure tubing containing saline, which is then connected to a pressure transducer and monitoring system. Typical transducers contain strain gauges (stretch wires or silicon crystals) that distort with changes in blood pressure. The strain gauges contain a variable resistance transducer and a diaphragm which links the fluid wave to electrical signals. When the

Table 18.1 Accepted indications for direct arterial blood pressure monitor

- Major surgery
- Major trauma
- Major vascular (i.e., carotid endarterectomy, aortic aneurysm)
- Cardiopulmonary bypass surgery
- Myocardial dysfunction (i.e., myocardial ischemia/infarct, heart failure, dysrhythmias)
- Uncontrolled/labile blood pressure (i.e., hypertension, hypotension)
- Inaccurate noninvasive monitor (i.e., morbid obesity)
- Sepsis/shock
- Pulmonary dysfunction

transducer diaphragm is distorted, there is a change in voltage across resistors of a Wheatstone bridge circuit (JPG 18.4). The transducer is constructed using such a circuit so that voltage output can be calibrated proportional to the blood pressure. Standard pressure transducers are calibrated to 5 μV/V excitation per mmHg [10]. Commonly, the electrical signals from such pressure monitoring systems are filtered, amplified, and displayed on a monitor, thus providing a typical arterial pressure waveform. It is important that the arterial pressure transducer be positioned and calibrated accurately at the level of the heart. Improper transducer height will result in inaccurate blood pressures; if the pressure transducer is positioned too high, the blood pressure is underestimated, while a lower positioned transducer will overestimate the actual blood pressure.

Common sites for intraarterial cannulation for arterial pressure monitoring are the radial, brachial, axillary, or femoral arteries. Although the ascending aorta is the ideal place to monitor arterial pressure waveforms, this is not practical in most clinical settings. However, it should be noted that pressure measurements in the more peripheral arteries become distorted when compared to central aortic pressure waveform (Fig. 18.12). Peripherally, the systolic blood pressure may be higher and diastolic blood pressure lower, while the mean arterial pressure is usually similar to central aortic pressure. The pressure waveform becomes more distorted as pressure is measured farther away from the aorta. This distortion is due to a decrease in arterial compliance and reflection and oscillation of the blood pressure waves. For example, an arterial pressure wave monitored from the dorsalis pedis will be significantly

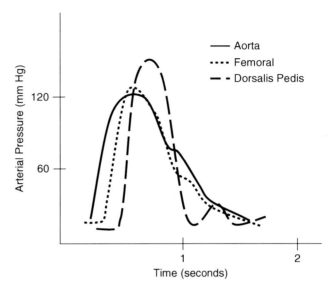

Fig. 18.13 A typical example of an arterial pressure waveform recorded from the ascending aorta. As the pressure monitoring site is moved more peripherally, the morphology of the waveform changes due to changes in arterial wall compliance as well as oscillation and reflection of the arterial pressure wave. Notice in the dorsalis pedis arterial waveform the absence of the dicrotic notch, overestimation of systolic blood pressure, and underestimation of diastolic pressure. Also note the presence of a small reflection wave

different from a central aortic wave when it is graphically displayed (Fig. 18.13). There is also a loss in amplitude or absence of the dicrotic notch, an increase in systolic blood pressure, and a decrease in diastolic blood pressure. One should also be aware of the possible appearance of a reflection wave as the blood pressure is monitored from a peripheral site. Importantly, risks associated with indwelling intraarterial pressure catheter include thrombosis, emboli, infection, nerve injury, and hematoma.

18.4.3 Pressure Transducer System

In clinical settings, arterial and venous blood pressures and waveforms are displayed by utilization of a pressure transducer monitoring system. A typical pressure transducer monitoring system includes: (1) an indwelling intravascular catheter; (2) pressure tubing; (3) a pressure transducer; (4) stopcock and flush valve; (5) a high pressure fluid bag; and (6) a graphical display monitor and microprocessor (Fig. 18.14A, B).

The pressure wave derived from the transducer system is a summation of sine waves at different frequencies and amplitudes. The fundamental frequency (first harmonic) is equal to the heart rate. Therefore, at a heart rate of 120 beats/min, the fundamental frequency is 2 Hz. Since the

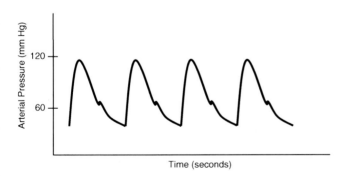

Fig. 18.12 An example of an arterial blood pressure wave from a typical optimally damped arterial blood pressure waveform. The peak portion of the waveform corresponds to the systolic blood pressure and the trough corresponds with the diastolic blood pressure. The dicrotic notch is associated with closing of the aortic valve. Information about cardiovascular function can be estimated from the waveform. The upstroke correlates with myocardial contractility. The downstroke and position of the dicrotic notch give information about systemic vascular resistance. The stroke volume is estimated by integrating the area under the curve

a

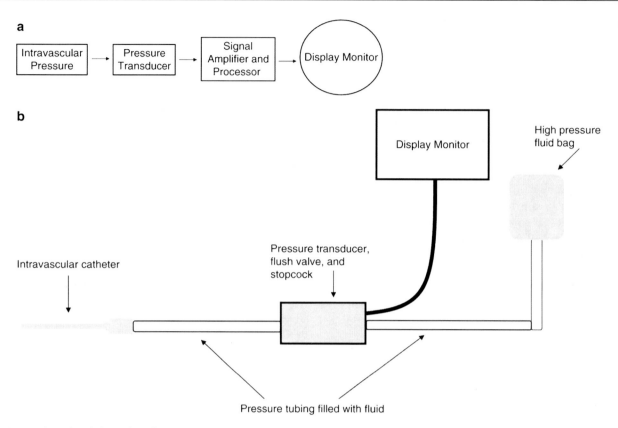

b

Fig. 18.14 (**a** and **b**) Schematics of a pressure transducer monitoring system (see text for details)

first ten harmonics of the fundamental frequency make significant contributions to the arterial waveform [11], frequencies up to 20 Hz make major contributions to the pressure waveform. It is generally considered for most recording systems that the maximum significant frequency in the arterial blood pressure signal is approximately 20 Hz [12].

All materials have a natural frequency, also known as "resonant frequency." The natural frequency of the monitoring system is the frequency at which the pressure monitoring system resonates and amplifies the actual blood pressure signal [12, 13]. If the natural frequency of the system is near the fundamental frequency, the blood pressure waveform will be amplified, giving an inaccurate pressure recording. The natural frequency is defined by the following equation [14]:

$$\mathrm{fn} = (d/8) * (3/\pi L\pi \mathrm{Vd})^{1/2}$$

$$\varsigma = (16n/d^3) * (3LVd/\pi\rho)^{1/2} \text{ (damping coefficient)}$$

where fn = natural frequency, d = tubing diameter, n = viscosity of fluid, L = tubing length, ρ = density of fluid, and Vd = transducer fluid volume displacement.

In order to increase accuracy of the blood pressure waveform, the natural frequency needs to be increased while the amount of distortion is reduced. The optimal natural frequency should be at least ten times the fundamental frequency, which is then greater than the tenth harmonic of the fundamental frequency [11, 12]. Therefore, the natural frequency should be greater than 20 Hz. In clinical settings, the input frequency is usually close to the monitoring system's natural frequency, which ranges from 10 to 20 Hz. When the input frequency is close to the natural frequency, the system amplifies the actual pressure signal. Ideally, the natural frequency should exceed the maximum significant frequency in a blood pressure signal which is about 20 Hz [12]. An amplified system typically requires damping to minimize distortion; an underdamped system will result in amplification, while an overdamped system will result in reduced amplification.

The ability of the system to extinguish oscillations through viscous and frictional forces is the damping coefficient (ς) [15]. Some degree of damping may be required to prevent overamplifications of blood pressure waveform. It is considered that more damping is required especially in patients with higher heart rates, such as neonates. At higher heart rates, the tenth harmonic of the fundamental frequency will approach the natural frequency and the waveform is amplified. Overamplification, or ringing, can be adjusted by increasing the damping coefficient. Specifically, in an overamplified system, a connector with an air bubble can intentionally be placed in line with the pressure transducer; the air bubble damps the system to diminish ringing.

The accuracy of pressure transducers is considered optimal in the following situations: low compliance of the pressure catheter and tubing, low density of fluid in the pressure tubing, and short tubing with a minimal number of connectors. Note that a suboptimal pressure system may produce an underdamped or overdamped pressure waveform; an underdamped waveform will overestimate systolic blood pressure, while an overdamped waveform will underestimate systolic blood pressure. Damping occurs when factors such as compliance of tubing, air bubbles, and blood clots decrease the peaks and troughs of the pressure sine waves by absorbing energy and diminishing the waveform. In an underdamped system, the pressure waves generate additive harmonics, which may also lead to an overestimated blood pressure. In an overdamped system, a pressure wave may be impeded from adequately propagating forward. Overdamping may occur due to air bubbles in the pressure lines, kinks, blood clots, low flush bag pressures, and multiple stopcocks or injection ports. This often results in underestimation of systolic blood pressure and overestimation of diastolic blood pressure. Fortunately, the mean arterial pressure is minimally affected by dampening (Fig. 18.15).

Optimal pressure waveforms can be obtained when there is balance between the degree of damping and distortion from the pressure tubing system. A simple way to

assess damping is to observe the results from a high pressure fluid flush. In the flush test, the pressure transducer system is flushed and the resulting oscillations (ringing) are observed. In an optimally damped system, a baseline results after one oscillation (Fig. 18.16). In an overdamped system, the baseline is reached without oscillations and the waveform is blunted. In an underdamped system, the flush test results in multiple oscillations before the waveform reaches baseline.

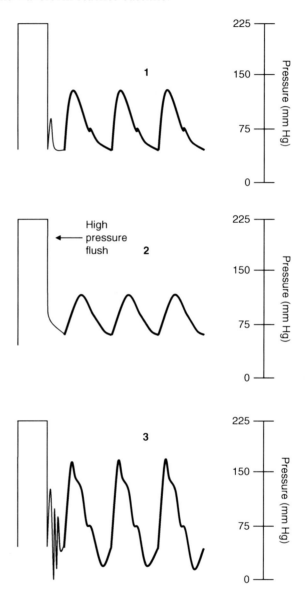

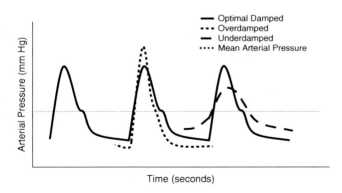

Fig. 18.15 Effects of damping on the arterial pressure waveform. In an underdamped pressure monitoring system, the pressure wave overestimates the systolic blood pressure and underestimates the diastolic blood pressure. In an overdamped system, the pressure wave underestimates the systolic blood pressure and overestimates the diastolic blood pressure. The mean arterial pressure remains essentially unchanged

Fig. 18.16 An example of a high pressure flush test. (1) In an optimally damped pressure monitoring system, the pressure wave returns to baseline after one oscillation. (2) In an overdamped system, the wave returns to baseline without any oscillations. The systolic blood pressure is underestimated and diastolic pressure overestimated. (3) In an underdamped system, the wave oscillates multiple times before returning to baseline. The arterial wave is amplified. The systolic pressure is overestimated and diastolic pressure underestimated. The mean arterial pressure usually is not significantly affected by overdamping or underdamping

18.4.4 Transducer Catheters

Common clinical methods to monitor arterial and venous pressures utilize a pressure transducer system that requires a fluid-filled system. Transducer catheters such as Millar catheters (JPG 18.5) monitor pressures directly from a sensor incorporated within the tip of the catheter. A sensor (JPG 18.6) placed directly at the end of the catheter allows direct and constant measurement of pressures, thus eliminating the intrinsic inaccuracies of a fluid-filled system (previously described in this chapter).

In general, transducer catheters are more accurate than conventional fluid-filled systems. Motion artifact is nearly eliminated and the issues of overdamped and underdamped systems are not present. Accurate pressure readings can be obtained with the catheter at any height; readings are not affected by the height of the pressure transducer as in the conventional system. With transducer catheters, there is no time delay since pressure is monitored directly at the source. Compared to the conventional fluid system, transducer catheters have high inherent fidelity (>10 MHz).

18.5 Central Venous Pressure Monitoring

An estimate of intravascular volume status and right heart function can be assessed with a central venous pressure catheter. Central venous pressure is ideally considered as the mean venous blood pressure at the junction of the right atrium and the inferior and superior venae cavae. The central venous pressure (Tables 18.2 and 18.3) is an estimate of right heart filling pressures and may be used to assess right heart function and circulating blood volume. The central venous pressure is dependent upon multiple factors such as intravascular volume, functional capacitance of veins, and status of the right heart. A limitation of central venous pressure monitoring is that it does not give direct information about the left heart function. Indications for central venous catheter placement may include monitoring of cardiac filling pressures, administration of drugs, and/or rapid infusion of large amounts of fluids (Table 18.4). A typical central venous pressure kit is shown in JPG 18.7. It is critical to properly calibrate and position the pressure transducer system at the level of the right atrium. Since the numeric value of central venous pressure is small (2–12 mmHg), minor changes in transducer height will cause significant inaccuracies in central venous pressure assessment.

There are multiple sites for placement of central venous catheters. Common sites used in clinical practice are the internal jugular and subclavian veins (JPG 18.8). Central venous access can also be accomplished by placement of a long catheter via the antecubital, external jugular, and femoral veins. Complications of central venous catheter placement may include inadvertent arterial

Table 18.2 Relative intracardiac pressures in the healthy heart

Pressures	Mean	Range
Left atrium	8	4–12
Left ventricle systolic	125	90–140
Left ventricle end-diastolic	8	4–12
Right atrium	5	2–12
Right ventricle systolic	25	15–30
Right ventricle end-diastolic	5	0–10
Pulmonary artery systolic	23	15–30
Pulmonary artery diastolic	10	5–15
Pulmonary capillary wedge	10	5–15
Mean pulmonary artery	15	10–20

Table 18.3 Cardiac hemodynamic parameters (with normal ranges)

Hemodynamic parameter	Derived formula	Range
CO	HR × SV	4–6 L/min
CI	CO/BSA	2.6–4.3 L/min/m^2
SV	CO × 1000/HR	50–120 mL/beat
SI	SV/BSA	30–65 mL/beat/m^2
SVR	(MAP − CVP) × 80/CO	800–1400 dyne s/cm^5
SVRI	(MAP − CVP) × 80/CI	1500–2300 dyne s/cm^5/m^2
PVR	(PAP − PCWP) × 80/CO	140–250 dyne s/cm^5
PVRI	(PAP − PCWP) × 80/CI	240–450 dyne s/cm^5/m^2
LVSWI	1.36 (MAP − PCWP) × SI/100	45–60 g m/m^2
RVSWI	1.36 (PAP − CVP) × SI/100	5–10 g m/m^2

BSA = body surface area; CI = cardiac index; CO = cardiac output; CVP = central venous pressure; HR = heart rate; LVSWI = left ventricular stroke work index; MAP = mean arterial pressure; PAP = pulmonary artery pressure; PCWP = pulmonary capillary wedge pressure; PVR = pulmonary vascular resistance; PVRI = pulmonary vascular resistance index; RVSWI = right ventricular stroke work index; SI = stroke index; SV = stroke volume; SVR = systemic vascular resistance; SVRI = systemic vascular resistance index.

Table 18.4 Relative indications for using a central venous pressure catheter

- Large fluid shifts
- Vascular access
- Infusion of medication
- Venous blood sampling
- Major trauma and surgery
- Monitoring of intravascular volume status
- Aspiration of venous air embolus

puncture (i.e., carotid and subclavian arteries), venous air embolism, pneumothorax, chylothorax, loss of guidewire, nerve injury, cardiac dysrhythmias, and/or infections. There are multiple types of central venous catheters ranging from a single lumen to multiple lumen (double, triple, quad) catheters. Typically, multilumen catheters have slower flow rates due to the smaller radii of these lumens; recall that resistance to flow is proportional to the fourth power of the radius. After placement of a central venous pressure catheter, all ports must be aspirated and flushed to confirm proper intravascular placement of the catheter. In clinical practice, a chest x-ray is often obtained to confirm proper positioning of the catheter. If a pneumothorax develops after accidental puncture of a lung, it will also be evident on chest x-rays.

The central venous pressure waveform can provide important information about the mechanical events occurring during a cardiac cycle (Fig. 18.17). An *a* wave is caused by atrial contraction which occurs after the P wave on the ECG. The *c* wave occurs during the start of

ventricular systole as the tricuspid valve is pushed up toward the right atrium. The next portion of the waveform is the *x* descent, which represents the tricuspid valve being pulled down toward the right ventricle in late systole. The *v* wave correlates with passive filling of the right atrium while the tricuspid valve is closed. The *y* descent completes the waveform and represents the opening of the tricuspid valve, passive emptying of the right atrium, and filling of the right ventricle during diastole. Again it should be noted that the central venous pressure waveform provides information primarily concerning the right heart. Yet, the same waveform can be observed for the left heart by recording the pulmonary capillary wedge pressure from a pulmonary artery catheter (discussed later in this chapter). The central venous pressure waveform is affected by respirations, thus it should be read at end expiration. Central venous pressure value is typically defined as the mean venous pressure at the end of exhalation during spontaneous or controlled ventilation. At end expiration, the intrathoracic pressure is closest to atmospheric pressure.

There are multiple clinical conditions that will affect the recorded central venous pressure waveform. For example, tricuspid stenosis may result in large ("cannon") *a* waves (Fig. 18.18) as the right atrium contracts and pushes blood past a stenotic valve. Abnormal cardiac nodal rhythms, ventricular arrhythmias, or heart block will result in cannon *a* waves, as the atrium and ventricle are not synchronized and the atrium may be contracting against a closed tricuspid valve. Large *a* waves may also occur during situations where the resistance to right

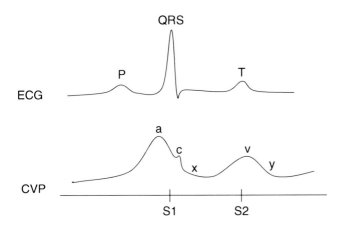

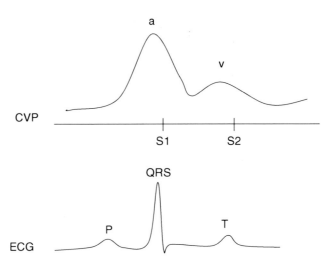

Fig. 18.17 A typical example of a central venous pressure waveform consisting of *a, c,* and *v* waves and *x* and *y* descents. The *a* wave is associated with atrial contraction. The *c* wave occurs as the tricuspid valve bulges up toward the right atrium during early ventricular systole. The *v* wave is associated with passive filling of the right atrium with closed valve. The *x* descent corresponds to the tricuspid valve being pulled down toward the right ventricle during late systole. The *y* descent corresponds with opening of the tricuspid valve as the right atrium begins to empty. CVP = central venous pressure; ECG = electrocardiogram

Fig. 18.18 An example of cannon *a* waves. A severely stenotic tricuspid valve or a junctional rhythm (atrium contracting against a close tricuspid valve) causes a large *a* wave. The mechanical events of the waveform must be correlated with the electrical events of the ECG

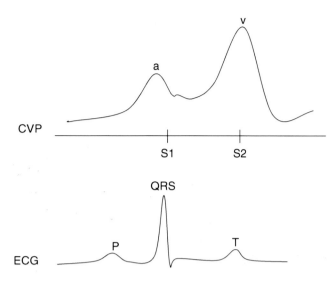

Fig. 18.19 An example of cannon *v* waves. An incompetent tricuspid valve (tricuspid regurgitation) abolishes the *x* descent and causes cannon *v* waves, as volume from the right ventricle backflows into the right atrium during ventricular systole. CVP = central venous pressure; ECG = electrocardiogram

atrium emptying is significantly increased, as in tricuspid and pulmonary valve stenosis, right ventricular hypertrophy, and/or pulmonary artery hypertension. Regurgitant valve disorders such as tricuspid regurgitation will result in large *v* waves (Fig. 18.19), representing overfilling of the atrium. Specifically, the large *v* wave occurs as blood volume from the right ventricle backflows into the right atrium past the incompetent tricuspid valve during systole. A noncompliant right ventricle, as in ischemia and heart failure, may also result in large *v* waves. During atrial fibrillation, *a* waves are absent due to ineffective atrial contractions. Again, similar waveforms for the left heart are seen from a pulmonary capillary wedge pressure waveform. Diagrams of "cannon" *a* and *v* waves are displayed in Figs. 18.18 and 18.19.

18.6 Pulmonary Artery Pressure Monitoring

The pulmonary artery catheter was first introduced into clinical practice by Swan and Ganz [16]. Since its introduction, the pulmonary artery catheter is often used in the management of critically ill patients and in those undergoing major cardiac surgery (Table 18.5). The effectiveness of pulmonary artery catheter monitors and their effect on patient morbidity and mortality continues to be debated and researched [17]. Current modifications also allow for continuous monitoring of pulmonary artery pressure, cardiac output, central venous pressure,

Table 18.5 Relative indications for using a pulmonary artery catheter

- Major organ transplant (liver, heart, lung)
- Cardiopulmonary bypass surgery
- Pulmonary hypertension
- Sepsis/shock
- Aortic aneurysm surgery
- Heart failure (right and/or left heart)
- Pulmonary embolus

See ASA Guidelines for more detailed indications and contraindications [35].

mixed venous oxygen saturation (SvO_2), and pulmonary capillary wedge pressure (Fig. 18.20 and JPG 18.9).

One of the advantages of the pulmonary artery catheter is that blood pressure information associated with the left heart may also be obtained via the pulmonary capillary wedge pressure. Under conditions of normal pulmonary physiology and left ventricular function and compliance, the pulmonary capillary wedge pressure is proportional to the left ventricular end-diastolic pressure, which is proportional to left ventricular end-diastolic volume. Left ventricular preload is best measured by left ventricular end-diastolic volume:

$$CVP{\sim}PAD{\sim}PCWP{\sim}LAP{\sim}LVEDP{\sim}LVEDV$$

where CVP = central venous pressure, PAD = pulmonary artery diastolic pressure, PCWP = pulmonary capillary wedge pressure, LAP = left atrial pressure, LVEDP = left ventricular end-diastolic pressure, and LVEDV = left ventricular end-diastolic volume.

Typically, after establishing central venous access, a pulmonary artery catheter is "floated" into the pulmonary artery with the catheter balloon inflated (see SWANP. mpg on the Companion CD; Visible Heart Viewer). The location of the pulmonary artery catheter balloon is monitored by analysis of the waveform as the catheter is floated from the vena cava to the right atrium, to the right ventricle, and ultimately into the pulmonary artery (Fig. 18.21). Once the catheter is in the pulmonary artery, it is advanced further until the balloon wedges into a distal arterial branch (smaller diameter) of the pulmonary artery (Fig. 18.22). The resultant mean pressure and waveform is the pulmonary capillary wedge pressure. Under normal physiologic conditions, this pressure correlates well with the left atrial pressure. However, the pulmonary artery catheter balloon should not be kept inflated for a long duration or kept in a wedged position due to the possibility of causing pulmonary artery rupture. Note that whenever the catheter is advanced, the balloon (JPG 18.10) should be inflated, and when it is pulled back the balloon should be deflated. The balloon on most pulmonary artery catheters holds a specific

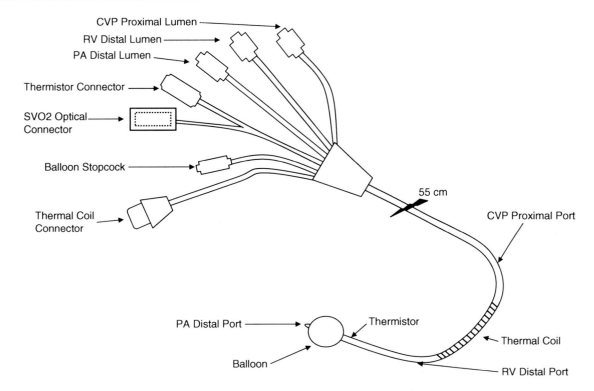

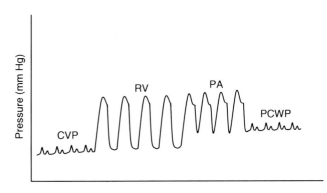

Fig. 18.20 A diagram of a typical pulmonary artery catheter with continuous cardiac output and mean venous oxygen saturation monitoring capabilities. Notice the addition of the thermal coils, thermistors, and optical components to the catheter. (Diagram courtesy of Sock Lake Group, LLC.) CVP = central venous pressure; PA = pulmonary artery; RV = right ventricle; SvO_2 = venous oxygen saturation

Fig. 18.21 A typical example of right heart blood pressure waveforms. As the pulmonary artery catheter is floated into the distal pulmonary artery, the morphology of the pressure waves changes as it goes through the chambers of the heart. CVP = central venous pressure; PA = pulmonary artery pressure; PCWP = pulmonary capillary wedge pressure; RV = right ventricle pressure

volume of air (1.5 mL). Exceeding this volume may result in balloon rupture and/or catastrophic pulmonary artery rupture. Most currently available catheter systems come with a balloon inflation syringe (built-in limiter) which minimizes the risk of such an error.

As with all pressure transducers, the pulmonary artery catheter pressure transducer must be accurately calibrated and zeroed prior to obtaining pressure readings. The pressure transducer should be zeroed at the level midway between the anterior and posterior chest at the level of the sternum; this is usually near the level of the right atrium. The pulmonary artery pressure should be obtained at end expiration (either during spontaneous or mechanical ventilation).

Proper positioning of the pulmonary artery catheter in the lung region is important in obtaining accurate pressure measurements. Since a greater portion of blood flow goes to the right lung (approximately 55%), the balloon of the pulmonary artery catheter most often floats to the right pulmonary artery. West et al. categorized three lung zones (I, II, and III) based on the correlation between pulmonary arterial pressure, alveolar pressure, and venous pressure [18]. Ideal placement of the pulmonary artery catheter requires the catheter tip to be in zone III. This is the area in the lung where blood flow is uninterrupted and therefore capable of transmitting the most accurate blood pressure; it is also the zone least affected by airway pressures. In order for the pulmonary capillary wedge pressure to best correlate with left atrial pressures, the distal tip of the catheter should be in a patent vascular bed. If the catheter tip is in the area of lung where alveolar pressure is greater than perfusion

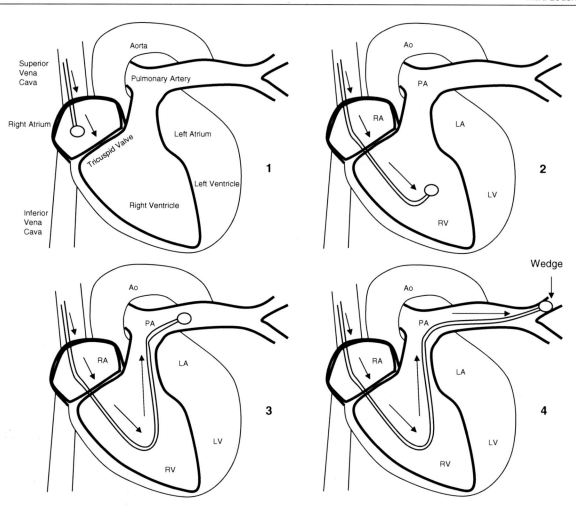

Fig. 18.22 Floating a pulmonary artery catheter through chambers of a heart until the balloon wedges in the distal pulmonary artery. (Diagram courtesy of Sock Lake Group, LLC.) Ao = aorta; LA = left atrium; LV = left ventricle; PA = pulmonary artery; RA = right atrium; RV = right ventricle

pressure, the pulmonary capillary wedge pressure will reflect the alveolar pressure, and not left atrial pressure. Controlled mechanical ventilation utilizing positive end-expiratory pressure decreases the size of West zone III and may affect correlation of pulmonary capillary wedge pressure and left atrial pressure [13]. Other clinical settings in which pulmonary capillary wedge pressure may not accurately reflect left atrial pressure include patients with pulmonary vascular disease, mitral valve disease, chronic obstructive pulmonary disease, and/or those being administered positive end-expiratory pressure [19]. It is possible to convert zone III into zone II, and even zone I, with major increases in pulmonary alveolar pressure, such as positive pressure ventilation and positive end-expiratory pressure [20]. Again, conditions such as positive pressure ventilation, obstructive and restrictive lung disease, and cardiac diseases (i.e., valvular and altered ventricular compliance, tachycardia, and pneumonectomy) are situations where pulmonary capillary wedge pressure does not accurately correlate with left ventricular end-diastolic pressure [21, 22], and hence left ventricular end-diastolic volume.

The pulmonary capillary wedge pressure waveform is similar to the central venous pressure waveform, and occurs at a similar time point within the cardiac cycle. Myocardial changes (i.e., myocardial ischemia), which commonly occur in compliance, and valvular disease will affect the waveform. Large *v* waves occur with mitral regurgitation, myocardial ischemia, papillary muscle dysfunction, and infarction (Fig. 18.19). Large *v* waves may look similar to the pulmonary artery waveform. To prevent errors in interpreting pulmonary capillary wedge pressure and pulmonary artery pressure, the waveform must be viewed and correlated with the ECG tracing. The *v* wave will always occur after the QRS complex and peak systemic arterial waveform and will not have a dicrotic notch. The pulmonary artery waveform has a dicrotic notch. A large *a* wave typically occurs in patients with mitral stenosis and/or left ventricular hypertrophy.

Pulmonary artery catheters may be contraindicated in patients with known abnormal anatomy of the right heart, such as tricuspid and pulmonic valve stenosis or masses in the right heart. Such catheters may also be contraindicated in patients with left bundle branch block of the myocardial conduction system; floating the pulmonary artery catheter through the right heart may cause right bundle branch block and increase the risk of developing complete heart block. The existence of cardiac pacer leads is not a contraindication, but may make placement of a pulmonary artery catheter difficult (see SWANP.mpg on the Companion CD; Visible Heart Viewer). Care also must be taken when removing such a catheter. Reported complications associated with pulmonary artery catheters include cardiac arrhythmias, heart block, pulmonary artery rupture, infection, and/or pulmonary infarction [23]. During cardiac surgery such as lung and heart transplant, it is possible to have the pulmonary artery catheter inadvertently sutured in the surgical field. Note that any resistance to catheter removal must alert the clinician to the above possibility.

18.7 Cardiac Output/Cardiac Index Monitoring

Determining cardiac output is now considered vital when managing any critically ill patient, in particular those with severe cardiac disease, pulmonary disease, and/or multi-organ failure. Cardiac output is the total blood flow by the heart measured in liters per minute (L/min); in an average adult, cardiac output is approximately 5–6 L/min. Cardiac output is often equated with global ventricular systolic function. Any increase in demand for oxygen delivery is usually accomplished with an increase in cardiac output. Furthermore, increasing cardiac output is an important factor in oxygen delivery. Cardiac output is dependent upon heart rate and stroke volume. In a normal heart, stroke volume is dependent upon preload, afterload, and contractility. Note that myocardial wall motion abnormalities and/or valvular dysfunction will also affect stroke volume.

Starling's law describes the relationship between cardiac output and left ventricular end-diastolic volume (Fig. 18.3). As preload is increased, the cardiac output increases in direct proportion to the left ventricular end-diastolic volume until an excessive preload is reached. At this point, increases in left ventricular end-diastolic volume do not result in increased cardiac output and may actually decrease it.

Due to variations in body size and weight, cardiac output is frequently expressed as a cardiac index. Cardiac index is equal to cardiac output divided by body surface area and has a normal range of 2.5–4.3 L/min/m^2:

$$CO = HR \times SV$$

$$CI = CO/BSA$$

where CO = cardiac output, HR = heart rate, SV = stroke volume, CI = cardiac index, and BSA = body surface area.

The equation for cardiac output can also be derived by rearranging the oxygen extraction equation. Oxygen extraction is the product of cardiac output and the difference between arteriovenous oxygen content:

$$VO_2 = CO \times (CaO_2 - CvO_2)$$

where VO_2 = oxygen extraction, CO = cardiac output, CaO_2 = arterial oxygen content, and CvO_2 = venous oxygen content.

Rearranging the oxygen extraction equation allows calculation of cardiac output:

$$CO = VO_2/(CaO_2 - CvO_2)$$

A limitation of the Fick method is that frequent blood samples from the arterial and venous circulation are required. Expiratory gas must also be analyzed to measure oxygen consumption.

Cardiac output can also be measured by utilizing an indicator (dye) dilution technique or a thermodilution technique. In the indicator dilution technique, a nontoxic dye (e.g., methylene blue or indocyanine green) is injected into the right heart. The dye mixes with blood and goes out the pulmonary artery to the systemic circulation. A circulating arterial blood sample with diluted indicator dye is collected and measured using spectrophotometric analysis. Repeat cardiac output measurements utilizing the indicator dilution technique are limited due to increasing concentrations of dye with each subsequent measurement.

The thermodilution method to measure cardiac output is a modification of the indicator dilution technique initially described by Fegler [24] in 1954. Thermodilution techniques are not considered to be affected by recirculation, as are the indicator dilution techniques. Typically, the distal tips of the pulmonary artery catheters contain thermistors that detect temperatures of the blood. The more proximal portion of the pulmonary artery catheter contains an opening that allows for injection of fluid such as normal saline or D_5W. The injected solution may be at an ambient temperature or iced. An iced solution increases the temperature difference, and therefore the signal-to-noise ratio [25], thus it is considered better than an injectate at room temperature. A computer program within the monitoring system commonly calculates the cardiac output utilizing the thermodilution cardiac output equation. The components of the equation include the following: specific heat of blood, specific gravity of blood and injectate, volume of injectate, and area of blood temperature curve. A modified Stewart–Hamilton equation [26] can also be used to calculate cardiac output using this approach:

$$CO = V(Tb - Ti) \times K1 \times K2 / \int \Delta Tb(t)dt$$

where CO = cardiac output in L/min, V = volume of injectate (mL), Tb = initial blood temperature (°C), Ti = initial injectate temperature, $K1$ = density factor, $K2$ = computation constant, and $\int \Delta Tb(t)dt$ = integral of blood temperature change over time.

Cardiac output is inversely proportional to the area under the curve (Fig. 18.23).

Nevertheless, an accurate calculation of cardiac output requires both proper position of the pulmonary artery catheter and a consistent volume of injectate. Note that

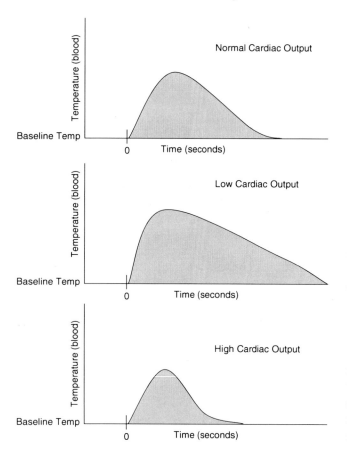

Fig. 18.23 An example of cardiac output monitoring. In this case, cardiac output is inversely proportional to the area under the thermodilution curve

situations such as tricuspid and pulmonic value regurgitation and intracardiac shunts will cause recirculation of blood, and thus result in the false elevation of cardiac output. The errors of intermittent bolus thermodilution techniques include valuable volumes and temperatures of injectate, technique of injection, and timing of injection with the respiratory cycle [27]. Cardiac output measurements are also affected by clinical conditions such as tricuspid insufficiency, intracardiac shunts, and/or atrial fibrillation [19].

More recently, continuous cardiac output monitoring has been made possible with advanced pulmonary artery catheters (JPG 18.11). Typically, continuous cardiac output monitors utilize a thermal coil which is positioned in the right ventricle; this coil intermittently heats the blood. Once the continuous cardiac output catheter and system reaches a steady state with its surroundings, the thermal coil intermittently heats blood. The temperature change of the surrounding blood is detected by a thermistor located at the distal tip of the pulmonary artery catheter; the recorded blood temperature varies inversely with cardiac output.

The accuracy of the system depends on the measurement of temperature differences from the injection port to the distal measurement thermistor. In the thermodilution technique, the volume of injectate must be constant (10 mL). Smaller amounts of cold solution reaching the thermistor will result in a higher cardiac output. Such detected differences may be caused by actual increased cardiac output, small amounts of injectate, warm indicator and/or injectate, a clot on the thermistor, or a wedged catheter. A calculated small cardiac output will result when the solution reaching the thermistor is too cold; this may occur if there is too large an amount of injectate, if the solution is too cold, if there is an actual decrease in cardiac output, and/or if the patient has an intracardiac shunt. A major limitation of continuous cardiac output method is its slow response time to acute changes in cardiac output [27, 28]. Although the response time may be slow, it is still faster in detecting cardiac output changes than the traditional intermittent thermodilution technique. Furthermore, continuous cardiac output monitoring is generally considered to be more accurate than the intermittent thermodilution technique [29, 30].

Noninvasive methods to measure cardiac output include Doppler modalities, transpulmonary dilution technique [31, 32], gas rebreathing technology [32, 33], and/or a bioimpedance [32, 34, 35] technique. Briefly, the noninvasive Doppler method to measure cardiac output is an esophageal Doppler monitor. As such, an esophageal Doppler probe is placed and an ultrasound beam is directed at the descending aorta. By knowing the cross-sectional area of the aorta and blood velocity, the stroke volume is calculated [32].

The transpulmonary dilution method for measuring cardiac output requires injections of an indicator (lithium or thermodilution) in the venous circulation (central or peripheral) and subsequent assessment of the indicator level of the systemic arterial circulation; a typical example is the lithium chloride solution technique [36–38]. Lithium chloride indicator is injected through a central or peripheral vein, and the plasma concentration of this indicator is measured via a lithium-specific electrode connected to the arterial line [39]. A concentration–time curve is generated and cardiac output is calculated from the area under the curve associated with the lithium ion concentrations [40].

The thoracic bioimpedance method measures cardiac output by detecting the change in flow of electricity with alteration in blood flow [31]. For thoracic bioimpedance, a low amplitude and high frequency current is transmitted and then sensed by sets of electrodes placed on both sides of the thorax and neck. The cardiac alterations in impedance (resistance to current flow) are analyzed and calculated as the blood volume changes for each heartbeat (stroke volume). The thoracic bioimpedance method of measuring cardiac output may be useful in clinical situations such as major trauma [41, 42] and cardiac disease [43].

Gas technology utilizing the measurement of carbon dioxide [32, 44] applies the Fick principle of oxygen consumption and cardiac output, but substitutes carbon dioxide production for oxygen consumption. By determining the change in CO_2 production and end-tidal CO_2, modification of the Fick equation can be applied to calculate cardiac output [45]:

$$CO = \Delta VCO_2 / \Delta EtCO_2$$

where CO = cardiac output, ΔVCO_2 = change in CO_2 production, and $\Delta EtCO_2$ = end-tidal CO_2.

It should be noted that the accuracy of the carbon dioxide rebreathing method to measure cardiac output is, at present time, inconclusive [45–48].

18.8 Mixed Venous Oxygen Saturation Monitoring

Mixed venous oxygen saturation monitoring (SvO_2) typically utilizes reflective spectrophotometric technology to measure the amount of oxygen in mixed venous blood. Yet, a true mixed venous blood sample is measured in the pulmonary artery. Systemic venous blood with different oxygen extraction ratios returns to the right atrium via the superior vena cava and inferior vena cava, mixes and equilibrates in the right ventricle, and flows out past the pulmonic valve to the pulmonary artery. As blood travels

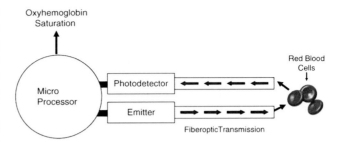

Fig. 18.24 An example of mixed venous saturation monitoring (SvO_2). Spectrophotometric technology such as pulse oximeter and mixed venous oxygen saturation monitors are utilized to measure the amount of oxygenated hemoglobin in circulating blood. A specific wavelength (infrared) is emitted and the reflected wavelength off the red blood cells is detected and processed

past the SvO_2, catheter light emitted from the catheter tip is reflected off the red blood cells and is detected by a photo detector. The difference in wavelengths of emitted and reflected light is processed to estimate SvO_2 (Fig. 18.24). Continuous venous saturation (SvO_2) monitoring has been made possible with the adaptation of a pulmonary artery catheter with fiberoptic technology (JPG 18.11). Such monitoring utilizes the principle of reflectance spectrophotometry which uses multiple wavelengths of transmitted light at specific intensities that is then reflected from red blood cells. For example, oxygenated hemoglobin absorbs most infrared light (940 nm) and reflects or transmits most red light (660 nm); this is the reason that oxyhemoglobin looks red and deoxyhemoglobin appears blue. The tip of the SvO_2 catheter emits light with specific wavelengths which measure both oxyhemoglobin and deoxyhemoglobin, as red blood cells flow past the tip of the catheter. The difference between absorption of light between saturated and desaturated hemoglobin results in the calculated SvO_2 value.

The SvO_2 equation is a modification of the Fick equation; SvO_2 is derived by rearranging the Fick equation as follows:

$$VO_2 = C(a-v)O_2 \times CO \times 10$$
$$SvO_2 = SaO_2 - VO_2 / DO_2$$
$$DO_2 = \text{volume of } O_2 \text{ delivered per minute}$$
$$= CO \times CaO_2 \times 10$$
$$VO_2 = \text{oxygen consumption per minute}$$
$$= C(a-v)O_2 \times CO \times 10$$
$$SaO_2 = \text{arterial } O_2 \text{ saturation}(1.0)$$
$$CaO_2 = 1.39 \times Hgb \times SpO_2 + 0.003 \times PaO_2$$

where VO_2 = oxygen consumption, CaO_2 = arterial oxygen content, CvO_2 = venous oxygen content, CO =

cardiac output, DO_2 = oxygen delivery, SaO_2 = arterial oxygen saturation, Hgb = hemoglobin, SpO_2 = oxygen saturation, and PaO_2 = partial pressure of arterial oxygen.

Accurate measurement of SvO_2 requires that vasoregulation be intact [49] and there must be a continuous flow of blood past the tip of the catheter. SvO_2 values may be incorrect if the tip of the pulmonary artery catheter migrates into the distal pulmonary artery and/or comes in contact with the arterial wall. Other causes of incorrect SvO_2 values include miscalibration of the microprocessor or light intensity that is too low (some sensor systems have incorporated intensity monitors). Note that the tip of the catheter must be in the pulmonary artery in order to have true mixed venous oxygen.

Mixed venous oxygen saturation (SvO_2) monitoring provides information about the balance between total body oxygen consumption and delivery. SvO_2 (0.65–0.75) measures the amount of oxygen not taken up by organs and tissues. Therefore, the lower the SvO_2, the higher the fraction extraction of oxygen by the tissues and a possible imbalance between oxygen consumption and oxygen delivery. SvO_2 is dependent upon arterial oxygen saturation, oxygen consumption, concentration of hemoglobin, and cardiac output. A significant change in SvO_2 may be caused by decreased oxygen delivery (decreased cardiac output and hemoglobin), increased oxygen consumption, or decreased arterial oxygen saturation. Continuous SvO_2 monitoring is useful in conditions where there is significant oxygen transport imbalance including severe cardiac and respiratory disease, sepsis, and/or dysfunctional oxygen transport [50]. During stable arterial oxygen content and consumption, SvO_2 reflects the relative cardiac output [51, 52]. Furthermore, monitoring of SvO_2 may provide vital information in the medical management of critically ill [53, 54] and/or cardiac surgery patients [55]. If SvO_2 drops during a period of increased oxygen demand, it may indicate inadequate tissue perfusion and oxygen delivery; this information would not be available with monitoring cardiac output only.

It is considered that SvO_2 may be a better measurement of myocardial performance than cardiac output alone. Acute decrease in SvO_2 below 0.65 indicates a disparity between oxygen delivery and oxygen consumption. A change in SvO_2 greater than ±0.1 is considered significant. Medical management of critically ill patients by implementing measures to keep SvO_2 normal is considered important for decreasing morbidity and mortality [39, 56]. Conditions where SvO_2 is greater than 0.75 include increased oxygen delivery and low oxygen consumption. SvO_2 may be elevated during septic shock, hyperoxygenation, cyanide toxicity, and in patients with arterial venous shunts [49, 50]. The increase in SvO_2 during sepsis is considered, in part, due to the loss of vasoregulation and yet

does not mean that organ tissues are being adequately oxygenated. It should be noted that under general anesthesia, the SvO_2 value is increased due to the decreased metabolic requirement for oxygen by tissues.

In clinical settings where a pulmonary artery SvO_2 catheter is not possible (i.e., pediatric patients), a central venous oxygen saturation ($ScvO_2$) monitor may be used. The advantage of $ScvO_2$ is that a pulmonary artery catheter is not required; only central venous access is needed. The $ScvO_2$ obtains venous oxygen saturation readings from the superior vena cava or right atrium. During normal physiologic and hemodynamic conditions, $ScvO_2$ correlates well with SvO_2 [57–59]. However, in critical illness and shock, the $ScvO_2$ does not accurately reflect the true SvO_2 [60–62] and, therefore, true SvO_2 can only be measured in the pulmonary artery in such cases [63]. Resuscitation and medical management of critically ill patients with a $ScvO_2$ monitor may provide benefits over conventional monitors such as vital signs and/or central venous pressure [60].

18.9 Flow Monitoring

While cardiac output is similar regardless of where it is measured within the heart, the flow profiles can change dramatically within different anatomical structures and disease states. Given a constant cardiac output, flow velocity increases with a smaller diameter vessel, with larger velocities seen at the center of the flow profile and with zero velocity at the vessel wall.

For example, flow through the cardiac valves is important for diagnosis of stenosis and regurgitation. Stenosis is defined as a narrowing of the orifice area of the valve. This can be caused by a variety of factors including sclerosis formation on leaflets and is characterized by abnormally high flow velocities through the valve. Regurgitation is defined as flow reversal through a valve and can be caused by annular dilatation, leaflet prolapse, and/or changes in chamber dimensions affecting the valve performance. While a small amount of regurgitation is normal (caused by valve closing called the "closing volume"), patients with pathologic regurgitation have abnormally high flows traveling retrograde across the valve orifice.

Clinical diagnoses of regurgitation and stenosis are typically done using echocardiography (see Chapter 20). Pulsed wave Doppler measures a frequency shift in the ultrasound waves to calculate a flow velocity. Color flow mapping allows for visualization of the flow through the valve. By standards, areas flowing toward the transducer head appear red, areas flowing away from the transducer head appear blue, and areas of regurgitation or turbulent flow appear in a third color, typically yellow or green. A

Table 18.6 Indications for diagnosing stenosis of the cardiac valves

	Jet velocity (m/s)	Pressure gradient (mmHg)	Orifice area (cm^2)
Aortic stenosis			
Mild	<3.0	<25.0	>1.5
Moderate	3.0–4.0	25.0–40.0	1.0–1.5
Severe	>4.0	>40.0	<1.0
Mitral stenosis			
Mild	<5.0	<30.0	>1.5
Moderate	5.0–10.0	30.0–50.0	1.0–1.5
Severe	>10.0	>50.0	<1.0
Tricuspid stenosis			
Severe	NA	NA	<1.0
Pulmonic stenosis			
Severe	>4.0	>60.0	NA

table of flow rates, pressure gradients, and orifice area measurements is available in Table 18.6 for the varying degrees of stenosis for each of the cardiac valves, as reported by the American College of Cardiology (ACC)/American Heart Association (AHA) guidelines [64]. Consult the ACC/AHA guidelines for diagnosing the severity of regurgitation.

In a research setting, several other methods are available for flow monitoring across the cardiac valves in an in vivo setting. Doppler sensors, using the same principles as echocardiography, are available in a number of forms, a c-ring transducer (transonic) being common. This flow probe takes frequency measurements, calculates a velocity from the measurement, and then multiplies the velocity by the area of the c-ring to determine the flow through the vessel. This type of sensor is useful for flows downstream of the aortic or pulmonary valves, but cannot be attached in the atrioventricular positions.

Electromagnetic sensors take advantage of Faraday's law of inductance to measure velocity of a conducting fluid, such as blood. A rapidly reversing magnetic field is produced and, as the fluid moves through this field, a voltage is generated. This voltage is measured and translated into a frequency signal which is proportional to flow rate. They are capable of measuring the instantaneous velocity of a small area with high temporal resolution and can be attached to a catheter. The disadvantage of electromagnetic sensors is that the measurements are affected by catheter placement, the exact location of which can be difficult to determine through fluoroscopy.

Cardiac magnetic resonance can be utilized in both a clinical and research role to investigate flow through valves and major vessels. Phase contrast cardiac magnetic resonance enables the measurement of blood flow velocity across the cardiac valves and the great vessels with a high temporal and spatial resolution. As blood flows through the static magnetic field, the precession frequency changes in the hydrogen atoms of the tissue. This frequency change results in a dephasing effect on the magnetization of the atoms. The net dephasing of the atomic spins is a function of the velocity of the blood flow as well as the direction. This technique is used for clinical diagnosis of valvular regurgitation, aortic stenosis, and to investigate coronary flow. For more information on these methods, the reader is referred to Chapter 22.

Angiograms are utilized to observe acute flow through the coronary system. While this is a qualitative technique for flow monitoring, it is of clinical importance, particularly for the assessment of coronary blockages. In an angiogram, the patient is typically cannulated via a femoral artery and the catheter is fed into or near the coronary ostia. Contrast is then injected through the catheter and into the bloodstream. By imaging via fluoroscopy (continuous x-rays), the contrast can be observed traveling through the coronary system. Flow is considered interrupted anywhere that contrast cannot traverse, indicating a blockage in the coronary system. An arterial dissection of the left anterior descending coronary artery is shown in the Companion CD (JPG 18.12). The dissection is a tear in the tunica intima of the blood vessel, which allows blood into the space between the inner and outer layers of the vessel wall, resulting in vessel stenosis and possible occlusion. The area of the dissection is circled on the left of the image and the reduction in flow is visible downstream of the dissection. The image on the right shows the same artery after the vessel has healed.

Classification of blood flow using engineering terms is not a simple task. Blood flow through vessels is typically laminar, but partial occlusions can lead to turbulence downstream of the occlusion. This phenomenon is utilized in blood pressure measurements (see Korotkoff sounds). Flow through or near a cardiac valve becomes quite a bit more complicated, as it is neither laminar nor turbulent. Yoganathan et al. classify the pulsatile flow of blood through cardiac valves as "borderline turbulent flow," characterized by regions of flow reversal, 3D separation, and vortex formation, with borderline turbulent flow being defined as unsteady laminar flow with more than one temporal frequency excited. Yet, they further describe the flow to transition into a fully turbulent state during peak systole [65].

18.10 Implantable Monitoring

In both the research and clinical settings, the ability to more optimally and continuously monitor hemodynamic properties is being realized. Furthermore, devices are being developed for researchers who work with small animals, for clinical researchers, and for physicians to monitor their patients without clinical visits. These devices may consist of sensors that transmit data to an implantable loop recorder, where the information is stored until it is collected by the researcher or physician by telemetry or other means.

An implantable loop recorder is a valuable tool for researchers conducting chronic studies and for clinicians. For example, data can be collected continuously when investigating properties that occur only rarely or change slowly over time. Clinically, implantable loop recorders that gather ECG data are used for diagnosis of patients with unexplained syncope, near syncope, episodic or recurrent palpitations, and seizure-like events. The use of an implantable loop recorder has diagnosed patients in which standard tilt table testing has failed to induce syncopy [66–68] and is now advised for management of patients with syncopy [69, 70]. Two examples of implantable loop recorders such as the ones described here are the Sleuth (Transoma Medical, Inc., Arden Hills, MN) and the Reveal Plus (Medtronic, Inc., Minneapolis, MN).

Perhaps the most advanced implantable hemodynamic monitoring system to date is the investigational device called Chronicle (Medtronic, Inc.). It is a pressure sensor equipped lead that is implanted in the right ventricle to provide continuous hemodynamic monitoring of heart rate, right ventricular systolic pressure, right ventricular diastolic pressure, right ventricular pulse pressure, maximum right ventricular dP/dt, and/or estimated pulmonary artery diastolic pressure [71, 72]. The data storage period of this device can be adjusted with the desired sampling rate, but can also be reprogrammed as desired.

Another application of implantable sensors is the monitoring of patients with congestive heart failure. Signs and symptoms of congestive heart failure are not well correlated with the disease status [73, 74], and investigational devices combining pacing capabilities with monitoring capabilities have been implanted in ambulatory patients with congestive heart failure to monitor parameters such as the mixed venous oxygen saturation and right ventricular pressures. The feasibility of these devices has been shown [75], but clinical validation studies are ongoing.

However, implantable monitors are only as valuable as the information they collect and the manner and ease in which that information is transferred to those interpreting it. Collection of the data is less of an issue in a research setting, where the researcher can personally ensure the data are retrieved at the proper time and in the desired format. Clinicians, on the other hand, could have a large number of patients with implantable monitors who reside in a large geographic area. In addition, numerous home telemonitoring units are in use to gather data from patients with implantable devices and send the data to a location where it can be processed and interpreted by their physicians. Examples of telemonitoring systems include the LATITUDE® Patient Management system (Boston Scientific, Inc., Natick, MA) and the CareLink® network (Medtronic, Inc.).

18.11 Summary

Advanced methods and technology continue to develop for the assessment of cardiac hemodynamics. Such monitoring can be used acutely; however, many new technologies are being developed for chronic monitoring of the cardiac patient (e.g., employing miniaturized implantable sensors). In this chapter, we provided a general overview of several devices and/or systems that can be used either clinically or experimentally to monitor cardiac performance. However, it should be reiterated that to best understand how the output of such devices can be used for the assessment of cardiac function, one needs to first possess an in-depth understanding of underlying basic cardiac physiology.

References

1. Sengupta PP, Khandheria BK, Korinek J, et al. Apex-to-base dispersion in regional timing of left ventricular shortening and lengthening. J Am Coll Cardiol 2006;47:163–72.
2. Ratcliffe M, et al. Use of sonomicrometry and multidimensional scaling to determine the three-dimensional coordinates of multiple cardiac locations: Feasibility and initial implementation. IEEE Trans Biomed Eng 1995;42:587–97.
3. Gorman JH III, Gupta KB, Streicher JT, et al. Dynamic three-dimensional imaging of the mitral valve and left ventricle by rapid sonomicrometry array localization. J Thorac Cardiovas Surg 1996;112:712–25.
4. Meyer S, et al. Application of sonomicrometry and multidimensional scaling to cardiac catheter tracking. IEEE Trans Biomed Eng 1997;44:1061–7.
5. Geddes LA, Baker LE. The specific resistance of biological material—A compendium of data for the biomedical engineer and physiologist. Med Biol Eng 1967;5:271–93.
6. Baan J, van der Velde ET, de Bruin HG, et al. Continuous measurement of left ventricular volume in animals and humans by conductance catheter. Circulation 1984;70:812–23.
7. van der Velde ET, van Dijk AD, Steendijk P, et al. Left ventricular segmental volume by conductance catheter and cine-CT. Eur Heart J 1992;13 Suppl E:15–21.
8. White PA, Redington AN. Right ventricular volume measurement: Can conductance do it better? Physiol Meas 2000;21:R23–41.
9. Hettrick DA, Battocletti J, Ackmann J, Linehan J, Warltier DC. In vivo measurement of real-time aortic segmental volume using the conductance catheter. Ann Biomed Eng 1998;26:431–40.
10. Gardner RM. Accuracy and reliability of disposable pressure transducers coupled with modern monitors. Crit Care Med 1996;24:879–82.

11. Skeehan TM, Thys DM. Monitoring of the cardiac surgical patient. In: Hensley FA, Martin DE, eds. A practical approach to cardiac anesthesia. 2nd ed. Boston, MA: Little, Brown and Company, 1995:102.

12. Gorback MS. Considerations in the interpretation of systemic pressure monitoring. In: Lumb PD, Bryan-Brown CW, eds. Complications in critical care medicine. Chicago, IL: Year Book, 1988:296.

13. Shasby DM, Dauber IM, Pfister S, et al. Swan-Ganz catheter location and left atrial pressure determine the accuracy of wedge pressure when positive end expiratory pressure is used. Chest 1980;80:666–70.

14. Snyder JV, Carroll GC. Tissue oxygenation: A physiologic approach to a clinical problem. Curr Probl Surg 1982;19:650.

15. Stanley TE, Reves JG. Cardiovascular monitoring. In: Miller RD, ed. Anesthesia. 4th ed. Boston, MA: Churchill Livingstone, 1994:1167.

16. Swan HJC, Ganz W, Forrester J, Marcus H, Diamon G, Chonette D. Catheterization of the heart in man with use of a flow-directed balloon-tipped catheter. N Engl J Med 1970;283:447–51.

17. Practice guidelines for pulmonary artery catheterization. Anesthesiology 2003;99:989–1014.

18. West JB, Dollery CT, Naimark A. Distribution of blood flow in isolated lung; relation to vascular and alveolar pressures. J Appl Physiol 1964;19:713–24.

19. Wesseling KH. Finger arterial pressure measurement with Finapres. Z Kardiol 1996;3:38–44.

20. Brandstetter RD, Grant GR, Estilo M, Rahim R, Sing K, Gitler B. Swan-Ganz catheter: Misconceptions, pitfalls, and incomplete user knowledge–an identified trilogy in need of correction. Heart Lung 1998;27:218–22.

21. Wittnich C, Trudel J, Zidulka A, Chiu RC. Misleading "pulmonary wedge pressure" after pneumonectomy: Its importance in postoperative fluid therapy. Ann Thorac Surg 1986;42:192–6.

22. Van Aken H, Vandermeersch E. Reliability of PCWP as an index for left ventricular preload. Br J Anesth 1988;60:85–9S.

23. Stanley TE, Reves JG. Cardiovascular monitoring. In: Miller RD, ed. Anesthesia. 4th ed. Boston, MA: Churchill Livingstone, 1994:1184–5.

24. Fegler G. Measurement of cardiac output in anesthetized animals by thermodilution method. Q J Exp Physiol 1954;39:153.

25. Pearl RGB, Rosenthal MH, Mielson L, et al. Effect of injectate volume and temperature on thermodilution cardiac output determination. Anesthesiology 1986;64:798.

26. Reich DL, Moskowitz DM, Kaplan JA. Hemodynamic monitoring. In: Kaplan JA, Reich DL, Konstaelt SN, eds. Cardiac anesthesia. 4th ed. Philadelphia, PA: WB Saunders Co, 1999.

27. Burchell SA, Yu M, Takiguchi SA, Ohta RM, Myers SA. Evaluation of a continuous cardiac output and mixed venous oxygen saturation catheter in critically ill surgical patients. Crit Care Med 1997;25:388–91.

28. Poli d Figueiredo LF, Malbouisson LMS, Varicoda EY, et al. Thermal filament continuous thermodilution cardiac output delayed response limits its value during acute hemodynamic instability. J Trauma 1999;47:288–93.

29. Mihaljevi T, vonSegesser LK, Tonz M, et al. Continuous versus bolus thermodilution cardiac output measurements: A comparative study. Crit Care Med 1995;23:944–9.

30. Mihm FG, Gettinger A, Hanson CW, et al. A multicenter evaluation of a new continuous cardiac output pulmonary artery catheter system. Crit Care Med 1998;26:1346–50.

31. Della RG, Costa MG, Pompei L, et al. Continuous and intermittent cardiac output measurement: Pulmonary artery catheter versus aortic transpulmonary technique. Br J Anaesth 2002;88:350–6.

32. Pamley CL, Pousman RM. Noninvasive cardiac output monitoring. Curr Opin Anaesthesiol 2002;15:675–80.

33. Christensen P, Clemensen P, Andersen PK, et al. Thermodilution versus inert gas rebreathing for estimation of effective pulmonary blood flow. Crit Care Med 2000;28:51–6.

34. Imhoff M, Lehner JH, Lohlein D. Noninvasive whole-body electrical bioimpedance cardiac output and invasive thermodilution cardiac output in high-risk surgical patients. Crit Care Med 2000;28:2812–8.

35. Shoemaker WC, Wo CC, Bishop MH, et al. Multicenter trial of a new thoracic electrical bioimpedance device for cardiac output estimation. Crit Care Med 1994;22:1907–12.

36. Linton RA, Band DM, Haire KM. A new method of measuring cardiac output in main using lithium dilution. Br J Anaesth 1994;71:262–6.

37. Linton R, Band D, O'Brian T, et al. Lithium dilution cardiac output measurement: A comparison with thermodilution. Crit Care Med 1997;25:1767–8.

38. Kurita T, Morita K, Kato S, et al. Comparison of the accuracy of the lithium dilution technique with the thermodilution technique for measurement of cardiac output. Br J Anaesth 1997;79:770–5.

39. Rivers E, Nguyen B, Havstad S, et al. Early goal-directed therapy in the treatment of severe sepsis and septic shock. N Engl J Med 2001;345:1368–77.

40. Band DM, Linton RA, Jonas MM, et al. The shape of indicator dilution curves used for cardiac output measurement in man. J Physiol 1997;498:225–9.

41. Shoemaker WC. New approaches to trauma management using severity of illness and outcome prediction based on noninvasive hemodynamic monitoring. Surg Clin North Am 2002;82:245–55.

42. Shoemaker WC, Wo CC, Chan L, et al. Outcome prediction of emergency patients by noninvasive hemodynamic monitoring. Chest 2001;120:528–37.

43. Drazner MH, Thompson B, Rosenberg PB, et al. Comparisons of impedance cardiography with invasive hemodynamic measurements in patients with heart failure secondary to ischemic or nonischemic cardiomyopathy. Am J Cardiol 2002;89:993–5.

44. Binder JC, Parkin WG. Non-invasive cardiac output determination: Comparison of a new partial-rebreathing technique with thermodilution. Anaesth Intensive Care 2001;28:427–30.

45. Maxwell RA, Gibson JB, Slade JB, et al. Noninvasive cardiac output by partial CO_2 rebreathing after severe chest trauma. J Trauma 2001;51:849–53.

46. Tachibana K, Imanaka H, Miyano H, et al. Effect of ventilatory settings on accuracy of cardiac output measurement using partial CO_2 rebreathing. Anesthesiology 2002;96:96–102.

47. Botero M, Lobato EB. Advances in noninvasive cardiac output monitoring: An update. J Cardiothorac Vasc Anesth 2001;15:631–40.

48. Kotake Y, Moriyama K, Innami Y, et al. Performance of noninvasive partial CO_2 rebreathing cardiac output and continuous thermodilution cardiac output in patients undergoing aortic reconstruction surgery. Anesthesiology 2003;99:283–8.

49. Keech J, Reed RL II. Reliability of mixed venous oxygen saturation as an indicator of the oxygen extraction ratio demonstrated by a large patient data set. J Trauma 2003;54:236–41.

50. Snyder JV, Carroll GC. Tissue oxygenation: A physiologic approach to a clinical problem. Curr Probl Surg 1982;19:650.

51. Jain A, Shroff SG, Jnicki JS, et al. Relation between venous oxygen saturation and cardiac index. Nonlinearity and normalization for oxygen uptake and hemoglobin. Chest 1991;99:1403–9.

52. Inomata S, Nishikawa T, Taguchi M. Continuous monitoring of mixed venous oxygen saturation for detecting alterations in cardiac output after discontinuation of cardiopulmonary bypass. Br J Anaesth 1994;72:11–6.

53. Rivers E, Nguyen B, Vastad S, et al. Early goal-directed therapy in the treatment of severe sepsis and septic shock. N Engl J Med 2001;345:1368–77.

54. Kraft P, Steltzer H, Hiesmayr M, et al. Mixed venous oxygen saturation in critically ill septic shock patients: The role of defined events. Chest 1993;103:900–6.

55. Waller JL, Kaplan JA, Bauman LI, et al. Clinical evaluation of a new fiberoptic catheter oximeter during cardiac surgery. Anesth Analg 1982;61:676–9.

56. Vedrinne C, Bastien O, De Varax R, et al. Predictive factors for usefulness of fiberoptic pulmonary artery catheter for continuous oxygen saturation in mixed venous blood monitoring in cardiac surgery. Anesth Analg 1997;85:2–10.

57. Goldman RH, Klughaupt M, Metcalf T, et al. Measured central venous oxygen saturation in patients with myocardial infarction. Circulation 1968;38:941–6.

58. Berridye JC. Influence of cardiac output on correlation between mixed venous and central venous oxygen saturation. Br J Anaesth 1992;89:409–10.

59. Davies GG, Mendehall J, Symrey T. Measurement of right atrial oxygen saturation by fiberoptic oximetry accurately reflects mixed venous oxygen saturation in swine. J Clin Monit 1988;4:99–102.

60. Rivers EP, Ander DS, Powell D. Central venous oxygen saturation monitoring in the critically ill patient. Curr Opin Crit Care 2001;7:204–11.

61. Lee J, Wright F, Barber R, et al. Central venous oxygen saturation in shock: A study in man. Anesthesiology 1972;36:472–8.

62. Scheinman MM, Brown MA, Rapaport E. Critical assessment of use of central venous oxygen saturation as a mirror of mixed venous oxygen in severely ill cardiac patients. Circulation 1969;40:165–72.

63. Edwards JD, Mayall RM. Importance of the sampling site for measurement of mixed venous oxygen saturation in shock. Crit Care Med 1998;26:1356–60.

64. Bonow RO, Carabello B, de Leon AC, et al. ACC/AHA guidelines for the management of patients with valvular heart disease. Executive summary. A report of the American College of Cardiology/American Heart Association task force on practice guidelines (committee on management of patients with valvular heart disease). J Heart Valve Dis 1998;7:672–707.

65. Yoganathan AP, Chandran KB, Sotiropoulos F. Flow in prosthetic heart valves: State-of-the-art and future directions. Ann Biomed Eng 2005;33:1689–94.

66. Brignole M, Sutton R, Menozzi C, et al. Lack of correlation between the responses to tilt testing and adenosine triphosphate test and the mechanism of spontaneous neurally mediated syncope. Eur Heart J 2006;27:2232–9.

67. Deharo JC, Jego C, Lanteaume A, Djiane P. An implantable loop recorder study of highly symptomatic vasovagal patients: The heart rhythm observed during a spontaneous syncope is identical to the recurrent syncope but not correlated with the head-up tilt test or adenosine triphosphate test. J Am Coll Cardiol 2006;47:587–93.

68. Moya A, Brignole M, Menozzi C, et al. Mechanism of syncope in patients with isolated syncope and in patients with tilt-positive syncope. Circulation 2001;104:1261–7.

69. Strickberger SA, Benson DW, Biaggioni I, et al. AHA/ACCF scientific statement on the evaluation of syncope: From the American Heart Association councils on clinical cardiology, cardiovascular nursing, cardiovascular disease in the young, and stroke, and the quality of care and outcomes research interdisciplinary working group; and the American College of Cardiology foundation: In collaboration with the heart rhythm society: Endorsed by the American Autonomic Society. Circulation 2006;113:316–27.

70. Brignole M, Alboni P, Benditt DG, et al. Guidelines on management (diagnosis and treatment) of syncope-update 2004. Executive summary. Eur Heart J 2004;25:2054–72.

71. Adamson PB, Magalski A, Braunschweig F, et al. Ongoing right ventricular hemodynamics in heart failure: Clinical value of measurements derived from an implantable monitoring system. J Am Coll Cardiol 2003;41:565–71.

72. Reynolds DW, Bartelt N, Taepke R, Bennett TD. Measurement of pulmonary artery diastolic pressure from the right ventricle. J Am Coll Cardiol 1995;25:1176–82.

73. Stevenson LW, Perloff JK. The limited reliability of physical signs for estimating hemodynamics in chronic heart failure. JAMA 1989;261:884–8.

74. Wilson JR, Hanamanthu S, Chomsky DB, Davis SF. Relationship between exertional symptoms and functional capacity in patients with heart failure. J Am Coll Cardiol 1999;33:1943–7.

75. Bennett T, Kjellstrom B, Taepke R, Ryden L. Development of implantable devices for continuous ambulatory monitoring of central hemodynamic values in heart failure patients. Pacing Clin Electrophysiol 2005;28:573–84.

Chapter 19
Energy Metabolism in the Normal and Diseased Heart

Arthur H.L. From and Robert J. Bache

Abstract This chapter reviews the metabolic pathways involved in transferring the chemical energy stored in dietary carbon substrates (primarily glucose and fatty acids) into adenosine triphosphate (ATP) and the regulatory systems that integrate the functions of these pathways and make them responsive to changes in energy demand. Normal cardiac function depends upon both the adequate delivery of carbon substrates and oxygen to the heart by the coronary circulation and the ability of the heart to extract and metabolize these substrates at rates sufficient to support a wide range of ATP demands. The effects of several physiological states and disease processes on cardiac metabolism are also discussed and the concept that the diseased heart may be energy limited is presented. Lastly, an example of a new therapeutic approach, based on a detailed understanding of an inherited metabolic pathway abnormality, emphasizes the importance of detailed knowledge of energetic pathways.

Keywords Myocardial metabolism · Adenosine triphosphate · Myocardial blood flow · Glucose metabolism · Fatty acid metabolism · Oxidative phosphorylation

19.1 Introduction

Although this chapter is devoted to a discussion of myocardial metabolism, the reader should understand that ultimately all energy-requiring biological processes in our biosphere are dependent upon capture of solar energy and its entrapment in molecules that can be used to fuel biological processes such as cardiac contraction. The synthesis by plants of molecules such as glucose from CO_2 and H_2O is powered by the sun via the process of photosynthesis. Photons radiated by the sun are trapped by chlorophyll and used to drive the synthesis of adenosine triphosphate (ATP). ATP has two phosphate bonds with high levels of stored chemical energy (Fig. 19.1). The energy released by breakdown of the terminal high-energy phosphate bond is captured and used to drive the synthesis of glucose. Hence, a portion of the energy derived from the sun is ultimately stored in the form of chemical bonds resident in the chemically stable glucose molecule. The chemical energy stored in glucose can be released in a controlled fashion by enzyme-catalyzed reactions to drive the synthesis of other species of molecules including fatty acids (another convenient storage molecule for chemical energy) as well as for the resynthesis of ATP. Because animals are unable to convert solar energy to a storable form of chemical energy, most animal life is ultimately powered by the photosynthetic process in plants. The ingestion of plants supplies animals with usable forms of stored chemical energy. Even carnivores ultimately depend on energy storage compounds that have passed up the food chain from plants. The general aim of this chapter is to discuss processes involved in the transfer of chemical bond energy contained in the ingested energy storage molecules that we call food into ATP, which is the common energy currency of the heart and other biologic tissues.

In the myocardium, as in other biologic tissues, most energy-requiring processes use ATP as the immediate source of energy. Hydrolysis of the terminal phosphate bond of ATP releases energy that can be captured and used to drive energy-requiring processes such as protein synthesis, muscle contraction, and/or ion transport. The ability of the heart to pump blood to the pulmonary and systemic circulations is dependent on the availability of

A.H.L. From (✉)
University of Minnesota, Cardiovascular Division, Center for Magnetic Resonance Research, 2021 6th St. SE, Minneapolis, MN 55455, USA
e-mail: fromx001@umn.edu

This work was supported by NIH grants HL33600, HL58840, HL20598, and HL21872 and Veterans Administration medical research funds.

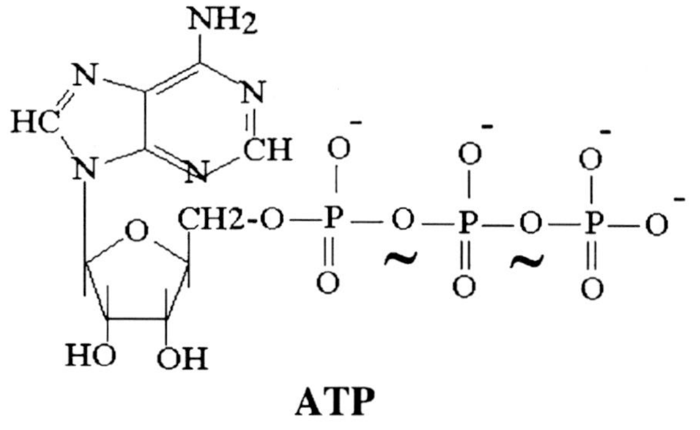

ATP

Fig. 19.1 Adenosine triphosphate (ATP). ATP is the major source of chemical energy used to power the reactions that support contractile and other processes in myocardium and all other living tissues. The $\sim$ symbol is used to designate a phosphate bond that has a very high level of stored chemical energy. Although ATP contains two $\sim$ phosphate bonds, it is the hydrolysis of the terminal phosphate bond that releases the energy that directly powers cellular processes

ATP. Because tissue stores of ATP are modest, continuous synthesis is required to maintain ATP levels sufficient to drive energy-requiring processes. Importantly, the energy required for ATP synthesis is derived from the controlled breakdown of the chemical bonds in carbohydrates (glucose) and fatty acids.

The primary purposes of this chapter are to: (1) describe mechanisms for delivery of carbon substrate and oxygen to the heart; (2) describe the biochemical pathways that transfer chemical bond energy in carbon substrates to ATP in the healthy heart and how these pathways are regulated and capable of responding to increasing ATP demand; and (3) discuss some of the alterations in these processes that occur in the diseased

heart. The reader should understand that this relatively brief summary of myocardial metabolism is, by necessity, a superficial overview of the individual topics discussed. For those readers wishing to review some of the major topics in greater detail, a list of recent references (primarily current topical reviews and research reports, and also several standard texts) is provided at the end of this chapter.

19.2 Myocardial Blood Flow

Blood containing carbon substrates and oxygen is delivered into human and most animal hearts by two coronary arteries that originate from the proximal aorta and then subdivide and course over the surface of the heart (epicardium) (see Chapter 6). These arteries arborize into progressively smaller branches, then progress inward to penetrate the epicardium and supply blood to the myocardium (Fig. 19.2). In the left ventricle, the heart muscle (for descriptive purposes) is arbitrarily subdivided into transmural layers termed the subepicardium (outermost layer), the midmyocardium, and the subendocardium (innermost layer). The coronary arterial tree terminates in muscular vessels 60–150 mm in diameter termed "arterioles." The arterioles are the major locus of resistance to blood flow, and contraction or relaxation of the smooth muscle in the walls of the arterioles (vasomotion) provides the mechanism for control of the rate of blood flow into the myocardium. Each arteriole supplies an array of capillaries, thin-walled tubes comprised of a single layer of endothelial cells, across which most of the exchange of nutrients, oxygen, and metabolic waste products occurs. At their terminal

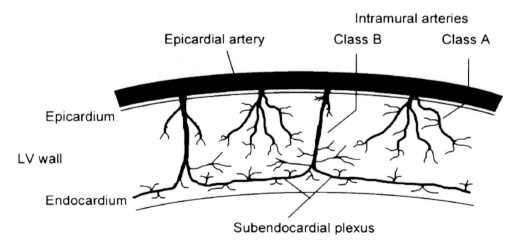

Fig. 19.2 Transmural distribution of the coronary arterial system. The large epicardial conductance arteries supply shallow and deep branches to the subepicardium and subendocardium, respectively. These perforating vessels arborize to create the arteriolar network that supplies the myocardial capillary bed. LV = left ventricle.

Reprinted from Duncker DJ, Bache RJ. Regulation of coronary vasomotor tone under normal conditions and during acute myocardial hypoperfusion. Pharmacol Ther 2000;86:87–110, with permission from Elsevier

end, capillaries coalesce into venules, the initial component of the cardiac venous system that conducts blood back into the venous circulation primarily through the coronary sinus, which drains into the right atrium. For more details of the coronary circulation, see Chapter 7.

19.2.1 Regulation of Myocardial Blood Flow

Coronary blood flow is highly regulated and responds appropriately to subtle or large changes in energy requirements of the myocardium. The principal work of the heart is muscle contraction that generates the pressure that drives blood through the arterial system of the body. Elevation of cardiac ATP expenditure during exercise or other stresses increases myocardial demand for oxygen and carbon substrates. In clinical practice, there is often a need to assess the effects of changes in the rate of myocardial energy expenditure on cardiac performance (e.g., during exercise stress testing). Since routine measurement of myocardial oxygen consumption is not practical, a rough estimate of the change in the energy demands of the heart can be obtained as the product of systolic blood pressure and the times per minute that pressure generation occurs (heart rate), termed the "rate–pressure product." This measurement provides a simple estimate of changes in the metabolic requirements of the heart resulting from different cardiac work states.

The coronary circulation operates on the principle of "just-in-time" delivery of oxygen and carbon substrates. In other words, coronary blood flow is regulated to be only minimally greater than required to meet the ambient metabolic demands of the heart. Furthermore, the heart extracts 70–80% of the O_2 from the blood as it flows through the coronary capillaries. Because of this high level of basal oxygen extraction, there is little ability to increase oxygen uptake by means of increased extraction of oxygen from the blood. As a result, increases in myocardial energy requirements during exercise or other stress must be satisfied by essentially parallel increases in coronary blood flow. Since ATP and oxygen stores in the myocardium are relatively small, the response time for the increase in coronary flow during an increase in cardiac work must be rapid (i.e., a few seconds). From these considerations, it is clear that highly responsive signaling systems must exist, which connect myocardial metabolic processes to vasomotor activity in the resistance vessels that control coronary blood flow. Interestingly, to date, these signaling systems are not fully understood despite intense study over the last 75 years.

19.2.2 Biologic Signals Regulating the Coronary Circulation

The regulatory signals that increase blood flow in response to increases in cardiac work can be classified as having feedback or feed-forward characteristics; the final common response to these signals is relaxation of the vascular smooth muscle cells comprising the resistance vessels that control coronary flow (Fig. 19.3). Several

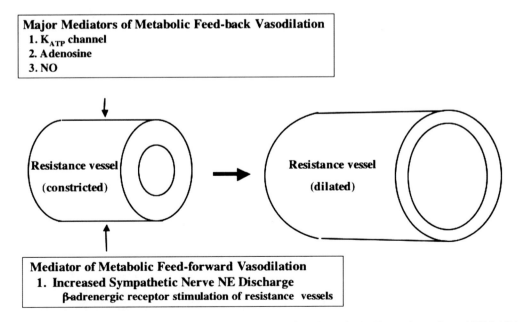

Major Mediators of Metabolic Feed-back Vasodilation
1. K_{ATP} channel
2. Adenosine
3. NO

Resistance vessel (constricted)

Resistance vessel (dilated)

Mediator of Metabolic Feed-forward Vasodilation
1. **Increased Sympathetic Nerve NE Discharge**
   β-adrenergic receptor stimulation of resistance vessels

Fig. 19.3 Major feedback and feed-forward mechanisms underlying metabolic vasodilatation of resistance vessels are depicted (see text for discussion). K_{ATP} channel = ATP-inhibited potassium channel; NO = nitric oxide

major feedback mechanisms resulting from increased cardiomyocyte metabolism (including adenosine, nitric oxide, and other less defined signals) cause opening of ATP-sensitive potassium channels (K_{ATP}) on the sarcolemma of smooth muscle cells of the coronary arterioles. Opening of these channels allows potassium to escape from the cytosol of the smooth muscle cells, resulting in hyperpolarization (increased negativity) of the cell membrane. The increased negativity of the membrane causes sarcolemmal voltage-dependent calcium channels to close; as a result, calcium entry is reduced, the muscle relaxes (vasodilation), and hence coronary blood flow increases. In addition to effects on the K_{ATP} channels, adenosine (a product of ATP utilization in the cardiomyocyte) also has potent, direct dilator effects on arteriolar smooth muscle. Another metabolic feedback signal is nitric oxide generated by the vascular endothelium. Mechanotransduction of flow-induced shear forces exerted on the endothelial cells augments nitric oxide synthesis. In addition to causing potassium channel opening, nitric oxide also initiates direct relaxation processes in vascular smooth muscle. It is important to note that this brief discussion does not include all of the known feedback mechanisms involved in regulation of coronary blood flow.

Increases in cardiac sympathetic nerve activity (i.e., during exercise) activate a feed-forward mechanism for control of coronary blood flow, which augments the local metabolic vasodilator influences. The sympathetic neurotransmitter norepinephrine activates α- and β-adrenergic receptors on vascular smooth muscle cells. Activation of α-adrenergic receptors causes modest constriction of the large coronary arteries; however, since these arteries function as conduit vessels that offer little resistance to blood flow, this has little effect on coronary flow. However, activation of β-adrenergic receptors on the coronary arterioles results in relaxation (vasodilation) of the small resistance vessels; the resultant decrease in coronary resistance causes a feed-forward increase in blood flow that is independent of local metabolic mechanisms and augments the increase in coronary blood flow during exercise.

Pharmacological studies have shown that simultaneous blockade of the coronary K_{ATP} channels, adenosine, and nitric oxide pathways significantly decreases myocardial blood flow in the resting animal. Moreover, the increase in coronary flow that normally occurs during exercise is severely blunted, resulting in a perfusion–metabolism mismatch that is accompanied by evidence of ischemia even in the normal heart. Hence, activation of these three pathways appears to be the primary means by which metabolic vasodilatation is achieved in the heart. However, in the normal situation or in the healthy heart, blockade of any one of these mechanisms for smooth muscle relaxation will elicit compensatory (i.e., increased) activation of the other pathways to minimize changes in coronary blood flow.

19.2.3 Blood Flow in the Diseased Heart

Coronary blood flow in the diseased heart can be limited by: (1) partial or complete obstruction of the large coronary arteries (e.g., atherosclerotic disease); (2) decreased responsiveness of the signaling systems relating blood flow to myocardial energy requirements; and/or (3) increases in extravascular mechanical forces acting to compress the small vessels in the wall of the left ventricle. In the case of obstructive coronary disease, a moderately narrowed vessel may only restrict blood flow during periods of increased work and blood flow demand (i.e., it reduces vasodilator reserve), while a severely narrowed vessel may limit blood flow even when the subject is at rest. In the presence of a moderate coronary obstruction, the arteriolar bed can maintain adequate blood flow by metabolic signaling-based arteriolar vasodilatation. That is, a decrease in small vessel resistance can compensate for the increased resistance caused by a coronary artery stenosis. However, when the capacity for vasodilation of the arterioles has been exhausted, any further increase in cardiac work cannot induce an increase in blood flow and the myocardium supplied by the narrowed vessel will become ischemic. There is also adequate evidence that malfunction of metabolic signaling pathways in the arteriolar resistance vessels (e.g., in patients with non-obstructed large coronary arteries) can cause myocardial ischemia.

In the normal heart, blood flow to the inner layers of the left ventricle occurs principally during diastole. This is because tissue pressures in the wall of the left ventricle during systole are so great that inner layer arterioles are squeezed shut by the extravascular compressive forces produced by cardiac contraction. Diastolic left ventricular tissue pressures are also greatest in the subendocardium. As the heart fails and/or becomes hypertrophied, these extravascular compressive forces increase as left ventricular filling pressure increases. Slowing of myocyte relaxation also shortens the duration of the diastolic interval, and thus limits coronary flow reserve, in the hypertrophied or failing heart. In the normal heart, autoregulatory (i.e., metabolic vasodilatation) processes cause arteriolar vasodilation in the subendocardium to compensate for systolic underperfusion. However, increases in left ventricular diastolic pressure in the failing heart may compress the arteriolar bed in the inner myocardial layers sufficiently to overwhelm autoregulatory mechanisms, particularly those that normally maintain adequate subendocardial blood flow. Since subendocardial blood flow occurs predominantly during diastole, tachycardia also acts to impede blood flow in the subendocardium by shortening the interval of diastole. Thus, even in the absence of obstructive coronary artery disease, functional abnormalities can limit blood flow to the inner myocardial layers of the diseased heart. These abnormalities are often associated with a reduction in ATP synthetic capacity in the subendocardium. Thus, the extravascular forces that act on the small coronary vessels embedded in the myocardium cause the subendocardium to be the region of the ventricular wall that is most vulnerable to hypoperfusion and ischemia.

19.3 Intermediary Metabolism and Bioenergetics in the Normal Heart

Glucose and fatty acids are generally the main substrates consumed by the heart, with fatty acid consumption predominating under most circumstances (Fig. 19.4). Exceptions to this statement will be discussed later.

19.3.1 Glucose Metabolism

Figure 19.5 shows a flowchart for glucose metabolism. Glucose enters the cardiomyocyte via the sarcolemmal glucose transport proteins, GLUT 1 (which is insulin independent) and GLUT 4 (which predominates and is insulin dependent). Once in the cell, glucose is phosphorylated to glucose-6-phosphate by the enzyme hexokinase. Since glucose-6-phosphate is membrane impermeable, it is effectively trapped within the cell. Glucose-6-phosphate can enter the glycogen synthesis pathway (glycogen is a macromolecular polymeric storage form of glucose), the pentose monophosphate shunt (which will not be further discussed), or it can undergo molecular rearrangement via the enzyme phosphohexose isomerase to form fructose-6-phosphate and continue on through the glycolytic series of reactions. A second phosphorylation of fructose-6-phosphate via phosphofructokinase generates fructose-1,6-bisphosphate. Each of these phosphorylations consumes one molecule of ATP. Dihidroxyacetone phosphate is then split into glyceraldehyde-3-phosphate and dihydroacetone phosphate by the enzyme aldolase. These two products are in constant exchange with each other via the enzyme phosphotriose isomerase. Glyceraldehyde-3-phosphate is phosphorylated to form 1,3-bisphosphoglycerate by the enzyme glyceraldehyde-3-phosphate dehydrogenase. The phosphate bond in the 1 position is a high-energy-containing bond (signified by the $\sim$P symbol); this reaction also simultaneously reduces NAD^+ to nicotinamide adenine dinucleotide (NADH). Cytosolic oxidation of NADH and transport of the two removed electrons and H^+ into the mitochondrial matrix then occur via the malate–aspartate shuttle (not shown in Fig. 19.5). In the

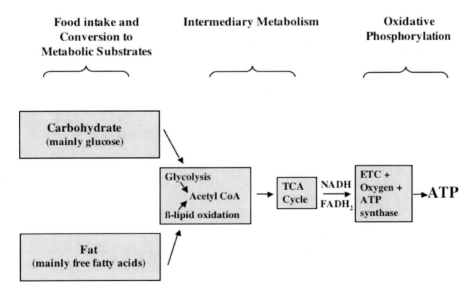

Fig. 19.4 A general overview of carbon substrate metabolism in the heart. First, ingested food is broken down into usable carbon substrates, primarily amino acids (not major contributors to ATP synthesis), glucose, and fatty acids. The pathways that convert amino acids and other molecules to glucose are not shown. Glucose and fatty acids are processed (via intermediary metabolic processes) to yield the reducing equivalents, NADH and FADH$_2$, which supply the energy necessary to power oxidative phosphorylation. The latter process, which occurs within the mitochondria in the presence of oxygen, supplies almost all of the ATP synthesized and utilized in the heart. ATP = adenosine triphosphate; ETC = electron transport chain; FADH$_2$ = flavin adenine dinucleotide; NADH = nicotinamide adenine dinucleotide; TCA = tricarboxylic acid

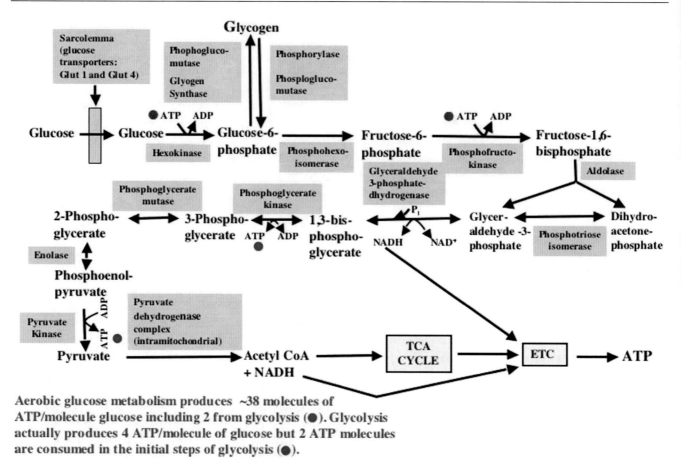

Aerobic glucose metabolism produces ~38 molecules of
ATP/molecule glucose including 2 from glycolysis (●). Glycolysis
actually produces 4 ATP/molecule of glucose but 2 ATP molecules
are consumed in the initial steps of glycolysis (●).

Fig. 19.5 Flowchart of cellular uptake of glucose and the pathways through which glucose metabolism proceeds. See text for discussion. ADP = adenosine diphosphate; ATP = adenosine triphosphate;

ETC = electron transport chain; NADH = nicotinamide adenine dinucleotide; TCA = tricarboxylic acid

mitochondrial matrix, NAD^+ is reduced to NADH, which can be utilized by the mitochondria to generate ATP (to be discussed later). In the next reaction, the high-energy phosphate bond in 1,3-bisdiphosphoglycerate is transferred to adenosine diphosphate (ADP) to form ATP and 3-phosphoglycerate via the enzyme phosphoglycerate kinase. The latter molecule is converted to 2-phosphoglycerate by the enzyme phosphoglycerate mutase. Enolase, another cytosolic enzyme, then converts 2-phosphoglycerate to the ~P-containing molecule phosphoenolpyruvate. The latter is converted to pyruvate by the enzyme pyruvate kinase. During this reaction, the ~P in phosphoenolpyruvate is transferred to ADP to form a second ATP molecule. Pyruvate can then enter the mitochondria to be further metabolized by the pyruvate dehydrogenase (PDH) complex of enzymes. Both the pyruvate dehydrogenase complex, which converts pyruvate to acetyl CoA (and NAD^+ to NADH), and the tricarboxylic acid (TCA) cycle that metabolizes acetyl CoA are located within the mitochondria (Figs. 19.5, 19.6A, and 19.7). Within the mitochondria, another metabolic pathway

for pyruvate exists. The enzyme pyruvate carboxylase converts pyruvate to oxaloacetate, which is a TCA cycle intermediate (Figs. 19.6A and 19.10). The significance of the latter reaction will be discussed later.

Within the cytosol, pyruvate can be converted to lactic acid by lactic acid dehydrogenase (LDH). Lactate is then exported from the cell via the monocarboxylic acid transporter (Figs. 19.5, 19.6A, and 19.15). This reaction results in the oxidation of NADH to NAD^+ and, as will be shown, this reaction is critical when the availability of oxygen to the cardiomyocyte is limited. Conversely, under aerobic conditions, lactate can be transported into the cardiomyocyte by the monocarboxylic acid transporter to be converted to pyruvate by LDH. The LDH-catalyzed reaction also reduces NAD^+ to NADH, and the reducing equivalents from NADH can be transferred into the mitochondrial matrix by the malate–aspartate shuttle. The pyruvate generated is then available for processing by PDH.

During glycolysis of one glucose molecule, two pyruvate molecules, four ATP molecules, and two NADH

A

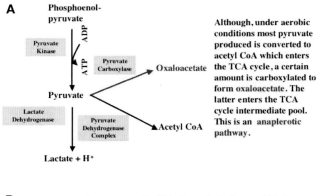

Although, under aerobic conditions most pyruvate produced is converted to acetyl CoA which enters the TCA cycle, a certain amount is carboxylated to form oxaloacetate. The latter enters the TCA cycle intermediate pool. This is an anaplerotic pathway.

B

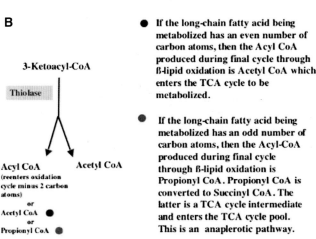

● If the long-chain fatty acid being metabolized has an even number of carbon atoms, then the Acyl CoA produced during final cycle through ß-lipid oxidation is Acetyl CoA which enters the TCA cycle to be metabolized.

● If the long-chain fatty acid being metabolized has an odd number of carbon atoms, then the Acyl-CoA produced during final cycle through ß-lipid oxidation is Propionyl CoA. Propionyl CoA is converted to Succinyl CoA. The latter is a TCA cycle intermediate and enters the TCA cycle pool. This is an anaplerotic pathway.

Fig. 19.6 Anaplerotic and cataplerotic processes. Anaplerotic processes are those that supply substrate used to maintain the TCA cycle intermediate pool size. In contrast, cataplerotic processes remove substrates from the TCA cycle intermediate pool and decrease its size. The balance between these two processes determines the TCA cycle pool size. **A** shows how glucose (via its metabolic product pyruvate) contributes to anaplerosis. **B** shows how β-oxidation of odd-numbered carbon-chain fatty acids contributes to anaplerosis. (Note that readers may want to review Fig. 19.13, a flowchart for β-lipid oxidation, before examining Fig. 19.6B, which depicts the terminal reaction of β-lipid oxidation). ADP = adenosine diphosphate; ATP = adenosine triphosphate; TCA = tricarboxylic acid

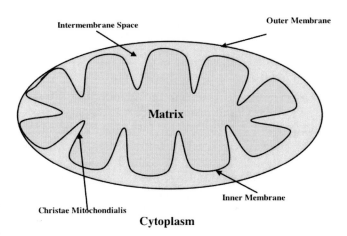

Fig. 19.7 Major features of mitochondrial morphology. See text for discussion

molecules are produced. However, because two ATP molecules are consumed early in the glycolytic pathway, the net production of ATP is two molecules/glucose molecule. As previously indicated, pyruvate and NADH are utilized in the mitochondria for oxidative generation of ATP. Complete metabolism of one glucose molecule (i.e., including oxidation of the products of glycolysis in mitochondria) results in the formation of many additional ATP molecules (36) than does glycolysis alone (2). However, under conditions when mitochondrial function is severely oxygen limited, the oxidative contribution to ATP synthesis is lost and only two ATP molecules can be formed from each glucose molecule.

19.3.2 The Mitochondrion

Mitochondria, which are the primary site of ATP synthesis in most mammalian cells, contain the β-lipid oxidation pathway enzymes, the TCA cycle enzymes, the electron transport chain, and the F_1F_0-H^+-ATPase (also called F_1F_0-ATP synthase or ATP synthase). To better understand the location of these systems, mitochondrial structure will be briefly reviewed (Fig. 19.7). The inner mitochondrial membrane contains the electron transport chain, F_1F_0-H^+-ATPase, the adenine nucleotide translocase, and other transporters. The mitochondrial matrix contains the TCA cycle enzymes, β-lipid oxidation enzymes, and other enzymes and reactants. The cristae are invaginations that markedly expand the surface area of the inner membrane and, thereby, the amount of enzymes that can be associated with the inner membrane. The membrane-bound components of the enzyme pathways are positioned to optimize the flow of substrates through their reaction sequences. The mitochondrial outer membrane forms a boundary between the cellular cytoplasm and the mitochondrial intermembrane space. The intermembrane space contains creatine kinase, which is important for high-energy phosphate transport out of mitochondria (Figs. 19.7, 19.11, and 19.13), and cytochrome c, a component of the electron transport chain. The importance of the intermembrane space to oxidative ATP synthesis will be discussed subsequently.

19.3.3 Fatty Acid Metabolism

Figure 19.8 presents a flowchart for the β-lipid oxidation pathway. Dietary long-chain, nonesterified, free fatty acids (NEFAs) are usually the predominant cardiac

Fig. 19.8 Flowchart depicting the cellular uptake of free fatty acids and the pathways through which their metabolism proceeds. See text for discussion. ATP = adenosine triphosphate; CPT 1 = carnitine palmitoyl- transferase 1; CPT 2 = carnitine palmitoyl- transferase 2; ETC = electron transport chain; FADH$_2$ = flavin adenine dinucleotide; FFA = free fatty acids; NADH = nicotinamide adenine dinucleotide; TCA = tricarboxylic acid

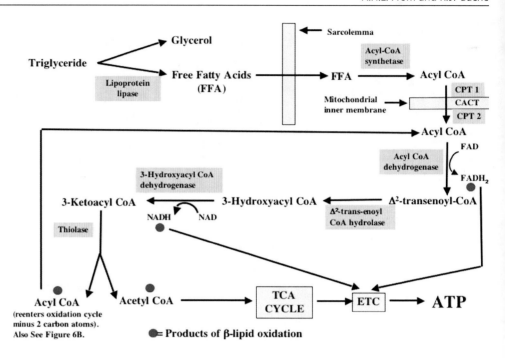

substrate. They are transported in the blood bound to plasma albumin, other lipoprotein moieties, or in the form of triacylglycerol, which is also bound to albumin. The latter can be broken down to release NEFAs by an enzyme present in the plasma and at the surface of the capillary and cardiomyocyte. After dissociating from albumin, NEFAs are transported into the cardiomyocyte by sarcolemmal fatty acid transport proteins. Within the cell, NEFAs are bound to fatty acid-binding proteins, which provide solubility. Once in the cell, NEFAs are either reesterified and stored as triglycerides or activated by acyl CoA synthetase (which requires the presence of free CoA and ATP) to form a long-chain acyl CoA. Because long-chain acyl CoA cannot readily diffuse through the mitochondrial inner membrane, it is converted to long-chain acyl carnitine by carnitine palmitoyl-transferase 1 at the outer surface of the inner mitochondrial membrane and then transported across the inner membrane by carnitine–acylcarnitine translocase (which also transports free carnitine liberated by carnitine palmitoyl-transferase 2 back into the intermembrane space). The long-chain acyl carnitine is then converted back to acyl CoA at the inner surface of the mitochondrial inner membrane by carnitine palmitoyl-transferase 2. Long-chain acyl CoA is then processed by a sequence of enzyme-catalyzed reactions that comprise the β-lipid oxidation pathway. If the long-chain acyl CoA has an even number of carbon atoms, then the final products of the last cycle (i.e., of a four-carbon acyl CoA molecule) through the β-oxidation sequence are two

acetyl CoA molecules (Fig. 19.6B). However, if the long-chain acyl CoA has an odd number of carbon atoms, then the products of the last cycle (i.e., of a five-carbon acyl CoA molecule) through β-oxidation are one acetyl CoA and one propionyl CoA. Unlike acetyl CoA, propionyl CoA cannot enter the TCA cycle. However, propionyl CoA is readily converted to succinyl CoA, which is a TCA cycle intermediate (Fig. 19.6B). Hence this pathway contributes to the maintenance of the TCA cycle intermediate pool size. Thus, both pyruvate molecules produced from glucose and odd-numbered fatty acid molecules that undergo complete β-oxidation contribute to the maintenance of the TCA intermediate pool. Processes that add molecules to the TCA intermediate pool are termed "anaplerotic" (Figs. 19.6A, B), and those that remove intermediates from the pool are called "cataplerotic." The importance of these processes to TCA cycle function will be illustrated in a clinical example to be presented later.

The products of complete β-oxidation of a fatty acid are acetyl CoA (and propionyl CoA if the chain has an odd number of carbons), NADH, and flavin adenine dinucleotide (FADH$_2$). Yet, consumption of these products by the TCA cycle and the electron transport chain cannot occur in the absence of oxygen. Thus, β-oxidation cannot occur under anoxic or ischemic conditions. Therefore, markedly ischemic myocardium does not support either pyruvate- or fatty acid-derived ATP synthesis, and the only remaining source of ATP synthesis is anaerobic glycolysis.

19.3.4 Regulation of Carbon Substrate Metabolic Pathways

Myocardial glycolysis is regulated at several levels (Fig. 19.9A); the first is entry of glucose into the cell. In heart and skeletal muscle, this process is largely dependent on the activity of the GLUT 4 glucose transporter. The quantity of the GLUT 4 transporter in the plasma membrane is determined by the action of insulin on its sarcolemmal receptor, the activation of which triggers migration of GLUT 4 from cytoplasmic stores to the plasma membrane. Increased levels of

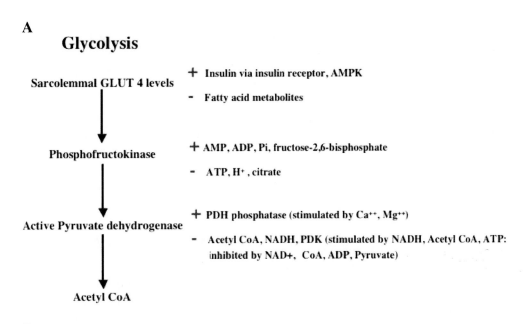

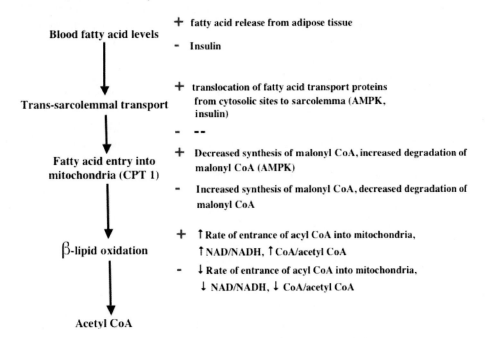

Fig. 19.9 A Major regulatory sites in the glycolytic pathway (including pyruvate dehydrogenase, which is immediately distal to the glycolytic sequence). **B** Major regulatory sites in the fatty acid metabolic pathway (including β-lipid oxidation). ADP = adenosine diphosphate; AMP = adenosine monophosphate; AMPK = adenosine monophosphate-activated kinase; ATP = adenosine triphosphate; CPT 1 = carnitine palmitoyl-transferase 1; NADH = nicotinamide adenine dinucleotide; PDH = pyruvate dehydrogenase

fatty acid metabolites inhibit insulin receptor activation, as noted below. Because blood glucose levels are generally well defended by an organism, glucose availability is not usually limiting to transport. Plasma membrane GLUT 4 levels are also enhanced during increased myocardial work states, which induce elevation of cytosolic adenosine monophosphate (AMP) and ADP. AMP then activates AMP-dependent protein kinase (AMPK), which also causes increased GLUT 4 trafficking to the plasma membrane. The subsequent reactions of the glycolytic sequence (and glycogen breakdown) are also activated by a number of factors including increased cytosolic Ca^{2+}, AMPK, protein kinases A and C, PI3K, and fructose 2,6-bisphosphate, as well as AMP and ADP. These reactions are inhibited by increased levels of ATP, increased cytosolic levels of H^+, and/or citrate. Because increased free fatty acid metabolism tends to increase mitochondrial citrate synthesis, increased citrate exiting the mitochondria can inhibit glycolysis. The first step of oxidative glucose metabolism (the decarboxylation of pyruvate to form acetyl CoA) by PDH is also highly regulated by PDH kinases and phosphatases, and a high level of β-lipid oxidation causes inactivation of PDH by stimulating its phosphorylation by specific kinases. The regulatory pathways are complex and discussed in more detail in several references cited at the end of the chapter.

Fatty acid metabolism has two major regulatory sites (Fig. 19.9B). The first is at the level of fatty acid transport through the plasma membrane; transport occurs by means of transport proteins in the membrane (major path) and via free diffusion through the plasma membrane (minor path). This process is mainly regulated by the blood concentrations of fatty acids, i.e., that fatty acid uptake is blood level dependent. This means that if the rate of fatty acid utilization is slower than the uptake rate, cardiomyocytes will accumulate fatty acids. The latter are mainly stored as triglycerides. Excess lipid accumulation can be damaging to cardiomyocytes (and other cells as well). The second regulatory site is at the level of long-chain fatty acid transport into mitochondria. As discussed above, long-chain acyl CoA must be converted to long-chain acyl carnitine at the outer mitochondrial membrane by the enzyme carnitine palmitoyl-transferase 1. This enzyme is inhibited by malonyl CoA, a molecule produced by acetyl CoA carboxylase in response to increased cytosolic levels of acetyl CoA. The latter occurs as a result of increased fatty acid or pyruvate oxidation by the mitochondria, although this overall signaling pathway is complex. Hence increased fatty acid oxidation or high blood concentrations of lactate (by virtue of increasing cytosolic pyruvate levels) will activate malonyl CoA

synthesis and thereby limit fatty acid uptake and oxidation by mitochondria. This explains why lactate (and exogenously supplied pyruvate; see below) is able to compete successfully with fatty acids for mitochondrial oxidation. Activation of AMPK by an increased cardiac work state or ischemia can directly inhibit acetyl CoA carboxylase and thereby reduce malonyl CoA levels. This will relieve inhibition of carnitine palmitoyl-transferase 1 and facilitate fatty acid entry into mitochondria. The rate of mitochondrial fatty acid or pyruvate oxidation (assuming no limitation of transport into mitochondria) is, of course, ultimately controlled by the rate of consumption of the products of these metabolic pathways. The latter is determined by the rate at which the cell utilizes ATP (see below for discussion of this point). A more detailed discussion of the regulation of fatty acid metabolic pathways and of how malonyl CoA levels are controlled is available in references cited at the end of this chapter.

19.3.5 Myocardial Carbon Substrate Selection

The primary carbon substrates (Fig. 19.4) taken up and metabolized by the myocardium are free fatty acids and glucose. The heart also readily takes up and metabolizes pyruvate, lactate, and ketone bodies, but usually the relatively low blood concentrations of these substrates limit their utilization. However, during intense exercise, which is associated with marked elevation of blood lactate content, or during periods when blood levels of ketone bodies are elevated, utilization of these substrates increases markedly at the expense of glucose and fatty acid utilization. A more detailed discussion of the regulation of blood levels of these substrates exceeds the scope of this chapter, yet a few orienting comments are appropriate with regard to glucose and fatty acid utilization patterns. Blood glucose levels are maintained within a narrow range (~4–5 mM) in non-diabetic subjects. Glucose homeostasis reflects a balance between the alimentary uptake of glucose, glucose release from the liver (which can synthesize glucose or release glucose from the glycogen storage pool), and removal of glucose from the blood by various organs. Glucose uptake is strongly influenced by the pancreatic secretion of insulin, a hormone that enhances glucose transport into the cells of many tissues (especially skeletal and cardiac muscle).

The heart has often been called an "omnivore" because of its capacity to consume virtually any available carbon substrate. Glucose is transported into the cardiomyocyte by a family of sarcolemmal glucose transport proteins; of these, the predominant transporter (GLUT 4) is insulin dependent. Fatty acids enter myocytes via sarcolemmal fatty acid transport proteins, and lactate and pyruvate are taken up by the sarcolemmal monocarboxylic acid transporter. Utilization of glucose by the heart is largely regulated by the availability of fatty acids in the blood. Thus, in the fasted state, blood fatty acid levels are high and fatty acids are the predominant cardiac substrate despite normal blood glucose levels. This is because increased fatty acid levels suppress glucose uptake and its utilization in heart and skeletal muscle. In contrast, during vigorous exercise, blood lactate levels can rise markedly and compete with the myocardial metabolism of fatty acids and glucose despite the presence of substantial blood levels of the latter substrates. Similarly, after a carbohydrate meal, blood glucose levels rise and this will elicit insulin secretion. Insulin stimulates glucose uptake by the heart, skeletal muscle, and other tissues and also causes blood fatty acid levels to decrease. As a result, myocardial glucose consumption increases and fatty acid consumption decreases. Of interest, fatty acids, pyruvate, and lactate are the most favored substrates when the relative blood concentrations of all of the substrates are experimentally equalized. Physiological switching of substrates does not affect myocardial performance.

19.3.6 The TCA Cycle

Acetyl CoA is the carbon substrate consumed by the TCA cycle. Acetyl CoA is produced both by glycolysis and by β-lipid oxidation, as described above. Figure 19.10 shows the individual reactions of the TCA cycle. In the first step of the cycle, acetyl CoA contributes two carbon atoms to oxaloacetate to form citrate and free CoA; this reaction is catalyzed by the enzyme citrate synthase. Citrate then enters a sequence of reactions that ultimately generate two molecules of CO_2 and four reducing equivalents in the form of NADH (three) and $FADH_2$ (one). One high-energy phosphate molecule (GTP) is also produced, which can be utilized or converted to ATP. During this process, citrate (a six-carbon molecule) is stepwise decarboxylated and ultimately converted back to oxaloacetate, a four-carbon molecule which, when condensed with a new acetyl CoA, reinitiates the sequence of reactions just described. The reducing equivalents generated, NADH and $FADH_2$, deliver electrons to the electron transport chain. Rate-limiting enzymes of the TCA cycle are the pyruvate dehydrogenase complex (which precedes but is not really a component of the TCA cycle), isocitrate dehydrogenase, and α-ketoglutarate; these enzymes are highly regulated as will be discussed later. Interestingly,

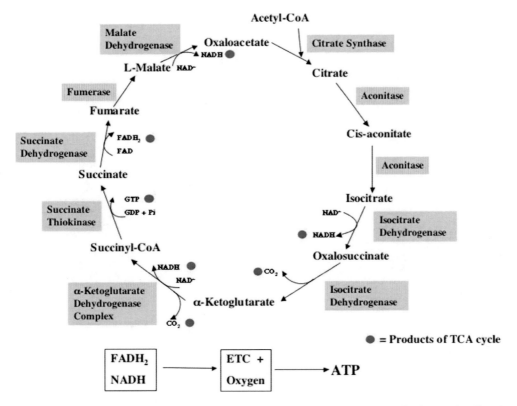

Fig. 19.10 Tricarboxylic acid (TCA) cycle. The *filled blue circles* are the products resulting from one turn of the TCA cycle. See text for discussion. ATP = adenosine triphosphate; ETC = electron transport chain; $FADH_2$ = flavin adenine dinucleotide; NADH = nicotinamide adenine dinucleotide; TCA = tricarboxylic acid

for elucidating the TCA cycle (also known as the Krebs cycle), Sir Hans Krebs was awarded the Nobel Prize in Medicine and Physiology in 1953.

19.3.7 The Electron Transport Chain and Oxidative Phosphorylation

The two substrates of the electron transport chain are NADH and $FADH_2$. These molecules are produced by glycolysis, β-lipid oxidation, and the TCA cycle as previously discussed. The electron transport chain (Fig. 19.11) is comprised of two freely diffusible compounds (ubiquinone, also known as coenzyme Q, which is confined to the mitochondrial inner membrane, and cytochrome c, which is located in the intermembrane space) and four multiprotein functional complexes (I, II, III, and IV), which are contained within the mitochondrial inner membrane. NADH interacts with the electron transport chain by transferring electrons to (and thereby reducing) complex I that, in turn, reduces coenzyme Q (ubiquinone). $FADH_2$ interacts with the electron transport chain by transferring electrons to complex II that, like complex I, also transfers its electrons to coenzyme Q. Reduced coenzyme Q then diffuses to complex III and transfers its electrons. Next, complex III reduces cytochrome c, which diffuses to complex IV and transfers electrons to this complex. The latter, when

reduced by four electrons, reduces O_2 to two O^{2-} ions. Each O^{2-} combines with two H^+ to form H_2O in an irreversible reaction.

During the process of electron transport, energy is released as electrons pass through the sequence of complexes. The purpose of electron transport chain complexes I, III, and IV is to capture this free energy and use it to pump H^+ from the mitochondrial matrix across the inner membrane into the intermembrane space (Fig. 19.11). These pumps create an electrochemical gradient comprised of an electrical potential and a chemical potential (the latter reflected by ΔpH) across the inner mitochondrial membrane. As a consequence of proton transport, the mitochondrial matrix is more negative than the intermembrane space. The F_1F_0-ATPase, which is also located in the inner mitochondrial membrane (Fig. 19.12), is the major pathway of H^+ return from the intermembrane space into the matrix. The energy released by the passage of H^+ down this electrochemical potential gradient is captured by the F_1F_0-ATPase and used to drive the reaction inorganic phosphate (Pi) + ADP → ATP. In this way, much of the energy released by the metabolism of glucose and fatty acids is transferred to the terminal high-energy phosphate bond of ATP. The concept of proton pumping into the intermembrane space, and the use of the electrochemical gradient thus formed to synthesize ATP, is known as the chemiosmotic theory. In recognition of his insight into how these processes function (ideas initially viewed as quite controversial), Sir Peter Mitchell was awarded the Nobel Prize in

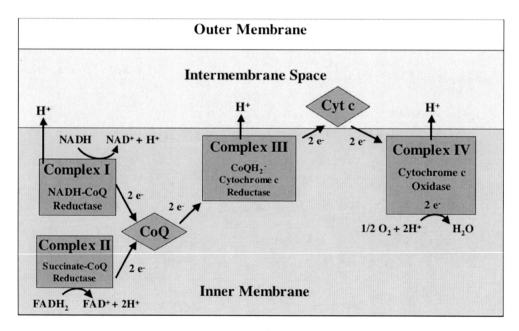

Fig. 19.11 Electron transport chain (ETC). See text for discussion. $FADH_2$ = flavin adenine dinucleotide; NADH = nicotinamide adenine dinucleotide

Fig. 19.12 Mechanism of oxidative phosphorylation and the transport of ATP from the mitochondrial matrix to the intermembrane space. See text for discussion. ADP = adenosine diphosphate; ANT = adenine nucleotide transporter; ATP = adenosine triphosphate; ETC = electron transport chain

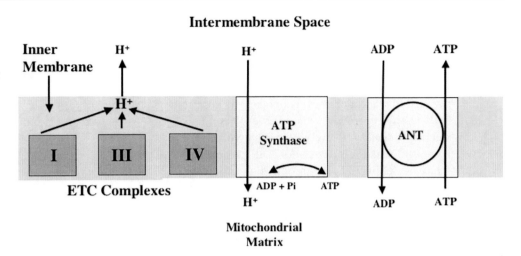

Chemistry in 1978. The production of ATP by mitochondria is termed oxidative phosphorylation; in virtually every human tissue (heart, brain, kidney, etc.), oxidative phosphorylation is the primary source of ATP generation.

To date, the precise mechanism by which the F_1F_0-H^+-ATPase generates ATP from its substrates (ADP and Pi) remains under investigation. However, a number of characteristics of the process are well established. For example, the F_1F_0-H^+-ATPase has been shown to be a near-equilibrium enzyme. In other words, the reaction can occur in both directions. However, it has also been shown both in isolated mitochondria, which are generating ATP under conditions of carbon substrate, ADP, and oxygen excesses, and in the perfused rat heart (and presumably in the in vivo heart as well), that the F_1F_0-H^+-ATPase operates far out of equilibrium so that virtually all fluxes are in the ADP + Pi → ATP direction. In the presence of abundant oxygen, the F_1F_0-H^+-ATPase is kinetically controlled by the concentrations of its immediate substrates (ADP and Pi) and the magnitude of the proton electrochemical potential gradient. Hence ADP levels alone can regulate the rate of ATP synthesis *as long as oxygen and carbon substrates are not limiting and the proton gradient is large.* However, in vivo regulatory mechanisms are far more complicated than those described by this simple scheme.

19.3.8 Regulation of the TCA Cycle, Electron Transport Chain, and Oxidative Phosphorylation and the Role of the Creatine Phosphate Shuttle

As pointed out, a simple kinetic regulatory scheme for oxidative phosphorylation with ADP availability controlling the ATP synthetic rates is valid when both oxygen and reducing equivalents are in excess. Under these conditions, the high proton electrochemical gradient will drive ATP synthesis until ADP falls to levels which are rate limiting. From this point on, ADP availability (i.e., the rate of ADP production) determines the steady-state rate of ATP synthesis. Therefore, because ADP is a product of ATP hydrolysis, the rate of ATP synthesis is determined by the rate of ATP hydrolysis (i.e., the rate of ATP utilization). This simple feedback regulation of ATP synthesis can be demonstrated in the perfused rat heart by providing a perfusate containing unphysiologically high concentrations of pyruvate or octanoate. Under these experimental conditions, myocardial ADP concentrations become low enough to kinetically regulate oxygen consumption; an increase in the rate of ATP utilization will cause ADP levels to rise which, in turn, stimulates an increase in the rate of oxygen consumption. In this construct, the increased rate of delivery of ADP to the F_1F_0-ATPase increases the rate of ATP synthesis, as long as ADP levels rise to values capable of supporting the new higher rate of ATP synthesis. In other words, ADP levels must increase concordantly with the rate of ATP synthesis. This type of regulation is well described by a single substrate Michalis-Menten kinetic model, as first reported by B. Chance and G.R. Williams more than 50 years ago.

However, in the in vivo large animal heart (e.g., dog, swine, or human, etc.) cytosolic unbound ADP levels (as estimated by means of ^{31}P magnetic resonance spectroscopy) are higher than those in the isolated perfused rat heart, and are well above the usual kinetic regulatory range described in studies of isolated mitochondria or perfused rat hearts. Further, in the in vivo large animal heart, ADP levels actually remain fairly constant even when increased rates of ATP utilization (increased cardiac work) drive substantial increases of myocardial oxygen consumption. Yet, this does not mean that ADP availability is not crucial to the rate of ATP synthesis.

When the rate of ATP expenditure is increased in normal myocardium, there is an obligatory identical increase in the rate of ADP delivery to mitochondria (once a new steady state is reached). To emphasize this point, the increase in the *rate of ADP delivery* to the ATP synthase (e.g., as myocardial work increases) is obligatory, despite the fact that a change in *steady-state ADP levels* is not.

The observation that ADP levels did not increase in the in vivo myocardium as the rates of ATP utilization and synthesis increase led to the recognition that additional regulatory systems are required to explain the data obtained in the in vivo models. Further, the overall regulatory processes must have very rapid response times with regard to facilitation of ATP synthesis. The latter is required because myocardial contents of ATP and creatine phosphate (another high-energy phosphate bond storage molecule which serves to buffer ATP levels) are only sufficient to support a few seconds of ATP expenditure in the absence of ATP synthesis. The reaction converting cytosolic ATP to phosphocreatine (catalysed by creatine kinase isozymes) is very rapid and near equilibrium; hence, the phosphocreatine energy reserve is immediately available to maintain ATP levels.

However the creatine kinase group of isozymes are thought to serve an additional important cellular function, i.e., the facilitation intracellular transport of ATP and ADP. This concept has been labeled the creatine kinase shuttle hypothesis (see Figure 19.13). It is based on the premise that the diffusion rates of ADP (and ATP) across the outer mitochondrial membrane and through the cytosol are relatively slow in relation to physiological demands. The creatine kinase shuttle is thought to facilitate the transfer of ATP from mitochondria to the sites of utilization and to also transfer ADP from sites of ATP utilization to mitochondria.

The adenine nucleotide transporter (ANT), which is not rate limiting, transports ADP from the mitochondrial intermembrane space to the mitochondrial matrix where it is rephosphorylated back to ATP. The ANT simultaneously transports newly synthesized ATP from the matrix to the intermembrane space. Within the intermembrane space, the mitochondrial isozyme of creatine kinase (MCK) transfers the terminal high-energy phosphate of ATP to creatine to form phosphocreatine. Phosphocreatine then diffuses into the cytosol and the ADP produced by this reaction in the intermembrane space is returned to the mitochondrial matrix by ANT, and is then rephosphorylated. The phosphocreatine which has diffused into the cytosol is then used as a high-energy phosphate donor for the rephosphorylation of cytosolic ADP by the cytosolic isozyme of creatine kinase. Because the cytosolic isozyme of creatine kinase has an extremely rapid turnover rate, the rapid (creatine kinase catalyzed) reactions

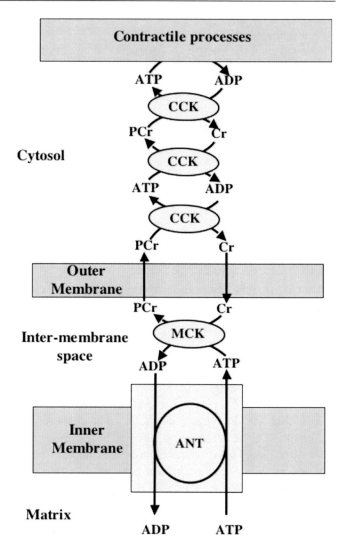

Fig. 19.13 A schematic of the proposed creatine kinase shuttle. See text for discussion. ADP = adenosine diphosphate; ANT = adenine nucleotide transporter; ATP = adenosine triphosphate; CCK = cytosolic creatine kinase; Cr = creatine; MCK = mitochondrial creatine kinase; PCr = phosphocreatine

between creatine phosphate and ADP, in effect, transport the terminal high-energy bonds of ATP to the sites of ATP utilization and the reverse reaction, in effect, transports ADP from the ATP hydrolysis site back to the mitochondrial outer membrane. In principle, "transport" of ADP and ATP by the shuttle is more rapid than that of the unfacilitated cytosolic diffusion rates of ADP and ATP molecules. Once the phosphocreatine leaving the mitochondria is used to rephosphorylate cytosolic AD, the creatine liberated from phosphocreatine diffuses into the mitochondrial inner membrane space to be rephosphorylated. As a result, cytosolic ADP levels (including those in proximity to the points of ATP utilization) are kept at low levels even if the rate of ATP utilization increases. The stability of ADP levels in the face of

Fig. 19.14 Pathways of Ca^{2+} entry and exit in the cardiomyocyte and several intracellular organelles relevant to excitation–contraction coupling and energy metabolism. The strong linkage between the stimulatory effects of intracellular [Ca^{2+}] ion contraction and ATP generation is also shown. See text for discussion. ATP = denosine triphosphate; LCC = l-type voltage-activated Ca^{2+} channel; RR = ryanodine receptor; SR = sarcoplasmic reticulum; TCA = tricarboxylic acid; TT = tubule

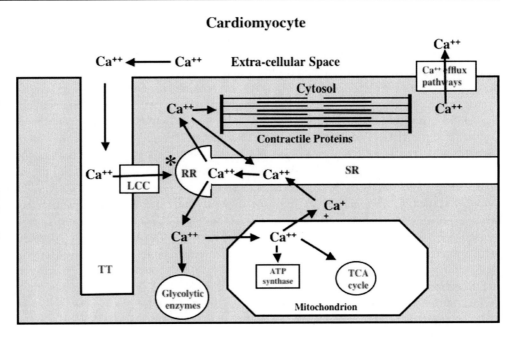

increasing ATP utilization permits ATP to maintain a high level of free energy that can be transferred to energy requiring cellular processes

A discussion of additional regulatory mechanisms for oxidative phosphorylation will be presented next, and readers can review the discussion of cardiomyocyte contraction mechanisms presented elsewhere in this book and briefly in Fig. 19.14 to refresh their understanding of cardiomyocyte Ca^{2+} dynamics.

During exercise, increased norepinephrine (from the sympathetic nerve fibers) and epinephrine (from the adrenal glands) release activates β-adrenergic receptors in cardiomyocytes. Their activation causes: 1) an increase of heart rate (by stimulating the sinoatrial node); and 2) an increase of Ca^{2+} entry per beat (i.e., increased size of the Ca^{2+} current) into the cytosol of the cardiomyocytes via the sarcolemmal voltage-dependent Ca^{2+} channel. This is further augmented by the increased heart rate (which reflects an increased number of Ca^{2+} channel openings/min). The increased Ca^{2+} entering the cytosol, together with β-adrenergic receptor mediated activation of sarcoplasmic reticulum Ca^{2+} sequestration, in turn, increases the sarcoplasmic reticulum Ca^{2+} store. The more fully loaded sarcoplasmic reticulum (which is the predominant source of "contraction initiating" Ca^{2+}) can then release more Ca^{2+} per beat into the cytosol, resulting in a larger systolic cytosolic Ca^{2+} transient. Both the increased frequency of Ca^{2+} transients (heart rate) and their larger size serve to increase the "average" Ca^{2+} level in the cytosol. Mitochondria normally transport Ca^{2+} both in and out of the matrix and maintain a "steady-state" matrix Ca^{2+} level that is related to average

cytosolic Ca^{2+}. In response to higher average cytosolic Ca^{2+} levels, mitochondrial Ca^{2+} uptake increases, resulting in an increase in the level of matrix Ca^{2+}. It is important to note that increased mitochondrial matrix Ca^{2+} has at least two primary effects on oxidative phosphorylation. First, as already mentioned, the TCA cycle has three rate limiting enzymes (PDH, isocitrate dehydrogenase, and α-ketoglutarate dehydrogenase) and the activities of these enzymes are regulated, in part, by mitochondrial matrix Ca^{2+} levels. Specifically, when these enzymes interact with Ca^{2+}, their sensitivities to their respective substrates are increased. This accelerates their reaction rates and increases the rates of acetyl CoA entry into and flux through the TCA cycle without requiring pyruvate, acetyl CoA levels, or immediate substrate levels of the TCA cycle pool to rise, provided that the rate of delivery of acetyl CoA to the TCA cycle is increased sufficiently to support the increased TCA cycle flux rate. Therefore, glucose uptake and glycolysis-mediated delivery of pyruvate to (and its rate of metabolism by) PDH must increase and/or the rates of fatty acid uptake and β-oxidative delivery of acetyl CoA to the TCA cycle must increase to support the increased rate of TCA cycle flux. As noted above, the rates of cellular substrate uptake, glycolytic flux, and β-oxidation also respond to metabolic signaling to produce the required increases in the rates of acetyl CoA production.

A major consequence of an increased TCA cycle flux is the more rapid generation of both mitochondrial NADH and FADH$_2$. The subsequent stimulation of the electron transport chain fluxes results not only from an increased rate of reducing equivalent generation, but also from stimulation of electron transport chain complex activities by other metabolic signals which are present during periods of increased ATP demand. Increased rates of electron transport chain fluxes will then result in an increased rate of H^+ pumping by the electron transport chain, which serves to maintain the electrochemical gradient across the inner mitochondrial membrane at a level adequate to support the increased rate of ATP synthesis. Additionally, the F_1F_0-ATPase is also regulated in that the fraction of this enzyme that is in the active state is increased by elevations of mitochondrial matrix Ca^{2+}. More specifically, an increased fraction of this enzyme in the active state is beneficial during periods of increased ATP synthesis, because an increased amount of active enzyme increases the rate of ATP synthesis without requiring ADP levels to rise, as long as the rate of ADP delivery to mitochondria increases appropriately (which it does when the rate of ATP utilization increases). To summarize, the major point to appreciate is that no matter how activated the carbon substrate metabolic pathways, the TCA cycle, the electron transport chain and ATP synthase are, ultimate control of respiration, electron flux, TCA cycle fluxes, and/or carbon substrate utilization ultimately resides in the rate of ATP utilization and the resulting rate of delivery of ADP to the mitochondrial matrix.

Taken together, these observations support the concept that increased average cardiomyocyte cytosolic Ca^{2+} levels (e.g., that occur during exercise) act as an important feed-forward signal for oxidative phosphorylation. This signal stimulates, in a parallel manner, ATP utilization by the contractile processes and ATP synthesis by the F_1F_0-ATPase as well as many preceding reactions in the energy generating scheme (Fig. 19.14). The net effects of these regulatory mechanisms (and additional feedback regulatory mechanisms which are not discussed) are to facilitate fluxes of basic food-derived carbon substrates through the metabolic sequences without requiring the cytosolic concentrations of the initial and intermediate substrates (including ADP) to increase. The rapid response time of this entire system also allows ATP levels to remain relatively constant despite wide and rapid fluctuations in the rate of ATP utilization. Since these mechanisms allow both ADP and ATP levels and the ATP/ADP ratio to remain stable at increased ATP synthetic rates, the free energy that can be released by ATP hydrolysis (ΔG ATP) and transferred to other reactions is maintained constant despite the increased rate of ATP expenditure. Control theory as applied to the regulation of oxidative phosphorylation, glycolysis, β-lipid oxidation, and the TCA cycle has been the subject of detailed study; for further discussion of this topic refer to the references listed at the end of this chapter.

19.4 Metabolism in Abnormal Myocardium

19.4.1 Ischemic Myocardium

The most common cause of inadequate myocardial ATP synthesis is ischemia, and the most frequent cause of myocardial ischemia is occlusive coronary artery disease. "Demand ischemia" occurs when narrowed coronary arteries can conduct adequate blood flow to sustain aerobic metabolism in the dependent myocardium during basal levels of activity, but do not allow for sufficient increases in flow to meet increased demands for ATP production during states of increased cardiac work (as during exercise). This state accounts for the condition of stable and inducible angina pectoris; the patient is asymptomatic at rest or during mild exertion, but when the work of the heart exceeds the ability of a narrowed coronary artery to meet the increased blood flow demand, ischemia ensues and the patient experiences chest pain. In response to the symptom of chest pain, the patient will typically discontinue exercise. During the ensuing rest period, the cardiac work falls into the range where the narrowed coronary artery can meet the blood flow demand and the ischemia is relieved.

In contrast, "supply ischemia" occurs when the coronary artery narrowings are so severe that they limit blood flow in the absence of increased ATP demand, i.e., ischemia occurs even when the patient is at rest. Supply ischemia is generally caused by an acute narrowing or abrupt complete closure of coronary vessels; the latter often causes myocardial infarction. Less commonly, supply ischemia can occur as a result of coronary spasm, in which inappropriate (pathologic) vasoconstriction of an epicardial coronary artery causes transient total or near total occlusion of blood flow. Although the nature of the myocardial ischemic process is qualitatively similar in supply and demand ischemias, supply ischemia is generally more clinically severe. Because of the greater vulnerability of the inner myocardial layers of the left ventricle to blood flow reduction, mild ischemia is usually confined to the subendocardium; as the coronary obstruction becomes more severe, ischemia proceeds as a wavefront from subendocardium to subepicardium until the full myocardial wall is involved.

When myocardial blood flow is inadequate, the limited availability of both oxygen and carbon substrate may limit the ATP synthetic rate, but it is usually the oxygen deficiency that is most critical. This is because the myocyte has substantial carbon substrate reserves (i.e., glycogen and triglycerides), but is unable to store significant quantities of oxygen. Consequently, when coronary blood flow is insufficient to meet myocardial needs, the severity of the induced oxygen deficit, in turn, determines the extent of limitation of oxidative phosphorylation.

Obviously, the effect of oxygen limitation is confined to pathways supporting oxidative phosphorylation, whereas glycolytic ATP synthesis does not require oxygen (Figs. 19.5 and 19.9). During hypoxia or anoxia (i.e., when blood oxygen content is moderately or markedly reduced, but blood flow is not limited) or during ischemia (when blood flow is restricted, but blood oxygen content may be normal), electron transport within the electron transport chain slows or stops depending on the severity of the oxygen deficit. This is because electrons cannot be transferred from cytochrome oxidase to molecular oxygen (the terminal electron acceptor). In consequence, the pumping of H^+ from the mitochondrial matrix into the intermembrane space stops, because it depends on the energy liberated as electrons pass through the electron transport chain. As a result, the proton-motive force across the inner mitochondrial membrane begins to dissipate and mitochondrial ATP synthesis fails. If the dissipation of the H^+ gradient is marked, then the F_1F_0-H^+-ATPase begins to operate in the reverse direction, i.e., it converts ATP to ADP and uses energy liberated by ATP hydrolysis to pump H^+ back into the intermembrane space. This partially maintained H^+ gradient is dissipated to support crucial functions that support mitochondrial stability. One result is reversed electron flow through the electron transport chain. Hence, mitochondria can either synthesize ATP under physiological conditions or degrade ATP when oxygen is severely limited. Because the H^+ electrochemical potential is also used to energize other mitochondrial transport functions in addition to supporting ATP synthesis, mitochondrial degradation of ATP during periods of oxygen limitation may serve to preserve nonoxidative mitochondrial function for a time, at the expense of hastening the fall in cytoplasmic ATP levels.

Glycolysis, which, in principle, can proceed normally in the absence of oxygen, is also limited when blood flow is reduced during ischemia. Oxygen limitation causes cessation of forward electron transport chain function and, thereby, stops the mitochondrial oxidation of reducing equivalents generated by the TCA cycle and/or transferred from cytosolic NADH into mitochondria. Cytosolic NAD^+ is a substrate of glyceraldehyde phosphate dehydrogenase, and if the NADH generated by that reaction is not oxidized back to NAD^+ by the transfer of reducing equivalents into the mitochondria by the malate–aspartate shuttle or into cytosolic lactate by LDH (see below), the lack of NAD^+ will then inhibit glyceraldehyde phosphate dehydrogenase. Other factors limiting the rates of glycolytic ATP synthesis during ischemia are cytosolic accumulations of lactate and hydrogen ions (Figs. 19.5 and 19.15). Under conditions of normal coronary flow, the myocardium can rapidly export both of these ions even when the glycolytic rate is augmented.

Thus, a low oxygen content of coronary arterial blood does not limit lactate and H^+ export. In contrast, when the myocardium is ischemic, the capacity to export lactate and protons decreases in proportion to the severity of the blood flow reduction. Furthermore, the increase in cytosolic lactate concentration during ischemia can inhibit the conversion of pyruvate to lactate via LDH, so that pyruvate generated by glycolysis may have limited exit possibilities, since pyruvate oxidation is also inhibited. Because the conversion of pyruvate to lactate results in the oxidation of cytosolic NADH, the availability of NAD^+ to glyceraldehyde phosphate dehydrogenase is further reduced when rising cytosolic levels of lactate slow this reaction (Figs. 19.5, 19.9A, and 19.15). In contrast, during hypoxia, coronary flow is not restricted and glycolysis proceeds at a rapid rate because metabolic signaling activates both the rate-limiting glycolytic reactions and the transport of glucose into the myocyte. During moderate ischemia, when both glucose and oxygen delivery are impaired, myocyte glycogen stores are the main source of glucose for glycolysis. When glycogen stores are exhausted, the limited rates of glucose delivery to (and lactate clearance from) the ischemic myocyte control the rate of glycolysis.

These concepts have specific importance in patients with coronary artery disease, because they typically define the temporal boundary for viability of the ischemic myocardium. For example, in the moderately ischemic myocardium, contractile function rapidly decreases in response to: (1) decreased ATP availability; (2) accumulation of H^+ ions; and/or (3) other less well-defined factors. However, if residual coronary blood flow during ischemia is sufficient to permit some glycolysis (by allowing the export of some

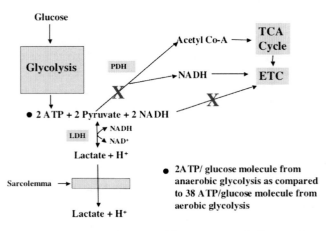

Fig. 19.15 Flowchart for anaerobic glucose metabolism. A *large red* X indicates metabolic pathways blocked during ischemia. See text for discussion. ATP = adenosine triphosphate; ETC = electron transport chain; LDH = lactic acid dehydrogenase; NADH = nicotinamide adenine dinucleotide; PDH = pyruvate dehydrogenase; TCA = tricarboxylic acid

lactate and H^+ and the import of some glucose), then modest ATP production may preserve viability for some time. In contrast, during acute total coronary occlusion, glycolysis is rapidly inhibited and myocyte death will occur. In other words, a level of coronary blood flow that is insufficient to maintain oxidative phosphorylation and contractile function may support glycolytic ATP production at a rate sufficient to sustain myocardial viability until appropriate medical or surgical treatment can restore blood flow to the ischemic myocardium.

19.4.2 Metabolism in Hypertrophied and Failing Hearts

During fetal life, the myocardium primarily metabolizes glucose rather than fatty acids. This pattern of metabolism is well suited to the low oxygen levels in fetal arterial blood; glucose metabolism requires less oxygen than fatty acid metabolism. Additionally, the lower cardiac work levels (lower blood pressure) in the fetus are adequately supported by ATP production through glycolysis and pyruvate oxidation. However, after birth, substrate preference of the heart (now in a higher oxygen environment and operating at a higher work load) rapidly shifts to the adult metabolic pattern, which is predominantly dependent on fatty acid oxidation. This change of substrate preference is considered to be the result of upregulated expression of genes controlling the transport of fatty acids into the myocyte and their subsequent metabolism in the cytosol and mitochondria. The upregulation in the expression of genes involved in fatty acid metabolism and oxidative phosphorylation is commonly referred to as the shift from a fetal to an adult gene expression pattern.

A chronic mechanical overload produced by hypertension, heart valve abnormalities, and/or destruction of a portion of the left ventricle by infarct often results in some degree of left ventricular dilation. In general, left ventricular wall tension (systolic and diastolic) increases as a consequence of the LaPlace relationship between pressure generation and chamber radius (and wall thickness). The increased wall tension then activates changes in the expression patterns of a number of genes involved in both myocyte growth (hypertrophy) and metabolism. This resultant increase in left ventricular wall thickness returns systolic wall stresses toward normal, often resulting in a prolonged period of compensated myocardial hypertrophy. However, chronic myocardial hypertrophy may be associated with important changes in energy metabolism, including reductions in HEP levels and alterations in carbon substrate preference with decreased utilization of free fatty acids

and increased dependence on glucose. This shift in the myocardial gene expression, which leads to increased glucose and decreased fatty acid utilization, is referred to as a reversion to the fetal gene expression pattern. Subsequently, reductions in the levels of molecules crucial to oxidative phosphorylation also occur. Although the increased glucose metabolism and decreased fatty acid metabolism associated with this reversion (to a fetal gene expression pattern) may have short-term energetic benefits (perhaps by modestly decreasing the oxygen cost of ATP synthesis), the overall ATP synthetic capacity of severely hypertrophied and failing myocardium is significantly reduced. Whatever the cause, the period of compensated hypertrophy in the chronically overloaded heart is often followed by a significant contractile dysfunction of the ventricular myocytes with ultimate progressive left heart dilation and dysfunction. At this point, the clinical syndrome known as "heart failure" is considered to have occurred.

Until recently, it has been unclear whether decreased ATP synthetic capacity in hypertrophied or failing cardiomyocytes can constrain contractile performance and, thereby, contribute to the progression to a decompensated state. The issue has been whether contractile dysfunction in the failing heart is caused primarily by a limited ability of the contractile apparatus to consume ATP or whether the reduced ability to produce ATP is also contributory. However, recent experimental data have shown that the upregulation of glucose metabolism that occurs in the hypertrophied or failing myocardium may not adequately compensate (from the standpoint of ATP synthetic capacity) for the downregulation of fatty acid metabolism that occurs in these hearts. Interestingly, transgenic mice that overexpressed a cardiomyocyte sarcolemmal glucose transporter (which caused an increase in glucose uptake and metabolism) were far less likely than non-transgenic mice to develop cardiac decompensation or die when subjected to chronic pressure overload of the left ventricle (induced by surgical narrowing of the ascending aorta). These findings imply that augmentation of glucose uptake is beneficial to the chronically overloaded heart and that the fetal shift in gene expression (substrate preference) that normally occurs in this condition may be insufficient to compensate for the bioenergetic abnormalities present in the hypertrophying myocardium.

The above discussion of cardiac dysfunction considers the possibility that acquired defects in the overloaded cardiomyocyte may limit ATP synthesis sufficiently to constrain mechanical function. Yet, abnormalities of left ventricular function can also add an ischemic component to the metabolic abnormalities of hypertrophied and failing myocardium even in the absence of occlusive coronary artery disease. As discussed earlier, increased ventricular filling pressures and tachycardia in the abnormal heart can limit the ability of myocardial blood flow (especially in the subendocardium) to increase normally in response to an increased metabolic rate. Hence in the chronically overloaded heart, both acquired intrinsic abnormalities of the cardiomyocytes and superimposed limitations of blood flow can act together to compromise cardiomyocyte ATP synthetic capacity and thus further impair overall cardiac function.

19.4.3 Primary (Genetic) Myocardial Metabolic Abnormalities

As described above, changes in gene expression in the hypertrophied or failing cardiomyocyte can cause various abnormalities of myocardial metabolism that, in turn, act to constrain contractile function. However, "primary" (genetically determined) abnormalities of carbon substrate metabolism or oxidative phosphorylation can also cause myocyte hypertrophy and/or failure. Interested readers can refer to the references at the end of this chapter for more information on such defects. A dramatic example of one such abnormality and a successful therapeutic approach for treatment of this metabolic defect based on sound biochemical principles have recently been reported and will be discussed below.

An inherited deficiency of the enzyme very long-chain acyl CoA dehydrogenase (VLCAD) is known to be associated with cardiomyopathy and skeletal muscle myopathy (Fig. 19.16). This enzyme is the first component of the β-lipid oxidation sequence. Because most dietary fatty acids are of the long-chain type, the deficiency of VLCAD results in a markedly increased cardiac dependence on glucose for ATP generation. The fact that even upregulated glucose metabolism cannot adequately support cardiac function is indicated by the development of progressive myopathy (although the cytosolic accumulation of long-chain fatty acids, which cannot be fully metabolized, also contributes to the myopathy). The classical treatment for this condition has been to replace the long-chain fatty acids in such an individual's diet with even-numbered short- or medium-chain length fatty acids such as octanoate or decanoate. Importantly, the short-chain fatty acids bypass the metabolic roadblock, because the medium- and short-chain acyl CoA dehydrogenases are normal in these patients. This therapeutic strategy induces increased fatty acid utilization and causes clinical improvement, but unfortunately in many such patients, cardiac and skeletal muscle myopathies may persist.

The question remains, "Why feeding even-numbered short-chain length fatty acids does not fully correct the muscle defects in these patients despite the augmentation of acetyl CoA delivery to the TCA cycle?". To answer this, it should be recalled that VLCAD deficiency causes

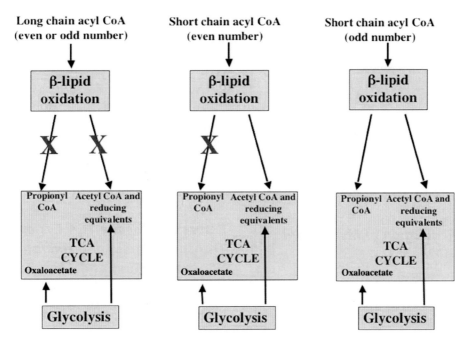

Fig. 19.16 Effects of very long-chain acyl dehydrogenase deficiency on the metabolism of long-chain fatty acids (even and odd numbered), short-chain fatty acids (even numbered), and short-chain fatty acids (odd numbered). Only the last one can also supply anaplerotic substrate to the TCA cycle. A *large red* X indicates metabolic pathways that cannot be used by a specific type of free fatty acid. See discussion in text. TCA = tricarboxylic acid

limitation of metabolism of both even- and odd-numbered long-chain fatty acids; hence both acetyl CoA and propionyl CoA delivery to the TCA cycle are limited. Although the metabolism of even-numbered short-chain fatty acids supplies acetyl CoA, it does not supply the anaplerotic substrate propionyl CoA. Consequently, even-numbered short-chain fatty acids cannot correct the defect in the anaplerotic delivery of substrate to the TCA cycle and, therefore, are unable to correct a possible decrease in TCA intermediate pool size resulting from propionyl CoA deficiency (Fig. 19.6B). Following this logic, dietary supplementation with an odd-numbered short-chain fatty acid would be expected to permit β-lipid oxidation to supply both acetyl CoA and propionyl CoA. In fact, when patients were treated with the short-chain, seven-carbon fatty acid, heptanoate, they showed marked improvement in both skeletal muscle and cardiac abnormalities. Hence this disorder can be effectively managed by understanding the basic biochemical defect and prescribing a biochemical treatment strategy that compensates for this defect.

19.5 List of Abbreviations

AMPK	adenosine monophosphate-activated kinase
AMP	adenosine monophosphate
ADP	adenosine diphosphate
ATP	adenosine triphosphate
FADH$_2$	flavin adenine dinucleotide
LDH	lactic acid dehydrogenase
NADH	nicotinamide adenine dinucleotide
NEFA	nonesterified free fatty acids
PDH	pyruvate dehydrogenase
TCA	tricarboxylic acid
VLCAD	very long-chain acyl CoA dehydrogenase

General References and Suggested Reading

References for Regulation of Myocardial Blood Flow

Ishibashi Y, Duncker DJ, Zhang J, Bache RJ. ATP-sensitive K + channels, adenosine, and nitric oxide-mediated mechanisms account for coronary vasodilation during exercise. Circ Res 1998;82:346–59.

Gorman MW, Tune JD, Richmond KN, Feigl EO. Feedforward sympathetic coronary vasodilation in exercising dogs. J Appl Physiol 2000;89:1892–902.

Duncker DJ, Bache RJ. Regulation of coronary vasomotor tone under normal conditions and during acute myocardial hypoperfusion. Pharmacol Ther 2000;86:87–110.

Standard Biochemistry Texts

Murray RK, Granner DK, Mayes PA, Rodwell VW, eds. Harper's illustrated biochemistry. 27th ed. New York, NY: Lange Medical Books/McGraw-Hill, 2006.

Berg JM, Tymoczko JL, Stryer L, eds. Biochemistry. 6th ed. New York, NY: W.H. Freeman & Co., 2006.

References for Glucose and Fatty Acid Metabolism and Regulation of Glycolysis and Fatty Acid Metabolism

Coven DL, Hu X, Cong L, et al. Physiological role of AMP-activated protein kinase in the heart: Graded activation during exercise. Am J Physiol Endocrinol Metab 2003;285:E629–36.

Nickerson JG, Momken I, Benton CR, et al. Protein-mediated fatty acid uptake: Regulation by contraction, AMP-activated protein kinase, and endocrine signals. Appl Physiol Nutr Metab 2007;32:865–73.

Roden M. How free fatty acids inhibit glucose utilization in human skeletal muscle. News Physiol Sci 2004;19:92–6.

Stanley WC, Recchia FA, Lopaschuk GD. Myocardial substrate metabolism in the normal and failing heart. Physiol Rev 2005;85:1093–129.

References for Myocardial Substrate Selection

Lehman JJ, Kelly DP. Transcriptional activation of energy metabolic switches in the developing and hypertrophied heart. Clin Exp Pharmacol Physiol 2002;29:339–45.

Drake AJ, Haines JR, Noble MI. Preferential uptake of lactate by the normal myocardium in dogs. Cardiovasc Res 1980;14:65–72.

Drake-Holland AJ, Van der Vusse GJ, Roemen TH, et al. Chronic catecholamine depletion switches myocardium from carbohydrate to lipid utilisation. Cardiovasc Drugs Ther 2001;15:111–7.

References for the TCA Cycle, Electron Transport Chain, and Oxidative Phosphorylation and Their Regulation

From AH, Zimmer SD, Michurski SP, et al. Regulation of the oxidative phosphorylation rate in the intact cell. Biochemistry 1990;29:3731–43.

Ludwig B, Bender E, Arnold S, Huttemann M, Lee I, Kadenbach B. Cytochrome C oxidase and the regulation of oxidative phosphorylation. Chembiochem 2001;2:392–403.

Brand MD, Curtis RK. Simplifying metabolic complexity. Biochem Soc Trans 2002;30:25–30.

Kushmerick MJ, Conley KE. Energetics of muscle contraction: The whole is less than the sum of its parts. Biochem Soc Trans 2002;30:227–31.

Zhang J, Murakami Y, Zhang Y, et al. Oxygen delivery does not limit cardiac performance during high work states. Am J Physiol 1999;277:H50–7.

Territo PR, Mootha VK, French SA, Balaban RS. Ca(2+) activation of heart mitochondrial oxidative phosphorylation: Role of the F(0)/F(1)-ATPase. Am J Physiol Cell Physiol 2000;278:C423–35.

Hochachka PW. Intracellular convection, homeostasis and metabolic regulation. J Exp Biol 2003;206:2001–9.

Das AM. Regulation of the mitochondrial ATP-synthase in health and disease. Mol Genet Metab 2003;79:71–82.

Levy C, Ter Keurs HE, Yaniv Y, Landesberg A. The sarcomeric control of energy conversion. Ann N Y Acad Sci 2005;1047:219–31.

Maack C, O'Rourke B. Excitation-contraction coupling and mitochondrial energetics. Basic Res Cardiol 2007;102:369–92.

References for Modeling of Energetic Function

Cortassa S, Aon MA, O'Rourke B., et al. A computational model integrating electrophysiology, contraction, and mitochondrial bioenergetics in the ventricular myocyte. Biophys J 2006;91:1564–89.

Saks VA, Kuznetsov AV, Vendelin M, Guerrero K, Kay L, Seppet EK. Functional coupling as a basic mechanism of feedback regulation of cardiac energy metabolism. Mol Cell Biochem 2004;256–257:185–99.

Saks V, Dzeja P, Schlattner U, Vendelin M, Terzic A, Wallimann T. Cardiac system bioenergetics: Metabolic basis of the Frank-Starling law. J Physiol 2006;571:253–73.

Korzeniewski B. Parallel activation in the ATP supply-demand system lessens the impact of inborn enzyme deficiencies, inhibitors, poisons or substrate shortage on oxidative phosphorylation in vivo. Biophys Chem 2002;96:21–31.

Korzeniewski B. Theoretical studies on the regulation of oxidative phosphorylation in intact tissues. Biochem Biophys Acta 2001;1504:31–45.

Aimar-Beurton M, Korzeniewski B, Letellier T, Ludinard S, Mazat JP, Nazaret C. Virtual mitochondria: Metabolic modelling and control. Mol Biol Rep 2002;29:227–32.

Reference for High-Energy Phosphate Shuttles

Dzeja PP, Terzic A. Phosphotransfer networks and cellular energetics. J Exp Biol 2003; 206:2039–47.

References for Metabolism During Ischemia

Stanley WC, Recchia FA, Lopaschuk GD. Myocardial substrate metabolism in the normal and failing heart. Physiol Rev 2005;85:1093–129.

Sambandam N, Lopaschuk GD. AMP-activated protein kinase (AMPK) control of fatty acid and glucose metabolism in the ischemic heart. Prog Lipid Res 2003;42:238–56.

References for Metabolism in Hypertrophied and Failing Myocardium

Ning XH, Zhang J, Liu J, et al. Signaling and expression for mitochondrial membrane proteins during left ventricular remodeling and contractile failure after myocardial infarction. J Am Coll Cardiol 2000;36:282–7.

Lehman JJ, Kelly DP. Transcriptional activation of energy metabolic switches in the developing and hypertrophied heart. Clin Exp Pharmacol Physiol 2002;29:339–45.

Young ME, Laws FA, Goodwin GW, Taegtmeyer H. Reactivation of peroxisome proliferator-activated receptor alpha is associated with contractile dysfunction in hypertrophied rat heart. J Biol Chem 2001;276:44390–5.

Liao R, Jain M, Cui L, et al. Cardiac-specific overexpression of GLUT1 prevents the development of heart failure attributable to pressure overload in mice. Circulation 2002;106: 2125–31.

Stanley WC, Recchia FA, Lopaschuk GD. Myocardial substrate metabolism in the normal and failing heart. Physiol Rev 2005;85:1093–129.

Ashrafian H, Frenneaux MP, Opie LH. Metabolic mechanisms in heart failure. Circulation 2007;116:434–48.

References for Inherited Defects in Myocardial Metabolism

Roe CR, Sweetman L, Roe DS, David F, Brunengraber H. Treatment of cardiomyopathy and rhabdomyolysis in long-chain fat oxidation disorders using an anaplerotic odd-chain triglyceride. J Clin Invest 2002;110:259–69.

DiMauro S, Schon EA. Mitochondrial respiratory-chain diseases. N Engl J Med 2003;348:2656–68.

Mochel F, DeLonlay P, Touati G, et al. Pyruvate carboxylase deficiency: Clinical and biochemical response to anaplerotic diet therapy. Mol Genet Metab 2005;84:305–12.

Roe CR, Mochel F. Anaplerotic diet therapy in inherited metabolic disease: Therapeutic potential. J Inherit Metab Dis 2006;29: 332–40.

Chapter 20
Introduction to Echocardiography

Jamie L. Lohr and Shanthi Sivanandam

Abstract The use of ultrasound to provide noninvasive evaluation of cardiac structure and function was a revolutionary advancement in cardiac care in the late 20th century. Today, echocardiography allows for detailed serial examinations of: (1) heart development; (2) cardiac structure and function; and (3) changes in normal physiologic states and pathologic conditions. The goals of this chapter are to: (1) provide the reader with a brief overview of the types of echocardiography in clinical use today; (2) review the basic physical principles that underlie this clinical tool; and (3) demonstrate how echocardiography can be used to assess cardiac structure and function.

Keywords Echocardiography · Ultrasound imaging · M-mode echocardiography · 2D imaging · Doppler ultrasound · Color Doppler flow mapping · Tissue Doppler imaging · Transvaginal echocardiography · Transthoracic echocardiography · Transabdominal echocardiography

20.1 Introduction

The use of ultrasound to provide noninvasive evaluation of cardiac structure and function was a revolutionary advancement in cardiac care in the late 20th century [1]. Development of the field of echocardiography has allowed detailed serial examinations of the development, structure and function of the human heart in normal physiologic states and in pathologic conditions. Echocardiography has increased the diagnostic accuracy of noninvasive evaluation and provides a tool for the monitoring of cardiac diagnostic and therapeutic procedures. The goals of this chapter are to: (1) provide the reader with a brief overview of the types of echocardiography in clinical use today; (2) review the basic physical principles that underlie this clinical tool; and (3) demonstrate how echocardiography can be used to assess cardiac structure and function.

Prior to the 1970s, diagnoses of congenital and acquired heart disease were achieved by the combination of physical examination, electrocardiography (EKG), and invasive cardiac catheterization. Unfortunately, clinical examination and EKG are often not very specific diagnostic tools. Furthermore, cardiac catheterization, while greatly augmenting noninvasive clinical information, can be a stressful and risky procedure, particularly in the very young or critically ill patient. Initial attempts at imaging the heart using reflected sound waves were made in the 1950s, with improvement in the experimental technology and its initial clinical application in the 1960s [1]. During the 1970s, simple motion-mode (M-mode) or linear images were available to define cardiac structures, but these were not adequate for providing great diagnostic detail in complex congenital heart disease. During the 1980s, the technologies to provide two-dimensional real-time imaging of the heart were developed, and this subsequently revolutionized noninvasive evaluation of cardiac structures and their function. In the late 1980s, techniques of Doppler ultrasound, including color mapping, were developed, which greatly extended the analyses of cardiac function and associated hemodynamics [1]. By the late 1980s, many cardiac defects could be diagnosed accurately and repaired completely without invasive testing by employing echocardiography.

20.2 Physical Principles of Echocardiography

20.2.1 Ultrasound Imaging of Tissues

Echocardiography uses the properties of sound waves to differentiate tissues of varied density in the human body.

J.L. Lohr (✉)
University of Minnesota, Division of Pediatric Cardiology, Department of Pediatrics, MMC 94, 420 Delaware Street SE, Minneapolis, MN 55455, USA
e-mail: lohrx003@umn.edu

P.A. Iaizzo (ed.), *Handbook of Cardiac Anatomy, Physiology, and Devices*, DOI 10.1007/978-1-60327-372-5_20,

Sound travels in mechanical waves with speeds dependent on both the density and the elastic properties of the medium in which it is traveling [2]. This property of tissue is termed its "acoustic density." Ultrasound waves, which are used in medical applications, have frequencies that are higher than those audible to the human ear. Ultrasound frequencies are generally over 20,000 cycles/s, or Hertz, and most cardiac applications are performed using frequencies in the range of two to ten million Hertz, or 2–10 megaHertz (MHz). When a sound wave, which is generated by electrical stimulation of at least one piezoelectric crystal, travels through an interface between two tissues of varied acoustic density, such as myocardium and blood, a portion of the energy is reflected backward (the reflected wave) and the rest travels forward through the next tissue (the refracted wave). The reflected wave is received by the transducer, turned back into electrical energy, amplified, and displayed [1]. If there is too much variance between the acoustic density of the tissues being imaged (as in air-filled lung and myocardium or bone and myocardium), the entire ultrasound wave is reflected and the cardiac structures cannot be clearly imaged [1]. The amount of reflected wave detected during ultrasound imaging depends not only on the acoustic characteristics of the interface but also on the angle of incidence or interrogation. An ultrasound beam which encounters a flat surface that is perpendicular to the beam will reflect a wave in the direction of the transmitted sound. In contrast, a beam that is parallel to a structure or that encounters an irregularly shaped structure, as is common in tissue imaging, will be reflected with a degree of scatter that is proportional to the angle of incidence [2].

20.2.2 Resolution of Structures

The ability of cardiac ultrasound to provide anatomical resolution depends on the wavelength of the sound used. The speed of transmission, the frequency, and the wavelength are related by the following equation:

$$c = f \times \lambda, \text{ or } \lambda = c/f,$$

where c = the speed of sound in the medium, f = the frequency of the wave (in Hertz or cycles per second), and λ = the wavelength. Thus, a higher frequency transducer will produce a smaller wavelength and improved resolution along the path of the beam, also termed "axial resolution" [1]. According to Geva, axial resolution is generally two times the wavelength used, so that a 3.5 MHz transducer has a wavelength of 0.43 mm and

an axial resolution of 0.86 mm, while a 7.5 MHz transducer (commonly used in pediatric imaging) has a wavelength of 0.2 mm and axial resolution of approximately 0.4 mm [1]. Unfortunately, the use of high-frequency transducers is limited because the smaller wavelength cannot penetrate as deeply into tissue, and they are therefore less useful for cardiac imaging in the larger adult heart. Lateral resolution in echocardiography is impacted by the diameter of the beam width, which is a function of the transducer size, shape, and focal plane, as well as the frequency [1].

20.3 Imaging Modalities

20.3.1 M-Mode Echocardiography

M-mode, or motion-mode, echocardiography was the first type of ultrasound used for clinical cardiovascular imaging. Its use today is primarily limited to assessment of valve motion and for reliable and reproducible measurements of chamber size and function [1, 3]. In M-mode echocardiography, a narrow ultrasound beam is pulsed rapidly in a single plane through the heart, and the movements of the structures in that single plane are plotted against time with very high temporal and axial resolution. M-mode echocardiography can be used to assess dynamic changes in cardiac wall thickness, aortic root size, chamber sizes, and/or ventricular function. In general, left ventricular function is quantitated using M-mode by determining the percent of fractional shortening of the left ventricle, which is calculated using the following equation:

$$\text{SF}(\%) = \frac{\text{LVEDD} - \text{LVESD}}{\text{LVEDD}} \times 100$$

where SF = shortening fraction, LVEDD = left ventricular end-diastolic dimension, and LVESD = left ventricular end-systolic dimension. Normal values vary with age and range from 35–45% in infants to 28–44% in adolescents and adults [4, 5].

20.3.2 Two-Dimensional Imaging

Two-dimensional imaging provides arcs of imaging planes by employing multiple ultrasound beams to offer a cross-sectional view of the heart. Currently, two-dimensional imaging provides the majority of information about cardiac structure and function in routine clinical studies. Two-dimensional imaging requires the presence of multiple beams of ultrasound interrogation in a single transducer, and several types of transducers are available to achieve this. Transducers available for two-dimensional imaging include mechanical (a sweeping or rotating ultrasound beam), phased array (multiple independently controlled sources), and linear array (a line of crystals simultaneously generating a beam of ultrasound). Today, phased array transducers are most commonly used due to their: (1) small size; (2) ability to provide simultaneous two-dimensional and M-mode or Doppler imaging; and (3) improved control of focal length for a more uniform image throughout the field of view [6]. In addition to using two-dimensional imaging for viewing anatomic detail, left ventricular function can be quantitated by this mode, e.g., using an estimated left ventricular ejection fraction. This method, which has been shown to correlate well with angiographic estimates of ventricular function, takes advantage of the conical shape of the left ventricle to estimate end-diastolic and end-systolic ventricular volumes from tracings of two-dimensional images using Simpson's biplane rule [3]. The ejection fraction is then calculated as follows:

$$EF\,(\%) = \frac{LV\,EDV - LV\,ESV}{LV\,EDV} \times 100$$

where EF = ejection fraction, LVEDV = left ventricular end-diastolic volume, and LVESV = left ventricular end-systolic volume.

Normal values for ejection fractions are approximately 55–65%, and cardiac outputs can be estimated by multiplying the volume ejected with each beat (stroke volume) by the heart rate, using the equation:

$$CO = HR \times SV$$

where CO = cardiac output, HR = heart rate, and SV = stroke volume.

20.3.3 Doppler Ultrasound

The Doppler principle, described by Christian Johann Doppler in 1843, states that the frequency of transmitted sound is altered when the source of the sound is moving [2]. The classic example is the change in pitch of a train whistle as it moves, getting higher as it approaches the receiver and lower as it moves away from it. This change in frequency, or Doppler shift, also occurs when the source of sound is stationary and the waves are reflected off a moving target, including red blood cells in the vasculature. The shift in frequency is related to the velocity of the moving target, as well as the angle of incidence, and can be described by the equation:

$$F_d = \frac{2(f_0)(V)\cos\phi}{C}$$

where F_d = the observed Doppler frequency shift; f_0 = the transmitted frequency; C = the velocity of sound in human tissue at 37°C (approximately 1560 m/s), V = blood flow velocity, and ϕ = the intercept angle between the ultrasound beam and the blood flow. Using this principle, Doppler ultrasound can be used to noninvasively estimate the velocities of blood flow in the human heart and vasculature. Using a modified Bernoulli equation where pressure drop is equal to four times the velocity squared ($4V^2$), Doppler ultrasound can also be used to estimate chamber pressures and gradients and thus to provide significant noninvasive hemodynamic data.

20.3.4 Continuous Wave Doppler

Continuous wave Doppler is performed by using a single transducer with two separate elements for transmission and reception of sound waves, so that there is continuous monitoring of the Doppler shift. This technique allows detection of very high-velocity blood flow, but does not allow localization of the site of the velocity shift along the line of interrogation [1].

20.3.5 Pulse Wave Doppler

Pulse wave Doppler uses bursts of ultrasound alternating with pauses to detect Doppler shift in a localized region. The timing between the generation of the ultrasound wave and detection of the reflected wave determines the depth of interrogation. Pulse wave Doppler is useful to measure velocity changes in a region defined by two-dimensional echocardiography; however, the spatial resolution limits the velocity shifts detected. In general, the maximal velocity shifts that are detectable are one half of the Doppler sampling rate (pulse repetition frequency); this is designated the "Nyquist limit" [1]. The maximal sampling rate is determined by the distance of the sampling site from the transducer and the transducer frequency, so that sampling from a transducer position nearer to the region to be interrogated and using a lower frequency transducer will improve the detection and localization of higher velocity flow [1].

20.3.6 Color Doppler Flow Mapping

Color Doppler flow mapping uses the principles of pulsed Doppler to examine multiple points along the scan lines. The mean velocities and directions of these signals are calculated and then displayed and superimposed upon a two-dimensional image. By convention, flow directed toward the transducer is red and flow directed away from the transducer is blue. Accelerated or turbulent flow is typically given a different color, e.g., yellow and green. Color flow mapping is valuable because of the large amount of information that can be obtained in a single image. It can also aid in the localization of flow acceleration, quantitation of valvar regurgitation, visualization of intracardiac shunting, and/or assessment of arterial connections. Information obtained from color Doppler can also be refined by pulse wave Doppler and continuous wave Doppler interrogation.

20.3.7 Quantification of Pressure Gradients Using Doppler Shift Measurements

Today, quantification of pressure gradients using Doppler echocardiography can provide hemodynamic information that could previously be obtained only by invasive cardiac catheterization. Specifically, the Bernoulli equation [3, 7] is employed, which defines the relationship between velocity shift across an obstruction and the pressure gradient caused by the obstruction. For practical purposes, the proximal velocity is neglected and the simplified equation becomes pressure difference = (distal velocity)^2 × 4. This is a valuable way to estimate pressure drops across obstructive valves and/or pressure differences between chambers (based on the velocity of valvar regurgitation or intracardiac shunting).

20.3.8 Myocardial Performance Index

The "myocardial performance index" is a noninvasive Doppler measurement of global ventricular function that incorporates both systolic and diastolic function and may be applied to either the right ventricle (RV) or left ventricle (LV) [8]. The myocardial performance index (or Tei index) is defined as the ratio of the sum of the isovolumic contraction time and isovolumic relaxation

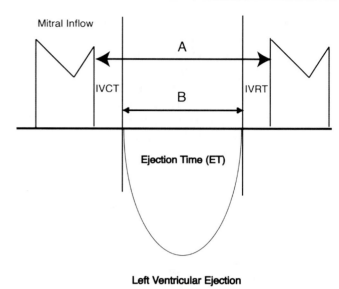

$$\text{Tei Index} = \frac{(\text{IVCT} + \text{IVRT})}{\text{ET}} = \frac{\text{A} - \text{B}}{\text{ET}}$$

Fig. 20.1 Diagrammatic representation of the myocardial performance index, or Tei index. The Tei index is the sum of the isovolumetric contraction time (IVCT) and isovolumetric relaxation time (IVRT) divided by the ejection time (ET). Adapted from Pellet et al. [8]

time divided by the systolic ejection time (Fig. 20.1). The index is easily measured with high reproducibility and is important in the assessment of global performance, as the active energy cycles of contraction and relaxation occur during ICVT and IVRT. The Tei index is independent of heart rate and blood pressure and can be a useful tool to evaluate myocardial function in different clinical situations [8].

20.3.9 Tissue Doppler Imaging

Tissue Doppler imaging is an extension of conventional Doppler flow echocardiography that measures myocardial motion and velocity [9] (Fig. 20.2A). Myocardial velocity information can be displayed as a pulse tissue Doppler signal and data color-coded and displayed in real time. Color Doppler allows for visual semiquantitation of myocardial motion superimposed on conventional M-mode and two-dimensional images. Velocity data from a region of interest can be arranged to obtain spectral displays of tissue velocity. The graphic display includes one positive systolic deflection and two negative diastolic waveforms. The systolic waveform is preceded by the regional isovolumic contraction time, and the

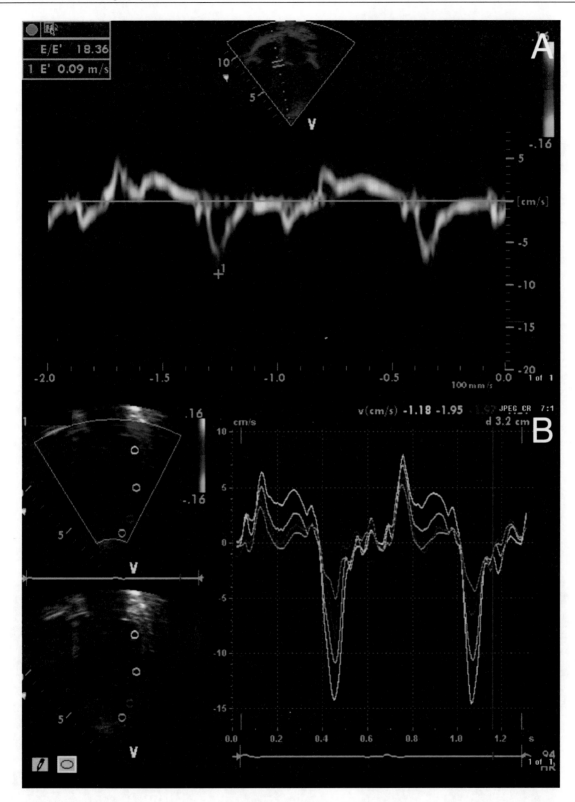

Fig. 20.2 Tissue Doppler imaging. (**A**) Pulse wave tissue Doppler provides a spectral display of peak tissue velocity. (**B**) Tissue Doppler velocity data for the quantification of asynchrony from apical four-chamber view. Sample volumes are in the lateral free wall segment

diastolic waves are preceded by regional isovolumic relaxation time; the first diastolic deflection represents the early rapid filling phase of diastole, which is followed by a period of diastasis, and a second late active filling phase of diastole due to atrial contraction (Fig. 20.2B).

20.4 Clinical Applications of Cardiac Ultrasound

20.4.1 Transvaginal and Transabdominal Fetal Echocardiography

The human fetal heart is fully developed and functional by 11 weeks after conception. Using transvaginal ultrasound, the structure and functional characteristics of the fetal heart can be observed as early as 9 weeks of gestational age [10]. This technique remains the most useful type of fetal cardiac imaging until approximately 16 weeks of gestation. At that time, transabdominal imaging becomes the preferred method (Fig. 20.3). Fetal imaging is routinely performed at 16–20 weeks of gestational age, and image quality improves until about 24–28 weeks of gestation [10]. The quality of fetal cardiac images can be reduced by loss of amniotic fluid, maternal body habitus, fetal bone density, and/or the fetal position. M-mode, two-dimensional, and Doppler ultrasound techniques are useful for the analyses of the anatomy and function of the fetal heart, as well as for the diagnoses and monitoring of fetal arrhythmias. In general, fetal echocardiography has contributed to: (1) improved understanding of the natural history of many forms of congenital heart disease; (2) improved monitoring and obstetric care of fetuses with structural heart diseases and arrhythmias; and (3) attempts at in utero correction of valvar abnormalities [11, 12]. For more information on heart development and congenital defects, refer to Chapters 3 and 9.

20.4.2 Transesophageal Echocardiography

Transesophageal echocardiography allows imaging of the heart from either the esophagus or stomach, which improves image resolution by eliminating much of the acoustic interference from the lungs and chest wall, while at the same time allowing for a reduced distance of the ultrasound source from the heart. Transesophageal imaging is commonly performed using either a biplane probe (two single plane arrays set at perpendicular planes) or a rotating single array probe that provides multiple planes of view (an omniplane probe). Today, transesophageal probes come in sizes appropriate for use in adults,

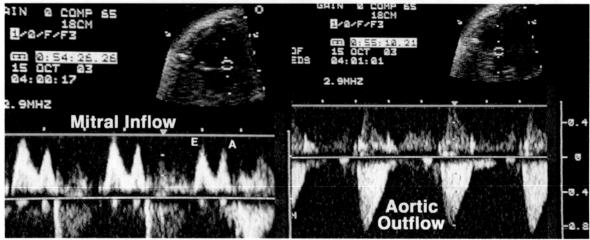

Fig. 20.3 Fetal echocardiogram at approximately 24 weeks gestation. Four-chamber views are shown with pulse wave Doppler analysis of mitral inflow and aortic outflow. Mitral inflow is characterized by two waves, an E wave representing passive filling of the left ventricle in diastole and an A wave representing active filling of the ventricle with atrial systole. Doppler flows are less than 1 m/s indicating unobstructed blood flow, and the interval between aortic outflow signals is approximately 0.5 s indicating a fetal heart rate of 120 beats/min

children, and/or infants. Transesophageal echocardiography is used when improved resolution is required or when transthoracic windows are unavailable, as is typical in the operating room or cardiac catheterization laboratory [3]. It also has become a routine form of intraoperative monitoring during open-heart surgery and is specifically useful to detect complications or incomplete repairs prior to separation from cardiopulmonary bypass [13]. Additionally, it is a useful adjunct to interventional cardiac catheterization procedures. Transesophageal echocardiography typically requires sedation or anesthesia and thus adequate patient monitoring. Furthermore, it is significantly more invasive than standard transthoracic echocardiography and can be complicated by airway compromise and/or dysphagia [3, 14, 15].

20.4.3 Transthoracic Echocardiography

Transthoracic echocardiography is the most common method for cardiac imaging. It is noninvasive, can be performed in any cooperative patient, and only rarely requires sedation or anesthesia. Yet, images obtained are limited by patient size and can be complicated by interference from soft tissues, bone, or lung. The transthoracic echocardiogram is performed from standard anatomic windows on the chest (Fig. 20.4) and typically

requires the use of multiple transducers at varied ultrasound frequencies to maximize the two-dimensional image resolution and Doppler ultrasound information obtained. Most commonly, images are obtained by trained and licensed cardiac sonographers and then interpreted by a cardiologist.

20.4.4 Standard Transthoracic Examination

The standard transthoracic cardiac echocardiogram includes images from parasternal, apical, suprasternal notch, and subcostal imaging windows (Fig. 20.4). Two-dimensional sectors are imaged in each window to provide appropriate cardiac anatomic details and functional analyses. While scanning for anatomical detail, the highest frequency transducer set at the lowest depth possible is used to maximize image resolution. Two-dimensional images are then used to guide Doppler ultrasound interrogations, often with a lower frequency transducer that will optimize Doppler information. Two-dimensional images are also used to guide M-mode measurements of chamber sizes and function and, with this mode, Doppler gradients are calculated across valves and shunts to maximize the hemodynamic information obtained.

The standardized transthoracic echocardiograms can be obtained by scanning at four regions on the chest wall: the parasternal window, apical window, subcostal region, and suprasternal notch (Fig. 20.2). Parasternal long axis views are used to obtain "long axis" images of the left side of the heart, including the left atrium, left ventricle, and aorta (Fig. 20.5). A subtle tilt of the transducer inferiorly from this position gives views of the right atrium, tricuspid valve, and right ventricle, and tilting leftward brings the pulmonary valve and main pulmonary artery into view. Turning the transducer and scan plane by 90° results in short axis views of the heart in planes from the base of the heart (region of the aorta, tricuspid, and pulmonary valves) to the apex (Fig. 20.6A–D). M-mode measurements of the left-sided chambers are best obtained from parasternal short axis windows and can then be used to assess chamber sizes and function (Fig. 20.6E, F). Apical windows are employed to reveal standard four-chamber views of the left atrium, mitral valve, left ventricle, right atrium, tricuspid valve, and right ventricle (Fig. 20.7A, B). This view sends the ultrasound beam parallel to the septal structures, so it is not adequate to assess the integrity of the atrial or ventricular septums. Tilting the transducer anteriorly results in a five-chamber view that allows excellent visualization of the left

Standard Transthoracic Echocardiographic Windows

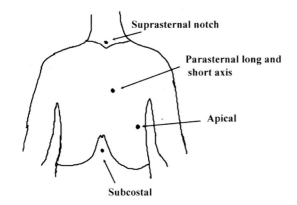

Fig. 20.4 Diagram of the chest showing transducer position for standard transthoracic echocardiographic windows. A typical examination in a cooperative patient is performed in a standard order: parasternal, apical, subcostal, and then suprasternal notch views. Perpendicular imaging planes can be obtained from each position by rotating the transducer 90°

Parasternal Long Axis Views

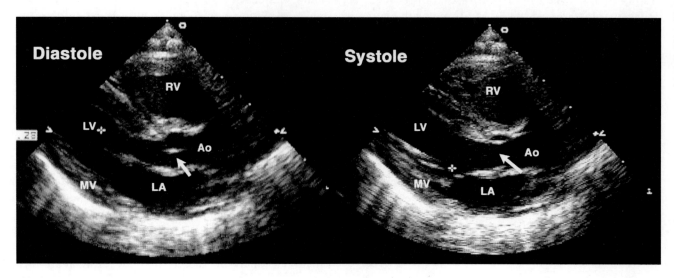

Fig. 20.5 Transthoracic parasternal long axis views in a newborn infant. These views demonstrate the long axis of the left side of the heart. **Frame 1** is in diastole with an open mitral valve to accommodate left ventricular filling and a closed aortic valve (*arrow*).

Frame 2 is in systole with an open aortic valve (*arrow*) and a closed mitral valve (*). *White dots* on the sector border represent centimeter marks. Ao = aorta; LA = left atrium; LV = left ventricle; MV = mitral valve; RV = right ventricle

ventricular outflow tract and aorta. Doppler gradients across the mitral, tricuspid, and aortic valves can readily be obtained from this view (Fig. 20.7C), and the velocity of a detected tricuspid valve regurgitation can be used to estimate right ventricular and pulmonary artery systolic pressures.

Subcostal views are particularly useful in patients with lung disease or in those who have had recent open-heart surgery. From subcostal images, the orientation of the heart in the chest and the major vascular connections can still be well established. Subcostal views also provide excellent visualization of the intraatrial septum (Fig. 20.8A) and four-chamber views in patients with poor apical windows. Suprasternal notch views are most useful for visualization of the aortic arch, its branching vessels, and the descending thoracic aorta (Fig. 20.8C), as well as for determining the Doppler shifts across the aortic valve. This view is also important to use for patients in whom one wants to exclude vascular abnormalities including coarctation of the aorta.

20.5 Emerging Techniques in Cardiac Ultrasound

To date, the use of ultrasound for cardiac imaging and investigation of hemodynamics has been seen as revolutionary in the diagnoses and treatment of heart disease.

Currently, ultrasound techniques available for use on a limited clinical or investigational basis include intravascular ultrasound, three- and four-dimensional imaging, and embryonic cardiac imaging. Intravascular ultrasound uses catheters with ultrasound transducers mounted on the tips. These transducers are capable of cross-sectional imaging or true sector imaging using phased array ultrasound transducers mounted on their tips [3, 16]. As such technology has improved, relatively small catheters and high-frequency transducers are now available for imaging of the aorta and pulmonary arteries, aortic and pulmonary valves, and even within the coronary arteries. Coronary artery imaging has been particularly useful in heart transplant patients as a means to detect intimal thickening associated with chronic rejection [17] and in patients with Kawasaki syndrome who develop coronary artery aneurysms [3]. Intravascular ultrasound has also been used for intracardiac monitoring of interventional procedures [16]. Three-dimensional imaging technology has recently been enhanced so that cardiac images can be displayed in real time (also called four-dimensional imaging). Thus, three- and four-dimensional images are useful for re-creation of movable three-dimensional images needed to assist with surgical planning [1]. Unfortunately, currently available large transducer sizes and slow image processing capabilities make three- and four-dimensional imaging inappropriate for routine cardiac ultrasound examinations [7]. Lastly, ultrasound

Parasternal Short Axis
Two Dimensional Images and M-Mode

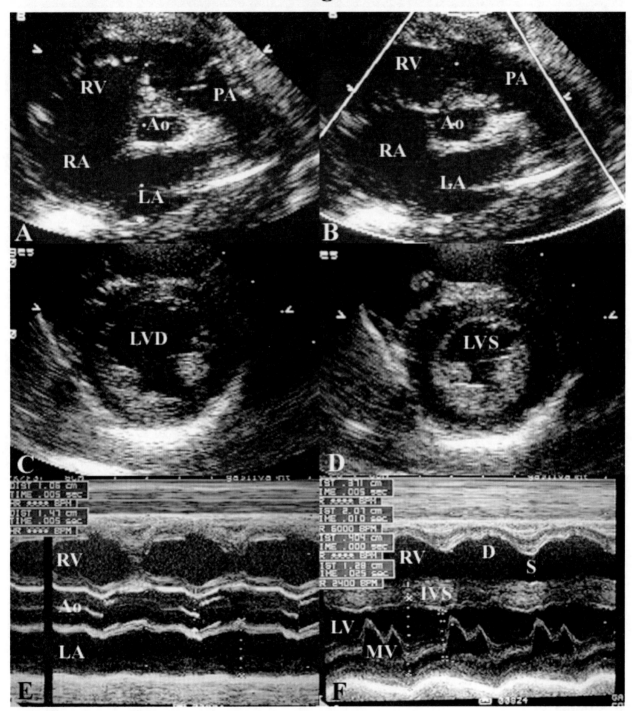

Fig. 20.6 Two-dimensional and M-mode images obtained from parasternal short axis views. **Panel A** shows a view through the base of the heart in diastole. **Panel B** shows the same imaging plane in systole, with the pulmonary valve open. M-mode measurements of the right ventricle, aorta, and left atrium (**Panel E**) are obtained in this plane. **Panel C** demonstrates a cross-sectional or short axis view of the left ventricle at the level of the papillary muscles in diastole, and **Panel D** is at the same plane in systole.

This is the appropriate level for quantification of left ventricular function by shortening fraction. **Panel F** shows an M-mode recording at the level of the mitral valve, a plane just above that seen in **Panels C** and **D**. Abnormalities of mitral valve motion can be demonstrated in this plane. Ao = aorta; D = diastole; IVS = interventricular septum; LA = left atrium; LVD = left ventricle, diastole; LVS = left ventricle, systole; PA = main pulmonary artery; RA = right atrium; RV = right ventricle; S = systole

Apical Four Chamber Views
with Pulse Wave Doppler

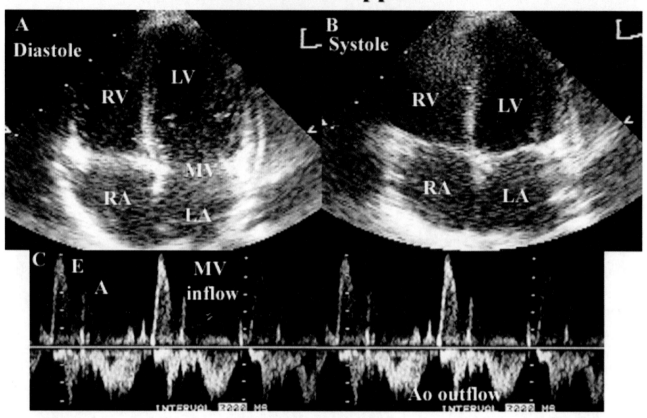

Fig. 20.7 **Panel A** illustrates a two-dimensional apical four-chamber view of the heart in diastole (open mitral valve) and **Panel B** shows the same imaging plane in systole (closed atrioventricular valves). The pulsed wave Doppler tracing shown in **Panel C** demonstrates mitral inflow toward the transducer (above the baseline) and aortic outflow away from the transducer (below the baseline). The mitral valve inflow tracing shows passive filling of the left ventricle during early diastole (E) followed by active filling of the left ventricle in late diastole with the onset of atrial contraction (A). Aortic outflow occurs in systole. LA = left atrium; LV = left ventricle; MV = mitral valve; RA = right atrium; RV = right ventricle

imaging technology has been improved so that the heart can be studied during embryonic development. For example, pregnant mice can be anesthetized and undergo fetal cardiac imaging as early as 8–9 days after conception so that the anatomy and blood flow patterns can be observed during both normal and abnormal cardiac development [18–20].

20.6 Summary

The development and application of clinical echocardiography has allowed for the thorough, accurate, noninvasive, real-time evaluation of cardiac structure and function. To date, transthoracic echocardiography is a mainstay of cardiac diagnoses and monitoring in both adult and pediatric patients. Advances in two-dimensional imaging allow significant anatomic detail to be visualized, especially in smaller patients, and Doppler ultrasound allows direct visualization of altered flow patterns and noninvasive investigation of hemodynamics. The use of transesophageal echocardiography, although slightly more invasive, has become routine when improved resolution and intraprocedural monitoring are required. New Doppler methods have improved quantification of regional and diastolic myocardial function. Future directions include increased utilization of intravascular ultrasound for diagnosis and monitoring of interventional procedures, improvement in three-dimensional ultrasound techniques that will make them appropriate for routine imaging, and the use of embryonic imaging to study normal and abnormal heart development.

Subcostal and Suprasternal Notch Two Dimensional Images

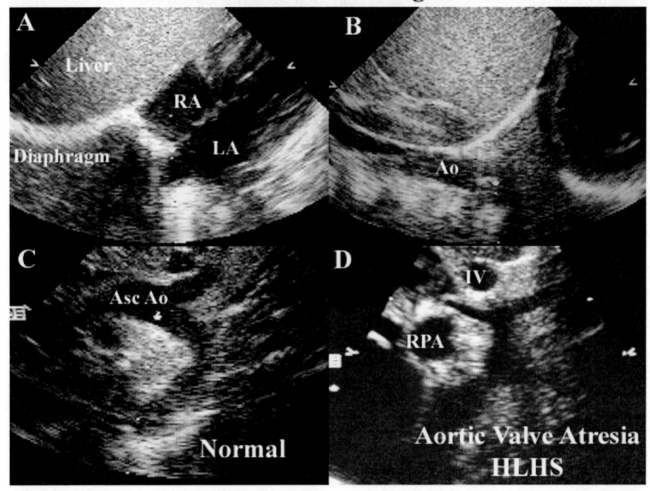

Fig. 20.8 Two-dimensional images from subcostal windows (**A, B**) and suprasternal notch windows (**C, D**). Subcostal views provide orientation of the heart relative to the abdominal organs as in **Panel A**, which shows a rightward liver and leftward cardiac apex. Subcostal windows also provide excellent four-chamber views as well as short axis views of the interatrial septum in smaller individuals, as shown in **Panel A**. **Panel B** is a subcostal view showing the descending thoracic aorta at the level of the diaphragm. **Panel C** is a suprasternal notch view of a normal aortic arch. **Panel D** shows the severe hypoplasia of the ascending aorta seen in a patient with hypoplastic left heart syndrome (HLHS) caused by aortic atresia. Ao = aorta; AscAo = ascending aorta; IV = innominate vein; LA = left atrium; RA = right atrium; RPA = right pulmonary artery

Acknowledgments The author would like to thank Jim Berry, Kim Berry, and Jay Hall for providing the images shown in this chapter and Kim Berry and Jay Hall for review of this manuscript.

References

1. Geva T. Echocardiography and Doppler ultrasound. In: Garson A, ed. The science and practice of pediatric cardiology. Philadelphia, PA: Williams and Wilkins, 1998:789–843.

2. Vermilion RP. Basic physical principles. In: Snider R, Serwer G, Ritter S, eds. Echocardiography in pediatric heart disease. St. Louis, MO: Mosby-Year Book, 1997:1–10.

3. Snider R, Serwer G, Ritter S, eds. Echocardiography in pediatric heart disease. St. Louis, MO: Mosby-Year Book, 1997.

4. Colan SD, Parness IA, Spevak PJ. Developmental modulation of myocardial mechanics: Age and growth related alterations in afterload and contractility. J Am Coll Cardiol 1992;19:619–29.

5. Gutgessel HP, Paquet M, Duff DF, McNamara DG. Evaluation of left ventricular size and function by echocardiography: Results in normal children. Circulation 1977;56:457–62.

6. Vermilion RP. Technology and instrumentation. Echocardiography. In: Snider A, ed. Pediatric heart disease. St. Louis, MO: Mosby-Year Book, 1997:11–21.

7. Danford DA, Murphy DJ Jr. Basic foundations of echocardiography and Doppler ultrasound. In: Garson A, ed. The science and practice of pediatric cardiology. Philadelphia, PA: Williams and Wilkins, 1998:539–58.

8. Pellet AA, Tolar WG, Merwin DG, Kerut EK. The Tei index: Methodology and disease state values. Echocardiogr J CV Ultrasound Allied Tech 2004;21:669–72.

9. Knebel F, Reibis RK, Bondke HJ, et al. Tissue Doppler echocardiography and biventricular pacing in heart failure: Patient selection, procedural guidance, follow-up, quantification of success. Cardiovasc Ultrasound 2004;2:doi:10.1186/1476-7120-2-17.

10. Allan L. The normal fetal heart. In: Allan L, ed. Textbook of fetal cardiology. London, UK: Greenwich Medical Media Limited, 2000:55–91.

11. Tworetzky W, Marshall AC. Balloon valvuloplasty for congenital heart disease in the fetus. Clin Perinatol 2003;30:541–50.

12. Tulzer G, Artz W, Franklin RC, Loughna PV, Mair R, Gardiner HM. Fetal pulmonary valvuloplasty for critical pulmonary stenosis or atresia with intact septum. Lancet 2002;360:1567–8.

13. Randolph GR, Hagler DJ, Connolly HM, et al. Intraoperative transesophageal echocardiography during surgery for congenital heart defects. J Thorac Cardiovasc Surg 2002;124:1176–82.

14. Stevenson JG. Incidence of complications in pediatric transesophageal echocardiography: Experience in 1650 cases. J Am Soc Echocardiogr 1999;12:527–32.

15. Rousou JA, Tighe DA, Garb JL, et al. Risk of dysphagia after transesophageal echocardiography during cardiac operations. Ann Thorac Surg 2000;69:486–9.

16. Ziada KM, Tuzcu EM, Nissen SE. Application of intravascular ultrasound imaging in understanding and guiding percutaneous therapy for atherosclerotic coronary disease. Cardio Rev 1999;7:289–300.

17. Costello JM, Wax DF, Binns HJ, Backer CL, Mavroudis C, Pahl E. A comparison of intravascular ultrasound with coronary angiography for evaluation of transplant coronary artery disease in pediatric heart transplant recipients. J Heart Lung Transplant 2003;22:44–9.

18. Srinivasan S, Baldwin HS, Aristizabal O, Kwee L, Labow M, Turnbull DH. Noninvasive, in utero imaging of mouse embryonic heart development with 40-MHz echocardiography. Circulation 1998;98:912–8.

19. Zhou YQ, Foster FS, Qu DW, Zhang M, Harasiewic KA, Adamson SL. Applications for multifrequency ultrasound biomicroscopy in mice from implantation to adulthood. Physiol Genomics 2002;10:113–26.

20. Insight through In Vivo Imaging, Vevo 660 System Product Information, Visualsonics 3080 Yonge Street, Suite 6020, Box 89, Toronto, Canada. (Accessed May 20, 2008, at www.visualsonics.com).

Chapter 21
Monitoring and Managing the Critically Ill Patient in the Intensive Care Unit

Greg J. Beilman

Abstract The need for monitoring of patients has grown as the health care system has developed the ability to care for more critically ill patients. Monitors serve several purposes including identification of shock and abnormal cardiac physiology, evaluation of cardiovascular function, and/or to allow for optimizing titration of therapy. An important function of an effective monitoring device is reliable detection of abnormal physiology. Despite much research on the use of monitoring techniques in critical care, there is little evidence of improved outcome related to use of monitors. Mainstays of invasive monitoring in the ICU include central venous pressure monitoring and arterial pressure monitoring, with pulmonary arterial monitoring reserved for occasional patients with multisystem disease. Recent trends in monitoring have included development of less invasive monitoring techniques that yield a number of cardiovascular parameters potentially useful to clinicians. New noninvasive measures of tissue perfusion (StO_2, sublingual capnometry) have significant potential in identification and treatment of pathophysiologic states resulting in inadequate tissue perfusion. Developers of new monitors, despite regulatory requirements that are less stringent than those of drug manufacturers, will increasingly be expected to demonstrate clinical efficacy of new devices. In the final analysis, the most important "monitor" is a caring health care provider at the patient bedside carefully evaluating the patient's response to intervention and therapy.

Keywords ICU monitoring · Near infrared spectroscopy · Pulse waveform contour analysis · Sublingual capnometry · Pulmonary artery catheter

All exact science is dominated by the idea of approximation
Bertrand Russell, 1870–1972

G.J. Beilman (✉)
University of Minnesota, Department of Surgery, MMC 11,
420 Delaware St. SE, Minneapolis, MN, USA
e-mail: beilm001@umn.edu

21.1 History

The treatment of shock is closely related to health care workers' experience during times of war. Ambroise Pare, a French military surgeon practicing during the 16th century first described ligature to control bleeding in 1545. Experiences during World War I resulted in a clear understanding of the need for operative interventions for bowel perforation, with this operative intervention available due to the accessibility of general anesthetics. The discovery of blood types by Karl Landsteiner in 1901 (for which he received the Nobel Prize in 1930) enabled the safe and practical use of blood transfusions by medical providers during World War II, thus allowing resuscitation of combat-injured casualties. Advances utilized in the Korean War included new surgical techniques such as vascular anastomosis and new medical therapies including renal dialysis. Use of positive pressure ventilation and renal dialysis was broadened during the Vietnam War due to development of complications of resuscitation in patients with previously nonsurvivable injury, including acute respiratory distress syndrome and/or renal failure.

The first described use of an intensive care unit (ICU) as a separate area to care for patients was in the early 1950s, as a result of a poliomyelitis epidemic in Denmark. The first coronary care unit was established in Kansas City, KS, in the early 1960s with the observation that new techniques of cardiopulmonary resuscitation could reduce mortality in patients suffering myocardial infarction. Their use expanded to postsurgical patients during the mid 1960s as more complicated surgery mandated a closer observation of patients and more aggressive intervention of the patients' physiology in the ICU.

As our ability to care for sicker patients has improved, the need for better monitoring techniques has also advanced. The first "monitors" were the five senses of the physician. Lanneac described the first stethoscope as an extension of the sense of hearing in the late 18th century. The development of neurosurgery as a specialty in the early 20th century and the need to monitor blood pressure during these operations led to development of the sphygmanomometer. The need to monitor the physiology of astronauts in space led to capability for continuous EKG and other types of monitors. ICU monitoring techniques developed over the last three decades have resulted in a significant improvement in our overall understanding of cardiac physiology and pathophysiology. One such device was the flow-directed balloon-tipped pulmonary artery catheter, also known as the Swan–Ganz catheter. The last two decades have seen a plethora of invasive and noninvasive monitoring tools developed for critical care use. Despite these tools, the most important tool available to the clinician remains his/ her five senses, mandating a careful examination of patients from a daily, routine basis.

21.2 Goals of Monitoring

Diagnosis of Shock: Many monitoring strategies relate to identification of shock, thus an important issue is the clinical definition of shock. In the final analysis, shock can be simply defined as inadequate oxygen delivery to given tissues, resulting in decreased adenosine triphosphate (ATP) production and flux at the mitochondrial level related to decreased oxidative phosphorylation. Therefore, the ideal monitor for diagnosis of shock would thus be able to identify the rate of ATP production and turnover. Unfortunately, to date, such a monitor does not exist for routine clinical use; hence, clinicians use common clinical end points to identify shock and other associated abnormalities in patients. A list of commonly used clinical monitoring end points is listed in Table 21.1. It requires an astute clinician to balance the sometimes contradictory findings during evaluation of the patient and to develop an appropriate treatment strategy. An important component of this process is frequent reevaluation of the patient to determine results of the initial intervention. Importantly, a response to intervention contradictory to initial evaluation should prompt reconsideration of the initial diagnosis.

Table 21.1 Commonly used clinical end points of resuscitation

Heart rate
Blood pressure
Mentation
Skin perfusion
Urine output 50 cc/h
Normal lactate/acid–base status
Appropriate response to therapeutic interventions

Evaluation of Cardiac Function: Another reason for consideration of invasive monitoring is for continuous evaluation of cardiac outcome. In particular, serious illness in patients with underlying cardiac disease (e.g., cardiomyopathy, congestive heart failure, congenital heart disease) may require a careful titration of therapy to prevent decompensation. Situations that commonly result in invasive monitoring of patients include serious infectious episodes, planned major operations, and/or decompensation of the underlying disease.

Titration of Vasoactive Therapy: Many patients receive invasive monitoring due to hemodynamic instability (i.e., hypotension or severe hypotension) or due to the need to titrate vasoactive therapy for other therapeutic purposes (e.g., optimization of cerebral perfusion in patients with neurologic insult). Most vasoactive agents have short half-lives, requiring frequent titration of therapy to achieve monitoring targets. This need mandates accurate, continuous monitoring of blood pressure (or other end point), typically via an invasive route (see Chapter 16).

An important, but frequently unstated, reason for invasive monitoring in the critically ill patient is to allow a more definitive diagnosis and/or end point for treatment. This more definitive observation after initial evaluation may allow ongoing management of the patient's issues away from the bedside, allowing the clinician to perform other duties.

21.3 Monitors: Do They Help?

Despite the common reliance on monitors in the modern ICU, a number of monitoring end points commonly used have not demonstrated consistent benefit with respect to patient outcome, including continuous EKG monitoring, pulse oximetry, pulmonary artery catheters, and/or intracranial pressure monitoring. For example, with regard to pulse oximetry, Pedersen et al. in the Cochrane database systems review of 2003 [1] noted that "the conflicting subjective and objective results of the studies, despite an intense methodological collection of data from a relatively large population (>20,000 patients) indicates that the value of perioperative monitoring with pulse oximetry is questionable in relation to improved quality outcomes effectiveness and efficacy." The same can be said regarding pulmonary artery catheters. Shah et al. [2] noted that "despite almost 20 years of randomized controlled trials, a clear strategy leading to improved survival with a pulmonary artery catheter has not been devised."

One nuance with regard to monitors is that the use of such devices will not change the outcome for a fatal disease if there is no treatment available for the disease [3].

For instance, while you can monitor the progression of end-stage organ function in a patient with metastatic cancer, it is unlikely that utilizing a monitor to guide therapy in such a patient will affect the ultimate survival outcome of the patient.

On the other hand, one positive bit of evidence demonstrating beneficial effects for physiologic monitoring relates to the significant decrease in anesthesia-related deaths over the last two decades. Anesthesia care is currently highly dependent on multiple physiologic monitors. As monitors have become increasingly utilized during anesthesia, the anesthesia-related mortality rate of 1 per 20,000 anesthetics reported in the late 1970s has decreased to a rate of 1 in 300,000 anesthetics at the turn of the century. Most knowledgeable clinicians in this area would agree that much of this decrease in mortality is related to both better understanding of pathophysiology and more widespread use of continuous monitoring.

21.4 Invasive Monitoring Techniques in the ICU

21.4.1 Central Venous Pressure (CVP) Monitoring

Pressure monitoring in a central venous location, using a central venous catheter, is likely the most frequently utilized invasive monitoring technique in current ICUs. Central venous catheters allow an estimate of "cardiac preload" (Fig. 21.1) and are typically placed via the internal jugular or subclavian venous route (Fig. 21.2). These

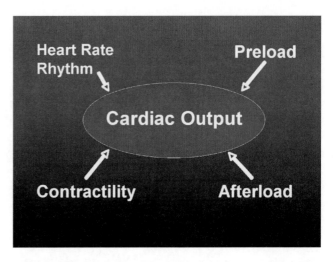

Fig. 21.1 Determinants of cardiac output. Cardiac output is related to appropriate diastolic filling of the left ventricle (preload), resistance of outflow (afterload), contractility (force of contraction), and cardiac rate and rhythm

monitors are very accurate for the identification of situations in which cardiac output is affected by a low preload. However, the assumption is made when monitoring central venous pressures that this value is proportional to pulmonary artery pressure which is proportional to left atrial pressure which is proportional to left ventricular end-diastolic volumes. Unfortunately, there are many common conditions in ICU patients that can elevate CVP that do not relate to increased filling of the left ventricle, including pneumonia, positive pressure ventilation, acute respiratory distress syndrome, pulmonary emboli, and/or others. Thus, one should have a strong concern for the situation in which a high CVP does not correlate with the clinical condition of the patient.

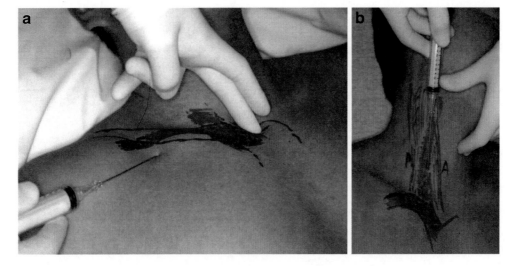

Fig. 21.2 Representation of cannulation of central veins with access needle by subclavian (**A**) or internal jugular (**B**) routes. *Blue* color on this human volunteer denotes location of veins, *red* on Fig. 21.2B denotes location of the sternocleidomastoid muscle

21.4.2 Arterial Blood Pressure Monitoring

Arterial blood pressure monitoring can be performed using both noninvasive and invasive techniques. Noninvasive monitors have progressed significantly over the years and currently allow a hands-off approach to intermittent measurement of blood pressure (Fig. 21.3). Unfortunately, it is difficult to measure blood pressure more frequently than every 5 min due to both patient comfort and potential for induced pressure sores. In situations where more frequent measures are necessary, invasive catheters placed percutaneously into a peripheral artery are utilized (Fig. 21.4). Typically, continuous

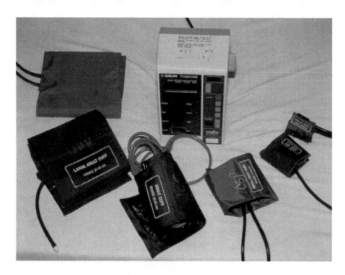

Fig. 21.3 Example of noninvasive blood pressure monitor with various size cuffs for a range of patient sizes

blood pressure is measured using an arterial line or catheter placed in one of several positions (most commonly radial or femoral arteries). Like CVP monitoring, there are assumptions built into blood pressure monitoring that are occasionally incorrect. Importantly, the assumption that a normal arterial blood pressure has excluded the presence of shock may be false, since afterload may be increased due to low cardiac output. This results in a normal blood pressure but inadequate oxygen delivery to tissues. For more details on noninvasive blood pressure monitoring, see Chapter 16.

21.4.3 Pulmonary Artery Catheter

The pulmonary artery catheter revolutionized the ability of clinicians to understand the physiology of the cardiovascular system during critical illness. This catheter was first described by Drs. Swan and Ganz in 1970 [4] and was rapidly incorporated into clinical practice. To a large extent, it is responsible for the specialty of critical care (Fig. 21.5). The pulmonary artery catheter is inserted via the central venous access approach through the femoral vein, subclavian vein, or the internal jugular vein. The balloon-tipped catheter floats through the right atrium and right ventricle with the balloon inflated and then is wedged into a smaller branch of the pulmonary artery. The pressure measurement obtained during this maneuver is known as the pulmonary artery occlusion pressure, or "wedge pressure." This catheter allows for a more accurate measure of intravascular volume than CVP

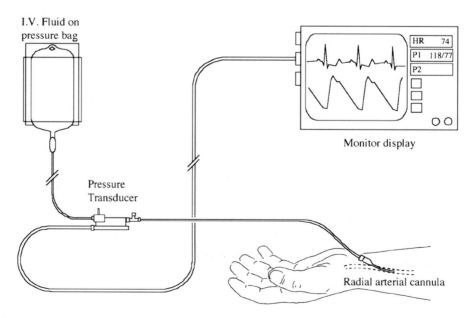

Monitor display

Radial arterial cannula

Fig. 21.4 Arterial line placed into radial artery. The line is attached to a pressure transducer which measures blood pressure and allows

slow flush of intravenous fluid though the line. This line can also be utilized for sampling of arterial blood

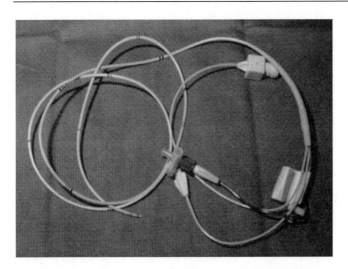

Fig. 21.5 Pulmonary artery catheter. This catheter has an inflatable balloon at the tip, allowing the catheter to be carried through the right heart and into the pulmonary artery during insertion

artery wedge pressure. Additionally, using these catheters, cardiac output can be measured either continuously or intermittently using a Fick thermodilution technique. Briefly, cold saline is infused through the catheter at a position proximal to the tip. The temperature is concurrently monitored via a thermistor at the tip of the catheter, and the rate at which the temperature decreases and then returns to normal and integration of this change allows for calculation of cardiac output. Additional measures of oxygen kinetics including oxygen delivery (DO_2) and oxygen consumption (VO_2) can be determined using the cardiac output and values measured from arterial and mixed venous blood samples (Table 21.2). Information obtained from the pulmonary artery catheter has significant diagnostic value, since this information can be utilized to distinguish among the various types of shock (Table 21.3). Nonetheless, given the lack of positive outcomes of several large trials using the pulmonary artery catheter in the last decade [5], the frequency of use of this catheter in the ICU has significantly decreased. Despite decreased use, the pulmonary artery catheter is still occasionally indispensable to assist in evaluation and titration of therapy of the patient with multisystem disease. For

because it bypasses the situations that can falsely elevate CVP. Since the pulmonary artery system is a high-flow low-resistance system, those conditions which falsely elevate pulmonary artery pressure do not affect pulmonary

Table 21. 2 Calculations for invasive hemodynamic measurements

Hemodynamic formula	Normal
$CI = CO/BSA$	$2.8–4.2\ l/min/m^2$
$SV = CO/HR$	$60–90\ ml/beat$
$MAP = DBP + 1/3\ (SBP − DBP)$	$80–120\ mmHg$
$SVR = [(MAP − CVP)/CO] \times 80$	$900–1400\ dynes\ cm\ s^3$
$SVRI = (MAP − CVP)/CI$	$1900–2400\ dynes\ cm\ m^3$
$PVR = [(MPAP − PAOP)/CO] \times 80$	$100–250\ dynes\ cm\ s^3$
Arterial oxygen content:	$21\ ml/100\ ml$
$CaO_2 = (SaO_2)\ (Hb \times 1.34) + PaO_2\ (0.0031)$	
Venous oxygen content:	$15\ ml/100\ ml$
$CvO_2 = (SvO_2)\ (Hb \times 1.34) + PvO_2\ (0.0031)$	
Oxygen consumption:	$225–275\ ml/min, 3.5\ ml/kg/min, 110\ ml/min/m^2$
$VO_2 = CO\ (CaO_2 − CvO_2) \times 10$	
(VO_2 not indexed, indexed by weight, BSA)	
Oxygen delivery: $DO_2 = CO\ (CaO_2) \times 10$	$1000\ ml/min$
Oxygen extraction ratio: $O_2ER = VO_2/DO_2$	$22–30\%$

BSA = body surface area; CI = cardiac index; CO = cardiac output; CVP = central venous pressure; DBP = diastolic blood pressure; Hb = hemoglobin; HR = heart rate; MAP = mean arterial pressure; MPAP = mean pulmonary artery pressure; PAOP = pulmonary artery occlusion pressure; PVR = peripheral vascular resistance; SBP = systolic blood pressure; SVR = systemic vascular resistance; SVRI = systemic vascular resistance index; SV = stroke volume

Table 21. 3 Changes in cardiac preload, systemic vascular resistance, and cardiac output in various causes of shock

Type of shock	PAOP	SVR	CO	Prime mover
Hemorrhagic	Decreased	Increased	Decreased	Decreased preload
Septic	Unchanged	Decreased	Increased	Decreased SVR
Cardiogenic	Increased	Increased	Decreased	Decreased CO
Neurogenic	Unchanged	Decreased	Increased	Decreased SVR

CO = cardiac output; PAOP = pulmonary artery occlusion pressure; SVR = systemic vascular resistance; prime mover = variable primarily responsible for shock in clinical syndrome.

additional discussion of Swan–Ganz catheters and a movie clip of its use, see Chapter 18.

21.4.4 Complications of Invasive Monitors

A major issue with all invasive monitors involves complications such as those related to insertion, infectious complications, and/or complications associated with an indwelling catheter. Insertion complications can result when the catheter (1) is placed in the wrong vessel; (2) creates a pneumothorax; or (3) causes bleeding related to coagulopathy or inappropriate dilation of a vessel (Fig. 21.6). Furthermore, centrally placed catheters can allow air within the central circulation, occasionally resulting in stroke [6]. Unfortunately, catheter line infections are common and represent a major source of hospital morbidity. Typical infection rates for central venous catheters are in the range of 3–5 infections per 1,000 patient catheter days. Thus, it is important to remove central venous catheters at the point where they are no longer necessary. Since indwelling catheters are made of a foreign material, there is risk of both thrombosis and embolus [7]. Both of these risks are well described in the literature, and attempts to decrease these risks with heparin bonding or using other coatings are prevalent.

21.5 Less Invasive Monitoring Techniques

There are many new monitors making their way into daily clinical use. The utility of these monitors varies widely depending on clinician experience and understanding of monitoring end points, patient populations chosen for study of these monitors, and the clinical relevance of these monitors. The two questions clinicians should ask themselves when evaluating any new monitoring strategy are the following: (1) Does this monitoring system give the information needed to make a decision about the patient's status that is clinically relevant? and (2) How should the clinician intervene related to the results of the monitor? If results from the monitoring system are not clinically relevant or do not allow decisions to be made with respect to intervention, then the monitor is likely not useful for patient care.

21.5.1 Cardiac Hemodynamics

There are several new measurements available allowing less invasive measurement of cardiac hemodynamics.

21.5.1.1 Pulse Contour Wave Processing

Newer, less invasive measures of cardiac hemodynamics include pulse contour wave processing (PiCCO, LiDCO, etc.). The PiCCO monitor utilizes intermittent arterial thermodilution with beat-to-beat analysis of the arterial pulse waveform to provide several hemodynamic parameters. Yet, this monitoring approach requires both a central arterial catheter (e.g., femoral or axillary) and a central line [8]. The LiDCO monitor also uses pulse contour analysis and is calibrated using a dye dilution technique utilizing lithium chloride as an indicator. This approach requires only a peripheral venous line and an arterial catheter [9]. These newer techniques also allow evaluation of preload using different calculated measures including stroke volume variation, pulse pressure variation, and others. These measures of preload have been demonstrated to correlate with fluid responsiveness in a number of settings [10].

21.5.1.2 Ultrasonography/Echocardiography

Ultrasonography and echocardiography have been used to measure flow volume and diameter of the aorta and left ventricular function as a noninvasive hemodynamic evaluation. The described methods include transthoracic or transesophageal echocardiograms. Transthoracic methods are less invasive but significantly less accurate, while transesophageal techniques require a sedated and/or mechanically ventilated patient. Subramaniam and coauthors suggest a method of rapid echocardiographic assessment using a standardized algorithm [11]. This approach uses transesophageal echocardiography for assessment but requires an experienced operator to prevent misinterpretation of findings. Various reports have demonstrated the potential utility of this noninvasive approach but, to date, this technique is finding limited use in ICUs in the United States, likely due to lack of training and experience with this technique for many ICU physicians. For more details on echocardiography and its uses, see Chapter 20.

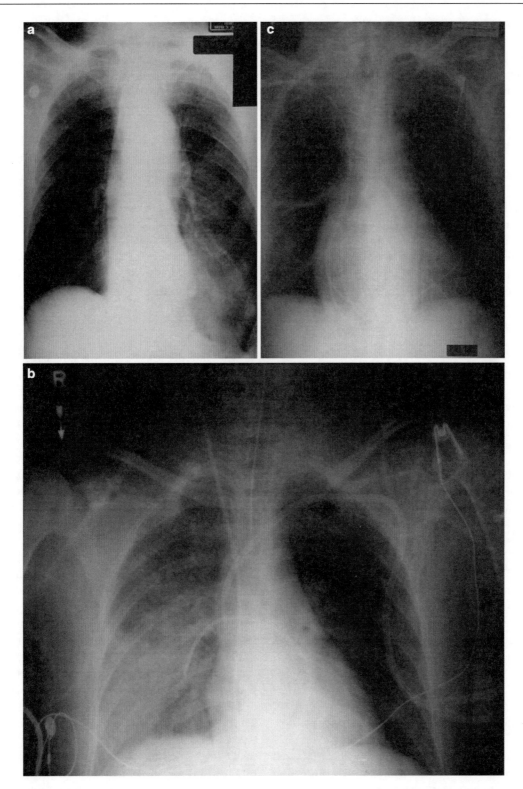

Fig. 21.6 Complications associated with insertion of central access and pulmonary artery catheter, including (**a**) right pneumothorax; (**b**) pulmonary hemorrhage due to distal migration of pulmonary artery catheter; and (**c**) knotting of pulmonary artery catheter in right ventricle

21.5.1.3 CO₂ Partial Rebreathing Technique

The CO_2 partial rebreathing technique can be used via a modified Fick technique in mechanically ventilated patients. The NiCCO device (Respironics, Murrysville, PA) allows measurement of cardiac output using this method. The technique involves measurement of end-tidal CO_2 obtained before and during rebreathing periods. The ratio of the change in end-tidal CO_2 allows a noninvasive estimate of cardiac output [12]. This technique is limited by the fact that the calculation includes blood flow perfusing ventilated portions of the lung and excludes any blood flow bypassing ventilated alveoli. Therefore, this can result in a significant underestimation of cardiac output, but can be corrected by making an estimate of shunt fraction (the amount of blood flow bypassing ventilated alveoli). A number of studies in ICU patients have demonstrated limitations of the current technique that reduce its utility at the current time [13].

21.5.1.4 Arterial Blood Pressure Measures

There are several noninvasive continuous or near-continuous blood pressure monitoring systems under development. These systems capitalize on oscillometric or tonometric techniques to determine blood pressure in a noninvasive fashion. To date, this technology has not progressed to the point of replacement of invasive blood pressure monitoring with these techniques [14].

21.5.2 Perfusion Monitors

There are a number of recently developed noninvasive measures of regional tissue perfusion, including near-infrared spectroscopic measurement of StO_2, sublingual and other capnometry methods, and the use of the $ScvO_2$ catheter.

21.5.2.1 Reflectance Near-Infrared Spectroscopy

Reflectance near-infrared spectroscopy has been utilized to measure peripheral tissue hemoglobin saturation (StO_2). This technology capitalizes on the near-infrared spectral changes of hemoglobin during oxygenation. Whereas pulse oximetry signals (SpO_2) are gated to measure saturation of arterial blood, the signal with StO_2 is derived from the average of small vessel hemoglobin saturation in the tissue bed of interest (arterioles, capillaries, and venules) and thus is proportional to both oxygen delivery to the tissue bed and, importantly, oxygen consumption in this tissue bed. Various animal studies have demonstrated the correlation of StO_2 with global oxygen delivery [15]. A recently published human trial in severely injured trauma patients has identified a StO_2 of less than 75% during the first hour after arrival in the emergency department to be as good a predictor as other commonly used clinical variables for development of multiple organ failure and mortality [16]. Yet, complications with regional changes in cutaneous blood flow need to be further studied. Note that additional human trials are ongoing in a variety of settings with promising results [17].

21.5.2.2 Capnometry

In shock states, it is common to see redistribution of flow away from the gastrointestinal tract, resulting in increased gastrointestinal mucosal pCO_2. Many investigators have demonstrated this effect in both septic and hemorrhagic shock [18, 19]. Unfortunately, techniques to measure pCO_2 in the gastrointestinal tract have been limited by the efforts involved in appropriate placement of catheters within that area. This has led to the development of sublingual capnometry, capitalizing on the fact that the oral tissues are embryologically continuous with the gastrointestinal tract. This technique has the potential to allow rapid information regarding adequacy of tissue perfusion in critically ill patients; however, clinical studies utilizing this technology are lacking at this time.

21.5.2.3 Central Venous O₂ Saturation Monitors

The measurement of mixed venous oxygen saturation in either the pulmonary artery (SvO_2) or the right atrium ($ScvO_2$) has been studied as a reflection of resuscitation of patients in a variety of settings [20–22]. This technique has the potential advantage both of yielding an end point for resuscitative efforts, and intravenous access. Since a decreased cardiac output and a resultant decrease in oxygen delivery to tissues will result in increased peripheral tissue extraction of oxygen from circulating blood, a low $ScvO_2$ in a critically ill patient has typically carried the implication that the patient is suffering from inadequate cardiac output. One potential shortcoming of this technique is the lack of sensitivity related to mixing of venous blood returning from organs with high and low metabolic needs, resulting in a falsely high reading. Despite these theoretic concerns, a recent study by Rivers and colleagues [20] used $ScvO_2$ as an end point of resuscitation in a group of septic patients presenting to an emergency department and demonstrated improved survival in patients who received interventions designed to improve $ScvO_2$ levels to greater than 70% (defined as early goal-directed therapy). These findings have resulted in incorporation of early goal-directed therapy into protocols for treatment of patients with severe sepsis or septic shock. Recent observations have been contradictory [23], however, and large multicenter trials are ongoing to confirm these earlier results.

21.6 Monitor Development

In the United States, medical devices are regulated by the Food and Drug Administration (FDA) [24]. Medical devices are separated into one of three classes based on the risk of the device, with Class I being lowest risk. Class I devices are subjected to the least regulatory control since they present minimal potential harm for the user. Examples of Class I devices include bandages, examination gloves, and handheld surgical instruments. Class II devices are classified by medical specialty "panels," with regulations dependent on the assigned panel. For instance, noninvasive blood pressure monitors are found under the cardiovascular classification; many monitoring devices will be within this class. For FDA approval, such monitoring devices need to measure what the manufacturer says the device should measure, the device must be safe, but there is no specific obligation to demonstrate efficacy. Finally, Class III devices are defined as those that support or sustain human life, are of substantial importance in preventing impairment of human health, or which present a potential unreasonable risk of illness or injury. These devices typically require premarket approval by scientific review to demonstrate safety and effectiveness. Examples of Class III devices are replacement heart valves or silicone-filled breast implants.

There will continue to be a significant need for new monitoring of the critically ill patient. The ideal new monitor would be noninvasive and measure a primary parameter of clinical use such as cardiac contractility, preload, and tissue oxygen utilization or mitochondrial function. Despite a "lower bar" set by regulatory agencies within the Unites States and elsewhere, because of concerns regarding resource utilization and evidence of recent negative monitoring trials, clinicians increasingly desire evidence of benefit. Demonstrated benefits may include less invasive measurement of a useful clinical parameter, identification of groups at high risk for complications, or improvement in outcomes utilizing strategies that include monitoring results (though this is less likely).

21.7 Conclusions

The need for monitoring of the critically ill patient has grown as the health care system has developed the ability to care for progressively more compromised and elderly patients. Monitors serve several purposes including (1) the identification of shock and abnormal cardiac physiology; (2) the evaluation of cardiovascular function; and (3) to allow titration of therapy. An important function of an effective monitoring device is reliable detection of abnormal physiology. Despite much research on use of monitoring techniques in critical care, there is little evidence of improved outcome related to routine use of monitors. To date, the mainstays of invasive monitoring in the ICU include central venous pressure monitoring and arterial pressure monitoring, with pulmonary arterial monitoring reserved for occasional patients with multisystem disease. Recent trends in monitoring have included development of less invasive monitoring techniques that yield a number of cardiovascular parameters potentially useful to clinicians. New noninvasive measures of tissue perfusion (StO_2, sublingual capnometry) have significant potential in identification and treatment of pathophysiologic states resulting in inadequate tissue perfusion. Developers of new monitors (despite what is currently considered as regulatory requirements that are less stringent than those of drug manufacturers) will increasingly be expected to demonstrate clinical efficacy of new devices. In the final analysis, the most important "monitor" is a caring health care provider at the patient bedside evaluating the patient's response to intervention and therapy.

References

1. Pedersen T, Dyrlund Pedersen B, Møller AM. Pulse oximetry for perioperative monitoring. Cochrane Database Syst Rev 2003;3:CD002013.
2. Shah MR, Hasselblad V, Stevenson LW, et al. Impact of the pulmonary artery catheter in critically ill patients: Meta-analysis of randomized clinical trials. JAMA 2005;294:1664–70.
3. Berthelsen PG. Double jeopardy. Acta Anaesthesiol Scand 2006;50:391–2.
4. Swan HJ, Ganz W, Forrester J, Marcus H, Diamond G, Chonette D. Catheterization of the heart in man with use of a flow-directed balloon-tipped catheter. N Engl J Med 1970;283:447–51.
5. Harvey S, Young D, Brampton W, et al. Pulmonary artery catheters for adult patients in intensive care. Cochrane Database Syst Rev 2006;3:CD003408.
6. Brouns R, De Surgeloose D, Neetens I, De Deyn PP. Fatal venous cerebral air embolism secondary to a disconnected central venous catheter. Cerebrovasc Dis 2006;21:212–4.
7. Kirkpatrick A, Rathbun S, Whitsett T, Raskob G. Prevention of central venous catheter-associated thrombosis: A meta-analysis. Am J Med 2007;120:901.e1–13.

8. Hamzaoui O, Monnet X, Richard C, Osman D, Chemla D, Teboul JL. Effects of changes in vascular tone on the agreement between pulse contour and transpulmonary thermodilution cardiac output measurements within an up to 6-hour calibration-free period. Crit Care Med 2008;36:434–40.

9. Costa MG, Della Rocca G, Chiarandini P, et al. Continuous and intermittent cardiac output measurement in hyperdynamic conditions: Pulmonary artery catheter vs. lithium dilution technique. Intensive Care Med 2008;34:257–63.

10. Belloni L, Pisano A, Natale A, et al. Assessment of fluid-responsiveness parameters for off-pump coronary artery bypass surgery: A comparison among LiDCO, transesophageal echocardiography, and pulmonary artery catheter. J Cardiothorac Vasc Anesth 2008;22:243–8.

11. Subramaniam B, Talmor D. Echocardiography for management of hypotension in the intensive care unit. Crit Care Med 2007;35:S401–7.

12. Jaffe MB. Partial CO_2 rebreathing cardiac output operating principles of the NICO system. J Clin Monit Comput 1999;15:387–401.

13. Nilsson LB, Eldrup N, Berthelsen PG. Lack of agreement between thermodilution and carbon dioxide-rebreathing cardiac output. Acta Anaesthesiol Scand 2001;45:680–5.

14. Findlay JY, Gali B, Keegan MT, Burkle CM, Plevak DJ. Vasotrac arterial blood pressure and direct arterial blood pressure monitoring during liver transplantation. Anesth Analg 2006;102:690–3.

15. Taylor JH, Mulier KE, Myers DE, Beilman GJ. Use of near-infrared spectroscopy in early determination of irreversible hemorrhagic shock. J Trauma 2005;58:1119–25.

16. Cohn SM, Nathens AB, Moore FA, et al. StO$_2$ in Trauma Patients Trial Investigators. Tissue oxygen saturation predicts the development of organ dysfunction during traumatic shock resuscitation. J Trauma 2007;62:44–54.

17. Creteur J, Carollo T, Soldati G, Buchele G, De Backer D, Vincent JL. The prognostic value of muscle StO$_2$ in septic patients. Intensive Care Med 2007;33:1549–56.

18. Creteur J, De Backer D, Sakr Y, et al. Sublingual capnometry tracks microcirculatory changes in septic patients. Intensive Care Med 2006;32:516–23.

19. Marik PE. Sublingual capnometery: A non-invasive measure of microcirculatory dysfunction and tissue dysoxia. Physiol Meas 2006;27:R37–47.

20. Rivers E, Nguyen B, Havstad S, et al. Early Goal-Directed Therapy Collaborative Group. Early goal-directed therapy in the treatment of severe sepsis and septic shock. N Engl J Med 2001;345:1368–72.

21. Collaborative Study Group on Perioperative ScvO$_2$ Monitoring. Multicentre study on peri- and postoperative central venous oxygen saturation in high-risk surgical patients. Crit Care 2006;10:R158.

22. Vedrinne C, Bastien O, De Varax R, et al. Predictive factors for usefulness of fiberoptic pulmonary artery catheter for continuous oxygen saturation in mixed venous blood monitoring in cardiac surgery. Anesth Analg 1997;85:2–10.

23. van Beest P, Hofstra J, Schultz M, Boerma E, Spronk P, Kuiper M. The incidence of low venous oxygen saturation on admission to the intensive care unit: A multi-center observational study in The Netherlands. Crit Care 2008;12:R33.

24. Food and Drug Administration (FDA) regulation of medical devices. (Accessed May 5, 2008, at http://www.fda.gov/cdrh/devadvice/3132.html#class_1).

Chapter 22
Cardiovascular Magnetic Resonance Imaging

Michael D. Eggen and Cory M. Swingen

Abstract Cardiovascular magnetic resonance imaging (MRI), or simply cardiac MR, is considered the "gold" standard for noninvasively characterizing cardiac function and viability, having 3D capabilities and a high spatial and temporal resolution. This imaging modality has proven to be an invaluable tool in diagnosing complex cardiomyopathies. Several clinical uses of cardiac MR include: (1) measuring myocardial blood flow; (2) the ability to differentiate between viable and nonviable myocardial tissue; (3) depicting the structure of peripheral and coronary vessels (magnetic resonance angiography); (4) measuring blood flow velocities (MR velocity mapping); (5) examining metabolic energetics (MR spectroscopy); (6) assessing myocardial contractile properties (multislice, multiphase cine imaging, MR tagging); and/or (7) guiding interventional procedures with real-time imaging (interventional MRI). Considering the expansive capabilities of cardiac MR, a condensed review of the concepts and applications of cardiac MR are provided in this chapter.

Keywords MRI · CMRI · Magnetic resonance imaging · Myocardial viability · Myocardial perfusion · Myocardial function · Morphology · Blood flow velocity · Fiber structure · Interventional MRI · Wall motion · Wall thickening · Myocardial strain

22.1 Introduction

"Magnetic resonance imaging" (MRI) of the heart has rapidly become very popular worldwide for its clinical versatility and flexibility, since it allows one to acquire information on anatomical structure and function simultaneously. An additional benefit of MRI is that patients are not subjected to any ionizing radiation or invasive procedures (e.g., catheterization). Recently, many specialized MR techniques have become available for cardiovascular imaging and thus may potentially replace other types of imaging modalities. As such, cardiac MR may become the "one-stop shop" for imaging, as it is able to: (1) measure myocardial blood flow; (2) differentiate viable from nonviable myocardial tissue; (3) depict the structure of peripheral and coronary vessels (magnetic resonance angiography); (4) measure blood flow velocities (MR velocity mapping); (5) examine metabolic energetics (MR spectroscopy); (6) assess myocardial contractile properties (multislice, multiphase cine imaging, MR tagging); and/or (7) guide interventional procedures with real-time imaging (interventional MRI). The capabilities of MRI as a tomographic imaging modality to capture, with high spatial resolution, the anatomy of 3D structures was already well appreciated before the first attempts were made to apply MRI to the heart. Cardiac motion, compounded by respiratory motion and turbulent blood flow in the ventricular cavities and large vessels, initially imposed formidable barriers to the acquisition of artifact-free images that could depict the cardiac anatomy with sufficient detail. It has taken well over a decade for cardiac MRI to mature to the point where it is currently being applied in routine fashion in the clinical setting. Therefore, in the future, other cardiac imaging modalities such as ultrasound imaging and nuclear imaging may be partially eclipsed by MRI for selected applications.

This chapter provides a condensed review of the basic principles of MRI and introduces the reader to some of the concepts and terminology necessary to understand the application of MRI to the heart. We then proceed to describe a wide range of cardiac applications of MRI, both in vivo and ex vivo, which should interest the biomedical engineer. While the capabilities of cardiac MRI are quite extensive, our choice of topics for this chapter is rather judicious, as cardiac MRI has evolved to the point where entire books are published on the subject.

C.M. Swingen (✉)
University of Minnesota, Medicine Cardiology Office, MMC 508, 420 Delaware St. SE, Minneapolis, MN 55455, USA
e-mail: swing001@umn.edu

P.A. Iaizzo (ed.), *Handbook of Cardiac Anatomy, Physiology, and Devices*, DOI 10.1007/978-1-60327-372-5_22,
© Springer Science+Business Media, LLC 2009

22.2 Overview of MRI

Magnetic resonance imaging works using the principle of nuclear magnetic resonance. That is, in the presence of a strong magnetic field (typically 1.5–3 tesla range for clinical systems), protons in the body are stimulated to emit radio waves. These radio waves are detected by an antenna, or coil, placed around the body region of interest and the signals are decomposed to reconstruct an image. We present a short summary of the basic concepts here and refer the reader to the overall literature for an in-depth examination.

22.2.1 Resonance

Inside the MRI scanner protons in the body align with the magnetic fields, similar to what happens to a compass needle placed in a magnetic field. These magnetic dipoles, if tipped away from the direction of the magnetic field, will precess about the direction of the static magnetic field (Fig. 22.1). This precession has a rotation frequency, ν_L, that is directly proportional to the magnetic field strength, B_0. For hydrogen nuclei, the precession frequency varies with field strength as

$$\nu_L = 42.6 [\text{MHz/tesla}] \cdot B_0 [\text{tesla}].$$

The precession frequency is also known as the "Larmor frequency." Tipping a nuclear magnetic moment away from the direction of the z-axis (B_0 direction) can be accomplished by applying an oscillating magnetic field, denoted by B_1, in a direction perpendicular to B_0. The radio frequency transmitter should be tuned to a frequency close to the Larmor frequency to elicit a resonant excitation. After a radio frequency excitation pulse, the static magnetic field, B_0, causes precession of the transverse magnetization component, which can be detected with an external coil as shown in Fig. 22.2. It is customary to refer to the magnetic fields that are oscillating at radio frequencies and turned on for brief durations as "radio frequency pulses." A pulse that tips the magnetic moment from the z-axis into the x–y plane is referred to as a "90° radio frequency pulse;" a pulse that inverts the orientation of the magnetic moment is called a "180° or inversion pulse." In general, the degree to which the spins are tipped into the transverse (x–y) plane is referred to as the "flip angle."

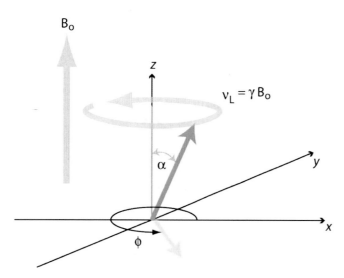

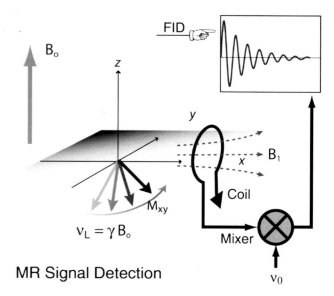

MR Signal Detection

Fig. 22.1 A single magnetic dipole moment in a static magnetic field of strength, B_0. It is customary to align the z-axis of a rectangular coordinate system with the direction of the externally applied static magnetic field, B_0. In this example, the magnetic moment, initially aligned with the applied magnetic field, was tipped away from the z direction by an angle α through application of an oscillating magnetic field (not shown). The oscillating magnetic field is kept on only for the time necessary to tip the magnetic dipole moment by a certain angle, α in this example. After turning the oscillating magnetic field off, the magnetic dipole moment precesses about the B_0 direction at a frequency, $\nu_L = \gamma \cdot B_0$, where γ is a constant, the gyromagnetic ratio, and represents a property of the nucleus. For ^{1}H nuclei, γ equals 42.6 MHz/tesla. The angle φ denotes the phase angle of the magnetization component in the x–y plane, orthogonal to the direction of B_0

Fig. 22.2 The transverse magnetization component of a nuclear dipole precesses at the Larmor frequency and produces an oscillating magnetic flux density that can be detected with a wire loop that is part of a resonant circuit. The induced voltage is amplified and mixed with the signal of an oscillator. The low-frequency component from the mixer is a free induction decay with frequency, $\nu_L - \nu_0$. Often two coils, oriented perpendicular to each other, are used to detect the signal from the M_x and M_y components of the transverse magnetization, which are in quadrature, i.e., they have a relative phase difference of 90°. By detection of the quadrature components, it is possible to determine the sign of the difference $\nu_L - \nu_0$, and by combination of the two signals, after phase shifting one by 90°, one improves the signal to noise by a factor of $\sqrt{2}$. FID = free induction decay; MR = magnetic resonance

Immediately after a radio frequency excitation, individual magnetic moments that were tipped into the transverse plane become in phase, i.e., they have the same phase angle. If all magnetic moments were to precess at exactly the same Larmor frequency, this phase coherence would persist. Residual magnetic field inhomogeneities, magnetic dipole interactions between neighboring nuclei, molecule-specific shifts of the precession frequency, and other factors produce a distribution of Larmor frequencies. The frequency shifts relative to a reference frequency can be tissue specific, as in the case of ^{1}H nuclei in fatty tissue. The spread of Larmor frequencies results in a slow loss of phase coherence of the transverse magnetization, i.e., the sum of all transverse magnetization components decays with time. The decay following a radio frequency excitation is called "free induction decay," and often has the shape of an exponential function with an exponential time constant denoted as T2, roughly on the order of ~0.1 to ~10^2 ms for ^{1}H nuclei in biological systems. In the presence of field inhomogeneities and other factors that cause a spread of Larmor frequencies, the transverse magnetization decay is further shortened. To distinguish the latter situation, one introduces a time constant, T2*, that is characteristic of the exponential decay of the transverse magnetization in "heterogenous" environments. It follows that T2* is always shorter than T2.

After any radio frequency excitation that tips the magnetization vectors away from the direction of the applied static magnetic field, B_0, the nuclear spins will, over time, realign themselves with the magnetic field to reach the same alignment as before the radio frequency excitation. This time constant is denoted as T1.

22.2.2 The Echo

A loss of phase coherence due to any spread in Larmor frequencies, for example, due to magnetic field inhomogeneities, can be (at least partially) reversed by applying a 180° pulse that flips the magnetization in the x–y plane such that the faster precessing spins now lag behind and the more slowly precessing spins are ahead, compared to spins precessing at the mean Larmor frequency. Once the echo amplitude peaks, the spread of Larmor frequencies again causes a loss of phase coherence. Multiple 180° pulses can be applied to repeatedly reverse the loss of phase coherence and thereby produce a train of spin echoes, referred to as "fast spin echo imaging." The decay of the spin echo amplitudes is governed by the decay constant T2, while a free induction decays with a characteristic time constant T2*, with T2* < T2. Importantly, for cardiac imaging applications, it is useful to note that the spin echo (and spin echo trains in particular)

provides a method to attenuate the signal from flowing blood, while obtaining "normal" spin echoes from stationary or slow-moving tissue.

Spin echoes provide an effective means of refocusing the transverse magnetization for optimal MR signal detection. A similar, but nevertheless different, type of echo-like effect can be achieved by applying two magnetic field gradient pulses of opposite polarity instead of a 180° radio frequency pulse. The first gradient pulse causes a rapid dephasing of the transverse magnetization; the second gradient pulse, of opposite polarity, can reverse this effect. An echo-type signal is observed and peaks at the point where the phase wrap produced by the first pulse is cancelled. This type of echo is called a "gradient echo."

A train of gradient echoes can be created by consecutive pairs of dephasing and rephasing gradient waveforms. The acquisition of multiple-phase-encoded gradient echoes after a single radio frequency excitation is useful for very rapid image acquisition, but is limited by the T2* decay of the signal.

A variation of the gradient echo technique that reestablishes phase coherence to the best possible degree before application of the next radio frequency excitation (i.e., the next phase-encoding step) can be used to produce a steady state. This allows the application of radio frequency pulses with fairly large flip angles. Instead of relying on T1 relaxation to return the magnetization from the transverse plane to the B_0 direction, the magnetization is toggled back and forth by the radio frequency pulses between the z-axis and the transverse plane. The attainable signal-to-noise ratio with this approach is significantly higher than with "conventional" gradient echo imaging. This type of gradient echo imaging is referred to in the literature by various acronyms—"steady-state free precession imaging," "TrueFISP," or "balanced fast field echo imaging." In particular, for cardiac cine studies, this technique has led to a marked improvement of image quality. Steady-state free precession (SSFP) works best with very short repetition times that, in turn, impose high demands on the gradient system of the MR scanner in terms of ramping gradients up and down.

22.2.3 Image Contrast

Biological tissues and blood have approximately the same density of ^{1}H nuclei, and spin-density images show poor contrast to differentiate, e.g., tissue from blood or fat from muscle. One of the most appealing aspects of MRI is the ability to manipulate the image contrast based on differences in the T1 or T2 relaxation times. For a gradient echo sequence, the T1 weighting is determined by the combination of flip angle and repetition time. Reducing repetition time or increasing the flip angle increases the T1 weighting in the image.

The T2* weighting of a gradient echo image is controlled by the time delay between the radio frequency pulse and the center of the readout window, i.e., the echo time TE. The T2 weighting of the spin echo signal is similarly determined by the echo time. In a fast spin echo sequence, one can use multiple echoes to read out the signal with different phase encodings for each echo. Controlling the T1 weighting through adjustment of repetition time and the flip angle imposes some limits that can be circumvented by applying an inversion pulse before the image acquisition and performing the image acquisition as rapidly as possible. The time between the inversion pulse and the start of the image acquisition controls the T1 contrast in this case. The image acquisition after the magnetization inversion is typically performed with a gradient echo sequence that uses small flip angles, i.e., the T1 contrast is controlled by the prepulse and the delay after the prepulse, instead of the repetition time and the flip angle, α, of the gradient echo image acquisition. Gradient echo imaging with a magnetization preparation in the form of a 180° or 90° radio frequency pulse is often the method of choice to acquire rapid T1-weighted images of the heart.

MR contrast agents, such as gadolinium, provide a further means for controlling the image contrast by injecting a compound with paramagnetic ions that reduce the T1 of blood and tissue permeated by the agent. The local T1 reduction depends on: (1) delivery of contrast agent to the tissue region through the blood vessels; (2) the degree to which the contrast agent molecules can cross barriers such as the capillary barrier; and (3) the distribution volume of the contrast agent within the tissue. The contrast seen after injection of such an agent can be used to determine pathology, such as the breakdown of the cardiac cell membranes and/or an above-normal concentration of contrast agent in infarcted myocardium.

22.3 Cardiac MR Techniques and Applications

22.3.1 Cardiac Morphology

The accurate depiction of cardiac morphology is important in most imaging applications. Numerous MR techniques have been developed and they are generally categorized based on the appearance of the intracardiac blood in the image, as either "black-blood" or "bright-blood" techniques.

"Spin echo" (SE) was the first sequence used for the evaluation of cardiac morphology; however, it was not until the advent of ECG gating that SE imaging became substantially more important by reducing motion artifacts associated with the beating heart. SE images are called "black-blood" images due to the signal void created by flowing blood, which provides very good contrast between the myocardium and the blood. Slower moving blood, particularly adjacent to the ventricular walls, however, can cause the blood signal to appear brighter, effectively reducing the quality of the image. So, presaturating with a radio frequency pulse and reducing the echo time (TE) is used to minimize the blood signal and increase the contrast in the image [1]. Although widely available, SE imaging is limited due to its poor temporal resolution and susceptibility to respiratory and other motion artifacts. Nevertheless, these problems have been overcome through the development of sequences with shorter acquisition times, so-called fast (or turbo) SE pulse sequences. Although soft tissue contrast is not as optimal, these sequences have become the frontline sequence for depiction of cardiac morphology (Fig. 22.3).

22.3.2 Global Cardiac Function

Global and regional assessments of ventricular function with MRI are very well established and have been shown

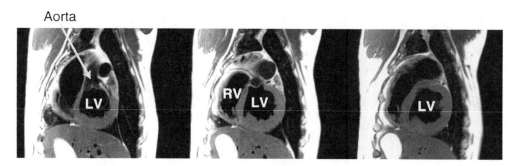

Fig. 22.3 Cardiac anatomy of a canine heart imaged with a T2-weighted fast spin echo sequence and in-plane resolution of 1.2 mm. Cardiac structures such as the left ventricle (LV), right ventricle (RV), and aorta are labeled. The signal from blood in the ventricular cavities was nulled by a magnetization preparation consisting of radio frequency inversion pulses. Furthermore, the use of an echo train (with seven spin echoes in this case) and a long effective echo time also causes attenuation of the signal from moving blood. These so-called black-blood imaging techniques are very useful for anatomical imaging to avoid image artifacts from flowing blood

to be accurate and reproducible compared with other imaging modalities for the calculation of volumes, masses, and derived parameters such as stroke volume and ejection fraction [2, 3]. Thus, it is now considered the gold standard for the evaluation of cardiac function and mass in numerous studies comparing different imaging modalities [4].

Cine loops are acquired to follow the changes in ventricular dimensions over the entire cardiac cycle and thus to assess cardiac function. The acquisition of each image in the cine loop is broken up into several "segments," and the image segments are acquired over consecutive heartbeats, as shown in Fig. 22.4. The acquisition of such image segments for each cardiac phase is subsequently synchronized with the heart cycle by gating of the encoding steps with the patient's electrocardiogram. This technique works well as long as the subject has a regular heartbeat. The final result of the segmented acquisition is a series of images, one for each phase of the cardiac cycle. These images can be played as a cine loop, e.g., to

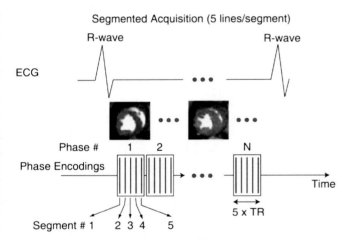

Segmented Acquisition (5 lines/segment)

Fig. 22.4 Illustration of the principle of segmented acquisitions of data, as used for imaging multiple phases of the cardiac cycle in ventricular function studies. The image acquisition is synchronized to the cardiac cycle by triggering of the pulse sequence with the R-wave on the ECG. The total number of phase encodings is split into five groups or segments in this example. The same five phase encodings are performed during each phase of one cardiac cycle. During the next R-to-R interval, five other phase encodings are performed for each cardiac phase. The R-wave-triggered acquisition of phase encodings is repeated k number of times to obtain a total of $k5$ phase encodings. The temporal extent of each cardiac phase is shown in the diagram by the boxes that contain the symbolic representations of the phase-encoded lines as vertical lines. The temporal resolution (TR) of the resulting cine loop is determined by the number of lines per segment (five in this example) and the repetition time for each phase-encoding step. Typical resolutions are on the order of 40–50 ms for resting heart rates and higher during inotropic stimulation of the patient's heart. The image acquisition is performed while the patient holds his/her breath. In this example the required duration of the breath hold would be k heartbeats, with k typically on the order of 10–20, depending on the heart rate

assess ventricular function. To increase the sharpness of the quality of images, clinicians ask patients to hold their breath during image acquisition. The segmented data acquisition approach always involves a tradeoff between temporal resolution (i.e., number of frames covering one R-to-R interval) and spatial resolution, as the image acquisition needs to be performed within a time short enough to allow for suspended breathing.

Typically, for the measurement of global cardiac function, "bright-blood cine MRI" is performed in multiple short-axis views, covering the heart from base to apex, using a multiphase, segmented k-space, "gradient echo" (GRE) sequence [5–7]. Yet, to date, GRE studies have suffered due to saturation effects in areas of low blood velocity, causing reduced contrast between blood and myocardium within the ventricular cavity [8]. In general, this problem causes difficulties in detection of the endocardial border, most dramatically in long-axis views of the heart where there is very minimal motion of blood through the imaging plane, as the majority of blood is moving within the image plane in these views as shown in Fig. 22.5A. Such problems associated with GRE cine imaging have recently been minimized with the advent of SSFP sequences (Fig. 22.5).

Although the concept of SSFP imaging has been described in the literature for many years, only recently has MR hardware developed to the point that these techniques have become practical and available on clinical scanners (e.g., those from multiple vendors) [9, 10]. Steady-state free precession sequences have dramatically improved contrast to noise, shortened acquisition times, and increased both spatial and temporal resolutions in comparison with previous GRE techniques [2, 11, 12]. These improvements have enhanced the detection of the epicardial and endocardial surfaces (delineation of trabeculation and papillary muscle), both manually and with automated detection schemes, resulting in improved accuracy and reproducibility for the quantification of cardiac mass and volumes [13, 14]. Scan times have been reduced as well, such that SSFP sequences for an entire 3D data set covering the heart can be acquired within a single breath-hold.

Steady-state free precession techniques are also employed in the emerging area of real-time MR imaging. Recently, real-time imaging techniques have been developed and improved such that they will be employed in future cardiac function studies, as well as in the emerging field of interventional imaging with MRI. These real-time sequences continuously acquire images of the heart with sufficiently high temporal resolution similar to fluoroscopy [15] without the need for ECG triggering or breath-holding, therefore making it possible to image patients with severe arrhythmias or heart disease. In the past,

Fig. 22.5 Comparison of end-diastolic long-axis views acquired with a segmented gradient echo sequence (**A**) and a steady-state free precession (SSFP) sequence (**B**). The SSFP technique provides significantly higher contrast to noise between intraventricular blood and myocardium, resulting in improved endocardial border definition throughout the cardiac cycle, as compared with the older gradient echo sequence

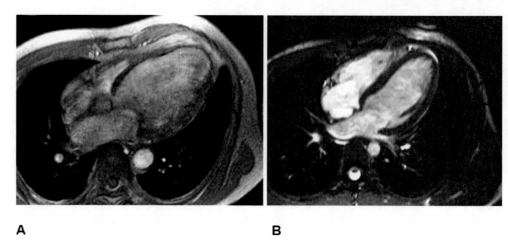

A   B

these were difficult requirements to fulfill with segmented k-space GRE or SSFP sequences. Furthermore, newly developed sequences implementing image reconstruction techniques with sensitivity encoding (SENSE) and simultaneous acquisition of spatial harmonics (SMASH) have reported imaging temporal resolutions down to 13 ms with a spatial resolution of 4.1 mm [16].

22.3.3 Regional Myocardial Function

Ventricular volumes and derived parameters such as stroke volume and ejection fraction are the most commonly used variables for the assessment of systolic function in the clinical setting; however, they have associated limitations related to the measurement of contractile properties of the heart. Furthermore, these descriptors of cardiac performance do not take into consideration the importance of regional contractile dysfunction, the degree and extent of which are important prognostic factors with ischemic heart disease, and/or following myocardial infarction [17–19]. It is generally accepted that quantitative estimates of wall motion and relative changes in wall thickening (expressed as percentage (%) of end-diastolic wall thickness) are useful for measuring regional function and are also more precise than the subjective visual wall motion scoring system which is commonly used in the clinic today [20, 21]. Wall motion changes and thickening are usually measured along the length of a centerline between the segmented endocardial and epicardial borders of the heart. They are further divided into myocardial segments of equal circumferential extent that are positioned relative to the location of an anatomical landmark such as the anterior–septal junction of the left ventricle and right ventricle. Dynamic changes in wall thickening can be considered as the radial

component of myocardial strain, defined as the percent change in dimension from a resting state. Such strain analyses have proven very useful for the assessment of regional contractile function in both animals and human patients [22–24].

Circumferential shortening and radial thickening are two components of myocardial strain typically assessed by MRI tagging [25–29]. This approach has a higher sensitivity to the identification of noncontracting regions of the myocardium compared to "conventional" cine MRI. As such, cine imaging of the heart can be combined with a series of magnetization preparation pulses that null the longitudinal magnetization along thin parallel stripes in the slice plane. The stripes or tags appear as black lines on the MR images and can be applied in two directions in a single slice, forming a grid pattern. This grid pattern is created immediately after the R-wave of the EKG and before acquisition of the segmented phase encodings (Fig. 22.4). The grid tags visible in the resulting images are "imbedded" in the tissue and are therefore distorted if any myocardial motion occurs. Thus, intramyocardial displacements and myocardial strain can be tracked through monitoring visible motion and deformation of the tag lines, respectively. Figure 22.6 shows an example of a myocardial grid pattern laid down at end-diastole and, in a second frame, the same pattern is recorded at end-systole with evident distortion of the tag lines due to myocardial contraction. The tag lines, created right after the R-wave, tend to fade during the cardiac cycle due to T1 relaxation, but for normal resting heart rates (e.g., 60–70 beats/min) the tag lines can persist long enough to allow visualization of cardiac motion over nearly the entire R-to-R interval. Importantly, tag lines in the ventricular blood pool disappear very quickly because of the rapid motion and mixing of blood in the ventricle; this effect is then useful for clearly defining the endocardial borders.

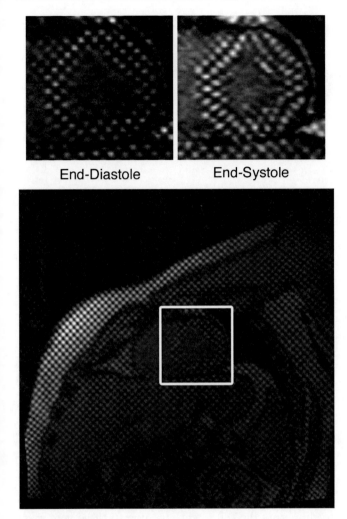

End-Diastole   End-Systole

Fig. 22.6 Images with spatial modulation of magnetization in the form of vertical and horizontal stripes in a human volunteer. The grid-tag lines spaced 6 mm apart were created immediately after the R-wave of the ECG. The *upper left* panel shows a magnified view of the heart during this initial phase. A second image is shown on the *upper right* for an end-systolic phase, with the distortion of the tag lines due to cardiac contraction clearly apparent. The tagging technique is equivalent to the implantation of intramyocardial markers. Tracking of the tag lines over the cardiac cycle allows determination of myocardial strains and has been shown to provide a sensitive method for assessing regional wall motion abnormalities

22.3.4 Myocardial Perfusion

Myocardial blood flow is assessed using very rapid MR imaging of the heart during the first passage of an administered contrast agent through the heart. T1 changes in the myocardium are directly proportional to the contrast agent concentration in the blood or tissue [30, 31], so that through the use of T1-weighted imaging techniques, myocardial territories affected by a coronary artery lesion can be both qualitatively and quantitatively evaluated. Furthermore, the myocardial territory affected by a coronary artery lesion may or may not show a perfusion deficit under resting conditions; however, during an imposed pharmacological stress, a stenotic vessel cannot respond (dilate) like a healthy vessel resulting in "vascular steal," a phenomenon in which increased blood flow to the myocardium is supplied by nonstenotic vessels [32]. Consequently, the relative blood flow is reduced through stenotic vessels resulting in a detectable perfusion deficit in the images; as such, both areas of reversible and nonreversible (scar) defects can be represented [33].

First pass perfusion imaging is typically performed using multislice fast gradient echo imaging, with saturation-recovery magnetization preparation obtained during the rapid administration (7 ml/s) of a small contrast agent dose (approximately 0.04 mmol/kg for the extracellular gadolinium agent Gd-DTPA). A saturation-recovery magnetization preparation consists of a nonslice selective 90° radio frequency pulse, followed by a gradient crusher pulse designed to dephase the transverse component of the magnetization [34]. This preparation drives the magnetization into a well-defined state, permitting the acquisition of a T1-weighted GRE signal that is independent of the properties of any previous relaxation delay, thus preventing fluctuations in the image signal intensities due to variations in the heart rate or ECG trace. Nevertheless, imaging is typically performed throughout the duration of 40–50 heartbeats to adequately capture the first pass of the injected contrast agent through the heart. With currently employed clinical 1.5 tesla MRI scanners (with state-of-the-art gradient coils and amplifiers producing gradient field amplitudes of 20–40 mtesla/m with slew rates up to 150 mtesla/m/s), this imaging can be done in approximately three to four slices for every heartbeat, with an in-plane image resolution of 2 mm or better.

Qualitative analyses of perfusion studies can be made by viewing the sequence of images as a movie loop and visually grading the rate of contrast enhancement in myocardial segments. However, qualitative assessments are highly observer dependent and thus are also subjective to misinterpretation based on image artifacts or variations in the image brightness due to the inhomogeneous detection of the MR signal by the surface coils. Therefore, in the future, a more quantitative technique based on the time course of signal intensity in the different myocardial segments of interest can provide an objective and robust method of analysis (Fig. 22.7).

22.3.5 Myocardial Viability

The ability to distinguish nonviable myocardium is of critical importance in the management of patients with

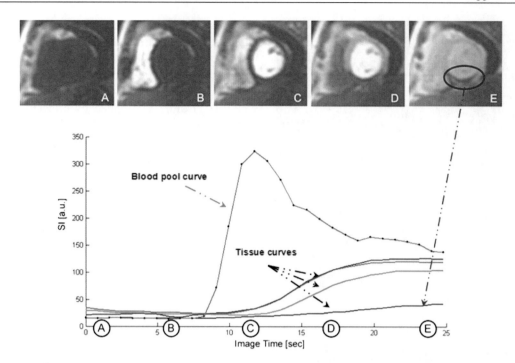

Fig. 22.7 A sample of images acquired using a fast T1-weighted gradient echo sequence during a bolus injection of 0.04 mmol/kg of the extracellular contrast agent Gd-DTPA is shown, with the resulting signal intensity curves for the left ventricular blood pool and several myocardial segments below. The first image in the series (**A**) shows a short-axis image of the heart prior to injection of the contrast agent. Following injection, the contrast agent quickly enters the right ventricle (**B**) and left ventricle (**C**) and then passes through the coronary and microcirculation (**D**, **E**) causing signal enhancement throughout the myocardium. This example shows a clear perfusion defect in the inferior wall of the left ventricle which can be seen in images **D** and **E** (*circled*) and also the corresponding tissue curve immediately following the first pass of the contrast through the left ventricle

both acute and chronic coronary artery disease syndromes; yet, this is complicated by the presence of both reversibly damaged and infarcted myocardium. Until very recently, thallium single proton emission computed tomography (SPECT) and positron emission tomography (PET) were the primary tools for evaluation of myocardial viability. However, with the development of delayed contrast-enhanced MRI (ce-MRI), the cardiac MRI method has quite dramatically and rapidly ascended into the forefront of viability imaging [35, 36]. In general, this technique has been shown to identify irreversibly damaged myocardium in both acute and chronic settings following a myocardial infarction and, in tandem with cine imaging, can be used to consistently predict reversibly damaged tissue that may benefit from revascularization and/or other therapies [37, 38]. Furthermore, with the availability of substantially higher spatial resolution than nuclear techniques, ce-MRI can detail the transmural extent of irreversibly damaged tissue and detect both small and large subendocardial defects not identified by either SPECT or PET [39, 40].

So-called delayed ce-MRI is performed following the intravenous administration of a gadolinium-chelate contrast agent; typical dosages for imaging viability are on the order of 0.1–0.2 mmol/kg. The contrast agents more readily cross the cell membrane due to the severe myocardial injury and loss of viability [33, 35, 41, 42]. After an appropriate delay (approximately 10–15 min), the contrast agent achieves approximate distribution equilibrium, and loss of functional viability and subsequent leakage of contrast agent result in T1-weighted signal enhancement because the distribution volume of the contrast agent is larger in the injured tissue compared to normal. Such imaging is typically performed under resting conditions using a breath-hold "inversion recovery" prepared and T1-weighted segmented GRE sequence. The appropriate inversion delay time following the inversion pulse (approximately 250 ms or less) results in signal nulling of viable myocardium. Note that, for the best results, appropriate inversion delay times are iteratively chosen for each patient. This results in images where the normal viable myocardium is dark, and nonviable, fibrotic, or scarred tissue has dramatically increased (hyperenhanced) signal intensity (Fig. 22.8). Typically, one or two signal averages are used with an in-plane image resolution of approximately 1.5 mm; this approach as a 2D sequence requires multiple breath-holds to encompass the left ventricle and can be typically accomplished in less than

Fig. 22.8 Example of an initial and follow-up MRI exam comparing the region of infarction (*arrows*) with wall thickness and contractility. The acute study at 2 days (*top*) shows evidence of microvascular obstruction within the infarct and reduced wall thickening in the anterior region, shown here by long-axis cine images. During the 3-month study (*bottom*), there is no longer a sign of microvascular obstruction within the infarct territory, diastolic wall thickness has decreased, and contractility has improved in regions adjacent to the infarcted territory

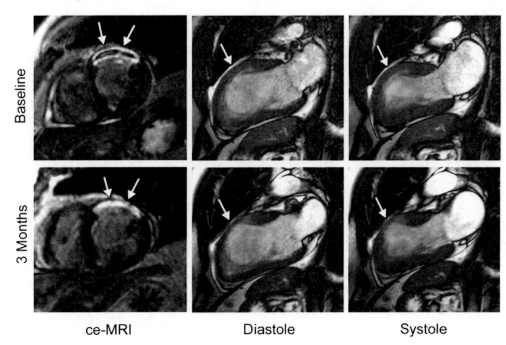

ce-MRI   Diastole   Systole

10 min. In addition, 3D approaches can also be used that cover the entire ventricle in a single, yet longer, breath-hold with comparable, but not as good, image quality.

While the delayed ce-MRI sequence is the most widely accepted approach for viability imaging with MRI, there are other less popular techniques that should be mentioned (e.g., imaging with the use of a manganese-based contrast agent). Manganese is a Ca^{2+} analog that is actively taken up by viable cells, thus in obtaining T1-weighted images, viable tissue is enhanced (bright) while nonviable tissue remains dark [43]. Manganese contrast agents are not currently being used in clinical cardiac imaging; however, this may provide an effective alternative method in the near future. MRI imaging of sodium or potassium are also effective methods with potential for imaging viability, but their use remains strictly a research tool due to the very limited availability of multifrequency MRI scanners for clinical use [44].

22.3.6 Blood Flow Velocity

A recorded MR signal can be represented in terms of a magnitude and a phase component. As such, MRI images can be analyzed to elicit the spatial variations of the signal magnitudes, but it is also possible to create maps showing the spatial variations of the signal phases. Furthermore, it has been shown that the phase of the signal is sensitive to the velocity of tissue or blood. The so-called phase contrast MRI technique uses the phases of the signals to

measure relative velocities. For an in-depth discussion of these methodologies, we refer the reader to the literature. Yet, an example of a phase contrast flow velocity measurement in an aorta is shown in Fig. 22.9, which has been used to calculate pulse wave velocities for measuring vessel stiffness [45].

22.3.7 Fiber Structure

22.3.7.1 Importance of Myofiber Orientation

The analysis of myocardial microstructure continues to be considered an important factor in better understanding underlying pathologies and/or associated arrhythmias. This is due to the fact that structural fiber arrangement is modified over the time course of various cardiomyopathies. In the healthy heart, it is generally accepted that cardiac muscle fibers or myofibers are arranged as counter-wound helices encircling the ventricular cavities and where fiber orientation is a function of their transmural location [46–48]. Furthermore, myofibers are predominantly organized in the base-apex direction at the epicardial and endocardial surfaces and rotate to a circumferential direction in the midwall. This counter-wound helical structure is considered to be responsible for the torsional or wringing motion of the left ventricle that serves three main mechanical functions: (1) equalizing myofiber strain and workload; (2) optimizing the volume of blood ejected during systole (stroke volume); and (3) storing torsional energy in the intracellular and

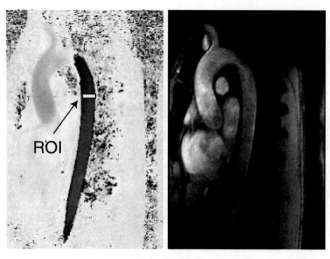

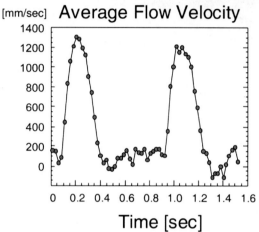

Fig. 22.9 Phase contrast imaging of the aorta in a human volunteer. Both the magnitude and phase images are shown. Images were acquired for 70 cardiac phases, covering approximately 2.5 heartbeats. A region of interest (*white box*) was placed on the phase images in the thoracic aorta to determine the variation of flow velocity in the vertical direction of the image plane. The variation of the velocity is shown in the graph. ROI = region of interest

extracellular matrices and, when released, increasing ventricular filling during diastole [49–56]. Therefore, cardiac fiber orientation can also be considered as a primary determinant of ventricular pump function.

22.3.7.2 Quantifying Fiber Structure with Diffusion Tensor MRI

More recently, "diffusion tensor" MRI (DTMRI) has been developed and employed as a nondestructive means to quantify 3D ventricular fiber orientation [46, 57–60]. The underlying principle in determining cardiac fiber orientation by DTMRI is that the fastest direction of water diffusion corresponds to the local myofiber orientation. Therefore, by obtaining a series of diffusion-weighted

images, the effective diffusion tensor of water in the myocardium can be estimated using a relationship between the measured echo attenuation in each imaging voxel and the applied diffusion-sensitizing gradient [61]. As such, diffusion-weighted pulse sequences are designed such that molecular displacements in the direction of the applied diffusion-sensitizing gradients will attenuate the echo signal, thus enabling the estimation of water diffusivity in a given direction. The strength of the diffusion weighting or b-value usually ranges from 500 to 1500 s/mm^2 in cardiac DTMRI. To date, the diffusion tensor, which is typically a symmetric 3×3 second rank tensor, is determined for each imaging voxel and represents the net 3D diffusion in the tissue. In order to determine the required six independent parameters of the diffusion tensor, at least seven images must be obtained for a given slice—six diffusion-weighted images applied in six noncolinear directions and one diffusion-independent image. However, it is also common today to estimate the diffusion tensor by applying multiple diffusion weightings in 12–16 directions. Nevertheless, ventricular fiber orientation can be obtained with DTMRI due to the anisotropic nature of water diffusion in the myocardium [62]. The fastest direction of diffusion or primary eigenvector of diffusion has been validated to coincide with the local longitudinal myofiber orientation, as water diffusion in the cross fiber directions is restricted by the cellular borders and laminar sheets in the myocardium [63, 64]. Note that the secondary and tertiary eigenvectors of diffusion correlate with the laminar sheet direction and sheet normal, respectively [58, 65, 66].

From a research perspective, it is also interesting to note that DTMRI can be used to obtain fiber orientation both in vivo and ex vivo [67, 68]. Currently, cardiac DTMRI is not a clinically employed cardiac MR protocol, as this imaging technique does not contribute to the diagnosis of cardiomyopathies. However, in concert with myocardial tagging, in vivo DTMRI does provide valuable insights into the myofiber structure–function relationship in the ventricles in both normal and diseased states. In general, the spatial resolution of diffusion imaging is dependent on the diffusion-sensitizing pulse sequence and magnetic strength of the scanner. For example, for in vivo diffusion imaging of large mammalian hearts in a 1.5 tesla magnetic field, a spatial resolution of approximately $3 \times 3 \times 3$ mm^3 can be expected [69]. For ex vivo diffusion imaging with high-field MRI scanners (3–9.4 tesla), a spatial resolution less than $1 \times 1 \times 1$ mm^3 can easily be obtained. An example of ex vivo DTMRI of a freshly cardioplegged and isolated human heart is shown in Fig. 22.10. The raw diffusion images are shown along with the fiber orientation projected into the imaging plane as determined by the primary eigenvector of diffusion for a midventricular slice.

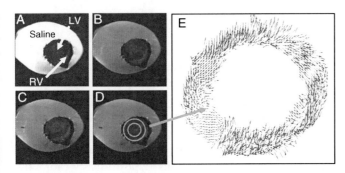

Fig. 22.10 Diffusion tensor MRI of a freshly excised normal human heart. The unfixed heart was submerged in saline and all air was removed prior to imaging. For the determination of cardiac fiber orientation, six diffusion-weighted images were acquired with one nondiffusion-weighted image (**A**) at the midventricular level. Three diffusion-weighted images are shown (**B, C, D**) acquired with diffusion gradients applied in three orthogonal directions. The left ventricular fiber orientation is projected onto the imaging plane (**E**) as determined by the primary eigenvector of diffusion or direction of fastest diffusion. Imaging parameters were as follows: field of view = 180×180 mm^2, matrix = 196×196, in-plane spatial resolution = 0.9×0.9 mm^2, b-value = 1000 s/mm^2; the slice thickness was 3 mm. LV = left ventricle; RV = right ventricle

22.3.7.3 Pathological Changes in Fiber Structure

It was recently reported that by using cardiac DTMRI in conjunction with phase contrast strain-rate imaging, Tseng et al. were able to determine that a state of fiber disarray exists in hypertrophic cardiomyopathy, which results in a disordered pattern of principle myocardial shortening. In the same study, these investigators observed that a positive correlation exists between fiber disarray and myocardial hypokinesis [69]. Additionally, several studies have attempted to quantify cardiac fiber architectural remodeling after the occurrence of myocardial infarction [70, 71]. In these reports, fiber disarrays and increases in diffusivity were evident in the infarcted regions; this was considered to be consistent with abnormal wall motion and/or cell death.

22.4 MRI and Biomedical Devices

22.4.1 Real-Time Imaging and Cardiovascular Interventions

To date, x-ray-based fluoroscopic techniques have been the gold standard for most invasive diagnostic and/or therapeutic applications relative to the heart. However, with the advent of ultrafast MRI and the development of MRI-compatible catheters and guidewires, the goal of achieving real-time guidance by MRI for cardiovascular interventions is emerging as a new alternative [72]. More specifically, the use of MRI for guided interventions

would minimize or even eliminate reliance on ionizing radiation and iodinated contrast agents, an advantage particularly for pediatric patients. To date, continuous improvements of MRI techniques and MRI scanner hardware have rendered it feasible to achieve the relative clinical fluoroscopic image rates of 5–15 images/s [73]. Thus, it is considered highly probable to use MRI for guiding interventional cardiovascular procedures, such as coronary catheterization [74] and cell or gene therapy delivery [15], with close to real-time image refresh rates. Initial interventional studies with MRI guidance have demonstrated the advantages of MRI, including: (1) the ability to image arbitrarily oriented cross-sections; (2) interactive steering of the image plane; and (3) excellent soft tissue contrast for the detection and visualization of lesions [75].

Several other technical advances have also been considered as crucial for advancing the possibility of performing interventional procedures under MRI guidance, including: (1) development of 1.5 tesla magnets with short bores that allow access to the groin area for catheter-based procedures; (2) LCD monitors that can be exposed to high magnetic fields to allow the operator to perform an intervention and control MRI scan parameters from a position right next to the magnet; and (3) development of catheter-based MRI antennae for localized intravascular signal reception and high-resolution imaging [76].

For MRI-guided cardiac interventions, one of the basic requirements is to visualize and track the catheters and devices used in the therapies while they are manipulated through the heart and vascular spaces [77]. In general, catheter-tracking techniques can be divided into two categories—active and passive. Active tracking of catheters and devices requires the instrument to receive or send a signal in order to identify its relative location. For example, a receiving coil can be incorporated into the device and thus connected to the scanner such that the position can be located based on the frequency of the received signal from the body coil. Passive tracking of catheters involves creating a signal void without interfering with the image quality of the tissue being imaged. This latter method can be achieved through the choices of materials incorporated into the catheter or device. For example, small amounts of titanium, gold, or copper can be deposited into the catheter tip in order to introduce a susceptibility artifact such that the tip of the catheter can be continuously tracked.

A recent development in the emerging field of MRI-guided cardiac interventions is the real-time delivery of transcatheter valves. Recently, McVeigh et al. demonstrated that a transcatheter bioprosthetic aortic valve could be delivered via a direct approach through the left ventricular apex in approximately 90 s with real-time interactive MRI guidance [78]. Importantly, immediately after the procedure, myocardial perfusion, blood flow through the valve, and ventricular function were assessed with MRI in order to verify proper placement of the valve. It is considered that this minimally invasive MRI-guided aortic valve replacement technique may prove to be a less morbid approach than conventional valve replacement surgeries, and thus may have added benefits for the very ill and/or elderly patient population.

To date, other reported MRI-guided cardiac interventions and applications include: (1) diagnostic cardiac catheterization; (2) electrophysiological recording/radio frequency ablation; (3) balloon dilation and stent placement; and (4) atrial septal defect closure [77]. For an in-depth discussion of the advantages and difficulties associated with these MRI-guided cardiac interventions, we refer the reader to the growing body of related literature (see also Chapters 29 and 33).

22.4.2 MRI Safety and Compatibility

Most currently used implantable devices contain metallic parts that would likely both seriously interfere with MR cardiac imaging and/or pose potential safety risks for the patient. More specifically, implanted devices with ferro-magnetic parts are considered a strict contraindication for cardiac MRI because of the potential associated hazards due to magnetic-induced movement, dislodgement, and/or heating effects. Although cardiac pacemakers are implanted in large numbers of patients, to date, there is no consensus whether or not pacemakers are MRI compatible or MRI safe. For example, the considered risks involved in scanning a patient with an implanted pacemaker include lead tip heating, which may damage the tissue resulting in a failure of the pacing pulse to capture the targeted tissue, and/or damage to the electrical circuitry inside the pacemaker. These risks, in turn, are also dependent on many variables including: (1) relative lead position; (2) pacemaker position; (3) manufacturer of the pacemaker; and/or (4) area of the body scanned. Despite these risks, it should be noted that case studies have been published in which patients with a cardiac pacemaker were scanned and no complications were observed [79]. In another example, Roka et al. used a 1.5 tesla MRI system to assist in finding the optimal left ventricular pacing site in a patient, based on myocardial viability during an upgrade to a biventricular pacing system [80]; they reported no malfunction in the pacemaker or changes in the relative pacing thresholds.

"MRI compatibility" can be quite simply defined as the property of a device not to interfere with imaging, e.g., by causing distortions of the magnetic field that cause signal loss. Note that a device may be MR compatible, but that does not necessarily mean it is "MR safe." The latter requires that the exposure to a strong static magnetic field, pulsing of the magnetic field gradients, and applications of radio frequency pulses do not cause any adverse effects to the patient. For example, the pulsing of the magnetic field gradients produces a changing magnetic flux that can induce current flow in lead wires which, in turn, may lead to tissue heating, and thus cell damage or death. Furthermore, the presence of metallic parts can also cause an inhomogeneous deposition of radio frequency power in the vicinity of the device, which could lead to broader radio frequency heating of tissue or blood. Therefore, to date, implanted cardiac pacemakers are a contraindication not only for MRI cardiac exams, but for MRI exams in general. It is noteworthy that one group of investigators reported that MRI imaging caused temperature elevations at pacing lead tips as high as 23.5°C at 0.5 tesla and 63.1°C at 1.5 tesla [81, 82]. As such, there has been some progress in the development of MRI safe cardiac pacemakers. Recently, one medical device manufacturer released an MRI safe pacing system for sale in Europe, and is seeking FDA approval for release in the United States (EnRhythm® MRI SureScan™ pacemaker and CapSureFix® MRI SureScan™ pacing leads, Medtronic, Inc., Minneapolis, MN). We can expect other medical device manufacturers to follow suit in the development of such devices in the future.

It is foreseen that a new set of MRI safety concerns may arise when such imaging is performed using intravascular coils [83, 84]. Such intravascular coils may, for example, be used to examine vulnerable plaque on vessel walls; localized heating in the vicinity of the coil could disrupt the plaque, thus causing catastrophic consequences. Note that heating strongly depends on the wavelength (MRI frequency), geometry of the body and the device, and placement of the body and device with respect to each other and within the MR system. On the other hand, one could also foresee potentially using this heating phenomenon to induce therapy itself (e.g., tumor ablation to lesion formation). For further information on MRI-compatible and MRI-safe biomedical devices and additional contraindications for cardiac MRI exams, we refer the reader to the growing body of literature on this topic.

22.4.3 Assessment of Biomedical Device Performance

Cardiac MRI also provides a unique opportunity to test, in vivo, the performance of implanted devices such as prosthetic heart valves and heart pacing devices (those that would be considered both MRI compatible and safe). For example, in patients with artificial aortic valves, the flow downstream from the implanted valve may be severely altered. These changes have been associated with an increased risk of thrombus formation and mechanical hemolysis. Therefore, the capabilities of MRI velocity mapping would be considered very useful for the noninvasive evaluation of the flow profiles in such patients with a mechanical valve prosthesis [85, 86]. For example, in one report, Botnar et al. found that peak flow velocity in the aorta was significantly higher in patients with a valvular prosthesis than in normal patients [87]. In that same study, the investigators also reported that diastolic mean flow was negative in patients after valve replacement, but not in controls. Furthermore, in instances where real-time MRI is used to guide the placement of a stented artificial valve, an assessment of the flow profile can be obtained immediately to determine the relative success of the implant procedure.

Interestingly, the usefulness of MRI for assessing the function of cardiac pacing devices has already been proven in experimental animal studies [88], although currently there exist hurdles for performing cardiac MRI on patients with such devices. For example, in our laboratory, we have quantified pacing-induced left ventricular dyssynchrony in swine paced from the right ventricular apex, a standard pacing lead implant site, using MR tissue

tagging. Figure 22.11 demonstrates that right ventricular apex pacing alters the mechanical activation pattern of the left ventricle, resulting in circumferential stretch in the lateral and posterior walls and regional variations in circumferential shortening in end-systole.

22.5 Quantitative Analysis of Cardiac MR

It is important to note that post-processing of cardiac MRI studies represents the stage at which the full potential of the cardiac MRI examination may be best realized. Postprocessing is comprised of two major steps: image postprocessing and data post-processing. The first step largely involves segmentation algorithms to delineate and extract features and structures of interest from the collected images. The second step consists mainly of applying mathematical and statistical methods to aid in a given diagnosis.

For many cardiac investigative protocols, the myocardium is the area of interest for analysis, so one needs to segment the myocardium from the rest of the image to extract further information, e.g., utilize contrast enhancement in a perfusion study or monitor systolic thickening of the wall for a MR cine study.

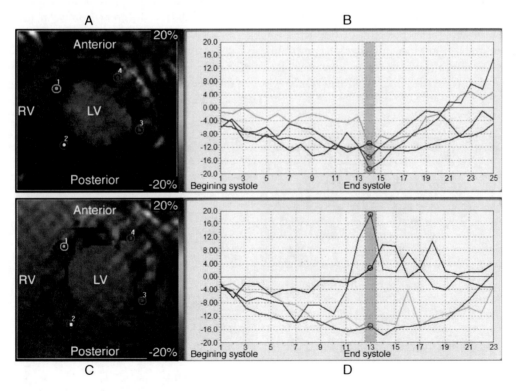

Fig. 22.11 Circumferential strain quantified by MR tissue tagging in a normal porcine heart (**A, B**) and after 6 weeks of cardiac pacing from the right ventricular apex in the same heart (**C, D**). Graphs (**B**) and (**D**) plot the circumferential strain values throughout the cardiac cycle prior to pacing and after 6 weeks of pacing at the specified probe locations in (**A**) and (**C**), respectively. Pacing from the right

ventricular apex caused regional disarray in cardiac strain in the left ventricle at end-systole (**C**) and throughout the cardiac cycle (**D**), in comparison to the same heart 6 weeks prior to the onset of pacing (**A, B**). Right ventricular apex pacing induces left ventricular dyssynchrony and results in poor left ventricular pump function. LV = left ventricle; RV = right ventricle

22.5.1 Ventricular Function

Quantitative analyses of relative ventricular function are also based on the segmentation of the myocardium. In general, this is achieved by drawing contours on the endocardial and epicardial borders of the myocardium (Fig. 22.12). In general, the ventricular volumes of interest are the end-diastolic and end-systolic volumes, as well as derived parameters such as the stroke volume and ejection fraction. Although ventricular volumes have been computed from differently orientated views of the heart, analyses of the short-axis views are most widely used in cardiac MRI due to their proven accuracy [89–92]. In the simplest case, myocardial segmentation is performed only for the images corresponding to the end-diastolic and end-systolic phases. The end-diastolic phase is defined as the phase containing the largest blood pool area in the left ventricle, whereas the end-systolic phase is identified as the image containing the smallest blood pool area (Fig. 22.13).

Once the end-diastolic and end-systolic phases are fixed, the contours are drawn in the images for the end-diastolic and end-systolic phases for all slices containing left ventricle. In images for a basal slice of the left ventricle, parts of the aorta and aortic valve may be visible. It should be noted that inclusion of contours above the mitral valve plane will significantly overestimate the values for myocardial mass and ventricular volume. Thus, the careful inclusion or exclusion of slices near the base of the heart for determination of the volumes at end-diastole and end-systole is of considerable importance for an accurate determination of the relative ventricular volumes. Once all contours are drawn and verified, the ventricular volume can be computed by simple slice summation using Simpson's rule with the slice thickness as the increment.

Recently, Young and colleagues [92] proposed an optimization method for speeding up the process of contour drawing by placing guide points on the endocardial and epicardial borders, instead of drawing continuous contours for both borders. The algorithm then automatically detects the myocardial borders by interpolation between the guide points. This user-friendly method reduces the burden of generating contours compared to the conventional tracing of the contours. Subsequently, Swingen et al. [93] modified the guide point technique by including feedback from continuously updated 3D models of the heart, to evaluate both the placement of guide points and the accuracy of the computed volumes. They showed that the combined use of short- and long-axis views results in more accurate estimates of the ventricular volumes and myocardial mass, compared to exclusive reliance on short-axis views [94] (Fig. 22.14).

Common parameters of interest for volumetric analyses are as follows:

- *Left ventricular mass:* The myocardial mass is obtained by multiplying the myocardial volume by the myocardial specific gravity (1.05). Myocardial volume is calculated as the difference between the epicardial and endocardial volumes. The normal mean for left ventricular mass is 92 ± 16 g/m^2 of body surface area.
- *Stroke volume:* The stroke volume is calculated as the difference between end-diastolic and end-systolic

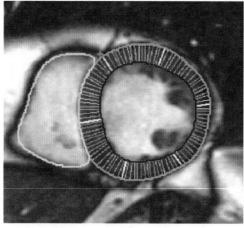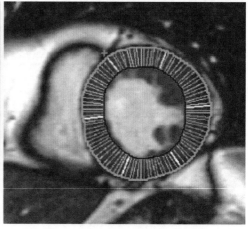

Fig. 22.12 Example of myocardial segmentation for two images corresponding to the end-diastolic (*left*) and end-systolic (*right*) phases in a patient with poor cardiac function. Contours are drawn around the blood pool demarking the endocardium and the epicardium. A contour is also drawn around the right ventricular blood pool. For this particular patient, the cross-section of ventricular cavity with the short-axis view changed significantly less than in a healthy normal. Also shown are chords connecting the endocardial and epicardial borders. The chords are orthogonal to a centerline between the two contours. The chords measure the true thickness of the myocardium as opposed to radial chords that emanate from the center of the left ventricle

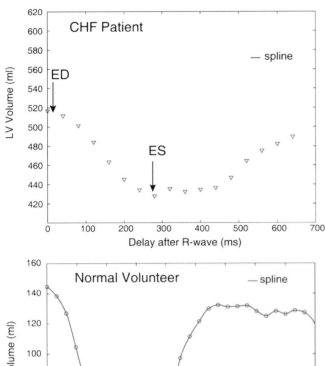

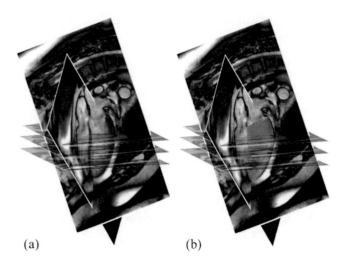

(a)   (b)

Fig. 22.14 A typical set of TrueFISP slices using a 3D analysis protocol (**a**) with co-registered long- and short-axis images (three of six short-axis images shown for clarity). Image set with 3D model of the left ventricle (**b**)

Fig. 22.13 Volume–time graph with the end-diastolic (ED) and end-systolic (ES) phases. The *upper graph* shows the variation of left ventricular (LV) volume over the cardiac cycle for a patient with congestive heart failure (CHF), and the *lower graph* is the same type of graph for a healthy volunteer. The CHF patient had an enlarged ventricle (i.e., large volume) and a very low ejection fraction. Because of the low ejection fraction, the *curve* in the CHF patient is relatively flat. Ventricular volumes were calculated by Simpson's rule from a set of short-axis images. The endocardial border had been traced on each cine frame to obtain a complete left ventricular volume versus time curve

blood or chamber volumes, and it represents the volume of blood ejected by a ventricle per heartbeat (in the absence of aortic regurgitation). Unless shunts and valvular regurgitation are present, the calculated stroke volumes of the two ventricles should be nearly equal. This is a rule of thumb for verification of the volume computation.

- *Ejection fraction:* This is the ratio of the ventricular stroke volume to the end-diastolic volume. The normal range is between 55 and 65%. An ejection fraction of less than 40% is considered to indicate impaired ventricular function.

- *Cardiac output:* This is the product of stroke volume and heart rate. It is a measure of the volume of blood ejected by the heart per beat. For an average adult, cardiac output is 4–8 l/min. Cardiac output is often corrected by normalization with respect to the body surface area.

22.5.2 Analysis of Wall Motion and Regional Myocardial Strain

22.5.2.1 Analysis of Relative Wall Motion

MRI wall motion analyses are typically performed to measure the changes in thickness of the left ventricular wall, from diastole to systole [95–100]. Wall motion abnormalities are commonly associated with many cardiac diseases, including dilated cardiomyopathy, end-stage valvular disease, and ischemic heart disease.

The assessment of relative myocardial wall thickness, thickening, and wall motion abnormalities proceeds from the MRI segmentation along the endocardial and epicardial borders. For example, a centerline can be drawn between the myocardial contours [101]; approximately 100 chords are then drawn orthogonal to the centerline at equal intervals to intersect the two myocardial contours (Fig. 22.12). With the centerline technique, the chords are optimally placed to measure the exact thickness of the transmural myocardium [101].

Parameters of interest for wall motion analyses include the following:

- *Myocardial thickness:* The lengths of the orthogonal chords, from the endocardial to the epicardial borders, measuring myocardial thicknesses.
- *Myocardial thickening:* Differences in end-diastolic and end-systolic thicknesses, as a percentage of end-diastolic thickness; these are measures of relative wall thickening and can be considered as the radial component of myocardial strain.

22.5.2.2 Analysis of Regional Myocardial Strain with Tagged MR Images

Although the time-consuming analyses of tagged MR images have been limiting factors for the widespread quantitative analyses of myocardial strains, a recently developed "harmonic phase" (HARP) MR technique permits fast and accurate analyses of strains from MRI tagging protocols [102–104]. The resultant analyses based on this technique are very fast, accurate, and observer independent since the myocardial strains are computed from information contained in the images, not the manual operator task of tracking the tagline intersections [105]. Figure 22.15 demonstrates a typical analysis of cardiac circumferential strain in three phases of the cardiac cycle using the HARP technique from data obtained from a human volunteer (HARP, Diagnosoft, Inc., Palo Alto, CA). The circumferential strain values peak at ~20% in the midwall where myofibers are predominately oriented in the plane of the cardiac short axis, consistent with the maximal amount of shortening permissible in a cardiac myocyte.

22.5.3 Perfusion Analysis

"Myocardial perfusion" is a measure of blood flow (e.g., ml/min) per unit mass of myocardial tissue. Myocardial

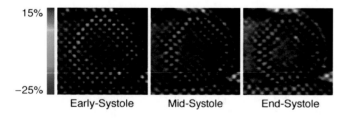

Fig. 22.15 Analysis of cardiac circumferential strain in a human volunteer for three phases of the cardiac cycle using the HARP technique for MR tissue tagging analysis (HARP, Diagnosoft, Inc., Palo Alto, CA). Circumferential strain in the images is indicated by the color palette. The grid-tag spacing used in this analysis was 6 mm

perfusion should ideally match the demand for oxygen in the myocardium. Commonly, perfusion is assessed at both rest and during stress to evaluate the capacity of the coronary circulation to increase blood flow above its baseline level, and thus match increases in oxygen demand. A ratio of the perfusion parameters, measured at stress and divided by the value for rest, will give a so-called perfusion reserve. In healthy individuals, myocardial blood flow increases approximately three- to fourfold above its baseline level with maximal vasodilation; with disease, the perfusion reserve decreases, and a flow reserve on the order of 2.5:1 is often used as the cutoff for deciding whether or not cardiovascular disease is present.

The analysis of myocardial perfusion can be carried to different levels of study, depending on the diagnostic needs and clinical resources available. One type of qualitative analysis associated with nuclear imaging is performed by visual comparison of the peak contrast enhancement in different myocardial segments during the first pass of the contrast medium through the left ventricle. The images are often viewed for this purpose in cine mode; delays in contrast enhancement and/or a reduced peak contrast enhancement relative to other myocardial sectors are then interpreted as signatures of locally reduced myocardial blood flow. However, to do so accurately, the absence of image artifacts is important if the analysis is purely qualitative and visual; if so, then no image post-processing is necessary. Nevertheless, a qualitative analysis does have limited capability to detect global reductions of myocardial perfusion, especially in patients with multiple vessel coronary artery disease.

A quantitative analysis of MRI perfusion studies commonly starts with image segmentation, similar to the procedure used for the analysis of cine studies. First, a technician typically segments one image with good contrast enhancement along the endocardial and epicardial borders of the left ventricle. These contours are then either copied to the remaining images in the data set or an automated algorithm is employed to identify the borders of the myocardium and this self-adjusts the contour positions. The latter approach is extremely useful (or even essential), as the number of images in a perfusion data set can be very large compared to a cine data set. In other words, the task of simply copying the contours to all other images would require extensive manual editing of the contour by the user. Unlike cine images, the myocardial boundaries can be slightly blurred in perfusion images due to the reduced spatial resolution and cardiac motion. Segmentation of myocardial perfusion images is therefore considered typically more challenging than for cine MR studies.

Once the myocardium is extracted by image segmentation, it is divided into smaller segments or sectors similar to those defined in cine wall motion analyses and

Fig. 22.16 Example of a typical graphical user interface software for analysis of perfusion studies. Segmentation contours are drawn by the user to define the endocardial and epicardial borders. Similar to the approach used for cine analysis, the analysis is carried out on a sector basis; in this case, 16 sectors have been defined. The drawn contours can be copied to other images for the same slice position in the perfusion study. After adjustment of the contours in each image, the software calculated the mean signal intensity in each myocardial sector. As a result, one can obtain graphs depicting the change in signal intensity in each myocardial sector as a function of image number or time (see inset panel)

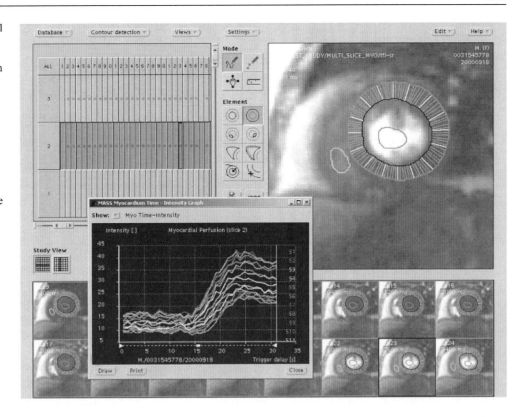

corresponding to the individual coronary supplied territories [106]. The signal intensity averages can be plotted versus the image number, or versus the time from the beginning of the perfusion scan. Various parameters that will characterize the contrast enhancement kinetics are computed from these signal intensity curves for assessing perfusion (see below). A typical interface with the software tool that can be used for analysis of MR perfusion studies is shown in Fig. 22.16.

As the perfusion images are acquired quite rapidly (<250 ms per image), there is often significant noise in the embedded images. Thus, to extract perfusion parameters, it is useful to perform some curve fitting to smooth out these signal intensity curves. One widely used method for this purpose is the gamma variate function [107], which approximates the first pass portion of the measured curves quite well. A gamma variate curve fitted to a signal intensity curve obtained from an MR perfusion study in a patient study is shown in Fig. 22.17. Nevertheless, there are certain constraints for the gamma variate analyses, e.g., it is best optimized only when the first pass portion of the curve is used (from the foot to the peak of the curve).

To date, a number of parameters have been proposed for a semi-quantitative assessment of perfusion. Commonly used parameters are as follows:

- *Percent peak enhancement:* The peak signal normalized by the derived average baseline signal, i.e., signal

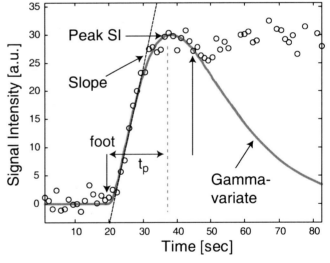

Fig. 22.17 Signal intensity curve for a myocardial sector in the lateral wall. Each of the data points (*round circles*) represents the mean signal intensity measured in the images for the user-defined myocardial sector. The images were acquired with a fast T1-weighted gradient echo sequence during injection of a 0.075 mmol/kg bolus of Gd-DTPA, an extracellular MR contrast agent. The gamma variate function can only be used to fit the portion of the tissue curve corresponding to the first pass of the contrast agent. The *gray curve* represents the best fit of gamma variate function to be part of the experimental data, covering the range indicated by the *vertical arrows*. The gamma variate fit was extrapolated to the end of the measurement range. In many cases, the end of the first pass and the appearance of the recirculation component can be best ascertained from the signal intensity changes observed in the left ventricular blood pool. Also shown are semi-quantitative perfusion parameters such as the slope, peak signal intensity, and the time from the foot to the peak (t_p)

before arrival of contrast agent expressed as a percentage.

- *Upslope:* The slope of the first pass segment primarily from the start of appearance of the contrast (foot) in the myocardium to the peak.
- *Time to peak:* The time from the foot to the peak of the curve.
- *Mean transit time:* The average time required for a unit volume of blood to transit through the region of interest. It can be determined as the ratio of blood volume in the region of interest to the blood flow through the region of interest. This value can be estimated from the gamma variate fit to the tissue curve.
- *Dynamic distribution volume:* The area under the signal intensity curve, often normalized by the area under the corresponding curve for the left ventricle.

More recently, the upslope parameter is increasingly becoming the most widely used parameter for a semi-quantitative evaluation of myocardial perfusion. The upslopes of the tissue curves are generally normalized by the upslope of the signal intensity curves for a region of interest in the center of the left ventricle, with the latter being considered as an arterial input in such analyses. The ratio defined as the normalized upslopes of the tissue curve measured for maximal vasodilation divided by the corresponding upslope value at rest has been proposed as a perfusion reserve index [108–111]. Yet, the perfusion reserve derived from the upslopes generally underestimates the actual ratio of blood flows for maximal vasodilation and rest by approximately 40% [112].

Our research group has shown that accurate myocardial blood flow estimates can be obtained by MRI methodologies, in comparison to invasive studies employing radioisotope labeled microspheres [113–116]; note that the latter are acknowledged as gold standards for the measurement of blood flow in tissues. MRI perfusion imaging may therefore play a pivotal future role in assessing novel therapeutic approaches for treating coronary artery disease, and automated quantitative analyses of MR perfusion measurements would play an essential role in this task.

22.5.4 Myocardial Scar Size

Myocardial infarct scar sizing and the identification of dysfunctional but potentially viable myocardium are the major prognostic indicators for the recovery of function after a myocardial infarction and have important clinical implications [117–120]. As such, myocardial infarct size measured using delayed ce-MRI has been shown to correlate well with histological measurements both in the acute and chronic settings [35, 121]. Furthermore, ce-MRI offers distinct advantages over other imaging modalities that either rely on the functional recovery of wall motion abnormalities to identify viability [17] or are not able to accurately depict smaller subendocardial infarctions [40]. Because of these advantages, ce-MRI is increasingly being used to quantify scar size in the acute and chronic setting and to predict the recovery of regional myocardial function using measurements of the segmental "transmural extent of infarction" (TEI) [37, 38, 122, 123]. Importantly, the exact measurement of infarct size with ce-MRI is of particular interest because both early revascularization and lytic therapy have been shown to lead to a reduced incidence of transmural infarctions, and also myocardial infarcts tend to be patchy [124, 125].

For the ce-MRI images, pixels containing nonviable myocardium have a signal intensity statistically greater (hyperenhanced) than a baseline sample from a remote normal region. Typically, hyperenhanced pixels have been classified as those with signal intensities greater than the mean + (2–6) standard deviations of a remote normal region [126, 127]. This threshold, whether manually or statistically defined, is highly subjective and highly dependent on the image quality and the noise present. Regions of signal hypoenhancement, associated with microvascular obstruction [33, 122] in the acute infarct

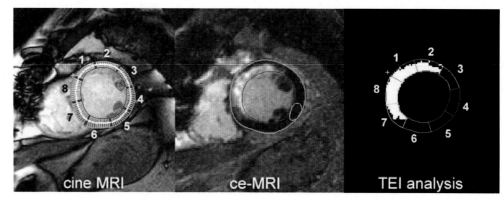

Fig. 22.18 Relative correspondence between the cine (*left*) image showing the 100 chords calculated using the centerline method (grouped into eight segments per slice) and contrast-enhanced MRI (ce-MRI) (*middle*) showing hyperenhanced scar region with the transmural extent of infarction (TEI) calculated in the eight segments (*right*)

case, are typically manually segmented and included as scar. The TEI can also be computed for each segment as the ratio (%) of scar to nonscar pixels (Fig. 22.18). Overall scar size is computed by summing the myocardial scar volume in each slice throughout the heart. Finally, infarct extent can be calculated as the scar volume divided by the myocardial volume.

22.6 Conclusions

For the biomedical engineer, cardiac MRI represents an opportunity to study the function of the heart and use these insights to design better biomedical devices. Due to the increasing relevance of cardiac MRI in the clinical arena, it will become even more important to address the challenges inherent in the use of cardiac MRI in patients with implanted devices. It should be noted that numerous topics such as MR coronary angiography and plaque imaging, although of great interest, have been left out of this overview of cardiac MRI.

Acknowledgment This work was supported in party by NIH grant #T32AR007612.

References

1. Pettigrew RI. Dynamic cardiac MR imaging. Techniques and applications. Radiol Clin North Am 1989;27:1183–203.
2. Bloomgarden DC, Fayad ZA, Ferrari VA, Chin B, Sutton MG, Axel L. Global cardiac function using fast breath-hold MRI: Validation of new acquisition and analysis techniques. Magn Reson Med 1997;37:683–92.
3. Sakuma H, Fujita N, Foo TK, et al. Evaluation of left ventricular volume and mass with breath-hold cine MR imaging. Radiology 1993;188:377–80.
4. Anand IS, Florea VG, Solomon SD, Konstam MA, Udelson JE. Noninvasive assessment of left ventricular remodeling: Concepts, techniques, and implications for clinical trials. J Card Fail 2002;8:S452–64.
5. Atkinson DJ, Edelman RR. Cineangiography of the heart in a single breath hold with a segmented turboFLASH sequence. Radiology 1991;178:357–60.
6. Bluemke DA, Boxerman JL, Atalar E, McVeigh ER. Segmented K-space cine breath-hold cardiovascular MR imaging: Part 1. Principles and technique. AJR Am J Roentgenol 1997;169:395–400.
7. Bluemke DA, Boxerman JL, Mosher T, Lima JA. Segmented K-space cine breath-hold cardiovascular MR imaging: Part 2. Evaluation of aortic vasculopathy. AJR Am J Roentgenol 1997;169:401–7.
8. Chien D, Edelman RR. Ultrafast imaging using gradient echoes. Magn Reson Q 1991;7:31–56.
9. Oppelt A, Graumann R, Barfuss H, Fischer H, Hartl W, Schajor W. FISP: A new fast MRI sequence. Electromedica (Engl. Ed.) 1986;54:15–8.
10. Zur Y, Wood ML, Neuringer LJ. Motion-insensitive, steady-state free precession imaging. Magn Reson Med 1990;16:444–59.
11. Pereles FS, Kapoor V, Carr JC, et al. Usefulness of segmented trueFISP cardiac pulse sequence in evaluation of congenital and acquired adult cardiac abnormalities. AJR Am J Roentgenol 2001;177:1155–60.
12. Plein S, Bloomer TN, Ridgway JP, Jones TR, Bainbridge GJ, Sivananthan MU. Steady-state free precession magnetic resonance imaging of the heart: Comparison with segmented k-space gradient-echo imaging. J Magn Reson Imaging 2001;14:230–6.
13. Francois CJ, Fieno DS, Shors SM, Finn JP. Left ventricular mass: Manual and automatic segmentation of true FISP and FLASH cine MR images in dogs and pigs. Radiology 2004; 230:389–95.
14. Shors SM, Fung CW, Francois CJ, Finn JP, Fieno DS. Accurate quantification of right ventricular mass at MR imaging by using cine true fast imaging with steady-state precession: Study in dogs. Radiology 2004;230:383–8.
15. Yang X, Atalar E, Li D, et al. Magnetic resonance imaging permits in vivo monitoring of catheter-based vascular gene delivery. Circulation 2001;104:1588–90.
16. Weiger M., Pruessmann KP, Boesiger P. Cardiac real-time imaging using SENSE. SENSitivity Encoding scheme. Magn Reson Med 2000;43:177–84.
17. Penicka M, Bartunek J, Wijns W, et al. Tissue doppler imaging predicts recovery of left ventricular function after recanalization of an occluded coronary artery. J Am Coll Cardiol 2004; 43:85–91.
18. Sanz G, Castaner A, Betriu A, et al. Determinants of prognosis in survivors of myocardial infarction: A prospective clinical angiographic study. N Engl J Med 1982;306:1065–70.
19. Weiss JL, Marino PN, Shapiro EP. Myocardial infarct expansion: Recognition, significance and pathology. Am J Cardiol 1991;68:35–40D.
20. Lieberman AN, Weiss JL, Jugdutt BI, et al. Two-dimensional echocardiography and infarct size: Relationship of regional wall motion and thickening to the extent of myocardial infarction in the dog. Circulation 1981;63:739–46.
21. Sasayama S, Franklin D, Ross J Jr, Kemper WS, McKown D. Dynamic changes in left ventricular wall thickness and their use in analyzing cardiac function in the conscious dog. Am J Cardiol 1976;38:870–9.
22. Azhari H, Weiss JL, Rogers WJ, Siu CO, Shapiro EP. A noninvasive comparative study of myocardial strains in ischemic canine hearts using tagged MRI in 3-D. Am J Physiol 1995; 268:H1918–26.
23. Gotte MJ, van Rossum AC, Twisk JWR, Kuijer JPA, Marcus JT, Visser CA. Quantification of regional contractile function after infarction: Strain analysis superior to wall thickening analysis in discriminating infarct from remote myocardium. J Am Coll Cardiol 2001;37:808–17.
24. Rickers C, Gallegos R, Seethamraju RT, et al. Applications of magnetic resonance imaging for cardiac stem cell therapy. J Interv Cardiol 2004;17:37–46.
25. Axel L, Goncalves RC, Bloomgarden D. Regional heart wall motion: Two-dimensional analysis and functional imaging with MR imaging. Radiology 1992;183:745–50.
26. Clark NR, Reichek N, Bergey P, et al. Circumferential myocardial shortening in the normal human left ventricle. Assessment by magnetic resonance imaging using spatial modulation of magnetization. Circulation 1991;84:67–74.
27. McVeigh ER. MRI of myocardial function: Motion tracking techniques. Magn Reson Imaging 1996;14:137–50.
28. McVeigh ER, Atalar E. Cardiac tagging with breath-hold cine MRI. Magn Reson Med 1992;28:318–27.
29. McVeigh ER, Zerhouni EA. Noninvasive measurement of transmural gradients in myocardial strain with MR imaging. Radiology 1991;180:677–83.

30. Koenig SH, Spiller M, Brown RD III, Wolf GL. Relaxation of water protons in the intra- and extracellular regions of blood containing Gd(DTPA). Magn Reson Med 1986;3:791–5.

31. Strich G, Hagan PL, Gerber KH, Slutsky RA. Tissue distribution and magnetic resonance spin lattice relaxation effects of gadolinium-DTPA. Radiology 1985;154:723–6.

32. Braunwald E, ed. Heart disease: A textbook of cardiovascular medicine. Philadelphia, PA: W.B. Saunders Company, 1997.

33. Lima JA, Judd RM, Bazille A, Schulman SP, Atalar E, Zerhouni EA. Regional heterogeneity of human myocardial infarcts demonstrated by contrast-enhanced MRI. Potential mechanisms. Circulation 1995;92:1117–25.

34. Tsekos NV, Zhang Y, Merkle H, et al. Fast anatomical imaging of the heart and assessment of myocardial perfusion with arrhythmia insensitive magnetization preparation. Magn Reson Med 1995;34:530–6.

35. Kim RJ, Fieno DS, Parrish TB, et al. Relationship of MRI delayed contrast enhancement to irreversible injury, infarct age, and contractile function. Circulation 1999;100: 1992–2002.

36. Simonetti OP, Kim RJ, Fieno DS, et al. An improved MR imaging technique for the visualization of myocardial infarction. Radiology 2001;218:215–23.

37. Bello D, Shah DJ, Farah GM, et al. Gadolinium cardiovascular magnetic resonance predicts reversible myocardial dysfunction and remodeling in patients with heart failure undergoing beta-blocker therapy. Circulation 2003;108:1945–53.

38. Kim RJ, Wu E, Rafael A, et al. The use of contrast-enhanced magnetic resonance imaging to identify reversible myocardial dysfunction. N Engl J Med 2000;343:1445–53.

39. Klein C, Nekolla SG, Bengel FM, et al. Assessment of myocardial viability with contrast-enhanced magnetic resonance imaging: Comparison with positron emission tomography. Circulation 2002;105:162–7.

40. Wagner A, Mahrholdt H, Holly TA, et al. Contrast-enhanced MRI and routine single photon emission computed tomography (SPECT) perfusion imaging for detection of subendocardial myocardial infarcts: An imaging study. Lancet 2003; 361:374–9.

41. Lekx KS, Prato FS, Sykes J, Wisenberg G. The partition coefficient of Gd-DTPA reflects maintained tissue viability in a canine model of chronic significant coronary stenosis. J Cardiovasc Magn Reson 2004;6:33–42.

42. Tong CY, Prato FS, Wisenberg G, et al. Measurement of the extraction efficiency and distribution volume for Gd-DTPA in normal and diseased canine myocardium. Magn Reson Med 1993;30:337–46.

43. Wendland MF, Saeed M, Bremerich J, Arheden H, Higgins CB. Thallium-like test for myocardial viability with MnDPDP-enhanced MRI. Acad Radiol 2002;9 Suppl 1:S82–3.

44. Kim RJ, Judd RM, Chen EL, Fieno DS, Parrish TB, Lima JA. Relationship of elevated 23Na magnetic resonance image intensity to infarct size after acute reperfused myocardial infarction. Circulation 1999;100:185–92.

45. Duprez DA, Swingen C, Sih R, Lefebvre T, Kaiser DR, Jerosch-Herold M. Heterogeneous remodelling of the ascending and descending aorta with age. J Hum Hypertens 2007;21: 689–91.

46. Hsu EW, Muzikant AL, Matulevicius SA, Penland RC, Henriquez CS. Magnetic resonance myocardial fiber-orientation mapping with direct histological correlation. Am J Physiol 1998;274:H1627–34.

47. LeGrice IJ, Smaill BH, Chai LZ, Edgar SG, Gavin JB, Hunter PJ. Laminar structure of the heart: Ventricular myocyte arrangement and connective tissue architecture in the dog. Am J Physiol 1995;269:H571–82.

48. Streeter DD Jr, Spotnitz HM, Patel DP, Ross J Jr, Sonnenblick EH. Fiber orientation in the canine left ventricle during diastole and systole. Circ Res 1969;24:339–47.

49. Ingels NB Jr. Myocardial fiber architecture and left ventricular function. Technol Health Care 1997;5:45–52.

50. Rijcken J, Bovendeerd PH, Schoofs AJ, van Campen DH, Arts T. Optimization of cardiac fiber orientation for homogeneous fiber strain at beginning of ejection. J Biomech 1997;30: 1041–9.

51. Rijcken J, Bovendeerd PH, Schoofs AJ, van Campen DH, Arts T. Optimization of cardiac fiber orientation for homogeneous fiber strain during ejection. Ann Biomed Eng 1999;27:289–97.

52. Sallin EA. Fiber orientation and ejection fraction in the human left ventricle. Biophys J 1969;9:954–64.

53. Tomioka H, Liakopoulos OJ, Buckberg GD, Hristov N, Tan Z, Trummer G. The effect of ventricular sequential contraction on helical heart during pacing: High septal pacing versus biventricular pacing. Eur J Cardiothorac Surg 2006;29:S198–206.

54. Tseng WY, Reese TG, Weisskoff RM, Brady TJ, Wedeen VJ. Myocardial fiber shortening in humans: Initial results of MR imaging. Radiology 2000;216:128–39.

55. Van Der Toorn A, Barenbrug P, Snoep G, et al. Transmural gradients of cardiac myofiber shortening in aortic valve stenosis patients using MRI tagging. Am J Physiol Heart Circ Physiol 2002;283:H1609–15.

56. Shapiro EP, Rademakers FE. Importance of oblique fiber orientation for left ventricular wall deformation. Technol Health Care 1997;5:21–8.

57. Tseng WY, Wedeen VJ, Reese TG, Smith RN, Halpern EF. Diffusion tensor MRI of myocardial fibers and sheets: Correspondence with visible cut-face texture. J Magn Reson Imaging 2003;17:31–42.

58. Helm PA, Tseng HJ, Younes L, McVeigh ER, Winslow RL. Ex vivo 3D diffusion tensor imaging and quantification of cardiac laminar structure. Magn Reson Med 2005;54:850–9.

59. Scollan DF, Holmes A, Zhang J, Winslow RL. Reconstruction of cardiac ventricular geometry and fiber orientation using magnetic resonance imaging. Ann Biomed Eng 2000;28: 934–44.

60. Geerts L, Bovendeerd P, Nicolay K, Arts T. Characterization of the normal cardiac myofiber field in goat measured with MR-diffusion tensor imaging. Am J Physiol Heart Circ Physiol 2002;283:H139–45.

61. Basser PJ, Mattiello J, LeBihan D. Estimation of the effective self-diffusion tensor from the NMR spin echo. J Magn Reson B 1994;103:247–54.

62. Garrido L, Wedeen VJ, Kwong KK, Spencer UM, Kantor HL. Anisotropy of water diffusion in the myocardium of the rat. Circ Res 1994;74:789–93.

63. Holmes AA, Scollan DF, Winslow RL. Direct histological validation of diffusion tensor MRI in formaldehyde-fixed myocardium. Magn Reson Med 2000;44:157–61.

64. Scollan DF, Holmes A, Winslow R, Forder J. Histological validation of myocardial microstructure obtained from diffusion tensor magnetic resonance imaging. Am J Physiol 1998;275:H2308–18.

65. Helm P, Beg MF, Miller MI, Winslow RL. Measuring and mapping cardiac fiber and laminar architecture using diffusion tensor MR imaging. Ann N Y Acad Sci 2005;1047:296–307.

66. Dou J, Tseng WY, Reese TG, Wedeen VJ. Combined diffusion and strain MRI reveals structure and function of human myocardial laminar sheets in vivo. Magn Reson Med 2003; 50:107–13.

67. Reese TG, Weisskoff RM, Smith RN, Rosen BR, Dinsmore RE, Wedeen VJ. Imaging myocardial fiber architecture in vivo with magnetic resonance. Magn Reson Med 1995;34:786–91.

68. Rohmer D, Sitek A, Gullberg GT. Reconstruction and visualization of fiber and laminar structure in the normal human heart from ex vivo diffusion tensor magnetic resonance imaging (DTMRI) data. Invest Radiol 2007;42:777–89.

69. Tseng WY, Dou J, Reese TG, Wedeen VJ. Imaging myocardial fiber disarray and intramural strain hypokinesis in hypertrophic cardiomyopathy with MRI. J Magn Reson Imaging 2006;23:1–8.

70. Chen J, Song SK, Liu W, et al. Remodeling of cardiac fiber structure after infarction in rats quantified with diffusion tensor MRI. Am J Physiol Heart Circ Physiol 2003;285:H946–54.

71. Wu MT, Tseng WY, Su MY, et al. Diffusion tensor magnetic resonance imaging mapping the fiber architecture remodeling in human myocardium after infarction: Correlation with viability and wall motion. Circulation 2006;114:1036–45.

72. Lardo AC. Real-time magnetic resonance imaging: Diagnostic and interventional applications. Pediatr Cardiol 2000;21:80–98.

73. Kerr AB, Pauly JM, Hu BS, et al. Real-time interactive MRI on a conventional scanner. Magn Reson Med 1997;38:355–67.

74. Serfaty JM, Yang X, Foo TK, Kumar A, Derbyshire A, Atalar E. MRI-guided coronary catheterization and PTCA: A feasibility study on a dog model. Magn Reson Med 2003;49:258–63.

75. Lardo AC, McVeigh ER, Jumrussirikul P, et al. Visualization and temporal/spatial characterization of cardiac radiofrequency ablation lesions using magnetic resonance imaging. Circulation 2000;102:698–705.

76. Atalar E, Bottomley PA, Ocali O, et al. High resolution intravascular MRI and MRS by using a catheter receiver coil. Magn Reson Med 1996;36:596–605.

77. Moore P. MRI-guided congenital cardiac catheterization and intervention: The future? Catheter Cardiovasc Interv 2005;66:1–8.

78. McVeigh ER, Guttman MA, Lederman RJ, et al. Real-time interactive MRI-guided cardiac surgery: Aortic valve replacement using a direct apical approach. Magn Reson Med 2006;56:958–64.

79. Nazarian S, Roguin A, Zviman MM, et al. Clinical utility and safety of a protocol for noncardiac and cardiac magnetic resonance imaging of patients with permanent pacemakers and implantable-cardioverter defibrillators at 1.5 Tesla. Circulation 2006;114:1277–84.

80. Roka A, Simor T, Vago H, Minorics C, Acsady G, Merkely B. Magnetic resonance imaging-based biventricular pacemaker upgrade. Pacing Clin Electrophysiol 2004;27:1011–3.

81. Sommer T, Vahlhaus C, Lauck G, et al. MR imaging and cardiac pacemakers: In-vitro evaluation and in-vivo studies in 51 patients at 0.5 T. Radiology 2000;215:869–79.

82. Achenbach S, Moshage W, Diem B, Bieberle T, Schibgilla V, Bachmann K. Effects of magnetic resonance imaging on cardiac pacemakers and electrodes. Am Heart J 1997;134:467–73.

83. Nitz WR, Oppelt A, Renz W, Manke C, Lenhart M, Link J. On the heating of linear conductive structures as guide wires and catheters in interventional MRI. J Magn Reson Imaging 2001;13:105–14.

84. Yeung CJ, Susil RC, Atalar E. RF safety of wires in interventional MRI: Using a safety index. Magn Reson Med 2002;47:187–93.

85. Houlind K, Eschen O, Pedersen EM, Jensen T, Hasenkam JM, Paulsen PK. Magnetic resonance imaging of blood velocity distribution around St. Jude medical aortic valves in patients. J Heart Valve Dis 1996;5:511–7.

86. Walker PG, Pedersen EM, Oyre S, et al. Magnetic resonance velocity imaging: A new method for prosthetic heart valve study. J Heart Valve Dis 1995;4:296–307.

87. Botnar R, Nagel E, Scheidegger MB, Pedersen EM, Hess O, Boesiger P. Assessment of prosthetic aortic valve performance by magnetic resonance velocity imaging. Magma 2000;10:18–26.

88. Wyman BT, Hunter WC, Prinzen FW, Faris OP, McVeigh ER. Effects of single- and biventricular pacing on temporal and spatial dynamics of ventricular contraction. Am J Physiol Heart Circ Physiol 2002;282:H372–9.

89. van der Geest RJ, de Roos A, van der Wall EE, Reiber JH. Quantitative analysis of cardiovascular MR images. Int J Card Imaging 1997;13:247–58.

90. van der Geest RJ, Lelieveldt BP, Reiber JH. Quantification of global and regional ventricular function in cardiac magnetic resonance imaging. Top Magn Reson Imaging 2000;11:348–58.

91. van der Geest RJ, Reiber JH. Quantification in cardiac MRI. J Magn Reson Imaging 1999;10:602–8.

92. Young AA, Cowan BR, Thrupp SF, Hedley WJ, Dell'Italia LJ. Left ventricular mass and volume: Fast calculation with guide-point modeling on MR images. Radiology 2000;216:597–602.

93. Swingen CM, Seethamraju RT, Jerosch-Herold M. Feedback-assisted three-dimensional reconstruction of the left ventricle with MRI. J Magn Reson Imaging 2003;17:528–37.

94. Swingen C, Wang X, Jerosch-Herold M. Evaluation of myocardial volume heterogeneity during end-diastole and end-systole using cine MRI. J Cardiovasc Magn Reson 2004;6:829–35.

95. Baer FM, Voth E, Schneider CA, Theissen P, Schicha H, Sechtem U. Comparison of low-dose dobutamine-gradient-echo magnetic resonance imaging and positron emission tomography with [18F]fluorodeoxyglucose in patients with chronic coronary artery disease. A functional and morphological approach to the detection of residual myocardial viability. Circulation 1995;91:1006–15.

96. Baer FM, Voth E, LaRosee K, et al. Comparison of dobutamine transesophageal echocardiography and dobutamine magnetic resonance imaging for detection of residual myocardial viability. Am J Cardiol 1996;78:415–9.

97. Nagel E, Lehmkuhl HB, Bocksch W, et al. Noninvasive diagnosis of ischemia-induced wall motion abnormalities with the use of high-dose dobutamine stress MRI: Comparison with dobutamine stress echocardiography. Circulation 1999;99:763–70.

98. Matheijssen NA, de Roos A, Doornbos J, Reiber JH, Waldman GJ, van der Wall EE. Left ventricular wall motion analysis in patients with acute myocardial infarction using magnetic resonance imaging. Magn Reson Imaging 1993;11:485–92.

99. Holman ER, Vliegen HW, van der Geest RJ, et al. Quantitative analysis of regional left ventricular function after myocardial infarction in the pig assessed with cine magnetic resonance imaging. Magn Reson Med 1995;34:161–9.

100. Nagel E, Fleck E. Functional MRI in ischemic heart disease based on detection of contraction abnormalities. J Magn Reson Imaging 1999;10:411–7.

101. Sheehan FH, Bolson EL, Dodge HT, Mathey DG, Schofer J, Woo HW. Advantages and applications of the centerline method for characterizing regional ventricular function. Circulation 1986;74:293–305.

102. Osman NF, Kerwin WS, McVeigh ER, Prince JL. Cardiac motion tracking using CINE harmonic phase (HARP) magnetic resonance imaging. Magn Reson Med 1999;42:1048–60.

103. Osman NF, McVeigh ER, Prince JL. Imaging heart motion using harmonic phase MRI. IEEE Trans Med Imaging 2000;19:186–202.

104. Osman NF, Prince JL. Visualizing myocardial function using HARP MRI. Phys Med Biol 2000;45:1665–82.

105. Kraitchman D, Sampath S, Derbyshire JA, Heldman AW, Prince JL, Osman NF. Detecting the onset of ischemia using real-time HARP. Proceedings of the International Society of Magnetic Resonance in Medicine 2001.

106. Cerqueira MD, Weissman NJ, Dilsizian V, et al. Standardized myocardial segmentation and nomenclature for tomographic imaging of the heart: A statement for healthcare professionals from the Cardiac Imaging Committee of the Council on Clinical Cardiology of the American Heart Association. Circulation 2002;105:539–42.

107. Thompson HK Jr, Starmer CF, Whalen RE, McIntosh HD. Indicator transit time considered as a gamma variate. Circ Res 1964;14:502–15.

108. Al-Saadi N, Nagel E, Gross M, et al. Noninvasive detection of myocardial ischemia from perfusion reserve based on cardiovascular magnetic resonance. Circulation 2000;101:1379–83.

109. Al-Saadi N, Nagel E, Gross M, et al. Improvement of myocardial perfusion reserve early after coronary intervention: Assessment with cardiac magnetic resonance imaging. J Am Coll Cardiol 2000;36:1557–64.

110. Panting JR, Gatehouse PD, Yang GZ, et al. Abnormal subendocardial perfusion in cardiac syndrome X detected by cardiovascular magnetic resonance imaging. N Engl J Med 2002;346:1948–53.

111. Schwitter J, Nanz D, Kneifel S, et al. Assessment of myocardial perfusion in coronary artery disease by magnetic resonance: A comparison with positron emission tomography and coronary angiography. Circulation 2001;103:2230–5.

112. Ibrahim T, Nekolla SG, Schreiber K, et al. Assessment of coronary flow reserve: Comparison between contrast-enhanced magnetic resonance imaging and positron emission tomography. J Am Coll Cardiol 2002;39:864–70.

113. Jerosch-Herold M, Hu X, Murthy NS, Rickers C, Stillman AE. Magnetic resonance imaging of myocardial contrast enhancement with MS-325 and its relation to myocardial blood flow and the perfusion reserve. J Magn Reson Imaging 2003;18:544–54.

114. Jerosch-Herold M, Seethamraju RT, Swingen CM, Wilke NM, Stillman AE. Analysis of myocardial perfusion MRI. J Magn Reson Imaging 2004;19:758–70.

115. Jerosch-Herold M, Swingen C, Seethamraju RT. Myocardial blood flow quantification with MRI by model-independent deconvolution. Med Phys 2002;29:886–97.

116. Jerosch-Herold M, Wilke N, Wang Y, et al. Direct comparison of an intravascular and an extracellular contrast agent for quantification of myocardial perfusion. Cardiac MRI Group. Int J Card Imaging 1999;15:453–64.

117. Baer FM, Theissen P, Schneider CA, et al. MRI assessment of myocardial viability: Comparison with other imaging techniques. Rays 1999;24:96–108.

118. Haas F, Haehnel CJ, Picker W, et al. Preoperative positron emission tomographic viability assessment and perioperative and postoperative risk in patients with advanced ischemic heart disease. J Am Coll Cardiol 1997;30:1693–700.

119. Lee KS, Marwick TH, Cook SA, et al. Prognosis of patients with left ventricular dysfunction, with and without viable myocardium after myocardial infarction. Relative efficacy of medical therapy and revascularization. Circulation 1994;90:2687–94.

120. Pagley PR, Beller GA, Watson DD, Gimple LW, Ragosta M. Improved outcome after coronary bypass surgery in patients with ischemic cardiomyopathy and residual myocardial viability. Circulation 1997;96:793–800.

121. Fieno DS, Kim RJ, Chen EL, Lomasney JW, Klocke FJ, Judd RM. Contrast-enhanced magnetic resonance imaging of myocardium at risk: Distinction between reversible and irreversible injury throughout infarct healing. J Am Coll Cardiol 2000;36:1985–91.

122. Beek AM, Kuhl HP, Bondarenko O, et al. Delayed contrast-enhanced magnetic resonance imaging for the prediction of regional functional improvement after acute myocardial infarction. J Am Coll Cardiol 2003;42:895–901.

123. Mahrholdt H, Wagner A, Parker M, et al. Relationship of contractile function to transmural extent of infarction in patients with chronic coronary artery disease. J Am Coll Cardiol 2003;42:505–12.

124. Marino P, Zanolla L, Zardini P. Effect of streptokinase on left ventricular modeling and function after myocardial infarction: The GISSI (Gruppo Italiano per lo Studio della Streptochinasi nell'Infarto Miocardico) Trial. J Am Coll Cardiol 1989;14:1149–58.

125. Sheehan FH, Doerr R, Schmidt WG, et al. Early recovery of left ventricular function after thrombolytic therapy for acute myocardial infarction: An important determinant of survival. J Am Coll Cardiol 1988;12:289–300.

126. Gerber BL, Garot J, Bluemke DA, Wu KC, Lima JA. Accuracy of contrast-enhanced magnetic resonance imaging in predicting improvement of regional myocardial function in patients after acute myocardial infarction. Circulation 2002;106:1083–9.

127. Kolipaka A, Chatzimavroudis GP, White RD, O'Donnell TP, Setser RM. Segmentation of non-viable myocardium in delayed enhancement magnetic resonance images. Int J Cardiovasc Imaging 2005;21:303–11.

Part IV
Devices and Therapies

Chapter 23
A Historical Perspective of Cardiovascular Devices and Techniques Associated with the University of Minnesota

Paul A. Iaizzo and Monica A. Mahre

Abstract The University of Minnesota has a unique history relative to advances in cardiovascular research, surgery, and the development of medical devices. Interestingly, the completion of this textbook coincides with two important anniversaries in cardiovascular medicine and engineering at the university. First, it was 50 years ago, in 1958, upon the request of Dr. C. Walton Lillehei, that the first wearable, battery-powered pacemaker was designed and built by Earl Bakken (Medtronic, Inc.) and used on a patient. Second, 30 years ago, in 1978, the first human heart transplantation was performed at the university. In this chapter, we will review some of this history and how it has led to the creation of a dynamic medical device industry in the state of Minnesota.

Keywords Medical device development · Cross-circulation · Bubble oxygenator · Pacemaker · Heart valves

23.1 Introduction

The era from 1950 to 1967 was an incredible time of innovation at the University of Minnesota's Department of Surgery in the newly emerging fields of open-heart surgery and medical devices. There were many reasons for this, but most importantly: (1) the university had excellent facilities, including a unique privately funded 80-bed heart hospital for pediatric and adult patients (Fig. 23.1); and (2) the Department of Surgery was led by a chairman, Owen H. Wangensteen, MD, who "created the milieu and the opportunities for great achievements by many of his pupils" and was considered the "mentor of a thousand surgeons" (Fig. 23.2, Table 23.1) [1]. More

specifically, Dr. Wangensteen encouraged his medical students, residents, and junior faculty to "step out of the box," look at problems in different ways, and not assume that those who went before them had all the answers. He also believed strongly in collaborations with the basic science departments, specifically the Department of Physiology whose department head, Maurice Visscher, played an integral role in supporting both research and the clinical training of surgical residents. To that end, Wangensteen instituted a 2-year research program for all residents; this surgical Ph.D. program was the only one in the country at its inception. It should be noted that these students were required to take various advanced physiology courses offered through the Department of Physiology.

In the early 1950s, the innovative surge was credited to the fact that many surgical residents were returning from World War II, where they had experienced life and death situations when managing MASH units; "they had little or no fear of death" and their generation was not afraid of "pushing the envelope" to help patients. By today's standards, they would be viewed as "mavericks" or "cowboys," but, in fact, they had little to lose, not unlike the battlefield; their patients were dying and/or had little chance of survival without the novel techniques that were successfully implemented in Minnesota.

One of these young war-experienced surgeons was C. Walton Lillehei, who returned to the University of Minnesota in 1950 to complete his surgical residency after leading an Army MASH unit in both North Africa and Italy (Fig. 23.3). Lillehei was very bright (he also completed M.S. and Ph.D. degrees during this time) and was known as an impulsive maverick, always pushing to the next level of care for his clinical patients for whom he had great empathy. Lillehei and his team launched many surgical innovations during this period, primarily due to their hands-on research experience in the experimental dog laboratories; one site for this research was located in the basement of the Mayo Hospital building, just three

M.A. Mahre (✉)
University of Minnesota, Department of Surgery, B 172 Mayo, MMC 195, 420 Delaware St. SE, USA
e-mail: mahre002@umn.edu

A.

B.

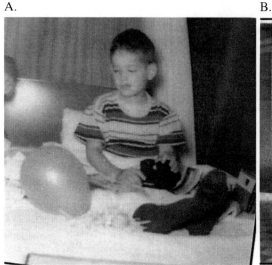

Fig. 23.1 John DiIorio (Dr. Iaizzo's cousin) was a young cardiac patient of Dr. Lillehei and his team, shown here in 1958 (**A**) in his hospital bed at the University Variety Club Hospital and then (**B**) leaving the hospital with his father

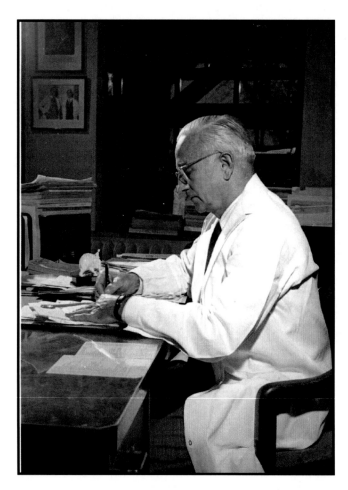

Fig. 23.2 "The Chief" Owen H. Wangensteen, the youngest Surgery Department chairman at age 31 years, served as chairman of the department from 1930 to 1967

floors below the main operating rooms. Today, this lab space houses the Visible Heart Laboratory under the direction of Dr. Paul Iaizzo.

Interestingly, prior to 1950, the heart was considered to be the core of human emotion, even the soul itself, with a role in human feelings toward others. When the medical profession eventually began to view the heart more physiologically, as a pump or machine within the body, researchers and clinicians began to develop new ways to repair and replace worn-out parts of the heart; innovations in the field of cardiac surgery then flourished (Table 23.2).

Such innovation became prominent at the University of Minnesota. For example, Dr. Clarence Dennis designed the first heart–lung machine for total cardiopulmonary bypass, which was subsequently tested successfully on dogs (Fig. 23.4). However, when Dennis and his team used the heart–lung machine in the clinical area for the first time on April 5, 1951, the patient died due to complications; a second patient also died during surgery from a massive air embolism. Not long after, Dr. Dennis moved his machine and most of his team to New York City [1].

Worldwide, one of the next major milestones in cardiac surgery was the first open-heart surgery performed using hypothermia, a procedure first attempted on September 2, 1952, by Dr. F. John Lewis and colleagues at the University of Minnesota (Fig. 23.5). This procedure, suggested by Dr. W.G. Bigelow of Toronto, lowered the body temperature of patients 12–15° to reduce their blood flow, thereby reducing the body's need for oxygen. Brain cells would die after 3–4 min at normal temperature

Table 23.1 Department of Surgery at the University of Minnesota: Chairs/Interim Chairs

Surgery Department chair/interim chair	Position	Years served
Arthur C. Strachauer	Department chair	1925, 1927–1929
Owen H. Wangensteen	Department chair	1930–1967
John S. Najarian	Department chair	1967–1993
Edward W. Humphrey	Interim chair	1993–1994
Frank B. Cerra	Interim chair	1994–1995
David L. Dunn	Department chair	1995–2005
David A. Rothenberger	Interim chair	2005–2006
Selwyn M. Vickers	Department chair	2006–present

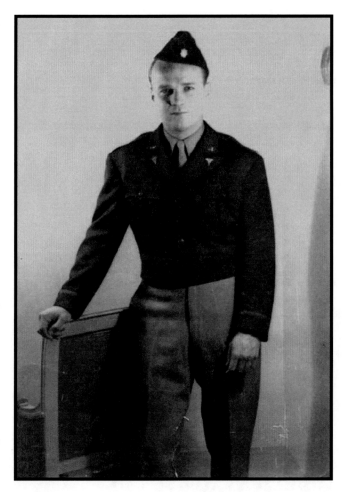

Fig. 23.3 Walt Lillehei in his Army uniform

procedures. One of the major drawbacks of this procedure at that time was the lack of any means to rewarm a cold, nonbeating heart [2].

From a historic perspective, another key milestone in cardiac surgery, though not accomplished at the University of Minnesota, occurred on May 6, 1953, when Dr. J. Gibbon closed an atrial septal defect using a pump oxygenator for an intracardiac operation. Although this first success with the pump oxygenator was well received, it aroused surprisingly little excitement or enthusiasm among cardiologists and cardiac surgeons at that time, likely because other centers had launched their own experiments with bubble oxygenators. Interestingly, Gibbon was never able to repeat his one clinical success; he ultimately became discouraged and did not use the pump oxygenator again.

During this era, "there was a common scenario, namely, good results with acceptable survival in the experimental animals but nearly universal failure when the same apparatus and techniques were applied to human beings [2]." Furthermore, it was written that "many of the most experienced investigators concluded with seemingly impeccable logic that the problems were not with the perfusion techniques or the heart–lung machines [2]. Rather, they came to believe that the 'sick human heart' ravaged by failure, could not possibly be expected to tolerate the magnitude of the operation required and then recover with good output, as occurred when the same machines and techniques were applied to healthy dogs [2]." It is important to consider that not only were these experimental animals typically healthy dogs, but that important anatomical differences (e.g., coronary anatomy) may also have been distinguishing factors (see Chapter 6).

23.2 Cross-Circulation

Extracorporeal circulation by controlled cross-circulation was introduced clinically on March 26, 1954, after much animal experimentation (Fig. 23.6). The use of cross-circulation for intracardiac operations was an immense departure from established surgical practice at

without oxygen, but hypothermia allowed Dr. Lewis and his research team (Drs. Mansur Taufic, C. Walton Lillehei, and Richard Varco) to successfully complete a 5½-min repair of the atrial septum on a 5-year-old patient. This was recognized as a landmark in the history of cardiac surgery; until this time, no surgeon had succeeded in opening the heart to perform intracardiac repair under direct vision. Hypothermia with inflow stasis proved to be excellent for some of the simpler surgical repairs, but it was not a viable option for more extensive cardiac

Table 23.2 University of Minnesota Milestones

1887	New standards requiring medical students to pass exams and gain medical examining board approval (led by Medical School Dean, Perry Millard)
1911	Minnesota became the first state to mandate hospital internships for medical students
1930s	Discovery of the link between cholesterol and heart disease (Ancel Keys)
1950	First adaptation of the mass spectrograph (Alfred Nier)
1951	First attempt to use a heart–lung machine (Clarence Dennis)
1952	First successful open-heart surgery using hypothermia (F. John Lewis)
1953	First jejunoileal bypass (Richard L. Varco)
1954	First open-heart procedure using cross-circulation (C. Walton Lillehei)
1954	First surgical correction of Tetralogy of Fallot (C. Walton Lillehei)
1955	First successful use of the bubble oxygenator (Richard DeWall)
1958	First use of a small, portable battery-powered pacemaker (Earl Bakken)
1963	First human partial ileal bypass (Henry Buckwald)
1966	First clinical pancreas transplant (William D. Kelly and Richard C. Lillehei)
1966–1968	First prosthetic heart valves (Lillehei–Nakib toroidal disc in 1966, Lillehei-Kaster pivoting disc in 1967, Kalke–Lillehei rigid bileaflet prosthesis in 1968)
1967	Bretylium, a drug developed by Marvin Bacaner, saved the life of Dwight Eisenhower
1967	World's first heart transplant (Dr. Christian Barnard, trained by C. Walton Lillehei)
1968	First successful bone marrow transplant (Robert A. Good)
1969	Invention of implantable drug pump (Henry Buckwald, Richard Varco, Frank Dorman, Perry L. Blackshear, Perry J. Blackshear)
1976	Medical Device Amendment to FDA Cosmetic Act
1977	First implant of St. Jude mechanical heart valve at University Hospital
1978	Human heart transplantation was performed at university
1978	Pediatric human heart transplantation was performed at University Hospital (Ernesto Molina)
1988	HDI/Pulse Wave® profiler founded (Hypertension Diagnostics, Inc., Jay Cohn, Stanley Finkelstein)
1993	Angel Wings® transcatheter closure device invented (Gladwin Das)
1994	First successful simultaneous pancreas–kidney transplant using a living donor (David Sutherland)
1995	Amplatzer® Occlusion Devices founded (AGA Medical Corp., Kurt Amplatz)
1997	First kidney–bowel transplantation (Rainer Gruessner)
1999	CardioPump Device evaluated (Keith Lurie et al.) 1999 Lillehei Heart Institute was established
2000	University's Medical School has produced more family doctors than any other institution in the United States
2003	Robotic cardiac surgery performed at the University of Minnesota (Kenneth Liao)
2005	Launch of free-access web site "Atlas of Human Cardiac Anatomy" (Visible Heart Laboratory; www.vhlab.umn.edu/atlas)
2006	Implant of left ventricular assist device using minimally invasive approach (Kenneth Liao) 2007 First Annual Bakken Surgical Device Symposium (Department of Surgery)

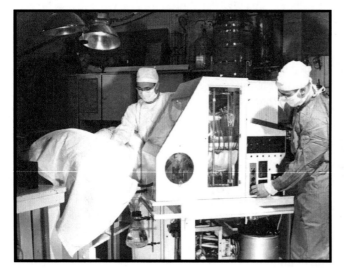

Fig. 23.4 Clarence Dennis with the first heart–lung machine at the University of Minnesota

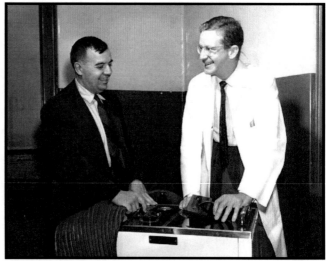

Fig. 23.5 In this 1952 photo, Richard L. Varco (*left*) and F. John Lewis stand behind the hypothermia machine that they used during the world's first successful open-heart surgery

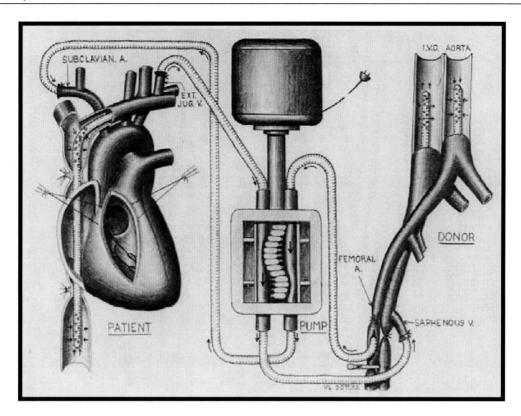

Fig. 23.6 Diagram of cross-circulation

the time and was considered as a major breakthrough that motivated numerous innovations in the area of open-heart surgery [3]. The thought of taking a normal healthy human being into the operating room to provide donor circulation was considered unacceptable and even immoral by some critics. The risks to the donors were: (1) blood incompatibility; (2) infection; (3) air embolism; and/or (4) blood volume imbalance. It should be noted that cross-circulation exists between a mother and her fetus.

From March 1955 onward, three additional bypass methods were introduced and successfully used, including: (1) perfusion from a reservoir of arterialized blood; (2) heterologous (dog) lungs as an oxygenator; and (3) the DeWall–Lillehei disposable bubble oxygenator [2]. Yet, many believe that the single most important discovery that contributed to the success of clinical open-heart operations was the realization of the vast discrepancy between the total body flow rate *thought* necessary and what was *actually* necessary. Lillehei and his team are credited with applying the findings of two British surgeons (Andreasen and Watson) who identified the "azygos factor"—the ability of dogs to survive up to 40 min without brain damage when all blood flow was stopped except through the azygos vein. Specifically, Morley Cohen and Lillehei hypothesized that when

blood flow was low, the blood vessels dilated to receive a larger share of the blood, while the tissues absorbed a much higher proportion of the oxygen as compared to normal circulation [2]. Previously, it was thought that basal or resting cardiac output at 100–160 ml/kg/min was safe maintenance during cardiopulmonary bypass. The azygos flow studies showed that 8–14 ml/kg/min maintained the physiological integrity of the "vital centers," but Lillehei added a margin of safety and set his basic perfusion rate at 25–30 ml/kg/min. This approach reduced excessive complications of blood loss, excessive hemolysis, abnormal bleeding, and/or renal shutdown [2].

Altogether, 45 patients (aged 5 months to 10 years) underwent open-heart surgery with cross-circulation at the university; prior to this surgery, these patients had lesions that were considered hopelessly unrepairable. Of this group, 49% of the patients lived to be long-term survivors (greater than 30 years) and lead normal productive lives; 11 of the female long-term survivors subsequently gave birth to a total of 25 children who were free from any congenital heart defects. In addition, all 45 donors survived, with only one donor experiencing a major complication.

It should be noted that during this period of time, an intense competition/collaborative relationship existed with the Mayo Clinic, the only other primary site where

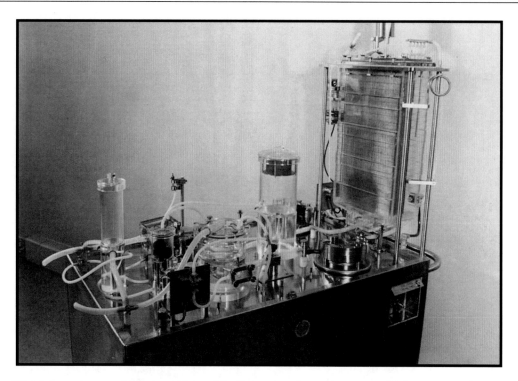

Fig. 23.7 Mayo Clinic's heart–lung machine was as big as a Wurlitzer organ; it cost thousands of dollars and required great skill to operate

open-heart surgery was being performed. Lillehei recalled in his interview to G. Wayne Miller (author of *King of Hearts*) that the Mayo Clinic operated 7 days a week, so on Saturdays when Lillehei's team was not scheduled for surgery, they would travel to the Mayo Clinic and watch Dr. John Kirklin and his colleagues (Miller, G.W., Transcriptions of audio tapes for *King of Hearts*, University of Minnesota Archives) [4]. Dr. Kirklin was successfully using a modification of the Gibbon heart–lung machine and, after observing his achievements, Lillehei began a slow transition away from cross-circulation and toward using a heart–lung machine of his own design (Fig. 23.7). In the beginning, Lillehei used the heart–lung machine for simpler, more straightforward cases and continued using cross-circulation for the more complicated cases. Although its clinical use was short-lived, cross-circulation is still considered today as an important stepping stone in the development of cardiac surgery.

23.3 Lillehei–DeWall Bubble Oxygenator

Importantly, John Gibbon, MD, from Boston, invented the cardiopulmonary bypass procedure and performed the first intracardiac repair using extracorporeal perfusion in 1953. His bubble oxygenator, which looked surprisingly like a computer, was manufactured and financed by IBM. His reported achievements stimulated rapid development of the knowledge base and equipment necessary for both accurate diagnoses of cardiac disease and successful intracardiac operations. Yet, at that time, it was recognized that the main problems with film oxygenators were: (1) poor efficiency; (2) excessive hemolysis; (3) large priming volumes; and (4) the development of bubbles and foam in the blood. All designs required blood flows of 2.2 $l/m^2/min$, usually three to four units of blood for priming, and another two units for the rest of the circuit. Furthermore, after each use, the machine had to be broken down, washed, rinsed in hemolytic solution, reassembled, resterilized, and reconfigured.

During this era, Richard DeWall came to work at the University of Minnesota as an animal attendant in Lillehei's research laboratory. It was noted that DeWall would manage the pump while the anesthesiologists would take breaks, and soon he began to take an interest in the problems associated with oxygenating blood. Eventually, Lillehei challenged DeWall to find a way to eliminate bubbles in the oxygenator procedure. Importantly, DeWall brought to fruition a dramatic technological breakthrough in 1955 by developing the first bubble oxygenator with a unique method for removing bubbles from the freshly oxygenated blood (Fig. 23.8). In DeWall's design, blood entered the bottom of a tall cylinder along with oxygen passed through sintered glass to create

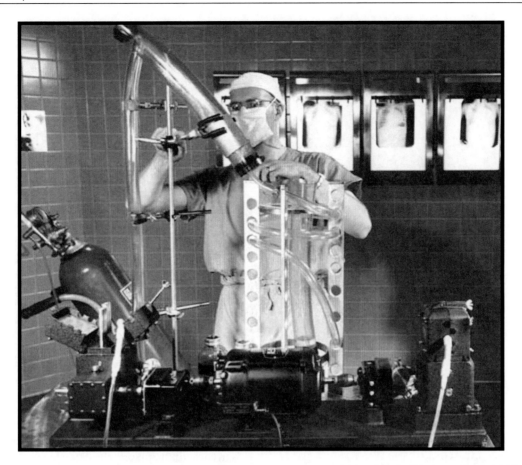

Fig. 23.8 University of Minnesota's bubble oxygenator cost $15 and was easy to use. Richard DeWall is shown here with his model in 1955

bubbles. As the bubbles and blood rose, gas exchange occurred at the surface of each bubble. At the top of the cylinder, arterialized bubble-rich blood passed over stainless steel wool coated with silicone antifoam; it then traveled through a long helical settling coil to allow bubbles to slowly rise and exit the blood.

Two important components in the "Lillehei–DeWall bubble oxygenator" were the tubing and the silicon antifoam solution. The tubing was Mayon polyethylene tubing (typically used in the dairy and beer industries and specifically in the production of mayonnaise), available from Mayon Plastics, a company whose CEO was a classmate of Lillehei's and a graduate of the university's chemical engineering program. The silicone antifoam solution, Antifoam A, was used to coat the tubing to prevent foaming of the liquids being transported.

The oxygenator was wonderfully efficient; animals (and later patients) did not show detectable effects of residual gas emboli. More importantly, this design eventually led to the development of a plastic, prepackaged, disposable, sterile oxygenator that replaced the expensive stainless steel, labor-intensive screen and film devices. An economic and reliable oxygenator had arrived and the medical industry began to think about disposable components for the heart–lung machine.

Two years after its introduction, the DeWall–Lillehei bubble oxygenator had been used in 350 open-heart operations at the University of Minnesota. DeWall steadily improved the device through three models, but it remained a very simple, disposable, heat-sterilizable device that could be built to accommodate only the amount of blood required for each patient and then discarded.

In 1956, another one of Lillehei's residents, Vincent Gott, developed a bubble oxygenator in which DeWall's helix design was flattened and enclosed between two heat-sealed plastic sheets (Fig. 23.9). This sheet bubble oxygenator proved to be the key to subsequent widespread acceptance of the device in open-heart surgery, because it could be easily manufactured and distributed in a sterile package, and it was inexpensive enough to be disposable. The University of Minnesota eventually licensed the rights to manufacture and sell the device to Travenol, Inc. With the bubble oxygenator and techniques developed by Lillehei and his colleagues, the University of Minnesota had become prominent for making the open-heart surgery possible and relatively safe [5].

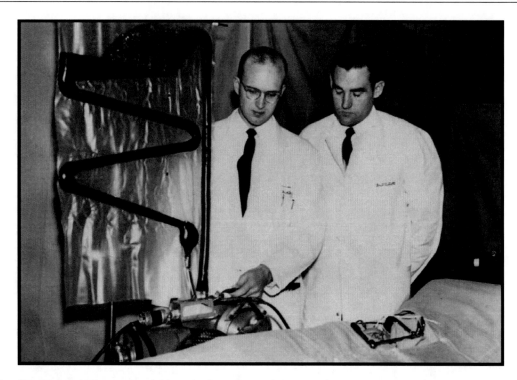

Fig. 23.9 Richard DeWall and Vincent Gott look at the first commercially manufactured sterile bubble oxygenator in 1956

23.4 Heart Block and the Development of the Pacemaker

An unexpected clinical consequence of the development of open-heart surgery was the discovery of a revolutionary new concept for treatment of complete "heart block." Heart block is typically defined as the inability of electrical impulses that begin high in the right atrium to reach the ventricles. Deprived of their normal signal, the ventricles may beat slowly on their own (escape rhythm) or not at all; any prolonged decrease in heart rate that limits a patient's normal activity typically results in heart failure. At that time, with the only existing treatment for complete block being positive chronotropic drugs or electrodes applied to the surface of the chest, there were no 30-day survivors.

Fortunately, in 1952, Paul Zoll, a cardiologist in Boston, invented the first pacemaker unit, which was a large tabletop external unit with a chest electrode. It was successfully used to resuscitate patients in the hospital, but required the transcutaneous delivery of 50–150 V, which was incredibly painful for children and typically left scarring blisters.

Complete heart block developed in more than 10% of Dr. Lillehei's early patients undergoing closure of ventricular septal defects (e.g., due to induced injury of the heart's conduction system by stitches), and hospital mortality was 100% in this group of patients. Early fatality

from heart block was completely eliminated with the use of a myocardially placed electrode in combination with an external plug-in electric stimulator [6]. This method of treatment, suggested by Dr. John A. Johnson, a professor of physiology at the University of Minnesota, required electrical stimuli of small magnitude (5–10 mA) and provided very effective control of the heart rate. Such an approach was almost painless, but it used an AC electrical source, thus limiting the mobility of the patient to the length of the extension cord employed. It was first used by Dr. Lillehei on a patient on January 30, 1957; subsequently, an 89% survival rate for patients with prior heart block was reported. More specifically, the pacemaker approach employed a multistrand, braided stainless steel wire in a Teflon sleeve that was directly implanted into the ventricular myocardium, with the other end brought through the surgical wound and attached to external stimulation. The pacemaker (pulse generator) was a Grass physiological stimulator borrowed from the university's Physiology Department. This procedure was designed for short-term pacing, with removal of the wires 1–2 weeks after the heart regained a consistent rhythm.

The surgical operating rooms in the 1950s were equipped with EKG and pressure-monitoring devices, and the vacuum tubes required frequent monitoring and maintenance to keep them running and calibrated. Hence, the University Hospital contracted a local electric equipment repair company, Medtronic Inc., to perform these tasks. It is reported that, following a disaster during which all electrical power service failed in the University Hospital due to a storm (October 31, 1957), Lillehei asked Medtronic's medical equipment expert, Earl Bakken, to design a battery-powered, wearable pacemaker to avoid heart block due to power failures and improve the patient's mobility. Bakken began this work in 1957, using a circuit modified from a diagram for a transistorized metronome from *Popular Electrons* as a model (Fig. 23.10). During this period, Bakken spent numerous hours working in the operating rooms alongside Lillehei, and they became great friends.

On April 14, 1958, the battery-powered wearable pacemaker was first used clinically, even though this was somewhat unplanned. Bakken's transistor pulse generator made a miraculous "overnight" transition from bench testing to clinical use. Bakken brought his first prototype to the Surgery Department's research lab, where researchers used it on an animal with an imposed heart block and it functioned as planned. Excited by this progress, Bakken went home for the evening; that night, Lillehei worked late in the hospital and paid a visit to the laboratory where he observed the battery-powered pacemaker performing well, and he took it off the animal and brought it upstairs to use it on a patient. The next day, when Bakken arrived back at the hospital, he was overwhelmed to see this device keeping a young child's heart beating.

It was this wearable, battery-powered invention that set the stage for further development in the cardiac pacing industry. For the next decade or so, it would become common practice to put new devices or prototypes (even fully implantable ones) into clinical use immediately and then iron out the imperfections later based on accumulation of clinical experience. This humanitarian practice developed because most of the early patients were close to death, and no other treatments existed [7]. Eventually, Medtronic, Inc., under Bakken's leadership, became the world's leading manufacturer of cardiac pacemakers beginning with the model 5800.

The first model of the 5800 pacemaker was black, but was quickly changed to white to look cleaner, more sanitary, or "hospital-like" (Fig. 23.11). Between 1959 and 1964, only a few hundred pacemakers were sold due to the reusability of the pacemaker and the short-term post-surgery focus; orders soared once the pacemaker became implantable and redefined for long-term pacing use (Fig. 23.12). Nevertheless, the 5800 pacemaker became

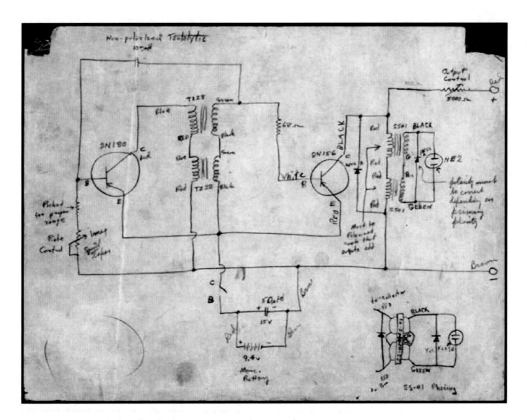

Fig. 23.10 Earl Bakken's original design for the battery-operated pacemaker

A
B

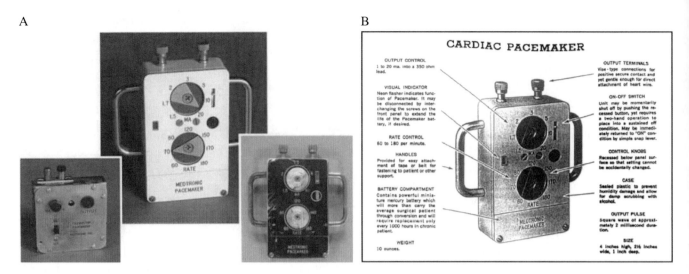

Fig. 23.11 (**A**) The first pacemaker prototype (*left*), the "Black Box" 5800 external pacemaker (the preliminary test model; *right*), and the "White Box" 5800 production model (*center*). (**B**) A page from the Medtronic catalog advertising the 5800 pacemaker

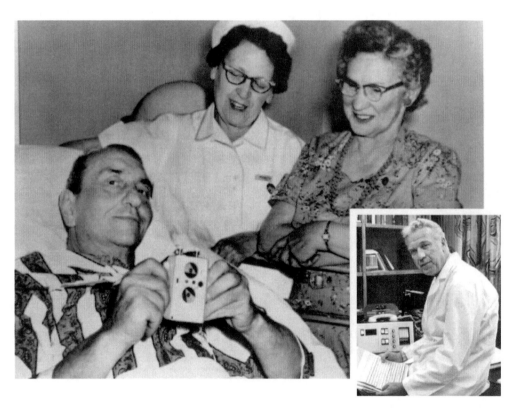

Fig. 23.12 Dr. Samuel Hunter (*inset*) and adult-pacing patient Warren Mauston. Dr. Hunter and Medtronic engineer Norman Roth developed a bipolar electrode that represented a major advance in pacing technology. First implanted in 1959, the Hunter–Roth lead helped contribute 7 years of life to a Stokes–Adams disease patient, Warren Mauston, in 1960

the symbol for Medtronic's shared belief in medical progress through technology; this was celebrated during an unveiling of a bronze statue of Earl Bakken holding the 5800 pacemaker at his retirement celebration in 1994. Years later, the 5800 was viewed by Lillehei as a technological watershed—it fostered interdisciplinary collaboration and exemplified the marriage of medicine and technology, long-lasting friendships, and mutual respect.

Both Lillehei and Bakken have named Professorships at the University of Minnesota. In addition, the Lillehei

Heart Institute was created at the university in 2002 to honor the past with a C. Walton Lillehei Museum while supporting the future through its Lillehei Scholar Program. The Lillehei Heart Institute is an interdisciplinary research institute within the Academic Health Center and Medical School, made possible by a generous gift from Kaye Lillehei, wife of C. Walton Lillehei. Dr. Daniel Garry, chief of the Cardiovascular Division of Medicine, was named director of the Lillehei Heart Institute in 2007, and Dr. Herbert Ward, current chief of Cardiothoracic Surgery, holds the position of associate director.

In December 2007, at a celebration of the 50th anniversary of the wearable, battery-powered pacemaker, the University of Minnesota awarded Earl Bakken with a honorary M.D. degree (Fig. 23.13). In the same month, the university's Department of Surgery hosted the "First Annual Bakken Surgical Device Symposium" to celebrate this legacy. Numerous key individuals joined this symposium (entitled "The Pacemaker: Past, Present, and Future") to speak about the history, current applications, and future direction of pacemaker

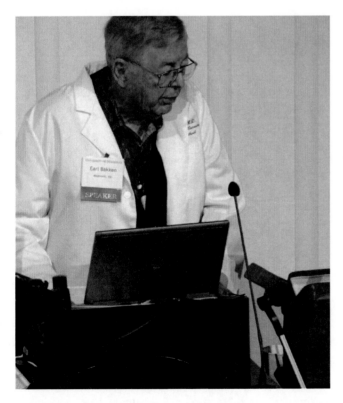

Fig. 23.13 Earl Bakken, the founder of Medtronic Inc., received a honorary M.D. degree from the University of Minnesota in 2007. He is shown here with his M.D. white coat and medical bag, presenting his historic prospective lecture at the "First Annual Bakken Surgical Device Symposium," hosted by the Department of Surgery at the University of Minnesota on December 13, 2007

technology, including Drs. Earl Bakken, Vincent Gott, Samuel Hunter, and David Benditt (Figs 23.9, 23.12, and 23.13).

23.5 Heart Valves

Initial development in the field of prosthetic heart valves involved the search for biologically compatible materials and hemologically tolerant designs; it is considered today that early successes could not have been achieved without the union of these two factors. At that time, as there was no satisfactory mechanism to scientifically achieve this goal, the trial-and-error method was used and much of this work was performed at the University of Minnesota. The development of prosthetic heart valves became the purview of numerous cardiovascular surgeons who often collaborated with engineers; to distinguish one valve from the others, each prosthesis often became identified and named after its surgeon developer [8].

It is notable that Lillehei and his colleagues developed four different valves: (1) a nontilting disc valve called the Lillehei–Nakib toroidal valve in 1967; (2) two tilting disc valves, the Lillehei–Cruz–Kaster in 1963 and the Lillehei–Kaster in 1970 (produced by Medical, Inc. in 1970 and eventually distributed by Medtronic, Inc. in 1974); and (3) a bileaflet valve, the Lillehei–Kalke in 1965 (manufactured by Surgitool in 1968 and used clinically by Dr. Lillehei at the New York Cornell Medical Center) (Fig. 23.14).

The St. Jude bileaflet valve was primarily designed by Chris Posis, an industrial engineer who approached Demetre Nicoloff, MD, a cardiovascular surgeon at the University of Minnesota. This valve had floating hinges located near the central axis of the rigid housing as well as an opening to the outer edge of each leaflet, leaving a small central opening (Fig. 23.15) [9]. Nicoloff first implanted this valve in October 1977, and it provided the foundation for the beginning of St. Jude Medical, Inc. Dr. Nicoloff was asked to serve as the medical director of the new company; however, he declined due to the demands of his clinical practice. Rather, he suggested that Dr. C.W. Lillehei become the medical director, a post that Lillehei held until his death in 1999 [8].

It is important to note that most of these past valve designs, as well as current designs, were evaluated in animal trials at the University of Minnesota. More specifically, Richard Bianco, director of Experimental Surgical Services, has been at the university for over 30 years working with a core of clinicians, scientists, and engineers

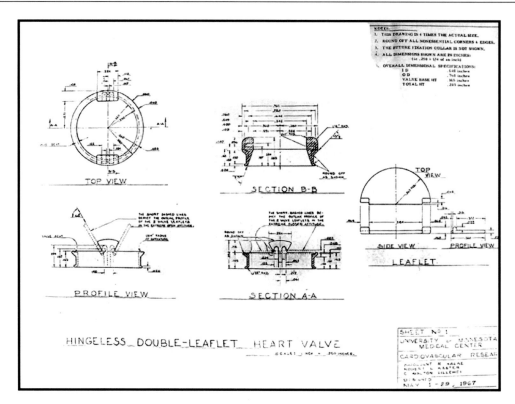

Fig. 23.14 The Lillehei–Kalke rigid bileaflet prosthesis (1968)

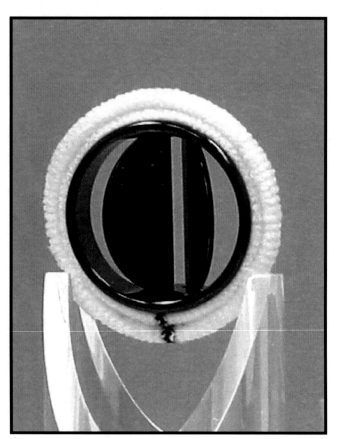

Fig. 23.15 St. Jude bileaflet prosthesis developed in 1976

on their designs, evaluations, and redesigns. For more details on such experimental trials, refer to Chapter 25. It should also be noted that Bianco organized the Second Annual Bakken Surgical Device Symposium, with the topic being "Heart Valves: Past, Present, and Future."

23.6 Other University-Affiliated Medical Devices

Many of the major breakthroughs in cardiac device development at the University of Minnesota occurred via associated collaborations with the Surgery Department. In more recent times, several more cardiovascular medical devices have been invented in areas other than the Department of Surgery, specifically the Departments of Medicine and Radiology. Examples of such devices and technologies include: (1) the compression/decompression cardiopulmonary resuscitation devices (Chapter 35); and (2) transcatheter closure devices, which are permanent cardiac implants designed to close defects between chambers of the heart (Chapter 34). The latter devices are self-expanding, self-centering umbrella-like devices whose design and shape varies, as does the exact mode of their deployment. They are implanted in the heart through catheters inserted into either the artery or vein in a cardiac catheterization laboratory. Transcatheter closure devices are intended to provide a less invasive alternative to open-heart surgery, which has been the standard of care.

23.7 FDA Regulates Medical Devices

Earl Bakken adopted the motto of his friend and colleague, Dr. Lillehei, for his initial method of device development—"Ready, Fire, Aim." In other words, devices were actually tested in humans; therefore, the transition from bench to bedside happened at an accelerated pace [7]. However, in 1976, the Medical Device Amendment to the Federal Food, Drug, and Cosmetic Act established three regulatory classes for medical devices, based upon the degree of control necessary to assure the safety and effectiveness of various types of devices. The most regulated devices are considered Class III which, by definition: (1) are devices designed to support or sustain human life; (2) are of substantial importance in preventing impairment of human health; or (3) present a potential unreasonable risk of illness or injury. All devices placed into Class III are subject to premarket approval requirements, including a scientific review to ensure the safety and effectiveness of the devices.

Under Medical Device Reporting in the FDA, all manufacturers, importers, and user facilities are required to report adverse events and correct them quickly. Although, since 1984, manufacturers and importers of medical devices have been required to report all device-related deaths, serious injuries, and certain malfunctions to the FDA, numerous reports show underreporting. Therefore, the Safe Medical Devices Act (SMDA) of 1990 was implemented; device user facilities must report device-related deaths to the FDA and the manufacturer. In addition, the SMDA requires that device user facilities submit reports to the FDA on an annual basis (FDA Modernization Act of 1998). In the past several years, recalls of defective pacing systems and leads have had a major effect on the medical device industry in the United States, resulting in dramatic shifts within the vitally affiliated companies.

23.8 LifeScience Alley

Spurred by the flurry of innovations from Minnesota inventors such as the pacemaker, bubble oxygenator, and artificial heart valve, Medical Alley was founded in 1984 as a nonprofit trade association to support the region's growing health care industry. "Medical Alley" recently merged with the Minnesota Biotechnology Industry Organization (MNBIO) and has been renamed "LifeScience Alley," an organization whose mission is to enable business success in the life sciences. LifeScience Alley serves the rich geographic area of health care-related organizations that extend from Duluth through Minneapolis/St. Paul and farther south to Rochester (see www.lifesciencealley.org); its reach has expanded beyond the Minnesota border into Canada, Wisconsin, Iowa, Illinois, and the Dakotas as well. This expanded territory is home to over 800 medical device manufacturers and thousands of health care-related organizations, making it one of the highest concentrations of businesses in this industry in the world.

LifeScience Alley was founded by Earl Bakken who pioneered the implantable pacemaker business through his company, Medtronic Inc., in the 1960s. Bakken remains on the LifeScience Alley Board of Directors to this day, and Don Gerhardt currently presides over the association. LifeScience Alley is a Minneapolis-based trade association that currently represents a membership of more than 500 health care-related companies and organizations. Its cohorts include a wide cross-section of businesses in the life sciences, including medical device and equipment manufacturers, agricultural and industrial bioscience organizations, pharmaceutical companies, health plans, insurers, hospitals and clinics, education and research institutions, government agencies and trade organizations, and a number of health-care services and consulting partners.

In 2001, LifeScience Alley announced a structural change that launched two "spin-off organizations"—Alley Institute and Alley Ventures. Alley Institute is a nonprofit affiliate that was created to directly address public health concerns. Its four core functions include the following:

1. Convener initiatives—gather broad expertise in the health care industry (i.e., payers, consumers, providers, manufacturers, other parties) to debate and develop creative solutions for key challenges such as measuring the cost-effectiveness of health care, helping the community understand how to address the fragmented health care system, encouraging more students to pursue health care careers to resolve the workforce shortage in the life science industry, or searching for options to improve end-of-life care.
2. Education—offer comprehensive continuing education programs for affiliates; additionally, interest groups meet monthly to learn about clinical studies, research and development, reimbursement, marketing, regulatory affairs, and manufacturing/quality issues in the life sciences arena.
3. Workforce development—cultivate new talent by offering scholarships in the life sciences (from undergraduate academic and technical classes to professional and graduate education) and develop programs

to expose young people to career options (i.e., internships, fellowships).

4. Research—commit to research efforts in the area of life sciences; for example, the Minnesota Palliative Care partnership, administered through Alley Institute, is currently working with a large self-insured organization to define a care model and finance model geared toward providing a palliative care benefit for employees.

The second "spin-off" organization, Alley Ventures, addresses the lack of early stage funding for emerging companies in the fields of medical technology, bioscience, and life sciences. Early stage funding is critical to getting innovative ideas launched, and Alley Ventures would like to be instrumental in accelerating the market entry and growth of portfolio companies. To achieve this end, the Alley Ventures Fund I was developed as a seed and early stage venture capital fund which is currently in the initial fund-raising stage.

Furthermore, LifeScience Alley is active in state legislative lobbying, informing public policy makers about the impact of Minnesota's thriving life sciences industry and supporting proposals to support growth of the life sciences industry. For example, in the 2008 Minnesota legislative session, LifeScience Alley worked with government affairs consultants to support proposals for a fast-track process to construct new bioscience labs, funding for college science/health-related facilities, stem cell research at the University of Minnesota, an investment tax credit for early stage companies, and initiatives that provide employers and individual purchasers with greater choice and flexibility in health care products, increased competition, and enhanced quality to control costs.

The year 2008 marks the seventh year that LifeScience Alley, in collaboration with the University of Minnesota's Biomedical Engineering Institute, has sponsored a poster session to showcase current biomedical engineering research. Graduates share posters, medical device prototypes, and bioengineering innovations on topics ranging from tissue engineering to cellular bioengineering to medical devices and diagnostic techniques. This interactive forum allows for dialogue and potential collaboration between students and industry professionals.

23.9 The Annual Design of Medical Device Conference at the University of Minnesota

The University of Minnesota's Institute for Engineering in Medicine, the Institute of Technology, the Academic Health Center, the Office of the President, and the Department of Mechanical Engineering hosted the eighth Annual Design of Medical Devices (DMD) Conference in April 2009. This annual conference includes 2 days of technical and clinical sessions and a 1-day Annual President's 21st Century Interdisciplinary Conference. The primary goals of this 3-day conference are to: (1) promote the medical device industry; (2) provide a forum to bring medical device designers, manufacturers, researchers, and representatives from the public sector together to share perspectives on medical devices; and (3) raise funds from corporate sponsorships to endow graduate fellowships in medical device design. The conference has grown to over 1000 participants from 12 different countries and 70 different companies or academic institutions.

23.10 The Institute for Engineering in Medicine and Center for Medical Devices

23.10.1 Institute for Engineering in Medicine

The Institute for Engineering in Medicine (IEM), which is jointly sponsored by the University's Institute of Technology and the Medical School, replaces the former Biomedical Engineering Institute. The primary mission of the IEM is to: (1) foster and support interdisciplinary research to solve medical problems or improve medical care for patients through engineering; (2) enhance university and industry relationships by identifying and fostering appropriate partnerships; and (3) leverage the strengths and expertise of affiliates for the benefit of Minnesota citizens. To date, the IEM has named associate directors of research, education, and outreach and has supported many successful collaborative research projects via its novel "What if" medical device idea campaign. This program is an initiative designed to encourage faculty from University of Minnesota Health Sciences and Institute of Technology to consider new or enhanced approaches to medical device design.

23.10.2 Center for Medical Devices

Under the direction of Professor Arthur Erdman, a new "Medical Devices Center" (MDC) was established by the University of Minnesota in 2006. The primary goal of this center is to strengthen interdisciplinary research among faculty in the health sciences field and engineering, specifically related to medical devices. The MDC has new core facilities, which include: (1) a computer aided design (CAD)/precision instrumentation laboratory;

(2) an electronic fabrication laboratory; (3) a mechanical prototyping facility; (4) a testing room—wet laboratory; (5) an anatomy–physiology SimPortal laboratory; and (6) a multipurpose room for modeling, assembly, demonstrations, or conferences. Recently, the MDC initiated a Fellows Program to recruit and hire four individuals across the medical engineering and clinical disciplines to form a functional team to develop novel medical technologies. In addition, as a subdivision of the MDC, Erdman leads the university's new Minimally Invasive Medical Technologies Center (MIMTeC), a National Science Foundation Industry/University Cooperative Research Center providing translational research that will enable medical device companies to bring the next generation of minimally invasive medical technologies to market.

23.11 Cardiovascular Physiology at the University of Minnesota

The Department of Physiology at the University of Minnesota has a rich history of performing basic cardiovascular research and establishing clinical collaborations within the institution. Not only have these individuals published many important basic research papers, but they have also been integrally involved in the training of many generations of cardiac physiologists, surgeons, and biomedical engineers.

One of the more notable chairmen of the Department of Physiology was Maurice Visscher, who was present during the Owen Wangensteen and C. Walton Lillehei eras. In 1936, Dr. Visscher returned to the University of Minnesota to succeed Dean Lyon as the head of physiology (Table 23.3). He first came to Minnesota in 1922 as a graduate student in physiology under the mentorship of Frederick Scott and satisfied the requirements for both Ph.D. and M.D. degrees in a 4-year period of time [10]. Interestingly, subsequent to his studies, Visscher served as a postdoctoral fellow in England at the University College London. While there, he worked under the advisement of the notable cardiac physiologist, Ernest Starling who, at that time, was near the end of his brilliant career (e.g., "Starlings law of the heart"). Together, in 1927, Starling and Visscher published a classic paper in which, using a heart–lung preparation (introduced by Starling in 1910), they reported that the oxygen consumption of the heart was correlated directly with its volume in diastole, without regard to the amount of work the heart was exerting in pumping blood [11, 12]. After Starling's death in 1927, Visscher continued research on this topic while serving as the Physiology Department chairman in Minnesota; his research was considered to shed valuable light on the mechanisms underlying heart disease due to coronary occlusion, in general. It has been described that Owen Wangensteen, having recognized how many of these findings were directly applicable to surgery, initiated collaborations with Visscher and the Physiology Department. To this extent, Wangensteen even initiated and conducted a regular "Physiology–Surgery Conference" that was considered "invaluable in acquainting surgical residents with the techniques of experimental physiology" [12]. Many also credit Wangensteen's academic philosophies for enabling the pioneering advancements in open-heart surgery and subsequent pacemaker technologies at the University of Minnesota. For example, Earl Bakken asked C. Walton Lillehei in 1997, "How did you have the courage to go ahead with these pioneering-type experiments?" Lillehei replied, "As I think, when I look back, that was part of the Wangensteen training system" [13]. He further elaborated, "[Wangensteen] was a unique person in many regards. One [aspect of his] uniqueness was his training system. He had a great faith in research, animal or other types of laboratory research. He felt that the results of his research gave the young investigator the courage to challenge accepted beliefs and go forward, which you would not have had, as I look back, as a young surgical resident. That's why many of the great universities didn't produce much in the way of innovative research, because they were so steeped in tradition. Wangensteen had a wide open mind. If research showed some value, then you should pursue it."

Table 23.3 Department of Physiology at the University of Minnesota: Chairs/Interim Heads

Physiology Department chair/interim head	Position	Years served
Richard O. Beard	Department chair	1889–1913
Elias P. Lyon	Department chair	1913–1936
Dr. Maurice B. Visscher	Department chair	1936–1968
Eugene Grim	Department chair	1968–1986
Richard E. Poppele	Interim head	1986–1988
Robert F. Miller	Department chair	1988–1998
Joseph DiSalvo	Interim head	1998–2002
Douglas Wangensteen	Interim head	2002–2008
Joseph M. Metzger	Department chair	2008–present

Table 23.4 Partial list of University of Minnesota physiologists (faculty and adjuncts) whose research is related to the cardiovascular area

Investigators	Era	Topics
Maurice Visscher	1930s	Coronary blood flow, oxygen delivery rate, and cardiac performance; autoregulation of coronary blood flow; medical research and ethics
Mead Cavert	1970s to 1980s	Clinical cardiology
Marvin Bacaner	1960s to 1990s	Antiarrhythmic, antifibrillatory, and hemodynamic actions of bethanidine sulfate
Irwin J. Fox	1970s to 1980s	Assessment of regional myocardial blood flows; arterial dilution curves
Victor Lorber	1950s to 1970s	Cellular junctions in the tunicate heart; regulation of energy liberation in the isolated heart
Michael Hoey	1980s to 2002	Cardiac ablation
Joseph DiSalvo	1990s to 2005	Chronic A–V block; properties and function of phosphatases from vascular smooth muscle
Steven Katz	1990s to present	The renin/angiotensin system and the failing heart
Paul Iaizzo	1990s to present	Intercardiac imaging within large mammalian isolated hearts
Robert Bache	2000s to present	Cardiac energetics
John Osborn	1990s to present	Autonomic response and the cardiovascular system; pathophysiology of hypertension
Scott O'Grady	1990s to present	Electrolyte transport in epithelia
Doris Taylor	2003 to present	Cardiac repair and regeneration
Joseph M. Metzger	2008 to present	Gene therapies for cardiovascular diseases
Daniel Sigg	2008 to present	Ischemic protection and biologics

The University of Minnesota has a rich history of basic and applied cardiac research. Noted in Table 23.4 are several of the physiologists who had full or adjunct appointments in the Physiology Department and worked on topics relevant to the cardiovascular system; these physiologists published many papers and/or served as advisors for numerous theses. Interestingly, the past few years have brought a renewed interest in refocusing the Physiology Department to again be a leader in the cardiovascular field. For example, the department has created novel educational outreach programs for the local cardiovascular industry and, just recently, added Professor Joseph M. Metzger as the new head of department which was recently renamed "Department of Integrative Biology and Physiology" (Table 23.3).

Dr. Lillehei believed that "What mankind can dream, research and technology can achieve." And with the support of the Lillehei Heart Institute, in collaboration with the Institute for Engineering in Medicine, the circle has been completed.

23.12 Summary

The University of Minnesota has a rich tradition of research and development in the fields of cardiovascular sciences and medical device design. Today, Minnesota has one of the highest densities of medical device companies in the world, and thus the university remains uniquely positioned to: (1) educate the next generation of employees for this industry; (2) be a strong academic collaborator to this industry by being an international leader in both basic and clinical cardiovascular research; and (3) serve the additional outreach mission of the university relative to cardiovascular sciences (e.g., partnering with Life-Science Alley and other such organizations). The rich legacy of the early pioneers in cardiovascular research, medicine, and surgery lives on at the University of Minnesota.

Acknowledgments We would like to thank Dee McManus for her assistance with this text and Karen Larsen at Medtronic for providing us with various photos.

References

1. Lillehei CW. The birth of open heart surgery: Then the golden years. Cardiovasc Surg 1994;2:308–17.
2. Lillehei CW, et al. The first open heart repairs of ventricular septal defect, atrioventricular communis, and Tetralogy of Fallot using extracorporeal circulation by cross-circulation. Ann Thorac Surg 1986;41:4–21.
3. Lillehei CW. A personalized history of extracorporeal circulation. Trans Am Soc Artif Intern Organs 1982;28:5–16.
4. Miller GW. King of hearts. New York, NY: Crown Publishers, 2000.
5. Moore M. The genesis of Minnesota's Medical Alley. UMN Medical Foundation Bulletin, Winter 1992.
6. Gott VL. Critical role of physiologist John A. Johnson in the origins of Minnesota's billion dollar pacemaker industry. Ann Thorac Surg 2007;83:349–53.
7. Rhees D, Jeffrey K. Earl Bakken's little white box: The complex meanings of the first transistorized pacemaker. In: Finn B, ed. Exposing electronics. Amsterdam, The Netherlands: Harwood Academic Publishers, 2000.
8. DeWall R. Evolution of mechanical heart valves. Ann Thorac Surg 2000;69:1612–21.
9. Villafana M. It will never work! The St. Jude valve. Ann Thorac Surg 1989;48:S53–4.

10. Visscher MB. A half century in science and society. Annu Rev Physiol 1969;1017:1–18.

11. Starling EH, Visscher MB. The regulation of the energy output of the heart. J Physiol Lond 1927;62:243–61.

12. Wilson LG, ed. Medical revolution in Minnesota: A history of the University of Minnesota Medical School. St. Paul, MN: Midewiwin Press, 1989.

13. Pioneers of the medical device industry in Minnesota: An oral history project, Earl E. Bakken and Dr. C. Walton Lillehei. Minnesota Historical Society Oral History Office, David Rhees (Interviewer), Minnesota Historical Society, 2002.

Additional Resources

U.S. Food and Drug Administration, Center for Devices and Radiological Health, website: www.fda.gov/opacom/7org.html

LifeScience Alley website: www.lifesciencealley.org

Rigby M. The era of transcatheter closure of atrial septal defects. Heart 1999;81:227–8.

Stephenson L, ed. State of the heart: The practical guide to your heart and heart surgery. Fort Lauderdale, FL: Write Stuff Syndicate, Inc., 1999.

Chapter 24
Pharmacotherapy for Cardiac Diseases

Anna Legreid Dopp and J. Jason Sims

Abstract Clinical trial design requires inclusion criteria that patients be on optimal medical therapy prior to enrollment or randomization, meaning that they are on medical regimens proven to be safe and effective and considered a standard in clinical practice for the particular disease state being studied. Only then can any clinical or statistical significance be determined between study groups. This chapter outlines optimal medical therapies for hypertension, acute coronary syndrome, myocardial infarction, heart failure, and/or arrhythmias.

Keywords Diuretics · Beta blockers · Angiotensin-converting enzyme inhibitors · Angiotensin receptor blockers · Calcium channel blockers · Antiplatelets · Anticoagulants · Aldosterone antagonists

24.1 Introduction

Chronic diseases claim seven out of ten or 1.7 million American lives every year and cause significant limitations on activities of daily living for nearly 90 million individuals [1]. Importantly, heart disease is considered as a chronic disease that is also the leading cause of death in the United States, accounting for 700,000 deaths annually or roughly 29% of all deaths [2]. Today, the most common form of heart disease is coronary heart disease (CHD), which occurs in 16 million Americans over the age of 20 years [3]; primary risk factors for CHD are listed in Table 24.1. This chapter will provide general pharmacotherapy treatment guidelines for the management of the following cardiac diseases: hypertension, acute coronary syndrome, myocardial infarction, heart failure, and/or arrhythmias.

A.L. Dopp (✉)
University of Wisconsin, 777 Highland Avenue, Madison, WI 58705, USA
e-mail: alegreiddopp@pharmacy.wisc.edu

24.2 Evidence-Based Medicine

In order to describe the drug therapy regimens for the above disease states, there needs to be a brief explanation of how general clinical guidelines are developed and applied. As such, evidence-based medicine is the process of conscientious, explicit, and judicious use of current best evidence in making decisions about the care of an individual patient [4]. Several expert working groups and agencies have developed systems for classifying evidence according to the scientific rigor of the study results available. For the purposes of this chapter, which focuses on pharmacotherapy for cardiac diseases, evidence levels developed by the American College of Cardiology (ACC)/American Heart Association (AHA) clinical data standards [5] will be primarily utilized for the discussion that follows (Table 24.2). In addition to evidence level designations, the ACC and AHA have developed a standardized classification system for recommending treatment regimens for various cardiovascular diseases (Table 24.3). Figure 24.1 is one example that incorporates the levels of evidence and classification of recommendations into one format to designate the estimate of certainty and size of treatment effect for the various standards and clinical guidelines available. For the purposes of this chapter, treatment recommendations will focus primarily on those that have a Class I or IIa classification.

24.3 Hypertension

Left untreated, hypertension will typically ignite a cascade of cardiovascular consequences; it is a leading risk factor for many of the specific cardiovascular diseases discussed in this chapter. Nearly 73 million people in the United States have high blood pressure [3], defined as systolic blood pressure >140 mmHg and diastolic blood pressure >90 mmHg and/or someone under treatment

P.A. Iaizzo (ed.), *Handbook of Cardiac Anatomy, Physiology, and Devices*, DOI 10.1007/978-1-60327-372-5_24,
© Springer Science+Business Media, LLC 2009

Table 24.1 Risk factors for coronary heart disease

Risk factor	Monitoring parameter	Statistic/supporting data
Increasing age	Men ≥ 55 years Women ≥ 65 years	83% of people who die of CHD are ≥65 years old
Heredity/family history	Primary male relative with first event before the age of 55 years; Primary female relative with first event before the age of 65 years	Primary refers to parent, child, or sibling
Smoking history	Any history of tobacco use	Risk of CHD is two to four times higher in smokers
Cholesterol	Elevated total cholesterol or LDL; Low HDL cholesterol	LDL goal ≤100 mg/dL if history of an event, diabetes, or presence of 2+ risk factors
High blood pressure/ hypertension	≥140/90 mmHg; On antihypertensive therapy	Goals of blood pressure will vary depending on presence of renal insufficiency or diabetes
Diabetes mellitus	Type 1 or Type 2	Considered a direct risk factor for CHD
Physical inactivity	Less than 30 min of activity the majority days of the week	Inactive lifestyle considered a risk factor
Obesity	Body mass index (BMI)* ≥30	Overweight = BMI of 25–29.9 Normal = BMI of 18.5–24.9 Underweight = BMI of <18.5

*BMI formula = [Weight (lb)/(height (in))^2] × 703
CHD = coronary heart disease

Table 24.2 American College of Cardiology/American Heart Association level of evidence designations

Level A	Data derived from multiple *randomized* clinical trials involving a large number of individuals
Level B	Data derived from a limited number of trials involving comparatively small numbers of patients or from well-designed data analysis of *nonrandomized* studies or *observational* data registries
Level C	Consensus of expert opinion was the primary source of recommendation

Table 24.3 American College of Cardiology/American Heart Association classification of recommendations

Class I	Conditions for which there is evidence and/or general agreement that a given procedure or treatment is beneficial, useful, and effective
Class II	Conditions for which there is conflicting evidence and/or a divergence of opinion about the usefulness or effectiveness of a procedure or treatment • Class IIa: Weight of evidence/opinion favors usefulness/efficacy • Class IIb: Usefulness/efficacy is less well established by evidence/opinion
Class III	Conditions for which there is evidence and/or general agreement that a procedure or treatment is not useful or effective and, in some cases, may be harmful

with an antihypertensive medication. Unfortunately, the incidence and prevalence of hypertension is on the rise in men, women, adolescents, and children. In addition, the role that ethnicity plays in the development of hypertension is rightfully gaining more research and clinical attention, e.g., African-Americans develop hypertension earlier in life and have higher average blood pressures than Caucasians [6]. Importantly, persons who are normotensive at the age of 55 years have a 90% lifetime risk of developing hypertension [7].

24.3.1 Goals of Therapy for Hypertension

Left untreated, hypertension can lead to target organ disease of not only the heart but also the cerebrovascular system, peripheral vascular system, kidneys, and/or eyes, eventually leading to consequences such as stroke, transient ischemic attacks, peripheral artery disease, chronic kidney disease, and/or retinopathy. Figure 24.2 illustrates the generally accepted continuum of hypertensive disease and, specifically, its effects on the myocardium.

The Seventh Report of the Joint National Committee on Prevention, Detection, Evaluation, and Treatment of High Blood Pressure [7] has added a "pre-hypertension" classification in an attempt to raise awareness and further prevent the progression to hypertension. Table 24.4 classifies typical blood pressure in adults. The ultimate goal of hypertension prevention and management is to reduce overall morbidity and mortality by achieving and maintaining a systolic blood pressure <140 mmHg and a diastolic blood pressure <90 mmHg. Patients with comorbid conditions, however, will require a greater reduction in blood pressure to prevent further complications of either disease. For example, the clinical management of patients with diabetes mellitus and patients with kidney disease should target a goal of <130/80 mmHg, and in patients with left ventricular dysfunction, one should try to consistently maintain a blood pressure of <120/80 mmHg [8].

24.3.2 Treatment Guidelines for Hypertension

Lifestyle modifications are considered as a key component in the treatment regimen for patients with hypertension.

SIZE OF TREATMENT EFFECT ⟶

	CLASS I *Benefit >>> Risk* Procedure/Treatment **SHOULD** be performed/ administered	CLASS IIa *Benefit >> Risk* *Additional studies with focused objectives needed* **IT IS REASONABLE** to perform procedure/administer treatment	CLASS IIb *Benefit ≥ Risk* *Additional studies with broad objectives needed; additional registry data would be helpful* Procedure/Treatment **MAY BE CONSIDERED**	CLASS III *Risk ≥ Benefit* *No additional studies needed* Procedure/Treatment should **NOT** be performed/administered **SINCE IT IS NOT HELPFUL AND MAY BE HARMFUL**
LEVEL A Multiple (3–5) population risk strata evaluated* General consistency of direction and magnitude of effect	■ Recommendation that procedure or treatment is useful/effective ■ Sufficient evidence from multiple randomized trials or meta-analyses	■ Recommendation in favor of treatment or procedure being useful/effective ■ Some conflicting evidence from multiple randomized trials or meta-analyses	■ Recommendation's usefulness/efficacy less well established ■ Greater conflicting evidence from multiple randomized trials or meta-analyses	■ Recommendation that procedure or treatment is not useful/effective and may be harmful ■ Sufficient evidence from multiple randomized trials or meta-analyses
LEVEL B Limited (2–3) population risk strata evaluated*	■ Recommendation that procedure or treatment is useful/effective ■ Limited evidence from single randomized trial or nonrandomized studies	■ Recommendation in favor of treatment or procedure being useful/effective ■ Some conflicting evidence from single randomized trial or nonrandomized studies	■ Recommendation's usefulness/efficacy less well established ■ Greater conflicting evidence from single randomized trial or nonrandomized studies	■ Recommendation that procedure or treatment is not useful/effective and may be harmful ■ Limited evidence from single randomized trial or nonrandomized studies
LEVEL C Very limited (1–2) population risk strata evaluated*	■ Recommendation that procedure or treatment is useful/effective ■ Only expert opinion, case studies, or standard-of-care	■ Recommendation in favor of treatment or procedure being useful/effective ■ Only diverging expert opinion, case studies, or standard-of-care	■ Recommendation's usefulness/efficacy less well established ■ Only diverging expert opinion, case studies, or standard-of-care	■ Recommendation that procedure or treatment is not useful/effective and may be harmful ■ Only expert opinion, case studies, or standard-of-care
Suggested phrases for writing recommendations†	should is recommended is indicated is useful/effective/beneficial	is reasonable can be useful/effective/beneficial is probably recommended or indicated	may/might be considered may/might be reasonable usefulness/effectiveness is unknown/unclear/uncertain or not well established	is not recommended is not indicated should not is not useful/effective/beneficial may be harmful

(left axis label) ESTIMATE OF CERTAINTY (PRECISION) OF TREATMENT EFFECT

Fig. 24.1 From the American College of Cardiology/American Heart Association, this figure incorporates the levels of evidence and classification of recommendations to designate the estimate of certainty and size of treatment effect for various standards and clinical guidelines available. Reproduced from Circulation, with permission from Lippincott Williams & Wilkins [15, p. e159]

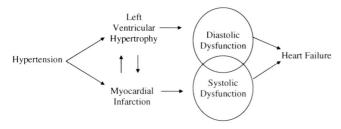

Fig. 24.2 Illustration of the generally accepted continuum of hypertensive disease and its effects on the myocardium

Table 24.4 Classification of blood pressure

Blood pressure classification	Systolic blood pressure (mmHg)		Diastolic blood pressure (mmHg)
Normal	<120	and	<80
Pre-hypertension	120–139	or	80–89
Hypertension			
Stage 1	140–159	or	90–99
Stage 2	≥160	or	≥100

Modifications such as smoking cessation, weight loss, increased physical activity, and decreased sodium intake have been shown to have a profound effect on lowering blood pressure and improving overall health (Table 24.5) [7]. In the situation of uncomplicated hypertension, a diuretic such as hydrochlorothiazide, which inhibits the absorption of sodium chloride in the distal convoluted tubule of the nephrons in the kidneys, is the initial drug of choice [9]. However, most patients will require two or more antihypertensive agents, such as a beta blocker, to achieve their goal blood pressure. Patients with one or more comorbid conditions such as ischemic heart disease, heart failure, diabetes, or kidney disease will have specific or compelling indications for alternative drug classes such as those shown in Table 24.6. See Fig. 24.3 for an example of a recommended hypertension treatment algorithm.

Table 24.5 Suggested lifestyle modifications

Lifestyle change	Suggested modification
Weight reduction	Maintain normal body weight (BMI 18.5–24.9)
DASH eating plan adoption	Consume diet of fruits, vegetables, low-fat dairy products; reduce amount of saturated and total fat
Dietary sodium restriction	Reduce dietary sodium intake to less than 2.4 g per day (6 g sodium chloride)
Physical activity	Engage in regular aerobic physical activity at least 30 min a day, most days of the week
Moderation of alcohol consumption	Men: limit consumption to no more than two drinks per day
	Women: limit consumption to no more than one drink per day

BMI = body mass index; DASH = dietary approaches to stop hypertension.

24.4 Acute Coronary Syndrome and Myocardial Infarction

Acute coronary syndrome is a blanket term used to describe any clinical symptoms associated with acute myocardial ischemia, including unstable angina, a ST-segment elevation myocardial infarction (STEMI), or a non-ST-segment elevation myocardial infarction (NSTEMI). It is estimated that nearly 1.7 million acute coronary syndrome hospital admissions occur annually, 500,000 of which are classified as STEMI [3]. The typical event that causes an imbalance between myocardial oxygen supply and demand occurs when a thrombus develops around an area where an atherosclerotic plaque has been disrupted, thereby blocking the arterial blood flow. Subsequently, the detection of biochemical cardiac markers such as troponin or the MB isoenzyme of creatine phosphokinase (CK-MB) indicates that myocardial cell death has occurred; they are not released in the setting of unstable angina [10]. An electrocardiogram can be utilized to differentiate between STEMI and NSTEMI.

24.4.1 Goals of Therapy for Acute Coronary Syndromes

The proper and immediate management for acute coronary syndrome is as complex as its differential diagnosis. Aside

from early recognition and response, goals of therapy are to remove the precipitating factor(s) causing the ischemia and minimize irreversible damage from occurring to the myocardial tissue. Importantly, patients are at a higher risk of death or worsening myocardial infarction if they have prolonged ischemic symptoms, clinical and ECG findings, and/or elevated biochemical cardiac markers [10, 11].

24.4.2 Treatment Guidelines for Acute Coronary Syndromes

Patients with unstable angina/NSTEMI should undergo an anti-ischemic therapy regimen that includes: (1) rapid vasodilation with nitroglycerin; (2) supplemental oxygen; (3) morphine sulfate for pain and agitation; (4) beta blockade; and (5) an ACE inhibitor for blood pressure control as needed [10]. If a patient has bradycardia or lung disease, then a calcium channel blocker with nodal cell inhibitory activity (diltiazem or verapamil) may be considered instead of a beta blocker. In addition to an anti-ischemia regimen, an antiplatelet and anticoagulation therapy should be initiated. Aspirin and heparin should be administered immediately and a glycoprotein IIb/IIIa receptor antagonist can be considered if ischemia persists or if a patient is deemed at high risk for immediate death or severe complications. It should be noted that low-molecular-weight heparin preparations have some advantages over unfractionated heparin. Specifically, enoxaparin (Lovenox®), a low-molecular-weight heparin, has consistently shown favorable benefits and is now the preferred preparation for anticoagulation therapy [12].

It is imperative to achieve myocardial reperfusion of STEMI patients within a timely manner to salvage as much viable myocardium as possible. Myocardial reperfusion can be achieved either with fibrinolytic pharmacologic therapy (tissue plasminogen activator, streptokinase, or urokinase) or through percutaneous coronary intervention. After reperfusion efforts, continued management is achieved through routine measures listed above including oxygen, nitroglycerin, aspirin, analgesia, beta blocker, and an ACE inhibitor [11].

The antiplatelet regimen for those patients undergoing a percutaneous coronary intervention and having a stent placed requires that the antiplatelet agents, aspirin, and

Table 24.6 Agents with compelling indications for the treatment of hypertension

Compelling indication	Diuretic	Beta blocker	ACE inhibitor	Angiotensin receptor blocker	Calcium channel blocker	Aldosterone antagonist
Heart failure	X	X	X	X		X
Post-myocardial infarction		X	X			X
High coronary heart disease risk	X	X	X		X	
Diabetes	X	X	X	X	X	
Chronic kidney disease			X	X		
Recurrent stroke prevention	X		X			

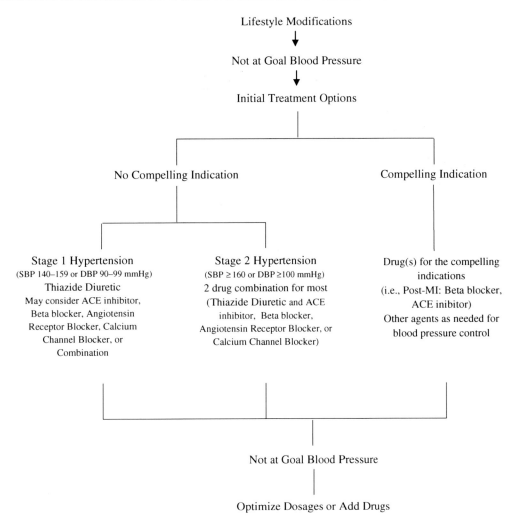

Fig. 24.3 Example of a recommended hypertension treatment algorithm. ACE = angiotensin-converting enzyme; DBP = diastolic blood pressure; MI = myocardial infarction; SBP = systolic blood pressure

clopidogrel (Plavix®) be given prior to the procedure. At a minimum, patients receiving a bare metal stent should take aspirin and clopidogrel daily for one month [13], and those receiving a drug-eluting stent should take both for up to 12 months due to the potential for late thrombosis complications [13, 14]. In addition and barring any contraindications, all patients discharged after a myocardial infarction should be placed on a beta blocker, ACE inhibitor, and aldosterone antagonist to minimize myocardial remodeling and other sequela [11].

24.5 Chronic Heart Failure

Chronic heart failure (CHF) is considered a major growing public health problem; over five million people in the United States [3] have been diagnosed with CHF and data indicate that it affects both men and women in equal proportions. It is defined as a complex clinical syndrome that can result from any structural or functional cardiac disorder

that impairs the ability of the ventricle to fill with or eject adequate blood volumes [15]. The incidence of CHF increases to 10 in 1,000 after the age of 65 years, and nearly 75% of all CHF cases have hypertension as a previously diagnosed medical condition [3]. Other risk factors for CHF are CHD, hyperlipidemia, and/or diabetes. Heart failure has several types of classifications such as ischemic or non-ischemic, diastolic or systolic, and acute or chronic. Efforts have been made to designate the severity of CHF by classification (New York Heart Association, NYHA; Table 24.7)

Table 24.7 New York Heart Association (NYHA) functional classification of heart failure

NYHA class	Definition
I	Patients with cardiac disease but *without limitations* of physical activity
II	Patients with cardiac disease resulting in *slight limitations* of physical activity
III	Patients with cardiac disease resulting in *marked limitations* of physical activity
IV	Patients with cardiac disease resulting in inability to carry on any physical activity without discomfort. *Symptoms present at rest*

Table 24.8 American College of Cardiology/American Heart Association staging in the evolution of heart failure

Stage	Definition
A	Patients with normal heart structure and function, no signs or symptoms of heart failure, and at increased risk for developing heart failure due to comorbid conditions (hypertension, coronary artery disease, diabetes) **(Asymptomatic risk)**
B	Asymptomatic patients with abnormal heart structure or function (left ventricular hypertrophy, enlarged, dilated ventricles, asymptomatic valve disease, previous myocardial infarction) **(Asymptomatic damage)**
C	Patients with abnormal structure or function and symptomatic heart failure **(Symptomatic damage)**
D	Patients with extremely abnormal and symptomatic heart failure despite optimal medical therapy and specialized interventions **(Extreme symptomatic damage)**

and staging ACC/AHA systems (Table 24.8). One is based primarily on physical assessment of symptoms (NYHA) and the other is based on the underlying cardiac disease. Unfortunately, mortality remains between 50 and 70% at five years for all classes of CHF and the cause of death is typically either sudden cardiac arrest or pump failure [15].

24.5.1 Goals of Therapy for Chronic Heart Failure

Chronic heart failure is a progressive disease in which initial compensatory mechanisms eventually become detrimental to the patient (Fig. 24.4). Therefore, pharmacologic treatment is aimed at those neurohormonal mechanisms, such as the renin–angiotensin–aldosterone system and sympathetic nervous system, which mediate the

progression of the disease. Goals of therapy include improving quality of life, reducing CHF symptoms and hospitalizations, and prolonging overall survival.

24.5.2 Treatment Guidelines for Chronic Heart Failure

Treatment decisions are largely guided by NYHA classification and to a lesser extent by the defined ACC/AHA disease stage (Table 24.9). To date, ACE inhibitors and beta blockers remain the cornerstone of therapy and are proven to provide significant morbidity and mortality benefit [16–19]. Initial doses for each agent are very low and titrated as tolerated over three to six months until goal dose is reached (Tables 24.10 and 24.11). Aldosterone antagonists have a role in treating patients with Class III and Class IV heart failure [20]. Fortunately, in circumstances where a patient has a contraindication or experiences an adverse event with an ACE inhibitor, an angiotensin receptor blocker can be substituted [21]. Other agents such as diuretics and digoxin can be given for symptom relief and to reduce hospitalizations. Currently, loop diuretics are the most potent class of clinically used diuretics and are the mainstay in volume control for CHF pharmacotherapy. In all such patients, fluid status is an important monitoring parameter; for example, fluid retention can blunt the response of ACE inhibitors and increase beta blocker adverse events, whereas fluid depletion can increase the risk of renal insufficiency. Importantly, both electrolyte levels and kidney function need to be monitored regularly when these agents are used in combination.

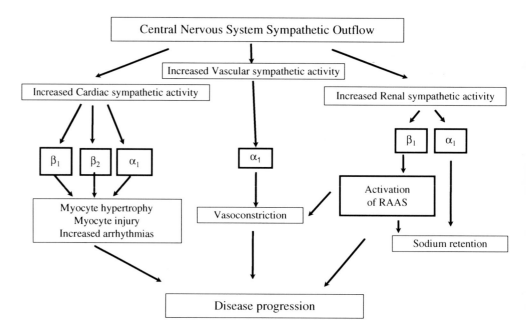

Fig. 24.4 Neurohormonal activation in heart failure. RAAS = renin–angiotensin–aldosterone system

Table 24.9 Chronic heart failure treatment guidelines based on NYHA classification

NYHA class	Pharmacotherapy options with morbidity and mortality benefit	Pharmacotherapy options for symptom management
I	ACE inhibitor	Diuretic
	Beta blocker	
II	ACE inhibitor	Diuretic
	Beta blocker	
III	ACE inhibitor	Diuretic
	Beta blocker	Digoxin
	Spironolactone	
IV	ACE inhibitor	Diuretic
	Beta blocker	Digoxin
	Spironolactone	Temporary intravenous inotropic support

ACE = angiotensin-converting enzyme.

Table 24.10 Angiotensin-converting enzyme (ACE) inhibitors with indications for chronic heart failure

Drug	Starting dose	Target dose
Captopril (Capoten®)	6.25 mg thrice daily	50 mg thrice daily
Enalapril (Vasotec®)	2.5 mg twice daily	10–20 mg twice daily
Fosinopril (Monopril®)	5–10 mg daily	40 mg daily
Lisinopril (Zestril®, Prinivil®)	2.5–5 mg daily	20–40 mg daily
Perindopril (Aceon®)	2 mg daily	8–16 mg daily
Quinapril (Accupril®)	5 mg twice daily	20 mg twice daily
Ramipril (Altace®)	1.25–2.5 mg daily	10 mg daily
Trandolapril (Mavik®)	1 mg daily	4 mg daily

Table 24.11 Beta blockers with indications for chronic heart failure

Drug	Starting dose	Target dose
Bisoprolol (Zebeta®)	1.25 mg once daily	10 mg once daily
Carvedilol (Coreg®)	3.125 mg twice daily	25 mg twice daily*
Metoprolol succinate (Toprol XL®)	12.5–25 mg once daily	200 mg once daily

*50 mg twice daily if patient weighs more than 85 kg.

24.6 Arrhythmias

Atrial fibrillation (AF), a supraventricular arrhythmia characterized by chaotic electrical activity in the atria, affects nearly two and a half million people in the United States alone [22], and its prevalence increases rapidly after the sixth decade of life [23]. Patients with AF often experience a lowered quality of life and frustration with currently available pharmacotherapy options for treatment; such agents offer marginal safety and efficacy. Risk factors for AF include hypertension, CHD, valvular disease, cardiomyopathy, chronic obstructive pulmonary disease, thyroid disease, electrolyte disturbances, alcohol abuse, and/or vagal stimulation. Clinically, AF is classified as "paroxysmal" (terminates spontaneously), "persistent" (terminates with chemical or electrical cardioversion), or "permanent" (refractory to any treatment).

Types of ventricular arrhythmias are premature ventricular complexes, nonsustained ventricular tachycardia, sustained ventricular tachycardia, and ventricular fibrillation. Each rhythm is complex and has a unique electrocardiography classification (see Chapter 26 for more details). Of late, "sudden cardiac arrest" and "sudden cardiac death" have gained more attention as they claim nearly 450,000 lives annually in the United States [24]. Ventricular fibrillation is the primary mechanism of sudden cardiac arrest, but evidence also attributes the elicitation of bradyarrhythmias, ventricular tachycardia, and torsades de pointes as additional mechanisms [25, 26].

24.6.1 Goals of Therapy for Arrhythmias

Importantly, atrial fibrillation has been linked with an increased risk of ischemic stroke by fivefold [27] and therefore the primary goal of pharmacotherapy in such patients is to prevent embolic events. Additional goals are to prevent tachycardia-induced cardiomyopathy, reduce symptoms of AF, and minimize adverse consequences of therapy [28]. Yet, risk factor awareness and minimization is the main goal in sudden cardiac arrest; risk factors are CHD, heart failure, or decreased left ventricular ejection fraction ($\leq30\%$), previous sudden cardiac arrest event, prior episode of ventricular tachycardia, hypertrophic cardiomyopathy, and/or long QT syndrome [29]. To date, beta blockers are the only antiarrhythmic drugs to have shown benefits in the primary prevention of sudden cardiac death; all other agents should be considered as adjuvant therapy to implantable cardioverter defibrillators [30–32].

24.6.2 Treatment Guidelines for Arrhythmias

All currently available antiarrhythmic drugs exert inhibitory activity on different phases of the action potential. In nodal tissue, type II and IV antiarrhythmic drugs control rate by decreasing calcium entry and therefore decreasing automaticity and associated conduction velocities in the depolarization phase. Type I and III antiarrhythmic drugs inhibit either sodium entry or potassium outflow, thereby decreasing automaticity and/or conduction velocities or increasing the refractory periods of the action potential. For a summary of these mechanisms, see Table 24.12. Figure 24.5A–F outlines commonly employed treatment algorithms for AF. In general,

Table 24.12 Antiarrhythmic drug mechanism of action

Type	Drug	Channel activity	Automaticity	Conduction velocity	Refractory period
Ia	Quinidine	Na^+ blocker	↓	↓	↑
	Procainamide*	K^+ blocker	↓	↓	↑
	Disopyramide		↓	↓	↑
Ib	Lidocaine	Na^+ blocker	↓	↓	—
	Mexiletine		↓	↓	—
Ic	Flecainide	Na^+ blocker	↓	↓↓	—
	Propafenone (Rythmol)		↓	↓↓	—
II	Beta blockers	Decreases Ca^{2+} (nodal cells)	↓	↓	—
III	Amiodarone	K^+ blocker Ca^{2+} (nodal cells)	↓	—	↑↑
	Dofetilide (Tikosyn)	K^+ blocker	—	—	↑↑
	Ibutilide (Corvert)	K^+ blocker	—	—	↑↑
	Sotalol (Betapace)	K^+ blocker Beta blocker (Ca^{2+} on nodal cells)	↓	—	↑↑
IV	Diltiazem Verapamil	Ca^{2+} blocker (nodal cells)	↓	↓	—

* Metabolized to *N*-acetylprocainamide (NAPA) which has class III activity.

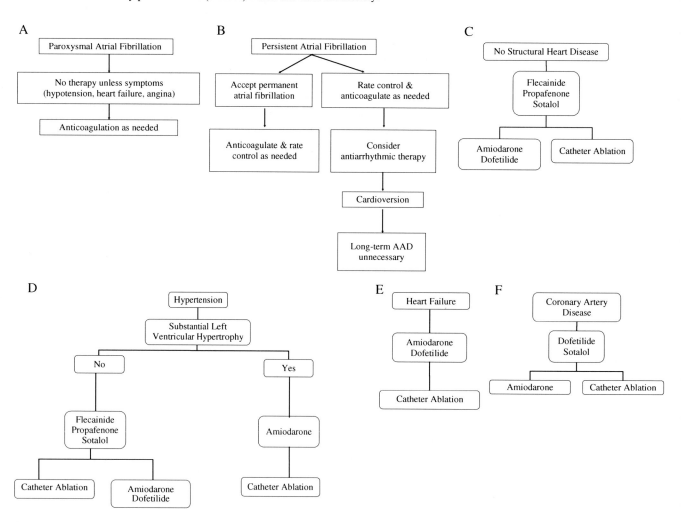

Fig. 24.5 Commonly employed treatment algorithms for atrial fibrillation: (**A**) newly diagnosed paroxysmal atrial fibrillation; (**B**) newly diagnosed persistent atrial fibrillation; (**C**) maintenance of normal sinus rhythm in patients without structural heart disease; (**D**) maintenance of normal sinus rhythm in patients with hypertension; (**E**) maintenance of normal sinus rhythm in patients with heart failure; (**F**) maintenance of normal sinus rhythm in patients with coronary artery disease

antiarrhythmic agents are used to either control ventricular rate or maintain normal sinus rhythm. Each strategy has important considerations for minimizing consequences of AF and thus burdensome symptoms.

Type III antiarrhythmic agents are used more frequently than type I agents in the setting of ventricular tachycardia/ventricular fibrillation. Amiodarone, a type III agent, is often used to decrease the frequency of supraventricular or ventricular arrhythmias in patients with an implantable cardioverter defibrillator to minimize defibrillation shock delivery [33].

24.7 Local Drug Delivery

Local drug delivery allows for a therapeutic concentration of a drug to be administered to a designated target without subjecting the rest of the body to potential adverse effects or toxic concentrations. Several methods for local drug delivery are already used in clinical practice. Transdermal delivery systems allow for localized penetration of a drug into the skin through a patch. Intrathecal drug pumps, through intraspinal catheters, deliver drugs to treat chronic pain and spasticity disorders with smaller doses of agents that traditionally would have been less effective and more sedating [34, 35]. Researchers have evaluated drug delivery into the pericardial space with antiarrhythmic agents and vasodilators and have found benefits such as enhanced efficacy, increased duration of action, lower doses, and less toxicity [36–38]. See Chapter 8 for an additional discussion of this topic.

24.7.1 Future Potential for Targeted Drug Delivery

Polymers being designed to allow for controlled, targeted release of drugs (i.e., technology used with drug-eluting stents) are successful in preventing vessel restenosis relative to that seen with bare metal stents. Similarly, drug-containing hydrogels placed next to a therapeutic target allow for controlled delivery [39]. As such, drug-eluting implants using these materials are intended to deliver a drug over a period of hours to months. In contrast, recent catheter technology has the potential for delivering a precise amount of drug to a very specific target while maintaining the efficiency of intravascular delivery but without obstructing blood flow [40]. These local drug delivery methodologies and more being developed will likely be utilized, as biologics and personalized medicine such as gene therapy begin to play a larger role in the treatment of cardiovascular diseases.

24.8 Summary

This chapter has provided a very brief overview of the pharmacotherapy decisions that have shown the most benefit in the current treatment of hypertension, acute coronary syndrome, heart failure, and arrhythmias. Guidelines and subsequent updates developed by experts in their respective areas of specialty should be consulted to develop an awareness of the optimal medical therapies including pharmacotherapy for the treatment of cardiovascular disorders.

24.9 List of Abbreviations

ACC	American College of Cardiology
AF	atrial fibrillation
AHA	American Heart Association
CHD	coronary heart disease
CHF	chronic heart failure
NSTEMI	non-ST-segment elevation myocardial infarction
STEMI	ST-segment elevation myocardial infarction

References

1. Centers for Disease Control and Prevention. (Accessed February 2008, at www.cdc.gov/heartdisease).
2. American Heart Association. (Accessed February 2008, at www.aha.org).
3. American Heart Association. Heart disease and stroke statistics: 2008 update. Dallas, TX: American Heart Association, 2008.
4. Sackett DL, Rosenberg WM, Gray JA, Haynes RB, Richardson WS. Evidence based medicine: What it is and what it isn't. BMJ 1996;312:71–72.
5. Radford MJ, Heidenreich PA, Bailey SR, et al. ACC/AHA 2007 methodology for the development of clinical data standards. Circulation 2007;115:936–43.
6. Hertz RP, Unger AN, Cornell JA, Saunders E. Racial disparities in hypertension prevalence, awareness, and management. Arch Intern Med 2005;165:2098–104.
7. Chobanian AV, Bakris GL, Black HR, et al. The seventh report of the Joint National Committee on prevention, detection, evaluation, and treatment of high blood pressure. JAMA 2003;289:2560–72.
8. Rosendorff C, Black HR, Cannon CP, et al. Treatment of hypertension in the prevention and management of ischemic heart disease: A scientific statement from the American Heart Association Council for High Blood Pressure Research and the Councils on Clinical Cardiology and Epidemiology and Prevention. Circulation 2007;115:2761–88.
9. Furberg CD, Wright JT, Davis BR, et al. Major outcomes in high-risk hypertensive patients randomized to angiotensin-converting enzyme inhibitor or calcium channel blocker vs diuretic: The Antihypertensive and Lipid-Lowering Treatment to Prevent Heart Attack Trial (ALLHAT). JAMA 2002;288:2981–97.

10. Braunwald E, Antman EM, Beasley JW, Califf RM, Cheitlin MD, Hochman JS. ACC/AHA guidelines for the management of patients with unstable angina and non-ST-segment elevation myocardial infarction. Circulation 2000;102:1193–209.

11. Antman EM, Anbe DT, Armstrong PW, Bates ER, Green LA, Hand M. ACC/AHA guidelines for the management of patients with ST-elevation myocardial infarction. Circulation 2004;110:588–636.

12. Antman EM, Morrow DA, McCabe CH, Murphy SA, Ruda M, Sadowski Z. Enoxaparin versus unfractionated heparin with fibrinolysis for ST-elevation myocardial infarction. N Engl J Med 2006;354:1477–88.

13. King SB III, Smith SC, Hirshfield JW, Jacobs AK, Morrison DA, Williams DO. 2007 focused update of the ACC/AHA/SCAI 2005 guideline update for percutaneous coronary intervention. Circulation 2008;117:261–95.

14. Steinhubl SR, Berger PB, Mann JT III, Fry ET, DeLago A, Wilmer C. Early and sustained oral antiplatelet therapy following percutaneous coronary intervention: A randomized controlled trial. JAMA 2002;288:2411–20.

15. Hunt SA, Baker DW, Chin MH, et al. ACC/AHA 2005 guidelines for the diagnosis and management of chronic heart failure in the adult. Circulation 2005;112:e154–235.

16. The SOLVD Investigators. Effect of enalapril on survival in patients with reduced left ventricular ejection fractions and congestive heart failure. N Engl J Med 1991;325:293–302.

17. The CONSENSUS Trial Study Group. Effects of enalapril on mortality in severe congestive heart failure: Results of the Cooperative North Scandinavian Enalapril Survival Study (CONSENSUS). N Engl J Med 1987;316:1429–35.

18. MERIT–HF Study Group. Effect of metoprolol CR/XL in chronic heart failure: Metoprolol CR/XL randomised intervention trial in congestive heart failure (MERIT-HF). Lancet 1999;253:2001–07.

19. Packer M, Coats AJ, Fowler MB, Katus HA, Krum H, Mohacsi P. Carvedilol Prospective Randomized Cumulative Survival Study Group: Effect of carvedilol on survival in severe chronic heart failure. New Engl J Med 2001;344:1651–58.

20. The RALES Investigators. Effectiveness of spironolactone added to angiotensin-converting enzyme inhibitor and a loop diuretic for severe chronic congestive heart failure (The Randomized Aldactone Evaluation Study [RALES]). Am J Cardiol 1996;78:902–07.

21. Granger CB, McMurray JJ, Yusef S, et al. Effects of candesartan in patients with chronic heart failure and reduced left-ventricular systolic function intolerant to angiotensin-converting-enzyme inhibitors: The CHARM-Alternative trial. Lancet 2003;362:772–76.

22. Go AS, Hylek EM, Phillips KA, et al. Prevalence of diagnosed atrial fibrillation in adults: National implications for rhythm management and stroke prevention: The AnTicoagulation and Risk Factors in Atrial Fibrillation (ATRIA) Study. JAMA 2001;285:2370–75.

23. Feinberg CD, Blackshear JL, Laupacis A, Kronmal R, Hart RG. Prevalence, age distribution, and gender of patients with atrial fibrillation: Analysis and implications. Arch Intern Med 1995;155:469–73.

24. Zheng ZJ, Croft JB, Giles WH, Mensah GA. Sudden cardiac death in the United States, 1989–1998. Circulation 2001;104:2158–63.

25. Luu M, Stevenson WG, Stevenson LW, Baron K, Walden J. Diverse mechanisms of unexpected cardiac arrest in advanced heart failure. Circulation 1989;80:1675–80.

26. Bayes de Luna A, Coumel P, Leclercq JF. Ambulatory sudden cardiac death: Mechanisms of production of fatal arrhythmias on the basis of data from 157 cases. Am Heart J 1989;117:151–60.

27. Singer DE, Albers GW, Dalen JE, Go AS, Halperin JL, Manning WJ. Antithrombotic therapy in atrial fibrillation: The Seventh ACCP Conference on antithrombotic and thrombolytic therapy. Chest 2004;126:429–56.

28. Fuster V, Rydén LE, Cannom DS, et al. ACC/AHA/ESC 2006 guidelines for the management of patients with atrial fibrillation. Circulation 2006;114:e257–354.

29. Zipes DP, Camm AJ, Borggrefe M, et al. ACC/AHA/ESC 2006 guidelines for management of patients with ventricular arrhythmias and the prevention of sudden cardiac death. J Am Coll Cardiol 2006;48:e248–346.

30. Buxton AE, Lee KL, Hafley GE, et al. The Multicenter Unsustained Tachycardia Trial Investigators. A randomized study of the prevention of sudden death in patients with coronary artery disease. N Engl J Med 1999;341:1882–90.

31. Bardy GH, Lee KL, Mark DB, et al. Amiodarone or an implantable cardioverter defibrillator for congestive heart failure. N Engl J Med 2005;352:225–37.

32. The Antiarrhythmics Versus Implantable Defibrillators (AVID) Investigators. A comparison of antiarrhythmic-drug therapy with implantable defibrillators in patients resuscitated from near-fatal ventricular arrhythmias. N Engl J Med 1997;337:1576–83.

33. Santini M, Pandozi C, Ricci R. Combining antiarrhythmic drugs and implantable devices therapy: Benefits and outcomes. J Intervent Cardiol Electrophysiol 2000;4:65–89.

34. Anderson VC, Burcheil K. A prospective study of long-term intrathecal morphine in the management of chronic nonmalignant pain. Neurosurgery 1999;44:289–300.

35. Albright LA, Gilmartin R, Swift D, Krach LE, Ivanhoe CB, McLaughlin JF. Long-term intrathecal baclofen therapy for severe spasticity of cerebral origin. J Neurosurg 2003;98:291–95.

36. Waxman S, Moreno R, Rowe KA, Verrier RL. Persistent primary coronary dilation induced by transatrial delivery of nitroglycerin into the pericardial space: A novel approach for local cardiac drug delivery. J Am Coll Cardiol 1999;33:2073–77.

37. Ujhelyi MR, Hadsall KZ, Eular DE, Mehra R. Intrapericardial therapeutics: A pharmacodynamic and pharmacokinetic comparison between pericardial and intravenous procainamide delivery. J Cardiovasc Electrophysiol 2002;13:605–11.

38. van Brakel TJ, Hermans JJ, Janssen BJ, van Essen H, Botterhuis N, Smits JF. Intrapericardial delivery enhances cardiac effects of sotalol and atenolol. J Cardiovasc Electrophysiol 2004;44:50–56.

39. Slepian MJ. Polymeric endoluminal gel paving: Therapeutic hydrogel barriers and sustained delivery depots for local arterial wall biomanipulation. Semin Interv Cardiol 1996;1:103–16.

40. Brieger D, Topal E. Local delivery systems and prevention of stenosis. Cardiovasc Res 1997;35:405–13.

Chapter 25
Animal Models for Cardiac Research

Richard W. Bianco, Robert P. Gallegos, Andrew L. Rivard, Jessica Voight, and Agustin P. Dalmasso

Abstract The modern era of cardiac surgery is largely considered to have begun in the animal research laboratories. Today, animal models continue to be used for the study of cardiovascular diseases and are required for the preclinical assessment of pharmaceuticals, mechanical devices, therapeutic procedures, and/or continuation therapies. This chapter was designed to provide readers and potential investigators with important background information necessary for the process of matching an experimental hypothesis to an animal species that will serve as an appropriate model for studying a specific cardiovascular disease or for testing a given medical device. A review of the current animal models used in cardiac research is provided and arranged by disease state. Critical factors to consider when choosing an appropriate animal model including cost, reproducibility, and degree of similarity of the model to human disease are discussed. Thus, this chapter can be utilized as a practical guide for planning of research protocols.

Keywords Animal model · Isolated cardiomyocytes · Isolated perfused heart · Valve disease · Atrial fibrillation · Myocardial ischemia · Heart failure · Heart transplantation · Mechanical device testing · Cardiomyoplasty · Stem cell research

25.1 Protocol Development

Several scientific governing bodies have developed guidelines and periodic review processes to ensure that animals are used in research in an ethical and scientifically appropriate manner. Investigators who plan to utilize animal subjects in their research should first familiarize themselves with the document entitled "Guide for the Care and Use of Laboratory Animals" prepared by the U.S. National Academy of Sciences [1]. In addition, investigators should use these guidelines in conjunction with accepted scientific methods in order to develop a standardized protocol for each research project. It is a required standard procedure that, prior to commencing research, a detailed protocol undergoes review and approval by the local institutional governing body responsible for the safety and ethical use of animals in research. In organizations in the United States where research using animals is performed, the standard governing body is known as the Institutional Animal Care and Use Committee or IACUC (see www.iacuc.umn.edu).

Both large and small animals have been extensively used in cardiovascular research. Yet, the choice of animal model should be primarily based on: (1) the scientific hypotheses; (2) the laboratory's capability to safely employ the model in the species chosen (i.e., appropriate animal housing and care, equipment, laboratory resources); and (3) the degree of the species similarity to the human anatomy. It is important to note that many of the best animal models can be expensive to establish and maintain; therefore, funding must be appropriate to complete the required number of animal experiments to satisfy a precalculated statistical power. Several obvious technical limitations for the use of small animals exist, for example, in the case of implanting mechanical devices such as heart valves. The animal species must be chosen to fit the device to be studied. Nevertheless, great strides have been made in both imaging (ultrasound and MRI) and miniaturizing electronic equipment (e.g., Transoma Medical, Arden Hills, MN) that can be used for monitoring physiological parameters, allowing for more intensive cardiac monitoring within small animal models. Nevertheless, in choosing the animal species, the researcher should attempt to match the physiological parameter to be investigated in the experimental animal to the

R.W. Bianco (✉)
University of Minnesota, Experimental Surgical Services,
Department of Surgery, MMC 220, 420 Delaware St. SE, 55455,
Minneapolis, MN, USA
e-mail: bianc001@umn.edu

corresponding human value to obtain results that are most clinically relevant. Note that many tables of physiological values are available for commonly used research animal species, and these should be used to assist in choosing the appropriate model [2, 3].

25.2 Spontaneously Occurring Animal Models of Congenital Cardiac Disease

Naturally occurring animal models of cardiac disease arise infrequently; importantly, when they do, they often occur with other associated congenital abnormalities that hinder breeding efforts. Furthermore, genetic manipulation of breeding stock for specific mutations has economical, ethical, and moral issues that preclude the development of such breeding lines. As a result, the commercial availability of animals for such specific research purposes is quite limited, necessitating the development of iatrogenic models in most cases. Nonetheless, even when some of those issues are of broad significance to all species, great strides have been made in the application of classical breeding techniques and, more recently, molecular engineering to develop breeding stocks of mice, and in some cases rats, that are available for different studies. Specifically, the use of transgenic mice and mice with gene deletions or other induced genetic changes has been considered essential for investigating pathophysiologic mechanisms of disease, including those of the cardiovascular system. Moreover, these genetically modified animals, in some instances, are useful for the initial in vivo testing of pharmaceuticals and/or certain devices.

25.3 Alternatives to Whole Animal Models

In some cases isolated cardiac cell lines in culture, segments of myocardium, or isolated heart models may provide an effective alternative to whole animal research. Isolated preparations have been particularly useful for the study of metabolic pathways, as the perfusate can be modified while the effluent can be easily collected for analysis. Additionally, functional measurements can be easily completed in this in vitro environment. Given the need to both reduce cost and limit the number of animals used in research, the attraction of using alternatives to whole animal models is strong. However, regulations typically do not permit the direct extrapolation of the experimental findings from isolated in vitro models to subsequent actual clinical trials. For example, in vitro studies often demonstrate whether a pharmaceutical

agent is potentially useful; however, the concentrations used may be either toxic or the agent may lack efficacy in the intact animal. Nevertheless, these alternatives are essential for initial studies pertaining to myocardial ischemia, transplantation, and/or pharmaceutical development.

25.3.1 Isolated Cardiomyocytes

The use of isolated cardiomyocytes has allowed researchers to eliminate confounding interactions with surrounding tissue elements; it has also allowed for measurement of intracellular changes at the single cell level. Yet, care must be taken to match the culture conditions to those of the intact organ to ensure both the quality and viability of the cells used [4, 5]. This simple model provides an important approach before the use of whole animals in early phase testing of experimental protocols, and is of particular interest for use in the testing of new pharmacological agents and/or gene therapies. Cardiac myocyte cultures can be obtained from freshly isolated tissue, differentiated embryonic stem cells or multipotent adult progenitor cells, or immortalized tumor cell lines such as HL-1 from the At-1 mouse [6]. Some functions of cardiac myocytes that can be examined include: (1) contractility, using optical or mechanical detectors; (2) specific RNA expression (e.g., using Q-PCR); and/or (3) membrane integrity, using release of lactate dehydrogenase, creatine phosphokinase, or troponin [5, 7–11].

25.3.2 Isolated Perfused Hearts

An isolated heart perfusion system replicates the physiological conditions outside of the body, allowing for easy access for measurement of the perfused effluent. Isolated in vitro perfusion studies have been performed using the entire heart or a portion of the heart (e.g., intraventricular septum, papillary muscle). Commercially available setups for such in vitro studies are available for the mouse, rat, and guinea pig hearts (ADInstruments, Colorado Springs, CO) (Fig. 25.1). Larger setups have also been described to accommodate canine, porcine, ovine, and human hearts. An excellent example of an application of the isolated heart model can be seen on the Atlas of Human Cardiac Anatomy website (www.vhlab.umn.edu/atlas) and on the Visible Heart website (www.visibleheart.com).

Several different methods for studying the isolated heart are possible—the Langendorff perfusion approach and the isolated working heart model [12, 13]. In the

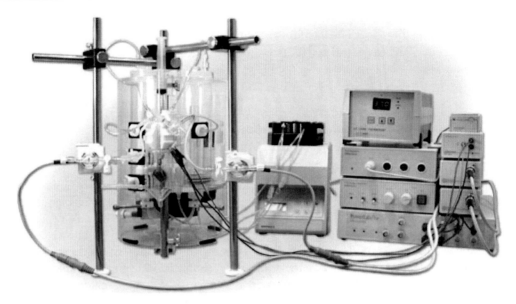

Fig. 25.1 ADInstruments Langendorff perfusion setup. Adapted from www.adinstruments.com

Langendorff system, constant pressure flow through an aortic cannula forces the aortic valve closed, and the perfusate passes through the coronary arteries without flowing through the left ventricle. This perfusion provides the myocardium with energy, allowing the heart to beat without flowing through the four chambers. This method was named after Oscar Langendorff who, in 1895, was the first to describe an experimental model of an isolated mammalian heart as a technique to assess its required contractile activity. The advantage of the Langendorff perfusion method is that measurement of EKG changes can be easily assessed, as well as measurement of metabolites that drain from the coronary sinus. Yet, the lack of flow in the left ventricle may limit its usefulness, i.e., minimal blood entering into the ventricle may promote clot formation, in turn, affecting the viability of the preparation. Additionally, the lack of flow in the ventricle may result in abnormal three-dimensional conformational changes in the heart that may cause coronary vascular compression. However, placement of a fluid balloon connected to a pressure transducer may allow for partial control of this problem, and may also be useful experimentally to assess changes in left ventricular function.

The major disadvantage of the Langendorff preparation is that it does not eject the perfusate from the left ventricle and is therefore a nonwork producing model. This problem was initially overcome by Neely, who used an isolated working heart which simulates physiological flow through the heart's four chambers [14]. In this model, the perfusate is supplied by a cannula inserted into the left atrium; outflow through the left ventricle is monitored, while left atrial pressure or aortic pressure is controlled. This setup is considered ideal for the study of pressure and flow in the aorta as well as the left and right ventricles.

25.3.3 Additional Problems with Isolated Perfused Heart Models

Both types of isolated heart preparations have problems in common that should be considered when attempting to extrapolate results to the in vivo condition. First, the isolation process used for these models requires global myocardial ischemia (a period of no perfusion). Typically, once the organ is reperfused, baseline data (heart rate, left ventricular pressure, coronary blood flow) must be collected after a stabilization period to ensure relative viability of the preparation. Clearly, both the ischemic time and stabilization time may influence research outcomes. Therefore, any results obtained must be carefully analyzed with reference to the preparation's baseline state as well as to the normal in vivo values, to avoid falsely attributing changes in cardiac function to the experimental protocol.

The composition of the perfusate can greatly impact the function and viability of the preparation in both of the aforementioned models. Early studies utilizing isolated heart models have employed whole blood as a perfusate [15]. However, significant problems with clotting and hemolysis may limit the time that the preparation remains viable. Saline compounds, which lack the potential for clotting and hemolysis, are considered useful alternatives to whole blood. However, such buffers have a lower colloid osmotic pressure and, coupled with the lower coronary vascular resistance, will typically result in progressive and severe edema; this results in interstitial edema formation and nonuniform perfusion. To extend the usefulness of the preparation, one can add osmotically active substances to the medium used for bathing and perfusing the preparation in an attempt to limit edema [16, 17]. Nevertheless, despite the technical difficulties associated with these models, isolated hearts have been used in research ranging from ischemia to transplant studies.

25.4 Animal Models in Valve Disease

The significant morbidity and mortality associated with heart valve disease has produced a highly lucrative and competitive market for manufactured prosthetic valves. Efforts to develop the ideal replacement heart valve have focused on producing a device that functions like the native valve (Table 25.1). To this end, certain basic principles of physics are fundamental in the design of mechanical valves, as evidenced by the evolution of various designs. The dynamics of blood flow through a tube with its specific viscosity is such that the flow is greatest in the center of the tube. Thus, any structure in the center

Table 25.1 Qualities of the ideal device for heart valve replacement

- Durable
- Does not leak
- Biologically inert
- Nonthrombogenic
- Facilitates laminar flow
- Easily implanted by the surgeon
- Quiet

of the valve (i.e., mechanical valve leaflets) will reduce the velocity through that valve (Fig. 25.2).

Guidelines for the design and testing of bio-artificial and/or mechanical heart valves have been established by the Center for Devices and Radiological Health of the Food and Drug Administration (FDA) and the International Standards Organization (ISO). The FDA has provided industry assistance in the form of guidance documents, advice, reporting, premarket approval, development of standards, and third-party reviews. Typically, prosthetic valve replacements are classified as either tissue (Fig. 25.3) or mechanical, yet, despite their common purpose, specific valve composition and function vary widely. Nevertheless, all valves must undergo performance-based testing to examine hydrodynamic performance (Table 25.2). For example, accelerated cyclic testing provides wear information, allowing for estimates of structural performance by providing data on fatigue, endurance limits, and damage tolerances of the valve (Table 25.2).

Importantly, the FDA requires the demonstration of both efficacy and safety of prototype heart valve replacements prior to final approval for human implantation. This is based on the principle that additional technical and biological information can be gained by observing the valve in actual use. As a result, animal studies remain a crucial component in the overall evaluation of replacement heart valves [18]. To date, all investigational valves undergo a preclinical animal study with valve implantation in the orthotopic or anatomically normal position

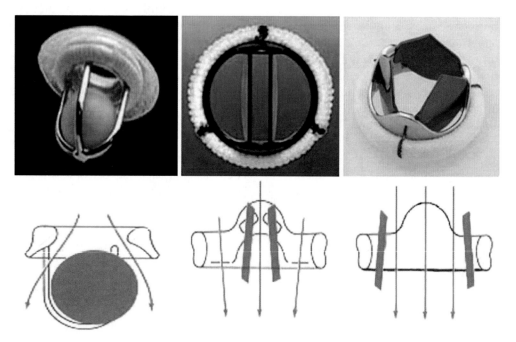

Fig. 25.2 Comparison of different valves with their flow characteristics. The evolution of the valve from the Starr–Edwards ball, the current standard bileaflet (St. Jude Medical, St. Paul, MN), and a novel trileaflet design (Triflow Medical Inc.) currently in development. Pictured below each valve is a stylized representation of the flow patterns across each valve reflecting the improvement in nonobstructive valve design

Fig. 25.3 The Medtronic Mosaic® stented tissue valve (Medtronic, Inc., Minneapolis, MN)

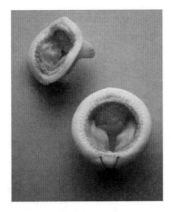

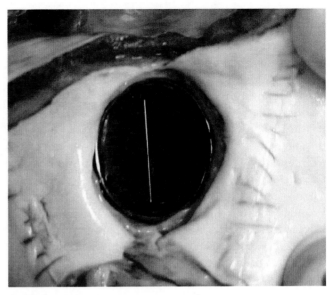

Fig. 25.4 Ovine model of a normal bileaflet valve implantation

Table 25.2 Mechanical valve fluid dynamic testing

- Forward flow testing
- Backflow leakage testing
- Pulsatile flow pressure drop
- Pulsatile flow regurgitation
- Flow visualization
- Cavitation potential
- Verification of the Bernoulli relationship

Source: "Replacement Heart Valve Guidelines," formulated by the U.S. Department of Health and Human Services, Food and Drug Administration, Center for Devices and Radiological Health.

(with a required 20-wk minimum period of evaluation). Specifically, the FDA looks for separate data from mechanical and biological valve studies. For example, mechanical valves generally place extreme shearing forces on the red blood cells and platelets, causing hemolysis and thrombosis that necessitate chronic anticoagulation after valve implantation. On the other hand, biologic valves place very low shear forces on the red blood cells and platelets, and thus there is no need for anticoagulation; however, they are sensitive to formation of calcium deposition, requiring the incorporation of some measures in their manufacturing that will attempt to prevent calcification after implantation. The lack of naturally occurring models of valve disease and the need for standardized models for FDA/ISO approval has led to the use of iatrogenic models of valve disease. To date, the ovine model has been used for producing a graded stenosis in the aortic and mitral valves by banding the aorta in young animals [19]. In contrast, aortic supravalvular stenosis, as well as aortic valvular stenosis, has been commonly induced in the canine model [20, 21]. Additionally, induction of mitral valve regurgitation in the canine is possible by placement of a shunt [22] or by incision of the chordae tendenae. Interestingly, experiments have also been performed to induce stenosis or regurgitation in the tricuspid and pulmonic valves [23]. However, most valve implantation studies approved for human use are completed in normal animals and their primary goals are to strictly examine valve performance (Fig. 25.4).

A principal advantage of employing the canine model is the large amount of background information available in the cardiovascular surgical literature. Historically, the dog was considered to be the gold standard for both acute and chronic models of valve replacement that was accepted by the FDA. Early success with the canine model in valve replacement identified the need for minimizing the risk of surgical infection at the time of prosthesis implantation. Specifically, the use of preoperative parenteral and postoperative topical antibiotics, strict sterile techniques, minimum numbers of operative arterial and venous lines, and short cardiopulmonary bypass times were all noted parameters to minimize the risk of bacterial valve implant seeding [24].

As described in Chapter 6, the anatomy of the porcine heart is most similar to that of the human heart in regard to the conduction system, coronary arteries, blood supply to the conduction system, and great vessels. In addition, the coagulation cascade of the swine is quite similar to that of humans. Despite these advantages, several problems have been identified in using this model for valvular research. First, the porcine heart is extremely sensitive to anesthesia, and surgical manipulation often results in postsurgical complications, arrhythmias, and/or even death. Second, the growth of young swine is rapid, resulting in heart size and physiological flow that is not constant over required follow-up periods over several months. Specifically, these alterations often result in fibrous sheathing and obstruction of the valve orifice, thrombus formation, or dehiscence (separation) of the sewing cuff. Finally, significant bleeding complications, due to application of anticoagulation therapy, and poor survival have limited the use of the pig in studying valve-related thrombosis [25].

The ovine model is currently accepted as the gold standard for valve replacement using defined survival surgeries that meet FDA requirements. Normal cardiovascular physiological parameters of sheep approximate those of humans in blood pressure, heart rate, cardiac output, and intracardiac pressure [26]. In addition, the anatomy of the adult heart provides valve orifice diameters that are similar to humans [27]. The use of animals of similar age and weight (8–12 months, 30–40 kg) allows for the testing of replacement valves using a single orifice size for comparison of valve performance to an appropriate standard. Although the heart and vessels are small in animals within this weight range, the sheep's relatively large left and right atria allow for straightforward surgical approaches to either the mitral or tricuspid valves.

In general, sheep as experimental animals allow for easy handing and long-term husbandry. Furthermore, juvenile sheep grow at a rate that does not cause excessive mitral or aortic stenosis during the postimplantation test periods, as compared to the porcine model [25]. However, specific attention to gastric decompression, perioperative antibiotics, sterile techniques, and minimally invasive interventions in the postoperative period will all increase the success of valve implantation studies in the ovine model [28].

25.4.1 Animal Models of Atrial Fibrillation for Preclinical Valve Testing

Given the increasing number of patients afflicted with atrial fibrillation worldwide, an animal model of the disorder is needed to predict valvular function and its effects on the natural course of the disease. For example, in one study, atrial fibrillation was associated with morbidity secondary to stroke (13%) and congestive heart failure (24%) despite anticoagulant treatment and independent of New York Heart Association (NYHA) functional classification, type of surgery, coronary artery disease, history of coronary artery bypass graft, or other cardiac risk factors [6]. Previous research has uncovered a number of cardiovascular structural and electrophysiological alterations associated with atrial fibrillation [18–21]. More specifically, the fibrillating heart will elicit a shorter refractory period at the right atrial appendage, shorter action potential duration, electrophysiological remodeling, and changes in gene expression [19, 21]. Myocardial remodeling leading to atrial enlargement appears to be a direct result of atrial fibrillation. From a structural standpoint, the fibrillating left atrium is larger, has relative stasis of blood particularly in the atrial appendage, and fails to give the "atrial kick" which comprises approximately 30% of ventricular filling. These characteristics also explain the increased thromboembolic risk and decreased cardiac output associated with atrial fibrillation.

25.4.2 Pacing-Induced Atrial Fibrillation

Control of the heartbeat using electrical stimulation is usually achieved using an intracardiac or transesophageal approach. Intracardiac pacing, subdivided into burst pacing and continuous pacing, is the most commonly used procedure for the induction of atrial fibrillation in the sheep model and in animal models overall. Rapid atrial pacing is the most common method of inducing atrial fibrillation for in vivo investigation. The transesophageal approach to pacing represents another possibility; however, it is used in humans and animal models primarily in the detection and assessment of irregular cardiac rhythms and coronary artery disease [29]. It should also be noted that implantable systems offer another alternative for the delivery of right atrial rapid pacing in order to induce atrial fibrillation in conscious animals [30].

25.4.3 Pharmacologic-Induced Atrial Fibrillation

Administration of catecholamines and acetylcholine perfused through the sinus node artery can induce atrial fibrillation. Isoproterenol (nonselective beta-adrenergic agonist) and adrenaline (alpha- and beta-adrenergic agonist) induce atrial fibrillation in dogs [31]. Atropine treatment prevented catecholamine-mediated atrial fibrillation, indicating a critical role of cholinergic tone in these atrial fibrillation episodes. Acetylcholine-mediated atrial fibrillation is facilitated by isoproterenol, which decreases the threshold of acetylcholine concentration required for atrial fibrillation induction and increases the atrial fibrillation duration. The focal delivery of these agents into atrial tissues can also cause episodic fibrillation.

25.4.4 Other Potential Atrial Fibrillation Models

Given that many genes are associated with cardiac contractility, it is reasonable to postulate that genetic engineering may have a potential role in the development of an atrial fibrillation model. The first important advance in this direction has been the identification of a genetic locus for familial atrial fibrillation on chromosome 10q22-q24 [32]. The discovery that the stem cell-derived cardiomyocytes have an intrinsic arrhythmic potential further leads to the question whether stem cell therapy could be the basis for a model of atrial fibrillation [33].

25.5 Animal Models in Myocardial Ischemia

Despite great advances in treatment options, atherosclerotic coronary vascular disease remains one of the leading causes of death worldwide. As a result, this disease continues to be an active area of cardiovascular research. Originally defined by the Greeks as a lack of blood flow, the modern definition of ischemia emphasizes both the imbalance between oxygen supply and demand as well as the inadequate removal of waste products. Impaired oxygen delivery causes a reduction in oxidative phosphorylation, resulting in myocardial dependence on anaerobic glycolysis for the production of high-energy phosphates. This shift in metabolism produces excess lactate which then accumulates in the myocardium. As impaired ATP production and acidosis prevail, there is a resultant decline in cardiac contractility. Ultimately, if ischemia is not reversed, myocardial infarction occurs with permanent cellular loss and impaired cardiac function. Multiple experimental techniques have been developed for the study of cardiac ischemia. Currently, scientists consistently use isolated myocytes to examine single cell responses, while isolated perfused hearts and whole animal models allow for a better understanding of the whole organ responses. Regardless of the model type, experimental animals remain a crucial tool in the area of research.

25.5.1 Experimental Methods for Creating Ischemia

The ideal model for ischemic investigations would theoretically be the intact chronically instrumented awake animal, as acute surgical trauma and anesthetic agents both depress cardiac function [2]. The awake animal model also has the advantage that it can be used in studies requiring physiological stress, e.g., stress produced by exercise. However, the high cost of the implanted transducers and probes as well as difficulties with measurement techniques often preclude the use of such an approach. To date, the majority of studies use anesthetized animal models for the study of ischemia in either closed or open chest models. Closed chest models have the advantage that

tissue trauma is minimized, but in such models, direct access to the heart for metabolite measurement is a major limitation. In contrast, the open chest preparation has the advantage that regional function and metabolism can be studied in detail. The open chest models suffer from drawbacks that include a greater susceptibility to temperature variations and a potential for surgical trauma that may considerably alter cardiac function (Fig. 25.5).

Multiple techniques have been used to create models of myocardial ischemia for research purposes, depending on whether the desired occlusion is to be permanent, temporary, or progressive. Methods to produce complete permanent occlusions include surgical coronary artery ligation or radiological embolization with microparticles. Furthermore, permanent or temporary partial coronary occlusions are commonly induced by ligation, balloon occlusion, or clamping. Typically, models of progressive coronary artery occlusions use either balloon/catheter occlusion or ameroid constrictors (Fig. 25.6). Regardless of the method chosen, the researcher must be aware that the concentric experimental lesions that are created differ from those of naturally occurring atherosclerotic coronary vascular disease which are typically eccentric. Normally, such eccentric stenoses remain vasoactive and are capable of altering coronary blood flow by changing their lumen diameter. It should be noted that no such vasoactivity remains in experimentally created concentric lesions which will prohibit humoral agents from altering regional coronary flow (Fig. 25.7).

Experience has shown that an induced occlusion of the left anterior descending coronary artery is favored over that in the left circumflex coronary artery for the production of regional myocardial ischemia. It is generally

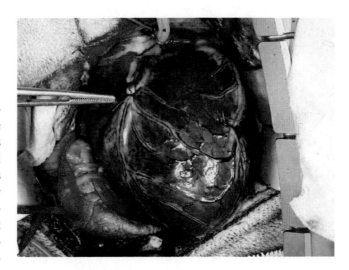

Fig. 25.5 Ligated left anterior descending coronary artery in an open chest canine model

Fig. 25.6 Ameroid occluder in the canine model. Photo courtesy of Michael Jerosh-Herold and Cory Swingen

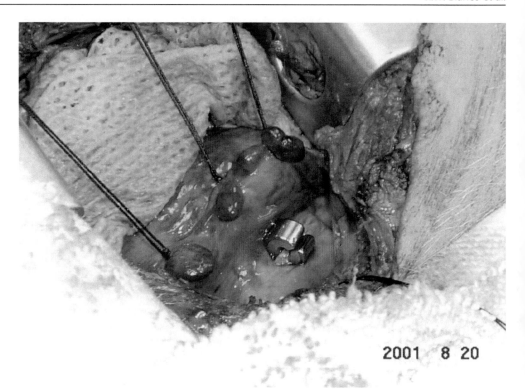

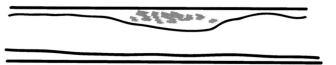

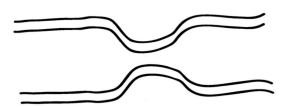

Fig. 25.7 (*Top*) An example of an eccentric vascular constriction as with coronary artery disease. (*Bottom*) A concentric lesion as created by experimental ligation or ameroid occlusion

accepted that occlusion of the left anterior descending coronary artery results in a larger area of myocardial ischemia, and therefore greater impairment of global left ventricular function. However, estimates of infarction size alone have not correlated well with ventricular function [34]. Thus it has been demonstrated that for the same amount of ischemic myocardium, the compensatory increase by the nonischemic myocardium is different for the left anterior descending coronary artery and the left circumflex coronary arteries [35]. Therefore, in an ideal model, both infarct size

and its location must be similar in order to achieve the same degree of impairment in left ventricular global function. If possible, one should also estimate the ischemic area at risk due to an imposed occlusion.

25.5.2 Localizing and Quantifying Myocardial Ischemia

Blood samples collected from the coronary sinus or from a regional coronary vein are commonly obtained and used for metabolic studies. Yet, such results must be interpreted with the knowledge that these samples include blood from adjacent noninjured myocardium. However, the use of coronary venous samples for studying metabolism is decreasing because of new approaches using microdialysis, MRI, nuclear magnetic resonance spectroscopy, and positron emission tomography [36–38].

The size and location of myocardial infarction can be determined by triphenyltetrazolium chloride (TTC) staining, which has been the gold standard for quantifying the extent of myocardial infarction in pathological specimens [39] (Fig. 25.8). In addition, the assessment of localized tissue blood flow using microspheres (radioactive or colored) remains another important standard. However, newer noninvasive methods of determining blood flow in the live animal that allow for repeated follow-up determinations are being developed and improved upon, including spectroscopy and MRI.

Fig. 25.8 Triphenyltetrazolium chloride (TTC) staining in canine infarct model showing paleness of myocardium in left anterior coronary artery distribution

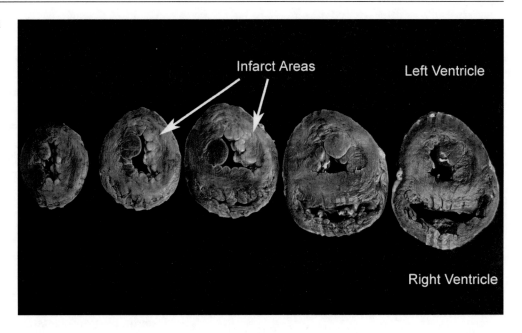

Infarct Areas

Left Ventricle

Right Ventricle

25.5.3 Specific Animal Models for Ischemia Investigations

Both large and small animal models have been developed for the study of myocardial ischemia. Advantages of large animal models are their similarity in physiology to humans and ease of instrumentation, and disadvantages include significantly greater care and cost issues that may make small animal models more attractive, particularly when large numbers of animals are required to achieve significant statistical power.

The dog has been the most frequently utilized species for in vivo studies of chronic ischemia because dogs have a well-developed coronary collateral circulation, similar to humans with chronic ischemia (progressive heart failure). Furthermore, dogs are easy to handle and lack significant growth as adults, which allows long-term follow-up. However, the significant variability in coronary collateral circulation may hamper efforts to create consistent sizes of ischemic regions between animals, or may result in a minimized ischemic zone.

The pig heart is more similar to the relatively healthy human heart in that there is limited collateral blood flow; this makes the swine heart ideal for acute ischemia studies. However, long-term follow-up using the swine model, in general, is considered problematic; if juvenile animals are utilized, significant changes in animal weight will result in both increased difficulties with handling as well as alterations in basic cardiac physiology. More specifically, in consideration of heart to body weight ratios, in a healthy person the ratio is about 5 g/kg; for pigs weighing between 25 and 30 kg, the ratio is similar to that in humans, but for animals exceeding 100 kg, it is

only half that value [35]. Importantly, such ratio changes must be considered when interpreting experimental results.

Small animals have also been used as models for investigations of regional myocardial ischemia. However, it has been established that the collateral circulation of the rat is sparse and that of the rabbit may show intraspecies differences [40]. In turn, the guinea pig has such an extensive collateral network that normal perfusion is maintained after a coronary artery occlusion and often infarction does not develop. Another problem with using these animals is that the small vessel diameters may delay or prevent instantaneous reperfusion following transient vessel occlusion, which is further complicated by the inability to make quantitative assessments of coronary blood flow in these small vessels to verify reperfusion. Nevertheless, the use of small animal models for studying myocardial ischemia remains important, including recent studies using stem cells for treatment; see also Chapter 6 for additional details on the comparative coronary circulations.

25.6 Animal Models in Heart Failure and Transplantation

Alexis Carrel reported the first heterotopic transplantation (Table 25.3) of a canine heart connected to the neck vessels of another dog in 1905, but the transplant succumbed to massive clotting and the animal survived for only 2 h. Many years later, Richard Lower and Norman Shumway perfected an orthotopic transplantation

Table 25.3 Definition of graft types

Graft type	Definition
Autograft	Transplant from one site to another in the same individual
Isograft	Transplant from a donor to a genetically identical individual (monozygotic twin)
Syngraft	Transplant from a donor to a recipient with no detectable genetic difference (inbred strain)
Allograft (homograft)	Transplant from a donor to a genetically different individual of the same species
Xenograft (heterograft)	Transplant from a donor to a recipient of another species

technique in the canine and achieved heart graft survivals of up to 21 days. Translation of this research to clinical practice was first performed by Christian Barnard in 1967, but acceptable graft survival required further studies in animal models to overcome rejection by the host immune system.

Today, the successful treatment of end-stage cardiac failure is possible with organ transplantation. In addition, mechanical assist devices are employed for patients who may not initially qualify for transplantation. However, it is clear that too few suitable donor organs are available to meet the current needs (Fig. 25.9). This lack of a reliable and stable source of donor hearts serves as the main impetus for further research into: (1) stem cell therapy used before heart failure; (2) the means to expand cardiac donor pools; and (3) the use of mechanical assist devices and xenotransplantation.

25.6.1 Methods in Transplantation Research

Extensive research has been conducted in the field of cardiac transplantation (Fig. 25.10). "Orthotopic" heart transplantation (the placement of the donor heart in the anatomically correct position) was made possible only after the pioneering efforts of C. Walton Lillehei (refer to Heart Transplantation by Kirklin et al. [41] for a complete discussion of the surgical technique). Orthotopic transplantation is technically feasible using available cardiopulmonary bypass circuits in both the canine and porcine animal models and has often been chosen for the study of organ preservation, graft rejection immunology, immunosuppressive regimens, and/or ischemia/reperfusion injury [42–44].

"Heterotopic" cardiac transplantation places the heart in an anatomical location other than the mediastinum. A heart transplanted into the heterotopic position is performed by connecting the donor aorta to the recipient aorta, and the donor pulmonary artery to the recipient vena cava. As a result, blood flow is typically nonphysiologic; normal patterns are limited to the coronary arterial and venous system. Absence of significant flow in the ventricles, except for drainage of blood from the coronary sinus into its right ventricle, may promote clot formation and graft failure. Heterotopic transplantation is typically used for studies on ischemia/reperfusion injury [45], prevention of rejection and immunosuppression [46], xenotransplantation, and/or coronary vascular pathology [47]. Heterotopic heart transplantations are most commonly performed using small mammal models such as the mouse, rat, hamster, guinea pig, or rabbit; yet, additional skills with microsurgical techniques are then required. An advantage of this approach is that recipients may retain complete function of their native hearts whether or not the heterotopic donor hearts survive.

25.6.2 Specific Animal Models for Transplantation Research

The choice of an animal model for cardiac transplantation depends greatly upon the area of pathophysiological research. The following is a brief introduction to models that are currently used in this field.

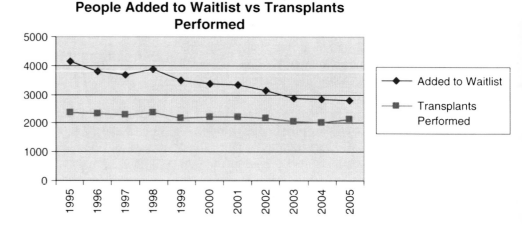

Fig. 25.9 Total number of United Network for Organ Sharing (UNOS) cardiac transplant waiting list registrants and donor hearts per year. Adapted from the UNOS database

Fig. 25.10 Orthotopic heart transplant drawing (original art by Martin E. Finch)

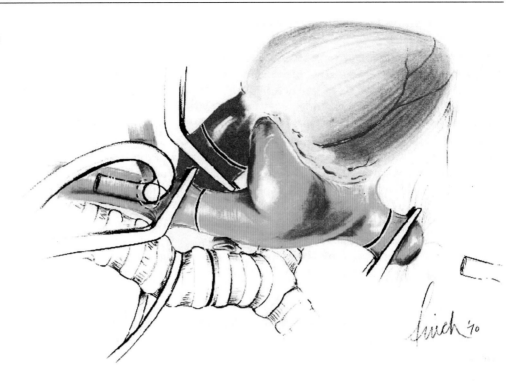

25.6.2.1 The Rodent Transplantation Model

The development of microsurgical techniques has allowed the performance of heart transplantation in rodents. Importantly, the use of rodents in transplantation research can dramatically reduce the costs associated with larger animal models. Typically, Lewis rats have been used for transplantation experiments related to ischemia and reperfusion, prevention of rejection, immunosuppression, and coronary vascular pathology. Because of the small size of rodents, the technique of heterotopic heart transplantation to the abdominal aorta and inferior vena cava, as described by Ono and Lindsey, has been used extensively [48].

Anatomically, the coronary artery blood flow in rodents differs somewhat from higher order mammals in that the left and right coronary arteries traverse the lateral wall of the right ventricle rather than the atrioventricular sulcus. In addition, the internal mammary arteries supply the atria with blood flow via the cardiomediastinal arteries. Some further disadvantages of the rodent model are that hemodynamic measurement of the transplanted hearts can be difficult and transplantation requires microvascular surgical techniques and a surgical microscope. Yet, an advantage of this model is its use for xenotransplantation experiments with grafts from mouse to rat, hamster to rat, guinea pig to rat, or hamster to guinea pig. In addition, preservation solutions can be fairly easily evaluated for the end points of survival, for histology, and/or

for high-energy phosphate analyses. Furthermore, the heterotopic rat transplant model has been extensively used in the pharmaceutical industry to evaluate the effectiveness of anti-rejection medications. More recently, the availability of transgenic or knock-out rodents continues to have a large impact in this area of research.

25.6.2.2 The Canine Transplantation Model

The anatomy of the canine heart is similar to that of the human heart (for more details, see Chapter 6). As mentioned above, the dog's heart has an extensive collateral circulation connecting the left and right coronary circulation. In contrast, nonathletic humans elicit few bridging collaterals. This collateral circulation in the dog is considered to be theoretically advantageous in heart transplantation experiments, as it may protect marginal areas of the heart from ischemia. From the perspective of an easy-to-employ model, dogs have a minimal amount of adipose tissue and their skin is loose, allowing tunneling of catheters if vascular access is needed postoperatively. Furthermore, the dog's relatively large thorax and mediastinum allow for clear visualization of the heart and great vessels. Thus, the canine model for heart transplantation is generally considered most easy to employ for animal studies on organ preservation, reperfusion injury, rejection studies, and/or posttransplant organ monitoring.

25.6.2.3 The Swine Transplantation Model

The porcine heart is often considered the most anatomically similar to the human heart. Specifically, as noted above, the porcine heart has few collateral vessels, and an end artery coronary anatomy predominates. Yet, cannulation for cardiopulmonary bypass may be difficult, and the right atrial tissue has typically been described as fragile or friable [2]. In addition, a surgical cut down for venous and arterial access may be required, secondary to the thick subcutaneous layer of adipose tissue. The pig transplantation model is also prone to postoperative wound infections, necessitating strict sterile techniques during cardiac surgery. Furthermore, juvenile pigs have a rapid rate of somatic growth, which can challenge long-term foreign body implantations. Physiologically, the porcine heart is considered to be prone to arrhythmias and is sensitive to physical manipulation. Bretylium tosylate can be given to limit such arrhythmias; however, ventricular fibrillation can be a recurrent problem following cardiopulmonary bypass [49]. The swine model is considered appropriate for heart transplantation, however, it is often described to be more suited to acute or short-term graft survival studies [50]. Ongoing projects to create a porcine heart with compatible tissue antigens to be used as a substitute for the human donor heart are exciting areas of research that will make the increased use of swine heart donors more likely. Thus, transgenic pigs that express human membrane-associated complement inhibitors in the vasculature have been used for studies of xenotransplantation in nonhuman primate recipients. Moreover, pigs with genetic deletions to prevent the expression of certain antigens that are involved in rejection are currently used as donors for nonhuman primates, making it possible to achieve significant prolongations of graft survival.

25.6.2.4 The Nonhuman Primate Transplantation Model

Researchers in the field of cardiac transplantation have used the nonhuman primate model extensively in developing both the technique of transplantation and the scientific background necessary for the survival of the donor heart [51, 52]. Numerous programs have successfully used the nonhuman primate in small and large cardiac transplant studies [53–55]. Yet, particular problems with the use of primates have been associated with their veterinary care requirements during preoperative and postoperative times, and thus appropriate facilities are needed. Furthermore, nonhuman primates are extremely susceptible to *Mycobacterium tuberculosis* and appropriate precautions must be taken to minimize the risk of infection. It should be noted that baboons are sensitive to stress and are apt to develop gastroenteritis and bacteremia after surgery, and handling of the baboon typically requires sedation. Nevertheless, the use of baboons and other nonhuman primates has many advantages as an experimental model in transplant research. First, the anatomy of baboons is similar to that of humans, except that the baboon heart has only two aortic arch vessels compared to the three found in humans. Second, the growth of the baboon can be controlled, and adult weights in the 20–30 kg range are maintained for 20–30 years. Additionally, physiologic characteristics of the baboon heart are similar to those of humans, allowing for the use of standard operative instrumentation. From a technical standpoint, the cardiac tissue of the nonhuman primate is not considered as friable or prone to serious arrhythmias as that of swine.

Adverse immunological responses in the primate are a main concern with xenotransplantation and also with anti-rejection treatments. Interestingly, the human ABO blood type system is applicable with simian tissue and saliva, but not with simian blood [56]. Tissue typing with the major histocompatibility system using primate tissue is also possible. Hyperacute rejection of a pig heart is inherent to xenotransplantation in this model because of the preexisting antibodies in the recipient. Specifically, the donor antigens on the surface of the endothelium of the donor's heart react with antibodies of the recipient, resulting in rejection upon subsequent activation of complement [57]. Inhibition of complement activation or depletion of complement factors was shown to abrogate cardiac xenotransplant rejection [58]. Heterotopic (nonanatomic and nonfunctional) heart transplantation in the nonhuman primate is an established surgical procedure appropriate for investigation of immunosuppressive drug therapies and study of immune reactions between the donor heart and recipient. Typical locations for heterotopic implantation of the donor heart include the neck or abdomen of the primate [59].

25.7 Animal Models for the Testing of Mechanical Devices

Maximizing surgical therapies in end-stage heart failure is a field of great interest. Recently, devices (i.e., ventricular assist devices) have become increasingly important because of the large numbers of patients presenting with end-stage heart failure. Interestingly, mechanical ventricular assist devices are filling a niche where they are both a "bridge to transplant" and a "destination therapy" at centers such as the University of Minnesota. Before any such device can be implanted into a human, the procedure requires years of high-level animal testing.

25.7.1 Animal Model Selection for Device Testing

Animal models are necessary for both research and development of mechanical devices such as the ventricular assist device and for training of the medical personnel involved in their use. The justification for use of a particular animal model is primarily based on: (1) the investigator's past and current success using a particular animal; (2) device size; and/or (3) the relative comparative anatomy. Careful selection of an appropriate model will decrease the difficulty of implanting such devices; devices designed for human use will require a comparably sized research animal for testing. For example, the sizes of in-line axial flow pumps (Fig. 25.11) have become relatively compact and have been implanted into the dog, sheep, and calf models [60, 61]. Larger pumps, based upon a moving diaphragm, still require a larger animal [62] (Figs. 25.12, 25.13, and 25.14); see Chapter 36 for more details.

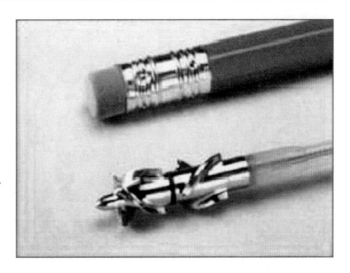

Fig. 25.11 Example of an axial flow pump impeller

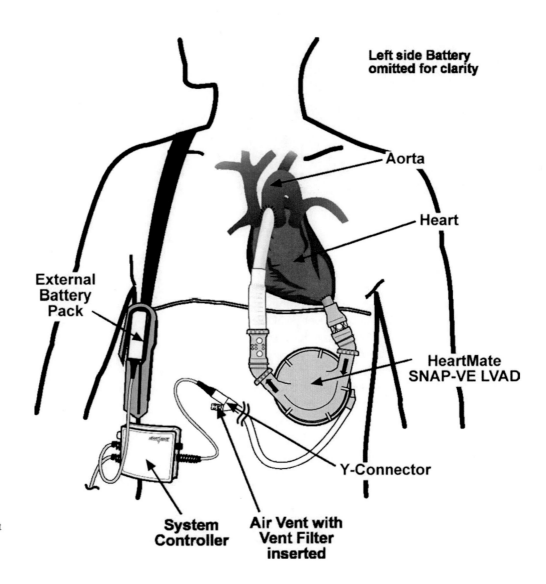

Left side Battery omitted for clarity

Aorta

Heart

External Battery Pack

HeartMate SNAP-VE LVAD

Y-Connector

System Controller

Air Vent with Vent Filter inserted

Fig. 25.12 Schematic of left ventricular assist device (LVAD) in human use

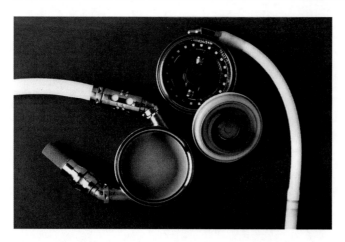

Fig. 25.13 Inside of typical left ventricular assist device (photo courtesy of Soon Park)

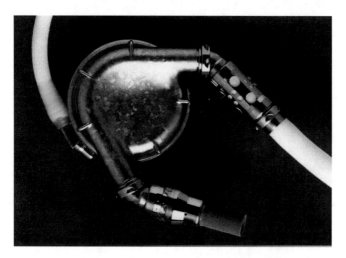

Fig. 25.14 Outside of typical left ventricular assist device (photo courtesy of Soon Park)

25.7.2 Federal Guidelines for Device Testing

Although ventricular assist device technology is a rapidly advancing field, the FDA has not yet published official guidance documents for such devices. However, the FDA does have specific evaluation criteria for the ventricular assist devices that are designed to identify possible hazards prior to clinical usage. Long-term reliability is a current issue of concern with such devices, as some patients waiting for a transplant survive longer, and destination therapy may become a reality for numerous device recipients. Consequently, long-term biocompatibility, thrombogenesis (long-term surface coating antithrombogenic integrity), bacterial infection, battery life, and hardware and software reliability have become important parameters for FDA evaluation of such devices. Ultimately, the ease of patient use related to ventricular assist devices is also of central importance.

25.8 Cellular Cardiomyoplasty

Cellular cardiomyoplasty, the process by which injured myocardium is repaired by cell transplantation, has significant clinical potential [63, 64]. Much of the excitement about cell-based therapy lies on the premise that repairing the injured heart will overcome the inherent limitations for the broad application of both organ transplantation and mechanical assist devices. A thorough review of the literature for stem cell-mediated cardiac therapy has been provided in Chapter 37, and thus will only be reviewed briefly in this section.

25.8.1 The Ideal Cell Population for Cardiomyoplasty

While advances in the field of cardiomyoplasty have recently been achieved with the advent of stem cell technology, the "ideal" population of cells that is able to effectively engraft damaged myocardium and restore cardiac function without improper differentiation to other contaminating cell types is still an issue of debate. Many cell types with the potential to repair the injured heart have been considered, including differentiated cells (fetal myocytes or satellite muscle cells) and undifferentiated cells (embryonic or adult stem cells). While pluripotent embryonic stem cells offer the promise of functional plasticity and the ability to differentiate into any cell type in vitro, extensive experimentation in vivo is still necessary to properly direct the formation of integrated, functional cardiac tissue at the site of injury without improper differentiation to form teratomas (tumors) or other noncardiac cell types. Multipotent tissue-specific cells that have already committed to a distinct lineage, such as hematopoietic stem cells, mesenchymal stem cells, and endothelial progenitor cells, have also produced encouraging results [65]. However, to date, the use of these cells often results in incomplete engraftment and a failure to restore cardiac function over time [66]. Regardless of the cell type used in cardiomyoplasty, it is clear that animal models will again play a crucial role in the translational research that will be necessary to advance this theory into clinical practice.

25.8.2 Animal Models for Stem Cell Research

Although multiple animal species have been used for the study of cellular cardiomyoplasty, most investigators have chosen acute ischemia as their experimental model of choice. However, while effective treatment options for acute ischemia do exist, only limited options are available for chronic myocardial ischemia. This observation strongly suggests that further development of the chronic ischemia models using cardiomyoplasty is warranted. As with most research, the experimental hypothesis will remain fundamental in choosing the correct animal model. However, the lack of appropriate stem cell lines in the desired species will add more limitations in selection. Fully characterizing cell lines are important and advantageous, so functional changes of the therapy are correctly attributed to the appropriate precursor cell.

The multiple types of stem cells available for the rodent, specifically the rat and mouse, have made small animal models effective for investigations of stem cell engraftments. However, the differences in myocardial perfusion and ventricular thickness may confer differences in nutrient supplies that would support engraftment in small animal models, but the results obtained may not be translatable to either large mammalian models or humans.

Ultimately, large animal models that better approximate the diseased human heart will be required to fully assess stem cell engraftment, differentiation, and/or functional improvement. Furthermore, large animal models, in general, are considered better suited for assessment of myocardial function via angiography, echocardiography, or MRI; however, to date, the limited availability of appropriate stem cell lines for use in these models has prevented the widespread use of large animal models. Nevertheless, stem cell lines are currently being developed for the pig, dog, and monkey at a number of institutions. More specifically, one lab has developed a canine model of cardiomyoplasty for chronic ischemia in which bone marrow-derived stem cells are used (Fig. 25.15). Two of this chapter's co-authors (Gallegos and Bianco) have demonstrated successful engraftment and statistically significant, sustained long-term improvement in regional myocardial function by MRI follow-up. Though successful, this first effort has resulted in additional questions that need resolution: (1) How and when should we deliver the cells? (2) How many cells should be implanted? (3) How often do cells need to be delivered? Much work has yet to be completed before one can be certain that stem cell therapies can be considered a viable treatment for various forms of myocardial disease.

25.8.3 Stem Cell Delivery Methods

Multiple methods of stem cell delivery have been investigated including direct myocardial injection, peripheral transfusion, and/or stem cell mobilization [67]. Direct epicardial–myocardial injection can be fairly consistently

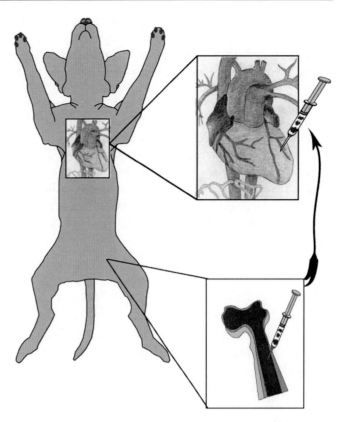

Fig. 25.15 Canine model for bone marrow-derived multipotent stem cell cardiomyoplasty (illustration courtesy of Kathy B. Nichols)

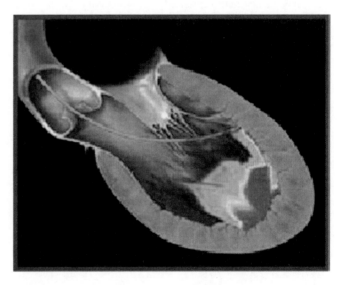

Fig. 25.16 Example of catheter-guided stem cell therapy for myocardial infarction. Adapted from http://www.texasheartinstitute.org/.html

completed intraoperatively during procedures such as coronary arterial bypass or valve operations. Endocardial injection will likely be completed by using commercially available, radiographically guided stem cell injection catheters (Fig. 25.16). Both transfusion and mobilization of resident stem cells offer the least invasive means of stem cell delivery, but require the availability of effective cellular homing signals to direct the correct location for engraftment. This latter hurdle could possibly be overcome by using guided direct myocardial injections, either surgically or via interventional catheter techniques. Available information suggests that multiple stem cell injections may be required to achieve full myocardial regeneration for therapeutic repair. As a result, the use of stem cell injection catheters may become the standard of practice. In addition, advanced imaging techniques such as MRI could be used to localize injured myocardium and direct, in real-time, stem cell injection catheters to the damaged area.

25.8.4 Stem Cell Engraftment Issues

The ability to track the implanted cell is critical not only to assess the potential of engraftment but also for later determination of differentiation and incorporation into the native tissue. Multiple techniques of cell labeling are currently under investigation including the use of viral gene transduction (e.g., DAPI, Green Fluorescent Gene, Lac Z), incorporation of dyes, and the use of metallic microparticles [68, 69]. For example, gene insertion can be fairly easily accomplished, i.e., allowing for fluorescence microscopy or Q-PCR identification of the stem cell. However, the exact insertion site into the DNA of the cell cannot currently be well controlled, introducing the possibility for nonexpression of the gene or potential disruption of normal cellular transcription and translation processes. The use of dyes incorporated into the cells by pinocytosis has been reported. The primary disadvantage of this technique has been the potential for dye incorporation into native cells in vivo. The use of metallic microparticles has received recent attention, since such particles may allow for real-time identification of cells by MRI imaging and later pathologically by staining. However, information about the potential disruption of cellular function and possible uptake in vivo by native cells has yet to be fully elucidated.

25.8.5 Functional Assessment of Stem Cell Therapies

Many efforts to demonstrate improvement in cardiac function following cellular cardiomyoplasty have been undertaken. Methods include pressure measurements, ultrasonic microcrystal placement, echocardiography,

and/or MRI. Regardless of the specific method used by the investigators, minimally significant long-term follow-up studies currently exist in the literature. Thus, we conclude that much more research is required before this approach can be applied to humans.

25.9 Summary

In preparing to embark on a preclinical study of a new cardiovascular device, procedure, drug, or therapy, it is important to carefully select the animal model. This can be done in consultation with your Institutional Animal Care and Use Committee or, if the investigator does not have appropriate experience in this area, by collaboration with an investigator who is experienced. Proper selection of the animal model in the protocol development will allow justification for the animal use and maximize the chances for a successful research outcome. New cardiovascular technologies will continue to be introduced in an environment of increasingly tighter regulations for animal and human safety. The use of animal models will continue to be important for testing new therapies before they are applied in clinical studies. Consultation with experienced centers of experimental research is recommended as additional assistance for preparing research protocols and completing the research necessary in preclinical studies. Experimental Surgical Services at the University of Minnesota provides such a service and is widely used for assessment of a variety of techniques and/or novel devices currently being developed globally by the medical industry.

References

1. tNRC Institute of Laboratory Animal Resources, and the National Academy of Sciences: Guide for the Care and Use of Laboratory Animals. National Academy Press. 3/96.
2. Gross DR, ed. Animal models in cardiovascular research. 2nd ed. Dordrecht, The Netherlands: Kluwer Academic Press, 1994:494.
3. Ettinger SJ. Congenital heart diseases. In: Ettinger SJ, Feldman EC, eds. Textbook of veterinary internal medicine: Diseases of the dog and cat. Philadelphia, PA: WB Saunders, 2000:737–87.
4. Haworth RA, Hunter DR, Berkoff HA, Moss RL. Metabolic cost of the stimulated beating of isolated adult rat heart cells in suspension. Circ Res 1983;52:342–51.
5. Spieckermann PG, Piper HM. Oxygen demand of calcium-tolerant adult cardiac myocytes. Basic Res Cardiol 1985;80:71–4.
6. Claycomb WC, Lanson NA Jr, Stallworth BS, et al. HL-1 cells: A cardiac muscle cell line that contracts and retains phenotypic characteristics of the adult cardiomyocyte. Proc Natl Acad Sci USA 1998;95:2979–84.

7. Niggli E. A laser diffraction system with improved sensitivity for long-time measurements of sarcomere dynamics in isolated cardiac myocytes. Pflugers Arch 1988;411:462–8.

8. Roos KP, Brady AJ, Tan ST. Direct measurement of sarcomere length from isolated cardiac cells. Am J Physiol 1982;242:H68–78.

9. Roos KP, Brady AJ. Individual sarcomere length determination from isolated cardiac cells using high-resolution optical microscopy and digital image processing. Biophys J 1982;40:233–44.

10. Murphy MP, Hohl C, Brierley GP, Altschuld RA. Release of enzymes from adult rat heart myocytes. Circ Res 1982;51:560–8.

11. Tung L. An ultrasensitive transducer for measurement of isometric contractile force from single heart cells. Pflugers Arch 1986;407:109–15.

12. Chinchoy E, Soule CL, Houlton AJ, et al. Isolated four-chamber working swine heart model. Ann Thorac Surg 2000;70:1607–14.

13. Hill AJ, Coles JA, Sigg DC, Laske TG, Iaizzo PA. Images of the human coronary sinus ostium obtained from isolated working hearts. Ann Thorac Surg 2003;76:2108.

14. Neely JR, Liebermeister H, Morgan HE. Effect of pressure development on membrane transport of glucose in isolated rat heart. Am J Physiol 1967;212:815–22.

15. Wicomb WN, Cooper DK, Barnard CN. Twenty-four-hour preservation of the pig heart by a portable hypothermic perfusion system. Transplantation 1982;34:246–50.

16. Dunphy G, Richter HW, Azodi M, et al. The effects of mannitol, albumin, and cardioplegia enhancers on 24-h rat heart preservation. Am J Physiol 1999;276:H1591–8.

17. Menasche P, Hricak B, Pradier F, et al. Efficacy of lactobionate-enriched cardioplegic solution in preserving compliance of cold-stored heart transplants. J Heart Lung Transplant 1993;12:1053–61.

18. Gallegos RP, Nockel PJ, Rivard AL, Bianco RW. The current state of in-vivo pre-clinical animal models for heart valve evaluation. J Heart Valve Dis 2005;14:423–32.

19. Taylor DE, Whamond JS. A method of producing graded stenosis of the aortic and mitral valves in sheep for fluid dynamic studies. J Physiol 1975;244:16–7P.

20. Su-Fan Q, Brum JM, Kaye MP, Bove AA. A new technique for producing pure aortic stenosis in animals. Am J Physiol 1984;246:H296–301.

21. Rogers WA, Bishop SP, Hamlin RL. Experimental production of supravalvular aortic stenosis in the dog. J Appl Physiol 1971;30:917–20.

22. Spratt JA, Olsen CO, Tyson GS Jr, Glower DD Jr, Davis JW, Rankin JS. Experimental mitral regurgitation. Physiological effects of correction on left ventricular dynamics. J Thorac Cardiovasc Surg 1983;86:479–89.

23. Swindle MM, Adams RJ, eds. Experimental surgery and physiology: Induced animals models of human disease. Philadelphia, PA: Williams & Wilkins, 1988.

24. Bianco RW, St Cyr JA, Schneider JR, et al. Canine model for long-term evaluation of prosthetic mitral valves. J Surg Res 1986;41:134–40.

25. Grehan JF, Hilbert SL, Ferrans VJ, Droel JS, Salerno CT, Bianco RW. Development and evaluation of a swine model to assess the preclinical safety of mechanical heart valves. J Heart Valve Dis 2000;9:710–9; discussion 719–20.

26. Barnhart GR, Jones M, Ishihara T, Chavez AM, Rose DM, Ferrans VJ. Bioprosthetic valvular failure. Clinical and pathological observations in an experimental animal model. J Thorac Cardiovasc Surg 1982;83:618–31.

27. Sands MP, Rittenhouse EA, Mohri H, Merendino KA. An anatomical comparison of human pig, calf, and sheep aortic valves. Ann Thorac Surg 1969;8:407–14.

28. Salerno CT, Droel J, Bianco RW. Current state of in vivo preclinical heart valve evaluation. J Heart Valve Dis 1998;7:158–62.

29. Yu WC, Chen SA, Lee SH, et al. Tachycardia-induced change of atrial refractory period in humans: Rate dependency and effects of antiarrhythmic drugs. Circulation 1998;97: 2331–7.

30. Au-Yeung K, Johnson CR, Wolf PD. A novel implantable cardiac telemetry system for studying atrial fibrillation. Physiol Meas 2004;25:1223–38.

31. Sharifov OF, Fedorov VV, Beloshapko GG, Glukhov AV, Yushmanova AV, Rosenshtraukh LV. Roles of adrenergic and cholinergic stimulation in spontaneous atrial fibrillation in dogs. J Am Coll Cardiol 2004;43:483–90.

32. Brugada R, Roberts R. Molecular biology and atrial fibrillation. Curr Opin Cardiol 1999;14:269–73.

33. Rivard AL, Suwan PT, Imaninaini K, Gallegos RP, Bianco RW. Development of a sheep model of atrial fibrillation for preclinical prosthetic valve testing. J Heart Valve Dis 2007;16:314–23.

34. Gallegos RP, Wang X, Clarkson C, Jerosch-Herold M, Bolman RM. Serum troponin level predicts infarct size. In: American Heart Association. San Antonio, TX: American Heart Association, 2003.

35. Verdouw PD, van den Doel MA, de Zeeuw S, Duncker DJ. Animal models in the study of myocardial ischaemia and ischaemic syndromes. Cardiovasc Res 1998;39:121–35.

36. McFalls EO, Baldwin D, Palmer B, Marx D, Jaimes D, Ward HB. Regional glucose uptake within hypoperfused swine myocardium as measured by positron emission tomography. Am J Physiol 1997;272:H343–9.

37. Headrick JP, Emerson CS, Berr SS, Berne RM, Matherne GP. Interstitial adenosine and cellular metabolism during beta-adrenergic stimulation of the in situ rabbit heart. Cardiovasc Res 1996;31:699–710.

38. Massie BM, Schwartz GG, Garcia J, Wisneski JA, Weiner MW, Owens T. Myocardial metabolism during increased work states in the porcine left ventricle in vivo. Circ Res 1994;74:64–73.

39. Lie JT, Holley KE, Kampa WR, Titus JL. New histochemical method for morphologic diagnosis of early stages of myocardial ischemia. Mayo Clin Proc 1971;46:319–27.

40. Winkler B, Binz K, Schaper W. Myocardial blood flow and infarction in rats, guinea pigs, and rabbits. J Mol Cell Cardiology 1984;16:48.

41. Kirklin JK, Young JB, McGiffin D, eds. Heart transplantation. New York: Churchill Livingstone, 2002:883.

42. Wicomb W, Cooper DK, Hassoulas J, Rose AG, Barnard CN. Orthotopic transplantation of the baboon heart after 20 to 24 hours' preservation by continuous hypothermic perfusion with an oxygenated hyperosmolar solution. J Thorac Cardiovasc Surg 1982; 83:133–40.

43. Tsutsumi H, Oshima K, Mohara J, et al. Cardiac transplantation following a 24-h preservation using a perfusion apparatus. J Surg Res 2001;96:260–7.

44. Fischel RJ, Matas AJ, Platt JL, et al. Cardiac xenografting in the pig-to-rhesus monkey model: Manipulation of antiendothelial antibody prolongs survival. J Heart Lung Transplant 1992;11:965–73; discussion 973–4.

45. Langman LJ, Nakakura H, Thliveris JA, LeGatt DF, Yatscoff RW. Pharmacodynamic monitoring of mycophenolic acid in rabbit heterotopic heart transplant model. Ther Drug Monit 1997;19:146–52.

46. Beschorner WE, Sudan DL, Radio SJ, et al. Heart xenograft survival with chimeric pig donors and modest immune suppression. Ann Surg 2003;237:265–72.

47. Perrault LP, Bidouard JP, Desjardins N, Villeneuve N, Vilaine JP, Vanhoutte PM. Comparison of coronary endothelial

dysfunction in the working and nonworking graft in porcine heterotopic heart transplantation. Transplantation 2002;74:764–72.

48. Ono K, Lindsey ES. Improved technique of heart transplantation in rats. J Thorac Cardiovasc Surg 1969;57:225–9.

49. Swindle MM, Horneffer PJ, Gardner TJ, et al. Anatomic and anesthetic considerations in experimental cardiopulmonary surgery in swine. Lab Anim Sci 1986;36:357–61.

50. Kozlowski T, Shimizu A, Lambrigts D, et al. Porcine kidney and heart transplantation in baboons undergoing a tolerance induction regimen and antibody adsorption. Transplantation 1999;67:18–30.

51. Goddard MJ, Dunning J, Horsley J, Atkinson C, Pino-Chavez G, Wallwork J. Histopathology of cardiac xenograft rejection in the pig-to-baboon model. J Heart Lung Transplant 2002;21:474–84.

52. DeBault L, Ye Y, Rolf LL, et al. Ultrastructural features in hyperacutely rejected baboon cardiac allografts and pig cardiac xenografts. Transplant Proc 1992;24:612–3.

53. Brenner P, Schmoeckel M, Reichenspurner H, et al. Technique of immunoapheresis in heterotopic and orthotopic xenotransplantation of pig hearts into cynomolgus and rhesus monkeys. Transplant Proc 2000;32:1087–8.

54. Kurlansky PA, Sadeghi AM, Michler RE, et al. Comparable survival of intra-species and cross-species primate cardiac transplants. Transplant Proc 1987;19:1067–71.

55. Lambrigts D, Sachs DH, Cooper DK. Discordant organ xenotransplantation in primates: world experience and current status. Transplantation 1998;66:547–61.

56. Wiener AS, Socha WW, Moor-Jankowski J. Homologous of the human A-B-O blood groups in apes and monkeys. Haematologia (Budap) 1974;8:195–216.

57. Kroshus TJ, Rollins SA, Dalmasso AP, et al. Complement inhibition with an anti-C5 monoclonal antibody prevents acute cardiac tissue injury in an ex vivo model of pig-to-human xenotransplantation. Transplantation 1995;60:1194–202.

58. Salerno CT, Kulick DM, Yeh CG, et al. A soluble chimeric inhibitor of C3 and C5 convertases, complement activation blocker-2, prolongs graft survival in pig-to-rhesus monkey heart transplantation. Xenotransplantation 2002;9:125–34.

59. Cramer DV, Podesta L, Makowka L, eds. Handbook of animal models in transplantation research. Boca Raton, FL: CRC Press, 1994:352.

60. Li X, Bai J, He P. Simulation study of the Hemopump as a cardiac assist device. Med Biol Eng Comput 2002;40:344–53.

61. Snyder TA, Watach MJ, Litwak KN, Wagner WR. Platelet activation, aggregation, and life span in calves implanted with axial flow ventricular assist devices. Ann Thorac Surg 2002;73:1933–8.

62. Mussivand T, Fujimoto L, Butler K, et al. In vitro and in vivo performance evaluation of a totally implantable electrohydraulic left ventricular assist system. ASAIO Trans 1989; 35:433–5.

63. Reffelmann T, Leor J, Muller-Ehmsen J, Kedes L, Kloner RA. Cardiomyocyte transplantation into the failing heart-new therapeutic approach for heart failure? Heart Fail Rev 2003;8:201–11.

64. Reffelmann T, Kloner RA. Cellular cardiomyoplasty—cardiomyocytes, skeletal myoblasts, or stem cells for regenerating myocardium and treatment of heart failure? Cardiovasc Res 2003;58:358–68.

65. Reffelmann T, Dow JS, Dai W, Hale SL, Simkhovich BZ, Kloner RA. Transplantation of neonatal cardiomyocytes after permanent coronary artery occlusion increases regional blood flow of infarcted myocardium. J Mol Cell Cardiol 2003;35:607–13.

66. Sakai T, Ling Y, Payne TR, Huard J. The use of ex vivo gene transfer based on muscle-derived stem cells for cardiovascular medicine. Trends Cardiovasc Med 2002;12:115–20.

67. Hill JM, Dick AJ, Raman VK, et al. Serial cardiac magnetic resonance imaging of injected mesenchymal stem cells. Circulation 2003;108:1009–14.

68. Kraitchman DL, Heldman AW, Atalar E, et al. In vivo magnetic resonance imaging of mesenchymal stem cells in myocardial infarction. Circulation 2003;107:2290–3.

69. Kraitchman DL, Sampath S, Castillo E, et al. Quantitative ischemia detection during cardiac magnetic resonance stress testing by use of FastHARP. Circulation 2003; 107:2025–30.

Chapter 26
Catheter Ablation of Cardiac Arrhythmias

Xiao-Huan Li and Fei Lü

Abstract The range of the resting sinus heart rate is 50–90 beats per minute (bpm); most average healthy individuals have resting rates in the 60–70 bpm range. *Bradycardia* (slow heart beat) is arbitrarily defined as any heart rate <60 bpm, and *tachycardia* (fast heart beat) as any rate >100 bpm. Disturbances of cardiac impulse formation and/or transmission comprise the principal mechanisms causing abnormalities of heart rhythm. In basic terms, these are classified as being either brady- or tachy-arrhythmias. The primary goals for treatment of arrhythmias are: (1) to alleviate symptoms and improve quality of life and; (2) to prolong patient survival. Pharmacologic treatment has been the mainstay for management of most cardiac arrhythmias, although implantable devices and ablation have become increasingly important. In recent years, nonpharmacologic therapy has begun to play an increasingly important role in curing many arrhythmias (catheter ablation) and preventing their life-threatening consequences (implantable cardioverter defibrillator therapy for both primary and secondary prevention of sudden cardiac death).

Keywords Ablation · Arrhythmia · Bradycardia · fibrillation · flutter · sudden cardiac death · Tachycardia

26.1 Introduction

Since it is fundamentally important to understand the mechanism underlying each individual cardiac arrhythmia for catheter ablation therapy, basic cardiac electrophysiology and individual arrhythmias are described first in this chapter. The normal heartbeat is initiated by pacemaker cells in the sinus node located in the right atrium, adjacent to its junction with the superior vena cava. These cells comprise a specialized, albeit somewhat diffuse, region of the right atrium called the sinus node. The rate and regularity of sinus node activity are determined by the intrinsic firing rate (automaticity) of the cells within the node and the influence of extrinsic factors on these cells, including autonomic neural tone, electrolytes, and drugs. The usual range of the resting sinus rate is 50–90 beats per minute (bpm), although rates as low as 35–40 bpm are common in fit (athletic) individuals. Most average healthy people have resting rates in the 60–70 bpm range. *Bradycardia* (slow heart beat) is a term used to refer to any heart rate <60 bpm and *tachycardia* (fast heart beat) indicates rates >100 bpm. Clearly, these definition boundaries are arbitrary.

Once generated by the sinus node cells, the cardiac electrical impulse traverses the atria by means of preferential conduction routes (determined by intra-atrial muscle band geography) to the atrioventricular (AV) node, which is the beginning of the true anatomic specialized conduction system in the ventricle (i.e., the His bundle, bundle branches, and penetrating Purkinje fiber network). Normally, impulse transit through the AV node is relatively slow (such delay accounts for the majority of the PR interval recorded on the surface electrocardiogram), thereby offering the opportunity for mechanical transfer of blood from the atria to the ventricles prior to initiation of ventricular activation (see Chapter 11).

26.2 Mechanism of Cardiac Arrhythmias

Disturbances of cardiac impulse formation and/or transmission comprise the principal mechanisms causing abnormalities of heart rhythm. In basic terms, these are classified as being either brady- or tachy-arrhythmias. Bradycardia may be "physiologic" in some individuals or it may be the result of either "sinus node dysfunction"

F. Lü (✉)
University of Minnesota, Department of Medicine, MMC 508, Minneapolis, MN 55455, USA
e-mail: luxxx074@umn.edu

P.A. Iaizzo (ed.), *Handbook of Cardiac Anatomy, Physiology, and Devices*, DOI 10.1007/978-1-60327-372-5_26,

(known still by some as "sick sinus syndrome") or AV conduction block (i.e., intermittent or permanent block of impulse transmission from the site of normal pacemaker activity in the atria through the specialized cardiac conduction system to the ventricles). Either of these conditions can be caused by intrinsic disease in the pacemaker cell or conduction system or by extrinsic factors such as medications or autonomic system disturbances.

The mechanisms underlying tachycardias are multiple and more complex than those causing bradycardias. Nevertheless, tachycardias can be classified as being due to either abnormally rapid impulse initiation (i.e., *abnormal automaticity* whether from the sinus node region or other subsidiary or abnormal pacemaker sites) or *abnormal impulse conduction*, or both (see Table 26.1).

The term "arrhythmia" is typically used to refer to disturbances of the normal heart rhythm. An exception to this rule is "sinus arrhythmia" which refers to the normal variation of the sinus rhythm associated with physiologic alteration of neural influence on sinus node cellular pacemaker automaticity. The most important cause of the later variation is the respiratory cycle, but other factors such as beat-to-beat changes in cardiac output (i.e., ventriculophasic feedback) may also contribute.

26.3 Clinical Presentation and Diagnosis

Arrhythmias can and often do occur in an apparently normal heart (e.g., premature atrial or ventricular beats, paroxysmal supraventricular tachycardias). However, the clinically important rhythm disturbances are more commonly associated with structural heart disease. Myocardial ischemia is the most important substrate for serious arrhythmias in the Western world, but other forms of cardiac dysfunction such as cardiomyopathies, valvular

heart disease, and certain genetically determined disorders (e.g., long QT syndrome, Brugada syndrome) are also to be considered. In certain regions of the world, infections remain an important cause of heart rhythm disturbance, such as rheumatic heart disease in Africa and Asia or Chagas disease in South America. In Western countries, viral illnesses and rare bacterial infections such as Lyme disease cause myocarditis or pericarditis, and are of particular concern in both children and adolescents.

The clinical presentation of cardiac arrhythmias may range widely from being completely asymptomatic or inducing mild symptoms (palpitations and anxiety) to syncope and even sudden cardiac death (SCD); the clinical impact is largely dependent on arrhythmia-induced hemodynamic changes. The electrophysiologic and hemodynamic consequences of a particular arrhythmia are primarily determined by: (1) the ventricular rate and duration; (2) the site of origin; (3) the underlying cardiovascular status (i.e., severity of associated heart and vascular disease); and/or (4) the promptness and completeness of autonomic nervous system response to the arrhythmia-induced "stress."

Some arrhythmias can be readily diagnosed by standard 12-lead electrocardiography (ECG), but the conventional 12-lead ECG is often too brief to detect transient rhythm problems. Consequently, other techniques are frequently required in order to establish an accurate diagnosis including: (1) prolonged ambulatory ECG monitoring (e.g., event monitors, Holter monitors, or mobile outpatient cardiac telemetry such as CardioNet® from CardioNet, Conshohocken, PA); (2) implantable loop recorders (Reveal® family, Medtronic, Inc., Minneapolis, MN or Sleuth® family, Transoma Medical Inc., St. Paul, MN); and (3) electrophysiologic testing. In selected cases, additional exercise stress testing and signal-averaged ECG recordings may also be used to assess an arrhythmia or the general susceptibility of a given patient to

Table 26.1 Mechanisms of tachycardias

Abnormal impulse initiation
  ☐ Automaticity
   • Enhanced normal automaticity: as seen in inappropriate sinus tachycardia and in some idiopathic ventricular tachycardias
   • Abnormal automaticity: as presumed to be the case in ectopic atrial tachycardia, accelerated junctional rhythm, and possibly certain idiopathic ventricular tachycardias
  ☐ Triggered activity
   • Early after-depolarization: as presumed to be the case in *Torsades de pointes*
   • Delayed after-depolarization: as seen in digitalis-induced or presumed to occur in certain exercise-induced arrhythmias

Abnormal impulse conduction
  ☐ Ectopic escape after block such as junctional escape
  ☐ Unidirectional block and reentry
   • Orderly reentry: macroreentry as seen in atrial flutter and microreentry as seen in atrial or ventricular tachycardia
   • Random reentry: as seen in atrial fibrillation
  ☐ Other concepts (reflection, phase 2 reentry, and anisotropic reentry)

arrhythmias. Other techniques have provided useful research information, but their value in daily practice remains to be fully defined at this time, such as: (1) analysis of heart rate variability; (2) relative baroreflex sensitivity; (3) assessment of QT dispersion or T-wave alternans; and/or (4) body surface potential mapping.

26.4 Treatment Considerations

The primary goals of treatment of arrhythmias are two-fold: (1) to alleviate symptoms and improve quality of life; and (2) to prolong individual survival. Pharmacologic treatment has been the mainstay for management of most cardiac arrhythmias although, in recent years, implantable devices and ablation have become increasingly important. In regard to antiarrhythmic drugs, many clinicians find it convenient to group them according to the old *Vaughn-Williams classification*. This classification is simple and has been widely used clinically, as it offers a means to keep the principal pharmacologic effects of drugs in mind (Table 26.2). A more comprehensive classification of antiarrhythmic drugs, termed *the Sicilian Gambit*, was introduced in 1991[1]. It is based on a more comprehensive consideration of the cellular basis of drug actions. However, neither scheme offers much help in the treatment of specific arrhythmias. Selection of antiarrhythmic drugs for a given patient should be individualized based on the arrhythmia being treated, the nature and severity of any underlying heart disease, the proposed drug's antiarrhythmic and proarrhythmic actions, and its potential side effects.

In patients with ischemia associated with left ventricular dysfunction, Class I antiarrhythmic agents should be avoided due to proarrhythmic risk (as well as the tendency of this class to exhibit marked negative inotropic effects). Class III drugs, on the other hand (i.e., amiodarone, sotalol, dofetilide), appear to have a neutral effect on survival in these patients and a lesser negative inotropic concern. Beta-blockers (Class II) are perhaps the only drugs that have been proven to prolong survival in patients with structural heart disease, but in terms of use for suppression of symptomatic arrhythmias, they are mainly useful for prevention of AV node- dependent reentrant supraventricular tachycardias (SVT). Nonpharmacologic interventions, such as catheter ablation for SVTs and implantable cardioverter defibrillator (ICD) therapy for primary and secondary prevention of sudden cardiac death (SCD), are considered the treatment of choice in these clinical settings. For more details on pharmacologic effects on the heart, see Chapters 24 and 27.

26.5 Tachyarrhythmias

26.5.1 Premature Complexes

Ectopic premature beats may originate from the atria, the AV junction, and/or the ventricles. Treatment of premature complexes is usually not necessary. If symptomatic, precipitating factors (such as alcohol, tobacco, and caffeine) should be identified and eliminated. Although anxiolytic agents and beta-blockers may be tried, they may result in troublesome side effects. Antiarrhythmic

Table 26.2 Vaughn-Williams classification[†]

Class I: Sodium channel blockers
- Class Ia: drugs that reduce V_{max} (phase 0 upstroke of action potential) and prolong action potential duration, such as quinidine, procainamide, and disopyramide
- Class Ib: drugs that do not reduce V_{max} and shorten action potential duration, such as lidocaine, mexiletine, and phenytoin
- Class Ic: drugs that predominantly slow conduction, moderately reduce V_{max}, and minimally prolong refractoriness, such as flecainide, propafenone, and moricizine

Class II: β-adrenergic receptor blockers
- β-blockers may be cardio- or β_1-selective, such as atenolol, esmolol, and metoprolol or noncardioselective, such as carvedilol, pindolol, and propranolol
- Some exert intrinsic sympathomimetic activity (acebutolol, bucindolol, and pindolol)
- Some have quinidine-like membrane stabilizing activity (acebutolol, carvedilol, and propranolol)
- D-Sotalol has strong Class III effect and has usually been regarded as a Class III agent

Class III: Potassium channel blockers (that prolong refractoriness, such as amiodarone, bretylium, dofetilide, ibutilide, and sotalol. Amiodarone has all the four class effects)

Class IV: Calcium channel blockers
- Dihydropyridine (almodipine and nefedipine)
- Nondihydropyridine drugs (diltiazem and verapamil)

[†]As discussed in the text, the utility of this classification in terms of selection of therapy is limited, but the grouping permits important toxicity issues to be more readily kept in mind, an important factor when choosing drugs for individual patients.

drugs may be used depending on the severity of symptoms and underlying cardiac disease, but avoidance of these drugs is the preferred strategy.

26.5.1.1 Atrial Premature Complexes (APCs)

Atrial premature complexes (APCs) are recognized on the ECG as early P-waves, with a P-wave morphology different from that of the sinus P-wave (Fig. 26.1a). Since the premature P-wave is often superimposed in the preceding T-wave, the T-wave preceding a premature beat should be carefully compared to other T-waves to identify any *buried P-waves*. APCs can conduct to the ventricles with a normal PR interval when AV junction is not refractory, or with a prolonged PR interval when AV junction is in its relative refractory period, or they can be blocked when the AV junction is in its *effective refractory period*. APCs almost always enter the sinus node and reset the sinus cycle length, resulting in an *incomplete compensatory pause* (the sum of pre- and post-APC intervals is less than that of two normal sinus PP intervals). They are frequently found in normal subjects and are usually asymptomatic; treatment is usually not necessary.

26.5.1.2 Multifocal Atrial Tachycardias

Multifocal atrial tachycardia, also called *chaotic atrial tachycardia*, is a relatively uncommon arrhythmia characterized by atrial rates between 100 and 130 bpm with marked variations in P-wave morphology (arbitrarily defined as at least three different P-wave contours). It often manifests as short bursts of tachycardia (Fig. 26.1d).

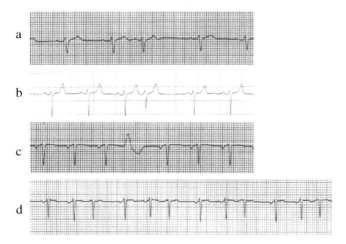

Fig. 26.1 Atrial (**a**), junctional (**b**), and ventricular (**c**) premature complexes, as well as multifocal atrial tachycardia (**d**)

Typically, multifocal atrial tachycardias occur in older patients with moderate-to-severe cardiopulmonary disease that may be especially elicited during an exacerbation. Treatment is difficult but should primarily be directed toward ameliorating the underlying disorders. If necessary, beta-blockers may be tried but, in the setting of concomitant pulmonary disease, this may be unwise. Verapamil or amiodarone may be considered as a second-line therapy. Amiodarone may be the most effective drug in this situation, but its multiple side effects (particularly pulmonary effects) are of concern, since many patients already have significant underlying pulmonary problems.

26.5.1.3 AV Junctional Premature Complexes

These complexes are recognized on the ECG as normal QRS complexes without a preceding P-wave (Fig. 26.1b). *Retrograde P-waves* (inverted in II, III, and aVF) may be seen after the QRS complexes, further supporting the diagnosis. AV junctional complexes are less common than APCs and are often associated with drug intoxication and cardiac disease. Most junctional beats have an incomplete compensatory pause (like an APC) because they generate a retrograde atrial activation that resets the sinus node. On rare occasions, a junctional premature beat may fail to conduct to either the atria or ventricles (*concealed junctional beats*), but results in refractoriness in the AV junction and blocks subsequent supraventricular beats.

26.5.1.4 Ventricular Premature Complexes (VPCs)

Ventricular premature complexes (VPCs) are recognized as wide bizarre QRS complexes which are not preceded by P-waves (Fig. 26.1c). In addition, they often fail to conduct retrogradely to the atria due to poor retrograde ventriculoatrial conduction in patients with heart disease who most often manifest VPCs. Thus, VPCs do not typically reset the sinus node, and the result is a *full compensatory pause* (the sum of pre- and post-APC intervals equals that of two normal sinus PP intervals). *An interpolated VPC* does not influence the following sinus beats, i.e., its occurrence is timed so as not to impair the next sinus beat from traversing the AV node and reaching the ventricles at the expected moment. VPCs may occur as a single event, but also occur in patterns of *bigeminy* (sinus beat and VPC alternating) and *trigeminy* (two sinus beats followed by a VPC). *Couplets* or *pairs* (two consecutive VPCs) and *nonsustained ventricular tachycardia* (arbitrarily defined as three or more consecutive VPCs at a rate of >100 bpm) are also relatively common observations during monitoring of patients with heart disease. These morphologies may be either *monomorphic* (*uniform*) or *polymorphic* (*multiform*).

VPCs often bear a fixed *coupling interval* (between the onset of VPC and the onset of its preceding sinus QRS complex). When there is a protected ventricular ectopic focus, the focus is constantly firing without being reset by sinus beats and is called *ventricular parasystole* which is characterized by varying coupling intervals, but these inter-intervals remain relatively fixed (i.e., variation <120 ms).

The relationship of VPCs to SCD is poorly defined. Frequent VPCs (>5–10 VPCs per minute) have been shown to be associated with increased risk of SCD. How-ever, it seems that suppression of VPCs using antiarrhyth-mic drugs does not reduce the risk of SCD in patients following myocardial infarction [2, 3]. This may indicate that mortality is primarily determined by the severity of underlying disease, and that the ectopy is an associated finding but not an independent determinant. Alterna-tively, any benefit derived from VPC suppression by con-ventional antiarrhythmic drugs may be counterbalanced by a drug-induced increment in mortality mainly due to negative inotropic effects and proarrhythmic effects of currently available antiarrhythmic medications.

At this time, pharmacological treatment of VPCs is aimed at alleviating symptoms rather than prolongation of survival. On the other hand, ablation of VPCs may eliminate the triggers or destroy the substrate for sus-tained ventricular arrhythmias; in this case, treatment of VPCs may improve survival.

26.5.2 Sinus Tachycardias

26.5.2.1 Physiological Sinus Tachycardia

Physiological sinus tachycardia represents a normal response to a variety of physiological (anxiety and exercise) and pathological stresses (fever, hypotension, thyrotoxico-sis, hypoxemia, and congestive heart failure). Sinus tachy-cardia rarely exceeds 200 bpm. It should not be treated for itself, but its causes must be explored (e.g., exercise, fever, anemia, hyperthyroidism) and some of these may require therapy (e.g., fever, anemia, hyperthyroidism).

26.5.2.2 Inappropriate Sinus Tachycardia (IST)

Inappropriate sinus tachycardia (IST) is characterized by an increased resting heart rate (often >100 bpm) and an exaggerated heart rate response to minimal stress. The tachycardia is usually associated with distressing

symptoms (palpitations, fatigue, anxiety, and shortness of breath). Unfortunately, their etiologies and underlying mechanisms are typically unclear.

Care must be taken in making a diagnosis of IST. First, it is not very common, but it may be observed after pre-vious cardiac arrhythmia ablation procedures or in the setting of symptoms suggestive of postural orthostatic tachycardia syndrome. When considering IST as a diag-nosis, it is crucial to exclude secondary sinus tachycardia and to correlate symptoms with tachycardia. Electrophy-siologic study can be used to exclude atrial tachycardia located close to the sinus node. Beta-blockers and calcium channel blockers can be used to treat IST, although typi-cally with imperfect results. Radiofrequency (RF) mod-ification of the sinus node can be considered if drug therapy fails, as is often the case.

26.5.3 Paroxysmal Supraventricular Tachycardias (PSVTs)

Paroxysmal supraventricular tachycardias (PSVTs) are a group of supraventricular tachycardias with sudden onset and termination. They are usually recurrent and often occur in otherwise seemingly healthy individuals.

26.5.3.1 Sinus Nodal Reentry Tachycardia

Sinus node reentry tachycardia is relatively rare (i.e., accounting for approximately 3% of all PSVTs), and tends to occur mainly in older individuals with other manifestations of sinus node disease. The average rate of sinus node reentry tachycardia is 130–140 bpm but its rate is quite labile, suggesting that autonomic influences may be at play. By definition, the P-wave morphology is iden-tical or very similar to the sinus P-wave. Vagal maneuvers can slow or terminate the tachycardia since it reenters within the region of the sinus node that is heavily influ-enced by vagal (parasympathetic) nerve endings. Sinus node reentry tachycardia should be suspected in "anxi-ety-related sinus tachycardia." Beta-blockers and calcium channel blockers (e.g., verapamil, diltiazem), as well as ablation, are treatment options.

26.5.3.2 Atrial Tachycardias (AT)

Atrial tachycardias (AT) refer to those tachyarrhythmias that arise in atrial tissue due to abnormal automaticity or reentry. They are classified separately from sinus node reentry or AV nodal reentry despite the fact that these latter tachyarrhythmias also arise within or predominantly utilize the "atria." A typical AT has an atrial rate of 150–200 bpm with a P-wave morphology that is usually different from that of sinus P-wave; AT accounts for 5–10% of all PSVTs.

Since ATs arise within and are sustained by atrial tissues alone, AV block may develop without interrupting the tachycardia. The latter is, in fact, one of the most valuable ways to distinguish ATs from other SVTs that are "AVN dependent" such as AV nodal reentry. ATs may be due to automaticity or triggered activity as well as reentry. Automatic AT has the following features: (1) it cannot be initiated or terminated by atrial stimulation; (2) the first P-wave of the tachycardia is the same as the subsequent P-waves of the tachycardia; (3) its rate often accelerates after initiation until it stabilizes (at 100–175 bpm), so-called *warm-up phenomenon*; (4) a premature atrial stimulation can reset automatic AT with a full or incomplete compensatory pause, usually accompanied by a constant return cycle; and (5) overdrive suppression is a hallmark of automaticity. Both reentrant and automatic AT can be cured by ablation.

26.5.3.3 AV Nodal Reentry Tachycardia (AVNRT)

AV nodal reentry tachycardia (AVNRT) is the most common of PSVTs (50–65%) and usually presents as a narrow QRS complex with regular rates between 120 and 250 bpm. In the absence of ventricular preexcitation (i.e., Wolff–Parkinson–White or WPW syndrome and related disorders), AVNRT and AV reentry tachycardia(AVRT, see below) using a concealed bypass tract account for >90% of all PSVTs.

A schematic of the AV nodal reentry circuit is shown in Fig. 26.2. In this disorder, retrograde P-waves may not be apparent in many instances because they are buried in the QRS complexes, or they appear as subtle distortions at the terminal parts of the QRS complex. As a rule, AVNRT can be reproducibly initiated and terminated by appropriately timed atrial extra stimuli; therefore this is routinely done as part of the diagnostic electrophysiologic study (EPS) in these patients. Spontaneous APCs that initiate AVNRT are usually associated with a prolonged PR interval. In intracardiac recordings during EPS, the onset of AVNRT is almost always associated with a prolonged AH interval. This, in turn, produces

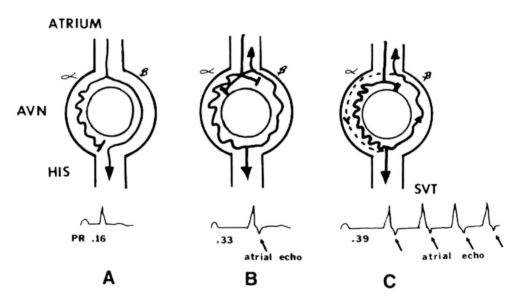

Fig. 26.2 Schema of the typical atrioventricular nodal reentry tachycardia. The atrioventricular node (AVN) has a slow pathway with short refractoriness and a fast pathway with long refractoriness. (**A**) During sinus rhythm, the impulse conducts to the ventricles through the fast pathway, yielding a normal PR interval. The impulse simultaneously goes down the slow pathway, but cannot conduct to the His bundle antegradely or retrogradely to the fast pathway since they are rendered refractory by the prior beat. (**B**) An atrial premature complex reaches the effective refractory period of the fast pathway and is blocked in the fast pathway. This atrial premature complex is able to conduct slowly down to the slow pathway, yielding a prolonged

PR interval. The delay in conduction over the slow pathway allows enough time for the fast pathway to recover and enables the impulse conducted from the slow pathway to continue over the fast pathway retrogradely to the atria, producing an atrial echo beat. At the same time, the returned impulse tries to conduct down over the slow pathway and fails due to unrecovered refractoriness of the slow pathway. (**C**) A sufficient early atrial premature complex occurs, producing a similar echo beat as in (**B**). However, the returned impulse is able to conduct down over the slow pathway, repeatedly producing another ventricular beat and atrial echo, i.e., supraventricular tachycardia (SVT). Reproduced from Ref. [4] with permission

sufficient conduction delay in the so-called slow AV nodal pathway (Fig. 26.2) to ensure recovery of the fast pathway and permit the fast pathway to conduct retrogradely back toward the atrium, thereby completing the reentry circuit. A critical balance between conduction delay and recovery of refractoriness in the two pathways is required to sustain the tachycardia. Simultaneous antegrade conduction to the ventricles and retrograde conduction to the atria often leads to the "retrograde" P-wave being buried in the QRS complex, as noted earlier. Furthermore, as a consequence of this physiology, in typical "slow–fast" AVNRT the RP interval is short (i.e., <80–100 ms) in AVNRT (Fig. 26.3). In contrast, in AVRT (i.e., a PSVT using an accessory AV connection such as in WPW syndrome), the ventricles and atria are activated sequentially and the RP interval is expected to be longer than 80 ms (Fig. 26.4).

Acute treatment to terminate AVNRT may include vagal maneuvers (e.g., carotid sinus massage, Valsalva maneuver), adenosine injections, administration of verapamil or diltiazem or beta-blocker, or electrical (direct current) cardioversion. The majority of these interventions are designed to interrupt AV nodal conduction transiently, thereby "breaking" the fragile reentry circuit. Drugs used for long-term prevention of AVNRT recurrence include digitalis (not recommended currently due to low efficacy), beta-blockers, calcium channel blockers, and Class Ia and Ic antiarrhythmic drugs. However, the most important advancement in

the treatment of AVNRT is transcatheter ablation (principally of the "slow" pathway region). It should be noted that catheter ablation, performed by experienced hands, cures AVNRT in almost 100% of cases with very low risk.

26.5.3.4 AV Reentry Tachycardia (AVRT) Using Concealed Accessory Pathway

AV reentry tachycardia (AVRT) is another common form of PSVT. Accessory conduction tissue remaining from embryonic development of the heart can create the substrate for reentry PSVT. The most common form of accessory pathway is that connecting the atria to the ventricles (i.e., an accessory AV connection). This connection is made up of working muscle tissue that is so small that it is usually invisible even during open-heart surgery. When these connections conduct in the antegrade direction (i.e., from atrium to ventricle), they necessarily modify the QRS configuration, usually by virtue of earlier than expected activation of part of the ventricular muscle (i.e., preexcitation). The classic case is the "delta" wave observed at the onset of the QRS in WPW syndrome.

In many cases, accessory connections only conduct in the retrograde direction (from ventricle to atrium) and are termed "concealed" accessory connections. In these cases, there is no apparent ECG footprint since ventricular

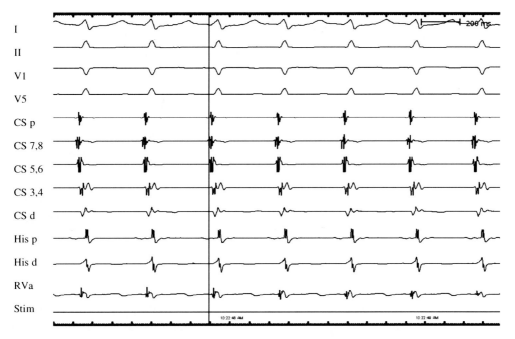

Fig. 26.3 Typical atrioventricular (AV) nodal reentry tachycardia. Since the tachycardia circuit is within the AV node, and it conducts simultaneously antegrade to the ventricles and retrograde to the atria, the time difference between ventricular and atrial activation is relatively short. The retrograde P-wave is often buried in QRS complex (RP interval is 0 ms), as shown in this case. I, surface ECG lead I; II, surface ECG lead II; V1, surface ECG lead V1; V5, surface ECG lead V5; CS, coronary sinus; d, distal; His, His bundle; p, proximal; RVa, right ventricular apex; Stim, stimulation

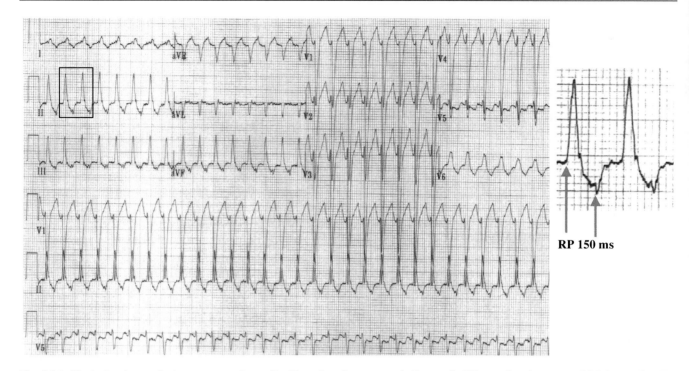

RP 150 ms

Fig. 26.4 Typical atrioventricular reentry tachycardia. Note that the retrograde P-wave is 150 ms after the onset of QRS complex (RP interval is 150 ms)

preexcitation does not occur. Nevertheless, since retrograde conduction can occur, a reentry tachycardia is possible. This form of accessory pathway most often occurs on the left side of the heart, and accounts for approximately 30% of all PSVTs. In general, the electrical impulses in this type of PSVT circulate in an antegrade direction through the AV node and retrograde through the concealed accessory pathway (Fig. 26.5). In other words, both the atria and ventricles are parts of the

reentry circuit. Since atrial activation always follows ventricular activation, the P-wave usually occurs after the QRS complex and the RP interval is relatively long (RP interval >80 ms, but usually in the range of 120 ms).

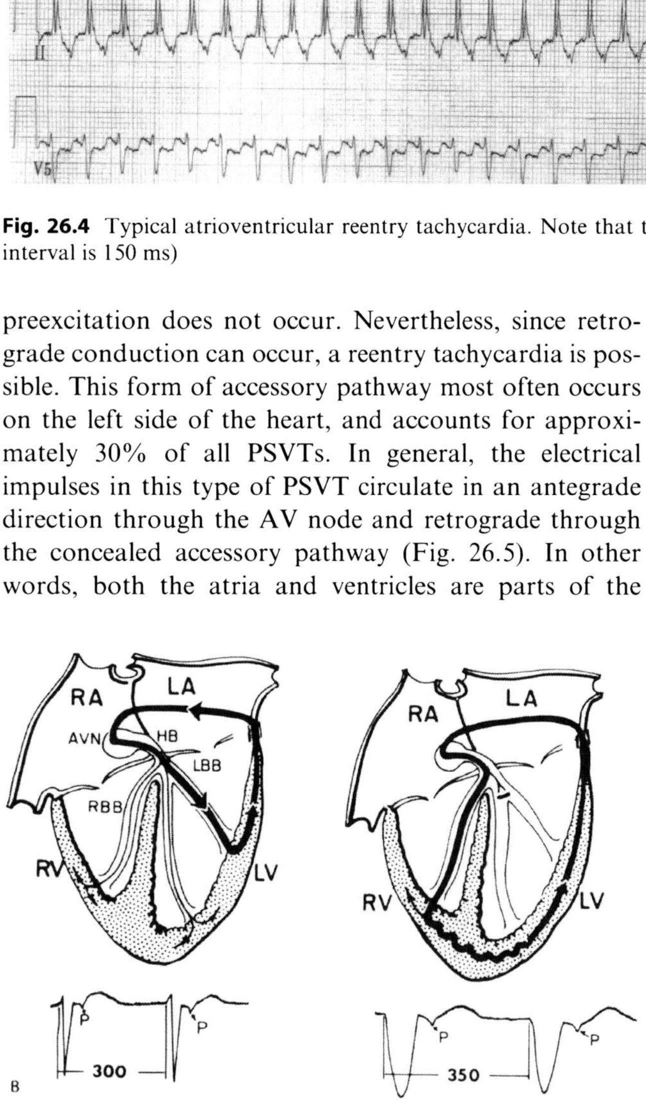

An AVRT can be initiated and terminated by either atrial or ventricular extrastimuli. Even when the His bundle is refractory, a VPC may be able to reset the atria by virtue of being transmitted to the atria through the accessory pathway(s). In contrast to the concentric atrial activation sequences in AVNRT, the atrial activation sequences in AVRT are eccentric when the accessory pathways are located at a distance from AV node. On occasion, however, the connection may be close to the AV node, making the distinction between the two arrhythmias clinically more challenging.

Medical treatment of an AVRT is similar to that of AVNRT. However, transcatheter ablation is highly effective for eliminating accessory AV connections and is often the preferred approach, especially in younger individuals. Mapping and ablation, thereby curing the problem, is effective in >95% of cases.

Fig. 26.5 Atrioventricular reentry tachycardia using a left-sided concealed accessory pathway (*left*). Left bundle branch block prolongs the tachycardia cycle length by 50 ms due to the conduction delay of the tachycardia circuit in the left ventricle (*right*). Reproduced from Ref. [4] with permission

26.5.3.5 Wolff–Parkinson–White (WPW) Syndrome and Related Preexcitation Syndromes

When there are one or more accessory AV pathways or connections that conduct in the antegrade direction, the ventricles may become overtly preexcited to a varying degree, as discussed earlier. The WPW syndrome is applied when palpitations/tachyarrhythmias occur in the setting of preexcitation. Tachycardias associated with WPW syndrome include: (1) *orthodromic reciprocating or reentry tachycardia,* in which the conduction path is antegrade through the normal AV conduction system and retrograde through the AV accessory pathways; (2) *antidromic reciprocating or reentry tachycardia*, in which the conduction path is antegrade through the AV accessory pathways and retrograde through the normal AV conduction system or another accessory connection; and (3) atrial flutter/fibrillation, in which there is activation of the ventricles antegradely through both the normal AV conduction system and AV accessory pathways. The ECG features of a typical AV connection in WPW syndrome (Fig. 26.6) are: (1) shortened PR intervals <120 ms during sinus rhythm; (2) widened QRS durations; and (3) the presence of delta waves (a slurred, slowly rising onset of the QRS). Note that the terminal QRS portion is usually normal, yet sometimes it is associated with secondary ST-T changes.

In addition to typical AV accessory pathways, other variants may exist, such as atriohisian, atriofascicular, nodofascicular, and/or nodoventricular fibers. For example, *Lown–Guang–Levine syndrome* is defined as a recurrent paroxysmal tachycardia or atrial fibrillation (AFib) associated with short PR intervals and a normal QRS complex.

Its presumed mechanisms include atriohisian fibers, preferential intranodal pathways or enhanced AV conduction, and posterior intranodal pathways or an anatomically small AV node. Apart from typical accessory connections found in WPW syndrome, there are other special forms of accessory AV connections (formerly termed *Mahaim fibers*) that were initially thought to be nodoventricular bypass tracts, but now include several types of connections such as atriofascicular, nodofascicular, nodoventricular, and fasciculoventricular fibers. The majority of these pathways are long right-sided atriofascicular or atrioventricular pathways between the lateral tricuspid and distal right bundle branch in the right ventricular free wall. These fibers almost represent a duplication of the AV nodal pathway and are typically capable of only antegrade conduction and decremental conduction property [5]. Therefore, only *"preexcited tachycardia"* can result. Often preexcitation is not initially apparent, but can be exposed by right atrial stimulation. Importantly, the associated ECG tends to exhibit a left bundle branch block type of morphology, with a leftward frontal axis similar to that associated with right ventricular apical pacing.

As a rule, accessory pathways conduct faster than the AV node, but have a longer refractory period and are thereby prone to block premature beats at longer coupling intervals (e.g., a premature beat will tend to block at a longer coupling

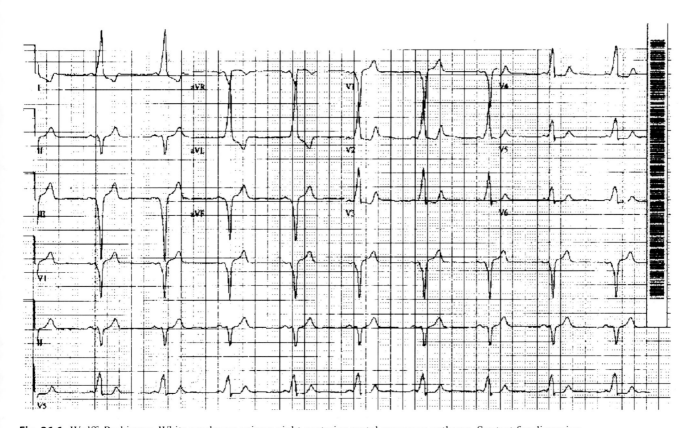

Fig. 26.6 Wolff–Parkinson–White syndrome using a right posterior septal accessory pathway. See text for discussion

interval than is the case for the AV node). However, accessory pathways can often sustain very high heart rates and this may be particularly hazardous during atrial fibrillation. Furthermore, accessory pathways do not usually manifest decremental conduction at faster pacing rates.

An incessant form of SVT has been recognized that is usually associated with a slow-conducting posteroseptal accessory pathway as its retrograde limb (the so-called permanent form of junctional reciprocating tachycardia). This tachycardia tends to be more often observed in children than in adults. Its sustained nature can result in deterioration of left ventricular function over time. Correct diagnosis is crucial to prevent subsequent heart failure, and ablation therapy in such patients is the treatment of choice.

The mere presence of an accessory pathway does not necessarily mean that it is involved in the mechanism of tachycardia in a given patient. Not infrequently, these pathways are innocent bystanders, yet during AFib they create additional stress on the heart by permitting conduction of very rapid rates to the ventricles. Further, multiple tachycardia mechanisms may reside in the same patient simultaneously. Thus, AV echoes or AVNRT may be present in 15–20% of patients after successful ablation of accessory pathways. Further, about 10% of patients with accessory AV connections have multiple connections.

It is estimated that 10–35% of patients with preexcitation will experience AFib at some point in time. In fact, AFib and atrial flutter may be the presenting arrhythmia in up to 20% of patients with accessory AV pathways. In patients with WPW syndrome, atrial tachyarrhythmias that conduct extremely rapidly (via the accessory pathway) to the ventricles may lead to syncope, ventricular fibrillation, or SCD. A grossly irregular RR interval with widened QRS complexes and extremely rapid ventricular rates should immediately suggest the presence of antegrade accessory AV pathway conduction that is associated with AFib (Fig. 26.7). Patients with AFib in the presence of an accessory pathway are at increased risk of developing ventricular fibrillation if the shortest preexcited RR interval during AFib is less than 250 ms. Intravenous procainamide is the acute treatment of choice for hemodynamically stable *preexcited AFib* (but it must be administered slowly to avoid inducing hypotension). Intravenous *AV nodal blocking agents*, such as digoxin and verapamil, are contraindicated in these patients because they may paradoxically enhance antegrade AV conduction via the accessory pathway resulting in hypotension or even cardiac arrest in extreme cases. Patients who are hemodynamically unstable require immediate DC (direct current) cardioversion. As noted earlier, it is likely that most episodes of AFib may result from degeneration of orthodromic AV tachycardia (*tachycardia-induced tachycardia*). In general, a successful ablation of the accessory AV pathway eliminates AFib in these patients. Furthermore, RF ablation of the accessory pathway is the long-term (curative) treatment of choice for symptomatic patients with WPW syndrome; it is safe and effective in more than 98% of patients.

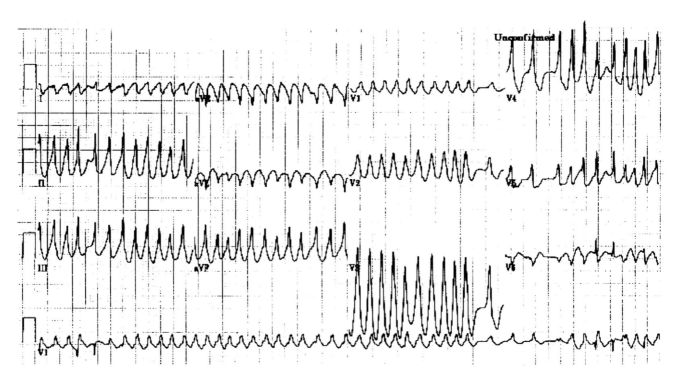

Fig. 26.7 Preexcited atrial fibrillation. See text for discussion

26.5.4 Atrial Flutter and Fibrillation

26.5.4.1 Atrial Flutter

Atrial flutter is characterized by an atrial rate between 250 and 350 bpm, usually accompanied by 2:1 AV conduction and thus resulting in a ventricular rate of approximately 150 bpm. Classical flutter waves (*F-waves*) are regular sawtooth-like deflections within the ECG, most prominent in the inferior leads and sometimes V1 (Fig. 26.8). A typical *F*-wave may appear to be similar to one generated by other atrial tachycardias with rates between 200 and 300 bpm. The flutter rate can be as low as approximately 200 bpm in some patients, particularly in the presence of antiarrhythmic drug therapy. Some atrial flutter episodes may be terminated by rapid atrial pacing (type I atrial flutter), but often this is not the case (type II atrial flutter). Although antiarrhythmic drugs may be useful to prevent recurrence of atrial flutter, they are less effective in conversion to sinus rhythm. In general, DC cardioversion (50–100 J) is most effective for termination of atrial flutter.

Typical atrial flutter is a macroreentrant rhythm confined to the right atrium. The tachycardia circulates around the atrium but passes through a relatively narrow isthmus of tissue between the inferior vena cava and the tricuspid valve annulus (cavotricuspid isthmus). Ablation-creating conduction block in this isthmus is highly effective and, as a result, the typical atrial flutter circuit can be easily ablated and recurrences prevented. Therefore, ablation is the treatment of choice for most of these patients. Although systemic embolization is less common in atrial flutter than in AFib, anticoagulation in atrial flutter should follow the guidelines for the management of Afib (see below) [6, 7].

26.5.4.2 Atrial Fibrillation (AFib)

In general, atrial fibrillation (AFib) is an uncoordinated atrial tachyarrhythmia characterized on the ECG by the absence of distinct P-waves before each QRS complex, the presence of rapid atrial oscillations (*F-waves*), and variable RR intervals (Fig. 26.9). *Paroxysmal* AFib is arbitrarily defined as being present when episodes last >2 min and <7 days, and are self-terminating in less than 48 h. *Persistent* Afib is defined by the need for intervention (usually cardioversion) to terminate the episode. An episode of AFib lasting longer than 7 days is termed *chronic*. If a number of attempts of cardioversion have failed or

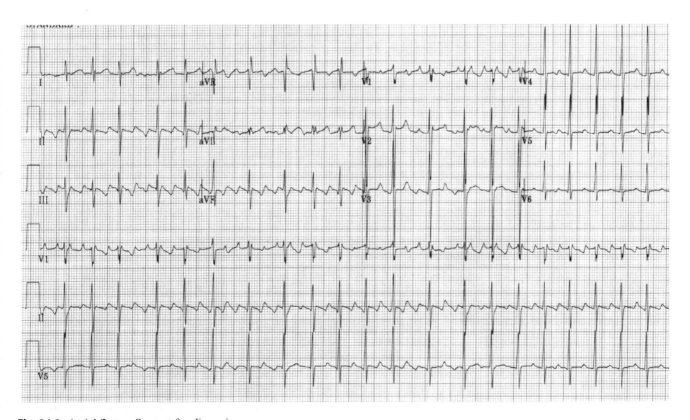

Fig. 26.8 Atrial flutter. See text for discussion

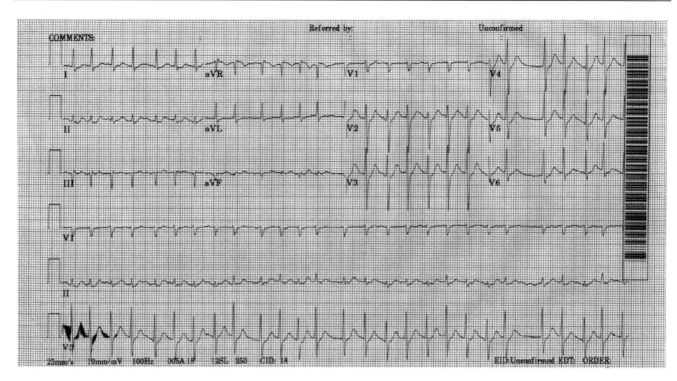

Fig. 26.9 Atrial fibrillation. See text for discussion

are not indicated in chronic forms (>1 year), AFib is regarded as *permanent*. When no prior history of AFib is available, the term *recent or new onset* is often used.

The relative incidence of AFib is strongly age dependent, with a substantial increase after the age of 50–60 years (6.2% in men and 4.8% in women of 65 years or older). In addition to age, other common cardiac precursors include a history of congestive heart failure, valvular heart disease, hypertension, and/or coronary artery disease. Nevertheless, rheumatic valvular disease, together with overt heart failure, is the most powerful predictor for AFib. As rheumatic heart disease has become less common in Western countries, heart failure alone has become the most important predisposing factor. The occurrence of AFib is common following acute myocardial infarction (10%) or cardiac surgery (~35%), except for heart transplantation in which it is rare. Usually, postoperative AFib is self-limited but often prolongs hospital stays and thus consequently has economic importance. Noncardiac precursors include thyrotoxicosis, anemia, and pulmonary pathology (e.g., infections, embolism) leading to hypoxemia. *Lone AFib* is said to be present when tachyarrhythmia occurs in the absence of underlying structural heart disease or transient precipitating factors.

The mechanisms underlying AFib include multiple wavelet reentry and/or focal enhanced automaticity. The atrial "rate" during AFib can range from 350 to 600 bpm. Due to *concealed AV nodal penetration* and subsequent

variable degrees of AV block, the characteristic *irregularly irregular* ventricular rate is usually between 100 and 160 bpm in untreated patients (those with normal AV conduction properties). *Aberrant conduction* may occur when a long ventricular cycle is followed by a short cycle (*Ashman phenomenon*). Importantly, AFib itself modifies atrial electrical properties in a way that promotes the occurrence and maintenance of the arrhythmia, a process termed *atrial electrical remodeling*.

Both branches of the autonomic nervous system may be involved in the initiation, maintenance, and termination of AFib in some patients. *Vagally mediated AFib* (parasympathetic) is relatively common, and is characterized by its onset during rest, especially in the middle of the night. *Adrenergically mediated AFib* (sympathetic) is much more rare, and is associated with elevated catecholamine states.

The major adverse clinical consequences of AFib include palpitations, impaired cardiac function, and/or increased risk of thromboembolism. Typical physical findings in such patients include (1) an irregularly irregular ventricular rhythm; (2) variations in the intensity of the first heart sounds; and (3) the absence of "a" waves in the jugular venous pulse. A peripheral *pulse deficit* (pulse rate less than heart rate) is often noted during a fast ventricular response due to insufficient ventricular filling that fails to open aortic valve. Importantly, patients with continuous rapid ventricular rates for a prolonged period are at risk of developing a *tachycardia-induced cardiomyopathy*, as was noted earlier in discussion of the permanent form of junctional reciprocating tachycardia.

The primary goals of therapies for AFib are improvement of symptoms, reduction of AFib-associated morbidities, and improvement in prognoses. The three basic tenets of therapy for AFib are: (1) control of ventricular rate response; (2) restoration and maintenance of sinus rhythm; and (3) prevention of thromboembolism.

A resting ventricular rate under 90 bpm and ventricular rates between 90 and 115 during moderate exercise are considered optimal. Commonly used medications for rate control include beta-blockers, calcium channel blockers, and digoxin (less often). Ablation of the AV node and the use of a pacemaker may be necessary in some cases to achieve adequate rate control.

Although controversial, most cardiologists still believe that, in general, sinus rhythm is preferable to AFib, as long as it can be achieved and maintained with relative safety. Approximately 50% of patients with recent onset of AFib will convert spontaneously to sinus rhythm within < 48 h. Potential precipitating factors should be sought and treated. Sinus rhythm can be restored pharmacologically or electrically. Class Ia, Ic, and III antiarrhythmic drugs all have the potential to restore sinus rhythm. Flecainide is a good choice for patients without coronary artery disease or significant left ventricular dysfunction; otherwise, class III agents should be used.

Currently, both ibutilide and flecainide have been shown to be effective in termination of AFib and atrial flutter. This is particularly true for patients with AFib following cardiac surgery or those not ideal for DC cardioversion. Approximately 50% of patients remain in sinus rhythm when treated with various Class I and III drugs (6 months to 3 years).

Single- or dual-site atrial pacing may be helpful for prevention of recurrences of paroxysmal AFib, but this is not recommended as the sole therapy. Implantable atrial defibrillators have been introduced for treatment of recurrent AFib, but they have not been as popular as initially thought. In fact, these two treatment strategies are rarely used now. The so-called surgical "Maze" procedure and catheter ablation may also be considered in patients with refractory arrhythmia. However, a catheter ablation procedure is preferred unless an open-heart surgery is planned for other reasons.

For elective cardioversion of AFib lasting >48 h, patients should be anticoagulated with warfarin (INR in the range of 2.0–3.0) for 3–4 weeks before and after cardioversion, regardless of their risk of embolization. Transesophageal echocardiography combined with short-term heparin infusion has gained acceptance as an alternative rapid preparation for DC cardioversion. *Atrial stunning* postcardioversion may create a favorable milieu for thrombogenesis, and embolization may occur despite a negative result on transesophageal echocardiography. Importantly, adequate anticoagulation is pivotal in preventing spontaneous embolism in patients with AFib. In addition to rheumatic mitral valve disease and prosthetic valves (mechanical or tissue valves), major risk factors for embolization in *nonvalvular AFib* include: (1) a prior history of ischemic stroke (or transient ischemic attack); (2) congestive heart failure or left ventricular dysfunction; (3) advanced age (>65–75 years); (4) hypertension; (5) coronary artery disease (particularly myocardial infarction); (6) diabetes; (7) left atrial thrombus; (8) thyrotoxicosis; (9) increased left atrial size (>50 mm); and/or (10) left atrial mechanical dysfunction. Patients with any risk factors for AFib should be treated with warfarin to achieve an INR 2.0–3.0 (target INR 2.5) (Table 26.3) [8]. Stroke risk stratification is often presented in the CHADS2 scheme (Cardiac failure, Hypertension, Age, Diabetes, Stroke [Doubled]). Anticoagulation therapy reduces stroke risk by 68% (4.5% versus 1.4%). Nevertheless, the major concern with anticoagulation therapy is bleeding, especially in elderly patients (>75 years), or when the patient's INR is >4.0. A complete guideline for management of AFib was recently published in 2006 [6]. In addition, the American College of Cardiology/American Heart Association physician consortium on clinical performance measures for adults with nonvalvular atrial fibrillation or atrial flutter was published in 2008 [7].

26.5.5 Ventricular Tachyarrhythmias

26.5.5.1 Ventricular Tachycardias (VT)

Although ventricular tachycardia (VT) can occur in a clinically normal heart, it generally accompanies some form of structural heart disease, particularly in patients with prior myocardial infarction. More specifically, fixed substrates (i.e., old infarct scars) are responsible for most episodes of recurrent monomorphic VT. Acute ischemia may play a more important role in the pathogenesis of polymorphic VT or ventricular fibrillation.

Table 26.3 Recommendations of anticoagulation therapy in atrial fibrillation by the American College of Chest Physicians

	No risk factors	With any risk factors
Age <65 years	Aspirin	Warfarin
Age 65–75 years	Aspirin/warfarin	Warfarin
Age >75 years	Warfarin	Warfarin

Modified from Ref. [8].

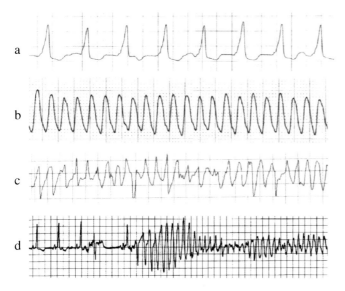

Fig. 26.10 Ventricular tachycardia (**a**), ventricular flutter (**b**), ventricular fibrillation (**c**), and Torsades de pointes (**d**). See text for discussion

VT is typically characterized on an ECG by a wide QRS complex tachycardia at a rate of >100 bpm (Fig. 26.10). Like VPCs, VTs can be monomorphic (Fig. 26.10a) or polymorphic. *Sustained VT* is defined as a VT that persists for >30 s or requires termination due to hemodynamic compromise. *Nonsustained VT* is defined as VT lasting >3 consecutive beats but less than 30 s. *Bidirectional VT* refers to VT that shows an alternation in QRS amplitude and axis. Nevertheless, the key marker of VT on an ECG is ventriculoatrial dissociation. Yet, capture and fusion beats support the diagnosis of VT. Finally, sustained VT is almost always symptomatic; the presentation, prognosis, and management of VT largely depend on the underlying cardiovascular state.

Among drugs available in most countries, procainamide and amiodarone are commonly used for acute termination of VT. However, procainamide is not advocated for long-term use due to its negative inotropic and other chronic adverse effects. In patients with heart disease, sotalol, dofetilide, and amiodarone are the principal longer-term drug therapies recommended. Implantable cardiac defibrillators (ICD), with and without amiodarone, are the most established long-term therapy for VT.

Ablation provides a cure for some normal heart VTs, bundle branch reentry VTs, and selected ischemic VTs. However, in patients with diminished left ventricular function, it may be prudent to place an ICD even after an apparently successful ablation. A complete guideline for management of ventricular arrhythmias was recently published in 2006 [9].

26.5.5.2 Ventricular Flutter and Ventricular Fibrillation

Electrocardiographically, *ventricular flutter* (Fig. 26.10b) usually appears as a "sine wave" with a rate between 150 and 300 bpm; it is essentially impossible to assign a specific morphology of these oscillations. In contrast, *ventricular fibrillation* (Fig. 26.10c) is recognized by grossly irregular undulations of varying amplitudes, contours, and rates, and is often preceded by a rapid repetitive sequence of VT. The spontaneous conversion of ventricular fibrillation to sinus rhythm is rare, and thus prompt electrical defibrillation is essential. Previously, there was interest in "antifibrillatory" drugs such as bretylium and bethanidine, but they have not proved popular among physicians, given the critical need for immediate effective treatment intervention. Longer-term prevention of SCD in these patients predominately depends on the clinical placement of ICDs.

26.5.5.3 Accelerated Idioventricular Rhythm

Accelerated idioventricular rhythm can be regarded as a type of slow VT with a rate between 60 and 110 bpm. This rhythm usually occurs in patients with acute myocardial infarction, particularly during reperfusion. Since the rhythm is usually transient without significant hemodynamic compromise, treatment is rarely required.

26.5.5.4 Torsades de Pointes (TdP)

When polymorphic VT occurs in the presence of prolonged QT intervals (congenital or acquired), it is termed *Torsades de Pointes* (TdP). This arrhythmia is often preceded by VPCs with a *long–short sequence* (Fig. 26.10d). TdP often presents with multiple nonsustained episodes causing recurrent syncope, but it also has a predilection to generate into ventricular fibrillation leading to SCD. Identification of TdP has important therapeutic implications because its treatment is completely different from that of common polymorphic VT. Magnesium, pacing, and isoproterenol can be used to treat TdP, as required. Left cervicothoracic sympathectomy has been proposed as a form of therapy for TdP in patients with congenital long QT syndrome. In addition, ablation of the VPCs preceding the onset of TdP may be an effective treatment for preventing multiple tachycardia episodes in these patients; however, an ICD is still recommended in most cases (Fig. 26.11).

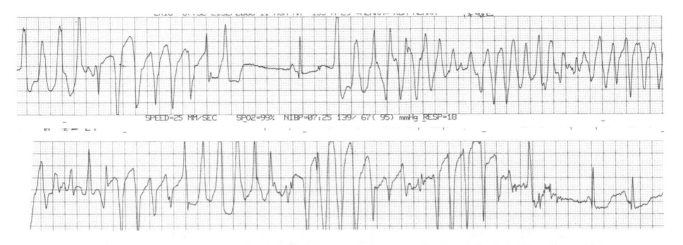

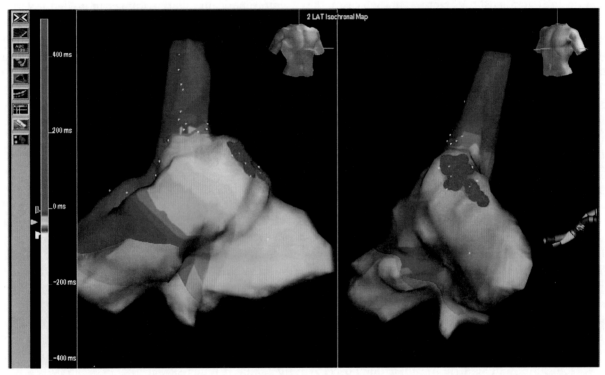

Fig. 26.11 Torsades de pointes. Successful catheter ablation of premature ventricular ectopics in the anteroseptal wall of the right ventricular outflow tract eliminates frequent episodes of Torsades de pointes (*top*) that are refractory to medical management. The *bottom* shows an activation map using the Ensite NavX system. The *red dots* indicate the ablation lesions

26.5.5.5 Nonparoxysmal Junctional Tachycardia

Nonparoxysmal junctional tachycardia, also called *accelerated junctional rhythm*, is recognized by a narrow QRS complex without a consistent P-wave preceding each QRS complex, and has a typical rate between 70 and 130 bpm, usually associated with a warm-up period at its onset. Nonparoxysmal junctional tachycardia frequently results from conditions that produce enhanced automaticity or triggered activity in the AV junction, such as inferior acute myocardial infarction, digitalis intoxication, and/

or post-valve surgery. Treatment should be primarily directed toward the underlying diseases.

26.6 Bradyarrhythmias

As discussed in the Introduction, bradycardia may result from either sinus node dysfunction or "*sick sinus syndrome*," or an AV conduction block. Acute treatment options for symptomatic bradycardia include atropine, isoproterenol, or temporary pacing. When the underlying cause is reversible, such as in the case of drug toxicity (e.g., excess digitalis or beta-blocker), temporary pacing and elimination of the offending agent is usually a sufficient therapy. However, if the cause is irreversible, the implantation of a permanent pacemaker is usually warranted.

26.6.1 Sinus Node Dysfunction (SND)

Normal sinus node function was discussed briefly earlier. Often sinus node performance deteriorates with age and/or age-related disease states, and the clinical syndrome of sinus node dysfunction (SND) emerges. In such cases, the clinical manifestations may be: (1) excessive sinus bradycardia; (2) alternating periods of bradycardia and atrial tachycardia; and/or (3) AFib. Additionally, the sinus node may simply become less responsive to physical exertion over time in terms of generating an appropriate heart rate; this is a special form of SND called "*chronotropic incompetence.*"

Sinus bradycardia is defined as sinus rates of <60 bpm. As mentioned above, sinus rates between 50 and 60 bpm may not be pathological in many subjects, e.g., the highly trained athlete. Yet, SND may manifest as either significant sinus bradycardia or abrupt and prolonged sinus pauses due to sinus arrest or sinus exit block. The typical resultant symptoms include fatigue, dizziness, confusion, exertional intolerance, diminished mental acuity, syncope, and/or congestive heart failure. Atrial tachyarrhythmias are particularly frequent in SND, and often alternate with periods of excessive bradycardia (*bradycardia-tachycardia syndrome*). SND may also present as various forms of sinoatrial exit block. On the surface ECG, only second-degree sinoatrial block (Wenckebach-type conduction from sinus node to atrium) can be diagnosed by observing progressive PP interval shortening prior to the blocked atrial impulse. First- and third-degree sinoatrial blocks cannot be recognized (absent specialized intracardiac recording techniques). It should be noted that Holter monitors and implantable event monitors are useful for confirming the suspected diagnosis of SND, particularly when bradycardia is associated with symptoms.

Carotid sinus massage is frequently performed when evaluating for SND. Although carotid sinus syndrome is not the same as SND, the two often coexist in the same patient. A sinus pause >3 s induced by a 5-s unilateral carotid sinus massage is usually considered clinically significant.

Since sinus rate can be slowed by vagal tone, *intrinsic heart rate* after complete autonomic blockage is often used to assess the integrity of sinus node function. Complete autonomic blockade can be achieved after intravenous propranolol (0.2 mg/kg) and atropine (0.04 mg/kg). Normal intrinsic heart rate can be determined by this equation: $118.1 - (0.57 \times age)$. An intrinsic heart rate <80 bpm in the elderly is usually suggestive of sick sinus syndrome. Furthermore, determining the sinus node recovery times (normal value <1,500 ms), corrected sinus node recovery times (normal value <550 ms), and, less frequently, the sinoatrial conduction times (normal value <125 ms) can be used in the electrophysiology laboratory to evaluate sinus node function when the initial clinical diagnosis is uncertain.

Pacemakers are the mainstay of therapy for treating symptomatic bradyarrhythmias in patients with SND. However, it is not uncommon that antiarrhythmic drugs are also needed to suppress the tachycardic component of the condition. In the latter case, the drugs may aggravate any tendency toward bradycardia, thereby further necessitating pacemaker therapy.

26.6.2 Atrioventricular (AV) Block

The clinical significance of AV block depends on: (1) the site of block; (2) the risk of progression to complete block; and (3) the subsidiary escape rate. When complete AV block occurs above the His bundle, the ventricular escape rhythm is believed to originate from the His bundle (40–60 bpm); this is usually called a *junctional escape rhythm* and the patient has an associated narrow QRS complex (although a bundle branch block appearance may occur if the patient has preexisting conduction system disease). When AV block occurs below the His bundle, the escape is generated in the distal His–Purkinje fibers and is much slower and less reliable (25–45 bpm); this is usually called *ventricular escape rhythm* with associated wide QRS complex. The *first-degree AV block* is characterized by a PR interval >0.20 s without drop of QRS complex following each P-wave (Fig. 26.12a).

AV conduction delay can occur at the right atrium, the AV node, and the His–Purkinje system. The *second-degree AV block* is present when some atrial impulses fail to conduct to the ventricles. In its classical form, *Mobitz type I* second-degree AV block (Fig. 26.12b) is characterized by progressive PR interval prolongation until an atrial impulse is blocked (*Wenckebach phenomenon*). Furthermore, after an incomplete compensatory pause, the Wenckebach cycle starts again with a shorter PR interval, compared with the PR interval prior to block. In some patients, the Wenckebach periodicity may be very long (greater than 6:5) and the progressive PR prolongation of the typical Mobitz I

Fig. 26.12 Atrioventricular (AV) block. The figures show first-degree (**a**), Mobitz type I second-degree (**b**), Mobitz type II second-degree (**c**), and third-degree AV block (**d**). See text for discussion

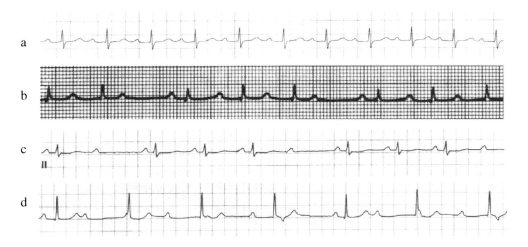

block becomes less apparent. Mobitz type I block is almost always located at the AV node, and the risk of developing complete AV block is low. In *Mobitz type II* second-degree AV block (Fig. 26.12c), AV conduction fails suddenly without a change preceding the PR interval. This type of block is usually due to His–Purkinje disease and is associated with a high risk of developing complete AV block; the escape rate is slow and unreliable. When two or more consecutive atrial impulses fail to conduct, *high-degree AV block* is present and pacemaker implantation is mandatory. The *third-degree AV block* (Fig. 26.12d) is complete AV block, and no atrial impulses can conduct to the ventricles. A permanent pacemaker is usually required in the third-degree AV block (whether congenital or acquired in origin). In this regard, dual-chamber pacing (i.e., pacing both the atrium and ventricle) has become widely accepted as the approach of choice for such patients.

26.7 Electrophysiological Study (EPS) and Catheter Ablation

The clinical EPS is important for evaluating a broad spectrum of cardiac arrhythmias. More specifically, it can help to: (1) assess the function of the sinus and AV nodes and the His–Purkinje system; (2) determine the characteristics of reentry tachycardias; (3) assess the efficacy of antiarrhythmic drugs and devices; (4) map the location of arrhythmogenic foci; and/or (5) ultimately define proper locations to ablate many forms of tachycardias. The EPS is performed in an *electrophysiology laboratory* which is, in many respects, similar to a conventional heart catheterization suite. The minimum equipment requirements for a comprehensive EPS include: (1) radiographic table; (2) fluoroscopy unit; (3) physiologic recording and analysis system; (4) programmable stimulator; (5)

RF generator and a variety of electrode catheters and introducers; (6) sterile working environment; and (7) monitoring and resuscitation equipment. Nevertheless, it is essential that a well-trained team experienced in dealing with a range of cardiac emergencies should be in place before such studies are undertaken.

EPS is usually performed on the patient in a fasting and antiarrhythmic drug-free state and in a sterilized fashion using various degrees of conscious sedation (such as fentanyl and midazolam), depending on the specific procedure. Typically, vascular access is obtained percutaneously through the femoral, subclavian, and internal jugular veins under local anesthesia using 1% lidocaine. Multiple electrode catheters are placed at key locations within the heart, such as the high right atrium close to the sinus node, the coronary sinus (for recording and stimulating the left atrium), the His bundle region, and the right ventricular apex. AH and HV intervals are routine baseline measurements of EPS (Fig. 26.13). A mapping and ablation catheter is also inserted when ablation is planned. The ablation catheter usually has a varying deflectable distal segment (1.5–3 in) with a distal electrode of 2.2 mm in diameter (7 French) and 4 or 8 mm in length. As such, physiological signals are usually digitized at 1,000 Hz and filtered between 30 and 500 Hz; pharmacological provocations, such as isoproterenol, are often required to facilitate induction of tachycardias.

The purpose of ablation is to destroy myocardial tissue by delivering electrical energy (or, in some cases, cryothermia or other forms of energy) over a distal electrode of a catheter placed on the endomyocardium at the arrhythmia substrate, i.e., the tissue integrally related to the initiation or maintenance of tachycardia. The first successful ablation using DC shocks in a human was performed in 1982. DC shocks have now been replaced by RF energy in the range of 100 KHz to 1.5 MHz. More recently, cryothermy has been introduced

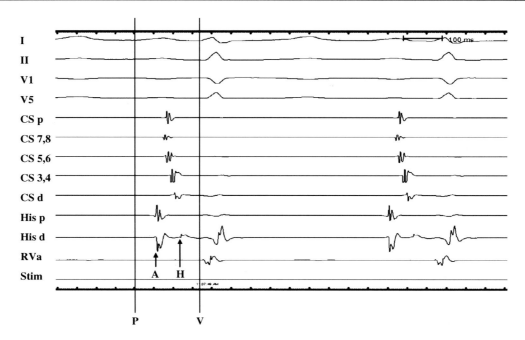

Fig. 26.13 Measurements in the His bundle electrogram. These measurements are important for evaluation of atrioventricular conduction. The AH interval, measured from the earliest reproducible rapid deflection of the atrial electrogram in the His recording to the onset of the His deflection, represents conduction time from the low right atrium at the interatrial septum through the atrioventricular node to the His bundle (atrioventricular node function). The HV interval, measured from the beginning of the His deflection to the earliest onset of ventricular activation (surface leads or intracardiac recordings), represents conduction time from the proximal His bundle to the ventricular myocardium (infra-His conduction function). I, surface ECG lead I; II, surface ECG lead II; V1, surface ECG lead V1; V5, surface ECG lead V5; A, onset of atrial activation; CS, coronary sinus; d, distal; H, onset of His activation; His, His bundle; p, proximal; P, onset of the P-wave; RVa, right ventricular apex; Stim, stimulation; V, onset of ventricular activation

in clinical practice. Lasers and microwave energy sources have been investigated and these methods continue to be of interest.

Since the RF portion of the electromagnetic spectrum is conducted through cardiac tissue, it generates resistive heat in the tissue under the tip of the ablation catheter (with the reference patch usually placed on the skin of the patient's thigh). Temperature at the tip of an ablation catheter is controlled between 50 and 70°C to avoid coagulation of blood and desiccation of tissue, which occurs when temperature reaches 100°C. Irreversible cellular damage and tissue death occur once tissue temperature exceeds 50°C. Application of such RF energy for 30–120 s results in a necrosis lesion of 4–5 mm in radius and 2–3 mm in depth. Note that the use of irrigated tip catheters can prevent excessive heating of the tip and allow greater power delivery, leading to larger and deeper ablation lesions.

Diagnostic EPS and ablative procedures are usually accomplished in a single session. Ablations of arrhythmias are usually indicated for reasons related to the patient's preference or refractoriness of arrhythmias to drug therapy. New technologies such as intracardiac echocardiography, nonfluoroscopic electroanatomical mapping, and noncontact endocardial activation mapping have significantly contributed to the advancements in interventional cardiac electrophysiology (see Chapter 29).

The general indications of ablation are summarized in Table 26.4. Note that polymorphic VT and ventricular fibrillation are usually not indicated for ablation using current ablative techniques. In general, RF ablation is now considered as an effective treatment for typical atrial flutter in addition to AVNRT and AVRT. AV junctional ablation plus pacemaker implantation is well accepted in controlling symptoms due to refractory AFib. Hybrid catheter-based RF ablative approaches, designed to isolate the pulmonary veins, together with other ablative strategies are exciting new approaches for drug-refractory AFib patients. In experienced hands, RF catheter ablation can eliminate spontaneous episodes of VT in up to two-thirds of patients after myocardial infarction [10]. At present, the catheter ablation of VT is largely adjunctive to amiodarone administration and the implantation of an ICD.

Complications of intracardiac ablation treatment, in general, can be related to: (1) the catheterization procedure, e.g., local vascular complications, vasovagal reactions, and perforation of the heart and vessels leading to tamponade and internal bleeding; (2) subclavian

Table 26.4 Indications for ablation of arrhythmias

- Atrial tachycardias
  - ☐ Inappropriate sinus tachycardia
  - ☐ Focal atrial tachycardia
  - ☐ Typical atrial flutter (type I)
  - ☐ Atypical atrial flutter (type II) *
- Atrial fibrillation
  - ☐ Atrioventricular nodal ablation for rate control
  - ☐ Pulmonary vein isolation*
  - ☐ Hybrid ablation techniques*
- Atrioventricular nodal reentry tachycardia
- Atrioventricular reentry tachycardia using concealed bypass tracts
- Wolff–Parkinson–White syndrome
- Ventricular tachycardia
  - ☐ Ischemic ventricular tachycardia (monomorphic, stable)
  - ☐ Ischemic ventricular tachycardia (monomorphic, unstable)*
  - ☐ Non-ischemic ventricular tachycardia (stable monomorphic)
  - ☐ Idiopathic ventricular tachycardia (including symptomatic ventricular premature complexes)
  - ☐ Bundle branch reentry tachycardia

*Ablation procedures are under investigation or whose clinical indications are undefined.

puncture, potentially resulting in pneumothorax, hemothorax, subclavian artery injury, branchial nerve injury, and/or subclavian arteriovenous fistula; (3) vascular complications, i.e., embolization, hypotension, myocardial infarction; and/or (4) RF ablation, in general, e.g., post-ablation pain, esophageal damage, phrenic nerve injury, AV block, or prolonged radiation exposure. It is important to note that the risk of complications is heavily dependent on the experience and skill of the operator, as well as the type of ablation procedure employed.

Ablation has been shown to be cost-effective in the management of drug-refractory PSVTs. The total charge for an outpatient ablation procedure is typically $10,000–$12,000. For ablation of the WPW syndrome, the cost is $6,600–$19,000 per quality-adjusted year of life gained.

26.7.1 Ablation of Inappropriate Sinus Tachycardia (IST)

Ablation of drug-refractory IST may be performed to eliminate the portion of the sinus node that generates the fast heart rate along the superior aspect of the crista terminalis. Due to the anatomical structure of the sinus node, multiple lesions over 3–4 cm along the crista terminalis are often required. 3D cardiac mapping and intracardiac echocardiography are useful in identification of the earliest activation site and the crista terminalis, respectively. The primary ablation goal is to achieve an approximately 30% reduction in maximal heart rate

during infusion of isoproterenol and atropine. Many of these patients have sustained improvement of symptoms. However, many such patients need additional ablation sessions in order to obtain more complete heart rate slowing. However, if it occurs, the complete ablation of the sinus node necessitates implantation of a pacemaker, but this is rare.

26.7.2 Ablation of Atrial Tachycardia

Right atrial tachycardias often originate along the length of the crista terminalis from the sinus node to the coronary sinus and AV node (*cristal tachycardia*), and they account for 80% of all ATs. Other sites of AT clustering include the pulmonary vein ostia, coronary sinus ostia, and/or the mitral and tricuspid valve rings. Appropriate identification of the earliest onset of the P-wave is critical for mapping. The "dancing catheter" or "pas de deux," pace mapping, and "destructive mapping" can be used for AT ablation. Mapping to the midseptum (particularly when the presystolic activity is not significantly early) or observing signals that are not fractionated or multiple sites that have similar activation time may suggest an origin of tachycardia in the left atrium, such as the pulmonary vein ostia. Diagnosis of anteroseptal AT is difficult but possible, and the arrhythmia can be ablated without causing AV block if undertaken with great care. Interestingly, it was recently noted that complications during such procedures, particularly damage to the specialized cardiac conduction system, can be minimized by using a cryothermia ablation system. Early data suggest that the average success rate of AT ablation is 91%, with a complication rate of 3% and recurrence rate of 9%. It is also noteworthy that the outcome of ablation of AT has been significantly improved by using a 3D mapping system. Nevertheless, complications associated with these procedures include sinus node dysfunction, AV block, phrenic nerve damage, and/or other common complications associated with catheter ablation (noted above).

26.7.3 Ablation of Atrial Flutter

26.7.3.1 Ablation of Typical Atrial Flutter

Endocardial mapping in patients with typical atrial flutter has confirmed that macroreentry occurs in the right atrium. Most often, typical atrial flutter rotates in a counterclockwise direction in the frontal plane, although clockwise rotation can also be observed. On 12-lead ECG (see Chapter 17), counterclockwise atrial flutter presents a stereotypical "sawtooth" pattern, an upright flutter wave in V1 and inverted flutter waves in the inferior leads and V6. In contrast, during clockwise rotation, flutter waves in V1 are inverted, while those in the inferior leads and V6 are upright. The macroreentrant circuit passes through a critical isthmus bounded by the inferior aspect of the tricuspid annulus, the ostium of the inferior vena cava, the ostium of coronary sinus, and the Eustachian ridge (*cavotricuspid isthmus*). During endocardial recording, a multielectrode catheter can be placed around the macroreentrant circuit adjacent to the tricuspid valve to evaluate rotation around the tricuspid annulus and through the isthmus. Linear lesions that transect this isthmus will typically block the reentry circuit and essentially cure typical atrial flutter. However, some atrial flutter circuits may not travel through this isthmus; consequently, it is important to confirm that the isthmus is critical to the maintenance of the flutter circuit by using pacing maneuvers to demonstrate *concealed entrainment*. In such complicated cases, 3D mapping systems may help to better identify the underlying tachycardia circuit and provide a more precise and effective way to complete a linear ablative lesion. An 8-mm tipped catheter and an irrigated tip catheter are more effective than (and as safe as) conventional catheters for atrial flutter ablation, and they can be useful in cases where a conventional 4-mm tipped catheter fails.

Currently, the success rate of typical atrial flutter ablation is >90% with the recurrence rate <10%. Confirmation of bidirectional isthmus block significantly reduces recurrence rates [11]. Our unpublished data suggest that unidirectional block with transisthmus conduction time >120 ms (preferably >150 ms) is sufficient to conclude a successful ablation of isthmus-dependent flutter; note that the transisthmus conduction time is measured during proximal coronary sinus pacing at 450 ms from the pacing spike to the low lateral wall of the right atrium at approximately 7 o'clock at the left anterior oblique view 50°. Ablation of Class Ic atrial flutter (atrial flutter which develops during Class Ic antiarrhythmic drug therapy for AFib) may be useful for drug-refractory AFib [12].

26.7.3.2 Ablation of Atypical Atrial Flutter

From an ablative viewpoint, the term *atypical atrial flutter* is sometimes used to describe any macroreentrant atrial tachycardia that does not utilize the cavotricuspid isthmus as a critical component of a tachycardia circuit. Therefore, atypical atrial flutter consists of a heterogeneous group of arrhythmias presenting with stable, flutter wave-like morphologies on 12-lead ECG. Techniques for ablation of atypical atrial flutters are continuing to evolve. Nevertheless, the key for successful ablation of atypical flutters is to identify and ablate the critical isthmus of the macroreentry flutter circuit arising from the right or left atrium. Yet, identifying this critical tissue is often challenging; 3D mapping systems and pacing maneuvers are usually used in concert to find these critical targets.

A proximal-to-distal coronary sinus activation sequence does not necessarily mean that the tachycardia is located in the right atrium, such as in perimitral annular reentry or periseptal reentry. For example, the following evidence suggests a left atrial origin:

1. Failure to demonstrate concealed entrainment at multiple right atrial sites.
2. No more than 50% of tachycardia cycle length cannot be mapped within the right atrium.
3. Passive conduction to the right atrium from the left atrium, with early septal activation in the right atrium, typically in the Bachman's bundle or the coronary sinus ostium.
4. Possible left–right atrial dissociation or conduction delays evidenced by a relatively fixed cycle length in the left atrium versus significant cycle length variations in the right atrium.

Special forms of atypical atrial flutter include: (1) upper loop reentry; (2) right atrial free wall flutter; (3) dual loop right atrial reentry; (4) left atrial macroreentry; and (5) left septal flutter.

26.7.3.3 Ablation of Incisional Atrial Tachycardia

Macro-reentrant atrial tachycardia occurs frequently following surgery for congenital and other heart diseases. The presence of multiple anatomic barriers (surgical incisions, patches, conduits, cavae, the coronary sinus ostium, and the pulmonary venous ostia) as well as atrial tissue damage (hypoxemia, ischemia, surgical scars, and fibrosis) all provide potential rich substrates for reentry. Furthermore, the partially successful Maze surgeries or RF ablative procedures for AFib may also leave substrates for intraatrial reentrant tachycardias (*"incisional reentry"*). The location for successful ablation varies from patient to patient and can be identified by concealed entrainment. In such patients, 3D mapping is useful in identifying and ablating the reentrant circuit. Recent data have shown that RF linear lesions transecting one or more protected isthmuses sustaining macroreentry are associated with acute success rates of 71–93%; however, recurrence rates may be as high as 40–46%. Nevertheless, these outcomes can be improved, especially when 3D mapping systems are employed.

26.7.4 Ablation of Atrial Fibrillation

In addition to ablation of the AV node for rate control, catheter ablation of AFib is useful, especially following the surgical Maze approach involving compartmentalizing the atrium. Yet, in general, this technique has proven problematic due to its long procedure time and unacceptably high thromboembolic complications. AFib ablation has evolved from ablation of the trigger to ablation of the total underlying substrates. More specifically, several catheter-based ablative techniques are currently available to provide symptomatic improvement in patients with drug-refractory AFib. Ablation of Afib is currently considered an investigational procedure but, nevertheless, has become quite widespread in electrophysiology clinical practice. It is generally thought that ablation of Afib should be limited to symptomatic patients with drug-refractory AFib. An "Expert Consensus Statement" on catheter and surgical ablation of AFib was published in 2007 [13].

26.7.4.1 AV Nodal Modification or Ablation for Rate Control

Catheter ablation of the AV junction and the concomitant insertion of a permanent pacemaker have been shown to be effective in achieving ventricular rate control in patients with drug-refractory AFib; this combination is superior to drug therapy alone for symptomatic relief in selected patients. This approach can also be used for rate control in patients with drug-refractory multifocal AT.

Importantly, it is well documented that pacing from the conventional right ventricular apex has detrimental effects on cardiac function. Rather, His bundle pacing is preferred since patients undergoing AV junctional ablation often already have severe left ventricular dysfunction. Unfortunately, His bundle pacing is technically difficult and not clinically feasible at the present time. We have demonstrated that isolation of a small area of atrial tissue surrounding the AV node is feasible by catheter RF ablation [14]. This procedure may be a useful alternative to conventional AV junctional ablation, as it can create complete AV block and, in effect, permit the "equivalent" of His bundle pacing after AV junctional ablation.

26.7.4.2 Catheter-Based Maze Procedure

Surgical treatment of AFib by compartmentalizing the atrium from an electrical transmission perspective is designed to preclude coexistence of multiple micro-reentry loops or fibrillatory waves, thereby extinguishing the arrhythmia while permitting maintenance of sinus node function, preservation of AV conduction, and restoration of atrial contractility. Surgical approaches include the modified Cox Maze procedure and the left atrial isolation procedure. The reported overall success rates in eliminating AFib are high (over 90%) with mortality rates of 2–3%. More recently, a catheter-based Maze procedure has been introduced and successfully employed. Fortunately, the technical difficulty in achieving stable linear conduction block has been improved by using new technology such as intracardiac echocardiography and a 3D mapping system. In patients with paroxysmal AFib, success rates with and without drug therapy, respectively, at 11 months follow-up were approximately 33 and 13% for linear ablation limited to the right atrium, and 85 and 60% for the biatrial approach. Due to rapid advances in the AFib ablation techniques targeting pulmonary vein isolation, the catheter-based Maze procedure is performed now by almost all clinical centers performing ablations.

26.7.4.3 Evolution of AFib Ablation

Focal Afib Ablation

One of the most significant recent advancements in transcatheter ablation of cardiac arrhythmias was the identification of patients with focal AFib [15, 16]. Focal sources of activity are critical for some patients with paroxysmal AFib, serving as either the main abnormality (focal drivers) or as the dominant trigger to induce repetitive episodes of AFib (focal triggers). A single rapidly discharging focus leads to fibrillatory conduction, mimicking the surface ECG features of AFib. Very early focal catheter ablation of AFib used activation mapping and pace mapping to identify sites of spontaneous firing that led to bursts of AFib.

Clinical experience has demonstrated that the pulmonary veins are the predominant sources of AFib triggers for many patients. More specifically, the left superior pulmonary vein is the most common focal source followed by the right superior, left inferior, and right inferior pulmonary veins, respectively. Initially, although acute success rates were quite high, the recurrences of AFib were unacceptably common. It is interesting to note that when investigators revisited the ablation of these patients, triggers were often found in other areas of the vein initially targeted and/or in remote veins. Because it appeared that either new triggers could arise in nonablated areas of veins or that these areas were arrhythmogenic but not realized during initial ablation, the technique of complete isolation of the pulmonary vein was developed as described below.

Segmental Ostial Isolation of Pulmonary Veins

To perform such a procedure, a circular mapping catheter is placed at the funnel-shaped opening of each vein to map electrical exit sites of the vein into the atrium [17]. Any segments with abnormal pulmonary potentials are then ablated until each pulmonary vein is completely isolated from the left atrium (segmental ostial isolation). It has been shown that electrical isolation of the pulmonary veins from the left atrium results in marked reduction or elimination of AFib. This may be accomplished by sequential elimination of the earliest breakthroughs at pulmonary venous ostia, or by empirically encircling and isolating the ostia. More recently, the use of saline-irrigated RF lesions has facilitated ablation procedures by successfully creating larger lesions. Success rates for catheter ablation of focal AFib may exceed 70%, however, multiple ablation sessions may be required to achieve this degree of drug-free arrhythmia control. In addition, saline irrigation may reduce charring and perhaps reduce the thromboembolic risk of this procedure. However, long procedure time, high recurrence rates (>50%), thromboembolism, and concerns about pulmonary vein stenosis remain problematic.

Circumferential Isolation of Pulmonary Veins

Concurrent with the development of segmental ostial isolation of the pulmonary veins, the circumferential approach has been developed which also employs electroanatomical mapping [18]. More specifically, RF ablation is performed circumferentially around each vein with the end point being the absence or dissociation of electrical signals within the encircling lesions.

Early attempts at electrical isolation of the pulmonary veins at their ostia occasionally caused pulmonary vein stenosis, necessitating angioplasty or stenting of the vein in some patients. This phenomenon has caused investigators to isolate the veins by using much larger circles with far greater diameters along the posterior left atrium, usually two larger circles encircling the left- and right-sided veins, respectively (Fig. 26.14) [19]. The wide circumferential isolation technique has significantly improved the successful rate of AFib ablation. Since macroreentry left atrial flutter as a complication following such isolation is relatively common (Fig. 26.15), many investigators now add more ablation lines along the roof of the left atrium as well as down to the mitral valve annulus from the left ablation circle [20]. Furthermore, some investigators also isolate the ostium of superior vena cava and the coronary sinus, and add an ablation line connecting the superior and inferior vena cava. Such techniques may isolate triggers as well as prevent arrhythmia propagation, analogous to the surgical Maze procedure. However, due to the extensive ablation lesions performed in such procedures, a fistula between the left atrium and esophagus may occur in rare cases; such patients with this rare complication often present with subacute infection and embolization following the AFib ablation procedure.

Substrate Ablation

This ablation technique is based on the assumption that AFib is more dependent on perpetuation of the arrhythmia in the diseased atria rather than initiation from the pulmonary veins. In such cases, complex fractionated atrial electrograms are sought and targeted for ablation [21, 22], often using 3D mapping systems. Both spot and linear ablation lesions may be used to ablate the regions with complex fractionated atrial electrograms.

Ablation of Autonomic Targets

It is well known that the autonomic nervous system plays a role in pathogenesis of AFib. It has been reported that ablation of ganglions in the atria may be associated with

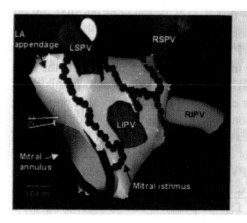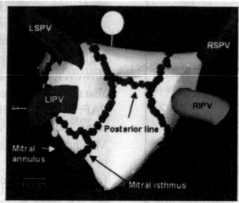

Fig. 26.14 Circumferential isolation of pulmonary veins for ablation of atrial fibrillation. Reproduced from Ref. [19] with permission. LA, left atrial; LIPV, left inferior pulmonary vein; LSPV, left superior pulmonary vein; RIPV, right inferior pulmonary vein, RSPV, right superior pulmonary vein

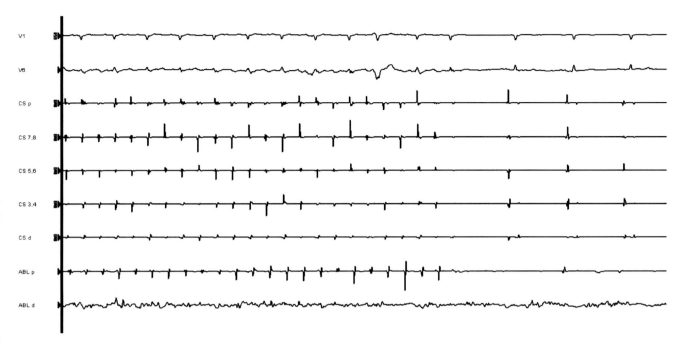

Fig. 26.15 Termination of atrial fibrillation during ablation. Atrial fibrillation is converted to left atrial flutter after circumferential isolation of all pulmonary veins. The flutter is terminated during the linear ablation in the roof of the left atrium. V1, surface ECG lead V1; V6, surface ECG lead V6; ABL, ablation; CS, coronary sinus; d, distal; p, proximal

higher likelihood of successful ablation of AFib [23]. The location of vagal innervation/ganglions is identified using stimulation/ablation-induced vagal effects, such as bradycardia or long pauses.

Hybrid Approach for Ablation of AFib

The increased success rate of the circumferential isolation has led investigators to attempt modifications of previous AFib ablation techniques, resulting in a hybrid approach (combination of two or more of above-mentioned techniques) for ablation of AFib.

Pooled data, analyzed from a series of publications of some 23,000 patients who underwent AFib ablation through 2005, provided evidence that ablation (including surgical ablation) for pulmonary vein isolation resulted in apparent elimination (no AFib recurrence at 6 months after initial ablation without antiarrhythmic drugs) or improvement with various definitions, in 75% of the cases [24]. In these reported cases, the average procedure time was 212 min and repeat procedures were required in 25% of cases. Noted complications included pulmonary vein stenosis (1.5%), cerebrovascular accidents (0.7%), transient ischemic attacks (0.5%), permanent pacer implants (8.5%, largely from surgical ablation), and others (5.2%) [24].

Ablation of AVNRT

The abnormal conduction circuit of most AVNRT is to proceed antegrade through the slow pathway and conduct retrogradely through the fast pathway (typical AVNRT). In a small number of patients (4%), the tachycardic circuit may run in an opposite direction (atypical AVNRT). The common characteristic of AVNRT is *dual pathways* or *dual physiology*, which is defined as a sudden increase of at least 50 ms in the AH interval, with a 10 ms decrease in the coupling interval of an atrial stimulus (Fig. 26.16). Dual pathway conduction curves can be elicited in a majority (85%) of patients with AVNRT, whereas dual physiology may exist in 25% of patients without AVNRT.

Ablation of AVNRT is usually aimed at ablating the slow pathway in the posteroinferior area of *the Koch's triangle* between the coronary sinus ostium and the tricuspid annulus (*posterior approach*) (Fig. 26.17) [25]. The A/V ratio for slow pathway ablation from the distal electrode pair in sinus rhythm should be less than 1 (starting from <0.25). Ablation of the fast pathway in the anterosuperior area of the Koch's triangle is rarely used due to increased risk of damage to normal AV conduction (*anterior approach*). For example, the reported risk of AV block is 1.0% with the posterior approach and 5.1% with the anterior

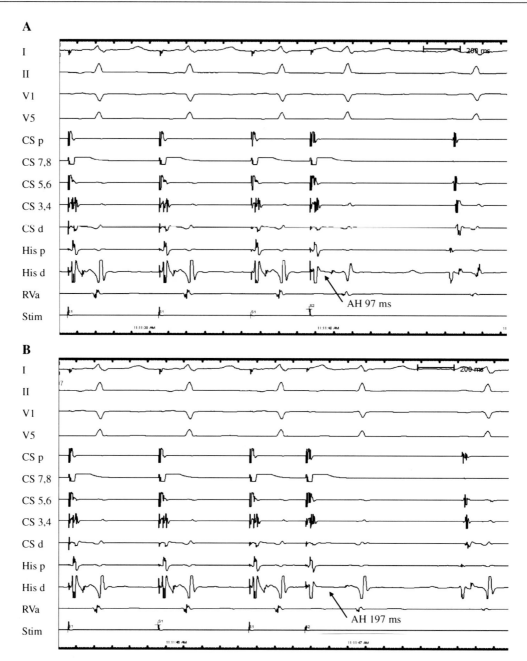

Fig. 26.16 Dual physiology (*jump*). An extrastimulus is delivered at different coupling intervals after 8-beat pacing at 500 ms from proximal coronary sinus. (**A**) AH interval is 97 ms following an extrastimulus with coupling interval of 320 ms. (**B**) AH is suddenly increased (*jumped*) by 100–197 ms at coupling interval of 310 ms. The sudden increase of >50 ms in AH interval associated with a 10 ms decrease in coupling interval is called a jump, indicating the presence of dual physiology of the atrioventricular node. I, surface ECG lead I; II, surface ECG lead II; V1, surface ECG lead V1; V5, surface ECG lead V5; CS, coronary sinus; d, distal; His, His bundle; p, proximal; RVa, right ventricular apex; Stim, stimulation

approach. Nevertheless, in experienced hands, the success rate of this procedure is almost 100%, with a recurrence rate of <3–5% and the risk of complete AV block of <1%. An accelerated junctional rhythm is to be expected with successful ablation of slow pathway conduction (100% in successful ablation versus 65% in unsuccessful ablation). Putative slow pathway potentials can be recorded during mapping. Residual slow pathway conduction or AV nodal echo beats may be present after successful AVNRT ablation and are not necessarily associated with increased recurrence during follow-up.

Recent experience on AVNRT ablation using a cryothermia ablation system has reported that the risk of

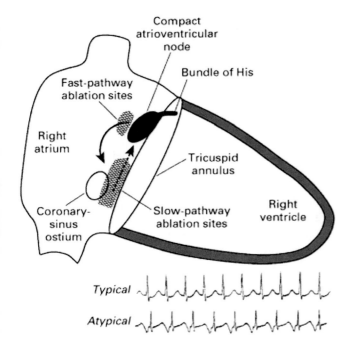

Fig. 26.17 The slow pathway (posterior) and fast pathway (anterior) ablation sites for atrioventricular nodal reentry tachycardia. Reproduced from Ref. [25] with permission. See text for discussion

complete AV block is approaching zero. It should be noted that patients with transient AV block during cryothermia ablation usually recover completely within minutes if ablation is terminated promptly when prolongation of PR interval or AV block is noted. To our knowledge, no such cases have developed significant AV conduction abnormalities during follow-up in these patients. Nevertheless, disadvantages of cryothermia ablation include: (1) it is more time-consuming in nature; and (2) there has been a small but somewhat higher recurrence rate than has been reported with RF energy therapy.

Ablation of Accessory Pathways (WPW Syndrome)

In general, the accessory pathways are left-sided in most patients. The approximate location of such accessory pathways can be typically determined from a surface ECG if preexcitation is present (Fig. 26.18) [26]. In any case, a preablation EPS is performed to determine the precise location of (and the relative number of) accessory pathways and their roles in inducible arrhythmias. Accessory AV pathways can exist at almost any site around the tricuspid and mitral annulus (with exception of where the mitral and aortic valve annuli coincide): free wall (anterolateral, lateral, and posterolateral) and septum (anteroseptal, midseptal, and posteroseptal). To date, multiple accessory pathways have been reported in 5–18% of ablation cases.

In the case of transcatheter ablation of left-sided accessory AV pathways, either the *retrograde transaortic approach* or *transseptal approach* can be used in conjunction with anticoagulation with heparin (target ACT 250–350 s). Ablation can be performed at atrial sites (during orthodromic AVRT or relatively fast ventricular pacing) or ventricular sites (during sinus rhythm or atrial pacing), targeting the earliest atrial or ventricular activation, respectively. Accessory AV pathways often cross the left AV groove obliquely with the atrial insertion closer to the coronary sinus ostium.

In contrast to the virtually invisible left-sided accessory AV connections, right-sided accessory AV pathways are often considered as more broad in nature. It is interesting to note that, when cardiac surgical ablation was done in the era prior to catheter treatment, the operator could often visualize the anomalous tissue as it crossed the tricuspid annulus. The site with the earliest atrial activation (retrograde conduction) or ventricular activation (antegrade conduction) is usually targeted for ablation.

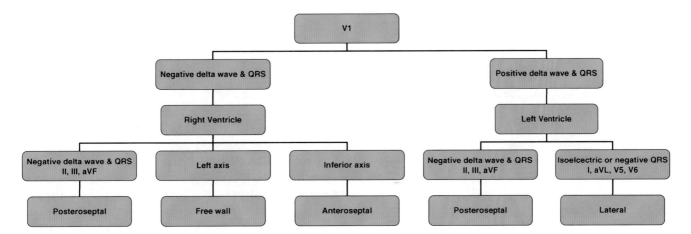

Fig. 26.18 Determination of the location of accessory pathways based on the delta wave and the QRS complex on surface 12-lead ECG. Reproduced from Ref. [26] with permission

Mechanical mapping (inhibition of accessory conduction by mechanical pressure) and a QS wave on unfiltered unipolar recordings may also be helpful. The optimal ablation site can best be found by direct recording of accessory pathway potentials and by monitoring stable fluoroscopic and electrical characteristics.

In general, the success rate of ablation for left free wall accessory pathways is 96% with a recurrence rate of 3–8% and complication rate of <6% (major complications 1.3%: tamponade 1.2%, AV block 0.5%, systemic embolization 0.08%, and death 0.08%). Ablation of right-sided accessory pathways is associated with a lower success rate (88%) and higher recurrence rates (up to 21% in earlier studies). On the other hand, the annual risk of natural SCD in WPW syndrome with symptomatic tachycardia is estimated to be 0.05–0.5%. Asymptomatic preexcitation also carries an increased risk of SCD [27], but this is not well defined and the uncertainty must be carefully discussed with the patient before recommending intervention in these cases.

26.7.5 Ablation of VT

26.7.5.1 VT in Clinically Normal Hearts

There are two main substrates for VT in a clinically normal heart: focal and reentrant. Focal VTs are commonly seen in patients without underlying organic heart disease (*idiopathic VT*). Idiopathic VT accounts for 10–15% of all diagnosed sustained VTs. Approximately 70% of idiopathic VT exhibits a left bundle branch block pattern, suggesting an origin in the right ventricle. These VTs almost uniformly show an inferior frontal plane axis, indicating an origin within the right ventricular outflow tract. *Arrhythmogenic right ventricular dysplasia/cardiomyopathy* should be suspected when other morphologies exist. The origin of idiopathic left VT is usually at the inferior left ventricular midseptum or apex in the region of the posterior fascicle or in the left ventricular outflow tract. Fortunately, RF ablation of these idiopathic VTs is curative in >90% of patients. In addition, it is common that isolated VPCs or nonsustained VT in a clinically normal heart can be ablated as well.

26.7.5.2 VT in Ischemic Heart Disease

Reentrant VTs usually occur in the presence of underlying organic heart disease, particularly in the event of prior myocardial infarction. Unfortunately, while mapping of these tachycardias is increasingly feasible with modern technology, the ability to undertake ablation of ischemic heart disease VTs remains limited due to their hemodynamic instability. At present, RF ablation for VT is predominately limited to hemodynamically stable tachyarrhythmias, although attempts have now been made to map unstable VTs under percutaneous hemodynamic supports. Yet, this latter group only accounts for 5–10% of ischemic VTs, or 20% of all ventricular tachyarrhythmias requiring clinical assessment. RF catheter ablation of VT after myocardial infarction may eliminate spontaneous episodes of VT in up to two-thirds of patients in experienced centers [10]. Furthermore, if one or two clinically documented VTs are targeted, successful ablation can be achieved in 71–76% [28] with serious complications in <2% of cases [25]. At present, catheter ablation of VT in patients following myocardial infarction is used primarily as an adjunctive to amiodarone and ICD therapy. Nevertheless, in the near future, more patients with VT may be eligible for RF ablation with new technologies such as noncontact endocardial activation mapping and electroanatomical mapping.

Entrainment is a very useful technique for assessing reentry tachycardia. *Entrainment* refers to the continuous resetting of reentry tachycardia circuit by pacing at a slightly faster rate than tachycardia, with the intrinsic rate of tachycardia resuming when the pacing is stopped. More specifically, each pacing stimulus creates a wave front that travels in an antegrade direction and resets the tachycardia to the pacing rate; a wave front propagating retrogradely in the opposite direction collides with the wave front of the previous beat.

26.7.5.3 Ablation of Bundle Branch Reentry Tachycardia

An uncommon form of VT that can be cured by RF ablation is bundle branch reentry tachycardia. The substrate for this form of reentry is usually a dilated cardiomyopathy associated with significant conduction system disease. Although cure of bundle branch reentry tachycardia can be easily accomplished by ablating the right bundle branch, long-term survival after RF ablation is limited by the almost uniform presence of severe left ventricular dysfunction. Therefore, in such cases, ICD therapy is usually needed. To date, the relative experience on ablation of VT in patients with structural heart diseases other than ischemia is limited, but the ablation technique is similar to those employed in other clinical settings.

26.8 New Technology in Cardiac Electrophysiology

26.8.1 Nonfluoroscopic Electroanatomical Cardiac Mapping—Carto™

Cardiac mapping is essential for understanding mechanisms of cardiac arrhythmias and for directing curative ablation procedures. Traditional endocardial mapping techniques are time-consuming, produce significant radiation exposure, and are limited by lack of 3D spatial information. One of the most important new advances in cardiac electrophysiology is a nonfluoroscopic electroanatomical cardiac mapping system (Carto™, Biosense Webster, Diamond Bar, CA). The Carto system uses an integrated, electroanatomical catheter-based technique that generates 3D geometry of the cardiac chambers. It is comprised of a miniature passive magnetic field sensor at the tip of a mapping catheter, an external ultra-low magnetic field emitter, plus a processing and display unit. The system uses magnetic technology to accurately determine the location and orientation of the mapping catheter while simultaneously recording the local electrogram from the catheter tip. By sampling electrical and spatial information from a variety of endocardial sites, the 3D geometry of the heart can be reconstructed in real time (with superimposed color-coded electrophysiological information) to generate an electroanatomical map (Fig. 26.19). Optimal mapping with the Carto system requires a stable rhythm and a fixed reference point.

Experience using the Carto system has provided an integrated look at cardiac electrophysiology and structure. The ability to provide enhanced spatial navigation and to guide RF ablation energy delivery to specific targets in the heart has significantly contributed to the management of many cardiac arrhythmias, such as AT, atypical atrial flutter, AFib, and VT. It has been reported that electroanatomic mapping using the Carto system during sinus

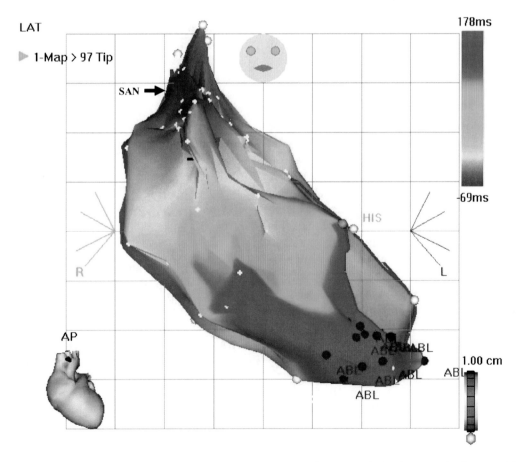

Fig. 26.19 3D right atrial activation map during sinus rhythm (anterior–posterior view) in a patient who underwent slow pathway ablation for typical atrioventricular nodal reentry tachycardia. The *color bar* shows the activation time, with the earliest activation at 69 ms before a reference signal in the coronary sinus (*red area*) and the latest activation at 178 ms after the reference (*purple area*). The *dark red dots* at the *bottom* are the ablation sites in the slow pathway area (ABL). The *yellow dot* indicates the location of the His bundle (HIS). The *arrow* indicates the location of the sinus node (SAN)

rhythm allows accurate 3D characterization of infarct architecture and helps to define the relationship between electrophysiological and anatomical abnormalities. This technique may prove useful in devising anatomically based strategies for ablation of VT (see Chapter 29).

26.8.2 Nonfluoroscopic Navigation and Mapping—EnSite® System

The EnSite® System provides nonfluoroscopic navigation of conventional electrophysiology catheters using the transmission of a 5.86 kHz locator signal to identify the 3D position of conventional catheter electrodes. The EnSite System initially used the EnSite Array catheter, which features an electrode array for noncontact mapping. However, the latest version of this system now also incorporates a second method of catheter navigation through the use of an EnSite NavX surface electrode kit that allows cardiac mapping similar to that of the Carto System.

For an EnSite array study, the system can be used to locate the position of electrodes on conventional electrophysiology catheters relative to the position of the EnSite electrode array. The array catheter consists of an 8-ml balloon mounted on a 9 French catheter; around the catheter is a woven braid of 64 wires, each with a single unipolar microelectrode in a pattern of eight columns by eight rows (see Chapter 29). Using the sensed voltage and respective array electrode location, the 3D position of the electrophysiology catheter electrode is located 100 times per second. Subsequently, by multiplexing the signal, the system can locate up to four electrodes at a reduced frequency (50 times per second). By locating a catheter as it is positioned at the outermost boundaries of a chamber, the system can generate detailed cardiac models that reflect the patient-specific size and shape of the chamber.

The EnSite array rapidly generates noncontact endocardial activation maps based on the electrical fields detected in the blood pool, with the potential to reduce procedure and fluoroscopy time and increase the efficacy of ablation through better appreciation of the arrhythmia mechanisms (Fig. 26.20). Using this approach, previously inaccessible and poorly tolerated VTs may become amenable to mapping and ablation because only one tachycardia beat is needed for an activation map of the tachycardia circuit. The mathematical technique used to enhance and resolve the far-field, low-frequency, and low-amplitude potentials is based on an inverse solution to Laplace's equation (using a boundary element method). By employing refined mathematical solutions, the noncontact mapping system is able to reconstruct and interpolate up to 3,360 electrograms simultaneously, covering virtually the entire endocardium of the chamber in which

a mapping catheter is deployed. Clinical studies have shown that this system is capable of reconstructing electrograms accurately at distances of up to 50 mm from the center of the mapping catheter [29]. However, overall accuracy decreases when the endocardium is farther than 34 mm from the center of the mapping catheter.

For an EnSite NavX study, the system locates the position of electrodes on conventional electrophysiology catheters which are connected to the EnSite System. Six electrode patches placed on the body surface form three orthogonal axes with the heart in the center. The patient interface unit sends a 5.86 kHz locator signal alternately from one surface electrode to another to create a transthoracic electrical field. Conventional electrophysiology catheters within this field sense the voltage of the locator signal on each axis between the pairs of surface electrodes. The voltage is used to calculate the relative position of each electrode simultaneously on each axis. By alternating the measurement between axes, the location of up to 64 intracardiac electrodes are determined 93 times per second. The electrodes are graphically organized on 3D renditions of catheter shafts, with a maximum of 12 definable catheter entities and a maximum of 20 electrodes definable on any one. The rendered catheters are oriented on the display relative to a user-selected positional reference electrode, to stabilize the display relative to the motion of the heart. In addition to nonfluoroscopic navigation, EnSite NavX can also be used to create detailed models of cardiac anatomy and superimpose color-coded maps of activation time, voltage, or fractionation levels, based on automated analysis of conventional waveforms (Fig. 26.11).

26.8.3 Intracardiac Echocardiography

Several recent studies have demonstrated that intracardiac echocardiography can be employed as a useful tool during RF ablation procedures [30]. More specifically, the potential benefits of direct endocardial visualization during RF ablative procedures include the following:

- Enhanced ability to guide ablative procedures and precise anatomical localization of the ablation catheter tip in relation to important endocardial structures (which cannot be visualized with fluoroscopy).
- Reduction in fluoroscopy time.
- Evaluation of catheter tip–tissue contact.
- Confirmation of lesion formation and identification of lesion size and continuity.
- Immediate identification of complications.
- A research tool to help in understanding the critical role played by specific endocardial structures in arrhythmogenesis.

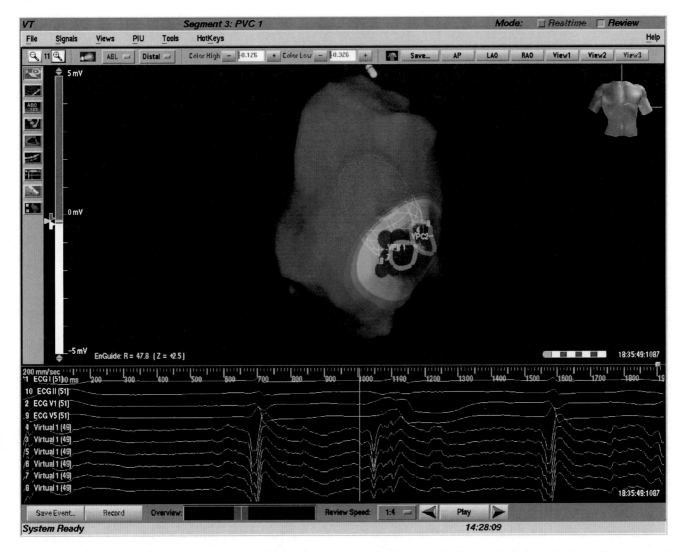

Fig. 26.20 EnSite array study for mapping ventricular ectopics in the left ventricle. The *red area* indicates the earliest activation site of an ectopic. Delivery of radiofrequency energy eliminates frequent ventricular ectopics in this patient. The *brown dots* represent ablation lesions

3D echocardiography is certainly useful and perhaps one of the ideal imaging techniques for cardiac electrophysiology. However, its overall quality must be improved before it becomes clinically applicable. Nevertheless, this is a field of active research and such systems will likely be available in the near future (see Chapter 20).

26.8.4 Magnetically Directed Catheter Manipulation

A recent intriguing development in the manipulation of intravascular electrode catheters for various EPS and mapping or ablation purposes involves the utilization of magnetic fields to direct malleable catheters. Yet, this technique (Stereotaxis, Inc., St. Louis, MO) requires catheterization laboratories fitted with large magnets at the bedside, as well as specially designed low-mass catheters capable of being directed by the magnetic field. The principal advantage in terms of mapping is the ability to turn tight corners since the catheters can be relatively supple and their movement is controlled by magnetic force without manual torque. Additionally, the operator can manipulate the catheter by a "joystick" from outside the laboratory, thereby reducing long-term radiation exposure to the operators. Finally, by retaining coordinates in memory, the system can bring the catheter back to a predetermined site with great accuracy.

26.9 Summary

Cardiac arrhythmias encompass a wide spectrum of abnormalities in electrical generation and conduction at all levels within the heart. They can be manifested as either tachycardia or bradycardia. The clinical significance of these cardiac arrhythmias is predominantly related to their associated hemodynamic consequences in addition to the increased risks of life-threatening consequences (e.g., SCD due to ventricular fibrillation). Both clinical and basic laboratory research have offered important insights into the mechanisms underlying various arrhythmias and have also provided valuable tools for their identification and treatment.

Historically, pharmacologic therapies have been widely used in the management of arrhythmias and, to a large extent, this remains true today. However, in recent years, nonpharmacologic therapies have begun to play an increasingly important role in curing many arrhythmias (e.g., catheter ablation) and preventing their life-threatening consequences (ICD therapy for both primary and secondary prevention of SCD). Nevertheless, our current understanding and available technologies in this field are far from ideal for the assessment and treatment of all cardiac arrhythmias. More specifically, we still strive to achieve a more thorough understanding of the underlying mechanisms of many arrhythmias and develop safer antiarrhythmic drugs (i.e., without negative inotropic or proarrhythmic effects). It is expected that, before long, the introduction of easier to use and more optimal imaging systems for interventional electrophysiology, and the clinical application of biological repairs of the pacemaker nodes and/or conduction abnormalities may substantially improve quality of care in patients with cardiac arrhythmias.

List of Abbreviations

AFib	atrial fibrillation
APC	atrial premature complex
AT	atrial tachycardia
AV	atrioventricular
AVNRT	atrioventricular nodal reentry tachycardia
AVRT	atrioventricular reentry tachycardia
bpm	beats per minute
DC	direct current
ECG	electrocardiography
EPS	electrophysiologic study
ICD	implantable cardioverter defibrillator
IST	inappropriate sinus tachycardia
PSVT	paroxysmal supraventricular tachycardia
RF	radiofrequency
SCD	sudden cardiac death
SND	sinus node dysfunction
SVT	supraventricular tachycardia
TdP	Torsades de Pointes
VPC	ventricular premature complex
VT	ventricular tachycardia
WPW	Wolff–Parkinson–White syndrome

References

1. Anonymous. The Sicilian Gambit. A new approach to the classification of antiarrhythmic drugs based on their actions on arrhythmogenic mechanisms. Task Force of the Working Group on Arrhythmias of the European Society of Cardiology. Circulation 1991;84:1831–51.
2. Anonymous. Preliminary report: Effect of encainide and flecainide on mortality in a randomized trial of arrhythmia suppression after myocardial infarction. The Cardiac Arrhythmia Suppression Trial (CAST) Investigators. N Engl J Med 1989;321: 406–12.
3. Anonymous. Effect of the antiarrhythmic agent moricizine on survival after myocardial infarction. The Cardiac Arrhythmia Suppression Trial II Investigators. N Engl J Med 1992;327: 227–33.
4. Josephson ME, ed. Clinical cardiac electrophysiology. Techniques and interpretations, 2nd ed. Malvern, PA: Lea & Febiger, 1993.
5. Benditt DG, Lu F. Atriofascicular pathways: Fuzzy nomenclature or merely wishful thinking? J Cardiovasc Electrophysiol 2006;17:261–65.
6. Fuster V, Ryden LE, Cannom DS, et al. ACC/AHA/ESC 2006 guidelines for the management of patients with atrial fibrillation—executive summary: A report of the American College of Cardiology/American Heart Association Task Force on Practice Guidelines and the European Society of Cardiology Committee for Practice Guidelines. J Am Coll Cardiol 2006;48:854–906.
7. Estes NA III, Halperin JL, Calkins H, et al. ACC/AHA/ Physician Consortium 2008 Clinical performance measures for adults with nonvalvular atrial fibrillation or atrial flutter: A report of the American College of Cardiology/American Heart Association Task Force on Performance Measures and the Physician Consortium for Performance Improvement. Developed in Collaboration with the Heart Rhythm Society. J Am Coll Cardiol 2008;51:865–84.
8. Laupacis A, Albers G, Dalen J, Dunn MI, Jacobson AK, Singer DE. Antithrombotic therapy in atrial fibrillation. Chest 1998;114:579–89S.
9. Zipes DP, Camm AJ, Borggrefe M, et al. ACC/AHA/ESC 2006 guidelines for management of patients with ventricular arrhythmias and the prevention of sudden cardiac death: A report of the American College of Cardiology/American Heart Association Task Force and the European Society of Cardiology Committee for Practice Guidelines. J Am Coll Cardiol 2006;48:e247–346.
10. Stevenson WG, Friedman PL, Kocovic D, Sager PT, Saxon LA, Pavri B. Radiofrequency catheter ablation of ventricular tachycardia after myocardial infarction. Circulation 1998;98:308–14.

11. Nabar A, Rodriguez LM, Timmermans C, Smeets JL, Wellens HJ. Isoproterenol to evaluate resumption of conduction after right atrial isthmus ablation in type I atrial flutter. Circulation 1999;99:3286–91.

12. Nabar A, Rodriguez LM, Timmermans C, van den Dool A, Smeets JL, Wellens HJ. Effect of right atrial isthmus ablation on the occurrence of atrial fibrillation: Observations in four patient groups having type I atrial flutter with or without associated atrial fibrillation. Circulation 1999;99:1441–45.

13. Calkins H, Brugada J, Packer DL, et al. HRS/EHRA/ECAS expert Consensus Statement on catheter and surgical ablation of atrial fibrillation: recommendations for personnel, policy, procedures and follow-up. A report of the Heart Rhythm Society (HRS) Task Force on catheter and surgical ablation of atrial fibrillation. Heart Rhythm 2007;4:816–61.

14. Lu F, Iaizzo PA, Benditt DG, Mehra R, Warman EN, McHenry BT. Isolated atrial segment pacing: An alternative to His bundle pacing after atrioventricular junctional ablation. J Am Coll Cardiol 2007;49:1443–49.

15. Haissaguerre M, Jais P, Shah DC, et al. Spontaneous initiation of atrial fibrillation by ectopic beats originating in the pulmonary veins. N Engl J Med 1998;339:659–66.

16. Chen SA, Tai CT, Tsai CF, Hsieh MH, Ding YA, Chang MS. Radiofrequency catheter ablation of atrial fibrillation initiated by pulmonary vein ectopic beats. J Cardiovasc Electrophysiol 2000;11:218–27.

17. Haissaguerre M, Shah DC, Jais P, et al. Electrophysiological breakthroughs from the left atrium to the pulmonary veins. Circulation 2000;102:2463–65.

18. Pappone C, Rosanio S, Oreto G, et al. Circumferential radiofrequency ablation of pulmonary vein ostia: A new anatomic approach for curing atrial fibrillation. Circulation 2000;102:2619–28.

19. Oral H, Scharf C, Chugh A, et al. Catheter ablation for paroxysmal atrial fibrillation: Segmental pulmonary vein ostial ablation versus left atrial ablation. Circulation 2003;108:2355–60.

20. Pappone C, Manguso F, Vicedomini G, et al. Prevention of iatrogenic atrial tachycardia after ablation of atrial fibrillation: A prospective randomized study comparing circumferential pulmonary vein ablation with a modified approach. Circulation 2004;110:3036–42.

21. Nademanee K, McKenzie J, Kosar E, et al. A new approach for catheter ablation of atrial fibrillation: Mapping of the electrophysiologic substrate. J Am Coll Cardiol 2004;43:2044–53.

22. Nademanee K, Schwab M, Porath J, Abbo A. How to perform electrogram-guided atrial fibrillation ablation. Heart Rhythm 2006;3:981–84.

23. Pappone C, Santinelli V, Manguso F, et al. Pulmonary vein denervation enhances long-term benefit after circumferential ablation for paroxysmal atrial fibrillation. Circulation 2004;109:327–34.

24. Fisher JD, Spinelli MA, Mookherjee D, Krumerman AK, Palma EC. Atrial fibrillation ablation: Reaching the mainstream. Pacing Clin Electrophysiol 2006;29:523–37.

25. Morady F. Radio-frequency ablation as treatment for cardiac arrhythmias. N Engl J Med 1999;340:534–44.

26. Zipes DP. Specific arrhythmias: Diagnosis and treatment. In: Braunwald E, ed. Heart disease: A text book of cardiovascular medicine, 5th ed. Philadelphia, PA: W.B. Saunders Company, 1997:640–704.

27. Triedman J, Perry J, Van Hare G. Risk stratification for prophylactic ablation in asymptomatic Wolff-Parkinson-White syndrome. N Engl J Med 2005;352:92–93.

28. Stevenson WG, Friedman PL. Catheter ablation of ventricular tachycardia. In: Zipes DP, Jalife J, eds. Cardiac electrophysiology from cell to bedside, 3rd ed. Philadelphia, PA: W.B. Saunders Company; 2000:1049–56.

29. Schilling RJ, Peters NS, Davies DW. Simultaneous endocardial mapping in the human left ventricle using a noncontact catheter: Comparison of contact and reconstructed electrograms during sinus rhythm. Circulation 1998;98:887–98.

30. Kalman JM, Olgin JE, Karch MR, Lesh MD. Use of intracardiac echocardiography in interventional electrophysiology. Pacing Clin Electrophysiol 1997;20:2248–62.

Chapter 27
Pacing and Defibrillation

Timothy G. Laske, Anna Legreid Dopp, and Paul A. Iaizzo

Abstract Currently most implanted pacing and defibrillation systems monitor and treat inappropriate cardiac rhythms. In general, these inappropriate rhythms result in cardiac outputs that are inadequate to meet metabolic demands, and thus can be life-threatening. In order to best understand the function of such pacing and defibrillation systems, the underlying physiologic situations indicated for their use must also be defined and understood. Furthermore, as with the design of any biomedical device or system, a "first-principles" understanding of the appropriate physiologic behavior is a prerequisite to the definition of the performance characteristics of the device. This chapter primarily aims to provide a basic understanding of the physiologic conditions that require intervention with pacing and/or defibrillation systems, as well as introduce technical information on these systems to provide the reader with a foundation for future research and reading on this topic.

Keywords Cardiac pacing · Defibrillation · Cardiac arrhythmia · Electrical stimulation · Drug interactions · Implantable pulse generator

27.1 Introduction

Currently, over 600,000 Americans have pacemakers and 150,000 have implantable cardioverter defibrillators (ICDs) [1].

In order to best understand the function of such pacing and defibrillation systems, the underlying physiologic situations indicated for their use must also be defined and understood. Furthermore, as with the design of any biomedical device or system, a "first-principles" understanding of the appropriate physiologic behavior is a prerequisite to the definition of the performance characteristics of the device. This chapter primarily aims to provide a basic understanding of the physiologic conditions that require intervention with pacing and/or defibrillation systems, as well as introduce technical information on these systems to provide the reader with a foundation for future research and reading on this topic. The information provided in this chapter is by no means comprehensive and thus should not be used to make decisions relating to patient care.

27.2 Cardiac Rhythms and Arrhythmias

27.2.1 Cardiac Function and Rhythm

Cardiac output (CO) is defined as the heart rate (HR, bpm) multiplied by the stroke volume (SV, liters), or $CO = HR \times SV$ (liters/min). Normally, the heart rate is determined by the rate at which the sinoatrial node (the "biologic pacemaker") depolarizes. In healthy individuals, the sinoatrial node maintains the appropriate heart rate to meet variable metabolic demands (e.g., increasing with exercise). More specifically, the sinoatrial nodal rate is modulated by: (1) sympathetic and parasympathetic innervation; (2) local tissue metabolites and other molecules; (3) neurohormonal factors; and/or (4) the perfusion of the nodal tissues. Stroke volume is the quantity of blood ejected from the heart during each ventricular contraction. The instantaneous stroke volume is governed by a number of factors including heart rate, degree of ventricular filling/atrial performance, atrial–ventricular synchrony, and/or myocardial contractility.

It is important to note that multiple physiologic and pathologic conditions exist that may result in an inappropriate cardiac output. These conditions need to be

T.G. Laske (✉)
University of Minnesota, Department of Surgery, and Medtronic, Inc., 8200 Coral Sea St. NE, MVS84, Mounds view, MN 55112, USA
e-mail: tim.g.laske@medtronic.com

P.A. Iaizzo (ed.), *Handbook of Cardiac Anatomy, Physiology, and Devices*, DOI 10.1007/978-1-60327-372-5_27,

defined to understand the functional requirements of pacing and defibrillation systems, and to motivate the logic behind the system features and performance characteristics.

27.2.2 Conditions of the Sinoatrial Node

Normal sinus rhythm	Sinoatrial nodal rate is appropriate for the current metabolic demand (see MPG 27.1)
Sinus bradycardia	A slow sinoatrial nodal rate, resulting in a slow heart rate which may or may not be functionally appropriate. $HR\downarrow \rightarrow CO\downarrow$
Sinus tachycardia	A fast sinoatrial nodal rate, resulting in a higher heart rate which may or may not be functionally appropriate. $HR\uparrow \rightarrow CO\uparrow$ (for excessive heart rates, $CO\downarrow$ due to reduced filling time)
Sick sinus syndrome	Unpredictable sinoatrial nodal rate. The rate is not appropriately coordinated with physiologic demand. $CO\uparrow$ or $CO\downarrow$
Chronotropic incompetence	Inappropriate response of the sinoatrial node to exercise. CO is too low for metabolic demands
Block	No sinoatrial nodal rhythm. The patient will have either no heart rate (asystole) or a rate defined by other regions within the heart. A rescue rhythm from the atrioventricular node normally occurs (40–60 bpm, a so-called "junctional rhythm") $HR = 0 \rightarrow CO = 0$ or $HR\downarrow \rightarrow CO\downarrow$

27.2.3 Conditions of the Atrioventricular Node

First-degree heart block	An atrioventricular interval >200 ms (normal atrioventricular interval is ~120 ms). $SV\downarrow \rightarrow CO\downarrow$
Second-degree heart block	Atrial and ventricular activity is not 1:1. Two types of second-degree block are defined: Mobitz types I and II Mobitz type I: "Wenckebach phenomenon." A ventricular beat is dropped after a progressive elongation of the atrioventricular interval. $HR\downarrow$ (missed beat) $\rightarrow CO\downarrow$ Mobitz type II: A ventricular beat is dropped without a progressive elongation of the atrioventricular interval. This is often an early indication of progressive disease of the conduction system. $HR\downarrow$ (missed beat) $\rightarrow CO\downarrow$

Third-degree heart block	No atrioventricular nodal conduction (conduction from the atrium to the ventricles). The atria contract at the sinoatrial nodal rate, and the ventricles are either asystolic or contract at a ventricular rescue rate (40–60 bpm). $HR\downarrow$ and $SV\downarrow \rightarrow CO\downarrow$

27.2.4 Arrhythmias

Atrial tachycardia/ flutter	High atrial rate of non-sinoatrial nodal origin. Not a physiologic rate, therefore decoupled from metabolic demand (see MPG 27.2). $HR\uparrow SV\downarrow \rightarrow CO\uparrow$ or $CO\downarrow$
Atrial fibrillation	Chaotic depolarization of the atrium. No atrial hemodynamic input to the ventricles and a nonphysiologic rate is conducted through the atrioventricular node to the ventricles. Ventricular output is decoupled from metabolic demand. Stasis of blood in the atria can result in clot formation and stroke (see MPG 27.3). $HR\uparrow SV\downarrow \rightarrow CO\uparrow$ or $CO\downarrow$
Ventricular tachycardia	High ventricular rate decoupled from sinoatrial nodal and atrial activity. This commonly results from a reentrant conduction loop or an ectopic foci (spontaneously beating region of myocardium). Ventricular rate is nonphysiologic, therefore decoupled from metabolic demand (see MPG 27.4). $HR\uparrow SV\downarrow \rightarrow CO\uparrow$ or $CO\downarrow$
Ventricular fibrillation	Chaotic depolarization of the ventricles. No organized heart rate (see MPG 27.5). $CO = 0$

27.3 Introduction to Implantable Pacing and Defibrillation Systems

For proper function and programming, implantable pacing and defibrillation systems require multiple components as well as external instruments. The implantable portion of the system is typically comprised of the implantable pulse generator (IPG or pacemaker) or an implantable cardioverter defibrillator (ICD or defibrillator) and the pacing and/or defibrillation leads. The IPG or ICD are most commonly implanted in a subcutaneous location in the left pectoral region. Depending on handedness, the condition of the upper venous system, the presence of other devices, and/or physician preference, the device may also be placed in the right pectoral region. The device may be placed in a submuscular location in situations where the physician is concerned about either erosion of the IPG or ICD through the skin (most common in thin, elderly, or very young patients) or for cosmetic reasons (to reduce

Fig. 27.1 Schematic of a typical implantable defibrillation system and the associated programmer. ICD, implantable defibrillation device

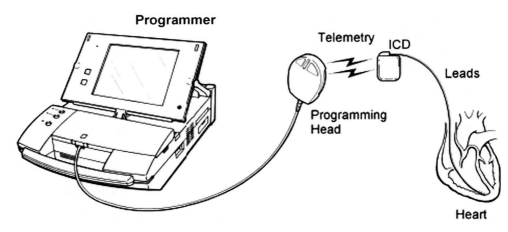

the obvious nature of the device). Another variation is to place the device in an abdominal location. This is commonly done in small children to avoid discomfort and/or interference with the motion of the arm since the device is often too large for a child's anatomy to accommodate.

In support of the implanted hardware, an external programmer is used to telemeter information to and from the programmable IPG. This allows the physician to set/reset parameters within the device and download information relating to the status of the patient and the device. A complete defibrillation system is shown schematically in Fig. 27.1 (pacing systems use a similar configuration).

Pacing and defibrillation systems can be implanted using several methods. Early systems used leads attached to the epicardial surface of the heart, with the IPG or ICD placed in the abdomen of the patient (due to their larger sizes). Although this technique is still used in certain clinical situations (i.e., neonates), a transvenous approach for attaching the leads to the heart and a pectoral placement of the IPG or ICD is far more common. The implantation technique for implantable pacing and defibrillation will be described to provide a more thorough understanding of the system requirements.

Following anesthesia and a sterile preparation of the incision site, typically one of two techniques are used to access the venous system for the implantation of transvenous leads. Accordingly, venous access is achieved through either a surgical "cutdown" to the cephalic vein (the jugular vein is also used, but this is rare) or a transcutaneous needle puncture into the subclavian vein. The "cutdown" involves a careful surgical dissection down to the vessel, placement of a cut through the vessel wall, and direct insertion of the lead into the vessel lumen. The subclavian puncture uses a needle to puncture the vessel, followed by passage of a guidewire through the needle. Subsequently, an introduction catheter (percutaneous lead introducer) with an internal dilator is forced over

the wire and into the vein. The dilator is removed, leaving the catheter behind. The lead is then inserted through the catheter (the "Seldinger Technique" can be viewed in MPG 27.6).

Following insertion into the vein, the lead(s) are advanced through the superior vena cava and into the right atrium for final placement in the right atrium, right ventricle, and/or the coronary sinus/cardiac veins (providing epicardial access to the left atrium and ventricle). Once positioned properly, the leads are secured in the desired location within the heart using either a passive or active means of fixation (see the section on leads). Next, an anchoring sleeve is used at the venous entry site to secure the lead into the vein and the surrounding tissue. This isolates the lead from mechanical forces outside of the vein, ensuring that adequate lead length remains within the heart to accommodate motion due to activity, respiration, and/or heart motion. Following lead implantation, the proximal terminal ends are connected to the IPG or ICD, which is then placed in a subcutaneous or submuscular pocket formed in the tissue. The implant site is then sutured closed, thus completing the implantation. Chest x-rays of a dual-chamber endocardial pacing system are shown in Fig. 27.2, and additional radiographic images of several pacing configurations are found in MPGs 27.7–27.12.

27.4 Cardiac Pacing

27.4.1 History

Discoveries relating to the identification of the electrophysiological properties of the heart and the ability to induce cardiac depolarization through artificial electrical stimulation are relatively recent. Gaskell, an electrophysiologist, coined the phrase "heart block" in 1882 and Purkinje first described the ventricular conduction system in 1845. Importantly, Gaskell also related the presence of

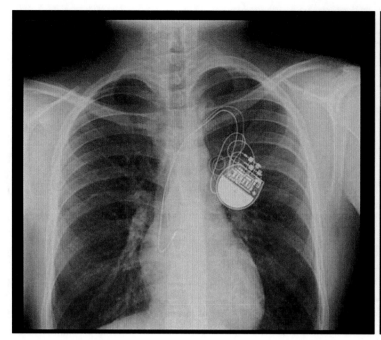
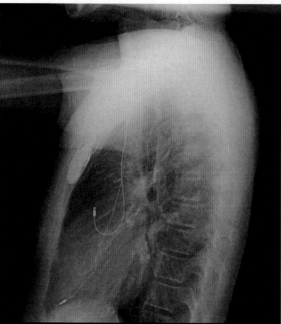

Fig. 27.2 Chest x-rays of an endocardial, dual-chamber pacing system in a young patient (anterior view on the *left*; lateral view on the *right*; Sainte-Justine Hospital, Montreal, Quebec, Canada, used with permission). The implantable pulse generator (IPG or pacemaker) is implanted in the left pectoral region. The superior lead is implanted in the right atrial appendage and the inferior lead is in the right ventricular apex

a slow ventricular rate to disassociation with the atria [2]. The discovery of the bundle of His is attributed to its namesake, Wilhelm His Jr. [3]. He described the presence in the heart of a conduction pathway from the atrioventricular node through the cardiac skeleton that eventually connected to the ventricles. Tawara later verified the existence of the bundle of His in 1906 [4]. He is also credited with being the first to clearly identify the specialized conduction tissues (modified myocytes) that span from the atrial septum to the ventricular apex, including the right and left bundle branches and Purkinje fibers.

The first known instance of electrical resuscitation of the heart was by Lidwell in 1929. Further, Hyman produced the first device for emergency treatment of the heart in 1932. Paul Zoll performed the first clinical transcutaneous pacing in 1952. Importantly for the pacing industry, the first battery-powered pacemaker was developed by Bakken and used in postsurgical pediatric patients by Lillehei in 1958 at the University of Minnesota (Fig. 27.3) [2, 5, 6].

27.4.2 Artificial Electrical Stimulation

In addition to the spontaneous contraction that occurs within the heart, artificial electrical stimulus (cardiac pacing) can be used to initiate myocardial contraction.

This stimulation, in the form of cardiac pacing, is routinely performed as a means to manage patients with cardiac arrhythmias and conduction abnormalities [7, 8]. Pacing induces myocardial contraction through the delivery of an electrical pulse to the patient's heart using an IPG ("pacemaker") and a cardiac pacing lead. The cardiac pacing lead acts as the electrical conduit for both stimulation and sensing, thus interfacing with the myocardial tissue. The electrical pulse is delivered in either a bipolar mode (involving cathodal and anodal electrodes on the lead) or in a unipolar mode (with a cathode on the lead and the IPG serving as the anode).

To initiate depolarization, an action potential must be created on a given volume of myocardium. As was described in previous chapters, a normal myocardial cell has a resting membrane potential of approximately –90 mV. The resting membrane potential is dominated by the concentration of potassium (K). A cellular action potential occurs when the resting membrane potential is shifted toward a more positive value (i.e., less negative value) to approximately –60 to –70 mV. At this threshold potential, the cell's voltage-gated Na channels open and begin a cascade of events. In artificial electrical stimulation (pacing), this shift of the resting potential and subsequent depolarization is produced by the pacing system.

Two theories describe the mechanism by which artificial electrical stimulation initiates myocardial depolarization. The "current density theory" states that a minimum

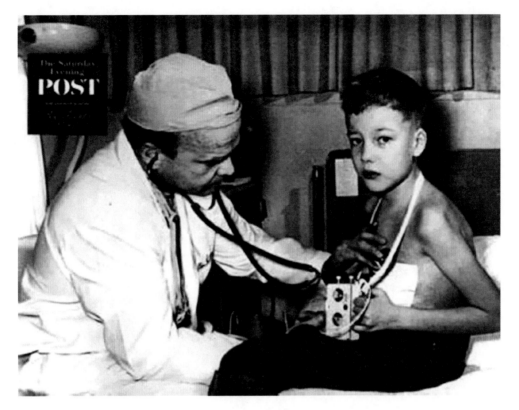

Fig. 27.3 Dr. C. Walton Lillehei with a patient being supported by a battery-powered, wearable pacemaker

current density (amp/cm^3) is required for stimulation of an excitable tissue. The "electric field theory" requires that a minimum voltage gradient (V/cm) be produced within the myocardium to initiate depolarization [9]. These two theories can, in part, be considered related, since the passage of current through the tissue (current density theory) will induce a potential difference across the cell membranes due to the limited conductivity of the tissue. Similarly, the creation of a potential within the tissue (electric field theory) will also induce a current. Regardless of the theoretical position taken regarding stimulation, the requirement for artificial stimulation is the shifting of the resting membrane potential from its normal value (typically –90 mV) toward a more positive value, until the depolarization threshold is reached.

The impedance associated with charge transfer from an IPG to the cardiac tissue is comprised of resistive (R) and reactive components (X_C, capacitive; X_L, inductive):

$$Z^2 = R^2 + (X_C + X_L)^2$$

The resistive term (R) includes the DC resistance associated with the conductors internal to the lead (R_C, cathodic conductor; R_A, anodic conductor), the cathode–tissue interface (R_{CT}), the anode–tissue interface (R_{AT}), and the tissue itself (R_T):

$$R = R_C + R_{CT} + R_T + R_{AT}$$

The capacitive term (X_C) is the sum of the capacitance of the cathode–tissue interface (C_{CT}) and the anode–tissue interface (C_{AT})

$$X_C = C_{CT} + C_{AT}$$

The inductance within the conductors and circuit is extremely small and this term is typically neglected. Ignoring inductance, the resulting equation for lead impedance is

$$Z^2 = R^2 + X_C^2$$

Schematic representations of the circuitry for bipolar and unipolar pacing systems are shown in Figs. 27.4 and 27.5. In these figures, the electric circuit for the delivery of energy to the myocardium is described as a simple RC circuit in which the IPG acts as the voltage/charge source and the lead conductors, electrodes, and cardiac tissue act as the load. Figure 27.4 depicts a bipolar pacing circuit in which the cathode and anode both reside on the pacing lead. Figure 27.5 represents the circuitry associated with a unipolar pacing system. In this case, the circuit is still

Fig. 27.4 Bipolar pacing circuit, including an implantable pulse generator and a pacing lead. Resistances: R_C, cathodic lead conductor; R_{CT}, cathode–tissue interface; R_T, tissue; R_{AT}, anode–tissue interface; R_A, anodic lead conductor. Capacitances: C_{CT}, cathode–tissue interface; C_{AT}, anode–tissue interface

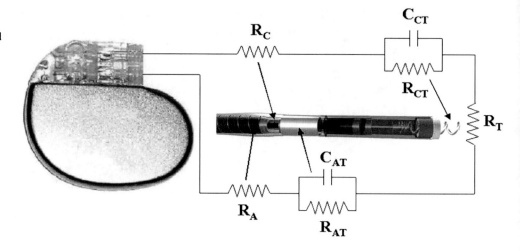

Fig. 27.5 A pacing circuit (unipolar type) which includes an implantable pulse generator and a pacing lead. Resistances: R_C, cathodic lead conductor; R_{CT}, cathode–tissue interface; R_T, tissue; R_{AT}, anode–tissue interface. Capacitances: C_{CT}, cathode–tissue interface; C_{AT}, anode–tissue interface

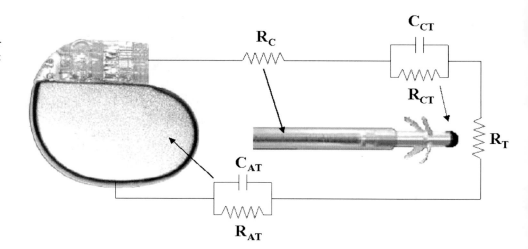

bipolar but the anode is the housing of the IPG; the term "unipolar" refers to the polarity of the lead.

Typical pacing circuit impedances range from 400 to 1,500 Ω. Approximately 80% of the total impedance is at the tissue interface; as an example, this will result in a 0.8 V drop at the tissue interface when a 1.0 V pacing pulse amplitude is used. Using the aforementioned impedances (400–1,500 Ω), a pacing output of 1.0 V produces currents of 2.5 and 0.67 mA, respectively.

To date, the most common pacing stimulation waveform used to electrically activate the myocardial tissue is an exponentially decaying square wave. An active recharge is also commonly included at the trailing edge of the stimulation pulse to reduce the post-pace polarization on the electrodes by balancing the charge delivered. The stimulating portion of the waveform is characterized by its amplitude (V) and width (ms). A relationship exists between the amplitude and pulse width that will be required for depolarization ("pacing") of the tissue. This relationship, termed a "strength duration curve," is most commonly plotted as shown in Fig. 27.6.

Terminology relating to the strength–duration curve includes the rheobase and chronaxie values. Rheobase is the threshold voltage at an infinitely long pulse width and chronaxie is the threshold pulse width at two times the rheobase voltage. The output of a clinical IPG is commonly set at twice the voltage threshold corresponding at the chronaxie pulse width, thus insuring a safety margin [9].

27.4.3 Indications for Pacing

Pacing and defibrillation systems are designed to maintain appropriate cardiac rhythms to maximize the patient's safety and quality of life. With the exception of cases of sudden cardiac death where an external defibrillator is clearly required, the determination of when to use a pacing or implantable defibrillation system can be complex. This section will describe the current classification of indications for pacing and provide a few practical

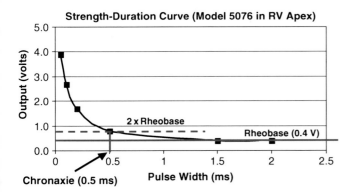

Fig. 27.6 A typical strength–duration curve for cardiac pacing. This particular curve was obtained using a Medtronic model 5076 bipolar pacing lead positioned in the right ventricular (RV) apex of a canine. In this plot, chronaxie and rheobase were 0.5 ms and 0.4 V, respectively

examples of these indications and the decision process associated with choosing the appropriate system for a given patient's condition.

The indications for either pacing or defibrillation therapies are commonly classified in the standard ACC/AHA (American College of Cardiology/American Heart Association) format as follows [10]:

Class I	Conditions for which there is evidence and/or general agreement that a given procedure or treatment is beneficial, useful, and effective
Class II	Conditions for which there is conflicting evidence and/or a divergence of opinion about the usefulness/efficacy of a procedure or treatment
Class IIa	Weight of evidence/opinion is in favor of usefulness/efficacy
Class IIb	Usefulness/efficacy is less well established by evidence/opinion
Class III	Conditions for which there is evidence and/or general agreement that a procedure/treatment is not useful/effective and, in some cases, may be harmful

Cardiac pacing can be used for both temporary and permanent management of heart rhythms and function. Although the permanent pacing systems are the most well known, there are numerous indications for temporary pacing. The most commonly utilized temporary pacing systems are transcutaneous wires that are stitched directly into the myocardium and connected to an external stimulator. Such a system is usually a small portable unit, but it can be a console. Common indications for temporary pacing include postsurgical heart block, heart block following an acute myocardial infarction, pacing for post/intraoperative cardiac support, pacing prior to implantation of a permanent pacemaker, and/or pacing during a pulse generator exchange.

The primary indication for the implantation of a permanent pacing system (pacemaker and leads) is to chronically eliminate the symptoms associated with the inadequate cardiac output due to bradyarrhythmias. Typical causes of these bradyarrhythmia are: (1) sinus node dysfunction; (2) acquired permanent or temporary atrioventricular block; (3) chronic bifascicular or trifascicular block; (4) hypersensitive carotid sinus syndrome; (5) neurocardiogenic in origin; and/or (6) side effect due to a drug therapy. The type of pacing system to be employed is dependant on the nature and location of the arrhythmia, the patient's age, previous medical/surgical history, as well as additional medical conditions.

For conditions related to dysfunction of the sinoatrial node, an IPG with atrial features is commonly used in combination with a lead placed in (or on) the atrium. When management of the ventricular rate is required, a device with ventricular functionality and a ventricular lead are used. When management of the rhythms of both the upper and lower chambers of the heart is required, a dual-chamber system is implanted.

Two clinical situations are outlined below to illustrate common indications for pacing, as well as the decision tree that is often used to determine the type of pacing system for the particular indication. The indications for pacing in a patient with sinus node dysfunction are found in Table 27.1 and the decision tree in Fig. 27.7 [11]. The indications for pacing in an adult with acquired atrioventricular block are found in Table 27.2 and the decision tree in Fig. 27.8 [11]. As an example, a patient with symptomatic chronotropic incompetence would have a Class I indication for pacing (Table 27.1). Since this is related to dysfunction of the sinus node, Fig. 27.7 would then be used to determine the type of pacing system required. In this situation, a rate response system (a pacing system that responds to patient activity/exercise) would clearly be desired. If atrioventricular synchrony were also required, a rate-responsive ventricular pacemaker would be implanted (mostly commonly a DDDR system; see the next section on the standard coding system and Table 27.3).

27.4.4 NASPE/BPEG Codes

In order to describe the function of a pacing system in a standardized manner, the North American Society of Pacing and Electrophysiology (NASPE; now the Heart Rhythm Society) and British Pacing and Electrophysiology Group (BPEG) have developed a standard coding system [12]. This code describes the pacing system's functionality using a multi-letter designation. The first four letters are typically

Table 27.1 Indications for permanent pacing in sinus node dysfunction

Class I	1.	Permanent pacemaker implantation is indicated for SND with documented symptomatic bradycardia, including frequent sinus pauses that produce symptoms (Level of Evidence: C)
	2.	Permanent pacemaker implantation is indicated for symptomatic chronotropic incompetence (Level of Evidence: C)
	3.	Permanent pacemaker implantation is indicated for symptomatic sinus bradycardia that results from required drug therapy for medical conditions (Level of Evidence: C)
Class IIa	1.	Permanent pacemaker implantation is reasonable for SND with heart rate less than 40 bpm when a clear association between significant symptoms consistent with bradycardia and the actual presence of bradycardia has not been documented (Level of Evidence: C)
	2.	Permanent pacemaker implantation is reasonable for syncope of unexplained origin when clinically significant abnormalities of sinus node function are discovered or provoked in electrophysiological studies (Level of Evidence: C)
Class IIb	1.	Permanent pacemaker implantation may be considered in minimally symptomatic patients with chronic heart rate less than 40 bpm while awake (Level of Evidence: C)
Class III	1.	Permanent pacemaker implantation is not indicated for SND in asymptomatic patients (Level of Evidence: C)
	2.	Permanent pacemaker implantation is not indicated for SND in patients for whom the symptoms suggestive of bradycardia have been clearly documented to occur in the absence of bradycardia (Level of Evidence: C)
	3.	Permanent pacemaker implantation is not indicated for SND with symptomatic bradycardia due to nonessential drug therapy (Level of Evidence: C)

SND, sinus node dysfunction. Adapted from ACC/AHA/HRS Guidelines, Epstein et al. [11].

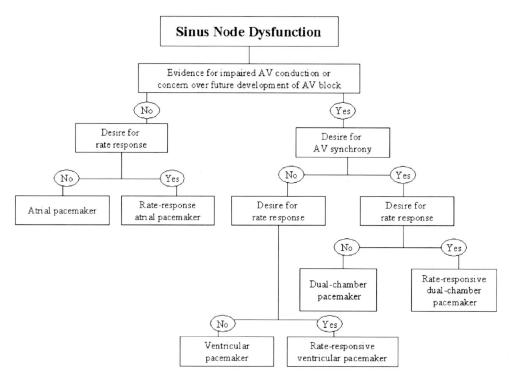

Fig. 27.7 A typical decision tree employed for determining proper therapy when the implantation of a pacemaker for sinus node dysfunction is being considered. AV, atrioventricular. Adapted from ACC/AHA/HRS Guidelines, Epstein et al. [11]

used, although this practice is evolving as new pacing features and indications are being developed. In the four-letter code system, the first letter indicates the pacing activity (A, atrial pacing; V, ventricular pacing; D, dual-chamber pacing; O, no pacing), the second letter indicates sensing (A, atrial sensing; V, ventricular sensing; D, dual-chamber sensing; O, no sensing), the third letter indicates the reaction to a sensed event (I, inhibit pacing; T, trigger pacing; D, inhibit and trigger; O, no reaction to sensing), and the fourth letter is used to describe unique device functionality (R, rate responsive, for example). Thus, a VVIR system would pace the ventricles (V—), sense ventricular activity (-V–), inhibit or withhold pacing upon detection of a sensed event in the ventricle (–I-), and provide rate response to manage chronotropic incompetence (—R) See Table 27.3 for a more complete explanation of the coding system.

Table 27.2 Recommendation for permanent pacing in acquired atrioventricular block in adults

Class I	1. Permanent pacemaker implantation is indicated for third-degree and advanced second-degree AV blocks at any anatomic level associated with bradycardia with symptoms (including heart failure) or ventricular arrhythmias presumed to be due to AV block (Level of Evidence: C)
	2. Permanent pacemaker implantation is indicated for third-degree and advanced second-degree AV blocks at any anatomic level associated with arrhythmias and other medical conditions that require drug therapy that results in symptomatic bradycardia (Level of Evidence: C)
	3. Permanent pacemaker implantation is indicated for third-degree and advanced second-degree AV blocks at any anatomic level in awake, symptom-free patients in sinus rhythm, with documented periods of asystole greater than or equal to 3.0 s or any escape rate less than 40 bpm, or with an escape rhythm that is below the AV node (Level of Evidence: C)
	4. Permanent pacemaker implantation is indicated for third-degree and advanced second-degree AV blocks at any anatomic level in awake, symptom-free patients with AF and bradycardia with 1 or more pauses of at least 5 s or longer (Level of Evidence: C)
	5. Permanent pacemaker implantation is indicated for third-degree and advanced second-degree AV blocks at any anatomic level after catheter ablation of the AV junction (Level of Evidence: C)
	6. Permanent pacemaker implantation is indicated for third-degree and advanced second-degree AV blocks at any anatomic level associated with postoperative AV block that is not expected to resolve after cardiac surgery (Level of Evidence: C)
	7. Permanent pacemaker implantation is indicated for third-degree and advanced second-degree AV blocks at any anatomic level associated with neuromuscular diseases with AV block, such as myotonic muscular dystrophy, Kearns–Sayre syndrome, Erb dystrophy (limb-girdle muscular dystrophy), and peroneal muscular atrophy, with or without symptoms (Level of Evidence: B)
	8. Permanent pacemaker implantation is indicated for second-degree AV block with associated symptomatic bradycardia regardless of type or site of block (Level of Evidence: B)
	9. Permanent pacemaker implantation is indicated for asymptomatic persistent third-degree AV block at any anatomic site with average awake ventricular rates of 40 bpm or faster if cardiomegaly or LV dysfunction is present or if the site of block is below the AV node (Level of Evidence: B)
	10. Permanent pacemaker implantation is indicated for second- or third-degree AV blocks during exercise in the absence of myocardial ischemia (Level of Evidence: C)
Class IIa	1. Permanent pacemaker implantation is reasonable for persistent third-degree AV block with an escape rate greater than 40 bpm in asymptomatic adult patients without cardiomegaly (Level of Evidence: C)
	2. Permanent pacemaker implantation is reasonable for asymptomatic second-degree AV block at intra- or infra-His levels found at electrophysiological study (Level of Evidence: B)
	3. Permanent pacemaker implantation is reasonable for first- or second-degree AV blocks with symptoms similar to those of pacemaker syndrome or hemodynamic compromise (Level of Evidence: B)
	4. Permanent pacemaker implantation is reasonable for asymptomatic type II second-degree AV block with a narrow QRS. When type II second-degree AV block occurs with a wide QRS, including isolated right bundle branch block, pacing becomes a Class I recommendation (Level of Evidence: B)
Class IIb	1. Permanent pacemaker implantation may be considered for neuromuscular diseases such as myotonic muscular dystrophy, Erb dystrophy (limb-girdle muscular dystrophy), and peroneal muscular atrophy with any degree of AV block (including first-degree AV block), with or without symptoms, because there may be unpredictable progression of AV conduction disease (Level of Evidence: B)
	2. Permanent pacemaker implantation may be considered for AV block in the setting of drug use and/or drug toxicity when the block is expected to recur even after the drug is withdrawn (Level of Evidence: B)
Class III	1. Permanent pacemaker implantation is not indicated for asymptomatic first-degree AV block (Level of Evidence: B)
	2. Permanent pacemaker implantation is not indicated for asymptomatic type I second-degree AV block at the supra-His (AV node) level or that which is not known to be intra- or infra-Hisian (Level of Evidence: C)
	3. Permanent pacemaker implantation is not indicated for AV block that is expected to resolve and is unlikely to recur (e.g., drug toxicity, Lyme disease, or transient increases in vagal tone or during hypoxia in sleep apnea syndrome in the absence of symptoms) (Level of Evidence: B)

AV, atrioventricular; AF, atrial fibrillation; LV, left ventricle. Adapted from ACC/AHA/HRS Guidelines, Epstein et al. [11].

27.4.5 Implantable Pulse Generators

The IPG is an implantable computer with an integral pulse generator and battery. The componentry is typically encased within a hermetically sealed stamped titanium housing with the battery taking up approximately half of the device volume. The most common battery chemistry used in modern pacemakers is lithium iodide. Device longevity is typically 8–10 years, but may vary significantly depending on system utilization (Fig. 27.9). Electrically insulated feedthroughs connect the internal circuitry to an external connector block, which acts as the interface between the internal circuitry of the IPG and the leads. Typically today, the connector block consists of a molded polyurethane superstructure which houses metallic contacts. The contacts may be simple machined blocks or "spring-type" metallic beams. Most connector blocks employ set screws to ensure permanent retention of the leads and these may also enhance electrical contact. A cutaway view of an IPG can be found in Fig. 27.10, and the scheme for

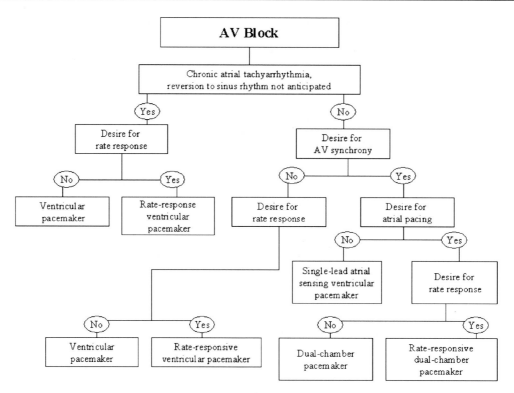

Fig. 27.8 A typical decision tree employed for determining proper therapy when the implantation of a pacemaker for atrioventricular (AV) block is being considered. Adapted from ACC/AHA/HRS Guidelines, Epstein et al. [11]

Table 27.3 NASPE/BPEG classifications for pacing and defibrillation systems

I	II	III	IV
Chamber(s) paced	Chamber(s) sensed	Response to sensing	Programmability/rate modulation
O, none	O, none	O, none	O, none
A, atrium	A, atrium	T, triggered	P, simple programmability
V, ventricle	V, ventricle	I, inhibited	M, multiparameter programmability
D, dual (A + V)	D, dual (A + V)	D, dual (T + I)	C, communication with programmer
			R, rate modulation

Roman numerals I–IV indicate the position in the coding. NASPE, North American Society of Pacing and Electrophysiology; BPEG, British Pacing and Electrophysiology Group. Adapted from Bernstein et al. [12].

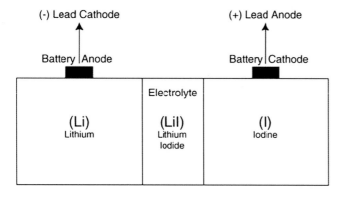

Fig. 27.9 Schematic of a lithium iodide battery. This is the most common chemistry used in modern pacemakers

connection between the IPG and the leads is shown in Fig. 27.11 and MPG 27.13.

27.4.6 Sensing Algorithms

In order to assess the need for therapeutic intervention, the pacing system must be able to accurately detect and interpret the various electrical activities of the heart. The instantaneous electrical activity of the heart, or electrogram (EGM), is recorded as a differential voltage measured between the bipolar electrode pair on the lead

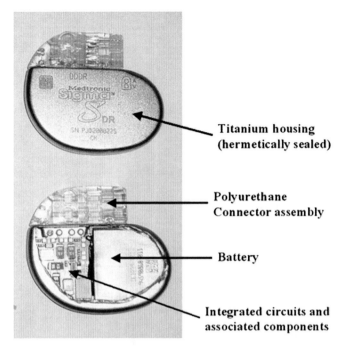

Fig. 27.10 Cutaway view of an implantable pulse generator (IPG or "pacemaker")

Titanium housing
(hermetically sealed)

Polyurethane
Connector assembly

Battery

Integrated circuits and
associated components

(bipolar lead) or between the cathode on the lead and the housing of the IPG (unipolar lead). This signal is then processed within the IPG and analyzed by the sensing algorithms. Typically, such signals are amplified, filtered, and rectified prior to undergoing analyses by the device (Figs. 27.12 and 27.13). The resulting signals are then passed through a level detector to determine if they exceed the minimum threshold for detection that was preprogrammed into the device by the clinician. The sensitivity setting (in mV) determines what is discarded as noise by the algorithm and which signals will be detected. An ideal sensitivity setting is one that will reliably detect the depolarization spike of the chamber (P-wave in the atrium; R-wave in the ventricle) while ignoring repolarization and other physiologic and non-physiologic signals.

Most rhythm management decisions are based on the heart rate detected. The modern IPG continuously measures the time from one sensed event to the next, and compares the interval to the rates and intervals programmed by the clinician. For example, if two atrial events occur with a separation of 1,500 ms (1.5 s), the heart rate is 40 bpm (HR = 60/measured beat-to-beat interval; 60/1.5 = 40 bpm). In order to understand the logic behind sensing algorithms and pacing timing diagrams, the terminology needs to be introduced. Table 27.4 includes the most commonly used terms and abbreviations. These terms will be freely used in further discussions of the logic behind pacing and defibrillation sensing and therapies without further explanation. This table will also provide the reader with the vocabulary required for interpreting and understanding current literature and publications on the topic.

The decision process and behavior of the typical pacing algorithm are usually described using a timing diagram (Fig. 27.14). An understanding of this diagram will provide the basis for the analysis of the behavior of pacing systems and will communicate the various parameters that the clinician and device manufacturer must be concerned with. The concepts associated with pacemaker timing are shown in Fig. 27.14; the information is presented in an alternate form in Fig. 27.15.

The actual behavior of pacing systems can deviate from their ideal for a number of reasons. For example, the pacing pulse can be of an inadequate energy to pace the chamber, losing capture on one or more beats (Fig. 27.16). Another undesired situation that commonly arises is oversensing. In this case, the device inappropriately identifies electrical activities as an atrial or ventricular event (Fig. 27.17). Clinically, this is resolved by reprogramming the device to a lower sensitivity. Conversely, if a system is undersensing, the sensitivity is increased. Assessment of the behavior of the pacing system is vastly simplified through the use of marker channels. These are shown below the electrograms in both Figs. 27.16 and 27.17. As such, the marker channel is used to report the overall behavior of the pacing system, allowing a quick assessment of the performance of the algorithms and device output levels.

Fig. 27.11 Schematic of the implantable pulse generator-to-lead interface. The IS-1 connector is the standard configuration for pacing. The DF-1 connector is the standard configuration for high-voltage defibrillation (see MPG 25.13)

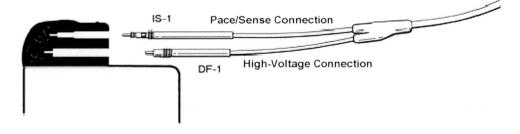

IS-1   Pace/Sense Connection

DF-1   High-Voltage Connection

Fig. 27.12 The electrogram amplification and rectification scheme that is used in most modern implantable pacing and defibrillation systems. EGM, electrogram

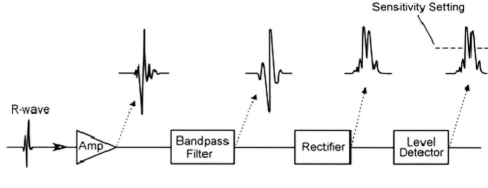

EGM Signal Processing

Fig. 27.13 Plot of electrical signals (amplitude and frequency) frequently encountered by pacing and defibrillation sensing algorithms. A bandpass filter for preferential detection of P-waves and R-waves is shown (*parabolic line*). This filter is designed to "reject" myopotentials and T-waves

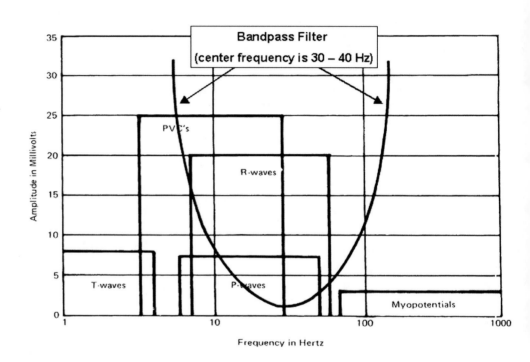

27.4.7 Drug Interactions with Pacing Systems

It is important to note that certain drug therapies have been reported to impact pacing system performances. Although it is rare for antiarrhythmic drugs to significantly effect pacing thresholds, they have been found to alter stimulation thresholds by inducing changes in the lead–myocardial interfacial conductivity and excitability. Additionally, they can slow the intrinsic sinus rates, which then necessitates pacing of the resultant bradycardia. In general, Class Ia drugs can increase pacing thresholds at toxic dosages; both sotalol and amiodarone can increase pacing thresholds while at therapeutic levels, but it is rarely clinically significant [13]. A summary of the more common administered drugs and their impact on pacing thresholds, action potentials, and the physiologic consequences of their action are found in Tables 27.5 and 27.6.

27.4.8 New Indications/Recent Clinical Trials

Today, single- and dual-chamber pacing systems have become the standard method of treating many bradyarrhythmias. Recent clinical evidence has raised interest in the selection of both the frequency at which patients are paced and the optimal site of stimulation [14]. It has long been known that pacing produces a nonphysiologic contraction pattern, but recent research has also indicated that potentially detrimental effects may result from long-term pacing [15–18]. Currently, alternate choices in ventricular stimulation sites are of particular interest due to the presumed physiologic and hemodynamic benefits. For example, pacing of the bundle of His is thought to produce a more physiologic contraction pattern, while additional evidence exists that there may also be hemodynamic benefits associated with right ventricular septal

Table 27.4 Pacing and timing abbreviations

AP, atrial pace

VP, ventricular pace

AS, atrial sense

VS, ventricular sense

AR, atrial refractory event

VR, ventricular refractory event

AEI, atrial escape interval—longest allowable interval between ventricular and atrial event (also called VA interval)

ARP, atrial refractory period

AV, atrioventricular

AV interval, longest allowable interval between atrial and ventricular event

LR, lower rate—slowest pacing rate allowed

LR interval, longest period of time allowed before delivery of a pacing stimulus

MS, mode switch

PAV, paced atrioventricular interval—longest allowable interval between paced atrial beat and paced or sensed ventricular beat

PMT, pacemaker-mediated tachycardia

PVAB, postventricular atrial blanking period

PVARP, postventricular atrial refractory period

SAV, sensed atrioventricular interval—longest allowable interval between sensed atrial beat and paced or sensed ventricular beat

TARP, total atrial refractory period (AV + PVARP)

UAR, upper activity rate (also called maximum sensor-indicated rate)

UR, upper rate—fastest pacing rate allowed

UR interval, shortest allowable interval between paced beats or a sensed and paced beat

UTR, upper tracking rate—fastest rate the ventricles may be paced in 1:1 synchrony with the sensed atrial rate (also called maximum tracking rate)

VA interval, time between ventricular and atrial event

VRP, ventricular refractory period

VSP, ventricular safety pacing

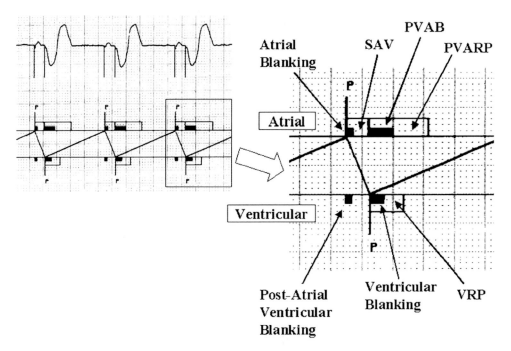

Fig. 27.14 A typical dual-chamber timing diagram, including sub-diagrams for the atrial and ventricular channels. The sequence of events begins with a paced atrial beat (P). This paced beat occurs when the maximum allowable interval between sensed atrial events is exceeded. For example, if the minimum rate is programmed to 60 bpm, an atrial pace will occur when a 1,000 ms interval between sensed events is exceeded. Immediately following this pacing pulse, both the atrial and ventricular sensing algorithms are blanked. This means that the threshold detector ignores all sensed activity. The system is blanked to avoid sensing the resultant atrial depolarization on the atrial channel, and the atrial pacing spike and the atrial depolarization on the ventricular channel. Concurrently in the

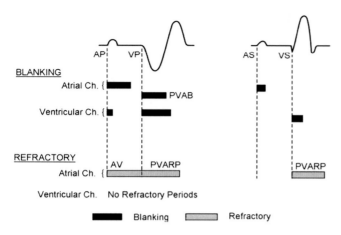

Fig. 27.15 Blanking and refractory periods. The *top trace* represents the electrocardiogram. The portion of the diagram on the *left* is a situation in which both the atrial and ventricular leads are pacing. The portion on the *right* is a situation where the system is sensing intrinsic atrial and ventricular activity (i.e., no pacing is occurring). AP, atrial pace; AS, atrial sense; AV, atrioventricular; PVAB, postventricular atrial blanking period; PVARP, postventricular atrial refractory period; VP, ventricular pace; VS, ventricular sense

and outflow tract pacing [15, 19–24]. In patients with heart failure and associated wide QRS complexes, biventricular pacing has been adopted [25, 26] (see MPG 27.14). Finally, current research in atrial pacing has largely focused on reducing atrial fibrillation, improving methods of pace terminating atrial tachycardias, and/or improving ventricular filling and atrial hemodynamics [27–29]. Recent research is even investigating the possibility of genetically engineering a biologic pacemaker [30].

27.5 Cardiac Defibrillation

Today, sudden cardiac arrest is one of the most common causes of death in developed countries; three million people experience sudden cardiac arrest worldwide, while the annual incidence in the United States is 300,000. Sudden

cardiac arrest claims more lives in the United States each year than the combination of deaths from AIDS, breast cancer, lung cancer, and stroke [31].

Several studies have identified multiple risk factors for sudden cardiac arrest, which include (1) coronary artery disease; (2) heart failure and/or decreased left ventricular ejection fraction; (3) previous events of sudden cardiac arrest; (4) prior episodes of ventricular tachycardias; (5) hypertrophic cardiomyopathies; and/or (6) long QT syndrome [32]. The combination of any three of these factors significantly increases the risk for sudden cardiac arrest. Ninety percent of sudden deaths occur in patients with two or more occlusions in their major coronary arteries [33].

27.5.1 History

The first documentation of ventricular fibrillation was noted in 1850 [34]. A little over a century later, in 1962, the first direct current defibrillator was developed. Ventricular fibrillation began to be recognized as a possible cause of sudden death in the 1970s and the first transvenous ICD was implanted in the 1990s. Since then, the medical device industry has provided dramatic reductions in ICD sizes, while simultaneously increasing safety, efficacy, battery longevity, diagnostics, and memory capabilities. Figure 27.18 shows the evolution in the size of one manufacturer's ICD models.

27.5.2 Tachyarrhythmias

The commonly recognized mechanisms that lead to tachyarrhythmias (tachycardias and fibrillation) include reentry circuits, triggered activities, and automaticity. Reentry is considered as the most common tachyarrhythmia mechanism. It can be described as an electrical loop within the myocardium that has a circular, continuous series of depolarizations and repolarizations (Fig. 27.19).

Fig. 27.14. (continued) atrium, a sensed atrioventricular (SAV) interval occurs. This is the longest interval that will be allowed by the device without a paced ventricular beat. The SAV is commonly programmed to 150 ms, and is set to optimize filling of the ventricle due to the atrial contraction. During a cardiac cycle, if the SAV value is reached (meaning an intrinsic ventricular beat does not occur within the programmed interval following the intrinsic or paced atrial beat), a ventricular pacing pulse is then delivered. This pacing pulse is again accompanied by blanking in both channels to avoid oversensing of the pacing pulse and the resultant ventricular depolarization. This interval is referred to as the postventricular

atrial blanking (PVAB) period on the atrial channel. Concurrently, the postventricular atrial refractory period (PVARP) occurs on the atrial channel in which the device attempts to avoid sensing of retrograde P-waves (i.e., atrial contractions conducted through the atrioventricular node in a retrograde manner) and the ventricular refractory period (VRP) occurs on the ventricular channel to avoid oversensing of T-waves. Following these intervals, the timing is repeated. If the atrial rate stays above the minimum programmed rate (the lower rate) and the SAV is never reached, the device will never pace unless inappropriate sensing occurs

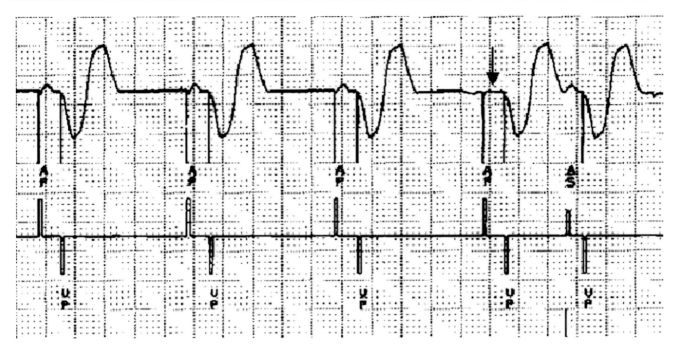

Fig. 27.16 An electrocardiogram (*above*) and pacemaker marker channel (*below*) printed from a programmer. Note the loss of capture on the atrial channel (indicated by the *arrow*); notice that no P-wave follows the pacing pulse

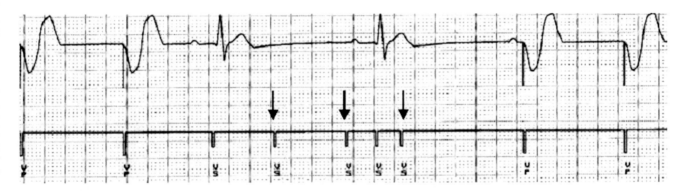

Fig. 27.17 An electrocardiogram (*above*) and pacemaker marker channel (*below*) printed from a programmer. Note the ventricular oversensing (indicated by the *arrow*); notice that no QRS complex is associated with the detected event

Table 27.5 Effect of antiarrhythmic drugs on pacing thresholds

Increase at normal drug levels	Increase at toxic drug levels	No increase
Flecainide	Quinidine	Lidocaine
Propafenone	Procainamide	Mexiletine
Amiodarone	Disopyramide	
Sotalol		

In general, there are three requirements for reentry to occur: (1) the presence of a substrate, for example, an area of ischemia or scar tissue; (2) two parallel pathways which encircle the substrate; and (3) one pathway that conducts slowly and one that exhibits unidirectional block. An impulse reaching the substrate is slowed by the unidirectional block and is allowed to slowly conduct down the slow pathway. As the impulse continues to move around the substrate, it conducts in a retrograde manner up the fast pathway and the impulse continues to conduct in a circular fashion.

Inappropriate atrial or ventricular tachycardias can be further classified as either hemodynamically stable or unstable. The level of hemodynamic compromise that occurs is typically considered to depend on both the rate and the pathway of the arrhythmia. In general, atrial tachycardias usually result in higher ventricular rates due to conduction through the atrioventricular node. As atrial rates increase, the rate conducted to the ventricles

Table 27.6 Antiarrhythmic drugs, action potential phases, and physiologic consequences

Class	Drug	Action potential phase	Physiologic consequence
Ia	Quinidine Procainamide Disopyramide	0	Decreases automaticity of the sodium channel Slows conduction velocity Prolongs refractory period
Ib	Lidocaine Mexiletine Tocainide Phenytoin	0	Decreases automaticity of the sodium channel May or may not slow conduction velocity Decreases refractory period
Ic	Flecainide Propafenone Encainide Moricizine	0	Decreases automaticity of the sodium channel Slows conduction velocity No effect on refractory period
II	Propranolol Atenolol Metoprolol	SA node	Decreases automaticity of nodal tissue Decreases conduction velocity Increases refractory period
III	Bretylium Sotalol Amiodarone Ibutilide Dofetilide	3	Increases refractory period No effect on conduction velocity No effect on automaticity
IV	Verapamil Diltiazem	SA node	Decreases automaticity of nodal tissue Decreases conduction velocity Increases refractory period

SA, sinoatrial.

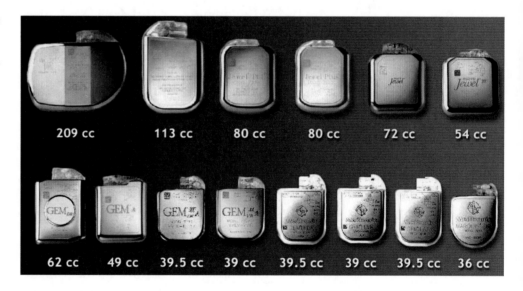

Fig. 27.18 The evolution of the implantable cardioverter defibrillator (ICD). Dramatic reductions in size have occurred, with simultaneous improvements in longevity, diagnostics, functionality, and memory

may or may not be 1:1, since the atrioventricular node has inherent limitations in its ability to conduct depolarizations. If, however, an abnormal pathway exists from the atria to the ventricles, then 1:1 conduction may be possible even at very high rates. Nevertheless, a patient's clinical risks are related to the level of hemodynamic compromise, with the most extreme case being ventricular fibrillation which, if not immediately reversed, most often results in death.

Triggered activity, or hyperautomaticity, is typically not consistently spontaneous and is a less common mechanism. Early and delayed afterdepolarizations seen in phases 3 and 4 of the action potential are associated with triggered activity. Automaticity is defined as the ability of the cell to depolarize spontaneously at regular intervals. However, in a diseased heart, often cells will exhibit abnormal automaticity that causes them to depolarize at rates faster than the intrinsic nodal rates.

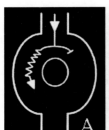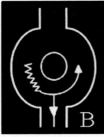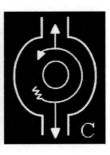

Fig. 27.19 Reentrant circuits. **Panel A**, unidirectional block; **Panel B**, slow conduction; **Panel C**, reentry circuit

Common symptoms observed in patients with tachyarrhythmias may include syncopal episodes, palpitations, fatigue, and/or dyspnea. Both invasive and noninvasive diagnostic tools are available for diagnosing tachyarrhythmias. The typical noninvasive procedures include: (1) a thorough patient interview; (2) blood work; (3) a 12-lead ECG; (4) tilt table testing; (5) holter monitoring; (6) exercise stress test; (7) echocardiography; (8) signal average ECG; and/or (9) SPECT/MuGA. Currently, an electrophysiological study using cardiac catheterization and insertable loop recorders is the most commonly used invasive diagnostic procedure.

Therapeutic interventions to manage tachyarrhythmias have a common objective of affecting the behavior of myocardial cells or the conduction of the electrical impulse in the diseased tissue. They include attempts to correct the underlying complication such as coronary reperfusion in the presence of a myocardial infarction, antiarrhythmic drugs to restore and maintain normal sinus rhythm, electrical therapies such as antitachycardia pacing, cardioversion, defibrillation, and lastly, ablation performed surgically or with the assistance of a catheter. The role of medical devices in the management of these arrhythmias will become clear as device function is described in subsequent text.

27.5.3 ICD Indications

As was the case for the pacing indications previously discussed, the indications for an ICD are also complex. The indications by class are shown in Table 27.7 [11].

27.5.4 External Cardiac Defibrillators

External defibrillators have become ubiquitous in most countries worldwide. In addition to traditional use in hospitals and by paramedics, these systems are now commonly found in many schools, public buildings, airplanes, and/or even homes. As with implantable cardioverter defibrillators, these systems are used to treat sudden cardiac death. These systems deliver high-voltage shocks (up to 360 J) directly to the chest of the patient, using either patches or paddles. One electrode is typically placed in the right pectoral region and the second in the left axilla for delivery of these energies (Fig. 27.20).

27.5.5 Implantable Defibrillators

Similar to a pacemaker, an ICD is a self-contained, implantable computer with an integral pulse generator and battery. In addition to providing pacing therapies for bradyarrhythmias and tachyarrhythmias, ICDs also deliver high-energy discharges. The major components of an ICD include (1) a battery; (2) electronic circuitry and associated components; (3) high-voltage capacitors; (4) high-voltage transformers; (5) a telemetry antenna; (6) a reed switch triggered upon application of a magnetic field; and (7) a connector block. To date, this componentry is most commonly housed within a hermetically sealed stamped titanium case. Feedthroughs connect the internal circuitry to an external connector block, which acts as the interface between the internal circuitry of the ICD and the leads. The connector block is commonly fabricated from a molded polyurethane superstructure, which houses metallic contacts for interconnection with the leads. The contacts may be simple machined blocks or "spring-type" metallic beams. Most connector blocks used today have set screws to ensure permanent retention of the leads. A cutaway view of an ICD can be found in Fig. 27.21.

Today, most ICDs will use one or two batteries with silver lithium vanadium oxide chemistry. A typical full charge of this type of battery is 3.2 V. As the ICD battery energy starts to deplete, the voltage will follow the path shown in Fig. 27.22 where there are two characteristic plateaus. The voltage is provided to the clinician upon device interrogation to determine if the battery is at beginning of life, middle of life, elective replacement indicator, or end of life [35]. Each manufacturer and each device from a given manufacturer will have its own elective replacement indicator voltage. This value is representative of the voltage current (V-C) drain from the circuitry, and is also related to the characteristics of the capacitor used. All devices should be replaced before end of life is reached. The longevity of such devices depends on the number of therapies delivered, but is typically between 6 and 8 years.

The primary function of the ICD's capacitor is the accumulation and storage of an adequate amount of energy to shock-terminate a fibrillating heart. As

Table 27.7 Indications for implantable cardioverter defibrillator (ICD) therapy

Class I	1.	ICD therapy is indicated in patients who are survivors of cardiac arrest due to VF or hemodynamically unstable sustained VT after evaluation to define the cause of the event and to exclude any completely reversible causes (Level of Evidence: A)
	2.	ICD therapy is indicated in patients with structural heart disease and spontaneous sustained VT, whether hemodynamically stable or unstable (Level of Evidence: B)
	3.	ICD therapy is indicated in patients with syncope of undetermined origin with clinically relevant, hemodynamically significant sustained VT or VF induced at electrophysiological study (Level of Evidence: B)
	4.	ICD therapy is indicated in patients with LVEF less than 35% due to prior MI who are at least 40 days post-MI and are in NYHA functional Class II or III (Level of Evidence: A)
	5.	ICD therapy is indicated in patients with nonischemic DCM who have an LVEF less than or equal to 35% and who are in NYHA functional Class II or III (Level of Evidence: B)
	6.	ICD therapy is indicated in patients with LV dysfunction due to prior MI who are at least 40 days post-MI, have an LVEF less than 30%, and are in NYHA functional Class I (Level of Evidence: A)
	7.	ICD therapy is indicated in patients with nonsustained VT due to prior MI, LVEF less than 40%, and inducible VF or sustained VT at electrophysiological study (Level of Evidence: B)
Class IIa	1.	ICD implantation is reasonable for patients with unexplained syncope, significant LV dysfunction, and nonischemic DCM (Level of Evidence: C)
	2.	ICD implantation is reasonable for patients with sustained VT and normal or near-normal ventricular function (Level of Evidence: C)
	3.	ICD implantation is reasonable for patients with HCM who have one or more major risk factors for SCD (Level of Evidence: C)
	4.	ICD implantation is reasonable for the prevention of SCD in patients with ARVD/C who have one or more risk factors for SCD (Level of Evidence: C)
	5.	ICD implantation is reasonable to reduce SCD in patients with long QT syndrome who are experiencing syncope and/or VT while receiving beta-blockers (Level of Evidence: B)
	6.	ICD implantation is reasonable for nonhospitalized patients awaiting transplantation (Level of Evidence: C)
	7.	ICD implantation is reasonable for patients with Brugada syndrome who have had syncope (Level of Evidence: C)
	8.	ICD implantation is reasonable for patients with Brugada syndrome who have documented VT that has not resulted in cardiac arrest (Level of Evidence: C)
	9.	ICD implantation is reasonable for patients with catecholaminergic polymorphic VT who have syncope and/or documented sustained VT while receiving beta-blockers (Level of Evidence: C)
	10.	ICD implantation is reasonable for patients with cardiac sarcoidosis, giant cell myocarditis, or Chagas disease (Level of Evidence: C)
Class IIb	1.	ICD therapy may be considered in patients with nonischemic heart disease who have an LVEF of less than or equal to 35% and who are in NYHA functional Class I (Level of Evidence: C)
	2.	ICD therapy may be considered for patients with long QT syndrome and risk factors for SCD (Level of Evidence: B)
	3.	ICD therapy may be considered in patients with syncope and advanced structural heart disease in whom thorough invasive and noninvasive investigations have failed to define a cause (Level of Evidence: C)
	4.	ICD therapy may be considered in patients with a familial cardiomyopathy associated with sudden death (Level of Evidence: C)
	5.	ICD therapy may be considered in patients with LV noncompaction (Level of Evidence: C)
Class III	1.	ICD therapy is not indicated for patients who do not have a reasonable expectation of survival with an acceptable functional status for at least 1 year, even if they meet ICD implantation criteria specified in the Class I, IIa, and IIb recommendations above (Level of Evidence: C)
	2.	ICD therapy is not indicated for patients with incessant VT or VF (Level of Evidence: C)
	3.	ICD therapy is not indicated in patients with significant psychiatric illnesses that may be aggravated by device implantation or that may preclude systematic follow-up (Level of Evidence: C)
	4.	ICD therapy is not indicated for NYHA Class IV patients with drug-refractory congestive heart failure who are not candidates for cardiac transplantation or CRT-D (Level of Evidence: C)
	5.	ICD therapy is not indicated for syncope of undetermined cause in a patient without inducible ventricular tachyarrhythmias and without structural heart disease (Level of Evidence: C)
	6.	ICD therapy is not indicated when VF or VT is amenable to surgical or catheter ablation (e.g., atrial arrhythmias associated with the Wolff–Parkinson–White syndrome, RV or LV outflow tract VT, idiopathic VT, or fascicular VT in the absence of structural heart disease) (Level of Evidence: C)
	7.	ICD therapy is not indicated for patients with ventricular tachyarrhythmias due to a completely reversible disorder in the absence of structural heart disease (e.g., electrolyte imbalance, drugs, or trauma) (Level of Evidence: B)

ARVD/C, arrhythmogenic right ventricular dysplasia/cardiopathy; CRT-D, cardiac resynchronization therapy device and defibrillator; DCM, dilated cardiomyopathy; HCM, hypertrophic cardiomyopathy; ICD, implantable cardioverter defibrillator; LV, left ventricle; LVEF, left ventricular ejection fraction; MI, myocardial infarction; RV, right ventricle; SCD, sudden cardiac death; VF, ventricular fibrillation; VT, ventricular tachycardia.

Adapted from ACC/AHA/HRS Guidelines, Epstein et al. [11].

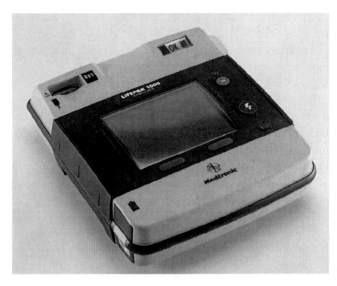

Fig. 27.20 An external cardiac defibrillator (LIFEPAK® 1000, Medtronic, Inc.)

each capacitor is required to maintain charge efficiency and therefore guarantee short charge times to allow rapid conversion of the arrhythmia [36]. The materials currently used in the capacitors slowly lose efficiency, especially when they are not used for a period of time due to a chemical decay process. This process (termed "deformation") is mitigated by conditioning the capacitors (termed "reformation"). Reforming of the capacitor should be performed regularly by charging the capacitor to its maximum capacity and leaving the charge on it until it gradually discharges the energy. Fortunately, reformation can be easily programmed at regular intervals in most modern devices (e.g., each 6 months) without affecting the patient.

27.5.6 Sensing and Detection

It is desirable for an ICD to be able to accurately sense ventricular rhythms that vary in amplitude, rate, and/or regularity, in order to distinguish between normal sinus rhythm, ventricular tachycardia, ventricular flutter, ventricular fibrillation, and/or supraventricular (atrial)

previously mentioned, a typical voltage of an ICD battery is 3.2 V, whereas the capacitor can store up to 800 V (delivering energies of 30–35 J). Periodic conditioning of

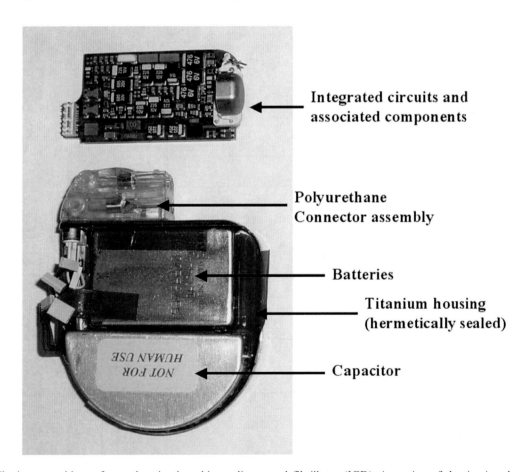

Integrated circuits and associated components

Polyurethane Connector assembly

Batteries

Titanium housing (hermetically sealed)

Capacitor

Fig. 27.21 The inner workings of a modern implantable cardioverter defibrillator (ICD). A portion of the titanium housing has been removed to expose the typical internal components

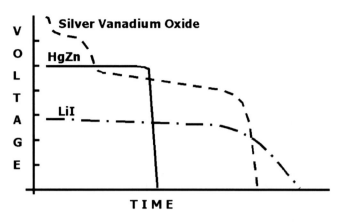

Fig. 27.22 A typical example of an implantable cardioverter defibrillator (ICD) depletion curve for a silver vanadium oxide battery. Lithium iodide and mercury zinc batteries included for comparative purposes

arrhythmias (see examples in Fig. 27.23). Current devices adjust their sensitivity on a beat-to-beat basis in order to sense fine waves of ventricular fibrillation and to avoid oversensing of intrinsic T-waves. If an ICD undersenses

(misses cardiac activity that it was intended to detect), the device may fail to treat ventricular flutter or may fail to treat a ventricular tachycardia, which subsequently may accelerate into ventricular fibrillation. If an ICD oversenses, overestimating the cardiac rate, it may deliver inappropriate therapy which will lead to patient discomfort or, more seriously, it may even induce a tachyarrhythmia.

The steps involved in sensing and detection are similar to those discussed previously for the pacemakers. In fact, almost all ICDs on the market today include the pacing algorithms described previously, with additional functionality/logic for detection and management of tachyarrhythmias. Arrhythmia detection typically occurs via the following steps: (1) sense the R-wave or P-waves; (2) measure the interval or cycle length between consecutive beats; and (3) compare the cycle length to prescribed detection zone intervals to classify the arrhythmia (Fig. 27.24). For the sake of simplicity, this chapter will focus on only two detection zones—the ventricular fibrillation and the ventricular tachycardia zones. A

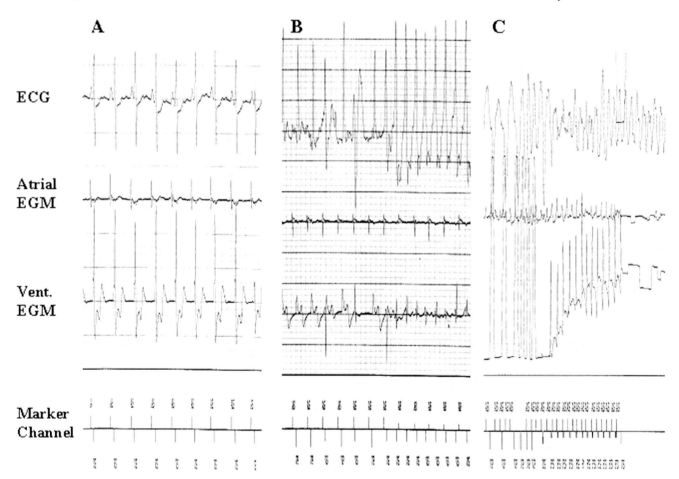

Fig. 27.23 Examples of recorded tachyarrhythmias and the associated device response (refer to the marker channel). **Panel A,** sinus rhythm; **Panel B,** spontaneous ventricular tachycardia; **Panel C,** atrial fibrillation resulting in ventricular fibrillation. ECG, electrocardiogram; EGM, electrogram

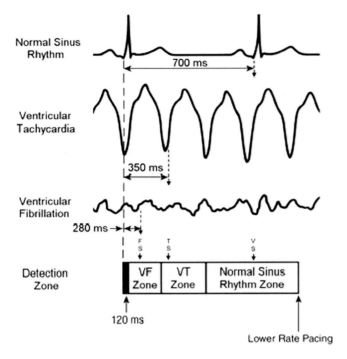

Fig. 27.24 Tachyarrhythmia detection intervals. The *top three traces* represent typical electrocardiograms that might be encountered by the device. The detection zones for ventricular fibrillation, ventricular tachycardia, and sinus rhythm are shown at the *bottom*. Note that an event with a cycle length of 700 ms is categorized as sinus rhythm, 350 ms as a ventricular tachycardia, and 280 ms as ventricular fibrillation. VF, ventricular fibrillation; VT, ventricular tachycardia

the arrhythmia. Most ICD designs employ two different counters when classifying whether an arrhythmia is ventricular fibrillation or ventricular tachycardia. The ventricular fibrillation counter uses a probabilistic approach. Since ventricular fibrillation waves are chaotic and vary in amplitudes and cycle lengths, the device will look for a programmed percentage of cycle lengths to fall within the fibrillation detection zone (e.g., 75%, Fig. 27.25) and if that criterion is met, the device will detect a given ventricular fibrillation and deliver the appropriate therapy. Ventricular tachycardias, on the other hand, usually have regular cycle lengths. A consecutive event counter is used which states that a programmed number of cycle lengths (e.g., 18 out of 18) needs to be within the tachycardia detection zone in order to classify the rhythm as a ventricular tachycardia. If one cycle length falls out of the tachycardia detection zone, the consecutive counter is reset to zero and the count begins again. Each ICD has the capability to redetect the same arrhythmia if the initial therapy was not successful. Redetection criteria will often be more aggressive (fewer number of beats sampled) than the initial detection criteria to ensure that subsequent therapies can be delivered quickly. An example of when the redetection criteria may not be as aggressive is in cases where the patient has a long QT interval and is prone to developing Torsades de Pointes which may spontaneously terminate.

Typical devices available today have the option of programming an additional detection zone, which is referred to as a "fast ventricular tachycardia" zone. This is a zone that can be programmed for those patients with a fast ventricular tachycardia who may benefit from antitachycardia pacing. Treating a fast ventricular tachycardia with antitachycardia pacing may decrease the number of high-voltage shocks delivered, increase the patient's quality of life, and prolong device longevity [37]. Evidence of the benefit of this therapeutic approach was seen in the Pain-FREE Rx trial which concluded that fast ventricular

fibrillation zone is commonly programmed to detect any interval faster than the interval prescribed by the clinician (e.g., 320 ms = 187.5 bpm). If a minimum number/percentage of beats is sensed within this interval, the rhythm will be detected as ventricular fibrillation and the device will treat the rhythm using the high-energy shock amplitudes preprogrammed by the clinician.

During the process of arrhythmia detection, the device counts the number of events in each of the detection zones and compares them to prescribed rules in order to classify

Fig. 27.25 An example of an implantable cardioverter defibrillator (ICD) device record including 16 consecutive beats and their classification. Since 12 of 16 events (75%) were within the ventricular fibrillation detection zone, the arrhythmia would be classified as ventricular fibrillation and high-voltage shocks would be delivered. ECG, electrocardiogram; VF, ventricular fibrillation; VT, ventricular tachycardia

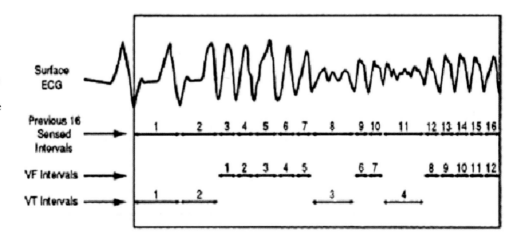

tachycardias with ventricular cycle lengths less than 320 ms could be terminated by antitachycardia pacing 3 out of 4 times with a low incidence of acceleration into ventricular fibrillation and syncopal episodes [37]. If a fast ventricular tachycardia zone is programmed, the device will always ensure that the most aggressive therapy is being delivered. For example, if a fast ventricular tachycardia is detected, the device will verify that no ventricular fibrillation intervals falls within that fast ventricular tachycardia zone before delivering antitachycardia pacing.

When targeting treatments of ventricular arrhythmias, it is important to verify that the arrhythmia is of a ventricular origin. Therefore, it is common that each manufacturer will have a unique algorithm for distinguishing a supraventricular tachycardia from a ventricular tachycardia. This is very important in order to avoid inappropriate shocking of a patient with sinus tachycardia due to exercise or an atrial arrhythmia (atrial fibrillation or atrial flutter).

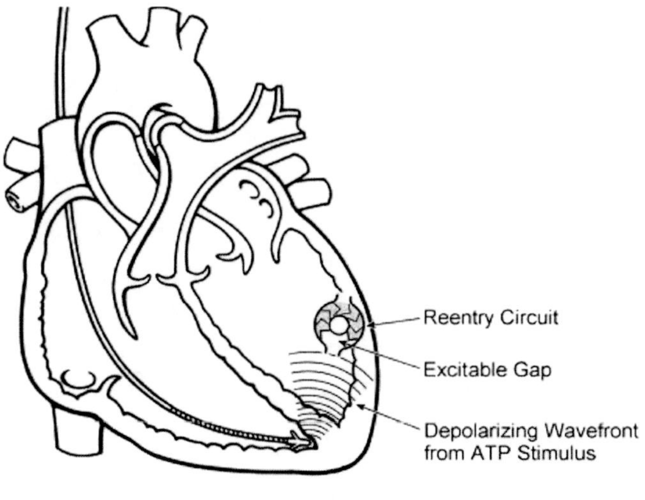

Fig. 27.26 Antitachycardia pacing therapy. A pacing stimulus is applied to entrain an excitable gap in the reentrant circuit. This disrupts the reentrant circuit and terminates the tachycardia. ATP, antitachycardia pacing

27.5.7 ICD Therapies

ICD therapies are programmed to ensure maximum patient safety, while attempting to deliver the lowest energy therapy (least painful and least impact on device longevity) that will terminate the arrhythmia. ICD therapies can be tiered, such that the device initially delivers low energies which are subsequently increased until the desired treatment is obtained. A typical delivery order is as follows: antitachycardia pacing (delivering the least amount of energy), followed by cardioversion, and finally by defibrillation. Nevertheless, each of these therapies can be programmed to the physician's preference.

Antitachycardia pacing is typically used in a clinical situation where one reentrant circuit is repeatedly activating the ventricles and causing a rapid, but regular ventricular tachycardia. The goal of the antitachycardia pacing therapy is to deliver, via a pacing stimulus, a depolarization wave into the area of the excitable gap (an area of repolarized tissue) of the reentry circuit. Recall that a reentrant circuit causes the majority of tachyarrhythmias. Thus, if a pacing pulse reaches the excitable gap before a new wave front of the reentrant circuit, the reentrant activity is terminated (Fig. 27.26).

Cardioversion and defibrillation shocks are high-energy shocks that are delivered between two or three high-voltage electrodes, one of which is typically the ICD itself (i.e., the titanium housing acts as an electrode). The goal of these shocks is to defibrillate a critical mass of the myocardial cells that are depolarizing at a rapid and irregular rate (Figs. 27.27 and 27.28), thus returning the heart to a normal rhythm.

Cardioversion can be described as a synchronized high-voltage shock, because the shock needs to be synchronized to an R-wave or the shock will not be delivered. Cardioversion shocks are used to treat ventricular tachycardias or regular fast ventricular tachycardias. Therefore, the shock is delivered on an R-wave that has been detected in the tachycardia detection zone. If the shock would happen to be delivered on a T-wave, the underlying arrhythmia could be dangerously accelerated into ventricular fibrillation, which is why a cardioversion shock will be aborted if it is not synchronized to an R-wave. The chaotic nature of ventricular fibrillation is treated by

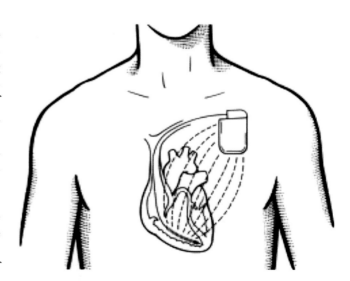

Fig. 27.27 Electric field between high-voltage electrodes during a shock; note that the implantable cardioverter defibrillator (ICD) is functioning as one of the electrodes

Fig. 27.28 Examples of successful defibrillation (*top electrogram*) and cardioversion (*lower electrogram*) therapies. VF, ventricular fibrillation; VT, ventricular tachycardia

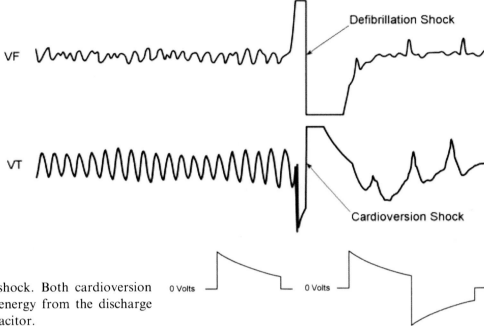

Fig. 27.29 Monophasic and biphasic shock waveforms

delivering an asynchronous shock. Both cardioversion and defibrillation gain their energy from the discharge of the ICD's high-voltage capacitor.

Depending on the manufacturer, each device will offer a number of programmable therapies per detection zone, again all of which can be programmed to physician preferences. Yet, importantly, the programming of the defibrillation therapy is typically based on a specific patient's defibrillation threshold. This threshold is defined as the minimum amount of energy needed to rescue the heart from the fibrillating state (various algorithms exist for determining this energy). The physician commonly will set the first defibrillation therapy at an energy output that is greater than the defibrillation threshold, to provide a margin of safety for the patient. A safety margin of at least 10 J greater than the defibrillation threshold is common. For example, if a patient's defibrillation threshold has been determined to be 15 J, the device will be programmed to deliver its first therapy at 25 J. Therefore, the maximum output of the device needs to be considered when assessing an appropriate safety margin. If a device has a maximum output of 35 J and the patient's defibrillation threshold is 27 J, there would only be an 8 J safety margin.

The relative shapes of shock waveforms delivered by the ICD have evolved over time. Early systems used a monophasic waveform delivered between a dedicated set of electrodes (i.e., delivered with a constant direction of current flow or polarity). Later, sequential monophasic shocks between selected pairs of electrodes were employed, since they were found to produce lower defibrillation thresholds in certain patients. Modern devices typically use a biphasic shock that reverses polarity during the discharge of the capacitors (Fig. 27.29).

The development of biphasic waveforms was considered as a significant improvement in ICD technology, and they have been almost exclusively used since the mid-

1980s [38]. The percentage of the drop in voltage, prior to termination of the waveform, is the current polarity, also known as "tilt." Tilt is measured from the instant the current starts to flow in one direction (leading edge) to the time that it ends its flow in that same direction (trailing edge). A tilt value can be measured for each direction that the current is flowing; typical tilts are between 50 and 65% (Fig. 27.30).

As mentioned previously, most modern ICDs also include pacemaker functionality. As a final summary of the similarities and differences between IPGs and ICDs, Table 27.8 is provided.

27.5.8 Pharmacologic Considerations in the Management of Tachyarrhythmias

In contrast to the relatively small effect that antiarrhythmic drugs typically have on pacing thresholds, the defibrillator threshold of an ICD may be significantly altered when used in conjunction with antiarrhythmic drug therapies. Nevertheless, there are several positive benefits that have been considered useful in the concomitant use of ICDs and antiarrhythmic drugs. For example, antiarrhythmic drugs may act to decrease the frequency and duration of sustained and nonsustained ventricular tachycardia events that would otherwise require a shock from an ICD. They can also slow the rate of the

Fig. 27.30 Determination of the percent tilt of a defibrillation waveform. LE, leading edge; TE, trailing edge

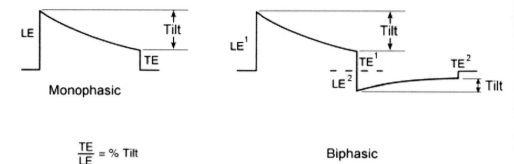

$$\frac{TE}{LE} = \% \text{ Tilt}$$

Table 27.8 Comparison of the principal differences between implantable pulse generator (IPG) and implantable cardioverter defibrillator (ICD)

ICD	IPG
Senses intrinsic rhythms, ventricular tachycardia/ ventricular fibrillation, and prefers to oversense	Senses intrinsic rhythms and prefers to undersense
Paces and shocks when appropriate	Paces when appropriate
Saves episode data	Rejects signals that occur at high rates
Battery requires high current capability for shocking	Battery optimized for long-term, low current use

Table 27.9 The impact of select antiarrhythmic drugs on defibrillation thresholds

Increase	Mixed effect	Decrease
Flecainide	Quinidine	Sotalol
Propafenone	Procainamide	Bretylium
Lidocaine	Amiodarone	
Mexiletine		

ventricular tachycardia to increase the efficacy of antitachycardia pacing, decreasing the need for shock therapy. Lastly and importantly, antiarrhythmic agents may lower defibrillation thresholds. Therefore, the use of antiarrhythmic drugs with ICDs can decrease the frequency and/or amplitude of therapeutic shocks, thereby increasing both patient comfort and prolonging battery longevity [39].

In addition to the benefits, there are also potentially undesired consequences associated with the concurrent use of ICDs and antiarrhythmic drugs [13]. Specifically, antiarrhythmic drugs may: (1) alter the detection of the arrhythmia leading to an increase in the duration of a tachyarrhythmia; (2) increase defibrillation thresholds, making it more difficult to successfully defibrillate the heart; (3) slow the rate of the tachyarrhythmia so much that it no longer falls within the detection zone for both antitachycardia pacing and shock; and/or (4) prolong the width of the QRS complex on the EKG, thus causing double counting and inappropriate shocks. The typical antiarrhythmic drugs that may affect defibrillation thresholds are: (1) Type I agents, those with sodium channel blocking activities and the membrane stabilization effects; (2) beta-blockers and calcium channel antagonists due to their effects on the nodal tissues; and (3) Type III agents which may either increase or decrease defibrillation thresholds after long-term therapy (Table 27.9).

Antiarrhythmic agents can also be proarrhythmic, which may even lead to an increased requirement for ICD therapies. Predisposing factors to proarrhythmias are: (1) electrolyte imbalances such as hypomagnesemia or hypokalemia; (2) underlying ventricular arrhythmias; (3) ischemic heart disease; and/or (4) poor left ventricular function. One of the most dangerous forms of proarrhythmia is considered to be Torsades de Pointes or "twisting of the points." Specifically, Torsades is a rapid form of polymorphic ventricular tachycardia that is associated with delayed ventricular repolarization. It should be noted that both inherited conditions such as long QT syndrome and the exposure to Type Ia or Type III antiarrhythmic drugs that prolong the refractory period on the cardiac action potential put patients at an increased risk of Torsades de Pointes.

27.5.9 New Indications/Recent Clinical Trials

This section will focus on some of the recent clinic trials assessing the value of ICD therapy. Clinical trials serve the important role of assessing therapeutic safety and efficacy for (1) determining the validity of current clinical indications; (2) discovering new indications for use; and/ or (3) driving reimbursement through identification of clinical value. Properly run clinical studies continue to play an important role in continuous improvement of patient outcomes. Yet, an important distinction to make here is that there are major differences between primary and secondary studies. Specifically, primary studies seek to find morbidity and mortality benefit in those patients who have not experienced an event. These studies identify a patient population that is considered "at risk" and attempt to determine means to treat such patients before they experience an event such as myocardial infarction or sudden cardiac arrest. In contrast, secondary studies evaluate posttreatment morbidity and mortality benefits to patient populations that have already suffered from an event (e.g., postmyocardial infarction patients or patients who have survived sudden cardiac arrest).

A recent example of an important clinical trial associated with the identification of the indications for ICD therapy is the Multicenter Automatic Defibrillator Implantation Trial (MADIT). This trial was instrumental in providing clinical evidence for identifying patients who would benefit from an ICD therapy. The clinical hypothesis stated "in patients with previous myocardial infarction and left ventricular dysfunction, prophylactic therapy with an ICD improves survival versus treatment with conventional medical therapy" [40]. The primary end point of the study was a reduction in total patient mortality and the secondary end points evaluated mortality associated with arrhythmias as well as cost effectiveness. Of 196 patients included in the study, there were 39 deaths in the conventional therapy arm and 15 deaths in the ICD group. The stated conclusions were that, in postmyocardial infarction patients at a high risk for ventricular tachycardia, prophylactic therapy with an ICD reduced overall mortality by 54% and arrhythmic mortality by 75% when compared with conventional therapy.

A follow-up to MADIT was the Multicenter Automatic Defibrillator Implantation Trial-II (MADIT-II). The purpose of this study was to investigate the effects of prophylactic implantation of an ICD on the survival of patients postinfarction who presented with significant left ventricular dysfunction (left ventricular ejection fraction ≤30%). The primary conclusion of this study was that prophylactic implantation of an ICD in such patients resulted in improved survival and decreased mortality by 28% after 3 years. Importantly, the noted benefits of this study have changed practice in that physicians now routinely implant an ICD in postmyocardial infarction patients with left ventricular dysfunction [41].

27.5.10 Pacing and Defibrillation Leads

Cardiac pacing and defibrillation leads are the electrical conduit between the IPG or ICD and the heart. Specifically, they transmit therapeutic energies to the cardiac tissue and return sensed information to the IPG or ICD for diagnostic and monitoring purposes. It is noteworthy

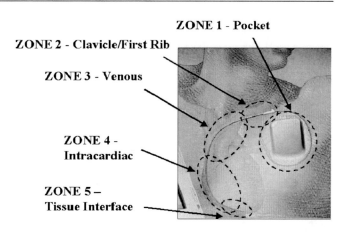

Fig. 27.31 The anatomic regions commonly spanned by transvenous endocardial pacing leads

that such leads must: (1) withstand the extremely harsh environment of the internal human body and its intense foreign body responses; (2) permanently span multiple anatomic and physiologic features, e.g., the moving body and heart (Fig. 27.31); and (3) undergo approximately 400 million heartbeat-induced deformations over each 10-year period within the heart (see MPG 27.15).

Leads can be placed either endocardially or epicardially, depending on the patient's indication, physician preference, and/or anatomic considerations. In the case of endocardial pacing systems (those implanted through the venous system to the endocardial surface of the cardiac chambers), the lead travels from subcutaneous tissue including muscle and fat into the blood stream. These leads then pass through the upper vasculature and finally are permanently placed within the beating heart. Today, the vast majority of pacing systems utilize endocardial leads (this lead placement technique can be viewed in MPG 27.6). In contrast, epicardial leads are attached directly to the surface of the heart and are routed through subcutaneous tissue to the ICD or IPG. Epicardial leads are most commonly used in pediatric patients and in adults with compromised venous accesses to their hearts. Typical implanted configurations for endocardial single- and dual-chamber pacing systems are shown in Fig. 27.32, endocardial defibrillation systems in Fig. 27.33 and MPG 27.16, and an epicardial defibrillation system with epicardial pacing leads in Fig. 27.34.

Modern leads are generally constructed of highly biostable and biocompatible polymers and metals. Configurations for the body of the leads (i.e., the portion traveling from the IPG or ICD to the distal electrodes) are chosen based on the number of circuits required as well as considerations relating to size, handling, and manufacturer preferences (Fig. 27.35). The electrodes for

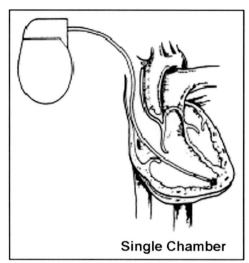
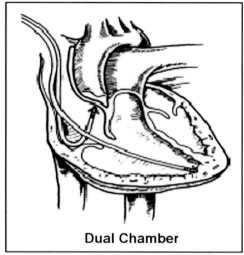

Fig. 27.32 Examples of single- and dual-chamber endocardial lead configurations

Fig. 27.33 Implanted configurations for two endocardial defibrillation systems with pectoral ICD placements. The single coil system (*left*) delivers the shock energy from the right ventricular coil to the ICD. The dual coil system (*right*) can deliver the energy from right ventricular coil to the ICD, or from the right ventricular coil to a superior vena cava coil and/or the ICD (See MPG 25.16). RV, right ventricle; SVC, superior vena cava

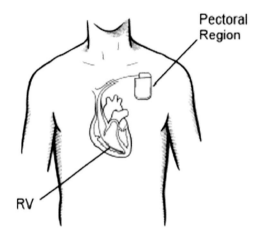

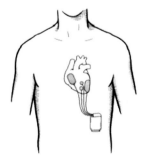
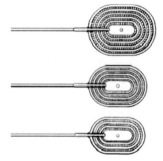
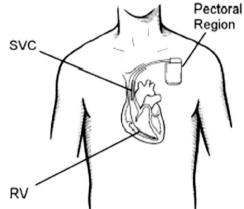

Fig. 27.34 Implanted configuration of an epicardial defibrillation system with an abdominal ICD placement. The system shown includes two unipolar epicardial pacing leads for stimulation and sensing as well as a pair of epicardial defibrillation patches

stimulation and sensing are designed to provide stable electrical performance acutely and chronically.

In order to provide stability at the cardiac–tissue interface, leads often use a mechanism for fixation to cardiac tissue and structures. Passive mechanisms for fixation include polymeric tines and shaped segments along the length of the lead. They are termed "passive" because they do not require an active deployment by the clinician. Common active means of fixation include helices, hooks, or barbs. Additionally, some epicardial leads require sutures to maintain a stable position. Finally, some leads have no fixation means whatsoever and count solely on lead stiffness to maintain locational stability when implanted within cardiac veins (Figs. 27.36, 27.37, 27.38, and 27.39). To view examples of leads placed within the Visible Heart® preparation, see the following movie clips: MPG 27.17 (active fixation pacing lead in human right atrium), MPG 27.18 (active fixation pacing lead in swine right atrium with simultaneous fluoroscopy), MPG 27.19 (tined passive fixation lead in swine right ventricle), MPG 27.20 (active fixation pacing lead in

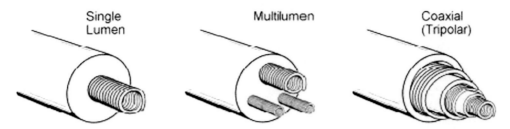

Single
Lumen

Multilumen

Coaxial
(Tripolar)

Fig. 27.35 Typical constructions used for cardiac pacing and defibrillation leads: (1) the single lumen design (*left*) has a central conductor surrounded by a polymeric insulation; (2) the multilumen design (*center*) uses an extruded polymer to insulate the conductors from one another and from the implanted environment; and (3) the coaxial design has conductors embedded within concentric layers of insulation. Today, the most commonly used insulation materials are silicones and polyurethanes and the conductors are usually coiled or cabled wires. Modern lead body diameters range from approximately 4 to 10 French (1 French = 1/3 of a millimeter)

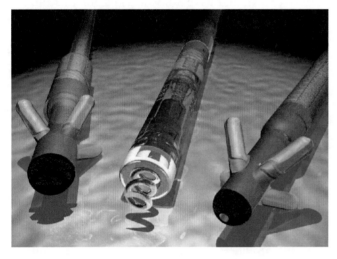

Fig. 27.36 Endocardial pacing leads: passive fixation leads (tined) are shown on the *left* and *right*. An active fixation lead (extendable, retractable helix) is shown in the *center*

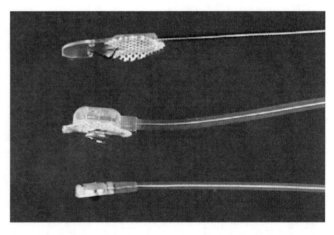

Fig. 27.37 Epicardial pacing leads: stab-in active fixation lead (*top*), active fixation lead with helical fixation (*middle*), and a hemispherical electrode secured by sutures (*bottom*)

human right ventricle), and MPG 27.21 (tined passive fixation defibrillation lead in human right ventricle).

Various electrode configurations have been utilized on a variety of commercially available leads. As described previously, unipolar pacing circuits use a lead with a single cathodal electrode, with the IPG serving as the anode. Bipolar pacing systems use electrodes placed distally on the lead as both the cathode and anode. Pacing leads commonly use a cylindrical electrode placed along the lead body (ring electrode) as the anode, while defibrillation leads may use a dedicated ring (the so-called "true bipolar" leads) or a defibrillation coil as the anode (an "integrated bipolar" lead). Defibrillation leads utilize electrodes with large surface areas, which allow for the delivery of high-energy shocks within and around the

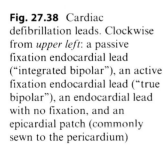

Fig. 27.38 Cardiac defibrillation leads. Clockwise from *upper left*: a passive fixation endocardial lead ("integrated bipolar"), an active fixation endocardial lead ("true bipolar"), an endocardial lead with no fixation, and an epicardial patch (commonly sewn to the pericardium)

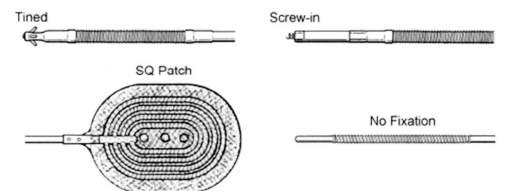

Tined

Screw-in

SQ Patch

No Fixation

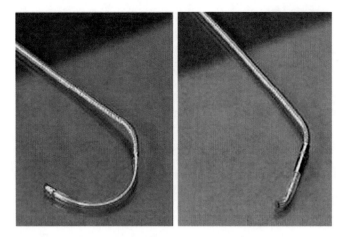

Fig. 27.39 Pacing leads designed for placement in the cardiac veins; they are shaped to enhance stability. The leads shown are primarily used in biventricular pacing systems for the management of heart failure patients with the appropriate clinical indications

heart. Defibrillation leads may be unipolar (defibrillation electrode only) or they may have a combination of defibrillation electrodes and pacing electrodes. The most common defibrillation lead configurations used today are shown in Figs. 27.38, 27.39, and 27.40. For examples of leads placed within the Visible Heart® preparation, see the following movie clips: MPG 27.22 (defibrillation lead in the right ventricle of a swine heart; ventricular fibrillation is induced with a shock on the T-wave and then converted to sinus rhythm with a high-energy shock), and MPG 27.23 (defibrillation lead in the right ventricle of a human heart; ventricular fibrillation is converted to sinus rhythm with a high-energy shock).

Typically, the portion of the lead that interfaces with the cardiac tissue has been designed to: (1) minimize

inflammatory responses; (2) provide low polarizations; (3) provide high capacitances and impedances; and/or (4) act as a fixation mechanism. This distal electrode is the most commonly used cathode but, in some cases, a similar electrode is used as the anode on a separate unipolar lead. To suppress inflammation, most modern electrodes incorporate a system for the delivery of an anti-inflammatory agent (e.g., dexamethasone sodium phosphate or beclomethasone); this helps to manage acute changes in the local tissue which will then aid in stabilizing pacing and sensing performances. Coatings are also applied to many pacing electrodes to produce a large surface area that is highly capacitive (i.e., to reduce battery drain), and have a low level of polarization following a pacing pulse (to avoid undersensing) (Fig. 27.41). Interestingly, the size of the pacing cathode has decreased over time, as a means to increase the cathode–tissue impedance and increase system efficiencies by reducing current drain (Figs. 27.42 and 27.43) [42].

27.6 Summary

This chapter has reviewed the basic methodologies and devices employed to provide pacing and/or defibrillation therapies to the patient with specific needs. A brief history was provided on the use of external electricity to deliver lifesaving therapies to the heart. Although significant progress has been made, future developments in materials, electronics, and communications systems (e.g., wireless) will allow ever increasing utility and patient value.

Fig. 27.40 Endocardial defibrillation leads. Various configurations are shown, including leads with active and passive fixation mechanisms, true and integrated bipolar pace/sense circuits, and/or single and dual defibrillation electrodes. The designs shown are typically placed in the right ventricle with the distal defibrillation coil within the right ventricular chamber and the proximal coil located in the superior vena cava

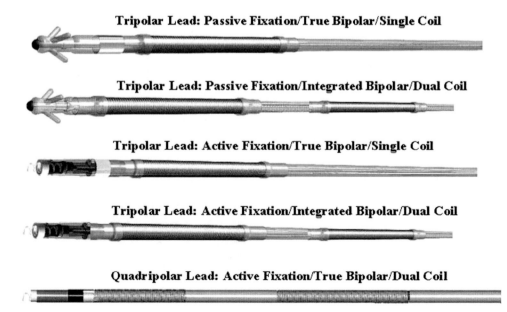

Tripolar Lead: Passive Fixation/True Bipolar/Single Coil

Tripolar Lead: Passive Fixation/Integrated Bipolar/Dual Coil

Tripolar Lead: Active Fixation/True Bipolar/Single Coil

Tripolar Lead: Active Fixation/Integrated Bipolar/Dual Coil

Quadripolar Lead: Active Fixation/True Bipolar/Dual Coil

Fig. 27.41 Common electrode coatings for high capacitance and low polarization. The *left panel* (**A**) shows a platinized surface at 20,000× and the *right panel* (**B**) a titanium nitride (TiN) surface at 20,000×

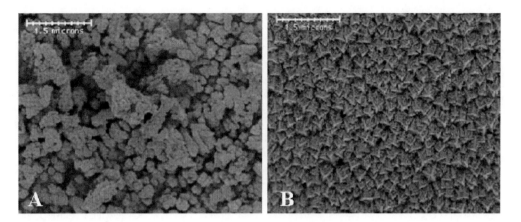

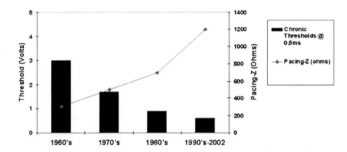

Fig. 27.42 Evolution of pacing lead impedances and pacing thresholds. Modified from Brabec et al. [42]

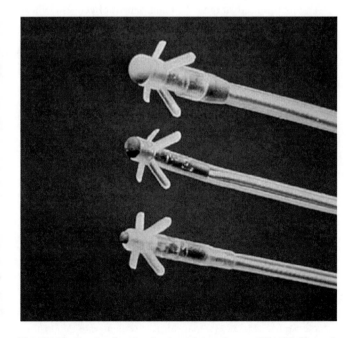

Fig. 27.43 Passive fixation leads with low (*top*; ~400–600 Ω), medium (*middle*; ~600–800 Ω), and high (*bottom*; ~800–1,200 Ω) impedance pacing cathodes

Companion CD Material

Section 27.2.2
MPG 27.1 (normal sinus rhythm)
Section 27.2.4
MPG 27.2 (atrial tachycardia)
MPG 27.3 (atrial fibrillation)
MPG 27.4 (ventricular tachycardia)
MPG 27.5 (ventricular fibrillation)
Section 27.3
MPG 27.6 (Seldinger Technique)
MPG 27.7 (biatrial pacing system)
MPG 27.8 (pacing post-mustard procedure)
MPG 27.9 (dual-chamber epicardial system)
MPG 27.10 (dual-chamber epicardial system)
MPG 27.11 (biventricular epicardial system)
MPG 27.12 (dual-chamber epicardial system)
Section 27.4.5
MPG 27.13 (connection between IPG and leads)
Section 27.4.8
MPG 27.14 (biventricular pacing)
Section 27.5.10
MPG 27.15 (pacing and defibrillation leads)
MPG 27.6 (Seldinger Technique)
MPG 27.16 (endocardial defibrillation system)
MPG 27.17 (active fixation pacing lead in human right atrium)
MPG 27.18 (active fixation pacing lead in swine right atrium with simultaneous fluoroscopy)
MPG 27.19 (tined passive fixation lead in swine right ventricle)
MPG 27.20 (active fixation pacing lead in human right ventricle)
MPG 27.21 (tined passive fixation defibrillation lead in human right ventricle)
MPG 27.22 (defibrillation lead in the right ventricle of a swine heart, ventricular fibrillation is induced with a shock on the T-wave and then converted to sinus rhythm with a high-energy shock)

MPG 27.23 (defibrillation lead in the right ventricle of a human heart, ventricular fibrillation is converted to sinus rhythm with a high-energy shock)

Acknowledgments We would like to thank Mike Leners for the development of procedural animations, Medtronic Training and Education for the use of various graphics, the Visible Heart® team for support in capturing the intracardiac footage, Monica Mahre for editorial support, LifeSource, and Drs. Anne Fournier and Suzanne Vobecky of Sainte-Justine Hospital, Montreal, Quebec, Canada, for the radiographic images.

References

1. Maisel WH, Sweeney MO, Stevenson WG, Ellison KE, Epstein LM. Recalls and safety alerts involving pacemakers and implantable cardioverter-defibrillator generators. JAMA 2001;286:793–99.

2. Furman S. A brief history of cardiac stimulation and electrophysiology–The past fifty years and the next century. NASPE Keynote Address, 1995.

3. His W Jr. Die Tatigkeit des embryonalen Herzens und deren Bedcutung fur die Lehre von der Herzbewegung beim Erwachsenen. Artbeiten aus der Medizinischen Klinik zu Leipzig 1893;1:14–49.

4. Tawara S. Das reizleitungssystem des saugetierherzens, Eine anatomisch-histologische studie uber das atrioventrikularbundel und die purkinjeschen faden, Jean, Germany: Gustav Fischer 1906;9–70:114–56.

5. Lillehei CW, Gott VL, Hodges PC, Long DM, Bakken EE. Transistor pacemaker for treatment of complete atrioventricular dissociation. JAMA 1960;172:2006–10.

6. Furman SC Walton Lillehei. Accessed November 25, 2003 from http://www.naspe.org/ep-history/notable_figures/walton_lillehei

7. Winters SL, Packer DL, Marchlinski FE, et al. Consensus statement on indications, guidelines for use, and recommendations for follow-up of implantable cardioverter defibrillators. PACE 2001;24:262–69.

8. Parsonnet V. Indications for Dual-chamber pacing. NASPE Position Statement, June 1, 1984.

9. Stokes KB, Kay GN. Artificial electrical stimulation. In: Ellenbogen KA, Kay GN, Wilkoff BL, eds. Clinical cardiac pacing. Philadelphia, PA: W.B. Saunders, 1995.

10. Gregoratos G, Cheitlin MD, Conill A, et al. ACC/AHA guidelines for the implantations of cardiac pacemakers and antiarrhythmia devices. JACC 1998;31:1175–209.

11. Epstein AE, DiMarcok JP, Ellenbogen KA, et al. ACC/AHA/HRS 2008 guidelines for device-based therapy of cardiac rhythm abnormalities. Circulation 2008;117:e350–408.

12. Bernstein AD, Daubert JC, Fletcher RD, et al. The revised NAPSE/BPEG generic code for antibradycardia, adaptive-rate, and multisite pacing. PACE 2002;25:260–64.

13. Fogoros RN. Antiarrhythmic drugs: A practical guide. Boston, MA: Blackwell Science, 1997:112.

14. Wilkoff BL, Cook JR, Epstein AE, et al. Dual-chamber and VVI Implantable Defibrillator Trial Investigators. Dual-chamber pacing or ventricular backup pacing in patients with an implantable defibrillator: The Dual-chamber and VVI Implantable Defibrillator (DAVID) Trial. JAMA 2002;288:3115–23.

15. Karpawich PP, Rabah R, Haas JE. Altered cardiac histology following apical right ventricular pacing in patients with congenital atrioventricular block. PACE 1999;22:1372–77.

16. Andersen HR, Nielsen JC, Thomsen PE, et al. Long-term follow-up of patients from a randomised trial of atrial versus ventricular pacing for sick-sinus syndrome. Lancet 1997;350:1210–16.

17. Lamas GA, Orav EJ, Stambler BS, et al. Quality of life and clinical outcomes in elderly patients treated with ventricular pacing as compared with dual-chamber pacing. Pacemaker Selection in the Elderly Investigators. N Engl J Med 1998;338:1097–104.

18. Lamas GA, Lee K, Sweeney M, et al. The mode selection trial (MOST) in sinus node dysfunction: Design, rationale, and baseline characteristics of the first 1000 patients. Am Heart J 2000;140:541–51.

19. Deshmukh P, Casavant DA, Romanyshyn M, Anderson K. Permanent direct His bundle pacing: A novel approach to cardiac pacing in patients with normal His-Purkinje activation. Circulation 2000;101:869–77.

20. Karpawich P, Gates J, Stokes K. Septal His-Purkinje ventricular pacing in canines: A new endocardial electrode approach. PACE 1992;15:2011–15.

21. Karpawich PP, Gillette PC, Lewis RM, Zinner A, McNamera DG. Chronic epicardial His bundle recordings in awake nonsedated dogs: A new method. Am Heart J 1983;105:16–21.

22. Scheinman MM, Saxon LA. Long-term His-bundle pacing and cardiac function. Circulation 2000;101:836–37.

23. Williams DO, Sherlag BJ, Hope RR, El-Sherif N, Lazzara R, Samet P. Selective versus non-selective His bundle pacing. Cardiovas Res 1976;10:91–100.

24. de Cock CC, Giudici MC, Twisk JW. Comparison of the haemodynamic effects of right ventricular outflow-tract pacing with right ventricular apex pacing: A quantitative review. Europace 2003;5:275–78.

25. Cleland JG, Daubert JC, Erdmann E, et al. CARE-HF Study Steering Committee and Investigators. The CARE-HF study (CArdiac REsynchronisation in Heart Failure study): Rationale, design and end-points. Eur J Heart Fail 2001;3:481–89.

26. Leclercq C, Daubert JC. Cardiac resynchronization therapy is an important advance in the management of congestive heart failure. J Cardiovasc Electrophysiol 2003;14:S27–S29.

27. Saksena S. The role of multisite atrial pacing in rhythm control in AF: Insights from sub-analyses of the dual-site atrial pacing for prevention of atrial fibrillation study. Pacing Clin Electrophysiol 2003;26:1565.

28. Leclercq JF, De Sisti A, Fiorello P, Halimi F, Manot S, Attuel P. Is dual-site better than single site atrial pacing in the prevention of atrial fibrillation? Pacing Clin Electrophysiol 2000;23:2101–07.

29. Kindermann M, Schwaab B, Berg M, Frohlig G. The influence of right atrial septal pacing on the interatrial contraction sequence. Pacing Clin Electrophysiol 2000;23:1752–57.

30. Miake J, Marban H, Nuss B. Biological pacemaker created by gene transfer. Nature 2002;419:132–33.

31. Malineni KC, McCullough PA. Sudden cardiac death. Accessed November 25, 2003 from http://www.emedicine.com/med/topic276.htm

32. Myerburg RJ, ed. Heart disease: A textbook of cardiovascular medicine, 5th ed. Philadelphia, PA: W.B. Saunders, 1997, Chapter 24.

33. Coronary Artery Disease Overview. Accessed November 25, 2003 from http://imaginis.com/heart-disease/cad_ov.asp?mode = 1

34. Electricity and the Heart: A Historical Perspective. Accessed November 25, 2003 from http://www.naspe.org/ep-history/timeline

35. Hayes DL, Lloyd MA, Friedman PA, eds. Cardiac pacing and dcfibrillation: A clinical approach. New York, NY: Blackwell Publishing, Inc., 2000:1–599.

36. Cummins RO. From concept to standard-of-care? Review of the clinical experience with automated external defibrillators. Ann Emerg Med 1989;18:1269–75.
37. Wathen MS, Sweeney MO, DeGroot PJ, et al. Shock reduction using antitachycardia pacing for spontaneous rapid ventricular tachycardia in patients with coronary artery disease. Circulation 2001;104:796–801.
38. Electricity and the Heart: A Historical Perspective. Accessed on November 26, 2003 from http://www.naspe.org/ep-history/timeline/1980s
39. Carnes CA, Mehdirad AA, Nelson SD. Drug and defibrillator interactions. Pharmacotherapy 1998;18:516–25.
40. Moss AJ, Hall WJ, Cannom DS, et al. Improved survival with an implanted defibrillator in patients with coronary disease at high risk for ventricular arrhythmia. Multicenter Automatic Defibrillator Implantation Trial Investigators. N Engl J Med 1996;335:1933–40

41. Kloner RA, Birnbaum Y, eds. Cardiovascular trials review, 7th ed. Shelton, Connecticut: Le Jacq Communications Inc., 2002:1065–66.
42. Brabec S, Laske TG. The evolution of bradycardia pacing electrodes. XII World Congress on Cardiac Pacing & Electrophysiology, 2003 (Hong Kong).

Additional Text Sources

Furman S, Hayes DL, Holmes DR, eds. A practice of cardiac pacing. New York, NY: Futura Publishing Company, Inc., 1993:1–753.
Ellenbogen KA, Kay GN, Wilkoff BL, eds. Clinical cardiac pacing. Philadelphia, PH: W.B. Saunders, 1995.

Chapter 28
Cardiac Resynchronization Therapy

Fei Lü

Abstract Congestive heart failure (CHF) has become a major health problem. Despite improved pharmacologic therapies, refractory symptoms and high mortality remain a challenge in such patients. There has been increased interest in the application of ancillary nonpharmacologic therapies for CHF management, such as implantable pacemakers, defibrillators, and/or left ventricular assist devices. Various methods of cardiac pacing are discussed and contrasted in this chapter, with the focus on biventricular pacing and cardiac resynchronization therapy for treatment of CHF. Cardiac resynchronization therapy has now become a part of standard therapy for patients with severe symptomatic CHF and intraventricular dyssynchrony.

Keywords Cardiac resynchronization therapy · Physiologic pacing · Cardiac function · Implantable cardioverter defibrillator · Mechanical remodeling · Biventricular pacing · His bundle pacing

28.1 Introduction

As other causes of premature death from heart disease have diminished, congestive heart failure (CHF) has become a major public health problem in the United States and elsewhere. Despite improved pharmacologic therapies, refractory symptoms and high mortality remain a challenge in patients with CHF [1]. As a consequence, there has been increased interest in the application of ancillary nonpharmacologic therapies for CHF management, such as implantable pacemakers, defibrillators, and/or left ventricular assist devices (e.g., see also Chapter 36).

Conventional cardiac pacing is often indicated for patients with CHF. Symptomatic chronotropic incompetence, sinus node dysfunction, and atrioventricular (AV) block, which are frequently present in such patients, are class I indications for cardiac pacing. Atrial fibrillation affects 10–30% of patients with CHF, and AV nodal ablation plus pacemaker insertion has been accepted as a standard therapy in patients with refractory symptomatic atrial fibrillation and uncontrolled ventricular rates. In addition, during the last decade, special attention has been paid to optimizing pacing modalities for patients with left ventricular (LV) dysfunction whenever ventricular pacing is required. Early studies suggested that dual-chamber pacing with a short AV delay was associated with improved cardiac function relative to the case with usual programmed AV delays; however, this observation needs to be further confirmed.

Traditionally, the ventricular pacing lead has been placed at the apex of the right ventricle (RV) due to both ease of placement and stability of the lead after implantation. Recent data clearly indicate that the RV apex is not an optimal pacing site, since RV apical pacing can be associated with deleterious changes in: (1) diastolic and systolic function; (2) myocardial perfusion; and/or (3) neurohumoral status in both animals and humans [2, 3]. Figure 28.1 shows a case of worsened hemodynamic changes that occurred during RV apical pacing compared to other ventricular sites [2]. The detrimental hemodynamic changes during RV apical pacing, which are mainly attributed to altered ventricular activation sequences and dyssynchronized contraction, are particularly important in the presence of concomitant LV dysfunction (Table 28.1). Minimizing RV pacing by use of longer AV delays or by LV-based pacing (LV pacing alone, biventricular pacing, or multisite ventricular pacing) has recently become the standard practice.

F. Lü (✉)
University of Minnesota, Department of Medicine, MMC 508, 420 Delaware St. SE, Minneapolis, MN, 55455, USA
e-mail: luxxx074@umn.edu

P.A. Iaizzo (ed.), *Handbook of Cardiac Anatomy, Physiology, and Devices*, DOI 10.1007/978-1-60327-372-5_28,
© Springer Science+Business Media, LLC 2009

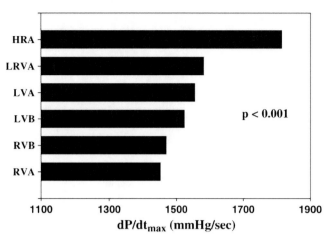

Fig. 28.1 Effects of ventricular pacing on myocardial contractility in normal hearts. Dp/dt$_{max}$ is used as a parameter of myocardial contractility. Cardiac contractility is decreased during ventricular pacing at any of these pacing sites (either single or biventricular pacing). Note that cardiac contractility during left ventricular or biventricular pacing is better than that during right ventricular pacing, but still significantly lower than atrial pacing at the same rate. Right ventricular apical pacing (RVA), left ventricular apical pacing (LVA), and biventricular apical pacing (LRVA) reduce maximal dP/DT$_{max}$ by 20, 14, and 13%, respectively, compared to high right atrial pacing (HRA). LVB, LV basal pacing; RVB, RV basal pacing. Reproduced from J Cardiovasc Electrophysiol 1999 with permission from Blackwell Publishing [2]

Table 28.1 Proposed mechanisms of adverse effects from right ventricular apical pacing

1. Paradoxical septal motion
2. Altered ventricular activation sequence
3. Impaired mitral or tricuspid apparatus function
4. Altered diastolic function
5. Diminished diastolic filling time
6. Increased serum catecholamine concentration

Compared to RV pacing, LV-based pacing alone is associated with better hemodynamics in many CHF patients with (widened QRS duration) and without (narrow QRS duration) intraventricular conduction delays. Consequently, the era of biventricular (Biv) pacing or cardiac resynchronization therapy (CRT) for CHF has ensued. For this reason, a fifth letter has been introduced to describe multisite pacing in the pacemaker mode (NBG) code [4]. CRT has now become a part of standard therapy for patients with severe symptomatic CHF and intraventricular dyssynchrony.

28.2 Physiologic Pacing

When using pacing for management of CHF, CRT should be considered as an integrated part of physiologic pacing. Because of the detrimental effects of right ventricular apical pacing on hemodynamics, methods to ensure more "physiologic" pacing are important, particularly in the presence of severe LV dysfunction. Components of physiologic pacing include: (1) improvement of appropriate chronotropic response (rate-responsive pacing); (2) preservation of atrial function (AV sequential pacing); (3) maintenance of optimal AV synchrony (AV delay); and (4) maintenance of normal ventricular activation sequences (e.g., with His bundle pacing or CRT).

Cardiac output is determined by heart rate and stroke volume. Traditionally, electronic pacing is mainly used to back up a key determinant of cardiac output, the heart rate. However, in addition to preserving heart rate, AV synchrony is equally important for maintenance of normal hemodynamics. More specifically, the consequences of AV dyssynchrony include: (1) diminished ventricular filling due to loss of consistent "atrial kick;" (2) potential mitral and tricuspid insufficiency; (3) pulmonary venous congestion secondary to atrial contraction against a closed mitral valve, leading to higher pressure in the pulmonary veins; and/or (4) inappropriate decrease in peripheral resistance due to atrial distension-induced autonomic activation (possibly caused by both atrial naturietic factor release and atrial wall mechnoreceptor activation).

The loss of the so-called "atrial kick" may reduce cardiac output in some patients by up to one-third (usually 15–30%). However, even if the AV synchrony is preserved, RV pacing-induced disturbance of spatiotemporal distribution of contraction may adversely affect ventricular function. The importance of synchronized ventricular electrical activation and contraction as manifested, albeit imperfectly by a narrow QRS complex, has been demonstrated. For instance, compared to typical RV apical pacing, RV pacing from alternate pacing sites on the interventricular septum (resulting in a narrower QRS duration) is significantly correlated with improved synchronization of LV contraction and also increased systolic function.

Figure 28.1 shows the maximal LV dP/dt (as an index of myocardial contractility) during high right atrial pacing, single ventricular pacing, and Biv pacing in normal hearts [2]. This clearly indicates that ventricular pacing, particularly RV apical pacing, is associated with reduced myocardial contractility. Furthermore, different pacing modes can significantly influence cardiac output during exercise in patients with sinus node dysfunction and normal AV node function without bundle branch block (Fig. 28.2) [5]. AAI pacing represents a pacing protocol associated with normal ventricular activation sequence and AV conduction (assuming no concomitant intraventricular conduction disturbance). DDD pacing maintains AV synchrony, but induces a disturbed

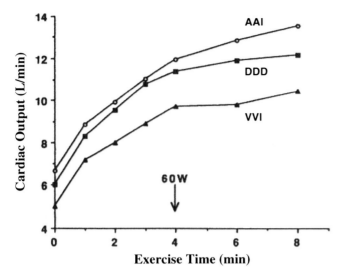

Fig. 28.2 Effects of pacing configurations on cardiac output during exercise in patients with sinus node dysfunction and normal atrioventricular node function without bundle branch block. See text for detailed discussion. Modified from Leclercq C et al. [5]

ventricular activation sequence (intraventricular dyssynchrony) when the RV is paced. VVI pacing has neither normal ventricular activation sequence nor AV synchrony; cardiac output is significantly lower during VVI pacing compared to either AAI or DDD pacing. Typically, at rest and during the initial part of exercise with lower workload, there is no significant difference in cardiac output between DDD and AAI pacing. However, AAI pacing is significantly better as exercise duration increases. These observations support the clinical importance of the maintenance of normal AV synchrony and intraventricular activation sequence.

28.2.1 Mechanisms of CRT

CRT is currently most commonly provided in an atrio-Biv pacing configuration, aimed at correcting ventricular dyssynchrony as well as providing optimal AV

Table 28.2 Potential mechanisms underlying cardiac resynchronization therapy

1.	Improved contraction pattern
2.	Improved interventricular synchrony
3.	Reduced paradoxical septal wall motion
4.	Improved left ventricular regional wall motion
5.	Reduced end-systolic volumes
6.	Improved maximal positive left ventricular dP/dt (contractility)
7.	Atrioventricular interval optimization
8.	Reduced mitral regurgitation
9.	Increased diastolic filling time
10.	Improved maximal negative left ventricular dP/dt (relaxation)

synchrony. Again, ventricular dyssynchrony can be associated with abnormal interventricular septal wall motion, reduced dP/dt, reduced diastolic filling time, and increased potential for diastolic mitral regurgitation. The underlying mechanisms of CRT benefit are proposed to include coordination of contraction, diminished valvular regurgitation, and preservation of AV synchrony in the absence of atrial fibrillation (Table 28.2). CRT may aid in shortening the pre-ejection period (principally by reducing LV electromechanical delay with a lesser reduction in isovolumic contraction time) and also shortening durations of LV systole with a consequent trend toward lengthening diastolic filling time. CRT devices also attempt to address AV synchrony and enhance interventricular synchrony as well as intraventricular synchrony (Fig. 28.3). In other words, CRT should be considered as the ultimate currently available physiologic pacing technique in CHF patients with intraventricular dyssynchrony. Increased LV filling time, decreased septal dyskinesis, and reduced mitral regurgitation all play an important role in CRT.

Although not originally designed to produce this potential benefit, the reduction of functional mitral regurgitation may play an important role in overall CRT. Furthermore, it seems that acute resolution of abnormal mitral valve tethering after CRT may not be caused by changes in mitral valve geometry, but rather by an increase in transmitral closing forces. Interestingly, in

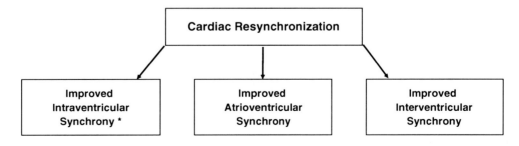

Fig. 28.3 Mechanisms underlying cardiac resynchronization therapy (CRT) or biventricular pacing

some patients, employing CRT reduces functional mitral regurgitation irrespective of LV remodeling reversal.

In general, the effects of CRT on diastolic function may be considered less important. Yet, limited data from animal [2] and human [6] studies have shown that Biv or multisite pacing may also be associated with better diastolic function (but limited) as well as dyssystolic function. It was also shown that CRT improves systolic function and systolic dyssynchrony, but has a neutral or limited effect on diastolic function and diastolic dyssynchrony; the LV reverse remodeling response was determined by the severity of prepacing systolic dyssynchrony, but not diastolic dyssynchrony or diastolic filling pattern [7].

28.2.2 Patient Population Eligible for CRT

Conduction delays within the AV node and the ventricles associated with idiopathic dilated or ischemic cardiomyopathy can contribute to LV dysfunction by impairing AV synchrony and the synchronous contraction and relaxation of the LV. It is estimated that approximately 30% of patients with severe CHF have some degree of intraventricular conduction disturbances characterized electrically by wide QRS complexes and mechanically by uncoordinated ventricular contraction and relaxation patterns. It has also been estimated that 10–20% of a general heart failure population and 13–35% of patients referred for initial cardiac transplantation evaluation may be eligible for CRT. To date, it is also considered that, in patients with an implantable cardioverter defibrillator (ICD), approximately 10–20% may be additionally eligible for CRT.

28.2.3 Effects of CRT on Cardiac Function

Both animal and human studies have shown that LV-based pacing, in the presence of an intrinsic intraventricular conduction delay, is associated with better cardiac function. To date, several clinical trials examining CRT for CHF patients without traditional indications for pacing have been published (Fig. 28.4, Table 28.3). The relative clinical effects of CRT on cardiac function can be best described by these clinical trials.

It is important to note that approximately a third of patients who meet the standard indications for CRT do not respond well to this therapy; in fact, cardiac function may even worsen in some patients with CRT. Yet, in the MIRACLE trial, the conditions of more patients in the group assigned to CRT were considered to have improved at the end of 6 months (67% versus 39% in the control group) and fewer were considered to have worsened (16% versus 27% in the control group) (P<0.001). Unfortunately, to date, there is no reliable means to predict which patient will respond to CRT. Although a prolonged QRS duration is widely used for selecting patients for CRT, baseline QRS duration essentially has limited predictive value regarding potential CRT benefit. On the other hand, to a limited extent, the Biv pacing-induced change in QRS duration may be useful in identifying patients who may respond to CRT. Many studies have shown that mechanical dyssynchrony is much more useful in identifying patients who will respond to CRT, although there is no universally agreed-upon definition for ventricular dyssynchrony.

The MUSTIC (Multisite Stimulation in Cardiomyopathy) study was an early, relatively small single-blind crossover study that opened the door for CRT [8]. It

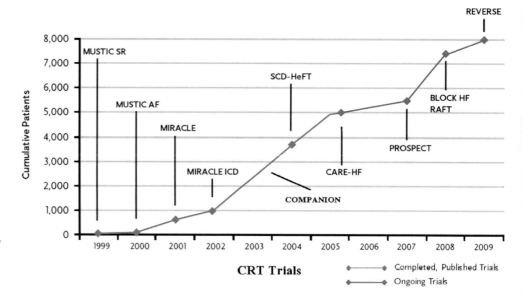

Fig. 28.4 Clinical trials on cardiac synchronization therapy (CRT). Courtesy of Medtronic, Inc. See text for the details of these trials

Table 28.3 Major clinical trials on cardiac resynchronization therapy

Title of study (n randomized)	NYHA class	QRS	Sinus	ICD	Status	Results
MIRACLE (n = 453)	III, IV	≥130	Normal	No	Published	+
MUSTIC SR (n = 58)	III	>150	Normal	No	Published	+
MUSTIC AF (n = 43)	III	>200	AFib	No	Published	+
PATH CHF (n = 41)	III, IV	≥120	Normal	No	Published	+
MIRACLE ICD (n = 369)	III, IV	≥130	Normal	Yes	Published	+
CONTAK-CD (n = 490)	II–IV	≥120	Normal	Yes	Published	+
COMPANION (n = 1,520)	III, IV	≥120	Normal	No	Published	+
PATH CHF II (n = 89)	III, IV	≥120	Normal	Yes	Presented	+
MIRACLE ICD II (n = 186)	II	≥130	Normal	Yes	Published	+
CARE-HF (n = 814)	III, IV	≥120	Normal	No	Published	+

AFib, atrial fibrillation; ICD, implantable cardioverter defibrillator; NYHA, New York Heart Association functional class

enrolled 67 patients from 15 centers in Europe. All patients had significant heart failure due to either idiopathic or ischemic LV systolic dysfunction, a left ventricular ejection fraction (LVEF) <35%, and an LV end-diastolic diameter (LVEDD) >60 mm. All patients were in sinus rhythm with QRS duration of >150 ms and had no standard indication for implantation of a pacemaker or defibrillator. Forty-eight patients completed the 6-month randomized crossover study. Compared to patients with no pacing, individuals with CRT increased their 6-min walk by 23%, peak oxygen uptake by 8%, and quality-of-life score by 32%, and decreased their hospitalization rates by two-thirds. The authors concluded that atrio-Biv pacing significantly improved exercise tolerance and quality of life in patients with chronic CHF and intraventricular conduction delay.

A follow-up study of the MUSTIC trial demonstrated that the benefits of CRT were sustained at 12 months [9]. Clinical improvement included a 5% increase in LVEF and a 45% reduction in mitral regurgitation. Forty-one patients with persistent atrial fibrillation were included in the follow-up study for the indication of a pacemaker due to bradycardia or AV nodal ablation for rate control. Similar clinical improvements were observed in this subset of patients with atrial fibrillation [9].

The InSync Registry was a prospective observational multicenter European and Canadian study that examined the safety and efficacy of CRT as a supplemental treatment for refractory CHF [10, 11]. Between August 1997 and November 1998, 103 patients were enrolled (with a mean LVEF of 22% and mean QRS duration of 178 ms). Over a follow-up period of 12 months, 21 patients died; the 12-month actual survival was 78%. Nine surviving patients were withdrawn from the study during long-term follow-up for miscellaneous reasons. At each point of follow-up over 12 months, a significant shortening of QRS duration was measured and significant improvements were observed in mean New York Heart Association (NYHA) functional class, 6-min walk distance, and quality-of-life score. In the 46 patients with complete echocardiographic data, LVEF

increased by 20% ($P = 0.006$), mitral regurgitation decreased by 26% ($P = 0.197$), and LV filling time increased by 12% ($P = 0.002$). These changes were accompanied by clinically relevant improvements in functional status and quality-of-life score, as well as a measurable increase in LV performance. The investigators concluded that long-term CRT can be safely and reliably achieved by transvenous synchronized atrio-Biv pacing.

The MIRACLE (Multicenter InSync Randomized Clinical Evaluation) study was a randomized, double-blind, controlled trial designed to assess CRT in patients with CHF [12]. The MIRACLE trial demonstrated that CRT resulted in significant clinical improvement in patients who had moderate-to-severe heart failure and intraventricular conduction delay. All patients studied were on stable medical therapy and had no traditional existing indication for a pacemaker or ICD. The inclusion criteria for the MIRACLE study were as follows: (1) moderate or severe CHF (in NYHA functional class III or IV and 6-min walking distance of ≤450 m); (2) LVEF ≤35%; (3) widened QRS duration ≥130 ms; and (4) LV dilation (LVEDD ≥55 mm). These criteria have now been widely adopted as standard indications for CRT.

Altogether, 571 patients were enrolled in the MIRACLE study [12] from November 1998 through December 2000 from 45 centers in the United States and Canada. A total of 453 patients (228 patients in the pacing therapy group and 225 patients in the control group without pacing) completed the 6-month follow-up study. The primary end points evaluated were the NYHA functional class, quality of life, and the distance walked in 6 min (the so-called "6-min walk test"). Compared to the control group, patients assigned to the CRT group experienced an improvement in the 6-min walk distance (+39 m versus +10 m, $P = 0.005$), NYHA functional class ($P < 0.001$), quality of life (–18.0 points versus –9.0 points, $P = 0.001$), time on the treadmill during exercise testing (+81 s versus +19 s, $P = 0.001$), and LVEF (+4.6% versus –0.2%, $P < 0.001$). In addition, fewer patients in the CRT group than control patients required hospitalization (8% versus 15%, $P<0.05$) or intravenous medications (7% versus 15%, $P<0.05$) for the treatment of heart failure. In general, there was a significant reduction in QRS duration (–20 ms versus 0 ms, $P<0.001$), LV end-diastolic dimension (–3.5 mm versus 0 mm, $P<0.001$), and mitral regurgitant jet area (–2.7 cm^2 versus –0.5 cm^2, $P<0.001$). In the intention-to-treat analysis, there were 16 deaths in the control group and 12 deaths in the CRT group. However, this study was not designed or powered to assess whether CRT improves survival in this patient population. Figure 28.5 shows the Kaplan–Meier estimates of the "time-to-death or hospitalization" for worsening heart failure in the control and CRT groups. It was concluded from the MIRACLE trial that in class III and IV systolic heart failure patients with intraventricular conduction delays: (1) CRT is safe and well tolerated; (2) CRT improves quality of life, functional class, and exercise capacity; and (3) CRT improves cardiac structure and function. Note that this study used combined mortality and hospitalization rather than mortality alone as an end point; this cannot be viewed as a substitute for true mortality rate.

ICD implantation has now been accepted for primary prevention of sudden cardiac death in patients with an LVEF $\leq$35% in the United States [13, 14]. Incorporating CRT in an ICD system (CRT-D) when indicated is feasible and also provides the possibility for improvement of CHF symptoms and survival. The MIRACLE ICD trial was designed to examine the efficacy and safety of combined CRT and ICD therapy in patients with severe CHF despite appropriate medical management [15]. This

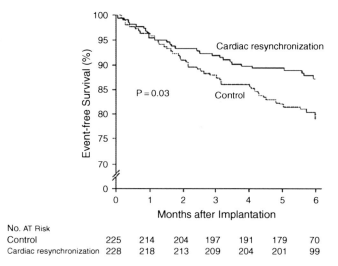

Fig. 28.5 Kaplan–Meier estimates of the time-to-death or hospitalization for worsening heart failure in the MIRACLE trial. The risk of an event was 40% lower in the resynchronization group compared to controls ($P-0.03$). Reproduced from Abraham et al. [12]. Copyright © 2002 Massachusetts Medical Society

randomized, double-blind, parallel-controlled trial was conducted from October 1999 to August 2001 in 369 patients with LVEF of 35% or less, QRS duration of at least 130 ms, at high risk of life-threatening ventricular arrhythmias, and in NYHA class III ($n=328$) or IV ($n=41$) despite optimized medical treatment. The primary double-blind study end points examined were changes between baseline and 6 months in (1) quality of life; (2) NYHA functional class; and (3) distance covered during a 6-min walk. Additional outcome measures included changes in exercise capacity, plasma neurohormones, LV function, and overall heart failure status; survival, incidence of ventricular arrhythmias, and rates of hospitalization were also compared. Of 369 randomized patients who received devices with combined CRT and ICD capabilities, 182 were controls (ICD activated, CRT off) and 187 were in the CRT group (ICD activated, CRT on). At 6 months, patients assigned to the CRT group elicited greater improvements in both median quality-of-life score and functional class than controls, but no difference in the distance walked in 6 min. Both treadmill exercise duration and peak oxygen consumption increased in the CRT group compared to controls. No significant differences were observed in changes in LV size or function, overall heart failure status, survival, and/ or rates of hospitalization. Proarrhythmia was not observed and arrhythmia termination capabilities were not impaired. It was concluded that CRT improved quality of life, functional status, and exercise capacity in patients with moderate-to-severe heart failure, a wide QRS interval, and life-threatening arrhythmias. These improvements occurred in the context of underlying appropriate medical management without proarrhythmia or compromised ICD function.

The CONTAK-CD trial enrolled 581 patients who also met conventional indications for ICD implantation [16]. Initially, patients were randomized (in a double-blind design) to either Biv or no pacing groups for 3 months and then crossed over to the opposite assignment for the next 3 months ($n=248$), but the scheme was later changed to a 6-month parallel control design ($n=333$). The primary end point analysis was a composite of mortality, heart failure hospitalizations, and episodes of ventricular arrhythmias, which was found to be not statistically significant. However, the 6-min walk test, NYHA class, and peak aerobic capacity were significantly improved with CRT, particularly in patients with NYHA class III/IV heart failure.

The COMPANION (Comparison of Medical Therapy, Pacing, and Defibrillation in Heart Failure) trial enrolled a total of 1,520 patients with advanced heart failure (NYHA class III or IV) due to ischemic or nonischemic cardiomyopathy and a QRS interval of at least

120 ms [17]. These patients were randomly assigned into a 1:2:2 ratio to receive optimal pharmacologic therapy alone (diuretics, angiotensin-converting-enzyme inhibitors, beta-blockers, and spironolactone) or in combination with CRT with either a pacemaker (CRT-P) or a pacemaker-defibrillator (CRT-D). The primary composite end point studied was the time to death or hospitalization for any cause. As compared to optimal pharmacologic therapy alone, CRT-P decreased the risk of the primary end point (hazard ratio, 0.81; $P = 0.014$), as did CRT-D (hazard ratio, 0.80; $P = 0.01$). The risk of the combined end point of death and hospitalization for heart failure was reduced by 34% in the CRT-P group ($P < 0.002$) and by 40% in the CRT-D group ($P < 0.001$), in comparison with the pharmacologic therapy group. There was a strong trend toward a reduction (by 24%) in the secondary end point of death from any cause ($P = 0.059$) in patients randomized with a CRT-P alone, and a CRT-D reduced the risk by 36% ($P = 0.003$). The investigators concluded that in patients with advanced heart failure and a prolonged QRS interval, CRT-P decreased the combined risk of death from any cause or first hospitalization and, combined with an implantable defibrillator (CRT-D), this significantly reduced mortality.

Altogether, 813 patients with NYHA class III or IV heart failure due to LV systolic dysfunction and cardiac dyssynchrony were enrolled in the CARE-HF (Cardiac Resynchronization-Heart Failure) trial [18]. These patients, who were receiving standard pharmacologic therapy, were randomly assigned to receive medical therapy alone or with CRT without defibrillators. The primary study end point was the time to death from any cause or an unplanned hospitalization for a major cardiovascular event; the principal secondary end point was death from any cause. These patients were followed for a mean time period of 29.4 months. The primary end point was reached by 159 patients in the CRT group, as compared to only 224 patients in the medical therapy group (39% versus 55%; $P < 0.001$). There were 82 deaths in the CRT group, as compared to 120 in the medical therapy group (20% versus 30%; $P < 0.002$). Also, CRT: (1) reduced the interventricular mechanical delay, the end-systolic volume index, and the area of the mitral regurgitant jet; (2) increased the LVEF; and (3) improved symptoms and quality of life ($P < 0.01$ for all comparisons), compared to the medical therapy group. The authors concluded that, in patients with CHF and cardiac dyssynchrony, CRT improves symptoms and patient's quality of life and reduces complications and the risk of death. Importantly, these pacing benefits are in addition to those afforded by standard pharmacologic therapy. More recently, a subsequent extended follow-up analysis of CARE-HF confirmed sustained CRT-P benefit [19].

28.2.4 Effects of CRT on Mechanical Remodeling

Cardiac myocytes are known to adapt to changes in hemodynamic load. *Ventricular remodeling* refers to changes in LV geometry, mass, and volume in response to myocardial injury or alterations in load. The extent of LV dilatation or remodeling after myocardial infarction or in patients with heart failure is a strong predictor of both morbidity and mortality. Angiotensin-converting enzyme inhibitors and β-adrenergic blockers, to some degree, reduce LV remodeling and thus improve survival in patients with LV dysfunction.

Chronic dyssynchronous electrical activation, such as long-term pacing or left bundle branch block, induces redistribution of cardiac mass. Furthermore, chronic RV apical pacing may adversely alter cellular growth, especially in the young, at the cellular and subcellular levels. These disturbances may contribute to diminished function observed clinically, such as increased myocardial perfusion defects and regional wall motion abnormalities, reduced LVEF, and diastolic dysfunction. Short-term RV apical pacing is associated with impaired LV pump function and relaxation. Additionally, long-term RV apical pacing may result in permanent impairment of LV function.

On the other hand, CRT has been shown to result in *reverse remodeling* in selected patients with CHF. In other words, CRT not only improves cardiac function but also slows down or reverses undesired electrical, mechanical, and anatomic progressive disease changes in selected patients. For example, chronic CRT may be associated with changes in axis without changes in QRS duration or lead dislocation, suggesting possible CRT-induced electrical remodeling. In one study, researchers demonstrated that 3 months of CRT was associated with reduced LV end-systolic and end-diastolic volume by 33 and 24%, respectively [20]. Another study using serial Doppler echocardiograms at baseline and at 6 and 12 months after CRT, in 228 patients enrolled in the MIRACLE trial, suggested that reverse LV remodeling and symptom benefits with CRT are sustained at 12 months in patients with NYHA class III/IV heart failure; this occurred to a lesser degree in patients with an ischemic versus a nonischemic etiology. Ischemic cardiomyopathy may reduce the potential for reverse remodeling by CRT; this is most likely due to the inexorable progression of ischemic disease. Patients with severe resting perfusion defects do not show significant improvement in LVEF or reduction in LV volumes despite clinical improvement. Yet, this may be correlated to the site as well as the extent of myocardial fibrosis developed from a previous infarction.

It is currently believed that effects of CRT on exercise tolerance and hemodynamics reach their plateau in

3 months in most patients, although delayed responses can also be seen. However, reverse remodeling may take longer (a year or more). More recent data show that LV reverse remodeling and beneficial echocardiographic changes were sustained throughout 2 years of follow-up.

28.2.5 Effects of CRT on Autonomic Activity

Sympathetic activity is commonly increased in patients with CHF, as evidenced by elevated levels of circulating norepinephrine levels and increases in adrenergic nerve outflow. Enhanced sympathetic responses in CHF may play an initial compensatory role in the early disease process; however, chronic adrenergic activation is associated with a vicious cycle that, in itself, will promote progression of the disease through multiple effects, including increased afterload, a direct "toxic" effect on the failing myocardium, increased myocardial oxygen demand, and increased susceptibility to ventricular arrhythmias. As such, elevated plasma norepinephrine levels have been shown to correlate with increased cardiac mortality rates and are a better prognostic predictor than LVEF itself. This has formed the pathophysiologic basis for β-blocker therapy in treatment of moderate CHF.

LV-based pacing has been shown to improve hemodynamics and decrease sympathetic nerve activity compared to RV pacing in patients with LV dysfunction, regardless of the QRS duration. CRT also results in a decrease in sympathetic nerve activity associated with improved hemodynamics, compared to intrinsic conduction in patients with LV dysfunction and intraventricular conduction delays. CRT significantly decreases the plasma concentrations of norepinephrine and N-terminal fragment of pro-brain natriuretic peptide, especially in dilated heart failure patients with the greatest sympathetic activation at baseline. Long-term CRT is often associated with decreased heart rate, suggesting that chronic CRT may have a positive impact on cardiac performance and mortality. Yet, the mechanism underlying the decrease in sympathetic activity by CRT is unclear, presumably due to reduction of sympathetic stimulation from cardiac dyssynchrony as well as the secondary effect following improvement of cardiac function provided by CRT. Since activation of sympathetic activity is directly associated with the severity of CHF, perhaps reversible sympathoinhibition may be used as a marker of the clinical response to CRT.

28.2.6 Effects of CRT on Cardiac Energetics

There is evidence that ventricular pacing is associated with increased myocardial oxygen consumption in hearts without intraventricular conduction delay [21]. Yet, CRT is reported not to increase myocardial oxygen consumption in patients with left bundle branch block [22, 23]. In contrast, dobutamine to achieve similar systolic changes induced by CRT significantly increased energy cost (Fig. 28.6). CRT also induces favorable changes in coronary and peripheral arterial function; changes in peripheral blood flow are related to patients' improvement and may be prognostically significant [24].

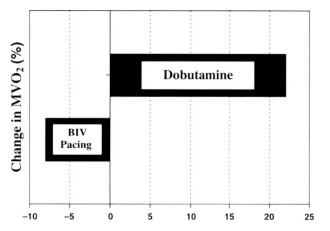
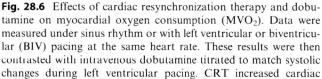
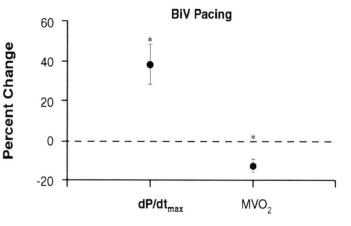

Fig. 28.6 Effects of cardiac resynchronization therapy and dobutamine on myocardial oxygen consumption (MVO_2). Data were measured under sinus rhythm or with left ventricular or biventricular (BIV) pacing at the same heart rate. These results were then contrasted with intravenous dobutamine titrated to match systolic changes during left ventricular pacing. CRT increased cardiac function with reduced MVO_2. In contrast, dobutamine raised dP/dt_{max} accompanied by a rise in per-beat MVO_2 ($P<0.05$ versus pacing). It was concluded that ventricular resynchronization by CRT in patients with left bundle branch block acutely enhances systolic function while modestly lowering energy cost

Long-term CRT is also considered to induce beneficial effects on myocardial efficiency at rest in patients with CHF; yet these effects are not directly associated with changes in myocardial perfusion or oxygen consumption. During dobutamine-induced stress, CRT does not affect functional parameters, but myocardial efficiency and metabolic reserve may be increased. Resting myocardial blood flow is unaltered by CRT despite an increase in LV function. In fact, the distribution pattern of resting myocardial blood flow becomes more homogeneous; hyperemic myocardial blood flow and, consequently, myocardial blood flow reserve are enhanced by CRT. This is consistent with our clinical impression that CRT significantly improves functional status regardless of the etiology of cardiomyopathy (ischemic or nonischemic) and without increasing mortality in ischemic patients. CRT-induced functional improvements are also shown to be associated with favorable changes in established molecular markers of CHF, including genes that regulate contractile function and pathologic hypertrophy [25].

28.2.7 Effects of CRT on Cardiac Arrhythmias

CRT may eventually alter the substrate responsible for ventricular arrhythmias and thus change the overall risk for ventricular arrhythmias. In addition, there is evidence that CRT may inhibit reentry, decrease the incidence of spontaneous ventricular arrhythmias (ectopy), and/or decrease inducibility of ventricular tachycardia. Appropriate ICD therapy occurs in approximately 21% of the primary prevention patients and 35% of the secondary prevention patients within 2 years after implant [26]. To date, there are limited data indicating that CRT reduces appropriate ICD therapy. Furthermore, in rare cases, CRT may suppress refractory ventricular tachycardia or electrical storm which is not well controlled by drugs or RV DDD pacing. It has been shown that Biv antitachycardia pacing may be more effective than RV antitachycardia pacing, but the role of Biv antitachycardia pacing remains controversial.

Although controversy exists, proposed mechanisms underlying these antiarrhythmic benefits of CRT are: (1) prevention of reentry; (2) improvement of cardiac function and myocardial perfusion; (3) reduction of sympathetic activity; and/or (4) decrease in ventricular dispersion of repolarization, including QT dispersion (Fig. 28.7). However, a pacing-induced increase in QT dispersion may predict sudden cardiac death following CRT [27]. Of interest is that epicardial LV pacing causes a much greater increase in spatial dispersion of ventricular repolarization than Biv pacing in CHF patients; as such, transvenous Biv pacing

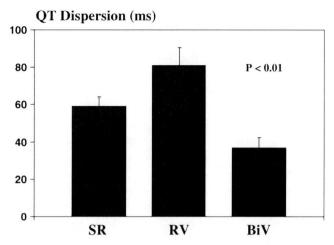

Fig. 28.7 Effect of biventricular pacing on QT dispersion. QT dispersion was measured in 10 heart failure patients treated with cardiac resynchronization therapy (6 males and 4 females, aged 62 ± 8 years and LVEF $19\pm7\%$). There was no significant difference in QT intervals between right ventricular (RV) pacing and sinus rhythm (SR) (437 ± 36 ms versus 426 ± 28 ms, $P=0.26$). QT intervals were significantly shorter during biventricular pacing (BiV) (407 ± 30 ms) than during RV pacing (437 ± 36 ms, $P<0.01$) and sinus rhythm (426 ± 28 ms, $P<0.01$). QT dispersion was significantly increased during RV pacing compared to sinus rhythm (81 ± 30 ms versus 59 ± 16 ms, $P<0.01$). BiV was associated with less QT dispersion (37 ± 17 ms) compared to sinus rhythm (59 ± 16 ms, $P=0.01$) and RV pacing (81 ± 30 ms, $P<0.01$). This was also true after correction of QRS durations. It seems that BiV pacing is associated with less QT dispersion, which may play a role in prevention of sudden cardiac death in heart failure patients treated with CRT [54]

may have a substantial advantage over epicardial LV pacing in minimizing the proarrhythmic perturbation of ventricular repolarization in association with CRT [28].

In rare cases, sustained ventricular arrhythmias requiring frequent ICD treatment may occur immediately following implantation of Biv devices. Temporarily turning off CRT may sometimes help reduce frequent ICD discharges. It is considered that, during CRT with ischemia, pacing at high-voltage output with a long interventricular delay is more likely to induce ventricular arrhythmias, particularly when left and right pacing results in a conduction pattern orthogonal to the ventricular myocardial fiber orientation. However, data from major randomized clinical trials involving the use of ICD and CRT-D devices showed that, regarding classified deaths, appropriate ICD therapies outnumbered control group sudden cardiac deaths by a factor of 2–3 in some studies [29]. Nevertheless, the potential proarrhythmic effects of CRT should be considered when CRT is employed.

To date, the question whether or not CRT reduces the incidence of atrial fibrillation remains undefined. Nonetheless, the beneficial effects of CRT are observed in some nonrandomized studies, particularly after AV nodal ablation.

28.2.8 Effects of CRT on Mortality

Sudden cardiac death accounts for up to half of death in patients with CHF; a significant number of patients may die suddenly despite improvement in cardiac function. A widened QRS duration is associated with increased mortality in patients with CHF [30]. Prior to the indication of ICD for primary prevention in CHF patients, it was estimated that approximately 20% of ICD patients had indications for CRT at the time of implantation.

Although most of the early studies were not designed or powerful enough to determine the effects of CRT on overall survival, it seems to be safe to implant CRT without a backup defibrillator (CRT-P). In support, current data (i.e., COMPANION trial and CARF-HF trial) suggest that CRT may decrease (or at least not increase) mortality rates in patients with CHF [17, 18]. The benefits of CRT persist at least 2.5–3 years postimplantation; reduction in mortality is due to fewer deaths from both worsening heart failure and sudden death [19].

A recently published multicenter longitudinal observational trial indicated that patients with advanced heart failure and a wide QRS complex, routinely treated with CRT, elicited a favorable long-term outcome that was reproducible at different centers [31]. This study was performed in 1,303 consecutive patients with ischemic or nonischemic cardiomyopathy, all on optimal pharmacologic therapy, treated from August 1995 to August 2004 at four European centers with CRT-P (44%) or with CRT-D for symptomatic heart failure and prolonged QRS duration. The leading cause of death in these patients was found to be heart failure.

A recent meta-analysis showed that CRT, in general, reduces mortality from progressive heart failure in patients with symptomatic LV dysfunction [32]. This finding suggests that CRT may have a substantial impact on the most common mechanism of death among patients with advanced heart failure. Pooled data from five trials (preliminary COMPANION data with CONTAK-CD, InSync ICD, MIRACLE, and MUSTIC) show a significant reduction in all-cause mortality [33]. Importantly, compared to optimal medical therapy, CRT alone reduces all-cause mortality in patients with advanced CHF, predominantly reducing worsening heart failure mortality [34].

At present, patients eligible for CRT are usually indicated for defibrillator implantation for primary prevention of sudden cardiac death, and thus CRT-P is rarely used in the United States. Due to the well-known fact that there is no ideal method with high predictive value for identifying high-risk patients, the safest strategy should be to advise a combined ICD-CRT device (CRT-D) for patients with indication for CRT. Total mortality is expected to be 20% lower with ICD backup (95% CI 42% lower to 17% higher) due to a protective effect against sudden cardiac death [31]. The InSync/InSync ICD Italian Registry showed that the annual total mortality rate was 10% during a 3-year follow-up after CRT [35]. It seems that ischemic etiology along with NYHA class IV is associated with higher risk of death. On the other hand, a 5% or more increase in LVEF after 3 months was associated with a better long-term survival [36].

28.2.9 Upgrade to Biv Pacing in Patients with Pacing-Induced CHF

Not only is spontaneous permanent left bundle branch block harmful to patients, but the iatrogenic variety produced by RV apical pacing during conventional permanent pacing may also be deleterious to some patients. In fact, RV apical pacing-induced dyssynchrony may lead, in some cases, to appearance or worsening of CHF symptoms. Alteration of activation pattern during RV pacing may lead to histological and functional remodeling of the LV, including inhomogeneous thickening of the ventricular myocardium and myofibrillar disarray, fibrosis, disturbances in ion-handling protein expression, myocardial perfusion defects, alterations in sympathetic tone, and/or mitral regurgitation. Mid- and long-term studies have demonstrated a progressive decline in LVEF and other indices of LV functional competence. Upgrading RV pacing systems to Biv resynchronization modalities is thus a theoretically promising option for paced patients with worsening HF; this has been demonstrated in a few non-randomized trials [37]. Yet, as with CRT, it is difficult to predict patients who will ultimately benefit from upgrading of RV pacing systems to Biv resynchronization modalities.

28.2.10 CRT After AV Nodal Ablation

Animal studies have demonstrated that LV-based pacing is associated with better hemodynamics in the presence or absence of complete AV block [2], potentially demonstrating the importance of LV-based pacing in patients after AV nodal ablation. Recent clinical studies have confirmed this observation.

Specifically, the PAVE study investigated the effects of Biv pacing in patients undergoing ablation of the AV node for management of atrial fibrillation with rapid ventricular rates [38]. This study enrolled 184 patients requiring AV node ablation who were randomized to receive a Biv pacing system (n = 103) or a RV pacing system ($n = 81$). Compared to patients receiving RV pacing at 6-month postablation, patients treated with CRT elicited a significant improvement in 6-min walk distance (82.9 ± 94.7 m versus 61.2 ± 90.0 m, $P = 0.04$) and LVEF (0.46 ± 0.13 versus 0.41 ± 0.13, $P = 0.03$), but no significant differences in the quality-of-life parameters. It appears that patients with LVEF $\leq 45\%$ or with NYHA class II/III symptoms have greater potential for improvements in their 6-min walk distance. It was concluded that for patients undergoing AV nodal ablation for fast atrial fibrillation, Biv pacing provides a significant improvement in the 6-min hallway walk test and LVEF compared to RV pacing. Note that these beneficial effects of CRT appear to be greater in patients with impaired systolic function or with symptomatic heart failure. The benefits of CRT in CHF patients with ventricular conduction disturbance and permanent atrial fibrillation sustain long-term (up to 4 years) improvements of LV function and functional capacity after AV nodal ablation; this was found to be similar to patients in sinus rhythm [39].

Although cardiac function during LV-based pacing is considered better than RV pacing, either LV or RV pacing is inferior to intrinsic AV conduction during sinus rhythm, atrial pacing, or His bundle pacing in the absence of intraventricular conduction delay or dyssynchrony [2]. In other words, LV pacing is associated with fewer detrimental effects on cardiac function compared to RV pacing. Thus, His bundle pacing should be preferred in patients following AV nodal ablation for refractory atrial fibrillation. We have recently developed a new technique for easy implantation of a pacemaker lead for His bundle pacing in this clinical scenario (Fig. 28.8) [40].

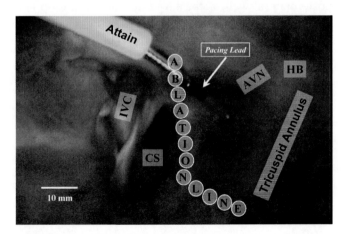

Fig. 28.8 Isolated atrial segment for His bundle pacing equivalent. A small segment of atrial tissue around the atrioventricular node (AVN) and His (HS) bundle is isolated using catheter ablation. Compared to pacing lead placement directly to the His bundle, it is relatively easier to place a lead within the isolated segment. Pacing from the isolated segment will activate the AV node and His–Purkinje system, achieving bundle pacing equivalent [40]. CS, coronary sinus; IVC, inferior vena cava

28.2.11 Application of CRT in Other Clinical Settings

Limited data that are currently available or show CRT may improve cardiac function in patients with right heart failure, functional mitral regurgitation, or bridging for cardiac transplantation. Yet, temporary epicardial LV (instead of conventional RV) pacing has shown to be beneficial in postcardiac surgical patients; this may particularly be useful as a temporary measure in cases of acute heart failure after cardiac surgery.

Several clinical trials are also underway to evaluate the potential of CRT in other heart failure populations as described in the following. Note that it will be several years, however, before the results of these trials become available.

1. The Biventricular versus Right Ventricular Pacing in Heart Failure Patients with Atrioventricular Block (BLOCK-HF) trial, sponsored by Medtronic, Inc. (Minneapolis, MN), is evaluating whether CRT can slow the progression of heart failure in patients with NYHA class I, II, or III heart failure and a traditional bradycardia indication for pacing.

2. The Resynchronization reVerses Remodeling in Systolic left Ventricular dysfunction (REVERSE) trial, sponsored by Medtronic, Inc., and the Multicenter Automatic Implantable Defibrillator Trial (MADIT)-CRT study, sponsored by Guidant Corporation, now Boston Scientific (St. Paul, MN), are investigating whether CRT is of benefit to patients with NYHA class I or II heart failure and a wide QRS complex.

3. CRT for CHF patients with narrow QRS complexes and coexisting mechanical dyssynchrony may result in LV reverse remodeling and improvement of clinical status. The amplitude of benefit is similar to the wide QRS group, provided that a similar extent of systolic dyssynchrony is selected [41]. Unfortunately, this observation has not been confirmed by other studies [42]. The Evaluation of Screening Techniques in Electrically-Normal, Mechanically-Dyssynchronous Heart Failure Patients Receiving CRT (ESTEEM) trial, sponsored by Boston Scientific, and the Resynchronization Therapy in Normal QRS Clinical Investigation (RETHINQ) trial, sponsored by St. Jude Medical Inc. (St Paul, MN), are evaluating the use of CRT in patients with significant heart failure and a narrow QRS but have echocardiographic evidence of dyssynchrony.

28.3 Optimal Pacing Configuration

28.3.1 Left Ventricular Versus Biventricular Pacing

Both Biv pacing and LV pacing alone for heart failure result in hemodynamic improvements, despite marked electromechanical differences. In general, LV pacing may result in more homogeneous but substantially delayed LV contraction, leading to shortened filling time and less reduction in postsystolic contraction. Yet, occasionally, single-site LV pacing provides even better hemodynamic responses both at rest and during exercise compared to Biv pacing.

Both interventricular and intraventricular dyssynchrony can cause prolonged QRS duration. However, intraventricular dyssynchrony may play a more important role in degradation of the hemodynamic status compared to interventricular dyssynchrony. This is probably why LV pacing provides similar clinical benefits to those induced by CRT (e.g., relative to RVA pacing). Nevertheless, the ultimate goal of CRT is to provide more cardiac synchrony and possibly subsequent hemodynamic benefits compared to LV pacing alone, as optimal A to V and V to V delays can be programmed (see below). Further, the technical difficulty in securing an LV lead in the coronary sinus (CS) may be a precaution against the use of LV pacing alone in a pacemaker-dependent patient.

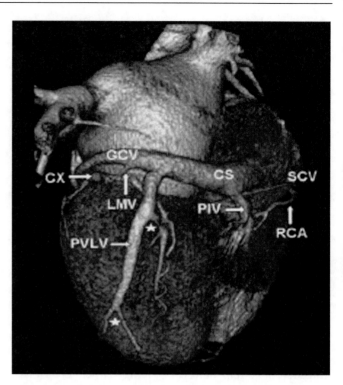

Fig. 28.9 Noninvasive visualization of the cardiac venous system using 64-slice computed tomography (posterolateral view). The first tributary of the coronary sinus (CS) is the posterior interventricular vein (PIV), running in the posterior interventricular groove. The second tributary of the CS is the posterior vein of the left ventricle (PVLV) with several side branches (*asterisks*). The next tributary is the left marginal vein (LMV). The great cardiac vein (GCV) will then continue as the anterior cardiac vein in the anterior interventricular groove. Also note the circumflex coronary artery (CX) and right coronary artery (RCA) [80]. SCV, small cardiac vein

28.3.2 Optimal Pacing Site

Pacing-induced changes in cardiac function depend importantly on the pacing site and timing relative to intrinsic activation. In several studies, it was reported that pacing from the high RV septum or RV outflow tract did not provide significant benefits compared to RV apical pacing [43, 44]. However, some pacing positions in the RV leading to the greatest QRS shortening may be associated with better beneficial outcomes [45].

Although LV pacing is associated with hemodynamic advantages compared to RV pacing, the optimal LV pacing sites are yet to be determined and will likely vary to some extent from patient to patient. During RV pacing, the posterior or posteroinferior base of the LV is usually the latest activation site. The PATH-CHF study showed that the mid-lateral wall of the LV may be the optimal site for CRT compared to other sites of the LV [46, 47]. To date, placement of a CS lead to a certain location of the LV depends importantly on the improvement of pacer lead technology. Currently, the lateral or

posterolateral wall of the LV is considered the optimal implanting site for CRT and should be targeted for CS lead placement. A posterior or lateral branch of the coronary venous system is available on retrograde CS venograms in a majority of patients (Fig. 28.9). However, optimizing the pacing site using epicardial leads may produce functional improvement up to 40% compared to random pace site selection.

Pacing at the anterior wall of the LV is associated with improved cardiac function and functional capacity, but is inferior to pacing at the posterolateral wall of the LV (Fig. 28.10) [48]. Yet, this improvement does not appear to dramatically influence mortality.

28.3.3 Optimal AV Delay

Optimal AV synchrony is fundamentally important to improve cardiac function mainly due to optimal ventricular filling and diminished systolic mitral and tricuspid

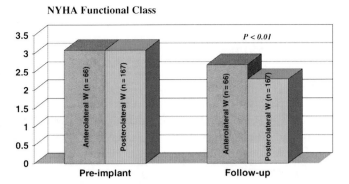

NYHA Functional Class

Fig. 28.10 Effects of coronary sinus lead position. Placement of the coronary sinus lead in the lateral and posterolateral branches is associated with significant improvement in functional capacity and greater improvement in left ventricular function compared to the anterior coronary sinus location. This improvement does not appear to influence mortality. Reproduced from J Cardiovasc Electrophysiol 2004 with permission from publisher [48]

regurgitation. This may contribute more to hemodynamic improvement than to correction of intraventricular conduction defects in some clinical settings. Thus, careful programming or subsequent reprogramming of the AV delays can be associated with significant hemodynamic benefits. Systolic performance of the dilated ventricle that depends on an elevated preload is critically affected by the appropriate timing of the AV delay during exercise. In contrast to normal pacemaker patients, the relatively short baseline AV delay in CRT should be prolonged at increased heart rates. However, this has to be balanced between LV filling and fusion of conducted and pacing signals.

The definition and techniques for adequate AV optimization remain to be fully investigated. In the MIRA-CLE trial, all patients underwent an AV optimization for optimal diastolic filling. Using a transmitral Doppler study, AV delays were adjusted to maximally prolong the LV diastolic filling time without truncating the A wave (i.e., atrial kick). This approach emphasizes the importance of AV optimization for ventricular filling, but draws attention away from improvement of overall cardiac function using CRT. Other methods used for AV optimization and programming include assessment of cardiac output, mitral regurgitation, aortic flow, and pulse pressure.

28.3.4 Optimal Interventricular Delay and Sequential Biv Pacing

Interventricular dyssynchrony contributes to impairment of cardiac function. Improved interventricular synchrony

provided by CRT is important for evaluating the efficacy of CRT. Since the location and degree of ventricular dyssynchrony is different amongst patients, it is more logical to provide an individualized synchronizing stimulation protocol or V–V timing for each patient. As such, tissue Doppler imaging, with tissue tracking that detects the segments with delayed longitudinal contractions and their locations, can be used to determine optimum interventricular delay programming during CRT. Yet, different degrees of fusion of paced activation and supraventricular conducted activation through the His–Purkinje system may influence intraventricular synchrony as well; this further implies the importance of AV optimization.

Compared to simultaneous Biv pacing, a sequential Biv pacing protocol may significantly improve LV systolic and diastolic performance. In one such comparative study, there was an associated and significant increase of LV dP/dt with no change in RV dP/dt with sequential Biv pacing [49]. Earlier activation of the RV was not beneficial in the majority of patients, and the highest LV dP/dt was achieved when the LV was stimulated before the RV (usually by 40 ms) [49]. Other studies showed that the V–V interval required for achieving maximal hemodynamic improvement by CRT may be less (with LV 10–20 ms earlier than RV) [50]. The InSync III study was a synchronization trial examining the safety of sequential RV and LV pacing. Echocardiographic optimization of sequential CRT (Medtronic InSync III, Model 8042) in 189 patients showed an improvement in stroke volume compared to simultaneous stimulation at baseline and at a 3-month follow-up [50]. In 88% (30/34) of the patients, these improvements were seen within a small range of V–V delays of ±20 ms and in 94% (32/34) within V–V delays of ±40 ms. In contrast, programming beyond this range reduced stroke volume below that of simultaneous Biv pacing. Importantly, at a 6-month follow-up, InSync III patients experienced greater improvement in the 6-min hall walk, NYHA functional class, and quality of life compared to controls [51]. Optimization of the sequential pacing increased (median 7.3%) stroke volume in 77% of patients; no additional improvement in NYHA functional class or quality of life was seen compared to the simultaneous CRT group; however, InSync III patients demonstrated greater exercise capacity.

In general, V–V timing is less important than A–V synchrony. Yet, optimal V–V timing-induced hemodynamic advantages might be of clinical significance in selected cases, such as non-responders to simultaneous Biv pacing.

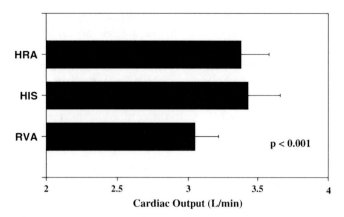

Fig. 28.11 Cardiac output during His bundle pacing (HIS) in normal hearts. There is a 12% increase in cardiac output during His bundle pacing compared to right ventricular apical (RVA) pacing. HRA, high right apical pacing. Reproduced from J Cardiovasc Electrophysiol 1999 with permission from Blackwell Publishing [2]

28.3.5 His Bundle Pacing

One of the main objectives underlying CRT is the correction of an abnormal ventricular activation sequence. If multisite pacing is truly able to improve cardiac function by resynchronizing the ventricular activation sequence, there should be no better pacing site than the His bundle, that is, in the absence of intraventricular conduction defects. Not surprisingly, His bundle pacing is associated with better cardiac function in a normal heart (Fig. 28.11). The benefit of His bundle pacing exists in the presence or absence of AV synchrony.

28.3.6 Other Pacing Modalities

Animal studies have shown that nonexcitatory stimulation (paired) improves LV function in an animal model with left bundle branch block, without affecting transmitral valve flow or subsequent LV diastolic function. Yet, the role of paired stimulation based on the postextrasystolic potentiation effect to augment ventricular function in the failing ventricle is inconclusive.

Early studies showed that *dual site* or *bifocal* RV pacing (apex and outflow tract) does not improve hemodynamics despite a narrowing QRS duration [52], since mechanical coordination plays a dominant role in global systolic improvement in LV-based pacing. Recent studies suggest that bifocal RV pacing may improve LV hemodynamics by decreasing the interventricular and intraventricular conduction delays in selected patients. When this pacing modality is used, the leads in the RV should be placed at the longest achievable distance. In general, it remains the consensus that Biv pacing is superior to bifocal RV pacing.

28.4 Implantation and Follow-Up of Biv Pacemakers

28.4.1 Implantation Considerations

The key portion of the procedure for implantation of a CRT device is the placement of the LV lead. Clinical studies on CRT in humans have mainly consisted of Biv pacing modalities with LV pacing transvenously via a CS lead or, less commonly, through a thoracotomy. It is usually necessary to target specific sites (posterolateral or lateral walls of the LV) to maximize hemodynamic benefits. However, limitations and variations of coronary vein anatomy, as well as patient safety, lead dislodgement, pacing thresholds, lead handling, and ease-of-use issues present technical challenges for current transvenous pacing lead designs; see Chapter 27.

During implantation, two views of CS venograms are usually obtained first to provide a "road map" of the venous anatomy and then to guide selection of CS leads. Several delivery systems (including steerable catheters, venogram balloon catheters, and guiding sheaths with different curves) have been developed. The current over-the-wire lead system has significantly reduced the implant failure rate and enabled clinicians to avoid other more invasive means of LV lead implantation. Additionally, use of a preshaped sheath may facilitate cannulation of the CS for implantation of CRT devices. Introduction of new delivering sheaths (various shapes, sheath-in-sheath, and side-hole) have improved successful CS lead placement rates. In some patients, CS angioplasty may be used for functional and structural CS stenosis.

Some investigators have implanted the LV lead through the transseptal approach for LV endocardial pacing. This seems more feasible in patients who require chronic anticoagulation, but it is not without potential thromboembolic risk. Epicardial placement into the anterior paraseptum, which may pace both ventricles synchronously and may increase cardiac output, is another practical but relatively untested approach. Like routine implantation of other pacers and defibrillators, it has been reported that Biv pacers can also be implanted in patients with elevated INRs; however, this is not routinely recommended, given bleeding risks.

If patients fail CS lead placement in our institution, we usually refer them for robotic-assisted epicardial LV lead placement through a minithoracotomy (see Chapter 32). Epicardial lead placement has been shown to be safe with benefits equivalent to those of CS leads. Finally, it is possible, in a patient with an existing right-sided device, that CRT can be achieved using two pacemakers and the triggered VVT mode [53].

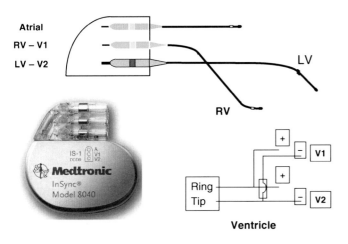

Fig. 28.12 Pacing configuration of Medtronic InSync pacemaker (model 8040). Courtesy of Medtronic, Inc. LV, left ventricle; RV, right ventricle

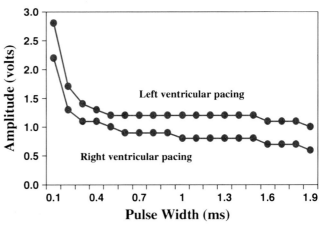

Fig. 28.13 The strength–duration curves. The strength–duration curves were measured in four patients during right ventricular apical pacing and during coronary vein left ventricular pacing with cardiac resynchronization therapy with a lead in the lateral wall of the left ventricle (Guidant, 4512). It appears that there is no substantial difference in the shape of the two curves, although pacing threshold was higher during coronary sinus pacing [54]

28.4.2 Intraprocedural Testing

The early CRT pacer (such as InSync model 8040 pacemaker, Fig. 28.12) has three lead outlets with a Y adaptor in the header for RV and LV leads. The combined sensing of the two ventricles (that may be separated by 80–150 ms) requires additional considerations in device programming to avoid double sensing. Currently, most commercially available LV leads are unipolar with a shared common ring bipolar sensing/pacing RV lead. The output of LV and RV leads is separated from each other and, during lead positioning, each threshold should be measured in a unipolar manner. Nevertheless, final thresholds should be determined using the intended pacing configuration after device connection. It is important to note that the pacing threshold for LV pacing from the CS is consistently higher compared to that during endocardial RV pacing (Fig. 28.13) [54]. It seems that the shape of the strength–duration curve during coronary vein LV pacing is not significantly different from that during endocardial RV pacing; the combined lead impedance is less than that of either lead and is typically in the range of 400 Ω. To date, note that a bipolar lead is usually thicker than a unipolar lead and may be used to minimize potential diaphragmatic stimulation and possibly to reduce high pacing threshold.

28.4.3 Risks and Complications

In the early implanting stage of CRT devices, of the 528 patients who underwent successful implantation in the MIRACLE study [12], the median duration of the procedure was 2.7 h (range of 0.9–7.3). Implantation of the system was unsuccessful in 8% of patients and was complicated by refractory hypotension, bradycardia, or asystole in four patients (two of whom died) and by perforation of the CS requiring pericardiocentesis in two others. Dissection or perforation of the CS or cardiac vein occurred in about 6%, and other serious complications (including complete heart block, hemopericardium, and cardiac arrest) presented in about 1.2% of patients [55]. Other complications included later lead revision (6%) and system explantation due to infection (1.3%). Other rare cases included malposition of the CS lead into the LV via a patent foramen ovale. The complication rate within 24 h following implantation was approximately 10% (mainly lead dislodgment of 2.2% and CS dissection/perforation of 2.1%). Lead dislodgement (2.8%) was the main complication between 24 h and 30 days after implantation [55].

A relatively recent analysis of the outcomes of transvenous CRT system implantation in 2,078 patients from the MIRACLE study, the MIRACLE ICD study, and the InSync III study has been published [56]. The implant attempt succeeded in 1,903 of 2,078 (91.6%) patients. Implant time decreased from 2.7 h in the MIRACLE study to 2.3 h in the InSync III study and from 2.8 h in the MIRACLE ICD study randomized phase to 2.4 h in the general phase. The implant procedure produced a 9.3% perioperative complication rate in MIRACLE trial patients, a 21.1% rate in the MIRACLE ICD study randomized phase patients, a 13.9% rate in the general phase patients, and an 8.8% complication rate in InSync

III study patients. A total complication rate of 11.7% was observed in MIRACLE trial patients, 11.9% in MIRACLE ICD study randomized phase patients, 11.0% in the general phase patients, and 8.6% in InSync III study patients. In all studies taken together, 8% of patients required reoperations to treat lead dislodgement, extracardiac stimulation, or infection during follow-up.

To date, transvenous CRT system implantation appears safe and well tolerated and has a high success rate; it will continue to improve with operator experience and the addition of new technologies [57]. It should be noted that extraction of LV CRT leads remains a concern, and published experience is rare. However, preliminary data show that CS leads (14±12 months old) can be safely extracted.

28.4.4 Follow-Up

"Pacemaker syndrome" has been reported with a CRT system. Frequent ICD discharges due to double sensing associated with Biv devices have also been well documented and were relatively common when a Y adaptor was used for both RV and LV sensing/pacing in the early devices. Fortunately, appropriate programming can prevent these episodes of inappropriate shocks.

In rare cases, a subsequent RV activation via antero-grade AV nodal conduction, sensed by the RV electrode, can trigger CRT and left atrial capture from CS lead, perpetuating an orthodromic pacemaker-mediated tachycardia in a patient in whom a Biv system is present without an atrial electrode. In these cases, because the left atrial threshold was often higher than the LV threshold in the CS, the problem could be resolved by lowering the output of the CS electrode.

Any loss of LV capture in patients with CRT devices may account for worsening heart failure and can be difficult to diagnose without a programmer. An electrocardiogram-based algorithm may be useful to initially detect loss of LV capture during CRT (Fig. 28.14) [58]. Loss of LV capture can be accurately detected by the ECG algorithm based on analysis of the R–S ratio on leads V_1 and I of the surface electrocardiogram with sensitivity of 94% and specificity of 93%.

Based on the follow-up data from the VENTAK CHF/CONTAK-CD CRT study in 443 patients, CRT is interrupted in 36% of the patients after successful implantation of a CRT-D device. Fortunately, CRT can be reinstituted in most patients and has a high long-term (2.5 years) retention rate (83%).

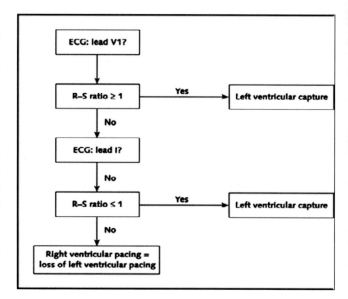

Fig. 28.14 An ECG-based algorithm to detect loss of left ventricular capture during biventricular pacing. Loss of left ventricular capture can be accurately detected by an algorithm based on analysis of the R–S ratio on lead V_1 and lead I of the surface ECG with sensitivity of 94% and specificity of 93%. Reproduced from Ann Intern Med 2005 with permission from publisher [58]

28.5 Prediction of CRT Efficacy

One of the most important and yet major challenges in the field of CRT pacing for CHF is the preimplant identification of patients who will benefit most from Biv pacing. To date, a majority of patients respond to Biv pacing (approximately two-thirds). For example, in the MIRACLE trial, Biv pacing was associated with more patients who improved (67% versus 39%) and fewer patients who worsened (16% versus 27%) at the end of 6-month follow-up, compared to controls [59]. Interestingly, significant placebo effects have been noted in CRT patients.

28.5.1 Clinical Variables

In general, demographic, clinical, and functional characteristics have limited value in predicting the effects of Biv pacing. Yet, there is some evidence that patients are more likely to benefit from Biv pacing when presenting with wider QRS durations and more advanced LV dysfunctions. Similarly, patients with echocardiographic evidence of more severe cardiac dyssynchronies and low systolic blood pressures gain greater benefit from CRT [60]. Reduced exercise times and peak VO_2 levels at rest may predict increasing peak oxygen consumption in response to CRT. However, it should also be noted that patients with a significantly enlarged heart or end-stage heart failure may not respond to Biv pacing, and some patients do not even tolerate the implantation procedure or Biv pacing at all. In general, it has been suggested that patients who have had a myocardial infarction, large scar tissues, a very low cardiac output, and no significant mitral regurgitation are not likely to improve with CRT. B-type natriuretic, which is commonly used for monitoring CHF, may be useful to monitor the efficiency of CRT; B-type natriuretic value independently predicts CRT response and has been shown to be superior to QRS duration reduction in identifying CRT responders [61]. Finally, reverse LV remodeling and symptom benefits with CRT have been shown to be sustained at 12 months in patients with NYHA class III/IV heart failure, but occur to a lesser degree in patients with an ischemic versus nonischemic etiology, most likely owing to the inexorable progression of ischemic disease [62].

28.5.2 12-Lead ECGs

The analysis of preimplantation ECGs in 110 patients in the MIRACLE ICD trial was shown to suggest some clinical and ECG variables that may be predictive of CRT efficacy [63]. In a univariate analysis, a dominant R wave in lead aVR, right bundle branch block, and evidence of prior anterior infarction were each associated with significantly lower improvements in peak oxygen consumption than their absence. In patients with complete right bundle branch block and drug-resistant heart failure, only patients with a right bundle branch block associated with a major left intraventricular dyssynchrony were found to be more likely to respond to CRT [63]. Alternative ECG criteria, including QRS duration, had no relationship with the outcome. Less mechanical dyssynchrony is commonly induced by RBBB than by LBBB in the failing hearts and, accordingly, the corresponding impact of CRT on the former is reduced. Therefore, RV pacing alone may be equally efficacious as Biv CRT in hearts with pure right bundle branch conduction delay [64].

In a multivariate model, only ECG evidence of prior anterior infarction was associated with outcome. In other words, ECG markers of anterior infarction and RV dilation may help identify patients unlikely to benefit from Biv pacing. Yet, the predictive value of such ECG analyses for CRT remains to be validated; in general, they may be more useful to predict CRT non-responders rather than CRT responders.

28.5.3 QRS Duration

It is generally accepted that mechanical, but not electrical, dyssynchrony is a better predictor of clinical efficacy of CRT, because increased QRS duration is not necessarily equivalent to mechanical dyssynchrony. Although a Biv pacing-induced reduction in QRS duration is commonly seen in CRT, such Biv pacing-induced QRS narrowing does not necessarily translate to maximal mechanical hemodynamic benefits. Animal and clinical studies have shown that improved mechanical synchrony and function do not have to require electrical synchrony [41, 65]. However, a high concordance is often observed between CRT-induced QRS shortening and clinical efficiency.

In general, patients with wider QRS duration are more likely to benefit from CRT, although both interventricular and intraventricular dyssynchrony increased with the increasing QRS duration, and the correlation between intraventricular mechanical and electrical dyssynchrony was weak. In a study of 86 patients, Auricchio et al. [66] demonstrated that patients with QRS duration <150 ms did not show any improvement in any end point with CRT (atrial-synchronized LV pacing). For patients with QRS duration >150 ms, peak VO_2 increased 2.46 ml/min/kg ($P<0.001$), anaerobic threshold increased 1.55 ml/min/kg ($P<0.001$), distance walked in 6 min increased 47 m ($P=0.024$), and quality-of-life score improved 8.1 points ($P=0.004$). Perhaps the main reason why patients with QRS duration <150 ms do not respond very well to CRT is due to currently available implanting techniques, which are characterized by both limited access to the LV and absence of detailed mapping of mechanical dyssynchrony.

As discussed earlier, it appears that CRT is beneficial in patients with narrow QRS complex and severe LV dyssynchrony, with similar improvement in symptoms and comparable LV reverse remodeling to patients with wide QRS complex. However, this has not been verified in larger patient cohorts [67]. Dyssynchrony can be observed in approximately a quarter of dilated cardiomyopathy patients with normal QRS duration, although its incidence is much higher in patients with prolonged QRS duration (86.7%).

28.5.4 Acute Hemodynamic Responses

Acute hemodynamic benefits can be expected at implantation. Importantly, although early hemodynamic testing does not always predict chronic effects of Biv pacing, observed acute hemodynamic improvements usually persist during long-term follow-up [68, 69]. Although decrease in QRS duration by CRT is not necessarily associated with improved cardiac function, responders usually have a more pronounced decrease in QRS duration with CRT. An acute increase in LVEF and a reduction in LV diastolic dimension, interventricular mechanical delay, and severity of mitral regurgitation are often observed in the responders (but not in non-responders). Such acute responses should be kept in mind until further concrete evidence of how to identify responders is available.

28.5.5 Pacing Sites

The ideal pacing site was briefly discussed above. In general, the posterolateral LV is the target for implantation of the LV pacing lead in current practice. Technically, it is relatively easy to place a CS lead into an anterior branch. It is noteworthy that hemodynamic benefits via anterior pacing are typically inferior to posterolateral pacing. Furthermore, several studies have shown that pacing the anterior wall may actually decrease cardiac function [70], although this is not universally true. Theoretically, in a non-responder who is being paced from the anterior LV, it may be best to reposition the lead into a posterolateral location transvenously or epicardially.

28.5.6 Evidence of Mechanical Dyssynchrony

At present, only echocardiographic image characteristics associated with LV dyssynchrony are generally accepted for prediction of CRT efficacy, although, in many centers, mechanical dyssynchrony is not routinely being assessed before implantation. As new echocardiographic imaging modalities such as tissue Doppler imaging, three-dimensional (3D) echocardiography, and speckle tracking echocardiography are further developed, they will be better able to quantify ventricular mechanical dyssynchrony. This is important for patients with large electromechanical dyssynchrony, as they benefit most from Biv pacing. For example, systolic synchronicity can be directly assessed using tissue Doppler imaging, which is highly accurate in predicting responders to therapy. For example, the combination of an LVEF >15% and a significant interventricular dyssynchrony (interventricular dyssynchrony >60 ms) at baseline will typically predict an improvement of LVEF of >5% at follow-up, with a sensitivity of 79% and a positive predictive value of 83% [71].

More recently, speckle tracking radial strain has been used to quantify dyssynchrony and has been shown to predict immediate and long-term responses to CRT; it also has potential for clinical application. In a study in 64 CHF patients undergoing CRT (aged 64 ± 12 years, LVEF $26 \pm 6\%$, QRS duration 157 ± 28 ms) and 10 normal controls, dyssynchrony from timing of speckle tracking peak radial strain was correlated with tissue Doppler measures in 47 subjects ($r = 0.94$) [72]. It predicted an immediate increase in stroke volume in 48 patients studied the day after CRT, with 91% sensitivity and 75% specificity. In 50 patients with long-term follow-up 8 ± 5 months after CRT, baseline speckle tracking radial dyssynchrony predicted a significant increase in LVEF with 89% sensitivity and 83% specificity [72]. Patients in whom LV lead position was concordant with the site of latest mechanical activation by speckle tracking radial strain had an increase in LVEF from baseline to a greater degree ($10 \pm 5\%$) than patients with discordant lead position ($6 \pm 5\%$, $P<0.05$).

28.5.7 Activation Map of the LV

It would be ideal to map the optimal pacing site followed by assessment of mechanical synchrony, as well as hemodynamic responses prior to placement of an LV lead. Unfortunately, preimplant mapping of optimal pacing site is not currently performed routinely.

Theoretically, the benefits of CRT are achieved by electrical pacing of the ventricles. Therefore, a 3D activation map of the LV could appropriately be used for guiding lead placement and predicting outcomes. Some limited data available from patients undergoing CRT have shown that noncontact mapping can identify regions of slow conduction; significant hemodynamic improvements can occur when the site of LV pacing is outside these slow conduction areas [73]. Some investigators feel that failure of CRT to produce clinical benefits may reflect LV lead placement in regions of slow conduction (possible scars) which can be overcome by pacing in more normally activating regions. Data from 3D electromechanical mapping also suggest that the presence of a larger amount of LV area with late endocardial activation time and preserved LV myocardium may identify patients who have better acute improvement in systolic performance during LV stimulation [74].

The presence of cardiac diseases is commonly characterized by LV global mechanical delays and intraventricular dyssynchronized contractions, characterized mostly by further mechanical delays in the free wall region; these changes can occur even in those with normal QRS duration. Some studies have demonstrated that LV or Biv pacing may improve cardiac function in patients with normal QRS duration who have evidence of mechanical dyssynchrony. The timing of LV free wall electrical activation has been shown to be correlated with improved synchrony. Whether the timing of LV free wall electrical activation can be used for assessment of mechanical synchrony remains to be determined.

In one study, 3D mapping using a nonconstraining epicardial elastic sock showed that in hearts with delayed lateral contraction, optimized CRT could be achieved over a fairly broad area of LV lateral wall in both non-failing and failing hearts, with modest anterior or posterior deviation still capable of providing effective CRT [75]. Sites selected to achieve the most mechanical synchrony were generally similar to those that most improve global function, implicating the importance of wall motion analysis during CRT.

28.5.8 Atrial Arrhythmias

CRT may also achieve clinical benefit in patients who present with atrial fibrillation. The long-term CRT survival rates are comparable between patients who elicit sinus rhythm, compared to those who were in atrial fibrillation. However, the number of non-responders was greater among patients who had atrial fibrillation, suggesting the importance of trying to manage atrial arrhythmias in such patients.

28.5.9 Right Versus Left Atrial Pacing

Right atrial pacing leads to a delayed electrical and mechanical activation of the left atrium and, subsequently, compromised transmitral inflow during late diastole and impeded LV preload. Therefore, avoidance of right atrial pacing may result in a higher degree of LV resynchronization in a substantial prolongation of the LV filling period and also in improved myocardial performance. In some non-responders programmed to the DDD mode, it may be helpful to test the VDD pacing mode [76]. There have been recent attempts to perform Bachman bundle pacing to better synchronize atrial contractions.

28.6 Management of Non-Responders

Left ventricular synchrony is expected to be improved significantly immediately after Biv pacing in responders, while there may be no change in non-responders. It is important to assess any significant improvement of interventricular and intraventricular dyssynchrony in managing non-responders to see whether revision of the CS lead is needed in these patients. Currently mechanical dyssynchrony is the only generally accepted technique for predicting overall CRT efficacy. The following is the strategy for management of CRT patients for maximal CRT benefits at the University of Minnesota:

- Step 1. Better selection of candidates for CRT. Search for mechanical as well as electrical dyssynchrony.
- Step 2. Placement of LV pacing at posterolateral region of the LV. Ideally, mechanical and/or activation map of the LV should be used to identify the optimal location of LV pacing lead placement.
- Step 3. Assessment of acute hemodynamic responses at the implantation. This may be used to guide selection of implanting site.
- Step 4. Careful follow-up to ensure functional LV pacing all the time.
- Step 5. Optimization of AV delays immediately after implantation and during follow-up.
- Step 6. Optimization of VV delays immediately after implantation and during follow-up, particularly in non-responders.
- Step 7. Better control of atrial arrhythmias and other cardiac arrhythmias, including frequent atrial and ventricular ectopics.
- Step 8. Revision of LV lead as needed, such as a dislodged lead. In non-responders, reposition of a CS lead to posterolateral location may be needed. Surgical placement of an epicardial LV lead, i.e., if appropriate lateral cardiac vein either does not exist or cannot be accessed.
- Step 9. Turn off ventricular pacing in true non-responders or those with worsening cardiac function with CRT.
- Step 10. Reassessment of optimal medical therapy in all the patients, including treating cardiac diseases (such as ischemia) and managing noncardiac factors (such as renal failure).

28.7 Cost-Effectiveness of CRT

Analysis based on data from the CArdiac REsynchronization in Heart Failure (CARE-HF) trial has shown that treatment with CRT appears to be cost-effective at the notional willingness to pay threshold of €29,400 (20,000 pounds sterling) per quality-adjusted life year (QALY) gained [77]. This prospective analysis was based on intention-to-treat data from all patients enrolled in the CARE-HF trial at 82 clinical centers in 12 European countries. Specifically, 813 patients with NYHA class III or IV heart failure due to LV systolic dysfunction and cardiac dyssynchrony were randomized to CRT plus medical therapy ($n = 409$) or medical therapy alone groups ($n = 404$). During a mean follow-up of 29.4 months, CRT was associated with increased costs (€4,316, 95% CI: 1,327–7,485), survival (0.10 years, 95% CI: –0.01 to 0.21), and quality-adjusted life year (0.22, 95% CI: 0.13–0.32). The incremental cost-effectiveness ratio was €19,319 per QALY gained (95% CI: 5,482–45,402) and €43,596 per life-year gained (95% CI: –146,236 to 223,849). Note that these results were also sensitive to the costs of the device, procedure, and required hospitalization.

The analysis of the cost-effectiveness of CRT based on the COMPANION trial is interesting to review. Compared to optimal medical therapy, CRT alone (CRT-P) in the COMPANION trial had a cost-effectiveness ratio of $19,600 per QALY added, which is well within the range of other generally accepted interventions. The overall benefit of 0.71 QALYs resulted from the significant improvement in quality of life and the trend toward improved survival. On the other hand, the COMPANION trial data showed that the combined CRT-ICD (CRT-D) had only slightly better outcomes than CRT alone (3.15 versus 3.01 QALYs), but it cost much more ($82,200 versus $59,900). The cost-effectiveness measure calculated from these data is $160,000 per QALY, which is expensive compared to standard benchmarks. The COMPANION trial data suggest that adding ICD capability to a CRT device may not improve outcomes sufficiently to justify the considerable additional expense [78].

There is some evidence that savings in postimplant healthcare utilization (hospitalizations and pharmacologic therapy) may offset some of the device and procedural costs associated with CRT devices [79]. For example, in the Canadian analysis of resynchronization therapy in heart failure (CART-HF) study, which included 72 patients with NYHA class II–IV CHF requiring an ICD, patients were randomized to receive either CRT-D treatment or ICD treatment alone [79]. Medical resource utilization data were collected for 6 months following treatment and were applied to representative costs for the provinces of Quebec and Ontario. Resource utilization was subcategorized into pharmacologic therapy, physician visits, hospitalizations, adverse events, and productivity losses. Posttreatment, per patient costs for the CRT-D treatment group were less than the follow-up costs for patients receiving ICD treatment only in each province. Mean savings for patients receiving Biv therapy were CAD $2,420 in Quebec and CAD $2,085 in Ontario during the 6-month follow-up.

28.8 Future Perspective

The concept of physiologic pacing should always be kept in mind to maximize the benefits of cardiac pacing, particularly in the presence of LV dysfunction. The deleterious effects of ventricular (particularly RV) pacing have been established and should be avoided when possible. Left ventricular or Biv pacing should be considered whenever cardiac pacing is required to prevent subsequent electrical and mechanical remodeling, such as after AV nodal ablation.

CRT has been accepted for treatment of patients with moderate-to-severe CHF in the presence of intraventricular conduction delays. Mechanical, but not electrical, dyssynchrony is most predictive for assessment of CRT efficacy. Note that CRT, to date, is no more than an imperfect technique for partially correcting cardiac electrical dyssynchrony and associated mechanical dyssynchrony. Nonetheless, the beneficial effects of CRT will be maximized if the following important clinical and technical questions can completely be resolved:

1. How can we better select the potential responders to CRT?
2. What is the optimal pacing site for CRT in an individual patient?
3. How best do we determine the optimal AV delay?
4. How can we easily and most securely implant an LV lead?
5. What is the therapeutic mechanism underlying CRT?
6. Can CRT help to prevent heart failure progression?
7. What is the impact of CRT on arrhythmogenesis?
8. What is the impact of CRT on mortality?

List of Abbreviations

AV	atrioventricular
Biv	biventricular
CHF	congestive heart failure
CRT	cardiac resynchronization therapy
CRT-D	combination of cardiac resynchronization therapy and defibrillator
CRT-P	combination of cardiac resynchronization therapy and pacemaker
CS	coronary sinus

ICD	implantable cardioverter defibrillator
LV	left ventricular
LVEDD	left ventricular end-diastolic diameter
LVEF	left ventricular ejection fraction
NYHA	New York Heart Association
RV	right ventricular

References

1. Hunt SA, Baker DW, Chin MH, et al. ACC/AHA guidelines for the evaluation and management of chronic heart failure in the adult: Executive summary. A Report of the American College of Cardiology/American Heart Association Task Force on Practice Guidelines (Committee to Revise the 1995 Guidelines for the Evaluation and Management of Heart Failure): Developed in Collaboration With the International Society for Heart and Lung Transplantation; Endorsed by the Heart Failure Society of America. Circulation 2001;104:2996–3007.
2. Fei L, Wrobleski D, Groh W, Vetter A, Duffin EG, Zipes DP. Effects of multisite ventricular pacing on cardiac function in normal dogs and dogs with heart failure. J Cardiovasc Electrophysiol 1999;10:935–46.
3. Wilkoff BL, Cook JR, Epstein AE, et al. Dual-chamber pacing or ventricular backup pacing in patients with an implantable defibrillator: Te Dual Chamber and VVI Implantable Defibrillator (DAVID) Trial. JAMA 2002;288:3115–23.
4. Bernstein AD, Daubert JC, Fletcher RD, et al. The revised NASPE/BPEG generic code for antibradycardia, adaptive-rate, and multisite pacing. North American Society of Pacing and Electrophysiology/British Pacing and Electrophysiology Group. PACE 2002;25:260–64.
5. Leclercq C, Gras D, Le Helloco A, Nicol L, Mabo P, Daubert C. Hemodynamic importance of preserving the normal sequence of ventricular activation in permanent cardiac pacing. Am Heart J 1995;129:1133–41.
6. de Cock CC, Vos DH, Jessurun E, Allaart CP, Visser CA. Effects of stimulation site on diastolic function in cardiac resynchronization therapy. Pacing Clin Electrophysiol 2007;30:S40–42.
7. Yu CM, Zhang Q, Yip GW, et al. Are left ventricular diastolic function and diastolic asynchrony important determinants of response to cardiac resynchronization therapy? Am J Cardiol 2006;98:1083–87.
8. Cazeau S, Leclercq C, Lavergne T, et al. Effects of multisite biventricular pacing in patients with heart failure and intraventricular conduction delay. N Engl J Med 2001;344:873–80.
9. Linde C, Leclercq C, Rex S, et al. Long-term benefits of biventricular pacing in congestive heart failure: results from the MUltisite STimulation in cardiomyopathy (MUSTIC) study. J Am Coll Cardiol 2002;40:111–18.
10. Gras D, Mabo P, Tang T, et al. Multisite pacing as a supplemental treatment of congestive heart failure: preliminary results of the Medtronic Inc. InSync Study. PACE 1998;21:2249–55.
11. Gras D, Leclercq C, Tang AS, Bucknall C, Luttikhuis HO, Kirstein-Pedersen A. Cardiac resynchronization therapy in advanced heart failure the multicenter InSync clinical study. Eur J Heart Fail 2002;4:311–20.
12. Abraham WT, Fisher WG, Smith AL, et al. Cardiac resynchronization in chronic heart failure. N Engl J Med 2002;346:1845–53.
13. Moss AJ, Zareba W, Hall WJ, et al. Prophylactic implantation of a defibrillator in patients with myocardial infarction and reduced ejection fraction. N Engl J Med 2002;346:877–83.
14. Bardy GH, Lee KL, Mark DB, et al. Amiodarone or an implantable cardioverter-defibrillator for congestive heart failure. N Engl J Med 2005;352:225–37.
15. Young JB, Abraham WT, Smith AL, et al. Combined cardiac resynchronization and implantable cardioversion defibrillation in advanced chronic heart failure: The MIRACLE ICD Trial. JAMA 2003;289:2685–94.
16. CRM GC. Summary of safety and effectiveness CONTAK-CD system.
17. Bristow MR, Saxon LA, Boehmer J, et al. Cardiac-resynchronization therapy with or without an implantable defibrillator in advanced chronic heart failure. N Engl J Med 2004;350:2140–50.
18. Cleland JG, Daubert JC, Erdmann E, et al. The effect of cardiac resynchronization on morbidity and mortality in heart failure. N Engl J Med 2005;352:1539–49.
19. Cleland JG, Daubert JC, Erdmann E, et al. Longer-term effects of cardiac resynchronization therapy on mortality in heart failure [the CArdiac REsynchronization-Heart Failure (CARE-HF) trial extension phase]. Eur Heart J 2006;27:1928–32.
20. Lau CP, Yu CM, Chau E, et al. Reversal of left ventricular remodeling by synchronous biventricular pacing in heart failure. PACE 2000;23:1722–25.
21. Baller D, Wolpers HG, Zipfel J, Hoeft A, Hellige G. Unfavorable effects of ventricular pacing on myocardial energetics. Basic Res Cardiol 1981;76:115–23.
22. Nelson GS, Berger RD, Fetics BJ, et al. Left ventricular or biventricular pacing improves cardiac function at diminished energy cost in patients with dilated cardiomyopathy and left bundle-branch block. Circulation 2000;102:3053–59.
23. Ukkonen H, Beanlands RS, Burwash IG, et al. Effect of cardiac resynchronization on myocardial efficiency and regional oxidative metabolism. Circulation 2003;107:28–31.
24. Flevari P, Theodorakis G, Paraskevaidis I, et al. Coronary and peripheral blood flow changes following biventricular pacing and their relation to heart failure improvement. Europace 2006;8:44–50.
25. Vanderheyden M, Mullens W, Delrue L, et al. Myocardial gene expression in heart failure patients treated with cardiac resynchronization therapy responders versus nonresponders. J Am Coll Cardiol 2008;51:129–36.
26. Ypenburg C, van Erven L, Bleeker GB, et al. Benefit of combined resynchronization and defibrillator therapy in heart failure patients with and without ventricular arrhythmias. J Am Coll Cardiol 2006;48:464–70.
27. Chalil S, Yousef ZR, Muyhaldeen SA, et al. Pacing-induced increase in QT dispersion predicts sudden cardiac death following cardiac resynchronization therapy. J Am Coll Cardiol 2006;47:2486–92.
28. Harada M, Osaka T, Yokoyama E, Takemoto Y, Ito A, Kodama I. Biventricular pacing has an advantage over left ventricular epicardial pacing alone to minimize proarrhythmic perturbation of repolarization. J Cardiovasc Electrophysiol 2006;17:151–56.
29. Germano JJ, Reynolds M, Essebag V, Josephson ME. Frequency and causes of implantable cardioverter-defibrillator therapies: is device therapy proarrhythmic? Am J Cardiol 2006;97:1255–61.
30. Gottipaty VK, Krelis SP, Fei L, et al. Patients with congestive heart failure and permanent pacemaker have an increased risk of "non-sudden" death. J Am Coll Cardiol 1999;33:125A.
31. Auricchio A, Metra M, Gasparini M, et al. Long-term survival of patients with heart failure and ventricular conduction delay

treated with cardiac resynchronization therapy. Am J Cardiol 2007;99:232–38.

32. Bradley DJ, Bradley EA, Baughman KL, et al. Cardiac resynchronization and death from progressive heart failure: a meta-analysis of randomized controlled trials. JAMA 2003;289:730–40.

33. Salukhe TV, Dimopoulos K, Francis D. Cardiac resynchronisation may reduce all-cause mortality: meta-analysis of preliminary COMPANION data with CONTAK-CD, InSync ICD, MIRACLE and MUSTIC. Int J Cardiol 2004;93:101–03.

34. Rivero-Ayerza M, Theuns DA, Garcia-Garcia HM, Boersma E, Simoons M, Jordaens LJ. Effects of cardiac resynchronization therapy on overall mortality and mode of death: A meta-analysis of randomized controlled trials. Eur Heart J 2006;27:2682–88.

35. Gasparini M, Lunati M, Santini M, et al. Long-term survival in patients treated with cardiac resynchronization therapy: A 3-year follow-up study from the InSync/InSync ICD Italian Registry. Pacing Clin Electrophysiol 2006;29:S2–10.

36. Delnoy PP, Ottervanger JP, Luttikhuis HO, et al. Sustained benefit of cardiac resynchronization therapy. J Cardiovasc Electrophysiol 2007;18:298–302.

37. Dilaveris P, Pantazis A, Giannopoulos G, Synetos A, Gialafos J, Stefanadis C. Upgrade to biventricular pacing in patients with pacing-induced heart failure: can resynchronization do the trick? Europace 2006;8:352–57.

38. Doshi RN, Daoud EG, Fellows C, et al. Left ventricular-based cardiac stimulation post AV nodal ablation evaluation (the PAVE study). J Cardiovasc Electrophysiol 2005;16:1160–65.

39. Gasparini M, Auricchio A, Regoli F, et al. Four-year efficacy of cardiac resynchronization therapy on exercise tolerance and disease progression: The importance of performing atrioventricular junction ablation in patients with atrial fibrillation. J Am Coll Cardiol 2006;48:734–43.

40. Lu F, Iaizzo PA, Benditt DG, Mehra R, Warman EN, McHenry BT. Isolated atrial segment pacing: an alternative to his bundle pacing after atrioventricular junctional ablation. J Am Coll Cardiol 2007;49:1443–49.

41. Yu CM, Chan YS, Zhang Q, et al. Benefits of cardiac resynchronization therapy for heart failure patients with narrow QRS complexes and coexisting systolic asynchrony by echocardiography. J Am Coll Cardiol 2006;48:2251–57.

42. Beshai JF, Grimm RA, Nagueh SF, et al. Cardiac-resynchronization therapy in heart failure with narrow QRS complexes. N Engl J Med 2007;357:2461–71.

43. Blanc JJ, Etienne Y, Gilard M, et al. Evaluation of different ventricular pacing sites in patients with severe heart failure: Results of an acute hemodynamic study. Circulation 1997;96:3273–77.

44. Butter C, Auricchio A, Stellbrink C, et al. Should stimulation site be tailored in the individual heart failure patient? Am J Cardiol 2000;86:K144–51.

45. Alonso C, Leclercq C, Victor F, et al. Electrocardiographic predictive factors of long-term clinical improvement with multisite biventricular pacing in advanced heart failure. Am J Cardiol 1999;84:1417–21.

46. Auricchio A, Stellbrink C, Sack S, et al. The Pacing Therapies for Congestive Heart Failure (PATH-CHF) study: Rationale, design, and endpoints of a prospective randomized multicenter study. Am J Cardiol 1999;83:130D–35D.

47. Auricchio A, Klein H, Tockman B, et al. Transvenous biventricular pacing for heart failure: Can the obstacles be overcome? Am J Cardiol 1999;83:136D–42D.

48. Rossillo A, Verma A, Saad EB, et al. Impact of coronary sinus lead position on biventricular pacing: mortality and echocardiographic evaluation during long-term follow-up. J Cardiovasc Electrophysiol 2004;15:1120–25.

49. Perego GB, Chianca R, Facchini M, et al. Simultaneous vs. sequential biventricular pacing in dilated cardiomyopathy: An acute hemodynamic study. Eur J Heart Fail 2003;5:305–13.

50. Mortensen PT, Sogaard P, Mansour H, et al. Sequential biventricular pacing: Evaluation of safety and efficacy. Pacing Clin Electrophysiol 2004;27:339–45.

51. Leon AR, Abraham WT, Brozena S, et al. Cardiac resynchronization with sequential biventricular pacing for the treatment of moderate-to-severe heart failure. J Am Coll Cardiol 2005;46:2298–304.

52. Buckingham TA, Candinas R, Schlapfer J, et al. Acute hemodynamic effects of atrioventricular pacing at differing sites in the right ventricle individually and simultaneously. PACE 1997;20:909–15.

53. Ortega DF, Pellegrino GM, Barja LD, Albina G, Laino R, Giniger A. Biventricular pacing using two pacemakers and the triggered VVT mode. Pacing Clin Electrophysiol 2002;25:1534–35.

54. Lu F, Miller LW. Biventricular pacing for congestive heart failure. In: Iaizzo PA, ed. Cardiac anatomy, physiology and devices: A handbook for the biomedical engineer, 1st ed. Totowa, NJ: The Humana Press Inc., 2005:812–22.

55. Gras D, Bocker D, Lunati M, et al. Implantation of cardiac resynchronization therapy systems in the CARE-HF trial: Procedural success rate and safety. Europace 2007;9:516–22.

56. Leon AR, Abraham WT, Curtis AB, et al. Safety of transvenous cardiac resynchronization system implantation in patients with chronic heart failure: combined results of over 2,000 patients from a multicenter study program. J Am Coll Cardiol 2005;46:2348–56.

57. Reynolds MR, Cohen DJ, Kugelmass AD, et al. The frequency and incremental cost of major complications among medicare beneficiaries receiving implantable cardioverter-defibrillators. J Am Coll Cardiol 2006;47:2493–97.

58. Ammann P, Sticherling C, Kalusche D, et al. An electrocardiogram-based algorithm to detect loss of left ventricular capture during cardiac resynchronization therapy. Ann Intern Med 2005;142:968–73.

59. Abraham WT. Cardiac resynchronization therapy for heart failure: Biventricular pacing and beyond. Curr Opin Cardiol 2002;17:346–52.

60. Richardson M, Freemantle N, Calvert MJ, Cleland JG, Tavazzi L. Predictors and treatment response with cardiac resynchronization therapy in patients with heart failure characterized by dyssynchrony: A pre-defined analysis from the CARE-HF trial. Eur Heart J 2007;28:1827–34.

61. Lellouche N, De Diego C, Cesario DA, et al. Usefulness of preimplantation B-type natriuretic peptide level for predicting response to cardiac resynchronization therapy. Am J Cardiol 2007;99:242–46.

62. Sutton MG, Plappert T, Hilpisch KE, Abraham WT, Hayes DL, Chinchoy E. Sustained reverse left ventricular structural remodeling with cardiac resynchronization at one year is a function of etiology: Quantitative Doppler echocardiographic evidence from the Multicenter InSync Randomized Clinical Evaluation (MIRACLE). Circulation 2006;113:266–72.

63. Garrigue S, Reuter S, Labeque JN, et al. Usefulness of biventricular pacing in patients with congestive heart failure and right bundle branch block. Am J Cardiol 2001;88:1436–41, A8.

64. Byrne MJ, Helm RH, Daya S, et al. Diminished left ventricular dyssynchrony and impact of resynchronization in failing hearts with right versus left bundle branch block. J Am Coll Cardiol 2007;50:1484–90.

65. Leclercq C, Faris O, Tunin R, et al. Systolic improvement and mechanical resynchronization does not require electrical

synchrony in the dilated failing heart with left bundle-branch block. Circulation 2002;106:1760–63.

66. Auricchio A, Stellbrink C, Butter C, et al. Clinical efficacy of cardiac resynchronization therapy using left ventricular pacing in heart failure patients stratified by severity of ventricular conduction delay. J Am Coll Cardiol 2003;42: 2109–16.

67. Bleeker GB, Holman ER, Steendijk P, et al. Cardiac resynchronization therapy in patients with a narrow QRS complex. J Am Coll Cardiol 2006;48:2243–50.

68. Steendijk P, Tulner SA, Bax JJ, et al. Hemodynamic effects of long-term cardiac resynchronization therapy: Analysis by pressure-volume loops. Circulation 2006;113:1295–304.

69. Bleeker GB, Mollema SA, Holman ER, et al. Left ventricular resynchronization is mandatory for response to cardiac resynchronization therapy: Analysis in patients with echocardiographic evidence of left ventricular dyssynchrony at baseline. Circulation 2007;116:1440–48.

70. Butter C, Auricchio A, Stellbrink C, et al. Effect of resynchronization therapy stimulation site on the systolic function of heart failure patients. Circulation 2001;104:3026–29.

71. Toussaint JF, Lavergne T, Kerrou K, et al. Basal asynchrony and resynchronization with biventricular pacing predict long-term improvement of LV function in heart failure patients. Pacing Clin Electrophysiol 2003;26:1815–23.

72. Suffoletto MS, Dohi K, Cannesson M, Saba S, Gorcsan J III. Novel speckle-tracking radial strain from routine black-and-white echocardiographic images to quantify dyssynchrony and predict response to cardiac resynchronization therapy. Circulation 2006;113:960–68.

73. Lambiase PD, Rinaldi A, Hauck J, et al. Non-contact left ventricular endocardial mapping in cardiac resynchronisation therapy. Heart 2004;90:44–51.

74. Tse HF, Lee KL, Wan SH, et al. Area of left ventricular regional conduction delay and preserved myocardium predict responses to cardiac resynchronization therapy. J Cardiovasc Electrophysiol 2005;16:690–95.

75. Helm RH, Byrne M, Helm PA, et al. Three-dimensional mapping of optimal left ventricular pacing site for cardiac resynchronization. Circulation 2007;115:953–61.

76. Bernheim A, Ammann P, Sticherling C, et al. Right atrial pacing impairs cardiac function during resynchronization therapy: Acute effects of DDD pacing compared to VDD pacing. J Am Coll Cardiol 2005;45:1482–87.

77. Calvert MJ, Freemantle N, Yao G, et al. Cost-effectiveness of cardiac resynchronization therapy: Results from the CARE-HF trial. Eur Heart J 2005;26:2681–88.

78. Ward A, Guo S, Caro JJ. Cost-effectiveness of cardiac resynchronization therapy. J Am Coll Cardiol 2006;48:1283.

79. Bentkover JD, Dorian P, Thibault B, Gardner M. Economic analysis of a randomized trial of biventricular pacing in Canada. Pacing Clin Electrophysiol 2007;30:38–43.

80. Van de Veire NR, Schuijf JD, De Sutter J, et al. Non-invasive visualization of the cardiac venous system in coronary artery disease patients using 64-slice computed tomography. J Am Coll Cardiol 2006;48:1832–38.

Chapter 29
Cardiac Mapping Technology

Nicholas D. Skadsberg, Bin He, Timothy G. Laske, and Paul A. Iaizzo

Abstract In general, the methodologies for cardiac electrical mapping entail registration of the electrical activation sequences of the heart by recording extracellular electrograms. The initial use of cardiac mapping was primarily to better understand the normal electrical excitations of the heart. However, the focus in mapping over time has shifted to the study of mechanisms and substrates underlying various arrhythmias; these techniques have been employed to aid in the guidance of curative surgical and/or catheter ablation procedures. More recently, the advent and continued development of high-resolution mapping technologies have considerably enhanced our understanding of rapid, complex, and/or transient arrhythmias that typically cannot be sufficiently characterized with more conventional methodologies. For example, the ability to visualize endocardial structures during electrophysiology procedures has greatly advanced the understanding of complex cardiac arrhythmias in relation to their underlying anatomy. In addition, such technologies provide powerful tools in the subsequent treatment of cardiac patients, particularly with the promise of accurately pinpointing the source of arrhythmias and thereby providing possible curative treatments.

Keywords Cardiac mapping · Body surface potential mapping · Epicardial mapping · Endocardial mapping · Activation maps · Isopotential maps · Sequential mapping · Continuous mapping

29.1 Introduction and Background

The first recorded electrocardiogram (ECG) detailing the structure of atrioventricular conduction was made by Tawara nearly 100 years ago [1]. Soon thereafter, Mayer was the first to observe rhythmical pulsations in ring-like preparations of the muscular tissue of a jellyfish (*Scyphomedusa cassiopeia*) [2, 3]. In similar ring-like preparations of the tortoise heart, Mines was able to initiate circulating excitation by employing electrical stimulation [4]. Shortly thereafter, Lewis and Rothschild described the excitatory process in a canine heart [5], and after a delay due to the events of World War I, Lewis next reported the first real "mapping" experiment in 1920 [6]. These groundbreaking studies were the first attempts to illustrate and document electrical reentry in an intact heart, and these results have greatly influenced those who have continued to perform mapping studies. Hence, the field of "cardiac electrical mapping" was established. Soon afterwards, the idea of mapping arrhythmic activation encompassed an ever larger number of studies, including the early pioneering work of Barker et al. who performed mapping of the first intact human heart in 1930 [7]. Many research groups have continued along these lines of investigation, leading to many major discoveries in cardiac function as well as in the development of numerous systems to record such electrical activities in detail. One representative approach is the so-called body surface potential mapping [8], in which an array of electrodes is used to record and visualize the electrical potentials over the body surface. Much of the research performed to date has focused primarily on the mechanisms and substrates underlying various arrhythmias, and cardiac mapping has been employed to aid in the guidance of curative surgical and catheter ablation procedures [9–14]. More recently, the advent and continued development of high-resolution mapping technology has considerably enhanced our understanding of rapid, complex, and/or

N.D. Skadsberg (✉)
Medtronic, Inc., 8200 Coral Sea St. NE, Mounds View, MN 55112, USA
e-mail: nick.skadsberg@medtronic.com

P.A. Iaizzo (ed.), *Handbook of Cardiac Anatomy, Physiology, and Devices*, DOI 10.1007/978-1-60327-372-5_29,

transient arrhythmias that cannot be sufficiently characterized with more conventional methodologies.

29.2 Conventional Methodologies

Currently, approximately 10 million Americans annually are afflicted with cardiac arrhythmias (both ventricular and atrial), yet only a small percentage of these patients are expected to have electrophysiological (EP) mapping procedures. It is generally accepted that cardiac electrical mapping is critical in understanding the pathophysiological mechanisms that underlie arrhythmias as well as the mechanisms that control their initiation and sustenance. Furthermore, cardiac mapping is commonly used for evaluating the effect of pharmacological therapies and directing surgical and/or catheter ablation procedures in the clinical EP laboratory.

Mapping of the endocardial depolarization and repolarization electrical processes is considered critical for the selection of optimal therapeutic procedures. In particular, mapping of endocardial potential distribution and its evolution in time is required for precisely determining activation patterns, locating specific arrhythmogenic sites, and identifying anatomical areas of abnormal activity and/or slow conduction.

In short, the purpose of such advanced clinical cardiac mapping techniques is to better characterize and localize arrhythmogenic structures, and this can be accomplished by a variety of different methods. Thus, "cardiac mapping" is a broad term that encompasses many applications such as body surface potential maps (BSPMs), epicardial mapping, or endocardial mapping as well as approaches including activation maps and/or isopotential maps. Nevertheless, there are many fundamental similarities in all of these techniques.

Currently, the gold standard is the clinical EP study, which is primarily used to: (1) determine the source of cardiac arrhythmias; (2) support the management of treatment through pharmacological means; and/or (3) support nonpharmacological interventions such as implantable pacemakers, defibrillators, and/or radiofrequency (RF) ablation therapies (see also Chapter 26). More specifically, these methods are also used to assess the timing and propagation of cardiac electrical activities involving the 12-lead ECG and/or recordings of electrical activation sequences termed "extracellular electrograms." These signals are obtained by using multiple intravascular electrode catheters positioned at various locations within the heart. The technique of catheter-based mapping not only permits a better understanding of the underlying mechanisms of various arrhythmias but also serves as the basis for most of the emerging concepts for treatment,

namely ablative techniques. Subsequently, the need for more invasive arrhythmia surgery (e.g., maze procedures) has significantly decreased as a result of advances in (and increased use of) these particular catheter-based endocardial mapping and ablation methodologies [15].

Nevertheless, the EP study is not without limitations. The electrophysiologist can only record electrical activity from electrodes located on the surface of the catheter, which must be in contact with the chamber wall. Such electrode areas (mm in diameter) are relatively small in comparison to the heart's total surface area. Thus, to adequately obtain complete global electrical activation patterns, it often dictates the placement of multiple catheters at numerous locations within the chamber of interest. As a consequence, this process requires a considerable amount of time, thus leading to extensive use of fluoroscopy and exposing the medical staff and patients to undesirable levels of ionizing radiation [16].

Second, and perhaps more importantly, fluoroscopy does not sufficiently provide for the visualization of the complex 3D cardiac anatomy and soft tissue characteristics of a given heart's chambers (Fig. 29.1). As a direct result, the expedient and reproducible localization of sites of interest is often poor. More specifically, this inability to precisely relate EP information to a specific spatial location in the heart limits conventional techniques for employing RF ablation catheters for treatment of complex cardiac arrhythmias. Lastly, such techniques for mapping electrical potential activities from multiple sites do so sequentially over several cardiac cycles, without accounting for likely beat-to-beat variability in activation

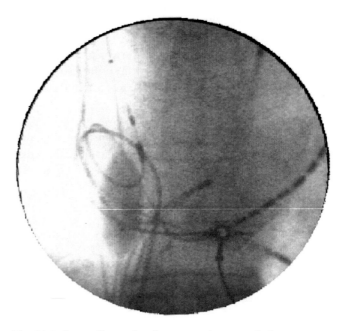

Fig. 29.1 Image illustrating fluoroscopy's poor soft tissue contrast

patterns. Despite these known limitations, electrophysiologists still use these conventional techniques as the "gold standard" for validation purposes.

29.3 Recent Developments

In an effort to overcome the limitations associated with conventional EP mapping techniques, considerable advances have been made with both invasive and noninvasive imaging of cardiac electrical activity. More specifically, several high-resolution mapping technologies have been developed that can function in a complementary role to conventional mapping techniques, or they can be used independently. These techniques can broadly be categorized into two primary technologies, each possessing unique advantages and disadvantages: (1) "sequential mapping;" and (2) "continuous mapping."

There are three distinct technologies that primarily comprise the first category (sequential mapping systems) including: (1) electroanatomical mapping, using the CARTO™XP System (Biosense Webster, Diamond Bar, CA); (2) the Real-Time Position Management system (RPM™, Boston Scientific Corporation, Natick, MA; and (3) the LocaLisa® system (Medtronic, Inc., Minneapolis, MN). Common to each system is the capability to collect 3D locations as well as their respective electrogram recordings in the target cardiac chamber, to create an accurate picture of the heart's electrical sequence.

"Continuous mapping" systems represent the second major mapping technology category, and typically consist of either basket or noncontact catheter mapping (NCM). Such systems allow for the recording of global data so that the rhythm can be characterized in only one to two cardiac beats. In general, basket catheter mapping technologies necessitate electrode contact with the chamber's walls in order to obtain sufficiently accurate reconstructed electrograms, whereas NCM simply needs to be placed in the blood pool of the chamber of interest. Yet, both methodologies overcome some of the limitations of fluoroscopy by allowing for the creation of accurate 3D intracardiac maps, hence providing new and unique insights on the specific diagnosis and treatment of complex arrhythmias.

Recently, exciting advancements have been made in the field of noninvasive imaging such that cardiac electrical activities are spatially represented over the 3D space of the heart. He and coworkers have pioneered the development of 3D cardiac electrical activity from bioelectric recordings [17–19]. The goal of such cardiac electrical imaging, also known as the "inverse problem" of electrocardiography, is to noninvasively image and visualize the electrical activity of the heart from BSPMs. Due to the high temporal resolution inherent in these bioelectric

measurements, the availability of bioelectric source imaging modalities provides much needed high temporal resolution in mapping functional status of the heart and, in turn, aids clinical diagnosis and treatment.

29.3.1 Sequential Mapping Systems

29.3.1.1 Electroanatomical Mapping Technologies

Principally, electroanatomical mapping utilizes ultra-low magnetic field technology in order to reconstruct 3D maps and activation sequences of the chamber of interest [20–22]. In short, the CARTO™ XP system uses one reference catheter (REFSTAR™), one mapping catheter (NAVISTAR™), and a pad that transmits three ultra-low magnetic fields (Fig. 29.2). Further, the amplifiers for the system are separate pieces of equipment that extract the

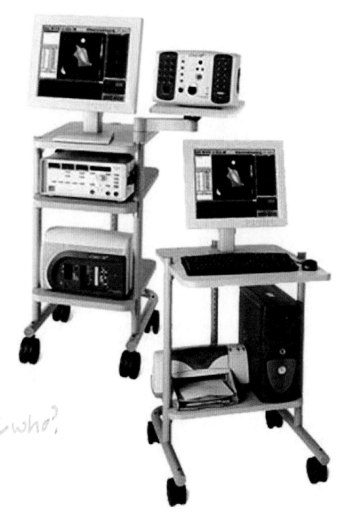

Fig. 29.2 CARTO™ sequential mapping system (Biosense Webster, Inc.)

information from the catheters and location pad, and then these data are sent to the workstation.

More specifically, three ultra-low magnetic fields are generated by coils in the locator pad positioned under the patient's bed. These ultra-low fields are detected by sensors in the distal tips of the mapping catheters, which are then positioned into the heart chamber(s) to be mapped under fluoroscopic guidance. Information within the magnetic fields such as amplitude, frequency, and phase of the field is subsequently used to determine the instantaneous spatial 3D position (x-, y-, and z-axes) and temporal characteristics (pitch, yaw, and roll) of the catheter's distal tip location within a chamber [7]. Catheters are then strategically placed at major anatomical landmarks (i.e., superior and inferior vena cavae, tricuspid valve annulus, coronary sinus ostium, crista terminalis, and His bundle for a right atrium map) to serve as reference points for the subsequently derived electroanatomic map. Recordings of the 3D locations of the catheter tips (via a triangulation calculation) and correlating electrograms from a multitude of points within the chamber are then sequentially recorded and used to reconstruct a 3D representation of the chamber.

After completion of the 3D reconstruction of the chamber's endocardial geometry, the timing of unipolar and bipolar electrogram signals, related to the fiducial point of the reference electrogram, allows for collection and display of activation times on the map in relation to the location of the catheter in the heart. To create the activation map, reconstructed locations on the map are typically color coded, with red and purple representing the regions of earliest and latest electrical activation, respectively, and yellow and green showing the intermediate activated areas. Local activation times are then represented on a normal color-scale sequence, where red is the earliest signal and purple is the latest recorded signal in reference to the chosen fiducial point. As a result, the sequential recording of different points by dragging the catheter along the endocardial walls of the chamber provides real-time, color-coded, 3D activation maps.

A relative voltage map displaying the peak-to-peak amplitude of the electrogram sampled at each site may also be produced and superimposed on the reconstructed chamber. Using custom software, all maps can be shown in single or multiple views concurrently, with the capability to be rotated in virtually any direction. As described, a second catheter equipped with a sensor in its distal tip is also positioned in the chamber of interest, and is used to identify small changes in the mapping catheter's relative position that may have been caused by respiration and/or patient movement. With CARTO™, the reference catheter is typically positioned on the back of the patient, not within the chamber.

Such electroanatomical mapping has experienced relatively widespread clinical use, and has also been utilized for the study of a variety of cardiac arrhythmias including atrial fibrillation [23], atrial flutter [24–27], ventricular tachycardia [28, 29], and atrial tachycardia [30, 31]. One of the primary reasons for the success of this method lies in its capability to return an ablation catheter to any endocardial location on a previous map of the chamber without relying on fluoroscopy. In most cases, the ablation catheter and mapping catheter are one in the same. This enables potential ablation target sites to be analyzed and treated in a single procedure, and provides the ability to precisely register the location of individual and/or linear RF lesions. In addition, the CARTO™ XP System allows for the construction of 20 different maps simultaneously and is considered to be quite practical for readily defining mechanisms of arrhythmias and optimal RF ablation strategies.

The reconstruction process using such a system can be generated in real time, however, due to the fact that this approach must sequentially acquire points, the process can be somewhat time-consuming [31, 32]; timing is governed by the number of points collected. Nevertheless, in practical use, the amount of time required to reconstruct a chamber's geometry relies on the comfort level of the physician manipulating the catheter and the knowledge of the individual participating at the workstation. It should be noted that other potential limitations associated with electroanatomical mapping include the inability to simultaneously acquire maps of different heart rhythms [32] as well as the potential for inaccurate mapping due to movement of the patient and/or catheter. As a direct result, an unstable rhythm may prove too complicated to delineate and, therefore, may not be a primary indication for this technology.

29.3.1.2 Real-Time Position Management Technologies

Previously, ultrasound ranging techniques have been utilized to accurately represent distance measurements (sizing) of the cardiac chambers and/or valves (e.g., see Chapter 20). More recently, this technological approach has been utilized to assess relative positions of catheters within the heart (i.e., Real-Time Position Management or RPM™ System). Such technologies have been used to facilitate RF catheter ablation procedures, as they allow for accurate and reproducible tracking of the mapping and ablation catheters. The RPM™ system consists primarily of an acquisition module and an ultrasound transmitter/receiver unit. Currently, the RPM™ system is capable of simultaneously processing seven position management catheters, 24 bipolar/48 unipolar electrogram signals, 12-lead ECG signals, and two pressure signals.

A typical procedure utilizing this system places two reference catheters and one mapping/ablation catheter percutaneously within the chamber of interest. In most cases, one of the reference catheters is positioned in the right atrial appendage or coronary sinus, and the other in the right ventricular apex. For specified ablation procedures, a 4-mm tip steerable catheter and RF ablation system are used. These reference and ablation catheters contain ultrasound transducers that are used to transmit and receive a continuous cycle of ultrasound pulses (558.5 kHz) to and from each other.

This approach derives the velocity of the transmitted signal by calculating the distance between the transmitting transducer and the associated time delay, assuming the speed of sound in blood is 1,550 m/s. To create a 3D map, a triangulation algorithm is then employed using signals sent back and forth between the catheters to establish a reference frame. A third catheter is then introduced into the same chamber and is tracked with relationship to the reference frame to locate and subsequently record its position. It is through this movement of the third catheter in the chamber that the 3D map is consequently created.

Initial benchtop validation studies using this system were performed and reported by de Groot et al. [33]. They described the use of the RPM™ system in a group of patients with various arrhythmias and demonstrated the system's feasibility, safety, and efficacy; the original system did not have the option of geometric reconstruction. Subsequently, Schreieck et al. evaluated the efficacy of a newly released version of the system, which included the option of 3D model reconstruction of the heart chambers for guiding mapping and ablation; they successfully studied 21 patients with different atrial and ventricular arrhythmias [34]. The currently available version of this system enables geometric reconstruction of all cardiac chambers, if desired.

There are a number of clinical advantages of the RPM™ system. First, it is an independent system which is capable of displaying a 3D map and recorded electrical activity on a single platform. In addition, the system incorporates cooled RF ablation methodologies which have been shown to improve lesion depth and efficacy [35]. Furthermore, the system allows for incorporation of activation times to the anatomic model to provide a real-time display of the distal catheter curve; it also stores information about the relative catheter positions. Importantly, this system minimizes the influence of body, cardiac, and/or respiratory motion on the reference field, and thus there is no need for skin or patch electrodes.

A major disadvantage of this technical approach is that it remains catheter specific (i.e., it is only able to use certain catheter types). Further limitations pointed out by Schreieck et al. include: (1) the need for placing at least three catheters in the heart for each electrophysiological study; (2) the lack of real-time display of the ablation catheter; (3) the inability to record intracardiac signals at the time of RF current delivery; (4) the potential for dislocation of the reference catheters due to roving catheter manipulation; and (5) a relatively undesired stiffness at the distal portion of the mapping/ablation catheter which could cause traumatic tissue injury [34].

29.3.1.3 LocaLisa® Technologies

Another technology that has been developed for real-time, 3D localization of intracardiac catheter electrodes within the chambers of the heart works on the principle that when an electrical current is externally applied through the thorax, a voltage drop occurs across the internal organs, including the heart. This particular voltage drop can then be recorded via standard catheter electrodes and subsequently used to determine electrode positions within a given 3D space.

Using similar physical properties, the LocaLisa® system (Fig. 29.3) delivers an external electrical field that is

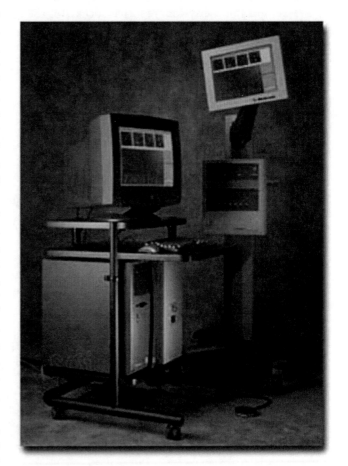

Fig. 29.3 The LocaLisa® mapping system (Medtronic, Inc.)

detected via standard catheter electrodes. This is achieved by sensing impedance changes between the catheter and reference points. Analogous to the Frank lead system, the electric field is applied in three orthogonal directions (x, y, and z) with different frequencies ($\sim$30 Hz) via three applied skin electrode pairs. This system then records the voltage potentials detected by the catheter's electrodes within the three electric fields, thus allowing for a defined coordinate system to be created.

These voltage potentials are next translated into a measure of distance relative to a fixed reference catheter, giving the user a 3D representation of the catheter location within the heart's chamber. Important catheter locations are subsequently recorded and represented as color-coded spots on a 3D grid, a process that requires a skilled operator's interpretation (Fig. 29.4). Individual catheter locations can be saved, annotated, and revisited later in the procedure.

Due to the fact that the system displays real-time electrode movements, catheter movements due to cardiac and respiratory cycles are similar to those observed with fluoroscopy. In initial human validation studies, the LocaLisa® system was described to provide clinically feasible and accurate catheter locations within the heart [36]. Developers of the system reported successful use in over 250 complex ablation procedures for both ventricular and supraventricular tachyarrhythmias. The novel capabilities of this system include: (1) its ability to use any general catheter to collect data; (2) relative improvements in the visualization of catheters in 3D space; and (3) a broad clinical applicability. Finally, this methodology can be applied with complex catheter designs such as multielectrode catheters, irrigated electrode catheters, and/or basket catheters [37–39].

29.3.2 Continuous Mapping Systems

29.3.2.1 Basket Catheter Mapping Technologies

In general, the limited mapping resolution of conventional catheters may be greatly overcome via the use of a multielectrode basket catheter. As such, basket catheter mapping was developed in the 1990s, and typical catheters contain 32–64 nickel or titanium electrodes that are 1–2 mm long and 1 mm in diameter (Fig. 29.5) [39, 40]. Depending on the basket catheter shape and radius, the interelectrode distance can vary between 3 and 10 mm. Regardless, the accuracy in reconstruction of the chamber's geometry and electrical activity created by the basket system relies on: (1) the number of splines on the basket; (2) the number of electrodes on each spline; and (3) the percentage of those electrodes which achieve

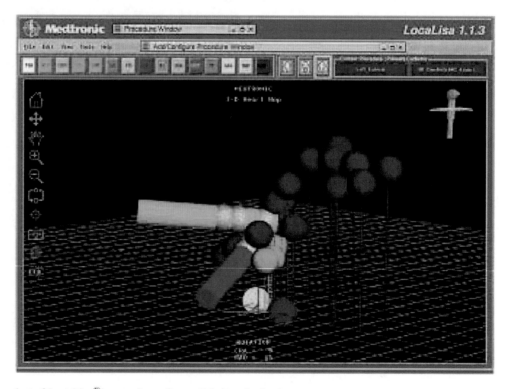

Fig. 29.4 Screen shot of LocaLisa®'s mapping software (Medtronic, Inc.)

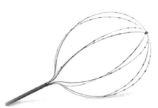

Fig. 29.5 Constellation® multielectrode basket catheter (Boston Scientific, Inc.)

adequate contact with the endocardial surface. It should be noted that, due to specific anatomic features of the chambers that do not allow complete endocardial coverage by the basket catheter electrodes, the quality of contact of all the electrodes with the endocardium cannot be ensured, and thus it is common that some anatomic regions cannot be adequately mapped.

The initial use of basket catheters was reported in a number of animal studies which were aimed at characterizing either atrial [39] and/or ventricular arrhythmias [40]. More specifically, Triedman et al. [41] reported studies in which they utilized a Webster-Jenkins catheter (Cordis Webster Inc., Baldwin Park, CA), a 5-spoke flexible ellipsoid with 25 bipolar electrode pairs, for the mapping of right ventricular activation patterns. Data were obtained from catheters placed into the right atria and ventricles of juvenile sheep which were eliciting either normal sinus rhythm or acute and chronic pathological sequelae [41]. They concluded that employing a basket catheter had the potential to provide rapid, nearly real-time, activation sequence maps which improved their understanding of the mechanisms of complex reentrant tachyarrhythmias. In addition, this approach was considered to provide assistance with the development of curative ablative therapies that are targeted for such abnormal rhythms.

Subsequently, Schalij et al. [42] reported on the first application of a basket catheter and resultant animation programs in 20 human patients with ventricular tachycardia. They reported that percutaneous endocardial mapping with basket catheters was feasible, of clinical value, and reasonably safe. Since then, basket catheter mapping has been employed in the study of numerous cardiac arrhythmias in various human populations [43–45].

Nevertheless, it should be noted that there are limitations associated with basket catheter mapping. First, the use of a basket catheter that is too large or small compared with the relative dimensions of the chamber of interest will result in poor quality of electrograms in terms of morphology, stability, and relations with the given anatomic structures. Second, it has been cited that the relative movement between the beating heart and the electrodes can be detrimental to the electrical reconstruction process or may even cause irritation of the myocardium. Third, the use of a basket catheter provides minimal specific anatomic information, and is typically unfavorable for clinical diagnosis and subsequent successful guidance of catheters in ablation procedures. Lastly, due to product size constraints, the basket catheter approach does not have the ability to map areas of the atrial appendage or pulmonary veins, which play major roles in the sustenance of atrial fibrillation.

29.3.2.2 Noncontact Mapping Technologies

Recently, NCM approaches have been more widely used in the clinical diagnosis and ablative treatment of complex cardiac arrhythmias, as described by Schilling et al. [11, 46, 47]. More specifically, one currently available product, the EnSite® 3000 noncontact mapping system (St. Jude Medical, St. Paul, MN) introduced by Taccardi et al. [48], is comprised of a catheter-mounted, inflatable multielectrode array, a reference patch electrode, amplifiers, and a workstation (Fig. 29.6). To date, this computerized data acquisition system has the capability for 100 analog inputs which include 64 inputs from the multielectrode array, a 12-lead surface ECG, 16 unipolar or bipolar catheter inputs, and/ or eight user-defined analog inputs.

Specifically, this system's EnGuide® locator technology utilizes a single use 9 French, 110 cm transvenous multielectrode array catheter (Fig. 29.7) consisting primarily of: (1) a polyamide-insulated wire braid with 64

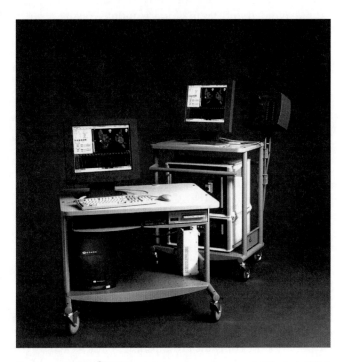

Fig. 29.6 EnSite® 3000 noncontact mapping system (St. Jude Medical, Inc.)

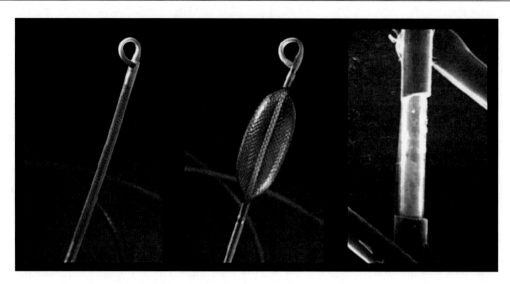

Fig. 29.7 Multielectrode array catheter (St. Jude Medical, Inc.)

laser-etched unipolar electrodes; (2) a 7.5 mL inflatable polyurethane balloon; and (3) distal and proximal E1 and E2 ring electrodes. Additionally positioned on the proximal end of the catheter is a handle and cable connector that allows the physician to deploy a balloon in the chamber of interest, providing the electrical connection from the array to the patient interface unit of the system.

Typically, the multielectrode array is inserted transvenously into the patient's chamber of interest over a standard 0.032″ guidewire. Once positioned within a given chamber, the multielectrode array wire braid is mechanically expanded and the balloon is inflated using a 50/50 contrast–saline solution. Next, a second catheter, termed the "roving" catheter, is introduced into the same chamber of interest. Following connection to the breakout box, the system's EnGuide® technology emits a low 5.68 kHz signal via the tip of the roving catheter that is detected by the E1 and E2 ring electrodes on the multielectrode array catheter. Subsequently, by determination of the locator signal angles and strengths, the system is able to compute the 3D relationship of the tip of the roving catheter to that of the multielectrode array catheter ring electrodes. In order to reconstruct the 3D "virtual" endocardium of the chamber, the roving catheter continues to emit the 5.68 kHz signal, as it is moved around the chamber by dragging the tip around the endocardial wall's contour. This approach employs a bicubic spline-smoothing algorithm to create the contour of the chamber's geometry.

A convex-hull algorithm is then utilized to omit the previously collected points that are inferior to the facets created during the collection process, so that the system essentially stores only the most distant points visited by the roving catheter (i.e., those from the endocardial surface during diastole). The roving catheter is used to locate the major anatomical locations associated with fluoroscopic imaging, and these anatomical landmarks are subsequently labeled on the reconstructed geometry to provide a frame of reference for the physician.

Once the geometry reconstruction is complete, the multielectrode array is used to detect and record the far-field intracavitary electrical potentials from the surrounding myocardium by employing an approximation method based on algorithms developed for inverse problems [49]. To further explain, the potentials in this field are typically lower in amplitude and frequency than the source potentials of the endocardium itself. Therefore, to improve accuracy and stability in reconstruction, a technique is used based on an inverse solution to Laplace's equation by the use of a boundary element method so that the resulting signals are used to reconstruct and display >3,300 "virtual" electrograms.

After the establishment of the chamber's voltage field, cardiac activation can be displayed as computed "virtual" electrograms or as isopotential maps. More specifically, these resulting isopotential maps are dynamic representations of the propagation of the electrical wave front. As such, the electrophysiological information is visually represented by color coding that describes voltage, ranging from red (representing regions of depolarized myocardium) to purple (representing regions electrically neutral) (Fig. 29.8A). Additionally, the system allows for the creation of a static representation of the electrical propagations via "isochronal maps" (Fig. 29.8B). Consequently, the color-coded EP information is representative of the time required to activate different regions of the chamber. In cases where ablation is employed, the EnGuide® technology aids in navigating RF catheters to the appropriate site with an accuracy of ±1 mm.

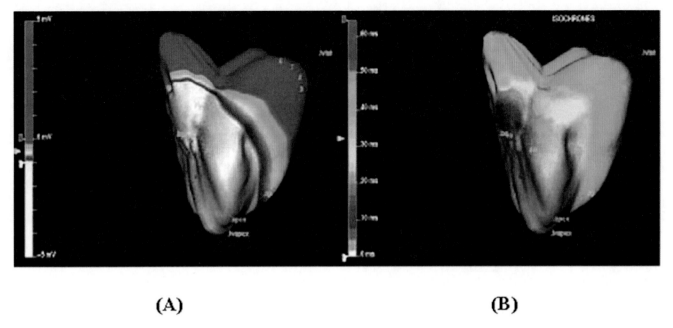

Fig. 29.8 Swine left ventricular (**A**) isopotential activation map and (**B**) isochronal activation map

The more recent EnSite NavX™ electrode-based navigation system uses externally applied high-frequency electric fields from cutaneous patches. It requires three pairs of skin patches, one for each of x-, y-, and z-axes, thus creating a 3D coordinate system. Therefore, the NavX™ system can, in theory, be used to perform EP studies and catheter ablation procedures without fluoroscopy [50]. With the NavX™ software system, it is also possible to import a 3D reconstruction of anatomy taken from a high-resolution computed tomographic scan performed prior to the procedure; this is then synchronized to the images so that 3D images and maps can be manipulated simultaneously [51].

Most recently, NCM has been utilized and validated in several clinical settings such as the evaluation and treatment of atrial flutter, atrial fibrillation [52–54], and/or ventricular tachycardia [55]. In such cases, this system has been used to aid in the identification of critical regions of slow conduction, to identify and then precisely return catheters to areas of interest in the chamber, and to subsequently visualize ablation lesion lines that have been created. Therefore, this system permits for the detailed reconstruction of global and local cardiac electrical events in a timely fashion within the EP lab. Most importantly, the system allows for a great deal of data to be recorded within the short duration of only one to two heartbeats, thus allowing the physician to adequately evaluate the origination, maintenance, and termination of nonsustained complex cardiac arrhythmias, pathways of reentrant activity, and/or electrical changes that may occur on a beat-to-beat basis.

Despite the vast number of advantages associated with NCM mapping, there are several current limitations worth noting. Background noise can greatly affect the quality of the recordings; this commonly originates from the surrounding environment or from the amplifier circuitry due to electrical fluctuations. In order to obtain optimally reconstructed electrograms, it has been documented that the distance from the area mapped to the multielectrode array should be less than 40 mm [46, 47, 56]; beyond this distance, there is an overall decrease in the accuracy of the reconstructed electrograms. NCM is only able to reconstruct the electrical activity on the endocardial surface of a given chamber, thus it is unable to identify subendocardial activation characteristics which may play a critical role in the successful identification of various arrhythmias and, hence, the subsequent therapy employed. The dimensions of the multielectrode array when in full profile are 1.8×4.6 cm^2, which can restrict mapping catheter manipulation when placed in particular areas of the heart, such as right and left atrial appendages. Lastly, despite several software updates, the system is still complex and quite expensive.

29.4 Noninvasive Cardiac Mapping

Significant and innovative advancements have been made in the noninvasive imaging of cardiac electrical activity. Ongoing research in this area is aimed at improving our overall understanding of the mechanisms of cardiac function and dysfunction, in turn, aiding clinical diagnosis and management of cardiac diseases. Employing such an approach allows clinicians the opportunity to precisely localize the arrhythmic substrate and study mechanisms prior to the intervention by solving the so-called "inverse problem." As a result, one can quickly focus therapy at the primary source of the arrhythmia and subsequently decrease the need for a lengthy EP procedure and, importantly, minimize fluoroscopy exposure to the patient and clinical staff.

The investigation of the epicardial potential inverse solution has garnered interest since the 1970s [57]. Recently the epicardial potential inverse solution has demonstrated the ability to reconstruct epicardial potentials in in vivo humans [58]. In addition, heart surface activation mapping, where activation maps over both the epicardial and endocardial surfaces are estimated from BSPMs, has been investigated [59].

Quite recently, He and coworkers proposed and developed the 3D cardiac electrical imaging (3-DCEI) approach for noninvasively imaging 3D cardiac electrical activity employing BSPMs [17–19, 60, 61]. In this 3D approach, cardiac electrical activity is estimated and visualized over the 3D myocardium by solving a linear or nonlinear inverse problem. This 3-DCEI approach was recently validated using 3D intracardiac mapping in both rabbit [62] and swine models [63].

The validation study of the 3-DCEI in the swine model [63] is reviewed below, as the swine represents perhaps the most similar model to humans. In brief, a heart excitation model and heart-torso volume conductor model were constructed based on preoperative MRI scans and prior physiological knowledge of the swine heart. The MR images were segmented to obtain detailed cardiac geometry and the cellular-automaton heart model. The entire heart excitation process could be simulated and the corresponding BSPMs were calculated by employing a boundary element method. A preliminary classification system was also employed to initialize the parameters of the heart-excitation model, and then model parameters were iteratively adjusted in an attempt to minimize any dissimilarity between the measured and heart-model-generated BSPMs until the convergent criteria were satisfied. In this swine validation study, we employed site-specific pacing and, for each pacing site, both the 3D location of the initiation site for electrical activation and the corresponding activation sequence throughout the ventricles were noninvasively estimated using the above procedure. In total, data from five right ventricular and five left ventricular pacing sites from control and heart failure animals were collected and, subsequently, sequences of 100 paced beats were analyzed. It was demonstrated that the averaged localized error of the right and left

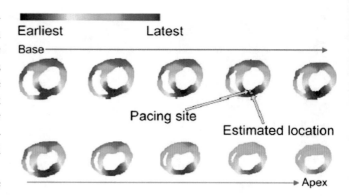

Fig. 29.9 An example of a 3D activation sequence imaged from noninvasive body surface potential maps in a control swine, following left ventricular pacing. Modified from Ref. [63]

ventricular sites was 7.3 ± 1.8 mm ($n = 50$) and 7.0 ± 2.2 mm ($n = 50$), respectively. The global 3D activation sequences throughout the ventricular myocardium were also derived. The endocardial activation sequences as a subset of the estimated 3D activation sequences were first compared with those reconstructed from simultaneously obtained data collected using an NCM system in order to validate the procedure. Figure 29.9 shows an example of the 3D activation sequence estimated from acquired BSPMs which were induced by ventricular pacing in a healthy animal. These promising results suggest that the 3-DCEI approach may, in the near future, provide a useful tool for both basic cardiovascular research and the clinical diagnosis and management of arrhythmias.

29.5 Future Directions

The mapping technologies developed and employed to date have revolutionized the clinical EP laboratory, and their use has led to numerous novel insights into mechanisms underlying all types of arrhythmias. Relative to the multicatheter approach, such technologies have improved resolution, 3D spatial localization, and/or rapid acquisition of the detailed characteristics of cardiac activation in both normal and diseased hearts. In general, these technologies employ novel computational approaches to accurately determine the 3D location of mapping catheters and anatomic-specific local electrograms. Acquired data of the relative intracardiac catheter position and recorded intracardiac electrograms are commonly used by such technologies to reconstruct, in real time, a representation of the 3D geometry of the cardiac chamber of interest.

Nevertheless, to date, such mapping systems are relatively expensive and generally not required for the diagnosis of more common clinical arrhythmias such as atrioventricular nodal reentry, accessory pathway-mediated tachycardia (Wolff–Parkinson–White syndrome and concealed pathways), or typical atrial flutter. Furthermore, it should be noted that other emerging technologies, such as intracardiac echocardiography [64], and the incorporation of high-resolution imaging modality data sets (such as CT or MRI) are considered useful adjuncts for more precise and rapid catheter positioning, perhaps even providing more reproducible catheter positioning toward specific intracardiac structures that are more difficult to identify for mapping or ablation. Yet, the mechanistic contribution of the newer cardiac mapping systems to treat various arrhythmias is likely to be well substantiated. Despite the theoretical clinical advantages highlighted by the discussed technologies, further prospective human clinical trials will ultimately need to be performed to provide further validation of their optimal clinical utility.

References

1. Tawara S. Das Reizleitungssystem des Säugetierherzens. Eine Anatomisch-Histologische Studie Über das Atrioventrikular-bündel und die Purkinjeschen Fäden, 1906.
2. Mayer AG. Rhythmical pulsation in scyphomedusae. Carnegie Institute of Washington, Washington, DC, 1906.
3. Mayer AG. Rhythmical pulsation in scyphomedusae. In: II. Papers from the Marine Biological Laboratory at Tortugas. Washington: Carnegie Institution, 1908:115–31.
4. Mines GR. On dynamic equilibrium in the heart. J Physiol (Lond) 1916;46:349–82.
5. Lewis T, Rothschild MA. The excitatory process in the dog's heart, II: The ventricles. Phil Trans R Soc Lond B Biol Sci 1915;206:181–266.
6. Lewis T, Feil S, Stroud WD. Observations upon flutter and fibrillation. II. The nature of auricular flutter. Heart 1920;7:191–346.
7. Barker PS, McLeod AG, Alexander J. The excitatory process observed in the exposed human heart. Am Heart J 1930;5:720–42.
8. Taccardi B. Distribution of heart potentials on dog's thoracic surface. Circ Res 1962;11:862–89.
9. Jackman WM, Wang XZ, Friday KJ, et al. Catheter ablation of accessory atrioventricular pathways (Wolff- Parkinson-White syndrome) by radiofrequency current. N Engl J Med 1991;324:1605–11.
10. Gasparini M, Coltorti F, Mantica M, Galimberti P, Ceriotti C, Beatty G. Noncontact system-guided simplified right atrial linear lesions using radiofrequency transcatheter ablation for treatment of refractory atrial fibrillation. Pacing Clin Electrophysiol 2000;23:1843–47.
11. Schmitt H, Weber S, Tillmanns H, Waldecker B. Diagnosis and ablation of atrial flutter using a high resolution, noncontact mapping system. Pacing Clin Electrophysiol 2000;23:2057–64.
12. Schilling RJ, Davies DW, Peters NS. Characteristics of sinus rhythm electrograms at sites of ablation of ventricular tachycardia relative to all other sites: A noncontact mapping study of the entire left ventricle. J Cardiovasc Electrophysiol 1998;9:921–33.
13. Sra J, Thomas JM. New techniques for mapping cardiac arrhythmias. Indian Heart J 2001;53:423–44.
14. Schumacher B, Jung W, Lewalter T, Wolpert C, Luderitz B. Verification of linear lesions using a noncontact multielectrode array catheter versus conventional contact mapping techniques. J Cardiovasc Electrophysiol 1999;10:791–98.
15. Calkins H, Langberg J, Sousa J, et al. Radiofrequency catheter ablation of accessory atrioventricular connections in 250 patients. Abbreviated therapeutic approach to Wolff- Parkinson-White syndrome. Circulation 1992;85:1337–46.
16. Wittkampf FH, Wever EF, Vos K, et al. Reduction of radiation exposure in the cardiac electrophysiology laboratory. Pacing Clin Electrophysiol 2000;23:1638–44.
17. He B, Wu D. Imaging and visualization of 3-D cardiac electric activity. IEEE Trans Information Tech Biomed 2001;5:181–86.
18. Li G, He B. Localization of the site of origin of cardiac activation by means of a heart-model-based electrocardiographic imaging approach. IEEE Trans Biomed Eng 2001;48:660–69.
19. He B, Li G, Zhang X. Noninvasive three-dimensional activation time imaging of ventricular excitation by means of a heart-excitation model. Phys Med Bio 2002;47:4063–78.
20. Ben-Haim SA, Osadchy D, Schuster I. Nonfluoroscopic, in vivo navigation and mapping technology. Nat Med 1996;2:1393–95.
21. Gepstein L, Hayam G, Ben-Haim SA. A novel method for nonfluoroscopic catheter-based electroanatomical mapping of the heart. In vitro and in vivo accuracy results. Circulation 1997;95:1611–22.
22. Shpun S, Gepstein L, Hayam G, Ben-Haim SA. Guidance of radiofrequency endocardial ablation with real-time three-dimensional magnetic navigation system. Circulation 1997;96:2016–21.
23. Pappone C, Oreto G, Lamberti F, et al. Catheter ablation of paroxysmal atrial fibrillation using a 3-D mapping system. Circulation 1999;100:1203–08.
24. Poty H, Saoudi N, Abdel Aziz A, Nair M, Letac B. Radiofrequency catheter ablation of type 1 atrial flutter. Prediction of late success by electrophysiological criteria. Circulation 1995;92:1389–92.
25. Sra J, Bhatia A, Dhala A, et al. Electroanatomic mapping to identify breakthrough sites in recurrent typical human flutter. Pacing Clin Electrophysiol 2000;23:1479–92.
26. Willems S, Weiss C, Ventura R, et al. Catheter ablation of atrial flutter guided by electroanatomic mapping (CARTO): A randomized comparison to the conventional approach. J Cardiovasc Electrophysiol 2000;11:1223–30.
27. Shah DC, Jais P, Haissaguerre M, et al. Three-dimensional mapping of the common atrial flutter circuit in the right atrium. Circulation 1997;96:3904–12.
28. Stevenson WG, Delacretaz E, Friedman PL, Ellison KE. Identification and ablation of macroreentrant ventricular tachycardia with the CARTO electroanatomical mapping system. Pacing Clin Electrophysiol 1998;21:1448–56.
29. Tomassoni G, Stanton M, Richey M, Leonelli FM, Beheiry S, Natale A. Epicardial mapping and radiofrequency catheter ablation of ischemic ventricular tachycardia using a three-dimensional nonfluoroscopic mapping system. J Cardiovasc Electrophysiol 1999;10:1643–48.
30. Kottkamp H, Hindricks G, Breithardt G, Borggrefe M. Three-dimensional electromagnetic catheter technology: electroanatomic mapping of the right atrium and ablation of ectopic atrial tachycardia. J Cardiovasc Electrophysiol 1997;8:1332–37.
31. Marchlinski F, Callans D, Gottlieb C, Rodriguez E, Coyne R, Kleinman D. Magnetic electroanatomical mapping for ablation of focal atrial tachycardias. Pacing Clin Electrophysiol 1998;21:1621–35.

32. Varanasi S, Dhala A, Blanck Z, Deshpande S, Akhtar M, Sra J. Electroanatomic mapping for radiofrequency ablation of cardiac arrhythmias. J Cardiovasc Electrophysiol 1999;10:538–44.

33. de Groot N, Bootsma M, van der Velde ET, Schalij MJ. Three-dimensional catheter positioning during radiofrequency ablation in patients: First application of a real-time position management system. J Cardiovasc Electrophysiol 2000;11:1183–92.

34. Schreieck J, Ndrepepa G, Zrenner B, et al. Radiofrequency ablation of cardiac arrhythmias using a three- dimensional real-time position management and mapping system. Pacing Clin Electrophysiol 2002;25:1699–707.

35. Soejima K, Delacretaz E, Suzuki M, et al. Saline-cooled versus standard radiofrequency catheter ablation for infarct-related ventricular tachycardias. Circulation 2001;103:1858–62.

36. Wittkampf FH, Wever EF, Derksen R, et al. LocaLisa: New technique for real-time 3-dimensional localization of regular intracardiac electrodes. Circulation 1999;99:1312–17.

37. Avitall B, Helms RW, Kotov AV, Sieben W, Anderson J. The use of temperature versus local depolarization amplitude to monitor atrial lesion maturation during the creation of linear lesions in both atria. Circulation 1996;94:I-558.

38. Borggrefe M, Budde T, Podczeck A, Breithardt G. High frequency alternating current ablation of an accessory pathway in humans. J Am Coll Cardiol 1987;10:576–82.

39. Jenkins KJ, Walsh EP, Colan SD, Bergau DM, Saul JP, Lock JE. Multipolar endocardial mapping of the right atrium during cardiac catheterization: Description of a new technique. J Am Coll Cardiol 1993;22:1105–10.

40. Eldar M, Ohad DG, Goldberger JJ, et al. Transcutaneous multielectrode basket catheter for endocardial mapping and ablation of ventricular tachycardia in the pig. Circulation 1997;96:2430–37.

41. Triedman JK, Jenkins KJ, Colan SD, Van Praagh R, Lock JE, Walsh EP. Multipolar endocardial mapping of the right heart using a basket catheter: Acute and chronic animal studies. Pacing Clin Electrophysiol 1997;20:51–59.

42. Schalij MJ, van Rugge FP, Siezenga M, van der Velde ET. Endocardial activation mapping of ventricular tachycardia in patients: First application of a 32-site bipolar mapping catheter electrode. Circulation 1998;98:2168–79.

43. Triedman JK, Jenkins KJ, Colan SD, Saul JP, Walsh EP. Intra-atrial reentrant tachycardia after palliation of congenital heart disease: Characterization of multiple macroreentrant circuits using fluoroscopically based three-dimensional endocardial mapping. J Cardiovasc Electrophysiol 1997;8:259–70.

44. Greenspon AJ, Hsu SS, Datorre S. Successful radiofrequency catheter ablation of sustained ventricular tachycardia postmyocardial infarction in man guided by a multielectrode "basket" catheter. J Cardiovasc Electrophysiol 1997;8:565–70.

45. Schmitt C, Zrenner B, Schneider M, et al. Clinical experience with a novel multielectrode basket catheter in right atrial tachycardias. Circulation 1999;99:2414–22.

46. Schilling RJ, Peters NS, Davies DW. Simultaneous endocardial mapping in the human left ventricle using a noncontact catheter: Comparison of contact and reconstructed electrograms during sinus rhythm. Circulation 1998;98:887–98.

47. Schilling RJ, Peters NS, Davies DW. Feasibility of a noncontact catheter for endocardial mapping of human ventricular tachycardia. Circulation 1999;99:2543–52.

48. Taccardi B, Arisi G, Macchi E, Baruffi S, Spaggiari S. A new intracavitary probe for detecting the site of origin of ectopic ventricular beats during one cardiac cycle. Circulation 1987;75:272–81.

49. Khoury DS, Taccardi B, Lux RL, Ershler PR, Rudy Y. Reconstruction of endocardial potentials and activation sequences from intracavitary probe measurements. Localization of pacing sites and effects of myocardial structure. Circulation 1995;91:845–63.

50. Tuzcu V. A nonfluoroscopic approach for electrophysiology and catheter ablation procedures using a three-dimensional navigation system. Pacing Clin Electrophysiol 2007;30:519–25.

51. Novak P, Macle L, Thibault B, Guerra P. Enhanced left atrial mapping using digitally synchronized NavX three-dimensional nonfluoroscopic mapping and high-resolution computed tomographic imaging for catheter ablation of atrial fibrillation. Heart Rhythm 2004;4:521–22.

52. Schilling RJ, Kadish AH, Peters NS, Goldberger J, Davies DW. Endocardial mapping of atrial fibrillation in the human right atrium using a noncontact catheter. Eur Heart J 2000;21:550–64.

53. Schneider MA, Ndrepepa G, Zrenner B, et al. Noncontact mapping-guided catheter ablation of atrial fibrillation associated with left atrial ectopy. J Cardiovasc Electrophysiol 2000;11:475–79.

54. Liu TY, Tai CT, Chen SA. Treatment of atrial fibrillation by catheter ablation of conduction gaps in the crista terminalis and cavotricuspid isthmus of the right atrium. J Cardiovasc Electrophysiol 2002;13:1044–46.

55. Strickberger SA, Knight BP, Michaud GF, Pelosi F, Morady F. Mapping and ablation of ventricular tachycardia guided by virtual electrograms using a noncontact, computerized mapping system. J Am Coll Cardiol 2000;35:414–21.

56. Kadish A, Hauck J, Pederson B, Beatty G, Gornick C. Mapping of atrial activation with a noncontact, multielectrode catheter in dogs. Circulation 1999;99:1906–13.

57. Barr RC, Spach MS. Inverse calculation of QRS-T epicardial potentials from normal and ectopic beats in the dog. Circ Res 1978;42:661–75.

58. Ramanathan C, Raja NG, Jia P, Ryu K, Rudy Y. Noninvasive electrocardiographic imaging for cardiac electrophysiology and arrhythmia. Nat Med 2004;10:422–28.

59. Tilg B, Fischer G, Modre R, et al. Model-based imaging of cardiac electrical excitation in humans. IEEE Trans Med Imag 2002;21:1031–39.

60. He B, Li G, Zhang X. Noninvasive imaging of ventricular transmembrane potentials within three-dimensional myocardium by means of a realistic geometry anisotropic heart model. IEEE Trans Biomed Eng 2003;50:1190–202.

61. Liu Z, Liu C, He B. Noninvasive reconstruction of three-dimensional ventricular activation sequence from the inverse solution of distributed equivalent current density. IEEE Trans Med Imag 2006;25:1307–18.

62. Zhang X, Ramachandra I, Liu Z, Muneer B, Pogwizd SM, He B. Noninvasive three-dimensional electrocardiographic imaging of ventricular activation sequence. Am J Physiol Heart Circ Physiol 2005;289:H2724–2732.

63. Liu C, Skadsberg N, Ahlberg S, Swingen C, Iaizzo P, He B. Estimation of global ventricular activation sequences by noninvasive 3-dimensional electrical imaging: Validation studies in a swine model during pacing. J Cardiovasc Electrophysiol 2008;19:535–40.

64. Lesh MD, Kalman JM, Karch MR. Use of intracardiac echocardiography during electrophysiologic evaluation and therapy of atrial arrhythmias. J Cardiovasc Electrophysiol 1998;9:S40–47.

Chapter 30
Cardiopulmonary Bypass and Cardioplegia

J. Ernesto Molina

Abstract This chapter describes the history and techniques of cardiopulmonary bypass, a process that effectually excludes the heart from the general circulation and leaves it empty so that it can accommodate open cardiac surgical intervention. Since its first implementation, cardiopulmonary bypass has improved significantly to become a very highly sophisticated, but reliably performed procedure. The near future promises even more improvements because research and innovations continue to make cardiac operations safer and more efficient.

With the advent of coronary bypass in the late 1960s and early 1970s, surgeons became increasingly interested in finding ways to protect the heart during the period of global ischemia via infusion of cold perfusates into the coronary circulation (i.e., cardioplegia). Therefore, this chapter further details the advantages and disadvantages of various cardioplegia solutions which have been developed at several separate institutions, including extracellular- and intracellular-type solutions.

Keywords Cardiopulmonary bypass · Cross-circulation · Anticoagulation · Heart–lung machine · Cardioplegia

30.1 Cardiopulmonary Bypass

Extracorporeal circulation and cardiopulmonary bypass are synonymous terms denoting a method by which the blood that usually returns directly to the heart is temporarily drained from superior and inferior vena cavae. The blood is diverted into a reservoir where it is oxygenated and subsequently returned to the patient's arterial circulation. This process effectually excludes the heart from the general circulation and leaves it empty so that it can accommodate surgical intervention (Fig. 30.1).

The breakthrough technologies that first allowed this type of open-heart operation were developed by two separate centers in the United States in the early 1950s. Importantly, Lillehei and Varco [1] at the University of Minnesota developed a cross-circulation technique. This technique utilized a human donor (usually the parent of a child undergoing cardiac surgery) who, in essence, functioned as an extracorporeal pump for the patient's circulatory system. This type of extracorporeal circulation also allowed the blood to be drained from the child's vena cava so that the surgical procedure could be performed within the empty heart. The subsequent development of the heart–lung machine by Gibbon [2] was considered revolutionary in that it eliminated the need for a support donor (a second patient). Gibbon's system has been improved since the mid-1950s and has gradually evolved into the standardized, but very complex and sophisticated, machine it is today.

The basic components of an extracorporeal circuit include: (1) a reservoir into which the patient's blood is diverted; (2) an oxygenator that replaces the function of the lungs; and (3) a pump that propels the oxygenated blood back into the patient's arterial circulation. In this manner, the machine bypasses both the heart and the lungs while maintaining the functions of other organs during surgical interventions within the heart.

30.1.1 Venous Drainage

The venous blood that is normally delivered to the right atrium is commonly diverted to the heart–lung machine, either by cannulating the veins themselves or by cannulating the right atrial chamber. Surgery performed in or through the right atrial chamber requires that both the right atrium and right ventricle be empty. To do so,

J.E. Molina (✉)
University of Minnesota, Division of Cardiothoracic Surgery, MMC 207, 420 Delaware St. SE, Minneapolis, MN 55455, USA
e-mail: molin001@umn.edu

P.A. Iaizzo (ed.), *Handbook of Cardiac Anatomy, Physiology, and Devices*, DOI 10.1007/978-1-60327-372-5_30,

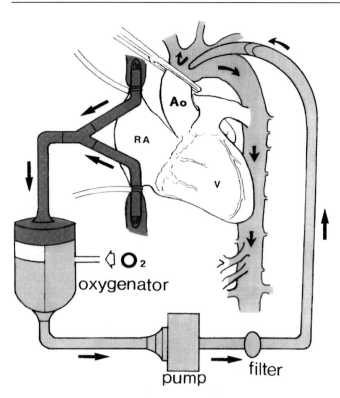

Fig. 30.1 Total cardiopulmonary bypass showing the venous cannulas in the superior and inferior vena cavae with constrictions placed around the respective veins. The venous blood is draining to the oxygenator and is propelled by the pump into the distal ascending aorta to maintain perfusion of the entire body. A cross-clamp is applied to the ascending aorta, and all chambers of the heart therefore are excluded from the perfusion system. Ao, aorta; RA, right atrium; V, ventricle

cannulas are placed directly into the superior and inferior venae cavae. Constricting tourniquets are then placed around the vein over the cannulas, and blood is diverted into the heart–lung machine (Fig. 30.1). These procedures constitute total cardiopulmonary bypass.

Venous cannulation is normally performed in one of two ways: (1) by placing a purse string suture either directly in the superior vena cava or in the right atrium or (2) by advancing the cannula into the superior vena cava. It should be noted that direct cannulation of the superior vena cava generally provides more room for any work that may need to be done inside the right atrium.

A modification of this type of bypass can be used when the cardiac chambers are not surgically entered, such as in coronary bypass operations involving procedures on the surface of the heart. In such cases, a single cannula is placed in the right atrium, or a double-staged cannula is placed with the tip of the cannula in the inferior vena cava and the side drainage holes positioned at the level of the right atrium. Coronary bypass surgery does not involve direct vision of the inside of the cardiac chambers, so there is no need to constrict the superior or inferior

venae cavae. When coronary bypass operations are undertaken simultaneously with cardiac valve repairs or replacements, total cardiopulmonary bypass is typically implemented.

30.1.2 Arterial Return

Once the blood has been oxygenated in the heart–lung machine, it is returned to the patient's general circulation via cannulas placed directly in the arterial system (Fig. 30.1). The most common method involves the placement of a cannula in the highest portion of the ascending aorta below the origin of the innominate artery. Depending on the type of surgery, other sites are also used, including cannulation of the femoral artery in the groin and infusion of the arterial system in a retrograde manner. The ascending aorta is cross-clamped at this point, so no systemic blood enters the coronary artery circulation. The heart is, therefore, totally excluded from the circulation. Thus the heart needs to be protected by using one of a number of methods to infuse cardioplegic solutions (see Section 30.2 in this chapter). Any blood remaining in the operative field is removed via cardiotomy suction lines which are used to aspirate it back to the heart–lung machine, where it reenters the bypass circulation with the rest of the removed blood.

In some operations involving the descending thoracic aorta, total cardiopulmonary bypass is not necessary. If the portion of the aorta that needs to be isolated lies between the left carotid artery and the diaphragm, only part of the total blood volume needs to be removed, and partial bypass can be implemented (Fig. 30.2). The blood is removed by the heart–lung machine via a cannula inserted into either the left atrium or left superior pulmonary vein. Then, the blood is infused back into the descending thoracic aorta beyond the level of distal aortic cross-clamping. Doing so allows the heart to continue to beat normally and helps maintain the viability of the proximal organs (head, neck, and arms), while the rest of the lower body is perfused and thus maintained by the pump. This technique is called *left heart bypass*, because it involves only removal of blood and decompression of the left side cardiac chambers. As shown in Fig. 30.2, after a descending thoracic aorta aneurysm operation is completed, the bypass is discontinued. The clamps which were placed to occlude the aorta in the arch and the descending portion are removed. The normal physiological perfusion of the body (which was interrupted during surgery without ever stopping the heartbeat) is thus reestablished.

In contrast, total cardiopulmonary bypass involves complete stoppage of the heart. After an operation

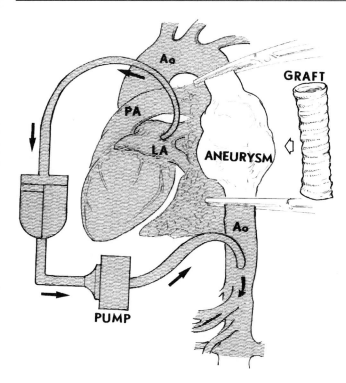

Fig. 30.2 Left heart bypass showing a cannula inserted in the left atrium draining approximately half of the cardiac output into the oxygenator through the pump, and reinfusing it in the distal aorta for perfusion of the abdominal organs. The excluded portion is only the descending thoracic aorta (between clamps). The left heart continues to beat and pumps half of the cardiac output to the head and upper organs. The graft is shown in the position in which it will be implanted after the aneurysm is resected. Ao, aorta; LA, left atrium; PA, pulmonary artery

applying total cardiopulmonary bypass and cardiac arrest, the aortic clamp is released allowing the general circulation to reperfuse the coronary arteries and to rewarm the heart. After the air is expelled from the cardiac chambers, the heart usually elicits ventricular fibrillation. Such fibrillation normally requires cardioversion with an electric shock administered directly to the heart by employing paddles that deliver currents that vary from 20 to 30 watts/sec. The patient is then ventilated using the endotracheal tube connected to the anesthesia machine, which reinflates the lungs. After the normal sinus rhythm of the heart is reestablished, the patient is gradually weaned off the extracorporeal circulation until the heart takes over full function. At this point the heart–lung machine is stopped, and all cannulas are removed and access areas closed.

In some complex surgical cases involving the aortic arch, separate independent perfusion of the arch vessels may require implementation, that is, in addition to the perfusion of the lower part of the body through the cannula inserted in the femoral artery. This situation places a great demand on the perfusionist operating the heart–lung machine. The perfusionist must monitor two

separate infusions to regulate pressures and make certain that a balance and sufficient perfusion is achieved in both the upper and the lower areas of the patient's body.

Another specialized bypass method that needs description is the *deep hypothermia and total circulatory arrest* technique. This type of total cardiopulmonary bypass employs a decreasing body temperature to very low levels (15–20°C); this is typically accomplished using heat exchangers installed in the heart–lung machine circuits. Circulation is stopped altogether when the proper temperature is reached, and the heart is emptied for several minutes with the entire volume of the patient's blood remaining in the reservoir of the heart–lung machine. The pump is then stopped and the arterial perfusion ceases. The venous return line, however, is left open to continue emptying the patient's blood volume completely into the reservoir of the heart–lung machine.

This technique is used in special cases to allow repair of very complicated conditions. The period of total circulatory arrest induced during deep hypothermia is usually less than 45 min [3, 4]. This time restriction is to insure that the patient does not suffer neurological deterioration or central nervous system damage during such global ischemia. As soon as the repair is completed, normal cardiopulmonary bypass is reestablished. The patient is gradually rewarmed to a normal core temperature of 37°C prior to removal from extracorporeal circulation. The use of such deep hypothermia always requires careful evaluation by the surgical team. In such clinical cases, the danger of inducing neurological damage must be weighed against the benefits of correcting a major cardiac anomaly.

30.1.3 Anticoagulation

To prevent the formation of clots during cardiopulmonary procedures, both within the body and in the extracorporeal heart–lung machine, it is necessary to anticoagulate the patient. The most common agent used for such anticoagulation is heparin. It is commonly administered intravenously before cannulation at a dose of 300 units/kg. There are two types of heparin: (1) the lung beef type which is extracted from a bovine source and (2) the porcine mucosal type which is from a swine source. Since the mid-1980s, the porcine mucosal heparin has been preferred because it is less likely to lead to thrombocytopenia and production of heparin antibodies in the patient, a condition known as HIT syndrome [5].

The effectiveness of anticoagulation therapy requires testing, usually by measuring the activated clotting time of the patient's blood. The result is expressed in seconds, with normal values ranging between 100 and 120 s.

Heparinization is deemed adequate when the activated clotting time runs above 300 s. At any time after such values are achieved, it is considered that the patient can undergo cannulation and be placed on extracorporeal circulation. Typically, the anticoagulant effects induced during such surgeries must be reversed postoperatively. Protamine sulfate is the drug of choice to neutralize the effects of the heparin and allow the patient to elicit normal clotting values. Yet, this drug is a macromolecule compound that may produce pulmonary vasoconstriction and severe hypotension [6, 7], particularly in diabetic patients. Nevertheless, such side effects are rare and, in most patients, this drug can be used safely, as it neutralizes the effects of heparin. Naturally, the amount of protamine necessary to achieve neutralization depends on the amount and timing of heparin administered. Initially, a test dose is given; if no reaction occurs, protamine is then administered in the appropriate amounts. Its effects are monitored by measuring activated clotting times until they return to a normal range. It should be noted that if any reaction or side effect occurs, additional treatments are commonly employed, such as the administration of epinephrine, calcium, steroids, or fluids [7].

Occasionally patients cannot be given heparin because they have developed heparin antibodies from previous exposure. Other anticoagulant agents are studied and occasionally used in such cases, including hirudin (Lepirudin) [8], a potent anticoagulant that is extracted from leaches and lampreys. Other drugs include the heparinoids [9] like Orgaran (Org10172, Organon Company, West Orange, NJ), for which a different monitoring protocol is implemented. Unfortunately, to date, no drug has been identified that can reverse the effects of Orgaran, thus it must be metabolized by the human body. For such patients bleeding is a constant, and often very difficult, postoperative complication.

If the cardiopulmonary bypass takes an extended time, coagulopathies often pose complications. In such cases, the body, primarily the liver, is unable to produce the appropriate clotting factors to reverse the anticoagulation status. Other factors that can contribute to coagulopathies include ischemia of the abdominal organs, particularly if necrosis occurs in the liver cells and/or in the intestine. Bleeding, therefore, can be a very serious and difficult complication to treat; administration of multiple coagulation factors, platelets, and cryoprecipitates may be required.

30.1.4 Temperatures of Perfusion

Since their inception, cardiopulmonary bypass and extracorporeal circulation have been implemented using some degree of hypothermia. Lowering core body temperature decreases the overall oxygen demands of body tissues, and a more desirable protective state during pulseless circulation is provided by the heart–lung machine.

Several degrees of hypothermia are commonly identifiable relative to extracorporeal circulation interventions. *Normothermia* indicates that core body temperature is between 35.5 and 37°C [10], *mild hypothermia* is between 32 and 35°C, and *moderate hypothermia* is between 24 and 32°C. An important distinction must be made between mild and moderate hypothermia. If the heart is perfused at mild levels (above 31°C), the heart will continue to beat although at a slower rate. This mild level of hypothermia allows surgical correction of some congenital anomalies without arresting the heart. An addition level of hypothermia used occasionally is *deep or profound hypothermia*, which was previously mentioned, and usually brings the body temperature below 20°C.

Currently, most open cardiac operative procedures are conducted under conditions somewhere between moderate and mild hypothermia. Some centers routinely use moderate hypothermia, while others employ normothermia [11, 12]. One reason to maintain normothermic perfusion is to avoid coagulopathies that may develop when body temperature is lowered to the moderate levels, and thus allow for normal function of the body's enzyme systems. Normothermic temperatures also enable the kidneys to respond better to diuretics.

Several reports have indicated the relative safety of normothermic perfusion [10–16], but an equal number have suggested complications with this modality [17, 18]. As a result, the spontaneous drifting to mild hypothermic levels is generally preferred. Deep or profound hypothermia is associated with the implementation of total circulatory arrest as mentioned before. With this level of hypothermia, body temperature is lowered to between 15 and 18°C. Such operations are thus usually prolonged given the time it takes to cool the body to those levels before surgery and also by the required time to rewarm it afterwards.

30.1.5 Perfusion Pressures

Under normal physiological conditions, the heart provides a pulsatile pressure and flow. The systolic pressure depends on the ventricular function. The diastolic pressure in normal states is primarily regulated by the blood volume and the vascular tonus. During cardiopulmonary bypass, the heart–lung machine facilitates pulseless perfusion; there is no systolic or diastolic pressure, but rather one steady mean pressure throughout the arterial circulatory system. Therefore, this pressure should be high enough to provide adequate blood oxygen to all organs of the body, particularly the brain and kidneys. Since the patient is typically hypothermic, the oxygen requirements are lower; the perfusion pressure is usually maintained around 70 mmHg. Occasionally, specifically in patients with severe obstructive carotid disease, a higher perfusion pressure is recommended to ensure proper perfusion of the brain. Nevertheless, this recommendation is somewhat debated because the brain is known to have its own regulatory system to maintain low resistance near obstructed areas [12, 14].

During cardiopulmonary bypass, if the patient shows decreased vascular tonus (despite adequate volume of fluid), vasoconstrictors are routinely used; a typical therapy is a bolus or drips of neosynephrine [10]. A decreased vascular tonus is common in septic patients with bacterial endocarditis, for whom an emergency operation sometimes is necessary to replace the affected valve and reverse the profound heart failure. In general, a mean perfusion pressure of around 70 mmHg during cardiopulmonary bypass should be maintained.

30.1.6 Hemodilution

Up to a certain level, hemodilution can be a desirable side effect of cardiopulmonary bypass. Lowering the hematocrit prevents "clumping" of the red cells or "sludging," thereby providing better circulation at the capillary level; viscosity of the circulating blood is decreased, on the other hand, to also ensure that oxygen is adequately delivered to the body's tissues during cardiopulmonary bypass. Hematocrit levels are monitored and maintained at a minimum between 22 and 26%. Toward the end of the bypass operation, typically the perfusionist deliberately removes some of the fluid from the patient's circulation to hemoconcentrate the blood toward more normal hematocrit levels [19, 20]; this rises to above 30% by the time the patient is removed from cardiopulmonary bypass. Subsequent diuresis and/or removal of red blood cells will further aid in reestablishing the hematocrit to normal levels.

Pulseless perfusion, as provided by the heart–lung machine, and hemodilution will both invariably lead to a transfer of fluid across the capillary walls into the third space (interstitial). Therefore, all patients develop, to some degree, peripheral third spacing or edema, which is particularly seen in children and usually requires several days to clinically resolve completely. In an attempt to avoid this condition, plasma expanders (such as albumin, hetastarch, dextran, and mannitol) are usually added to the priming solution of the heart–lung machine.

30.1.7 Heart–Lung Machine Basics

The basic components of the heart–lung machine include an oxygenator, a reservoir for the perfusion solution, a perfusion pump, line filters, two heat exchangers, and monitoring devices. Although the bubble oxygenator has been used for many years, it has been largely supplanted by the membrane oxygenator. The membrane oxygenator is associated with less trauma to red blood cells and is less likely to produce micro-bubbles that might pass into the patient's arterial system and cause air embolism. In addition, the newer centrifugal pumps (Fig. 30.3), like the Bio-Medicus (Medtronic, Inc., Minneapolis, MN) and the Performer® CPB (Medtronic, Inc.), offer a distinct advantage over the older roller-type pumps such as the standard DeBakey type. More specifically, the roller pumps use occlusive pressure to propel the blood within the tubing, and can cause damage to the red blood cells and dislodge debris from the tubing material. In contrast, the newer centrifugal pumps minimize trauma to the red blood cells, because the motion required to move the blood does not constrict the tubing.

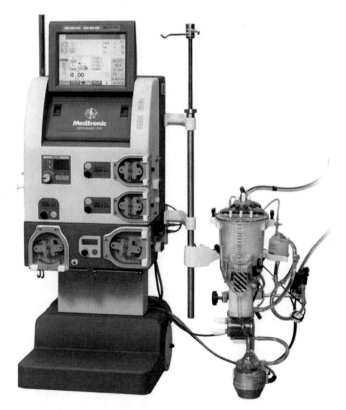

Fig. 30.3 Performer® CPB cardiopulmonary bypass machine manufactured by Medtronic, Inc. shows a smaller size adjustable to any position. Attached to the machine is the resting heart device which eliminates most of the large size reservoirs. It contains the filters and monitoring devices. All tubings are coated with Carmeda (see description in the text)

Although the classic heart–lung machine used gravity to drain the venous blood into the reservoir, modern machines like the Performer® CPB (Medtronic, Inc.) (Fig. 30.3) employ an active vacuum in a very small system that reduces significantly the use of the reservoir [21, 22]. This feature has significant clinical advantages, because it eliminates the large volume of fluid that is usually required to prime the heart–lung machine, most of which is taken by the reservoir. The Performer® CPB is smaller in size and can be placed closer to the operating table, saving tubing length, and it accommodates to any position. In addition, the tubing used for the heart–lung machine where the blood circulates has undergone significant improvement with the use of Carmeda [23, 24], which is a bioactive surface with which the inner side of the tubing is coated. Carmeda is bonded to the wall tubing, mimicking the human endovascular endothelium to reduce coagulation and inflammatory responses of the body due to the blood–material surface interaction. Therefore the doses of heparin, the common anticoagulant for extracorporeal circulation, can be reduced significantly. As a corollary, the risk for bleeding during or after surgery is significantly reduced. The Performer® CPB machine displayed in Fig. 30.3 incorporates multiple safety features consisting of alarm sensors for air bubbles, debris, pressure changes, and temperatures, making its use practically fool proof for protection of the patient.

The initial priming of the heart–lung machine is done with crystalloid solution. Currently, in our institution, Plasmalite is the preferred crystalloid solution to which albumin or hetastarch can be added. The latter two components help to maintain osmolarity and volume in the intravascular space and prevent peripheral third spacing, i.e., caused by leaking of fluid into the extravascular tissues producing edema. As the extracorporeal circulation is implemented, it leads to hemodilution, thus the blood of the patient mixes with the priming crystalloid solution used in the pump. However, pumps like the Performer® CPB automatically monitor the hematocrit of the patient and subtract the extra fluid from the circulation, leaving the patient at the end of the procedure with normal values of hematocrit and hemoglobin. The red cell sludging, which in the past was prevented by adding more heparin to the perfusate, is no longer needed, and the patient who usually was given 300 units/kg weight of heparin now requires only half of that amount without the occurrence of sludging. Once all the cannulas are inserted in the proper places and the connections are properly made, the surgeon gives the order to begin cardiopulmonary bypass and the planned operation is undertaken.

After the blood is oxygenated, it is passed through the heat exchangers that cool or rewarm it as necessary for a given stage of the operation. Typically, one heat exchanger provides temperature control for systemic perfusion to the patient's body, whereas a second exchanger controls the temperature within the cardioplegia line. In most current systems, the temperature within each circuit is separately controlled by a central regulatory unit. The blood is then filtered which helps prevent microembolization when it is returned to the patient's arterial system. In addition, two suction lines are employed to aspirate any blood from the operative field, thus recovering and returning the blood to the reservoir where it is oxygenated before being pumped back into the patient's arterial system.

The perfusionist needs to monitor the general circulation flow, the electrolyte parameters, the anticoagulation parameters, and the ultrafiltration system (which extracts fluids from the patient's arterial system to avoid over hydration). The perfusionist is also responsible for maintaining the proper pressures within each circuit and monitoring the temperature of the cardioplegic solution that will be used to protect the heart during the period of its exclusion from general circulation. Normally, at 15–20 min intervals, the perfusionist apprizes the surgeon of the elapsed time of perfusion and reinfuses the heart as necessary to maintain a temperature within the appropriate range (below 15°C). The perfusionist also remains in direct communication with the anesthesiologist to coordinate administration of any drugs or any other action necessary to maintain the balance of the patient's other organ systems. Finally, at the end of cardiopulmonary bypass, the perfusionist administers protamine in an amount sufficient to neutralize the effects of the heparin, thus returning the patient's coagulation system to normal function.

At the conclusion of the surgery, cardiopulmonary bypass is discontinued and the patient's heart resumes systemic blood circulation. A small volume of blood often remains in the pump and needs to be reinfused into the patient. This remaining blood is sometimes reinfused directly from the reservoir or it may be concentrated and reinfused later.

30.1.8 Heart–Lung Machine Priming

Before cardiopulmonary bypass is undertaken, the heart–lung machine needs to be primed. For an adult patient, the priming fluid consists of about 1,500 mL of fluid based on the basic crystalloid solution. Plasmalite is the preferred crystalloid solution to which albumin or hetastarch (about 500 mL for a normal-sized patient) is typically added. Doing so helps maintain osmolality and volume in the intravascular space, and helps prevent peripheral third spacing and edema. Red cell sludging usually is prevented within the system by the addition of extra

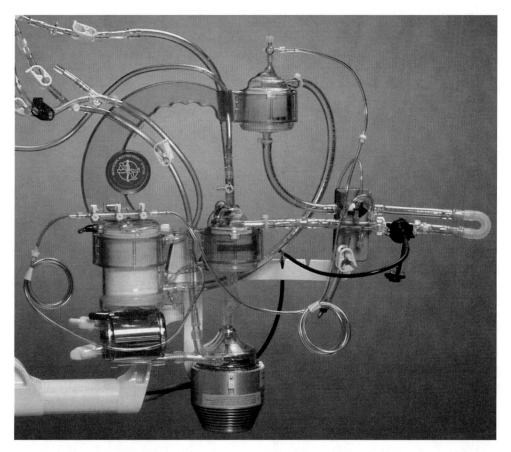

Fig. 30.4 Closeup image of the resting heart system showing the small reservoir in the center. The centrifugal pump is shown at the *bottom*. The rest are filters provided with alarm systems for air venting

heparin; however, with the new systems like the Performer® CPB (Medtronic, Inc.) this is no longer required. In the pediatric patient, ideally one should have much less volume than what is required in adults. In such cases, the so-called resting heart system provided by Medtronic, Inc. (Fig. 30.4) can be integrated into the regular Performer® CPB system to significantly reduce the entire volume needed for priming the pump. This integrated unit also provides for an automatic venous air removal and integrated air removal from the cardioplegic system. As mentioned before, at the end of the perfusion the blood is hemoconcentrated to normal levels by eliminating the extra fluid from the circulation and all the air is eliminated as well.

30.1.9 Hemodynamics

As cardiopulmonary bypass is implemented, the patient's blood pressure usually drops briefly as the blood is diverted from the heart to the heart–lung machine. This drop is precipitated by the cold (ambient) temperature of the fluid that was used to prime the machine and which the heart–lung machine has now introduced into the patient's aorta. This drop should last no more than a minute or two before the proper pressure and flow is reestablished. In general, it is preferable to maintain a systemic pressure of approximately 70 mmHg and flows between 1,500 and 2,500 mL m^2 of body surface area throughout the entire surgical procedure. If the systemic pressure tends to sag, which can happen because of various factors (e.g., loss of vascular tonus), the anesthesiologist and perfusionist must coordinate administration of vasoconstrictor agents (such as neosynepherine). If the pressure is too high, vasodilators are administered and/or the rate of perfusion is decreased to restore safe pressures.

Importantly, venous pressures and oxygen saturations should be monitored very carefully throughout the bypass procedure. An altered venous pressure is one of the most important indicators that a potential obstruction in the venous return has occurred, either at the level of the venous cannula or within the superior or inferior venae cavae. Such obstructions will often lead to major procedural complications if they are not monitored and immediately corrected. Typically the perfusionist reports any concern to the surgeon so that she/he can check whether any obstruction may exist. During cardiopulmonary bypass, the venous pressure should usually be near zero and saturation above 70% because all the blood is completely diverted into the heart–lung machine. Once the pressures are equilibrated, the temperatures must be maintained at the level of hypothermia that the surgeon has chosen.

The written records for the cardiopulmonary bypass are normally called *pump records*. They must contain all pertinent information including pressures, flows, temperatures, medications, periods of ischemia, and beginning and end times. Precise monitoring during cardiopulmonary bypass is extremely important especially in patients with compromised renal function (i.e., those who cannot produce urine to remove extra fluid from their own systems). In such patients, the most important electrolyte to monitor is potassium, which after any major operation usually rises above the normal level of 4.0–4.5 mEq/L. Potassium must be very strictly monitored to prevent associated severe bradycardia or cardiac arrest. A dialysis system can be used during cardiopulmonary bypass, if necessary, to prevent such serious complications. Even in large medical centers, patients who are normally on dialysis rarely receive potassium during cardiopulmonary bypass. In general, after weaning from cardiopulmonary bypass, most patients will display various degrees of bradycardia, usually because of the persistent effect of large amounts of β-blockers administered preoperatively. Few patients will elicit heartbeats greater than 80 beats/min when taken off cardiopulmonary bypass. All patients are commonly provided with a temporary pacemaker system postoperatively. This consists of wires placed on the surface of the heart (external leads) and connected to an external pacemaker unit. Based on many years of research and experience, the optimal post-cardiopulmonary heart rate has been determined as 90 beats/min in an adult; atrial pacing is set at that rate, with appropriate ventricular sensing. Such pacing is usually necessary for only 24–48 h which, in general, provides higher cardiac outputs and significantly improved hemodynamics, and allows the patient to eliminate the extra water that is usually third spaced during such an operation. Ventricular leads are routinely implanted in all patients as a very simple and safe prophylactic lifesaving measure [25]. This practice is highly advisable during the postoperative period because serious problems such as complete heart block are frequently unpredictable regardless of the patient's age or general health. If serious problems occur, there is no substitute for the ability to pace the ventricle immediately. Once the acute recovery period is over and the patient is stable (typically 5 days after surgery), the temporary pacemaker wires can usually be removed. In rare cases when heart block or severe bradycardia occurs, a permanent pacemaker system may be necessary to implant; see Chapter 27 for more details.

30.2 Cardioplegia

In the 1950s, the consensus among cardiac surgeons was that the results of the surgical methods were satisfactory [26]. Yet, numerous reports described low cardiac output syndromes occurring after surgical correction of congenital anomalies [27]. Unfortunately, at that time no definite connection was provided between the lack of proper myocardial protection during surgery and the potential for postoperative cardiac dysfunction and/or high mortality rates. Not until the advent of coronary bypass in the late 1960s and early 1970s were intraoperative myocardial infarctions or deaths clearly attributed to poor protection of the myocardium [28, 29]. At that time, several reports also noted that the levels of cardiac enzymes after surgery were significantly elevated indicating that additional myocardial damage had occurred even during the operation [29]. As a result, surgeons of that era showed an increasing interest in attempting to protect the heart during the period of global ischemia (aortic cross-clamping) via infusion of cold perfusates into the coronary circulation. Cold infusion of any solution into the heart separated from the total body perfusion is one of the methods known collectively as *cardioplegia*. After continued demonstration of its effectiveness, the use of hypothermic cardioplegia became quite widespread. In order to implement the use of cardioplegia, the general circulation to the coronary arteries must be interrupted. This is achieved by placing a vascular clamp across the aorta just above the coronary arteries; in this manner, as the heart is excluded from the general circulation, the infusion of cardioplegic solution is done in the aortic root entering in the coronary circulation to achieve a rapid and complete stoppage of the cardiac activity. Other modes of inducing cessation of cardiac activity employ chemical additions to perfusates or shocking the heart with electrical stimuli.

Yet, today many issues still need to be investigated concerning optimizing cardioplegic methodologies, such as: (1) what type of solution to use; (2) how much solution to inject; (3) how often to reinfuse the solution; (4) how long to extend global ischemia safely using cardioplegia approaches; and/or (5) how well a specific solution protects the energy reserves of the myocardium. As mentioned above, operative settings requiring the injection of cardioplegia involve aortic cross-clamping and

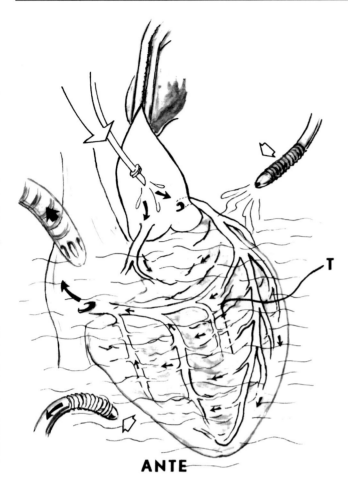

ANTE

Fig. 30.5 Antegrade cardioplegia (ANTE). The ascending aorta is cross-clamped and cardioplegia is infused into the root of the aorta. The solution runs through the coronary arterial system and leaves the heart via the coronary sinus in the right atrium. At the *upper right corner* is an irrigating catheter that provides continuous topical hypothermia. This solution is removed by the suction line at the lower left (*clear arrows*). T, temperature probe positioned in interventricular septum for monitoring purposes

coronary infusion (Fig. 30.5) of usually a cold chemical solution [30–34]. Some cardiac surgeons prefer to inject warm [35, 36] or tepid [37] solutions that have been mixed with chemical components (e.g., high potassium concentrations). Ideally normal myocardial cells require uninterrupted coronary perfusion. Therefore the principles of applying cardioplegia are aimed at: (1) conserving energy through the rapid induction of diastolic arrest; (2) slowing the metabolic demands and degenerative processes that inevitably follow global myocardial ischemia; and (3) preventing unfavorable ischemic changes. Extensive research over the past 30 plus years has provided several formulations of chemical components with or without cooling to obtain these three goals. Interestingly, the relative use of these solutions still varies widely, likely because they have been independently developed at several separate institutions.

30.2.1 Types of Solutions

Crystalloid solutions generally can be divided into two categories based on their approximate formulation—extracellular or intracellular. Extracellular solutions contain calcium and sodium, the primary determinants for transcellular calcium exchange. Cardioplegic cardiac arrest can still be achieved by extracellular solutions containing only moderate amounts of potassium or magnesium. Cold blood cardioplegia solution [32–38], the most commonly used throughout North America, is considered an extracellular ionic formula. The principle advantage to extracellular-type solutions is that they make it simpler to control equilibration characteristics within the ischemic myocardial tissue. Because no calcium or sodium variant exists in the extracellular fluid, subsequent replacement is easily achieved without any major reequilibration with the intracellular fluid. The disadvantage of extracellular solutions is that they are more easily washed out by noncoronary flow, but this effect can be counteracted by adding calcium channel blockers or procaine. Cardioplegic solutions that mimic intracellular ionic concentrations usually contain no sodium or calcium. Their advantage, at least in theory, is that their lack of sodium or calcium generates a large osmolar space which is available for other potentially protective components. In turn, this allows the solution to contain a high concentration of glucose, dextrose, mannitol, or histidine without excessive hyperosmolarity. Another advantage of intercellular-type solutions is that their minimal or reduced levels of extracellular calcium will limit contraction or restrict ischemia-induced calcium entry. The primary disadvantage of such solutions is that the lack of sodium and calcium may, under extreme conditions, predispose the heart to elicit the so-called calcium paradox. Another disadvantage is the potentially complex pattern of subsequent reequilibration then required. As Hearse et al. [39] pointed out, low-volume infusion of intracellular solutions offers good protection, but intermediate volumes offer only marginal protection, and high volumes may actually exacerbate injury to the myocardium.

Each of the described crystalloid cardioplegic solutions is considered to contain several components that have been "proven" by various researchers to provide enhanced protection. For example, in one study published by Hearse and colleagues [30], the effects of changing the composition of the simple cardioplegic solution when used during a 30-min period of ischemia were compared. It was shown that, at the end of a period of ischemia when no cardioplegia was used, the percentage of ventricular function recovery was practically nil, only about 3%. However, if potassium was added, the recovery increased to about 30%. Furthermore, if both potassium and magnesium were added, the recovery was even better (up to 68%). And if potassium, magnesium, and adenosine triphosphate were used in combination, the recovery reached 86%. Finally, if a combination of potassium, magnesium, adenosine triphosphate, creatine phosphate, and procaine was used, the recovery peaked at a dramatic 93%.

After using crystalloid cardioplegia alone for several years, it was considered whether mixing cold blood with the crystalloid solution would offer better protection than the crystalloid alone; it was suggested that the ability of the blood to carry oxygen to the tissues and its buffering capacity particularly if the period of ischemia was more than 90 min and, in such cases, the ventricular function was less than normal. Although the idea of protecting the heart with blood cardioplegia originated in the early 1950s with Ebert and colleagues [40], it was not until 20 years later when it was reintroduced by Buckberg and associates [32, 36, 38, 41, 42] that it became popular among most surgeons in the United States and throughout the world to use cold blood cardioplegia. Nevertheless, controversy persists regarding the "optimal" formulation to protect and prevent damage to the heart. The following solutions are some of the most commonly used for such procedures today.

30.2.2 St. Thomas II Solution

The formulation for the St. Thomas II solution (Plegisol: Abbott Laboratories, Abbott Park, IL) originated with the published research of Hearse, Braimbridge, Stuart, and Jynge [30, 39, 43, 44] from the St. Thomas Hospital in London. The basic vehicle was Ringers solution to which potassium chloride, procaine, and magnesium were added (Table 30.1).

St. Thomas II solution is an extracellular-type formulation. It is used extensively as an isolated clear cardioplegic solution and also as the base mix for the cold blood cardioplegic solution proposed by Buckberg and colleagues. It is usually injected into the root of the aorta at temperatures between 4 and 6°C (Fig. 30.5) depending on

Table 30.1 Composition of St. Thomas II solution

Sodium chloride	120 mmol/L
Potassium	16 mmol/L
Sodium bicarbonate	10 mmol/L
Calcium	1.2 mmol/L
Magnesium	16 mmol/L
Procaine	1 mmol/L
Osmolality	280 mOsm/kg H_2O
Oncotic pressure	0.4
pH	7.8

the surgeon's preference with an initial volume of about 1,000 mL for a 70 kg adult, followed by 100 mL infusions intermittently every 15–20 min. This method has long been combined with or without topical hypothermia to maintain the heart's temperature below 15°C. The size of the catheter used for its infusion and the pressure for injecting it are discussed in Section 30.2.8.

30.2.3 Birmingham Solution

Various extracellular solutions were also developed in the United States. Most solutions sought to attain relatively high extracellular concentrations of potassium as an arrest-inducing agent. More specifically, Birmingham solution was developed by Conti and colleagues [45]; its effectiveness was primarily demonstrated by the publications of Kirklin and colleagues [46]. The importance of the Birmingham solution is that glucose was included as a substrate for the myocardium (Table 30.2). The development of this solution gave origin to many other formulations that use the basic additions of glucose, potassium, and insulin.

Table 30.2 Composition of Birmingham solution

Sodium	100 mmol/L
Potassium	30 mmol/L
Calcium	0.7 mmol/L
Glucose	5 g/L
Chloride	84 mmol/L
Albumin	50 g/L
Mannitol	5 g/L
Osmolality	300–335 mOsm/L

30.2.4 Bretschneider Solution (Custodiol)

During the early 1960s and 1970s, Bretschneider in Goettingen, Germany, published his studies introducing HTK (histidine–tryptophane–ketoglutarate) also known as Custodiol crystalloid cardioplegic solution (Dr. F. Köhler Chemie GmbHD-6146 Alsbach-Hähnlein, Germany) [47, 48] (Table 30.3). This intracellular-type solution has also been shown to be very effective in protecting the heart during surgery. It has been used extensively in Germany since its introduction and has also been used widely throughout Asia, North Africa, and Latin America. It is used not only as a protective solution for the heart during periods of surgical ischemia but also as a preservation solution for hearts [49–51], livers, and kidneys [52] prior to transplantation. According to Preusse et al. [48], this solution must be provided in large amounts, between 3,000 and 4,000 mL per organ.

Table 30.3 Composition of Bretschneider (Custodiol) solution

Sodium	15 mM
Potassium	9 mM
Magnesium	4 mM
α-Histidine	180 mM
α-Histidine Hcl	18 mM
Calcium chloride	0.015 mM
Mannitol	30 mM
Tryptophane	2 mM
Ketoglutarate	1 mM
pH	7.1–7.2
Osmolality	295–325 mOsm/kg H_2O

Therefore, double cannulation of the right atrium with exclusion of this chamber must be implemented during surgery in order to allow opening of the atrium and to eliminate the large volume of solution from the coronary sinus orifice to prevent the fluid from reaching the general circulation (Fig. 30.6). For Custodiol solution to be most effective, the period of equilibration is crucial [47, 48]; that is, it takes about 7 min of infusion to equilibrate the extracellular and intracellular spaces before the patient's operation should proceed. This solution has also been used for both antegrade and retrograde (through the coronary sinus) perfusions. One of the considered significant advantages of this solution is its buffering capacity, which even surpasses the buffering properties of blood. Importantly, Custodiol solution needs to be stored at a specific temperature (12–16°C) to prevent denaturation of the components.

30.2.5 Glucose–Insulin–Potassium Solutions

Most of the research performed on glucose–insulin–potassium (GIK) solutions was done in the United States. Multiple formulations with these components have been widely used for the past 30 years. Studies by Hewitt et al. [53] and later by Lolley et al. [54] demonstrated that continuous infusion of a solution containing 278 mmol/L glucose, 20 mmol/L potassium, and 20 U insulin with 69 mmol/L mannitol dramatically improved myocardial protection. Those studies illustrated that the combination of glucose, insulin, and potassium improved anaerobic glycolysis and the washout of toxic substances. A slight modification of this basic solution, which included albumin to increase osmolality, was used extensively for many years at the University of Minnesota (Minneapolis, MN) [55–57] (Table 30.4). The only concern with the use of GIK solution is the inevitable degradation of its constituent insulin over time. Therefore GIK solutions must be prepared fresh for each use and cannot be stored for prolonged periods of time.

Many investigators contributed to the formulation of GIK solutions, among them Follete and coworkers [38] and Todd and Tyers [58]. We consider here that Roe et al.'s classical solution [34] also belongs in this category. The common denominator among these formulations is the use of dextrose as the basic vehicle. Multiple publications have shown protective effects. However when used alone, GIK solutions often provide insufficient protection

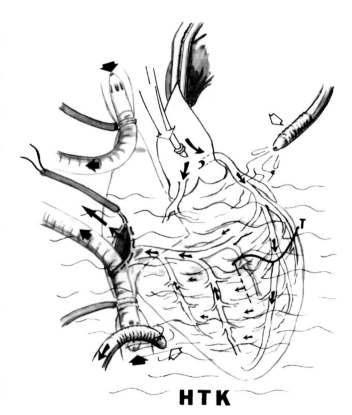

HTK

Fig. 30.6 Antegrade infusion of the Bretschneider (HTK, "Custodiol" solution containing histidine–tryptophane–ketoglutarate). The solution is infused in an antegrade manner into the aortic root while the aorta is cross-clamped. Because this method requires a large volume of solution, the right atrium is open and the solution exiting in the coronary sinus is aspirated and discarded. The superior and inferior vena cavae are individually cannulated to allow the right atrium to remain empty so that the HTK solution can be evacuated. Topical continuous hypothermia is shown with the irrigating cannula at the *upper right* and the suction catheter at the *lower left*. T, temperature probe

Table 30.4 Composition of crystalloid potassium insulin (University of Minnesota) solution

Dextrose	50 gm/1,000 mL
Sodium	3.5 mEq/L
Potassium	30 mEq/L
Chloride	30 mEq/L
Sodium bicarbonate	3.5 mEq/L
Regular insulin	10 units
Mannitol	12.5 g
Albumin	12.5 g
Osmolality	364 mOsm/L
pH	7.8
Oncotic pressure	3

Table 30.5 Components used to raise osmolality

Component	Oncotic pressure (mmHg)	Osmolality (mOsm)
Hespan (hetastarch) (6% in 0.9% saline solution)	18.4	311
Mannitol 25% (12.5 g/50 mL)	0.1	–
Albumin 25%	>200	239
Dextran (10% in dextrose)	130.2	319
Plasmanate (5% albumin)	16.86	239
Tris hydroxymethyl aminomethane (THAM)	–	370

Table 30.6 Composition of Buckberg's cold blood cardioplegic solution

5% Dextrose with ¼ normal saline	422 mL
Potassium chloride	2 mEq/mL
Tris hydroxymethyl aminomethane (THAM)	72 mL CPD 6
Diluent volume	500 mL
Blood hematocrit	22% = 500 mL
Osmolality	360 mOsm/kg
Potassium	22 mEq/L
pH	7.8
Calcium	0.3 mEq/L
Hematocrit	10%

during long periods of ischemia (i.e., beyond 120 min) or when the left ventricular function is marginal initially.

Several crystalloid solutions have been formulated without dextrose. The main difference among these is the basic vehicle which could be formulated with Ringers or Krebs–Henseleit. Potassium is commonly added at doses between 15 and 125 mmol/L. Some solutions in this group are the University of Wisconsin [50, 59] and Celsior [60] solutions, both of which are also used to preserve organs for transplantation. Several agents are considered available to help increase the osmolality of cardioplegic solutions (Table 30.5), for example, mannitol has been included in such solutions to stabilize osmolality and to act as a potential scavenger for oxygen radicals.

30.2.6 Additional Components

Other components have been added to crystalloid cardioplegic solutions by various investigators based on their own research. These include aspartate as the substrate to generate adenosine triphosphate [41]; glutamate as a substrate [42]; procaine as a membrane stabilizer [39, 44]; nifedipine to prevent calcium paradox [61]; phosphates as a base for adenosine triphosphate regeneration [62–64]; and/or steroids (methylprednisolone) as a cellular wall stabilizer [65–67]. Other elements found to help maintain an alkaline pH include Tris hydroxymethyl aminomethane (THAM), as advocated by Buckberg [32], and histidine as in the HTK solution.

30.2.7 Cold Blood Cardioplegia

The mixture of blood with crystalloid cardioplegia has become the most favored formulation for cardioplegia among cardiac surgeons both in the United States and throughout the world. It is considered superior to any other cardioplegic solution alone. The standard proportion of blood to crystalloid solution has remained fairly constant at 4:1 (4 parts of blood to 1 part of crystalloid cardioplegia), although some surgeons prefer a proportion of 8:1 in special circumstances. Nevertheless, as mentioned before, the actual formulation of the crystalloid portion varies across institutions [68].

Administration of cold blood cardioplegia in the proportions proposed by Buckberg (Table 30.6) can be easily accomplished using the appropriate equipment available as a kit. This contains the necessary caliber of tubing which is placed in a roller pump that automatically mixes the blood with the clear solution before injection into the root of the aorta (Fig. 30.7). As an example, the Performer CPB machine (Medtronic, Inc.) can accommodate any mixing proportion desired (4:1, 4:6, 4:8). The kit includes a heat exchanger which maintains the temperature of the solution between 4 and 6°C and allows the myocardial temperature to decrease even below 15°C. The significant advantage of cold blood cardioplegia is that it is considered to provide oxygen and nutrients to the ischemic myocardium and offer optimal buffering capacity. This mixture can be injected antegrade (in the root of the aorta) or retrograde (by coronary sinus cannulation using a self-inflating balloon to perfuse the entire heart) [69] (Fig. 30.8). Cold blood cardioplegia has endured many years of testing, both in its initial form of providing cardioplegia at cold temperatures and in its more recent adaptation to warm cardioplegia as promoted by Lichtenstein et al. [70]. The cold blood method is widely used in the pediatric population as well as for surgeries to correct all types of congenital anomalies.

30.2.8 Cardioplegia Administration

Our previous clinical work showed that cardioplegic solutions should be administered at a rapid rate and under moderate pressure [33–55]. Doing so shortens the

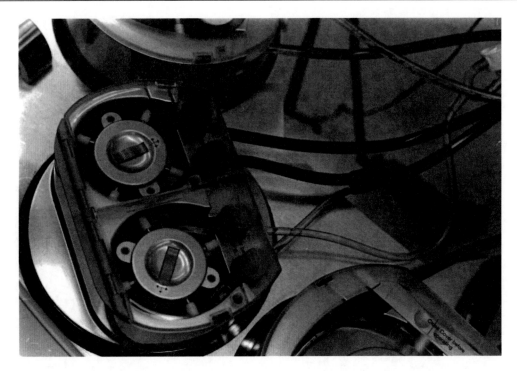

Fig. 30.7 Roller pumps of cardioplegia infusion system. The *upper pump* utilizes ¼ in tubing to move the blood, and the *lower pump* runs crystalloid cardioplegic solution using 1/16 in tubing. The blood and cardioplegic solution are automatically mixed in a 4:1 proportion in the outflow line before entering the ascending aorta

prearrest period, provides better flow distribution, and accelerates the decreasing myocardial temperature. In addition, rapid injection results in postoperative isoenzyme levels that are lower than those in patients who undergo slower cardioplegic injections [55].

Experimental studies on animals with normal coronary arteries have shown that low infusion pressures (less than 30 mmHg) and peak flow rates less than 125 mL/min result in a higher incidence of cellular ischemia, focal necrosis, and uneven flow distribution [57]. Consequently, patients with obstructive coronary disease who undergo low-pressure or low-volume cardioplegic injections will inevitably experience an increase in flow distribution problems.

Conversely pressures higher than 110 mmHg and peak flow rates greater than 1,500 mL/min may result in a higher incidence of mechanical and physical trauma to the vascular endothelium [57]. These higher levels, however, greatly enhance cellular protection. It should be noted that the use of high pressures in the aortic root in patients with coronary obstructions does not necessarily raise a concern. Rapid administration of cardioplegic solutions causes the temperature of the myocardium to fall rapidly within seconds to the protective range below 15°C and induces immediate cardiac arrest.

Cardioplegic solutions are most commonly administered via cannulas placed into the aortic root below the level of the aortic cross-clamp (Fig. 30.5). This site provides a normal antegrade flow to all areas of the heart. Several aortic valve procedures, however, require the aortic root to remain open for long periods of time. Therefore, infusion of cardioplegia can be done by direct injection into the coronary ostia by handheld cannulas, or in some cases, cardioplegic solution may be administered retrograde through the coronary sinus, while the valve repair is performed. This option also continuously protects the heart (Fig. 30.9). Yet, this approach has several limitations that are dependent on the degree of hypertrophy of the myocardium due to the preexisting condition. The delivery pressures in the coronary sinus must be intentionally kept below 50 mmHg to prevent possible injury of the veins. Such reduced pressures, however, may be insufficient to perfuse all areas of the heart. As a result, left ventricular dysfunction is occasionally observed after long periods of retrograde perfusion, even at myocardial temperatures below 15°C. In such cases, decompression of the left ventricular chamber is essential to facilitate the perfusion of all areas of the heart [71]. Therefore, some surgeons still prefer antegrade perfusion through the coronary orifices with the handheld cannulas, even though this may cause interruption in the flow of the operation. Over the past 30 years, the use of cardioplegic solutions should be noted as one of the most significant advances in cardiac surgery to increase the

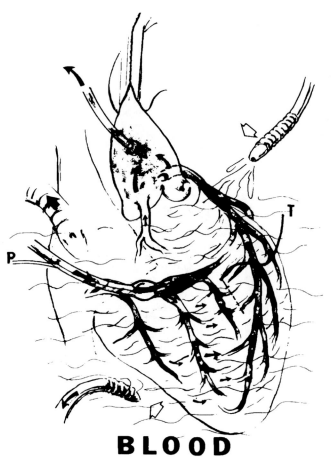

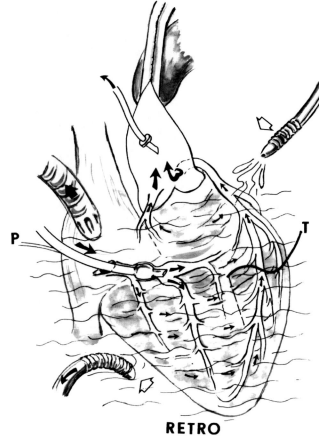

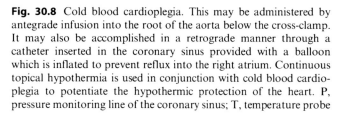

Fig. 30.8 Cold blood cardioplegia. This may be administered by antegrade infusion into the root of the aorta below the cross-clamp. It may also be accomplished in a retrograde manner through a catheter inserted in the coronary sinus provided with a balloon which is inflated to prevent reflux into the right atrium. Continuous topical hypothermia is used in conjunction with cold blood cardioplegia to potentiate the hypothermic protection of the heart. P, pressure monitoring line of the coronary sinus; T, temperature probe

Fig. 30.9 Retrograde (RETRO) administration of crystalloid cardioplegia. This is accomplished via the coronary sinus with a catheter provided with a balloon that is inflated to prevent reflux into the atrium. The solution eventually reaches the aortic root from where it is aspirated. It may also be allowed to drain into the left ventricle which is vented to the pump. Continuous topical hypothermia is again shown using cold saline over the heart. P, pressure line monitoring; T, temperature probe

safety of such operations. Continued research will look for optimal systems and methods to provide even better protection of the heart during cardiac surgery.

30.2.9 Adjunct Topical Hypothermia

The use of cardiac hypothermia has been one of the most important tools for increasing the safety of cardiac operations. The application of topical hypothermia in the form of ice slush was first introduced in the 1960s by Shumway, Lower, and Stofer [72, 73] and was used exclusively through the 1970s until the introduction of crystalloid cardioplegia. Topical hypothermia is considered to potentiate the use of all methods of cardioplegic perfusion, keeping the temperature of the heart in the safe

range to tolerate global ischemia. The heart can be effectively cooled externally by a continual flow of cold (6°C) saline or Ringers solution over the heart, eliminating the overflow solution using wall suction (Figs. 30.5 and 30.9). This technique is preferred to the older method of applying slush ice over the heart; the latter method has been blamed for causing frostbite lesions to the muscle and damage to the phrenic nerve, which runs along the pericardial sac. To avoid these problems, insulated pads have been designed to be placed around the heart to protect the phrenic nerves. Several types of plastic jackets were proposed and designed in the past, through which cold water was pumped continuously, while the jacket wrapped the heart entailing both ventricles. They are currently rarely used due to cumbersome application and crowding of the operative field. The topical cooling (whichever method is used) and the infusion of cold cardioplegia in the coronary circulation are discontinued when the operation is completed and rewarming of the patient begins. The aortic clamp placed in the ascending portion isolating the heart from systemic circulation is removed, and the heart receives the systemic warm blood from the body into the coronaries, reestablishing the normal perfusion of the organ. Once the heart temperature reaches 37°C and its function is reestablished, cardiopulmonary bypass is terminated and all cannulas are removed. Sometimes the normal beating of the heart reappears spontaneously but, if not, electrical cardioversion is implemented using internal paddles until a normal heartbeat is reestablished.

References

1. Lillehei CW, Cohen M, Warden HE, Varco RL. The direct-vision intracardiac correction of congenital anomalies by controlled cross circulation. Surgery 1955;38:11–29.
2. Gibbon JH. Application of a mechanical heart and lung apparatus to cardiac surgery. Minn Med 1954;37:171–80.
3. Bjork VO, Hultquist G. Contraindications to profound hypothermia in open-heart surgery. J Thorac Cardiovasc Surg 1962;44:1–13.
4. Brunberg JA, Reilly EL, Doty DB. Central nervous system consequences in infants of cardiac surgery using deep hypothermia and circulatory arrest. Circulation 1974;60(suppl 2):49–50.
5. Bell WR, Royall RM. Heparin-associated thrombocytopenia: A comparison of three heparin preparations. N Engl J Med 1980;303:902–07.
6. Fadali MA, Papacostas CA, Duke JJ, et al. Cardiovascular depressant effect of protamine sulfate: Experimental study and clinical implications. Thorax 1976;31:320–23.
7. Goldman BS, Joison J, Austen WG. Cardiovascular effects or protamine sulfate. Ann Thorac Surg 1969;7:459–71.
8. Greinacher A, Volpel H, Janssens U, et al. Recombinant hirudin (lepirudin) provides safe and effective anticoagulation in patients with heparin-induced thrombocytopenia: A prospective study. Circulation 1999;99:73–80.
9. Rowlings PA, Evans S, Mansberg R, Rozenberg MC, Evans S, Murray B. The use of a low molecular weight heparinoid (Org 10172) for extracorporeal procedures in patients with heparin dependent thrombocytopenia and thrombosis. Aus NZ J Med 1991;21:52–54.
10. Molina JE, Irmiter RJ, Vogelpohl DC, Nielsen KL, Callander D, Mueller R. Normothermic cardiopulmonary bypass for all cardiac operations. Cor Europ 1995;4:76–79.
11. Sing AK, Bert AA, Feng WC, Rotenberg FA. Stroke during coronary artery bypass grafting using hypothermic versus normothermic perfusion. Ann Thorac Surg 1995;59:84–89.
12. Lazenby WD, Ko W, Zelano JA, et al. Effects of temperature and flow rate in regional blood flow and metabolism during cardiopulmonary bypass. Ann Thor Surg 1992;53:957–64.
13. Nomoto S, Shimahara Y, Kumada K, Ogino H, Okamoto Y, Band T. Arterial ketone body ratio during and after cardiopulmonary bypass. J Thorac Cardiovasc Surg 1992;103:1164–67.
14. Croughwell ND, Frasco P, Blumenthal JA, Leone BJ, White WD, Reves JG. Warming during cardiopulmonary bypass is associated with jugular bulb desaturation. Ann Thorac Surg 1992;53:827–32.
15. Durandy Y, Hulin S, LeCompte Y. Normothermic cardiopulmonary bypass in pediatric surgery. J Thorac Cardiovasc Surg 2002;123:194.
16. Swaminathan M, East C, Phillips-Bute B, et al. Report of a substudy on warm versus cold cardiopulmonary bypass: Changes in creatinine clearance. Ann Thorac Surg 2001;72:1603–09.
17. Mora CT, Henson WB, Weintraub WS, et al. The effect of temperature management during cardiopulmonary bypass on neurologic and neuropsychologic outcomes in patients undergoing coronary revascularization. J Thorac Cardiovasc Surg 1996;112:514–22.
18. Craver JM, Bufkin BL, Weintraub WS, Guyton RA. Neurologic events after coronary bypass grafting: Further observations with warm cardioplegia. Ann Thorac Surg 1995;59:1429–33.
19. Naik SK, Knight A, Elliot M. A prospective randomized study of a modified technique of ultrafiltration during pediatric open-heart surgery. Circulation 1991;84(suppl III):422–31.
20. Davies MJ, Nguyen K, Gaynor JW, Elliot MJ. Modified ultrafiltration improves left ventricular systolic function in infants after cardiopulmonary bypass. J Thorac Cardiovasc Surg 1998;115:361–70.
21. Mahoney CB, Donnelly JE. Impact of closed versus open venous reservoirs on patient outcomes in isolated coronary artery bypass surgery. Perfusion 2000;15:467–72.
22. McCusker K, Vijay V, DeBois W, et al. MAST system: A new condensed cardiopulmonary bypass circuit for adult cardiac surgery. Perfusion 2001;16:447–52.
23. Aldea GS, Doursovnian M, O'Gara P, et al. Heparin-bonded circuits with a reduced anticoagulation protocol in primary CABG: A prospective randomized study. Ann Thorac Surg 1996;62:410–17.
24. Svenmarker S, Haggmark S, Jansson E, et al. Use of heparin-bonded circuits in cardiopulmonary bypass improves clinical outcome. Scand Cardiovasc J 2002;35:241–46.
25. Molina JE. Temporary dual-chamber pacing after open cardiac procedures. Medtronic News 1989;19:24–28.
26. Melrose DG, Dreyer B, Bentall HH, Baker JB. Elective cardiac arrest: Preliminary communication. Lancet 1955;2:21–22.
27. Helmsworth JA, Kaplan S, Clark LC Jr, McAdams AJ, Matthews EC, Edwards FK. Myocardial injury associated with asytole induced with potassium citrate. Ann Surg 1959;149:200–03.
28. Brewer DL, Bilbro RH, Bartel AG. Myocardial infarction as a complication of coronary bypass surgery. Circulation 1973;47:58–64.
29. Assad-Morell JL, Wallace RB, Elveback LR, et al. Serum enzyme data in diagnosis of myocardial infarction during or early after aorto-coronary saphenous vein bypass graft operations. J Thorac Cardiovasc Surg 1975;69:851–57.
30. Hearse DJ, Stewart DA, Braimbridge MV. Hypothermic arrest and potassium arrest: Metabolic and myocardial protection during elective cardiac arrest. Circ Res 1975;36:481–89.
31. Nelson RL, Goldstein SM, McConnell DH, Maloney JV, Buckberg GD. Improved myocardial performance after aortic cross-clamping by combining pharmacologic arrest with topical hypothermia. Circulation 1976;54(suppl III):11–16.
32. Buckberg GD, Olinger GN, Mulder DG, Maloney JV. Depressed postoperative cardiac performance: Prevention by adequate myocardial protection during cardiopulmonary bypass. J Thorac Cardiovasc Surg 1975;70:974–94.
33. Molina JE, Feiber W, Sisk A, Polen T, Collins B. Cardioplegia without fibrillation or defibrillation in cardiac surgery. Surgery 1977;81:619–26.
34. Roe BB, Hutchinson JC, Fishman NH, Ullyot DJ, Smith DL. Myocardial protection with cold ischemic potassium induced cardioplegia. J Thorac Cardiovasc Surg 1977;73:366–74.
35. Chocron S, Kaili D, Yan Y, et al. Intermediate lukewarm (20°C) antegrade intermittent blood cardioplegia compared with cold and warm blood cardioplegia. J Thorac Cardiovasc Surg 2000;119:610–16.

36. Rosenkranz ER, Vinten-Johansen J, Buckberg GD, Okamoto F, Edwards H, Bugyi H. Benefits of normothermic induction of blood cardioplegia in energy-depleted hearts, with maintenance of arrest by multidose cold blood cardioplegic infusions. J Thorac Cardiovasc Surg 1982;84:667–77.

37. Hayashida N, Ikonomidis JS, Weisel RD, et al. The optimal cardioplegic temperature. Ann Thorac Surg 1994;58:961–71.

38. Follete DM, Fey K, Becker H, et al. Superiority of blood cardioplegia over asanguineous cardioplegia: An experimental and clinical study. Chir Forum Exp Klin Forsch 1979;279–83.

39. Hearse DJ, Stewart DA, Braimbridge MV. Cellular protection during myocardial ischemia: The development and characterization of a procedure for the induction of reversible ischemic arrest. Circulation 1976;54:193–202.

40. Ebert PA, Greenfield LJ, Austen WG, Morrow AG. Experimental comparison of methods for protecting the heart during aortic occlusion. Ann Surg 1962;155:25–32.

41. Rosenkranz ER, Buckberg GD, Laks H, Mulder DG. Warm induction of cardioplegia with glutamate-enriched blood in coronary patients with cardiogenic shock who are dependent on inotropic drugs and intra-aortic balloon support. J Thorac Cardiovasc Surg 1983;86:507–18.

42. Beyersdorf F, Kirsh M, Buckberg GD, Allen BS. Warm glutamate/aspartate-enriched blood cardioplegic solution for perioperative sudden death. J Thorac Cardiovasc Surg 1992;104:1141–47.

43. Jynge P, Hearse DJ, Braimbridge MV. Myocardial protection during ischemic cardiac arrest. A possible hazard with calcium-free cardioplegic infusates. J Thorac Cardiovasc Surg 1977;73:848–55.

44. Harlan BJ, Ross D, Macmanus Q, Knight R, Luber J, Starr A. Cardioplegic solutions for myocardial preservation: Analysis of hypothermic arrest, potassium arrest, and procaine arrest. Circulation 1978;58(suppl I):114–18.

45. Conti VR, Bertranov EG, Blackstone EH, Kirklin JW, Digerness SB. Cold cardioplegia versus hypothermia for myocardial protection: Randomized clinical study. J Thorac Cardiovasc Surg 1978;76:577–89.

46. Kirklin JW, Conti VR, Blackstone EH. Prevention of myocardial damage during cardiac operations. N Eng J Med 1979;301:135–41.

47. Bretschneider J, Hubner G, Knoll D, Lohr B, Nordbeck H, Spieckermann PG. Myocardial resistance and tolerance to ischemia: Physiological and biochemical basis. J Cardiovasc Surg 1975;16:241–60.

48. Preusse CJ, Gebhard MM, Bretschneider HJ. Myocardial "equilibration processes" and myocardial energy turnover during initiation of artificial cardiac arrest with cardioplegic solution-reasons for a sufficiently long cardioplegic perfusion. Thorac Cardiovasc Surg 1981;29:71–76.

49. Preusse CJ, Schulte HD, Birks W. High volume cardioplegia. Ann Chirurg Gynaecol 1987;76:39–45.

50. Human PA, Holl J, Vosloo S, et al. Extended cardiopulmonary preservation: University of Wisconsin solution versus Bretschneider's cardioplegic solution. Ann Thor Surg 1993;55:1123–30.

51. Reichenspurner H, Russ C, Uberfuhr P, et al. Myocardial preservation using HTK-solution for heart transplantation. A multicenter study. Eur J Cardiothorac Surg 1992;7:414–19.

52. Groenewoud AF, Thorogood J. A preliminary report of the HTK randomized multicenter study comparing kidney graft preservation with HTK and Eurocollins solutions. Transplant Int 1992;5(suppl I):429–32.

53. Hewitt RL, Lolley DM, Adrouny GA, Drapanas T. Protective effect of glycogen and glucose on the anoxic arrested heart. Surgery 1974;75:1–10.

54. Lolley DM, Ray JF III, Myers WO, Sheldon G, Sautter RD. Reduction of intraoperative myocardial infarction by means of exogenous anaerobic substrate enhancement: Prospective randomized study. Ann Thor Surg 1978;26:515–24.

55. Molina JE, Gani KS, Voss DM. How should clear cardioplegia be administered? A method of rapid arrest with high flow and pressure. J Thorac Cardiovasc Surg 1982;84:762–72.

56. Molina JE, Gani KS, Voss DM. Pressurized rapid cardioplegia versus administration of exogenous substrate and topical hypothermia. Ann Thorac Surg 1982;33:434–44.

57. Molina JE, Galliani CA, Einzig S, Bianco R, Rasmussen T, Clack R. Physical and mechanical effects of cardioplegic injection on flow distribution and myocardial damage in hearts with normal coronary arteries. J Thorac Cardiovasc Surg 1989;97:870–77.

58. Todd GJ, Tyers GF. Amelioration of the effects of ischemic cardiac arrest by the intracoronary administration of cardioplegic solutions. Circulation 1975;52:1111–16.

59. Fremes SE, Zhang J, Furukawa RD, Mickle DA, Weisel RD. Cardiac storage with University of Wisconsin solution, calcium, and magnesium. J Heart Lung Transplant 1995;14:916–25.

60. Ackemann J, Gross W, Mory M, Schaefer M, Gebhard MD. Celsior versus Custodiol: Early postischemic recovery after cardioplegia and ischemia at 5°C. Ann Thor Surg 2002;74:522–29.

61. Nayler WG. Protection of the myocardium against postischemic reperfusion damage. The combined effect of hypothermia and nifedipine. J Thorac Cardiovasc Surg 1982;84:897–905.

62. Bolling SF, Bies LE, Gallagher KP, Bove EL. Enhanced myocardial protection with adenosine. Ann Thorac Surg 1989;47:809–15.

63. Sharov VG, Saks VA, Kupriyanov VV, et al. Protection of ischemic myocardium by exogenous phosphocreatine. J Thorac Cardiovasc Surg 1987;94:749–61.

64. Foker JE, Einzig S, Wang T. Adenosine metabolism and myocardial preservation. J Thorac Cardiovasc Surg 1980;80:506–16.

65. Vejlsted H, Andersen K, Hansen BF, et al. Myocardial preservation during anoxic arrest. Scand J Thorac Cardiovasc Surg 1983;17:269–76.

66. Rao G, King J, Ford W, King G. The effects of methylprednisolone on the complications of coronary artery surgery. Vasc Surg 1977;11:1–7.

67. Kirsh MM, Behrendt DM, Jochim KE. Effects of methylprednisolone in cardioplegic solution during coronary bypass grafting. J Thorac Cardiovasc Surg 1979;77:896–99.

68. The Warm Heart Investigators. Randomized trial of normothermic versus hypothermic coronary bypass surgery. Lancet 1994;343:559–63.

69. Menasche P, Kural S, Fauchet M, et al. Retrograde coronary sinus perfusion. A safe alternative for ensuring cardioplegic delivery in aortic valve surgery. Ann Thorac Surg 1982;34:647–58.

70. Lichtenstein SV, Ashe KA, El Dalati H, Cusimano RJ, Panos A, Slutsky AS. Warm heart surgery. J Thorac Cardiovasc Surg 1991;101:269–74.

71. Wechsler AS. Deficiencies of cardioplegia–the hypertrophied ventricle. In: Engelman RM, Levisky S, eds. A textbook of clinical cardioplegia. Mount Kisco, NY: Futura, 1982:381–439.

72. Shumway NE, Lower RR, Stofer RC. Selective hypothermia of the heart in anoxic cardiac arrest. Surg Gynec Obstet 1959;109:750–54.

73. Shumway NE, Lower RR. Topical cardiac hypothermia for extended periods of anoxic arrest. Surg Forum 1959;10:563–66.

Chapter 31
Heart Valve Disease

Ranjit John and Kenneth K. Liao

Abstract This chapter was designed to provide the reader with a brief overview of the current surgical treatment options for heart valve disease. Major topics of discussion are: (1) development of prosthetic valve replacements; (2) current issues with valve replacement; (3) major valvular diseases that affect humans in the Western world; and (4) recent advances in therapeutic options for valvular diseases.

Keywords Mechanical prosthetic valve · Biologic prosthetic valve · Aortic stenosis · Aortic sclerosis · Aortic regurgitation · Mitral stenosis · Mitral regurgitation · Tricuspid valve disease

31.1 Introduction

The function of the heart is to circulate blood in closed circuit to the lungs where blood is oxygenated and transported out to the body where oxygen provides fuel for cellular metabolism. To accomplish this task, blood is pumped by the right heart system from the body to the lungs. Once oxygenated in the lungs, blood is returned to the left heart where it is then pumped out to the body. Although described as a biologic pump, the heart is actually two biological pumps in series, composed of a right and left heart. Each unit of the heart is composed of an atrial and ventricular chamber, whose synchronized contractions result in the forward flow of blood out of the heart. Crucial to the appropriate function of the heart are four valves (the mitral, aortic, tricuspid, and pulmonic

valves) that function in concert to maintain forward flow of blood across the heart (Fig. 31.1). Diseases affecting the heart valves result in either obstruction to forward flow (stenosis) or reversal of flow across an incompetent valve (regurgitation). In either case, significant morbidity and mortality will result if no treatment is offered to the patient.

31.2 A New Frontier–Valve Replacement

Before 1950, the ability to safely and effectively operate on the human heart was considered an insurmountable goal. Attempts to operate to correct valvular diseases without stopping the heart resulted in severe, often fatal complications including uncontrollable bleeding and the introduction of air emboli [1]. The ability to maintain forward flow of blood while stopping the heart to allow the surgeon access to the valve would have to wait for the development of cross-circulation, and later for the perfection of the cardiopulmonary bypass procedure by Drs. C. Walton Lillehei, Richard L. Varco, and F. John Lewis at the University of Minnesota [2]. With this new technology, a new frontier in surgical options for the treatment of heart valve disease began to emerge. During the past several years, major advances have occurred in diagnostic techniques (i.e., imaging) and therapeutic interventions for valvular diseases as well as improved understanding of the natural history of both treated and untreated valvular disease (see Chapter 33).

31.2.1 Mechanical Prosthetic Valves

By 1961, Dr. Albert Starr and Lowell Edwards had successfully implanted the world's first mechanical valve into a human to replace a mitral valve that had been deformed

R. John (✉)
University of Minnesota, Division of Cardiovascular and Thoracic Surgery, Department of Surgery, MMC 207, 420 Delawaree St. SE, Minneapolis, MN 55455, USA
e-mail: johnx008@umn.edu

P.A. Iaizzo (ed.), *Handbook of Cardiac Anatomy, Physiology, and Devices*, DOI 10.1007/978-1-60327-372-5_31,

Fig. 31.1 Apical view of the
four heart valves—aortic,
mitral, pulmonic, and tricuspid

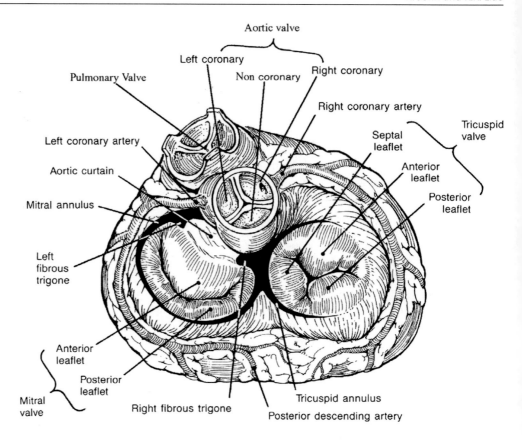

by rheumatic fever [3]. Initially, this steel ball and cage design was successful in approximately 50% of implantations. Major complications were soon recognized including: (1) clot formation resulting in embolic strokes; (2) significant noise; (3) red blood cell destruction; and/or (4) tissue in-growth causing subsequent valve obstruction. A complete history of the development of currently used mechanical prostheses is beyond the scope of this text. However, it is important to mention two key aspects of any successful new valve design: (1) improved valve hemodynamics and (2) reduced thrombogenic (or clot forming) potential. Efforts to optimize valve hemodynamic function date back to the development of the Lillehei/Kaster tilting disk valve which allowed blood to flow centrally through the valve. At that time, this new type of valve emphasized the requirement to design a valve that would reduce turbulent blood flow, reduce cell destruction, and minimize the transvalvular gradients [4]. A transvalvular gradient is defined as the pressure difference across the valve. Despite the advantages of a new steel tilting disk design, careful strict anticoagulation therapy was still required to reduce the risk of clot formation [5]. The next improvement of valves came with the development of the pyrolytic carbon valve leaflets. The nonthrombogenic weight and strength properties were determined by Drs. Jack Bokros and Vincent Gott.

Subsequently, pyrolytic carbon was used in the creation of a bileaflet valve, inspired by Dr. Kalke. This valve, originally manufactured by St. Jude Medical (St. Paul, MN), provided exceptional performance, and today this design remains the gold standard of mechanical valve designs [6]. To date, all patients with mechanical valves require anticoagulation, e.g., with oral warfarin therapy which reduces the risk of thromboembolism to 1–2% per year (Table 31.1) [7]. It should be noted that numerous studies have demonstrated that the risk of thromboembolism is directly related to the valve implant position, i.e., in the descending order of tricuspid, mitral, and aortic. In addition, this risk of emboli appears to be greatest in the early post-implant period, and then becomes reduced as the valve sewing cuff becomes fully endothelialized.

In general, management of anticoagulation must be individualized to the patient to minimize risk of thromboembolism and, at the same time, prevent bleeding complications. In situations where a patient with a valve prosthesis requires noncardiac surgery, warfarin therapy should be stopped only for procedures where risk of bleeding is substantial. A complete discussion of anticoagulation therapy is beyond the scope of this chapter; however, it is noted that several excellent reviews are available on this subject [7].

Table 31.1 Anticoagulation after prosthetic heart valves [7]

		Warfarin INR 2–3	Warfarin INR 2.5–3.5	Aspirin 80–100 mg
Mechanical prosthesis				
First 3 months post-implantation			+	+
After initial 3 months	Aortic valve	+		
	Aortic valve + risk factor		+	+
	Mitral valve		+	+
	Mitral valve + risk factor		+	+
Biological prosthesis				
First 3 months post-implantation			+	+
After initial 3 months	Aortic valve			+
	Aortic valve + risk factor	+		+
	Mitral valve			+
	Mitral valve + risk factor	+		+

31.2.2 Biological Prosthetic Valves

Because of the problems related to anticoagulation, a majority of subsequent valve research has focused on developing a tissue alternative that avoids the need for anticoagulation. From a historical perspective, Drs. Lower and Shumway performed the first pulmonary valve autotransplant in an animal model [8]. Later in 1967, Dr. Donald Ross completed the first successful replacement in a human. The "Ross Procedure" is a well-established method still used today to replace a diseased aortic valve with the patient's own pulmonary valve (Fig. 31.2). A donor tissue valve or homograft (Table 31.2) is then used as a prosthetic pulmonary valve. In general, tissue valves are significantly more biocompatible than their mechanical counterparts. These valves are naturally less thrombogenic, and thus the patient does not require aggressive anticoagulation. Specifically, a risk of <0.7% per year of clinical thromboembolism has been reported in valve replacement patients eliciting sinus rhythm without warfarin therapy [7]. Therefore, this treatment option is advantageous in clinical situations where the use of anticoagulation would significantly increase morbidity and mortality. Yet, to date, a potential major disadvantage of tissue valve implantation is early valvular degeneration as a result of leaflet calcification. Thus, methods for tissue preservation to prevent such calcifications are currently a major focus of research in this field.

31.2.3 Biological Versus Mechanical Valves

The choice of a mechanical or biologic valve for implant will typically depend on various factors: (1) the patient's

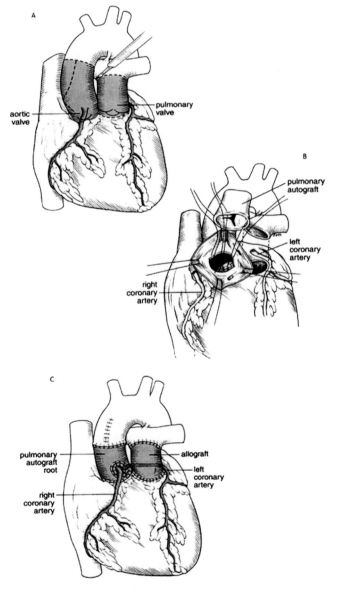

Fig. 31.2 Schematic drawing of the Ross procedure: (**A**) resection of the diseased aortic valve; (**B**) harvesting of native pulmonary valve; (**C**) implantation of the pulmonic valve in the aortic position and reimplantation of coronary arteries

Table 31.2 Tissue valve graft options: classification of bioprosthetic valves

Bioprosthetic valve	Description
Stented porcine valve (xenograft)	A three-leaflet valve supported by three artificial struts or stents to maintain leaflet structure and geometry
Stentless porcine valve (xenograft)	A length of porcine aorta including tissue below (proximal) and above (distal) the valve, called the "root"
Bovine pericardial valve (xenograft)	A three-leaflet valve created from bovine pericardium attached to a stented frame
Homograft	A human aortic valve and root
Autograft	A pulmonary valve and root excised from the patient and reimplanted in the same patient

current disease status; (2) the specific native valve involved; and/or (3) the surgeon's preference and experience. If these factors are not limiting, the choice of valve type should be based on the maximization of benefits over risks for the individual patient. Unfortunately, the ideal prosthetic valve that combines excellent hemodynamic performance and long-term durability without increased thromboembolic risk or the need for lifelong anticoagulation remains an illusion. In general, mechanical valves offer greater durability at the cost of requiring lifelong anticoagulation as well as the risk of thromboembolism. In contrast, bioprosthetic valves have a much lower thromboembolic risk without the need for anticoagulation, but elicit a higher risk for structural degeneration and thus potential need for reoperation. As such, mechanical valves are perhaps most well suited for the younger patient who does not desire future reoperations. Currently, mechanical valve replacement in the United States has been standardized and is commonplace, yielding satisfactory valve function that is quite reproducible from patient to patient. Furthermore, the flow gradients with newer bileaflet mechanical valves have dramatically improved from the early ball valve type; currently, a trileaflet valve is in the preclinical stages of development and may eventually not require anticoagulation therapy. In the interim, bioprosthetic or tissue valves offer a safe alternative for patients in whom the risk of anticoagulation is prohibitively high (e.g., elderly patients >70 years of age, women of childbearing years desiring pregnancy). Yet, the length of durability remains a serious concern for tissue valves, and thus a patient whose life expectancy is greater than that of the prosthesis will encounter the risk of another surgery for a second valve replacement. The current concept of a tissue replacement valve via a transcatheter-delivered procedure may dramatically change this clinical limitation.

It is important to note that two historic randomized clinical trials have compared outcomes between early generation tissue and mechanical valves—the Edinburgh Heart Valve trial and the Veteran Affairs Cooperative Study on Valvular Heart Disease [8–10]. Both trials showed increased bleeding associated with mechanical valves and increased reoperation with tissue valves. While the strength of these trials is a prospective randomized design, the disadvantages are that the valves used in these trials are currently obsolete. More recently, a large meta-analysis comparing mechanical versus bioprosthetic aortic valves found no difference in risk-corrected mortality regardless of patient age [11]. Based on this and other studies, the choice of valve should not be based on age alone. Clearly, there is a trend toward increasing use of bioprosthetic valves in younger patients; this is based on the fact that advances in tissue fixation and improved anti-calcification treatments have resulted in superior durability of the newer generation bioprosthetic valves. Specifically, third-generation bioprosthetic valves have been shown to have a greater than 90% freedom from structural generation at 12-year follow-up [12]. Furthermore, improvements in cardiac surgery including better techniques for myocardial preservation, less invasive procedures, as well as strategies for cardiac reoperation have significantly reduced the risks for cardiac reoperation. This has further allowed an increasing application of bioprosthetic valves in patients younger than 55–60 years old. In conclusion, in the absence of current randomized trials, physicians must make a choice based on existing data and individualize that choice based on patient-related factors such as age, lifestyle, tolerance for anticoagulation, and/or position of the replacement valve.

31.2.4 Prosthetic Heart Valve Endocarditis and Performance Tracking

All patients with prosthetic valves also need appropriate antibiotics for prophylaxis against infective endocarditis. Details of these therapies are beyond the scope of this chapter, but the reader is referred to guidelines published by a joint committee from the American Heart Association (AHA) and American College of Cardiology (ACC) for the applicable protocols. In addition, a registry has been established to track the long-term performance of all clinically approved implanted valve prostheses. Established standards were revised in 1996 and are briefly summarized in Table 31.3. As alluded to in Chapter 25, investigators seeking approval for all new valves must also

Table 31.3 Reportable valve prosthesis complications [8]

Complication	Description
Structural valvular deterioration	Any change in function of an operated valve resulting from an intrinsic abnormality, causing stenosis or regurgitation
Nonstructural dysfunction	Any stenosis or regurgitation of the operated valve that is not intrinsic to the valve itself, including inappropriate sizing, but excluding thrombosis and infection
Valve thrombosis	Any thrombus, in the absence of infection, attached to or near an operated valve that occludes part of the blood flow path or interferes with function of the valve
Embolism	Any embolic event that occurs in the absence of infection after the immediate perioperative period (new temporary or permanent, focal or global neurological deficit, and peripheral embolic event)
Bleeding event (anticoagulant hemorrhage)	Any episode of major internal or external bleeding that causes death, hospitalization, permanent injury, or requires transfusion
Operated valvular endocarditis	Any infection involving an operated valve, resulting in valve thrombosis, thrombotic embolus, bleeding event, or paravalvular leak

report any complications that occur in the preclinical animal testing phase to the appropriate regulatory authority.

31.3 Specific Valvular Diseases: Etiologies and Treatments

The remainder of this chapter is devoted to a generalized summary of the most common valvular diseases affecting patients in the Western world. Of the four heart valves, significant clinical disease can primarily affect all but the pulmonary valve. Yet, compromised function of this valve is noted to occur in the adult congenital heart patient who previously underwent reparative surgeries. Indications for diagnostic, therapeutic, and follow-up intervention will be discussed for each disease. Note that a complete evidence-based summary of recommendations for intervention and physical activity in individuals with valvular disease is available from several excellent reviews [13, 14].

31.3.1 Aortic Valve Disease

Anatomically, the normal aortic valve is composed of the annulus and the left, right, and noncoronary leaflets (sometimes referred to as "cusps") (Fig. 31.3). Diseases affecting these structures can be subdivided into aortic

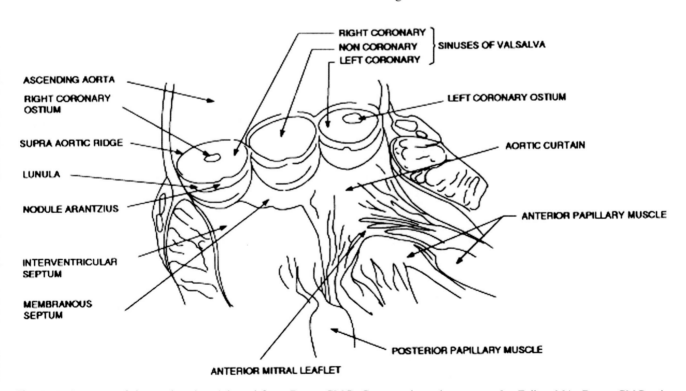

Fig. 31.3 Anatomy of the aortic valve. Adapted from Duran CMG. Conservative valve surgery. In: Zaibag MA, Duran CMG, eds. Valvular heart disease. New York, NY: Marcel Dekker, 1994:584

stenosis or regurgitation, or some combination thereof. Overall, aortic stenosis is considered a surgical disease with aortic valve replacement considered to be the standard of care. Treatment of aortic regurgitation is also typically surgical, though the exact method chosen will vary widely based on the etiology of the disease.

31.3.1.1 Aortic Stenosis

"Aortic stenosis" causes varying degrees of left ventricular outflow tract obstruction [15, 16]. The various etiologies of aortic stenosis are subdivided into acquired versus congenital. Regardless of the etiology, the most common cause of aortic stenosis in adults is calcification of a normal trileaflet or a congenital bicuspid aortic valve. Interestingly, among individuals under the age of 70, bicuspid aortic valve disease is the most common cause of aortic stenosis. These congenitally abnormal valves typically develop progressive fibrosis and calcification of the leaflets over several decades and can present for surgery at any time during an individual's life, depending on the degree of deformity and rate of progression of the narrowing. Patients over the age of 70 more typically elicit the so-called "senile aortic stenosis;" these valves start out as normal valves, but develop thickening, calcification, and stenosis with aging. In a patient with any degree of aortic stenosis, careful clinical follow-up is mandatory to follow the progression of stenosis, and typically surgery is indicated at the onset of any symptoms (see below). Congenital malformations (typically presenting in bicuspid aortic valves) result in a progressive fibrosis and calcification of the leaflets over several decades. The average rate reduction in valve orifice area has been estimated to be ~0.12 cm^2/year, and valve orifice area is typically used to grade the severity of valve stenosis (Table 31.4) [17]. Nevertheless, progression of aortic stenosis does vary significantly and the appearance of symptoms may not correlate well with the measured valve area. Therefore, careful clinical follow-up is mandatory, as it is difficult to predict an actual individual rate of stenotic progression. In general, aortic stenosis is graded into various categories of severity based on degrees of mean pressure gradient, aortic jet velocity, and/or valve area.

Valve stenosis may also be associated with progressive outflow tract obstruction, which can then cause additional increases in left ventricular pressure. As a result, concentric left ventricular hypertrophy is an early response, which assists initially in maintaining normal left ventricular systolic wall tension and ejection fraction [18]. However, once this response becomes functionally inadequate, afterload tends to increase which, in turn, results in a gradual reduction in overall ejection fraction (Fig. 31.4). In some patients, an initial ventricular hypertrophy itself may also be detrimental, producing subendocardial ischemia even in the absence of coronary artery disease [19, 20]. As such, this results in further systolic and diastolic left ventricular dysfunction and may predispose such patients to a potentially larger degree of myocardial ischemia and higher mortality [7, 15, 16, 21].

Although aortic stenosis may not produce symptoms early in its clinical course, in time symptoms of angina, syncope, heart failure, and/or even sudden death will develop. Although the latter are the classic symptoms of aortic stenosis, more subtle symptoms such as reduced effort tolerance, fatigue, and exertional dyspnea can also occur. Once symptoms are present, average survival is less than 2–3 years without intervention [15, 16, 22–27]. Furthermore, the mortality of patients with aortic stenosis, in the absence of surgical treatment, present with: (1) angina, 50% within 5 years; (2) syncope, 50% mortality within 3 years; and (3) heart failure, 50% mortality within 2 years. Therefore, a high degree of skepticism is necessary to make the diagnosis prior to the onset of symptoms to maximize patient outcome. In general, aortic stenosis can be detected early based on: (1) the presence of a

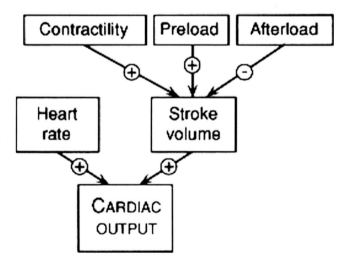

Fig. 31.4 Determinants of cardiac output include contributions from preload and afterload pressures, contractility, and heart rate. Adapted from Lilly LS, ed. Pathophysiology of heart disease. Philadelphia, PA: Lea & Febiger, 1993:149

Table 31.4 Degree of aortic stenosis [79]

	Valve orifice area (cm^2)	Peak aortic velocity (m/s)
Mild	>1.5	<3.0
Moderate	>1.0–1.5	3.0–4.0
Severe	<1.0	>4.0

systolic outflow murmur; (2) delayed/diminished carotid upstrokes; (3) sustained left ventricular impulse; (4) reduced intensity of the aortic component of the second heart sound; and/or (5) evidence of left ventricular hypertrophy on exam, chest x-ray, and/or EKG. Typically, echocardiography can be further used to confirm the diagnosis of aortic stenosis and also provide for the detailed assessment of: (1) the mean transvalvular pressure gradient; (2) derived valve area; (3) left ventricle size (degree of hypertrophy) and function; and/or (4) the presence of other associated valvular disease. For more details on the clinical use of echocardiography, the reader is referred to Chapter 20. It should also be noted that advances in magnetic resonance imaging may be applied in diagnosing such patients (see Chapter 22).

Physicians who follow patients with known aortic stenoses commonly perform an annual history and physical examination, and urge the patients to promptly self-report the development of any new symptoms. Although changes in valve area alone are not totally predictive, annual echocardiography is also useful to assess progression of ventricular hypertrophy and alterations in function. In any case, the development of any new symptoms (e.g., exertional chest discomfort, shortness of breath, or fainting spells) warrants additional clinical assessment, given that aortic stenosis progresses rapidly once such symptoms are present.

In patients being considered for aortic valve replacement secondary to aortic stenosis, cardiac catheterization is generally indicated in individuals >40 years of age to assess for any degree of significant coronary artery disease. Additional indications include the assessment of (1) hemodynamic severity of the aortic stenosis in situations where there is a discrepancy between clinical and echocardiographic findings and (2) situations where there is evidence of pulmonary hypertension or other valvular or congenital disease. Complete diagnostic evaluation should include: (1) the measurement of transvalvular flow (liters/min); (2) the determination of the transvalvular pressure gradient (mmHg); and (3) the calculation of the effective valve area (cm^2) [28].

Stress testing is recommended in patients with equivocal symptoms, and should only be carried out under close monitoring by a physician. Positive findings suggestive of hemodynamically significant aortic stenosis include the development of symptoms, limited exercise tolerance, and a blunted blood pressure response to exercise. In all such cases, surgical replacement of the aortic valve is indicated.

Medical therapy for aortic stenosis is primarily relegated to the prevention of endocarditis and the control of arterial hypertension. As most asymptomatic patients lead a normal life, no interventions are typically considered. Yet, there are some studies that have shown slowing of disease progression with statins. While there are theoretical benefits for the use of ACE inhibitors, studies so far have not shown significant benefits on disease progression [29, 30]. Nevertheless, once symptoms develop, prompt intervention should be offered to prevent morbidity and mortality. In some patients, interventional radiological therapy using balloon aortic valvotomy can effectively reduce the transvalvular pressure gradient. This procedure uses percutaneously inserted catheters advanced into the aortic valve, then a balloon is inflated to fracture calcific deposits and separate fused commissures [31, 32]. Though successful at providing clinical improvement, the post-procedure valve area rarely exceeds 1.0 cm^2, and aortic regurgitation is often created, thus increasing the burden on the left ventricle. To date, the rate of significant complications (10%) and symptomatic restenosis (6–12 months) unfortunately makes balloon valvotomy an undesirable substitute for aortic valve replacement in adults with aortic stenosis [7].

Aortic valve replacement is technically possible at any age, and is the treatment of choice for aortic stenosis in most adults [33]. Yet, the degree of stenosis mandating surgery in asymptomatic patients remains an issue of debate. Nevertheless, the degree of improvement following aortic valve replacement is directly related to preoperative left ventricular function; patients with a depressed ejection fraction caused by excessive afterload demonstrate significant improvement in left ventricular function after aortic valve replacement. Conversely, if depressed left ventricular function is caused by myocardial insufficiency, improvement in left ventricular function and resolution of symptoms may not be reversed after valve replacement. In general, survival is improved for patients undergoing aortic valve replacement, with the possible exception of a subset of patients with severe left ventricular dysfunction caused by coronary artery disease [34, 35]. In summary, in contrast to the dismal survival rate of patients with untreated severe aortic stenosis, the long-term survival of patients who have undergone aortic valve replacement approaches that in the normal population. Therefore, it is recommended that patients with severe aortic stenosis, with or without symptoms, who are undergoing coronary artery bypass surgery should undergo aortic valve replacement at the time of the revascularization procedure. Similarly, patients with moderate-to-severe aortic stenosis undergoing surgery for the replacement of other heart valves or an aortic root repair should also undergo aortic valve replacement as part of their overall surgical procedure. Hence, in the absence of contraindications, aortic valve replacement is indicated in virtually all symptomatic patients with severe aortic stenosis (Table 31.5).

Currently, there are two areas of major controversy in the management of aortic stenosis including: (1) the

Table 31.5 Aortic valve replacement in aortic stenosis [7]

- Symptomatic patients with severe aortic stenosis alone or
  - Undergoing coronary artery bypass surgery
  - Undergoing surgery on the aorta or other heart valves
- Patients with moderate aortic stenosis and
  - Undergoing coronary artery bypass surgery
  - Undergoing surgery on the aorta
  - Undergoing surgery on other heart valves
- Asymptomatic patients with severe aortic stenosis and left ventricular systolic dysfunction typified by
  - Abnormal response to exercise (e.g., hypotension)
  - Ventricular tachycardia
  - Marked or excessive left ventricular hypertrophy (>15 mm)
  - Valve area <0.6 cm^2
  - Prevention of sudden death without the findings listed

asymptomatic patient with severe aortic stenosis and (2) the patient with low ejection fraction with reduced gradient aortic stenosis [15, 16]. There is a low (1–2%) risk of sudden death or rapid progression to symptoms in the asymptomatic patient with severe aortic stenosis. Adverse clinical outcomes are more likely in the asymptomatic patient with severe aortic stenosis who demonstrates more rapid progression of hemodynamic parameters such as increase in aortic jet velocity greater than 0.3 m/s per year or a decrease in aortic valve area greater than 0.1 cm^2 per year. Therefore, other than in a small selected group of patients, the risks of surgery may still exceed any potential benefits in this group of patients, those with severe aortic stenosis with normal ventricular function who are truly asymptomatic. On the other hand, patients with low ejection fraction and reduced gradient aortic stenosis may present an even more challenging problem. The complexity partly lies in the difficulty to distinguish this entity from those patients with reduced ejection fraction and only mild-to-moderate aortic stenosis; the latter group will not benefit from aortic valve replacement. It should be noted that patients with severe aortic stenosis who present with reduced ejection fraction and reduced gradient will ultimately face an increased operative mortality. The use of dobutamine stress echocardiography to measure the pressure gradient and the valve area both during baseline and at stress can help determine the true severity of aortic stenosis [36]. It should be noted that, in general, patients with reduced ejection fraction with a low transvalvar gradient who have no response to stress such as inotropes have a poorer outcome even with surgery.

31.3.1.2 Aortic Sclerosis

"Aortic sclerosis" is a common finding in older patients and is present in approximately 25% of patients older

than 65 years [14, 15]. The classic findings of aortic sclerosis include focal areas of valve thickening with otherwise relatively normal leaflet mobility. It is important to note that, by definition, valvular hemodynamics are within normal limits in aortic sclerosis. In other words, other than the presence of a systolic murmur, there are no clinical signs or associated symptoms. Histologic findings in aortic sclerosis include focal subendocardial plaque-like lesions with accumulations of lipoproteins. The similarity of these findings to atherosclerosis suggests that both of these are in some way an age-related process.

Despite the lack of valve-related symptoms with aortic sclerosis, it is generally associated with an increased risk of cardiovascular mortality. This may be related to the development of coronary artery disease and, occasionally, to a progression to severe aortic stenosis. Thus, while symptoms in the patient identified with aortic sclerosis may be initially benign, these individuals warrant a close cardiovascular follow-up.

31.3.1.3 Aortic Regurgitation

Aortic regurgitation results from a structural defect in the aortic valve that allows for blood flow to reverse direction across the valve during diastole (i.e., re-enter the ventricle). The etiologies of aortic regurgitation are best discussed if one subdivides this disease into acute or chronic regurgitation (Table 31.6). The majority of such lesions result in chronic aortic regurgitation with insidious dilatation of the left ventricle. In contrast, lesions responsible for acute aortic regurgitation may result in sudden catastrophic elevation of left ventricular filling pressure, reduction in cardiac output, and/or sudden death.

Table 31.6 Etiologies of aortic regurgitation (subdivided by presentation time)

Acute	Chronic
Infective endocarditis	Idiopathic aortic root dilatation
Aortic dissection	Congenital bicuspid valves
Trauma	Calcific degeneration
	Rheumatic disease
	Infective endocarditis
	Systemic hypertension
	Myxomatous proliferation
	Ascending aortic dissection
	Marfan syndrome
	Syphilitic aortitis
	Rheumatoid arthritis
	Osteogenesis imperfecta
	Giant cell aortitis
	Ehlers–Danlos syndrome
	Reiter's syndrome
	Discrete subaortic stenosis
	Ventricular septal defects with aortic cusp prolapse

Chronic Aortic Regurgitation

Valve damage that results in progressively larger retrograde flow across the aortic valve produces the condition of "chronic aortic regurgitation." The patient's left ventricle responds to the volume load of aortic regurgitation with several compensatory mechanisms such as an increase in end-diastolic volume and a combination of eccentric and concentric hypertrophy [37]. The increased diastolic volume allows the ventricle to eject a larger total stroke volume, thereby initially maintaining stroke volume in the normal range. As a result, the majority of such patients remain asymptomatic for prolonged periods of compensation, during which time they maintain forward stroke volume within the normal ranges. Yet, after a while, the compensatory mechanisms become inadequate, and further increases in afterload result in reduced ejection fraction. Once the left ventricle can no longer compensate, patients typically present with symptoms of dyspnea and exertional angina, reflecting declining systolic function, elevated filling pressures, and/or diminished coronary flow reserve of the hypertrophied myocardium [38]. Several natural history studies have identified age and left ventricular end-systolic pressure (or volume) as predictive factors associated with higher risk of mortality in this clinical population (Table 31.7) [7].

Importantly, although the progression of asymptomatic aortic regurgitation is slow, approximately one-fourth of patients will develop systolic dysfunction, or even die, before the onset of warning symptoms [7]. Therefore, quantitative evaluation of left ventricular function with echocardiography is necessary, as a serial

history and physical exam alone are insufficient, in general.

The clinical diagnosis of chronic severe aortic regurgitation by a trained physician can be made on (1) the presence of a diastolic murmur (the third heart sound) and/or a rumble (Austin-Flint sign) on auscultation and (2) the detection of a displaced left ventricular impulse and wide pulse pressure [39, 40]. Similar to aortic stenosis, the chest x-ray and ECG will typically reflect left ventricular enlargement/hypertrophy and may also elicit evidence of conduction disorders. Echocardiography is then indicated to (1) confirm the diagnosis of aortic regurgitation; (2) assess valve morphology; (3) estimate the severity of regurgitation; (4) assess aortic root size; and (5) determine left ventricular dimension, mass, and systolic function. If the patient has severe aortic regurgitation and is sedentary, or has equivocal symptoms, exercise testing is helpful to assess the following: functional capacity, symptomatic responses, and/or the hemodynamic effects of exercise.

In patients who are symptomatic on initial evaluation, cardiac catheterization and angiography is considered indicated for the subsequent evaluation of coronary artery disease for possible revascularization therapy, if the echocardiogram is of insufficient quality to assess left ventricular function and the severity of aortic regurgitation. The ultimate aim of any serial evaluation of the asymptomatic patient with chronic aortic regurgitation is to detect the onset of symptoms and objectively assess changes in left ventricular size and function that may occur in the absence of physical symptoms (Fig. 31.3). Medical therapy for aortic regurgitation is primarily based on the use of vasodilating agents which are believed to improve forward stroke volume and reduce regurgitant volume; the use of such agents can often result in regression of left ventricular dilatation and hypertrophy.

Initial left ventricular systolic dysfunction in chronic aortic regurgitation is commonly associated with an increased afterload pressure, and is considered to be reversible following aortic valve replacement, i.e., with full recovery of left ventricular size and function [7]. However, depressed myocardial contractility (rather than volume overload) is responsible for the systolic dysfunction as the ventricle becomes more hypertrophic and dilatation progresses the chamber to a more spherical geometry. At this stage, neither return of normal left ventricular function nor improved long-term survival has been documented even after aortic valve replacement [7]. For patients with chronic aortic regurgitation, left ventricular systolic function and end-systolic size have been identified as the most important determinants of postoperative survival and normalization of left ventricular function following aortic valve replacement [7].

Table 31.7 Natural history of aortic regurgitation

Asymptomatic patients with normal left ventricular systolic function	• Progression to symptoms and/or left ventricular dysfunction	<6%/year
	• Progression to asymptomatic left ventricular dysfunction	<3.5%/year
	• Sudden death	<0.2%/year
Asymptomatic patients with left ventricular systolic dysfunction	• Progression to cardiac symptoms	>25%/year
Symptomatic patients	• Mortality rate	
	○ with angina	>10%/year
	○ with heart failure	>20%/year

Medical therapy with vasodilating agents is generally indicated for chronic therapy in patients with severe aortic regurgitation who have symptoms of left ventricular dysfunction and for whom surgery is not recommended because of either cardiac or noncardiac factors. The benefits of vasodilating agents are based on their potential ability to improve stroke volume and reduce regurgitant volume [41]. In general, the acute administration of vasodilating agents such as sodium nitroprusside, hydralazine, and nifedipine reduces peripheral vascular resistance and results in an immediate augmentation in forward cardiac output and a decrease in regurgitant volume. The ACC/AHA recommends three guidelines for the use of vasodilating agents in severe aortic regurgitation: (1) long-term treatment of patients with severe aortic regurgitation who have symptoms and/or left ventricular dysfunction who are considered poor candidates for surgery; (2) improvement in the hemodynamic profile of patients with severe heart failure symptoms and severe left ventricular dysfunction with short-term vasodilator therapy before proceeding with aortic valve replacement; and (3) prolong the compensated phase of asymptomatic patients who have volume overload, but have normal systolic function.

Acute Aortic Regurgitation

When damage to the aortic valve is acute and severe, the subsequent and sudden large regurgitant volumes that return into the left ventricle will decrease the functional forward stroke volume dramatically. In contrast to chronic aortic regurgitation, in such acute cases, there is no time for compensatory ventricular hypertrophy and dilatation to develop. As a result, the considered typical exam findings of ventricular enlargement and diastolic murmur associated with chronic aortic regurgitation are absent. Instead, the patient with acute aortic regurgitation presents with pronounced tachycardia, pulmonary edema, and/or potentially life-threatening cardiogenic shock.

Echocardiography, which is considered crucial in the initial workup of the acute aortic regurgitation patient, will likely demonstrate a rapid equilibration of aortic and left ventricular diastolic pressure and may provide some insights as to the etiology of aortic regurgitation. Echocardiography also allows for a rapid assessment of the associated valve apparatus, the aorta, and/or the relative degree of pulmonary hypertension (if tricuspid regurgitation is present). Transesophageal echocardiography is indicated when aortic dissection is suspected [42, 43] (see also Chapter 20). Importantly, acute aortic regurgitation resulting from aortic dissection is a known surgical emergency requiring prompt identification and management. Cardiac catheterization, aortography, and coronary angiography are considered as important components of such an evaluation of aortic dissection with acute aortic regurgitation and thus should be performed if these procedures do not unduly delay urgent surgery. Additionally, following trauma, computed tomographic imaging can be quite useful in obtaining the appropriate clinical status and underlying diagnosis.

Nevertheless, appropriate treatment of acute aortic regurgitation is dependent on the etiology and severity of the disease. For example, only antibiotic treatment may be required in a hemodynamically stable patient with mild acute aortic regurgitation resulting from infective endocarditis. Conversely, severe acute aortic regurgitation is a surgical emergency, particularly if hypotension, pulmonary edema, and/or evidence of low cardiac output are present. In such cases, temporary preoperative management may include the use of agents such as nitroprusside (to reduce afterload) and inotropic agents such as dopamine or dobutamine (to augment forward flow and reduce left ventricular end-diastolic pressure). Intraaortic balloon counterpulsation is contraindicated in such patients, and beta-blockers should be used cautiously because of their potential to further reduce output by blocking the compensatory tachycardia. Typically, mortality associated with acute aortic regurgitation is usually the result of pulmonary edema, ventricular arrhythmias, electromechanical dissociation, and/or circulatory collapse.

In general, aortic valve replacement is the treatment of choice in aortic regurgitation. In such cases of aortic disease, additional aneurysm repairs (Fig. 31.5) or aortic root replacements (Figs. 31.6, 31.7) need to be considered. Aortic root replacement with a homograft or autograft should be offered to patients in whom anticoagulation is contraindicated (e.g., elderly with risk, women of childbearing years) as the tissue valve graft does not require anticoagulation. In addition, patients with disease resulting from endocarditis benefit, as a homograft appears to have more resistance to subsequent infection. Finally, although the use of mechanical valves is effective, the prosthesis may impose a clinically relevant degree of stenosis in certain patients due to unavoidable size mismatch. Naturally, homografts and autografts are superior as they can be tailored to provide a larger outflow tract. In certain situations, repair of the aorta may involve the use of an artificial conduit using materials such as Dacron.

Careful post-aortic valve replacement follow-ups are necessary during the early and long-term postoperative course to evaluate both prosthetic valve and left ventricular function. An accepted excellent predictor of long-term success of aortic valve replacement is a reduction in left ventricular end-diastolic volume occurring within the

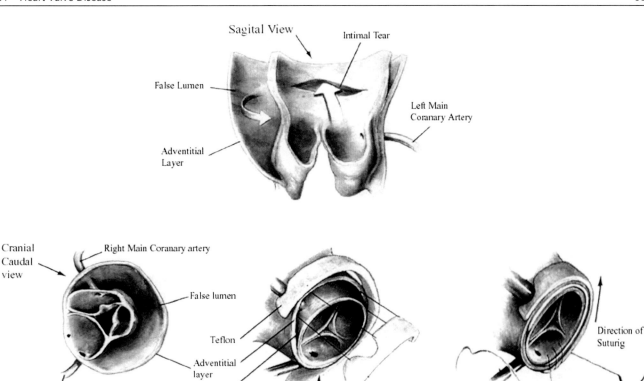

Sagital View

Intimal Tear

False Lumen

Left Main
Coronary Artery

Adventitial
Layer

Cranial
Caudal
view

Right Main Coranary artery

False lumen

Teflon

Adventitial
layer

False
lumen

Left Main Cooranary Artery

Teflon tailored
around coranaries

Direction of
Suturig

Fig. 31.5 Aortic aneurysm repair using a teflon felt reinforcement technique preserving the aortic valve and coronary arteries. From Yun KL and Miller DC. Operation for aortic root aneurysm or dissection. In: Operative techniques in cardiac and thoracic surgery. 1996:68–81

first 14 days after the operation. It should be emphasized that, in most patients, as much as 80% of the overall reduction in end-diastolic volume that will occur happens within this time period. In addition, the degree of regression in left ventricular dilatation typically correlates well with the magnitude of functional increases in ejection fraction [40]. Nevertheless, long-term follow-up should include an exam at 6 months post-aortic valve replacement, and then yearly examinations are recommended if the clinical course is uncomplicated. Note that serial postoperative echocardiograms after the initial early postoperative study are usually not indicated. However, repeat echocardiography is warranted at any point when there is evidence of: (1) a new murmur; (2) questions of prosthetic valve integrity; and/or (3) concerns about adequate left ventricular function.

Aortic Valve Disease Associated with Disease of the Ascending Aorta

Dilatation of the ascending aorta is a common cause of aortic regurgitation. It is well recognized that patients with bicuspid aortic valves also have disorders of the vascular connective tissue system, which can result in dilatation of the ascending aorta and/or aortic root even in the absence of hemodynamically significant valvular disease. The dilatation of the aorta can be progressive over time with an increased risk for aortic dissection. Currently, echocardiography is the primary diagnostic modality used for these patients. However, a more detailed anatomic study can be obtained with either computerized tomography or cardiac magnetic resonance imaging (see Chapter 22).

Regardless of the etiology of the dilated ascending aorta, the recommended indications for operative intervention include an aortic diameter >5.5 cm and growth of the aorta >0.5 cm/year. In patients with bicuspid aortic valves undergoing aortic valve replacement, repair of the aortic root or replacement of the ascending aorta is indicated if the diameter of the aorta is >4.5 cm. Note that aortic valve-sparing operations are feasible in many patients with dilatation of the aorta who do not have significant aortic regurgitation or aortic valve calcification. The techniques for aortic valve-sparing surgery have been pioneered by Yacoub and David [44, 45]. In early

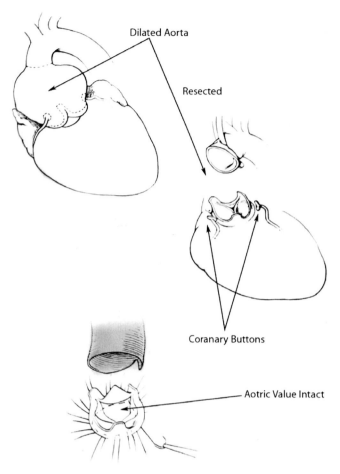

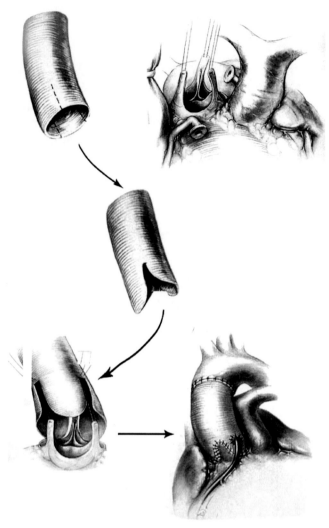

Fig. 31.6 David procedure for aortic root replacement. The dilated aorta is resected, sparing the aortic valve and coronary buttons. The repair is then completed with insertion of a graft with reimplantation of the coronary arteries. Adapted from Smedira, NG. Mitral valve replacement with a calcified annulus. In: Cox JL, Sundt TM III, eds. Operative techniques in cardiac and thoracic surgery. Philadelphia, PA: Saunders, 2003:2–13

Fig. 31.7 Aortic root replacement using Dacron graft as the technique used for correct sizing is demonstrated, for suturing in place to yield the final graft implantation along with coronary reimplantation. Adapted from Yacoub M. Valve-conserving operation for aortic root aneurysm or dissection. In: Operative techniques in cardiac and thoracic surgery. 1996:57–67

stages of this disease, the use of beta-adrenergic blocking agents may slow the progression of aortic dilatation.

Atlas of Human Cardiac Anatomy (http://www.vhlab.umn.edu/atlas).

31.3.2 Diseases of the Mitral Valve

Diseases of the mitral valve can be subdivided in a similar fashion as those affecting the aortic valve—stenosis and regurgitation. The general anatomy of the mitral valve consists of a pair of leaflets attached to the left ventricle by chordae tendinae. Normal mitral valve area ranges between 4.0 and 5.0 cm^2. However, in the case of mitral stenosis, symptoms do not typically develop until the functional valve area is reduced to <2.5 cm^2[46]. For more details on valve anatomy, the reader is referred to Chapters 4 and 5, the Visible Heart® Viewer CD, and the

31.3.2.1 Mitral Stenosis

Stenosis of the mitral valve orifice typically produces a funnel-shaped mitral apparatus described to resemble a "fish mouth," which then hinders normal diastolic filling of the left ventricle. In the past, roughly 60% of all patients with mitral stenosis presented with a history of rheumatic fever [47, 48]. Three typical pathological processes are observed in such patients: (1) leaflet thickening and calcification; (2) commissural and chordal fusions; or

(3) a combination of these processes [49, 50]. Yet, congenital malformations of the mitral valve, though rare, are usually responsible for mitral stenosis observed in infants and children [50]. Currently, women (2:1) account for the overall majority of mitral stenosis cases [47, 48, 51]. Other entities can also simulate the clinical features of rheumatic mitral stenosis, such as left atrial myxoma, infective endocarditis, and mitral annulus calcification in the elderly.

Mitral stenosis is normally a slowly progressive disease with a typical mean age of presentation of symptoms in the fifth to sixth decade of life [52, 53], with narrowing of the valve to <2.5 cm^2 before the development of symptoms. As the severity of stenosis increases, cardiac output becomes reduced even at rest and fails to increase with exercise. The relative degree of pulmonary vascular resistance also influences the development of symptoms. Diagnosis of mitral stenosis may be made solely on the presence of abnormal physical exam findings, or may be suggested by symptoms of fatigue, dyspnea, frank pulmonary edema, atrial fibrillation, and/or embolus [48]. In the asymptomatic patient, survival is 80% at 10 years, with 60% of these patients eliciting no progression of symptoms [7]. However, once symptoms related to pulmonary hypertension develop, to date, there remains a dismal 0–15% 10-year survival rate [7]. Common causes of death in the untreated patients with mitral stenosis are due to: (1) progressive heart failure (60–70%); (2) systemic embolism (20–30%); (3) pulmonary embolism (10%); or (4) infection (1–5%) [50, 51].

Shortness of breath (dyspnea) precipitated by exercise, emotional stress, infection, pregnancy, and atrial fibrillation are typically the first symptoms to present in patients with underlying mild mitral stenosis [54]. Yet, as the obstructions across the mitral valve increase, there will typically be progressive symptoms of dyspnea, as the left atrial and pulmonary venous pressures increase [55]. Increased pulmonary artery pressures and distension of the pulmonary capillaries can lead to pulmonary edema, which occurs as pulmonary venous pressure exceeds that of plasma oncotic pressure. Subsequently, the pulmonary arterioles will elicit vasoconstriction, intimal hyperplasia, and medial hypertrophy, which then further exacerbate pulmonary arterial hypertension.

Commonly, the diagnosis of mitral stenosis can be made based on patient history, physical examination, chest x-ray, and ECG. Nevertheless, at the initial examination, a patient may be asymptomatic although abnormal physical findings, including a diastolic murmur, may be present [52, 53]. In such patients, diagnostic imaging is recommended and currently the tool of choice is 2D and Doppler transthoracic echocardiography. Transesophageal echocardiography or cardiac catheterization is not required unless questions concerning diagnosis remain [7]. Yet, heart catheterization may be indicated to: (1) assess the potential for coronary artery disease or aortic valve disease; (2) assess pulmonary artery pressure; (3) perform balloon valvotomy; and/or (4) evaluate the situation when the clinical status of a symptomatic patient is not consistent with the echocardiography findings.

Typically, echocardiography is capable of providing an appropriate assessment of: (1) the morphological appearance of the mitral valve apparatus; (2) ventricular chamber size/function; (3) the mean transmitral gradient [56, 57]; (4) the relative functional mitral valve area; and (5) the pulmonary artery pressure [58]. In addition, if deemed necessary, noninvasive dobutamine or exercise stress testing can be completed with either the patient supine (using a bicycle) or upright (on a treadmill) to assess changes in heart rate and blood pressure in response to their overall exercise tolerance. Patients who are symptomatic with a significant elevation of pulmonary artery pressure (>60 mmHg), mean transmitral gradient (>15 mmHg), or pulmonary artery wedge pressure (>25 mmHg) on exertion have, by definition, hemodynamically significant mitral stenosis that may require further intervention [7].

In mitral stenosis, medical treatment is typically indicated for the prevention of emboli (10–20%), which is primarily associated with the onset of atrial fibrillation [47, 48, 59–61]. Atrial fibrillation ultimately develops in 30–40% of patients with symptomatic mitral stenosis and, importantly, ~65% of all embolic events occur within the first year after the onset of atrial fibrillation [47, 48]. The etiology behind atrial fibrillation is thought to be disruption of the normal conduction pathways caused by structural changes in the myocardium resulting from a pressure/volume overloaded atrium; in fewer cases, it may also result from rheumatic fibrosis of the atrium [53]. Development of atrial fibrillation associated with mitral stenosis occurs more commonly in older patients and has been associated with a decreased 10-year survival rate (25% versus 46%) [48, 51]. In addition to the thromboembolic potential, acute onset of atrial fibrillation can herald sudden deterioration in patients with mitral stenosis. This is considered as secondary to an acute reduction in left ventricular ejection fraction and elevated pulmonary artery pressures, which will result from loss of the atrial contribution to left ventricular filling. The urgent treatment for an acute episode of atrial fibrillation with a rapid rate typically consists of: (1) anticoagulation with heparin; (2) heart rate control (digoxin, calcium channel blockers, beta-blockers, or amiodarone); and/or (3) electrical cardioversion. It should be noted that in patients with atrial fibrillation for more than 24 to 48 h without anticoagulation, cardioversion is then associated with an increased risk of embolism. Today, in chronic or recurrent atrial fibrillation that is resistant to prevention or cardioversion, heart rate control (digoxin, calcium channel blockers, beta-blockers, or amiodarone) and long-term anticoagulation are considered as the mainstay of therapy [61, 62]. Yet, use of anticoagulation for patients with mitral stenosis who have not had atrial fibrillation or embolic events is not indicated due to the risk of bleeding complications.

The principle for treating symptomatic mitral stenosis rests on the alleviation of the fixed left ventricular inflow obstruction, thereby reducing the transvalvular gradient. Methods of disrupting the fused valve apparatus (open or closed mitral commissurotomy, or percutaneous mitral balloon valvotomy) or mitral valve replacement have both demonstrated significant postprocedural improvements in both symptoms and survival. The timing of intervention is commonly related to the severity of disease, while the method of intervention is chosen based on: (1) morphology of the mitral valve apparatus; (2) presence of other comorbid diseases; and/or (3) expertise at each specific clinical center. Significant calcification, fibrosis, and subvalvular fusion of the valve apparatus can make either commissurotomy or percutaneous balloon valvotomy less likely to be successful. It should also be noted that the presence of mitral regurgitation is a contraindication for valvotomy/commissurotomy and is considered best treated with mitral valve replacement.

Closed commissurotomy is a surgical technique that uses finger fracture of the calcified valve (Fig. 31.8). This procedure has the advantage of not requiring cardiopulmonary bypass, however, the operator is not afforded direct visual examination of the valve apparatus. In

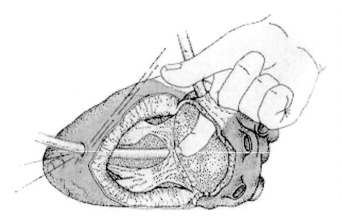

Fig. 31.8 Treatment of mitral stenosis using the finger fracture closed mitral commissurotomy technique. Adapted from Zipes DP, ed. Braunwald's heart disease: A textbook of cardiovascular medicine. Philadelphia, PA: W.B. Saunders Co., 1992:1016

contrast, open commissurotomy, which commonly employs cardiopulmonary bypass, has gained favor in the United States because it allows inspection of the mitral valve apparatus under direct vision. During this procedure, division of the commissures, splitting of fused chordae tendinae/papillary muscles, debridement of calcium deposits [7], and/or mitral valve replacement can be completed to attain optimal results. The 5-year reoperation rate following open commissurotomy has been reported to be between 4 and 7%, and the 5-year complication-free survival rate ranges from 80 to 90%.

However, more recently, both these operative techniques have given way to percutaneous balloon valvotomy. This is now the initial procedure of choice for the symptomatic patient with moderate-to-severe mitral stenosis, or those with favorable valve morphology and no significant mitral regurgitation and/or left atrial thrombus (Fig. 31.9). Immediate reduction in the transvalvular gradient (by at least 50–60%) is associated with gradual regression of pulmonary hypertension over several months [7]. If selected appropriately, 80–95% of patients undergoing this procedure will achieve a functional mitral valve area >1.5 cm^2 and a resultant decrease in left atrial pressure without complication. Yet, potential acute complications include mitral regurgitation (10%), atrial septal defect (5%), left ventricle perforations (0.5–4.0%), emboli formation (0.5–3%), myocardial infarctions (0.3–0.5%), and/or increased mortality (<1%) [63]. Currently, echocardiographic assessment of mitral valve morphology is the most important predictor of outcome for percutaneous balloon valvotomy. Patients with valvular calcification, thickened fibrotic leaflets with decreased mobility, and subvalvular fusions have a higher incidence of acute complications following balloon valvotomy and a higher rate of recurrent stenosis on follow-up. The presence of left atrial thrombus, detected by transesophageal echocardiography, is a relative contraindication and, at a minimum, warrants 3 months of oral warfarin anticoagulation in an attempt to resolve the thrombus prior to the planned procedure. A post-procedure echocardiogram, typically within 72 h after the procedure, is useful to assess postoperative hemodynamics, as well as to exclude significant complications such as mitral regurgitation, left ventricular dysfunction, and/or an atrial septal defect. However, recurrent symptoms have been reported to occur in as many as 60% of patients 9 years post-procedure [58, 64, 65]; it should be noted that recurrent stenosis accounts for symptoms in <20% of such patients [64]. In patients with an adequate initial result, progressive mitral regurgitation and development of other valvular or coronary problems are more frequently responsible for the subsequent presentation of symptoms [64]. Thus, in patients presenting with symptoms late after

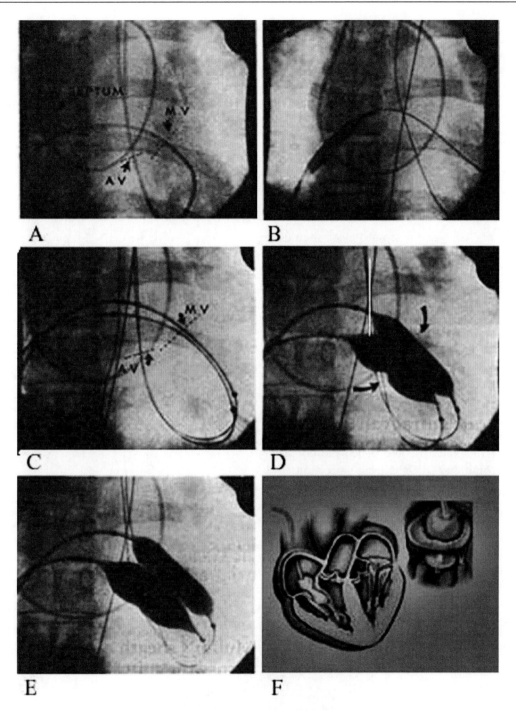

Fig. 31.9 Treatment of mitral stenosis using balloon valvotomy. Sequence of percutaneous mitral valvotomy: (**A**) floating balloon catheter in position across the atrial septum through the mitral and aortic valves. The tip is in the ascending aorta; (**B**) an 8 mm dilating balloon catheter enlarging the atrial septal puncture site; (**C**) two 20 mm dilating balloon catheters advanced into position across the stenotic mitral valve over two separate 0.038 in transfer guidewires; (**D**) partially inflated dilating balloon catheters across the mitral valve; note the "waist" produced by the stenotic valve (*arrows*); (**E**) fully inflated dilating balloon catheters in position across the mitral valve; (**F**) illustration of balloon commissurotomy technique. Adapted from www.rjmatthews.com and Braunwald's heart disease: A textbook of cardiovascular medicine (Zipes DP, ed. Philadelphia, PA: Saunders, 2003)

commissurotomy, a comprehensive evaluation is required to look for other causes.

Mitral valve replacement is an accepted surgical procedure for patients with severe mitral stenosis who are not candidates for surgical commissurotomy or percutaneous mitral valvotomy (Table 31.8, Figs. 31.10, 31.11). In addition, patients with recurrent severe symptoms, severe deformity of the mitral apparatus, severe mitral

Table 31.8 Mitral valve replacement for mitral stenosis [7]

- Moderate-to-severe mitral stenosis (mitral valve area <1.5 cm^2)
  - With NYHA functional Class III–IV symptoms
  - Who are not considered candidates for percutaneous balloon valvotomy or mitral valve repair
- Patients with severe mitral stenosis (mitral valve area <1 cm^2)
  - With severe pulmonary hypertension (pulmonary artery systolic pressure >60–80 mmHg)
  - With NYHA functional Class I–II symptoms who are not considered candidates for percutaneous balloon valvotomy or mitral valve repair

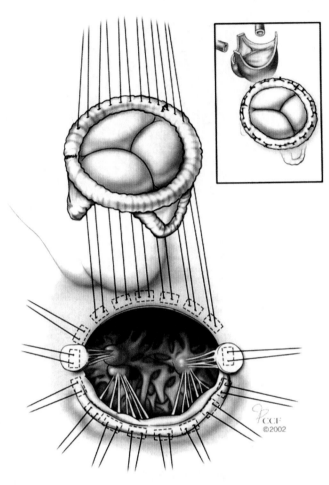

regurgitation, or a large atrial septal defect should be offered mitral valve replacement. The risks associated with mitral valve replacement are also highly dependent on age, left ventricular functional status, low cardiac outputs, presence of comorbid medical problems, and/or concomitant coronary artery disease. More specifically, morbidity and mortality associated with mitral valve replacement is directly correlated with age, with risk in a young healthy person of $<5\%$, increasing to as high as 10–20% in the older patient with concomitant medical problems or pulmonary hypertension. Mitral valve replacement can be further complicated by (1) the potential for embolic events; (2) the need for (and risk of) long-term anticoagulation therapy; and/or (3) the potential for valve thrombosis, dehiscence, infection, or malfunction.

Fig. 31.11 Mitral valve positioning into the mitral orifice. Adapted from Smedira NG, ed. Mitral valve replacement with a calcified annulus. In: Cox JL, ed. Operative techniques in thoracic and cardiovascular surgery. Philadelphia, PA: Saunders, 2003:2–13

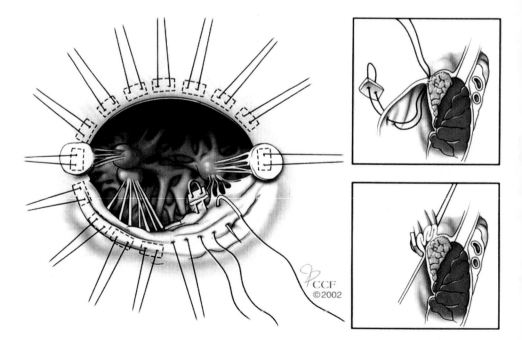

Fig. 31.10 Placement of circumferential sutures and plication of the anterior leaflet of the mitral valve. Adapted from Smedira NG, ed. Mitral valve replacement with a calcified annulus. In: Cox JL, ed. Operative techniques in thoracic and cardiovascular surgery. Philadelphia, PA: Saunders, 2003:2–13

31.3.2.2 **Mitral Regurgitation**

The common etiologies for mitral regurgitation include mitral valve prolapse secondary to myxomatous degeneration, rheumatic heart disease, coronary artery disease, infective endocarditis, or collagen vascular disease. As with aortic regurgitation, mitral regurgitation can be categorized as both acute and chronic presentation. In some cases, mitral regurgitation due to ruptured chordae tendinae or infective endocarditis may present as both acute and severe. Alternatively, mitral regurgitation may worsen gradually over a prolonged period of time. Yet, these very different presentations of mitral regurgitation are both treated with surgical intervention as dictated by the character of the symptoms presented.

Acute Severe Mitral Regurgitation

In acute severe mitral regurgitation, a sudden volume overload is imposed on the left atrium and the left ventricle is without time for typical compensatory hypertrophy. Thus, a sudden drop in forward stroke volume and cardiac output occurs (cardiogenic shock) in such a patient, with simultaneous pulmonary congestion. In severe mitral regurgitation, the hemodynamic overload often cannot be tolerated, and mitral valve repair or replacement must be performed urgently.

The acute nature of this form of mitral regurgitation results in patients who almost always present with symptoms upon a physical exam; they are typically positive for a holosystolic murmur and a third heart sound (see Chapter 16). Transthoracic echocardiography is commonly used to confirm the diagnosis and also to assess the general degree of disruption within the mitral valve apparatus. Furthermore, the use of transesophageal echocardiography is warranted if mitral valve morphology and regurgitation are still not clearly elucidated following transthoracic echocardiography. Note that it is the high level of detail provided by transesophageal echocardiography that is also helpful in demonstrating the anatomic cause of mitral regurgitation and, subsequently, directing successful surgical repair (see Chapter 20). Coronary arteriography is necessary before surgery in all patients >40 years of age, unless hemodynamic stability is of concern. If necessary, myocardial revascularization should be performed during mitral valve surgery in those patients with concomitant coronary artery disease [66, 67].

If the patient is not a candidate for surgery or if preoperative stabilization is required, medical therapy can help to diminish the relative amount of mitral regurgitation, thus increasing forward output and reducing pulmonary congestion; yet this therapy should be initiated promptly. However, in acute severe mitral regurgitation, medical therapy has a limited role and is primarily used to stabilize patients prior to surgery. In normotensive patients, nitroprusside has been used to increase the forward output not only by preferentially increasing aortic flow but also by partially restoring mitral valve competence as the left ventricular size diminishes [68, 69]. In hypotensive patients with severe reduction in forward output, aortic balloon counterpulsation can be employed to increase forward outputs and mean arterial pressures while, at the same time, diminishing mitral valve regurgitant volumes and left ventricular filling pressures. If infective endocarditis is the cause of acute mitral regurgitation, identification and treatment of the infectious organism are important to optimize successful clinical outcomes.

Chronic Asymptomatic Mitral Regurgitation

As with chronic aortic regurgitation, time for hypertrophy and chamber dilatation is typically present in the patient presenting with chronic severe mitral regurgitation [31, 70]. The dilatation, or increase in left ventricular end-diastolic volume, is a compensatory mechanism which permits an increase in total stroke volume and allows for restoration of forward cardiac output [71]. At the same time, an increase in left ventricular and left atrial size accommodates the regurgitant volume with a lower filling pressure; consequentially, symptoms of pulmonary congestion abate. Such patients with mild-to-moderate mitral regurgitation may remain without symptoms for several years with very little hemodynamic compromise. This compensated phase of mitral regurgitation is variable and can last several years. However, the prolonged burden of volume overload may eventually result in left ventricular dysfunction. At this time, contractile dysfunctions impair myocardial ejection and end-systolic volume increases; there may also be further left ventricular dilatations and increased left ventricular filling pressures. Therefore, correction of mitral regurgitation is generally recommended shortly following the diagnosis of severe mitral regurgitation, irrespective of the presence or absence of symptoms.

Initial diagnosis of chronic mitral regurgitation is commonly accomplished by physical exam which may demonstrate findings of left ventricular apical impulse displacement, indicating that mitral regurgitation is severe and chronic and has likely caused cardiac enlargement. Typically, ECG and chest x-ray can be useful to evaluate rhythm changes and heart sizes, respectively. Nevertheless, an initial echocardiogram, including Doppler interrogation of the mitral valve, is considered indispensable for the subsequent management of the patient with mitral regurgitation. Such an echocardiogram typically provides a baseline estimation of left ventricular and left atrial volume, an estimation of the left ventricular ejection fraction, and an approximation of the severity of regurgitation. Note that any presence of pulmonary hypertension is worrisome because it likely indicates advanced disease with a worsened prognosis [72]. Serial clinical follow-ups are used to assess changes in symptomatic status, left ventricular function, and/or exercise tolerance. Annual echocardiography is recommended once patients elicit a moderate mitral regurgitation. Left ventricular end-systolic dimensions (or volumes) can typically aid in the timing of mitral valve surgery. For example, an end-systolic dimension, which may be less load dependent than ejection fraction, should be <45 mm preoperatively to ensure normal postoperative left ventricular function [71, 73]. If patients become symptomatic, they should undergo mitral valve surgery even if left ventricular function is considered appropriately normal. Similar to acute mitral regurgitation, cardiac catheterization is considered indicated if: (1) there is discrepancy between clinical and noninvasive findings; (2) there is a need for preoperative coronary assessment for potential revascularization at the time of mitral valve replacement; and/or (3) an absence of chamber enlargement raises the question of the accuracy of the diagnosis, which should then be assessed with ventriculography at cardiac catheterization.

To date, there is no generally accepted therapy for asymptomatic patients with chronic mitral regurgitation. In such patients who develop symptoms but have preserved left ventricular function, surgery is considered as the most appropriate therapy. Atrial fibrillation is commonly associated with mitral regurgitation, and preoperative atrial fibrillation can be an independent predictor of reduced long-term survival after mitral valve surgery for chronic mitral regurgitation [74]. Atrial fibrillation should be treated with heart rate control (digitalis, calcium channel blockers, beta-blockers, or amiodarone) and anticoagulation to avoid embolism [75, 76]. Common predictors for the persistence of atrial fibrillation after successful valve surgery include the presence of atrial fibrillation for >1 year and/or a left atrial size >50 mm [77]. Although patients who develop atrial fibrillation also usually manifest other symptomatic or functional changes that would warrant mitral valve repair or replacement, today many clinicians would also consider the onset of episodic or chronic atrial fibrillation to be an indication, in and of itself, for valvular surgery [78, 79].

Three categories of surgical procedures are now in vogue for correction of mitral regurgitation: (1) mitral valve repair; (2) mitral valve replacement with preservation of part or all of the mitral apparatus; and (3) mitral valve replacement with prior removal of the mitral apparatus. Each procedure has its advantages and disadvantages as well as separate indications. In general, with the appropriate valve morphology and sufficient surgical expertise, mitral valve repair is the operation of choice. Yet, valve repair may require longer extracorporeal circulation time and may also occasionally fail, thus requiring mitral valve replacement. Valve calcification, rheumatic involvement, and anterior leaflet involvement all decrease the likelihood of an adequate repair, whereas uncalcified posterior leaflet disease is almost always repairable. The primary advantage of repair is the avoidance of anticoagulation and/or a rare prosthetic valve failure. In addition, postoperative left ventricular function and survival are improved with preservation of the mitral apparatus, as the mitral apparatus is considered essential for maintenance of normal left ventricular chamber shape, volume, and function [7]. Similar advantages are gleaned with the use of mitral valve replacement with preservation of the mitral chordal apparatus, except that it adds both the risks of deterioration inherent in tissue valves and the need for anticoagulation with mechanical valves. It is generally considered today that mitral valve replacement, in which the mitral valve apparatus is excised, should be performed only in circumstances when the native valve and apparatus are so distorted by the preoperative pathology (rheumatic disease, for example) that the mitral apparatus cannot be spared.

In an asymptomatic patient with normal left ventricular function, repair of a severely regurgitant valve may be offered as a means to: (1) preserve left ventricular size and function and/or (2) prevent the sequela of chronic mitral regurgitation (Fig. 31.12). Similarly, this approach has proven successful in the hemodynamically stable patient with newly acquired severe mitral regurgitation as the result of a ruptured chordae or recent onset of atrial fibrillation. The timing of surgery in asymptomatic patients is indicated by the appearance of echocardiographic indicators of left ventricular dysfunction (i.e., left ventricular ejection fraction <60% or left ventricular end-systolic dimension >45 mm). Mitral valve repair or replacement at this stage will likely prevent further deterioration in left ventricular function and thus improve survival [74]. Patients with symptoms of congestive heart failure, despite normal left ventricular function as determined by echocardiography (ejection fraction >60%, end-systolic dimension <45 mm), will likely require surgery. In both situations, mitral repair is preferred when possible. Mitral valve surgery is recommended for severe symptomatic mitral regurgitation with evidence of left ventricular systolic dysfunction; it is likely to both improve symptoms and prevent further deterioration of left ventricular function [80].

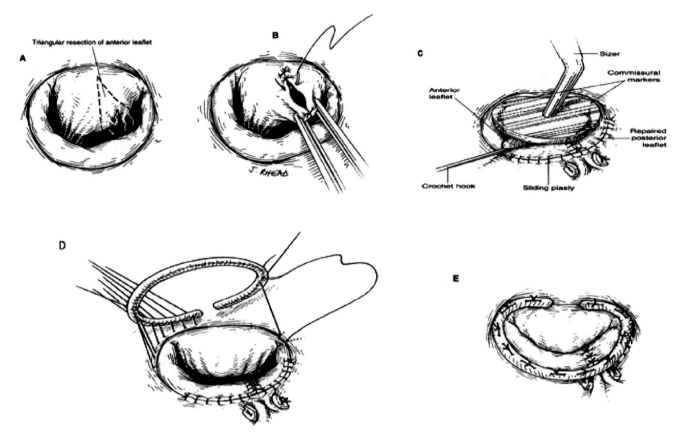

Fig. 31.12 Operative repair of the mitral valve using a technique developed by Carpentier. (**A**) Triangular resection of anterior leaflet; (**B**) anterior leaflet repair; (**C**) sizing of annulus; (**D**) annuplasty ring suture technique; and (**E**) completed repair. Adapted from Kirklin JW, ed. In: Cardiac surgery, 3rd ed. New York, NY: Churchill Livingstone, 2003:673–75

Ischemic mitral regurgitation is, by common definition, caused by left ventricular myocardial infarction, resulting in an associated papillary muscle dysfunction. The prognosis for such a patient with ischemic mitral regurgitation is substantially worse when compared with other etiologies [67, 81]. Following an acute infarction with the development of severe mitral regurgitation, hypotension and pulmonary edema often occur. Hemodynamic stabilization, usually with insertion of an intraaortic balloon pump, is completed preoperatively followed by coronary revascularization which only rarely improves mitral valve function. Unlike the case with nonischemic mitral regurgitation, it is more difficult to demonstrate a benefit of repair over replacement with ischemic mitral regurgitation. In general, operative mortality increases and survival is reduced in such patients >75 years of age with coronary artery disease, especially if mitral valve replacement must be performed [82]. In these patients, the goal of therapy is typically to improve the quality of life rather than prolong it, and medical therapy may be utilized to a greater extent to control cardiac symptoms.

31.3.3 Tricuspid Valve Disease

Tricuspid valve disease can be subclassified as regurgitation, stenosis, or a combination of both; it is most commonly the result of rheumatic fever, with rare cases attributed to infective endocarditis, congenital anomalies, carcinoid, Fabry's disease, Whipple's disease, or methysergide therapy [7]. Rheumatic tricuspid disease commonly presents as a combination of tricuspid stenosis and regurgitation. Furthermore, tricuspid disease commonly presents with concomitant mitral or aortic valve defects since acute rheumatic fever is also a common etiology for these disorders. It should be noted that right atrial myxomas or any type of large vegetations that produce an outflow tract obstruction will mimic stenosis; however, regurgitation may also result, as it often causes associated damage to the leaflet apparatus. Pure tricuspid regurgitation may result from rheumatic fever, infective endocarditis, carcinoid, rheumatoid arthritis, radiation therapy, anorectic drugs, trauma, Marfan's syndrome, tricuspid valve prolapse, papillary muscle dysfunction, and/or congenital disorders [7]. In addition, pressure/

volume overload conditions that do not cause direct damage to the leaflets themselves, such as those associated mitral stenosis and mitral regurgitation, typically cause ventricular enlargement, resultant tricuspid annular dilatation, and thus a sole tricuspid regurgitation [7].

The clinical features of tricuspid stenosis include auscultation of a tricuspid opening snap and a characteristic murmur. Auscultation may reveal a holosystolic murmur in the lower left parasternal region that may increase on inspiration (Carvallo's sign; see also Chapter 16). In rare instances, severe tricuspid regurgitation may produce systolic propulsion of the eyeballs, pulsatile varicose veins, or a venous systolic thrill and detectable murmur in the neck. Echocardiography is commonly used to (1) assess tricuspid valve structure and function; (2) measure annular size; (3) evaluate right pressures; and (4) rule out other abnormalities influencing tricuspid valve function. Systolic pulmonary artery pressure estimations, combined with information about annular circumference, further improve the accuracy of clinical assessment [7].

The etiology of tricuspid valve disease and the overall condition of the patient ultimately dictate the therapeutic approach. Tricuspid balloon valvotomy can be used to treat tricuspid stenosis; however, one must be aware of the potential for subsequently inducing severe tricuspid regurgitation. It has been documented that a poor long-term outcome is associated with right ventricular dysfunction and/or systemic venous congestion associated with severe tricuspid regurgitation [7]. In the situation where pulmonary hypertension is the underlying cause of tricuspid annular dilatation, medical management alone may result in substantial improvement of tricuspid regurgitation, and thus minimize the need for surgical intervention. Surgical options for treating tricuspid regurgitation include valve repair or valve replacement (Fig. 31.13). Today in the United States, the vast majority of diseased tricuspid valves are repaired. The basic techniques for tricuspid valve repair include bicuspidization, annular placation, and various types of annuloplasty, commonly using artificial rings. Tricuspid regurgitation annuloplasty is effective and can be optimized using intraoperative transesophageal echocardiography. Valve replacement with a low-profile mechanical valve or bioprosthesis is often necessary when the valve leaflets themselves are diseased, abnormal, or totally destroyed [83]. In both procedures, care must be taken to avoid causing damage to the heart's conduction system. In such cases, use of biological prostheses is preferred to avoid the high rate of thromboembolic complications known to occur with mechanical prostheses placed in the tricuspid position. Combined tricuspid and mitral valve procedures are often completed in the same

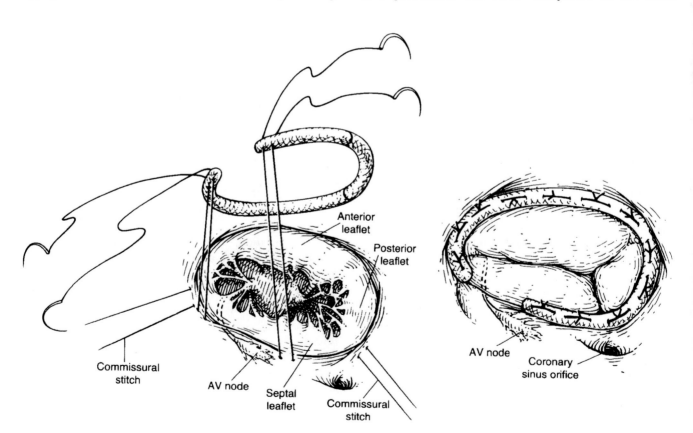

Fig. 31.13 Tricuspid annuloplasty procedure. AV = atrioventricular

interventions, as in the setting of rheumatic disease; however, to date, no long-term data regarding the value of such an approach exist. There is increasing awareness of the importance to correct tricuspid valve disease in the setting of associated cardiac diseases, most commonly mitral valve disease. In patients with associated conduction defects, insertion of a permanent epicardial pacing electrode at the time of valve replacement is also suggested.

31.4 Summary

The use of cross-circulation followed by the development of the bubble oxygenator for cardiopulmonary bypass was the turning point in the history of cardiac surgery. However, cardiac valvular surgery may be considered to still be in its infancy, with most of the major developments occurring only in the last 50 years. Tremendous advances in the field of cardiac surgery are certain to result from the numerous ongoing efforts of researchers and clinicians alike. This chapter was designed to give the reader an introduction to the complex nature of valve disease. Several excellent textbooks have been written that provide greater detail for each valve procedure discussed. Such reference texts are valuable for both the clinician and the engineer interested in understanding the etiology and the current treatment techniques for valve disease. Nevertheless, this basis of understanding, along with the use of further animal and clinical research, will allow for the development of the next generation of treatment options for heart valve disease. The reader is also referred to Chapters 32 and 33; these topics will have a dramatic impact in this field into the future.

References

1. Miller GW, ed. King of hearts. New York, NY: Times Books, 2000.
2. Bolman RM III, Black SM. Open cardiac repair under direct vision: F. John Lewis and the University of Minnesota. J Card Surg 2003;18:328–32, discussion 333.
3. Lewis RP, Herr RH, Starr A, Griswold HE. Aortic valve replacement with the Starr–Edwards ball-valve prosthesis. Indications and results. Am Heart J 1966;71:549–63.
4. Lillehei CW, Kaster RL, Coleman M, Bloch JH. Heart-valve replacement with Lillehei-Kaster pivoting disk prosthesis. NY State J Med 1974;74:1426–38.
5. Lillehei CW, Kaster RL, Bloch JH. New central flow pivoting disk aortic and mitral prosthesis. Clinical experience. NY State J Med 1972;72:1738.
6. Emery RW, Palmquist WE, Mettler E, Nicoloff DM. A new cardiac valve prosthesis: in vitro results. Trans Am Soc Artif Intern Organs 1978;24:550–56.
7. Bonow RO, Carabello BA, Kanu C, et al. ACC/AHA guidelines for the management of patients with valvular heart disease. A report of the American College of Cardiology/American Heart Association Task Force on Practice Guidelines. Circulation 2006;114:e84–231.
8. El Oakley R, Kleine P, Bach DS. Choice of prosthetic heart valve in today's practice. Circulation 2008;117:253–56.
9. Oxenham H, Bloomfield P, Wheatley DJ, et al. Twenty year comparison of a Bjork-Shiley mechanical heart valve with porcine bioprosthesis. Heart 2003;89:715–21.
10. Hammermeister K, Sethi GK, Henderson WG, Grover FL, Oprian C, Rahimtoola SH. Outcomes 15 years after valve replacement with a mechanical versus a bioprosthetic valve: Final report of the Veterans Affairs randomized trial. J Am Coll Cardiol 2000;36:1152–58.
11. Lund O, Bland M. Risk-corrected impact of mechanical versus bioprosthetic valves on long-term mortality after aortic valve replacement. J Thorac Cardiovasc Surg 2006;131:1267–73.
12. Bach DS, Metras J, Doty JR, Yun KL, Dumesnil JG, Kon ND. Freedom from structural valve deterioration among patients 60 years of age and younger undergoing Freestyle aortic valve replacement. J Heart Valve Diseases 2008;16:649–55.
13. Edmunds LH Jr, Clark RE, Cohn LH, Grunkemeier GL, Miller DC, Weisel RD. Guidelines for reporting morbidity and mortality after cardiac valvular operations. Ad Hoc Liaison Committee for Standardizing Definitions of Prosthetic Heart Valve Morbidity of The American Association for Thoracic Surgery and The Society of Thoracic Surgeons. J Thorac Cardiovasc Surg 1996;112:708–11.
14. Cheitlin MD, Douglas PS, Parmley WW. 26th Bethesda conference: Recommendations for determining eligibility for competition in athletes with cardiovascular abnormalities. Task Force 2: Acquired valvular heart disease. J Am Coll Cardiol 1994;24:874–80.
15. Carabello BA. Aortic stenosis. N Engl J Med 2002;346:677–82.
16. Freeman RV, Otto CM. Spectrum of calcific aortic valve disease: Pathogenesis, disease progression, and treatment strategies. Circulation 2005;111:3316–26.
17. Otto CM, Pearlman AS, Kraft CD, Miyake-Hull CY, Burwash IG, Gardner CJ. Physiologic changes with maximal exercise in asymptomatic valvular aortic stenosis assessed by Doppler echocardiography. J Am Coll Cardiol 1992;20:1160–67.
18. Krayenbuehl HP, Hess OM, Ritter M, Monrad ES, Hoppeler H. Left ventricular systolic function in aortic stenosis. Eur Heart J 1988;9:E19–23.
19. Marcus ML, Doty DB, Hiratzka LF, Wright CB, Eastham CL. Decreased coronary reserve: A mechanism for angina pectoris in patients with aortic stenosis and normal coronary arteries. N Engl J Med 1982;307:1362–66.
20. Bache RJ, Vrobel TR, Ring WS, Emery RW, Andersen RW. Regional myocardial blood flow during exercise in dogs with chronic left ventricular hypertrophy. Circ Res 1981;48:76–87.
21. Koyanagi S, Eastham C, Marcus ML. Effects of chronic hypertension and left ventricular hypertrophy on the incidence of sudden cardiac death after coronary artery occlusion in conscious dogs. Circulation 1982;65:1192–97.
22. Ross J Jr, Braunwald E. Aortic stenosis. Circulation 1968;38:61–67.
23. Schwarz F, Baumann P, Manthey J, et al. The effect of aortic valve replacement on survival. Circulation 1982;66:1105–10.
24. Sprigings DC, Forfar JC. How should we manage symptomatic aortic stenosis in the patient who is 80 or older? Br Heart J 1995;74:481–84.
25. Horstkotte D, Loogen F. The natural history of aortic valve stenosis. Eur Heart J 1988;9:E57–64.

26. Iivanainen AM, Lindroos M, Tilvis R, Heikkila J, Kupari M. Natural history of aortic valve stenosis of varying severity in the elderly. Am J Cardiol 1996;78:97–101.

27. Kelly TA, Rothbart RM, Cooper CM, Kaiser DL, Smucker ML, Gibson RS. Comparison of outcome of asymptomatic to symptomatic patients older than 20 years of age with valvular aortic stenosis. Am J Cardiol 1988;61:123–30.

28. Cheitlin MD, Alpert JS, Armstrong WF, et al. ACC/AHA guidelines for the clinical application of echocardiography. A report of the American College of Cardiology/American Heart Association Task Force on Practice Guidelines (Committee on Clinical Application of Echocardiography). Developed in collaboration with the American Society of Echocardiography. Circulation 1997;95:1686–744.

29. Rosenhek R, Rader F, Loho N, et al. Statins but not angiotensin-converting enzyme inhibitors delay progression of aortic stenosis. Circulation 2004;10:1291–95.

30. Rajamannan NM, Otto CM. Targeted therapy to prevent progression of calcific aortic stenosis. Circulation 2004;110:1180–82.

31. McKay RG, Safian RD, Lock JE, et al. Balloon dilatation of calcific aortic stenosis in elderly patients: Postmortem, intraoperative, and percutaneous valvuloplasty studies. Circulation 1986;74:119–25.

32. Safian RD, Mandell VS, Thurer RE, et al. Postmortem and intraoperative balloon valvuloplasty of calcific aortic stenosis in elderly patients: mechanisms of successful dilation. J Am Coll Cardiol 19987;9:655–60.

33. Tsai TP, Denton TA, Chaux A, et al. Results of coronary artery bypass grafting and/or aortic or mitral valve operation in patients > or = 90 years of age. Am J Cardiol 1994;74:960–62.

34. Smith N, McAnulty JH, Rahimtoola SH. Severe aortic stenosis with impaired left ventricular function and clinical heart failure: results of valve replacement. Circulation 1978;58:255–64.

35. Connolly HM, Oh JK, Orszulak TA, et al. Aortic valve replacement for aortic stenosis with severe left ventricular dysfunction. Prognostic indicators. Circulation 1997;95:2395–400.

36. Monin JL, Monchi M, Gest V, Duval-Moulin AM, Dubois-Rande JL, Gueret P. Aortic stenosis with severe left ventricular dysfunction and low transvalvular pressure gradients: Risk stratification by low-dose dobutamine echocardiography. J Am Coll Cardiol 2001;37:2101–07.

37. Grossman W, Jones D, McLaurin LP. Wall stress and patterns of hypertrophy in the human left ventricle. J Clin Invest 1975;56:56–64.

38. Nitenberg A, Foult JM, Antony I, Blanchet F, Rahali M. Coronary flow and resistance reserve in patients with chronic aortic regurgitation, angina pectoris and normal coronary arteries. J Am Coll Cardiol 1988;11:478–86.

39. Fortuin NJ, Craige E. On the mechanism of the Austin Flint murmur. Circulation 1972;45:558–70.

40. Parker E, Craige E, Hood WP Jr. The Austin Flint murmur and the A wave of the apexcardiogram in aortic regurgitation. Circulation 1971;43:349–59.

41. Miller RR, Vismara LA, DeMaria AN, Salel AF, Mason DT. Afterload reduction therapy with nitroprusside in severe aortic regurgitation: Improved cardiac performance and reduced regurgitant volume. Am J Cardiol 1976;38:564–67.

42. Smith MD, Cassidy JM, Souther S, et al. Transesophageal echocardiography in the diagnosis of traumatic rupture of the aorta. N Engl J Med 1995;332:356–62.

43. Cigarroa JE, Isselbacher EM, DeSanctis RW, Eagle KA. Diagnostic imaging in the evaluation of suspected aortic dissection. Old standards and new directions. N Engl J Med 1993;328:35–43.

44. Yacoub MII, et al. Results of valve sparing operations for aortic regurgitation. Circulation 1983;68:311–21.

45. David TE. Aortic valve-sparing operations for aortic root aneurysm. Semin Thorac Cardiovasc Surg 2001;13:291–96.

46. Gorlin R, Gorlin S. Hydraulic formula for calculation of the area of stenotic mitral valve, other cardiac values and central circulatory shunts. Am Heart J 1951;41:1–29.

47. Rowe JC, Bland EF, Sprague HB, White PD. The course of mitral stenosis without surgery: Ten- and twenty-year perspectives. Ann Intern Med 1960;52:741–49.

48. Wood P. An appreciation of mitral stenosis. I. Clinical features. Br Med J 1954;4870:1051–63.

49. Edwards JE, Rusted IE, Scheifley CH. Studies of the mitral valve. II. Certain anatomic features of the mitral valve and associated structures in mitral stenosis. Circulation 1956;14:398–406.

50. Roberts WC, Perloff JK. Mitral valvular disease. A clinico-pathologic survey of the conditions causing the mitral valve to function abnormally. Ann Intern Med 1972;77:939–75.

51. Olesen KH. The natural history of 271 patients with mitral stenosis under medical treatment. Br Heart J 1962;24:349–57.

52. Carroll JD, Feldman T. Percutaneous mitral balloon valvotomy and the new demographics of mitral stenosis. JAMA 1993;270:1731–36.

53. Selzer A, Cohn KE. Natural history of mitral stenosis: A review. Circulation 1972;45:878–90.

54. Hugenholtz PG, Ryan TJ, Stein SW, Abelmann WH. The spectrum of pure mitral stenosis. Hemodynamic studies in relation to clinical disability. Am J Cardiol 1962;10:773–84.

55. Braunwald E, Moscovitz HL, Amram SS, et al. The hemodynamics of the left side of the heart as studied by simultaneous left atrial, left ventricular, and aortic pressures; particular reference to mitral stenosis. Circulation 1955;12:69–81.

56. Holen J, Aaslid R, Landmark K, Simonsen S. Determination of pressure gradient in mitral stenosis with a non-invasive ultrasound Doppler technique. Acta Med Scand 1976;199:455–60.

57. Hatle L, Brubakk A, Tromsdal A, Angelsen B. Noninvasive assessment of pressure drop in mitral stenosis by Doppler ultrasound. Br Heart J 1978;40:131–40.

58. Currie PJ, Seward JB, Chan KL, et al. Continuous wave Doppler determination of right ventricular pressure: A simultaneous Doppler-catheterization study in 127 patients. J Am Coll Cardiol 1985;6:750–56.

59. Coulshed N, Epstein EJ, McKendrick CS, Galloway RW, Walker E. Systemic embolism in mitral valve disease. Br Heart J 1970;32:26–34.

60. Daley R, Mattingly TW, Holt CL, Bland EF, White PD. Systemic arterial embolism in rheumatic heart disease. Am Heart J 1951;42:566.

61. Abernathy WS, Willis PW III. Thromboembolic complications of rheumatic heart disease. Cardiovasc Clin 1973;5:131–75.

62. Adams GF, Merrett JD, Hutchinson WM, Pollock AM. Cerebral embolism and mitral stenosis: Survival with and without anticoagulants. J Neurol Neurosurg Psychiatry 1974;37:378–83.

63. Orrange SE, Kawanishi DT, Lopez BM, Curry SM, Rahimtoola SH. Actuarial outcome after catheter balloon commissurotomy in patients with mitral stenosis. Circulation 1997;95:382–89.

64. Higgs LM, Glancy DL, O'Brien KP, Epstein SE, Morrow AG. Mitral restenosis: an uncommon cause of recurrent symptoms following mitral commissurotomy. Am J Cardiol 1970;26:34–37.

65. Dahl JC, Winchell P, Borden CW. Mitral stenosis. A long term postoperative follow-up. Arch Intern Med 1967;119:92–97.

66. Cohn LH, Couper GS, Kinchla NM, Collins JJ Jr. Decreased operative risk of surgical treatment of mitral regurgitation with or without coronary artery disease. J Am Coll Cardiol 1990;16:1575–78.

67. Connolly MW, Gelbfish JS, Jacobowitz IJ, et al. Surgical results for mitral regurgitation from coronary artery disease. J Thorac Cardiovasc Surg 1986;91:379–88.

68. Chatterjee K, Parmley WW, Swan HJ, Berman G, Forrester J, Marcus HS. Beneficial effects of vasodilator agents in severe mitral regurgitation due to dysfunction of subvalvar apparatus. Circulation 1973;48:684–90.

69. Yoran C, Yellin EL, Becker RM, Gabbay S, Frater RW, Sonnenblick EH. Mechanism of reduction of mitral regurgitation with vasodilator therapy. Am J Cardiol 1979;43:773–77.

70. Carabello BA. Mitral regurgitation: basic pathophysiologic principles. Part 1. Mod Concepts Cardiovasc Dis 1988;57:53–58.

71. Zile MR, Gaasch WH, Carroll JD, Levine HJ. Chronic mitral regurgitation: Predictive value of preoperative echocardiographic indexes of left ventricular function and wall stress. J Am Coll Cardiol 1984;3:235–42.

72. Crawford MH, Souchek J, Oprian CA, et al. Determinants of survival and left ventricular performance after mitral valve replacement. Department of Veterans Affairs Cooperative Study on Valvular Heart Disease. Circulation 1990;81:1173–81.

73. Wisenbaugh T, Skudicky D, Sareli P. Prediction of outcome after valve replacement for rheumatic mitral regurgitation in the era of chordal preservation. Circulation 1994;89:191–97.

74. Enriquez-Sarano M, Tajik AJ, Schaff HV, Orszulak TA, Bailey KR, Frye RL. Echocardiographic prediction of survival after surgical correction of organic mitral regurgitation. Circulation 1994;90:830–37.

75. Blackshear JL, Pearce LA, Asinger RW, et al. Mitral regurgitation associated with reduced thromboembolic events in high-risk patients with nonrheumatic atrial fibrillation. Stroke Prevention in Atrial Fibrillation Investigators. Am J Cardiol 1993;72:840–43.

76. Beppu S, Nimura Y, Sakakibara H, Nagata S, Park YD, Izumi S. Smoke-like echo in the left atrial cavity in mitral valve disease: Its features and significance. J Am Coll Cardiol 1985;6:744–49.

77. Betriu A, Chaitman BR. Preoperative determinants of return to sinus rhythm after valve replacement. In: Cohn LH, Gallucci V, eds. Cardiac bioprosthesis. New York, NY: Yorke Medical Books, 1982:184–91.

78. Chua YL, Schaff HV, Orszulak TA, Morris JJ. Outcome of mitral valve repair in patients with preoperative atrial fibrillation. Should the maze procedure be combined with mitral valvuloplasty? J Thorac Cardiovasc Surg 1994;107:408–15.

79. Horskotte D, Schulte HD, Bircks W, Strauer BE. The effect of chordal preservation on late outcome after mitral valve replacement: A randomized study. J Heart Valve Dis 1993;2:150–58.

80. Bonow RO, Nikas D, Elefteriades JA. Valve replacement for regurgitant lesions of the aortic or mitral valve in advanced left ventricular dysfunction. Cardiol Clin 1995;13:73–83, 85.

81. Akins CW, Hilgenberg AD, Buckley MJ, et al. Mitral valve reconstruction versus replacement for degenerative or ischemic mitral regurgitation. Ann Thorac Surg 1994;58:668–75, discussion 675–76.

82. Enriquez-Sarano M, Schaff HV, Orszulak TA, Tajik AJ, Bailey KR, Frye RL. Valve repair improves the outcome of surgery for mitral regurgitation. A multivariate analysis. Circulation 1995;91:1022–28.

83. Silverman N. Tricuspid valve. In: Kaiser K, ed. Mastery of cardiac surgery. Philadelphia, PA: Lippincott-Raven, 1998:354–60.

Chapter 32
Less Invasive Cardiac Surgery

Kenneth K. Liao

Abstract To date, more and more cardiac surgeons are moving toward smaller incisions and the use of specialized less invasive surgical methodologies. The use of (and advances in) less invasive approaches or minimally invasive cardiac surgery can minimize or eliminate complications that may occur in conventional cardiac surgery. For example, for some surgeons, partial sternotomy and minithoracotomy have supplanted standard sternotomy as their preferred route for aortic valve and mitral valve surgeries.

Keywords Less invasive cardiac surgery · Cardiac robotic surgery · Minimally invasive cardiac surgery · Incision size · Laparoscopic surgery · Thoracoscope · Minithoracotomy · Partial sternotomy · Partial thoracotomy · Off-pump beating heart coronary artery bypass grafting surgery

32.1 Introduction

The history of cardiac surgery reflects a constant search by cardiac surgeons for safer and less invasive ways to treat their patients. Since Dr. F. John Lewis' pioneering operation in 1952, followed by Dr. C. Walton Lillehei's first successful series of intracardiac defect repairs in the mid-1950s, cardiac surgery as a surgical subspecialty has expanded dramatically. Notably, one of the most important technological innovations in cardiac surgery was the development and modification of a cardiopulmonary bypass machine. For years, this machine has been used extensively by cardiac surgeons. Its use enabled cardiac surgery, in general, to become a safe and reproducible daily routine in many hospitals across the country. Nowadays, though most cardiac operations are considered somewhat standardized, continued improvements as well as recognition of the importance of postoperative recovery and quality of life remain significant concerns for patients as well as physicians.

In recent years, there has been a major push to develop and provide "less invasive cardiac surgery" as standard care. It is generally recognized that all four of the major steps used in conventional cardiac surgery need to be considered when attempting to develop less invasive modifications: (1) gaining access to the heart through a full sternotomy or posterolateral thoracotomy; (2) supporting the vital organs through a cardiopulmonary bypass machine; (3) arresting the heart by administering cardioplegia; and (4) manipulating the ascending aorta during aortic cannulation, during cross- or side-clamping, and/or during proximal anastomosis in coronary artery bypass grafting. More specifically, manipulating the aorta can lead to strokes (e.g., plaque dislodgement) and/or other neurologic deficits. Unfortunately, any of these steps can impose significant risks or adverse effects. Furthermore, a large incision typically corresponds to greater pain, a noticeable scar, more complications, and/or a longer recovery time. Similarly, cardiopulmonary bypass has been known to trigger adverse inflammatory reactions and/or cause subsequent multiple organ dysfunction. Importantly, less invasive approaches or minimally invasive cardiac surgery can minimize or eliminate complications that may occur relative to each of the four steps commonly used in conventional cardiac surgery. This chapter focuses on less invasive methodologies commonly employed in adult cardiac surgical procedures.

32.2 Impact of Incision Size

For years, the physical and emotional impact of a large incision size on the patient has been ignored by most cardiac surgeons. Historically, adequate exposure of the

K.K. Liao (✉)
University of Minnesota, Division of Cardiovascular and Thoracic Surgery, Department of Surgery, MMC 207, 420 Delaware St. SE, Minneapolis, MN 55455, USA
e-mail: liaox014@umn.edu

P.A. Iaizzo (ed.), *Handbook of Cardiac Anatomy, Physiology, and Devices*, DOI 10.1007/978-1-60327-372-5_32,

target tissues or organs through large skin incisions took priority over concern about incision size; this mindset remained unchallenged until the early 1990s. Subsequently, with novel specially designed instruments and experience with laparoscopic surgery, it was demonstrated that those surgical procedures traditionally performed through large incisions could actually be accomplished with much smaller incisions. More recently, the patient benefits of small incisions have been clearly documented and these advantages include less pain, quicker recovery, lower infection rate, shorter hospital stays, and/or better quality of life [1, 2]. In some studies, fewer associated immune functional disturbances have also been reported [3]. Encouraged by positive results from the laparoscopic surgical community, some cardiac surgeons began to modify their approaches to perform less invasive cardiac surgery. Currently, a variety of approaches have been attempted: (1) thoracoscopies or minithoracotomies to replace thoracotomies; and (2) partial sternotomies, partial thoracotomies, or minithoracotomies to replace full medial sternotomies. Nevertheless, cardiopulmonary bypass support, if required, is typically established through cannulation in the peripheral vessels such as the femoral arteries, femoral veins, and internal jugular veins.

Various studies have reported advantages with smaller incisions or sternum sparing incisions in terms of pain, blood loss, postoperative respiratory function, time to recovery, infection, cosmesis, and/or 1-year survival rate [4–7]. However, one must also consider that the use of smaller incisions may have certain drawbacks. In order to have the same access and visualization as with larger incisions, special instruments and specialized surgical skills are required, and thus only selected patients may be considered as eligible. It should be specifically noted that, for surgeons, the initial learning curve to be able to perform such procedures clinically can be very steep. Nevertheless, smaller incisions are certainly very appealing to both patients and referring physicians. To date, more and more cardiac surgeons are moving toward smaller incisions and the use of these specialized less invasive surgical methodologies. For some surgeons, partial sternotomy and minithoracotomy have supplanted standard sternotomy as their preferred route for aortic valve and mitral valve surgeries.

32.3 Side Effects of Cardiopulmonary Bypass

Cardiopulmonary bypass procedures have become commonplace in cardiac surgical suites; however, capabilities to perform the same clinical procedure safely without its use would be desirable, for such bypass procedures are not performed without risks. More specifically, cardiopulmonary bypass has been associated with a complex systemic inflammatory reaction in the host patient. The hallmarks of this reaction are typically increased microvascular permeability in multiple organs, resulting in an increase in interstitial fluid, and the activation of humoral amplification systems. The complement system, including the kallikrein–bradykinin cascade, the coagulation cascade, the fibrinolytic cascade, and the arachidonic acid cascade, is activated. Inflammatory mediators, such as cytokines and proteolytic enzymes, are released (see also Chapter 30 for additional information on this topic).

In most classic cardiac cases where cardiopulmonary bypass is utilized, the heart is stopped to provide for a motionless field. Cardiac arrest is initiated with infusion of cardioplegia to the myocardium. Unfortunately, subsequent reperfusion of the heart can cause ischemic reperfusion injury to the myocardium.

Clinical manifestations of this systemic inflammatory reaction and myocardial ischemic reperfusion injury can be not only subtle, but also serious and even lethal in some patients. The incidence of this systemic reaction has been reported in 5–30% of cardiac surgery patients after cardiopulmonary bypass [8–13]. Importantly, this inflammatory response can affect multiple organs. More specifically, examples of this systemic response can vary from: (1) transient subtle cognitive impairment to a permanent stroke; (2) coagulopathy requiring transfusion of blood products to disseminated intravascular coagulation; (3) pulmonary edema to adult respiratory distress syndrome requiring prolonged ventilation support; (4) low cardiac output to acute heart failure requiring inotropic or mechanical circulatory support; and/or (5) transient kidney insult with increased creatinine to permanent kidney failure requiring hemodialysis. Any of these, or a combination thereof, commonly results in prolonged intensive care unit (ICU) stays requiring intense monitoring and often increased patient mortality (see Chapter 21). Importantly, the severity of these associated reactions tends to be related to cardiopulmonary bypass times, the patient's age, and/or comorbidities [11, 12].

To date, coronary artery disease remains as the leading cause of death for individuals living in developed countries. Despite widespread use of drug-eluting stents in treating coronary artery disease and sharply decreased patient volume for coronary artery bypass grafting (CABG), CABG operations still remain one of the most commonly performed cardiac procedures in the United States. Compared to percutaneous coronary artery interventions such as stenting, CABG has shown advantages of improved patient event-free survival and lower reintervention rate, especially in patients with multivessel coronary artery disease, diabetes, and decreased left ventricular function. Such benefits are attributed mainly to the use of in situ left internal mammary artery bypass to the left anterior descending artery (patency rate remains over 90% even after 15 years of implantation). Furthermore, the use of bilateral internal mammary arteries as bypass conduits has been shown to offer better patient survival rates and less reoperation rates when compared with the use of only the left internal mammary artery as a bypass conduit.

In the past 10 years, off-pump beating heart coronary artery bypass grafting surgery (OPCABG, a less invasive surgical approach) has entered the mainstream of clinical cardiac surgical practice. An increasing number of studies, including prospective randomized studies, have demonstrated that when compared to conventional CABG, OPCABG procedures result in: (1) lower incidences of postoperative neurologic deficits; (2) fewer blood transfusions; (3) shorter intubation times; (4) lower releases of cardiac enzymes; (5) fewer renal insults; (6) shorter ICU stays; (7) lower releases of cytokines IL8 and IL10; and/or (8) lower mortality [13–17]. It should be noted that the difference in these parameters between OPCABG and CABG procedures mostly range from 2 to 10%. In most OPCABG procedures, however, there has been the tendency to bypass fewer vessels which, in turn, may ultimately result in an incomplete revascularization. Moreover, certain anatomic locations and the nature of target coronary arteries may preclude safe and reliable anastomoses with OPCABG, e.g., arteries located in the posterolateral wall of hypertrophied hearts, intramyocardial arteries, and/or the severely calcified arteries. Furthermore, with today's available methodologies, OPCABG is more technically challenging for most cardiac surgeons. It should also be noted that emergency conversion of OPCABG to conventional CABG because of hemodynamic instability carries significantly higher morbidity and mortality rates than conventional CABG (i.e., about six times higher mortality) [18]; fortunately, the overall conversion is rare, at a rate of only 3.7%.

Though OPCABG surgery took off rapidly in the earlier part of the last decade, the initial enthusiasm for this procedure has tempered in recent years due to: (1) the lack of highly anticipated "drastic" clinical benefits of OPCABG over conventional CABG and (2) the additional technical challenges faced by surgeons. Currently, OPCABG comprises 20–25% of all CABG procedures performed in the United States, a percentage which has not changed much compared to 5 years ago. Although isolated centers perform virtually all CABG procedures off pump, in many centers, OPCABG is a seldom-used procedure. Such a large discrepancy appears to be related to the lack of effective education of practicing surgeons and the steep learning curve required to master the intricacies of performing OPCABG.

32.4 Effects of Manipulating the Aorta

Coronary artery disease is often considered as a component of an underlying systemic vascular disease. The same risk factors that contribute to coronary artery disease, such as smoking, diabetes, hypertension, and hyperlipidemia, also contribute to carotid artery disease and thus the atherosclerotic changes in the aorta; this is especially true for the ascending aorta. "Atheroma" within the aorta can present with calcified hard plaques or with "cheese-like" soft plaques, which can be both disrupted (dislodged) during: (1) cannulation of the ascending aorta for cardiopulmonary bypass; (2) cross-clamping in general; and/or (3) side-clamping of the ascending aorta for attachment of proximal anastomoses of bypassed grafts. Subsequently, these mobilized plaques can cause microembolization or macroembolization of brain vessels, resulting in neurologic deficits. Multiple episodes of microembolic events have been documented by transcranial Doppler studies during routine CABG surgery. The number of microembolic signals is reported to be related to the extent that the ascending aorta is manipulated [19]. Nevertheless, calcified areas of the aorta (or porcelain aorta) can be identified prior to the procedure by palpation and can be avoided during surgery, whereas soft plaques are typically unnoticed until they are disrupted during surgical manipulation. The overall incidence of plaque formation in the ascending aorta has been reported to be as high as 30% [20].

Recently, several methodologies have been described to avoid disrupting plaques when working in the region of the ascending aorta. For example, topical ultrasound devices have been used to identify hidden plaques, especially the soft types. In addition, a single aortic cross-clamp technique has been shown to reduce the risk of plaque disruption during conventional CABG surgery [21]. Similarly, aortic cross-clamping or side-clamping can be avoided by using proximal anastomotic devices during OPCABG. More recently, totally aortic "non-touch" techniques have been described that can be applied during OPCABG by using: (1) bilateral in situ internal mammary arteries; (2) sequential grafts; (3) in situ gastroepiploic arteries; (4) radial artery Y or T grafts from the internal mammary arteries; (5) radial artery or vein grafts from innominate, subclavian, or axillary arteries; and/or (6) descending thoracic aortic graft sites. Currently, non-touch techniques during OPCABG are gaining popularity, especially in high-risk patients

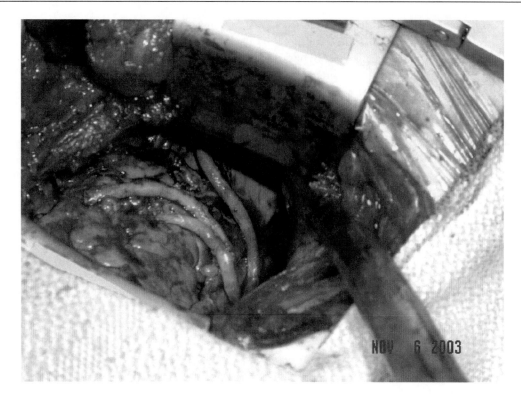

Fig. 32.1 Totally aortic "non-touch" technique in off-pump three vessel coronary artery bypass grafting surgery via left minithoracotomy; the inflow vein grafts come from the distal left subclavian artery in addition to the in situ left internal mammary artery graft

(Fig. 32.1). Nevertheless, to date, given the limited patient numbers and short follow-up times, the long-term graft patency rates for these later procedures remain unknown.

32.5 Technological Innovations

New technologies have played a crucial role in the evolution of less invasive cardiac surgeries. Importantly, they have changed the perceptions of cardiac surgeons regarding how cardiac surgery can or should be performed. With the help of new instruments specifically designed to meet the surgeon's need, less invasive cardiac surgical procedures once deemed impossible or impractical have now become reality, or even common practice, in some medical centers. These technological innovations have typically involved the following aspects of cardiac surgery.

32.5.1 Sternum Sparing Surgery, Minithoracotomy, and Thoracoscopy

Major advances in this area include the development of a cardiopulmonary bypass support system via peripheral access. Specifically, the application of suction to the

venous drainage has made possible aortic valve and mitral valve surgeries via partial sternotomy, as well as mitral valve surgery via a minithoracotomy. An early breakthrough device in this field was the HeartPort system (HeartPort, Redwood City, CA), which was composed of: (1) peripheral vessel-based cardiopulmonary bypass perfusion; (2) an endo aortic balloon occlusion catheter; (3) transvenously placed venting and cardioplegia cannulas; and (4) access ports for extra long and thin operating instruments. Though early use of the HeartPort system proved impractical in most cardiac operations, its potential to be less invasive has significantly changed the perceptions of both cardiac surgeons and medical engineers for utilizing and advancing future technologies. Furthermore, the concept of the HeartPort system led to numerous other technological modifications and innovations in the field of less invasive cardiac surgery. Such innovations include (1) development of small caliber multistage peripheral venous cannula; (2) safe application of vacuum-assisted venous drainage to ensure bloodless exposure inside the heart; (3) a small thin blade minithoracotomy retractor and atrial retractor; (4) development of the Chitwood aortic cross-clamp; (5) thoracoscopy or endoscopic robotics to assist in mitral valve repairs or replacements; and (6) liberal use of transesophageal echocardiography to guide the insertion of various intracardiac cannulas.

32.5.2 OPCABG Improvement

New instruments have also been developed to better position the heart during surgery and to stabilize and improve the visualization of target arteries. For example, an available left ventricle suction device applies –400 mmHg suction to the left ventricular apex and can hold the heart up in different positions. Now widely used in OPCABG surgery, it has less of an effect on the venous return as compared with the old "suture retraction" techniques. Similarly, focal myocardial stabilization devices have been developed to stabilize segments of target arteries; one such device has both suction and compressing effects on the topical epicardial tissue, and thus significantly decreases the motion of target arteries (Fig. 32.2). An additional noteworthy device for OPCABG surgery is the temporary intracoronary plastic shunt that can be inserted via arteriotomy to maintain blood flow to the distal myocardium during anastomosis, thus avoiding or minimizing ischemia time. Importantly, the use of such a shunt is considered to be crucial when the target artery supplies a large territory of myocardium. In order to facilitate the distal coronary anastomosis during OPCABG, especially in the anatomically difficult-to-reach areas, an innovative distal coronary artery anastomotic device (C-PortxA for open sternotomy approach and C-Port Flex A™ for minithoracotomy or endoscopic robotic approach; Cardica Inc., Redwood City, CA) was

developed and recently approved for clinical use by the Food and Drug Administration (FDA). The early clinical results using such a system are very encouraging [22].

32.5.3 Aortic "Non-touch" Techniques

Different proximal anastomotic devices or hand-sewn facilitators are being developed to avoid clamping on the aorta during OPCABG surgery. Of interest to note, the FDA-approved SJM Symmetry (St. Jude Medical, Inc., St Paul, MN) automated proximal connector, which allows the vein graft to be anastomosed to the aorta without side-clamping and suturing, was pulled off the market by St. Jude, Inc. after an alarmingly high incidence of premature vein graft stenosis or occlusion was noted. Early on, a detected drawback of this device was that proximal anastomosis needed to be performed first, making it difficult to assess the length of the vein graft when the distal anastomosis was then performed; moreover, a delivery device needed to be inserted into the lumen of the vein graft, which could denude the endothelium and subsequently affect long-term patency. Nevertheless, in time, new innovations will likely correct for these noted compromises. For example, one promising new proximal anastomotic device, the PAS-Port (Cardica, Inc.) recently obtained the European

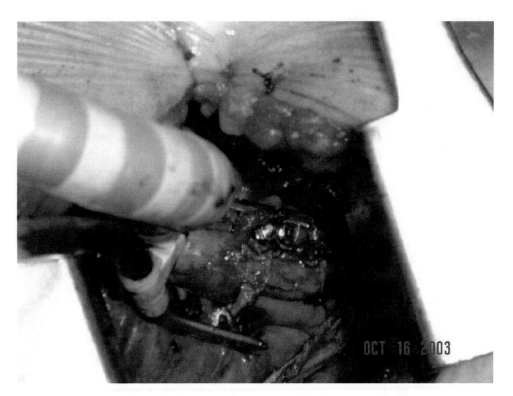

Fig. 32.2 An "octopus" myocardium stabilizing device is used to steady the coronary artery during direct bypass grafting anastomosis

Conformity (CE) mark for clinical use, and a multicenter clinical trial is currently being conducted for FDA approval. There is also Boston Scientific, Inc.'s Heart-string proximal seal system (Natick, MA), which is a facilitator for proximal hand-sewn suture anastomosis. More specifically, it is used to temporarily occlude the aortotomy during direct suture anastomosis of the proximal vein graft to the aortotomy; yet, to date, one of the major drawbacks with its use is that the suture can catch the device, requiring that the anastomosis be redone.

32.5.4 Endoscopic Robotics

Will operating rooms be devoid of cardiac surgeons in the near future? Perhaps yes, with the addition of robotics as a forefront technology. For example, Intuitive Surgical's da Vinci robotic system (Sunnyvale, CA) has improved significantly in the last decade and has made operating inside the chest cavity possible. Intuitive Surgical's second-generation system, which is smaller and more user friendly, also has a "third arm." Its 3D visualization, seven degrees of wrist motion, and capability to eliminate human hand tremors all help to facilitate fine cutting and suturing tasks. For those few surgeons that are currently using these sophisticated machines, it has made both internal mammary artery takedown and OPCABG surgery via thoroscopy or minithoracotomy easier (Fig. 32.3). Further, this technology has been used to repair atrial septal defects and mitral valves without sternotomy or thoracotomy. Importantly, the employment of such systems will lead the way in moving toward total endoscopic CABG surgery (Figs. 32.4 and 32.5).

Nevertheless, numerous complementary innovations have been required to allow for robotic surgery on the heart. For example, to make OPCABG surgery easier when it is performed via a minithoracotomy or via total endoscopic robotic approaches, an "endo suction device" and an "endo myocardium stabilizer" (Medtronic, Inc., Minneapolis, MN) have been developed to assist in the positioning the heart and stabilize the target artery through port accesses. Other devices that are currently being developed include proximal and distal anastomotic devices such as PAS-Port (Smiths Medical, Colonial Way, Watford, UK) and C-PortxA Flex and endo "U" clips.

Endoscopic robotics has greatly enhanced the surgeon's ability to perform OPCABG via thoracoscopy or minithoracotomy. Robotic-assisted OPCABG performed at our institution and others [23] has been associated with the following advantages: (1) less postoperative pain; (2) lower blood loss; (3) shorter length of hospital stays; and (4) fewer complications, when compared to conventional CABG, especially in elderly high-risk patients. In another application of robotic surgery (mitral valve repair and

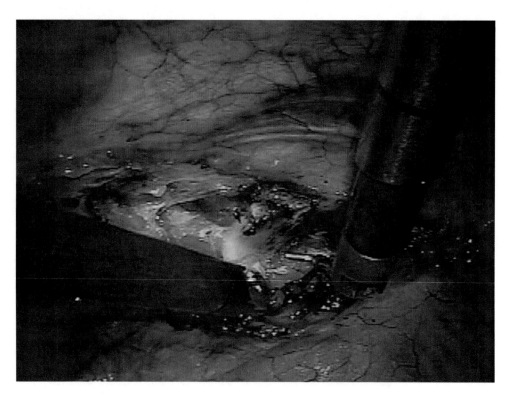

Fig. 32.3 Robotic arms operating inside the chest cavity to take down left internal mammary artery

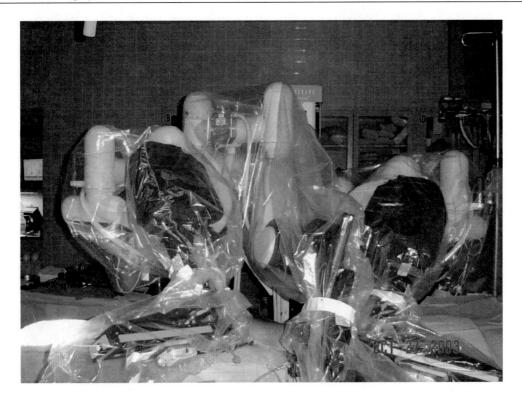

Fig. 32.4 Robotic arms in the operating room

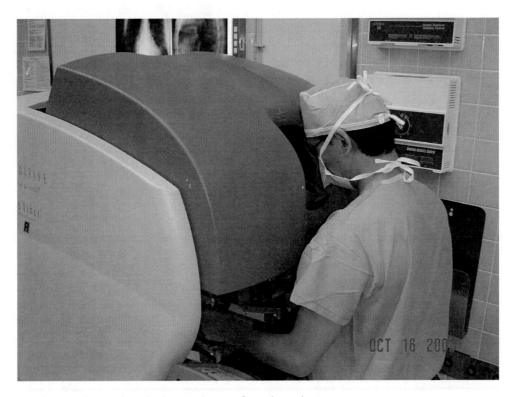

Fig. 32.5 The surgeon is operating on the robotic console away from the patient

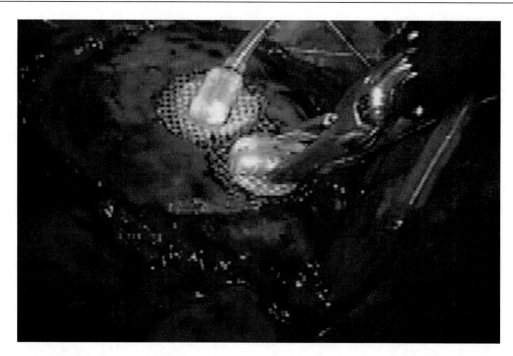

Fig. 32.6 Two left ventricular epicardial leads are placed by a robotic grasper in a patient who had previous coronary artery bypass grafting

replacement via thoracoscopy or minithoracotomy), when compared with standard sternotomy, major reduction in blood product utilization and length of hospital stay are observed while equivalence in complexity and success of mitral repairs is preserved [24]. Furthermore, the recent use of robotics to implant left ventricular pacing leads as part of cardiac resynchronization therapy for congestive heart failure has demonstrated the advantages of accurately locating the optimal pacing site and rapidly paving the epicardial leads, compared to the cath-lab percutaneous implantation [25] (Fig. 32.6).

32.6 Summary and Future Directions

The ultimate goal of less invasive cardiac surgery is to avoid cardiopulmonary bypass support, sternotomy, and thoracotomy, and rather to perform surgery through tiny incisions. A variety of specially designed instruments have been developed to make such procedures possible, including: (1) automated proximal and distal CABG anastomotic devices; (2) "endo myocardium stabilizers"; (3) "endo suture devices"; and (4) "endo vascular clamps." Furthermore, the da Vinci surgical robotic system has enabled use of such instruments inside the closed chest cavity. It is likely that, in the very near future, cardiac surgery will be performed utilizing only three to four key holes in the chest wall (Fig. 32.7).

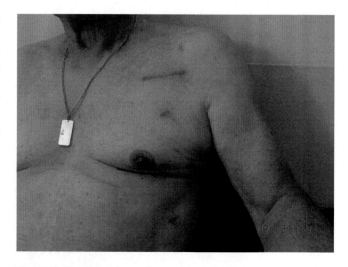

Fig. 32.7 Small incisions after multivessel off-pump sternum sparing coronary artery bypass grafting surgery

The following cardiac procedures will likely realize major advances in the near future with regard to becoming less invasive approaches: (1) total endoscopic robotic OPCABG using single or bilateral in situ internal mammary artery, with the help of flexible distal coronary artery anastomatic device; (2) hybrid robotic-assisted OPCABG and percutaneous stenting in the same patient who is being treated in the hybrid catheter lab/operating room (Fig. 32.8); (3) total endoscopic robotic mitral valve repair; (4) robotic-assisted left ventricular pacing lead implantation or hybrid electrophysiology ablation therapy; and/or

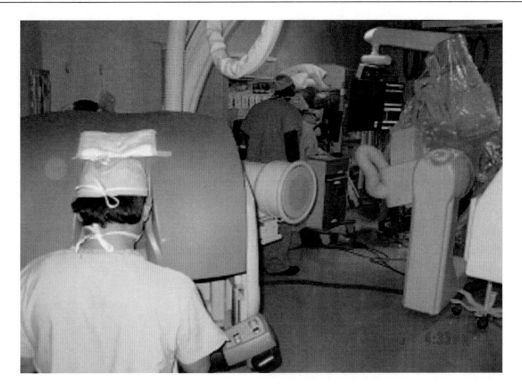

Fig. 32.8 Surgeon is performing robotic-assisted hybrid surgery in the catheter lab

(5) aortic valve replacement via percutaneous or transapical approaches in the hybrid catheter lab/operating room.

Companion CD Material

Figures 32.1–32.8

References

1. Grace PA, Quereshi A, Coleman J, et al. Reduced postoperative hospitalization after laparoscopic cholecystectomy. Br J Surg 1991;78:160–62.
2. Southern Surgeons Club. A prospective analysis of 1518 laparoscopic cholecystectomies. N Engl J Med 1991;324:1073–78.
3. Bruce DM, Smith M, Walker CBJ, et al. Minimal access surgery for cholelithiasis induces an attenuated acute phase response. Am J Surg 1999;178:232–34.
4. Szwerc MF, Benchart DH, Wiechmann RJ, et al. Partial versus full sternotomy for aortic valve replacement. Ann Thorac Surg 1999;68:2209–14.
5. Cosgrove DM, Sabik JF, Navia JL. Minimally invasive valve operations. Ann Thorac Surg 1998;65:1535–39.
6. Svensson LG. Minimally invasive surgery with a partial sternotomy "J" approach. Semin Thorac Cardiovasc Surg 2007;19:299–303.
7. Bakir I, Casselman FP, Wellens F, et al. Minimally invasive versus standard approach aortic valve replacement. A study in 506 patients. Ann Thorac Surg 2006;81:1599–604.
8. Zilla P, Fasol R, Groscurth P, et al. Blood platelets in cardiopulmonary bypass operations. J Thorac Cardiovasc Surg 1989;97:379.
9. Ko W, Hawes AS, Lazenby WD, et al. Myocardial reperfusion injury. J Thorac Cardiovasc Surg 1991;102:297.
10. Sladen RN, Berkowity DE. Cardiopulmonary bypass and the lung. In: Gravlee GP, Davis RF, Utley JR, eds. Cardiopulmonary bypass. Baltimore, MD: William & Wilkins, 1993:468.
11. Tuman KJ, McCarthy RJ, Najafi H, et al. Differential effects of advanced age on neurologic and cardiac risks of coronary artery operations. J Thorac Cardiovasc Surg 1992;104:1510.
12. Abel RM, Buckley MJ, Austen WG, et al. Etiology, incidence and prognosis of renal failure following cardiac operations: Results of a prospective analysis of 500 consecutive patients. J Thorac Cardiovasc Surg 1976;65:32.
13. Castillo FC, Harringer W, Warshaw AL, et al. Risk factors for pancreatic cellular injury after cardiopulmonary bypass. N Engl J Med 1991;325:382.
14. Cleveland JC, Shroyer AJ, Chen AY, et al. Off-pump coronary artery bypass grafting decrease risk-adjusted mortality and morbidity. Ann Thorac Surg 2001;72:1282–89.
15. Ascione R, Lloyd CT, Underwood MJ, Lotto AA, et al. Inflammatory response after coronary revascularization with or without cardiopulmonary bypass. Ann Thorac Surg 2000;69:1198–204.
16. Diegeler A, Doll N, Rauch T, et al. Humoral immune response during coronary artery bypass grafting: A comparison of limited approach, "off-pump" technique, and conventional cardiopulmonary bypass. Circulation 2000;102:III95–100.
17. Reston JT, Tregear SJ, Turkelson CM. Meta-analysis of short-term and mid-term outcomes following off-pump coronary artery bypass grafting. Ann Thorac Surg 2003;76:1510–15.
18. Edgerton JR, Dewey TM, Magee MJ, et al. Conversion in off-pump coronary artery bypass grafting: An analysis of predictors and outcomes. Ann Thorac Surg 2003;76:1138–42.

19. Stump DA, Newman SP. Embolic detection during cardiopulmonary bypass. In: Tegler CH, Babikian VL, Gomez CR, eds. Neurosonology. St. Louis, MO: Mosby, 1996:252–55.

20. Goto T, Baba T, Matsuyama K, et al. Aortic atherosclerosis and postoperative neurological dysfunction in elderly coronary surgical patients. Ann Thorac Surg 2003;75:1912–18.

21. Tsang JC, Morin JF, Tchervenkov CI, et al. Single aortic clamp versus partial occluding clamp technique for cerebral protection during coronary artery bypass: A randomized prospective trial. J Card Surg 2003;18:158–63.

22. Matschke KE, Gummert JF, Demertzis S, et al. The Cardica C-Port System: Clinical and angiographic evaluation of a new device for automated, compliant distal anastomoses in coronary artery bypass grafting surgery – A multicenter prospective clinical trial. J Thorac Cardiovasc Surg 2005;130:1645–52.

23. Poston RS, Griffith B, Bartlett. Superior financial and quality metrics with robotic – Assisted coronary artery revascularization (abstract); presented at the 128th annual American Surgical Association, New York, NY, April 26, 2008.

24. Woo YJ, Nacke EA. Robotic minimally invasive mitral valve reconstruction yields less blood product transfusion and short length of stay. Surgery 2006;140:262–67.

25. Liao K. Surgical implantation of left ventricular epicardial pacing leads for cardiac resynchronization therapy. In: Lu F, Benditt D, eds. Cardiac pacing and defibrillation – Principle and practice. Beijing China: People's Medical Publishing House, 2008.

Chapter 33
Transcatheter Valve Repair and Replacement

Alexander J. Hill, Timothy G. Laske, and Paul A. Iaizzo

Abstract Cardiac device technologies continue to advance at a rapid pace, with heart valve design and placement procedures being one of the major focus areas. Minimally or less invasive procedures to replace cardiac valves will enable an increasing number of individuals to receive this therapy, including the older and more frail individual or the adult patient with prior surgeries for repair of congenital defects. Transcatheter-delivered replacement valves for the four heart valves are either available on the market today or in development. This chapter provides a brief introduction of this rapidly emerging device area as well as general considerations related to delivering a device via catheter into the heart, e.g., percutaneous beating heart interventional procedures performed under fluoroscopic or echocardiographic guidance.

Keywords Transcatheter valve repair · Transcatheter valve replacement · Transcatheter-delivered valve system · Pulmonic valve · Aortic valve · Mitral valve · Tricuspid valve

33.1 Introduction

Transcatheter valve repair and replacement have the potential to reduce operative morbidity, expand the indication of valve replacement for nonsurgical candidates, and treat patients who have been declined for (or chose to decline) surgery. Catheter-based valve therapies are a relatively new entry into the medical practitioner's arsenal. Balloon valvuloplasty for aortic and mitral stenosis is perhaps the earliest incarnation of the current, rapidly changing environment. Cribier

demonstrated the technique of balloon aortic valvuloplasty in patients with calcific degenerative aortic stenosis in the 1990s. Although temporarily very successful, these patients often experienced restenosis of the aortic valve and worsening of symptoms. Balloon valvuloplasty was also a popular technique to treat post-rheumatic mitral stenosis but, with rheumatic fever essentially eliminated in developed nations, this technique is not currently in widespread practice. Similarly, pulmonic stenting with bare metal stents has been utilized as a treatment for patients with recurrent pulmonary stenosis due to repaired congenital heart malformations over the past two decades or so. Both types of treatment were radically changed when Andersen demonstrated the feasibility of the first transcatheter valve replacement in 1992 in animals [1]. While this device was not suitable for use in humans at that time (i.e., it required a 41 French delivery system), it sparked the minds of other inventors who soon expanded on the idea of a transcatheter-delivered valved stent.

The first report of a transcatheter valve replacement was in 2000 by Professor Philipp Bonhoeffer and colleagues in France who successfully delivered and implanted a valved stent in a right ventricle to pulmonary artery conduit of a patient with a congenital heart malformation [2]. Shortly thereafter, Cribier et al. reported on a transcatheter-delivered valve stent into the aortic position of a patient with degenerative calcific aortic stenosis [3]. Since that time, large and small medical device corporations, as well as individual inventors, have been developing techniques to treat valvular heart disease which can be delivered or affected via catheter. The main focus of these developments has been to treat the pulmonic and aortic valves with valve replacement, and treat the mitral valve with valve repair. Currently, there are approved devices in Europe and Canada for pulmonic and aortic valve replacement in select groups of patients. There are clinical trials investigating these devices in the United States, as well as clinical trials for mitral repair devices. In addition,

A.J. Hill (✉)
Departments of Biomedical Surgery, Medtronic, Inc., 8200 Coral Sea St. NE, MVS84, Mounds View, MN 55112, USA
e-mail: alex.hill@medtronic.com

P.A. Iaizzo (ed.), *Handbook of Cardiac Anatomy, Physiology, and Devices*, DOI 10.1007/978-1-60327-372-5_33,

to market released devices and formalized clinical trials, there are many devices which are currently being tested in animal and human feasibility trials around the world. These devices and trials will be discussed in greater detail in the following sections.

The development of transcatheter-delivered valve systems requires a combination of numerous technologies including access systems, delivery systems, a stent or support structure with a valve or repair system (i.e., a clip to capture native leaflets), closure systems, and imaging and/or navigation systems. Currently, transcatheter valve replacement stents can generally be classified as balloon-expandable or self-expanding. Balloon-expandable devices are typically made from materials such as stainless steel or platinum iridium alloys, while self-expanding devices are usually made from nitinol, a shape memory material. Valves are either bovine jugular vein valves or pericardial constructs. It should be noted that valvuloplasty is often recommended or employed prior to the placement of a transcatheter-delivered valve, but it is not necessarily required in transcatheter repair procedures. Additionally, if a minimally invasive surgical approach or procedure is employed, then additional specific technologies/devices are needed as well. Furthermore, depending on the valve design, a company may also be required to develop systems to load the valves within the delivery systems, e.g., crimping systems. Finally, many of these device developers are simultaneously creating training simulation systems for the delivery of each product type or procedural approach.

33.2 Pulmonic Valve

A transvenously delivered transcatheter pulmonic valve can be employed as a novel nonsurgical means to treat complications associated with congenital heart disease, such as pulmonary valve insufficiency. A minimally invasive surgical approach is also an option, if warranted, depending on individual patient history and/or other interventions that need to be performed. For example, Fig. 33.1 demonstrates that a transcatheter pulmonic valve could be delivered either transvenously (via the superior or inferior vena cava) through the tricuspid valve into position or via a transventricular puncture through the right ventricular wall.

The needs of congenital heart patients inspired the original creation of the transcatheter-delivered stented valve; as noted above; Philipp Bonhoeffer is the pioneer of this technology. One example of such a replacement system is the Melody® Transcatheter Pulmonary Valve

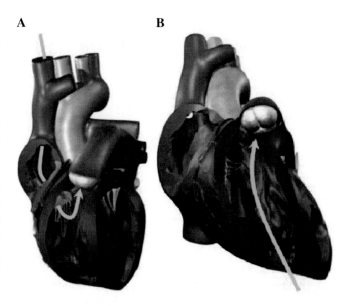

Fig. 33.1 Two potential approaches for the delivery of a transcatheter pulmonic valve: (**A**) transvenously into the right atrium, then through the tricuspid valve; or (**B**) transapically through the right ventricular wall. The latter approach would require a minimally invasive surgery

(Medtronic, Inc., Minneapolis, MN). The stent supporting the valve is composed of a platinum iridium alloy, which is expanded during delivery by balloons located within the delivery system. The valve is a bovine jugular vein valve which is sewn to the stent. The Melody valve is delivered using the Ensemble® Transcatheter Delivery System through the cardiovascular system, eliminating the need to open the patient's chest (Fig. 33.2). The

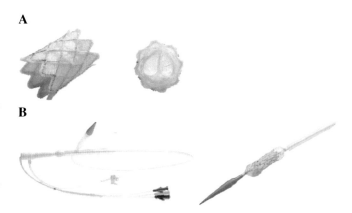

Fig. 33.2 The Melody® Transcatheter Pulmonary Valve and Ensemble® Transcatheter Delivery System have received CE Mark approval and are available for distribution in Europe. Additionally, a Medical Device License has been granted and the system is available for distribution in Canada. Products are not available for sale in the United States. The system consists of a bovine jugular valve vein sewn inside a platinum iridium stent (**A**) and delivered via a sheathed balloon-in-balloon delivery catheter (**B**)

overall procedure minimizes trauma and offers a quicker recovery than traditional surgical procedures. Furthermore, it is considered that such procedures (1) could help reduce the total number of surgeries that these patients would require in their lifetimes, e.g., by postponing time to surgery while restoring pulmonic function; (2) would allow for earlier intervention and potentially better outcomes for patients, while avoiding surgical complications; (3) avoid the risks of bleeding and infection associated with reoperation; and/or (4) reduce costs by avoiding postoperative intensive care [4, 5].

It is common that developers of these technologies partner with leading congenital interventional cardiologists and cardiac surgeons. Furthermore, managing these complex congenital heart disease patients requires a cohesive team approach. It is likely that such patients will be treated in the hybrid catheter lab/operating room by a team of healthcare professionals including a cardiologist and cardiac surgeon.

33.3 Aortic Valve

Currently, transcatheter aortic valve replacement is considered for select high-risk patients with severe calcific aortic stenosis that are not candidates for conventional valve replacement. This procedure has similar benefits as mentioned above, such as eliminating the need for cardiopulmonary bypass and shorter recovery times. It is conceivable that a transcatheter aortic valve could be delivered by one of four different approaches: (1) transarterially (e.g., via the femoral artery); (2) transseptally via the right heart; (3) transatrially through the left atrial wall or a port in the atrial appendage; or (4) transapically through the left ventricular wall (Fig. 33.3). Currently, the transarterial and transapical approaches are the most widely adopted. In current practice, the *transapical* approach through the left ventricular wall (myocardium) requires a minimally invasive surgery (see Chapter 32),

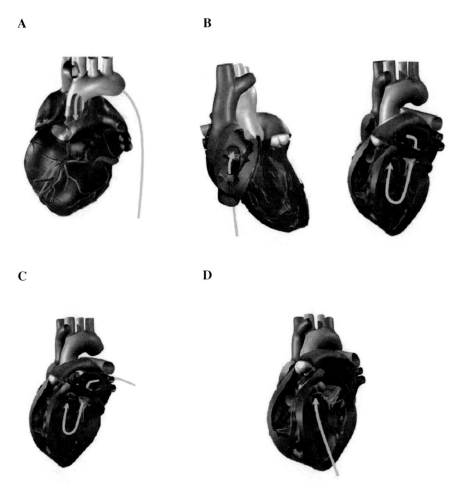

Fig. 33.3 Four potential approaches for the delivery of a transcatheter aortic valve or repair tool: (**A**) transarterially (e.g., via femoral artery access); (**B**) transseptally from the right heart (transvenous access) into the left atrium, then through the mitral valve; (**C**) transatrially through the left atrial wall or through a port in the left atrial appendage, then through the mitral valve; or (**D**) transapically through the left ventricular wall. The latter two approaches would currently require a minimally invasive surgical procedure

yet it likely provides the most direct anatomical approach. On the other hand, this approach requires closure of the myocardium post delivery and, if the delivery system is large, this can be challenging. As technology advances, the need for minimally invasive surgery with this approach may be eliminated. The *transseptal* approach, which has the advantage of employing transvenous access for the delivery system, has the potential drawback that if the system passing through the interatrial wall is large, the physician may create a septal defect which will require repair (see Chapter 34). Additionally, the system must make a turn of approximately 180 degrees in the left ventricle after passing through the mitral valve to be positioned in the aortic valve, a maneuver that can be technically challenging. Anatomically, inferior access via a femoral vein is considered advantageous due to the proximity of the inferior vena caval ostium and the fossa ovalis, which is the preferred transseptal puncture location. The *transarterial* approach involves femoral artery access and retrograde navigation of the delivery system through the aorta to the aortic root. This approach can be challenging due to: (1) the size of the patient's arteries; (2) the tortuosity of the arteries and aorta; and (3) the degree of calcification in the aorta, some of which can potentially be knocked free by the delivery system; however, it is still the preferred route by most interventional cardiologists. It has been reported that rapid ventricular burst pacing can be employed to facilitate transcatheter heart valve implantation. Pacing rates were between 150 and 220 bpm with durations of 12 ± 3 s; pacing was relatively well tolerated ($n = 40$) when cautiously used. Rapid pacing was associated with a rapid and effective reduction in systemic blood pressure, pulse pressure, transvascular flow, as well as cardiac and catheter motion [6].

As can be observed in Fig. 33.3, the potential pathways/approaches to place a transcatheter-delivered valve in the aortic position are quite varied and have dramatic differences in the angles and anatomical features that would be required to be navigated within or through (e.g., vessels, chamber walls, valves, or chordae tendinae). Due to this complexity, the flexibility of the delivery system (with the loaded valve within it) will be a major factor to consider when selecting a delivery approach; furthermore, the patient's cardiac anatomy is a major consideration. This is true for the delivery of the system and also for the positioning of the valve stent into the aortic position, as one must prevent obstruction to the ostia of the coronary arteries.

Currently, there are several transcatheter aortic valves available for clinical use, in clinical trial or in animal testing. The Corevalve® ReValving™ System (Medtronic, Inc., Minneapolis, MN) and the SAPIEN transcatheter valve by Edwards Lifesciences (Irvine, CA) are in clinical trials, and several hundred devices have been implanted in patients worldwide (Fig. 33.4). More specifically, for the transarterial placement of the SAPIEN transcatheter heart valve, the surgeon uses the RetroFlex delivery system, whereas she/he uses the Ascendra delivery system for a transapical placement. The Corevalve® ReValving™ System is also delivered via a transarterial or transapical approach in a specialized delivery catheter. In addition, there are several smaller companies that have developed (and continue to develop) competing technologies, such as those from Direct Flow Medical, Inc. (Santa Rosa, CA) and Heart Leaflet Technologies Inc. (Maple Grove, MN). Nevertheless, nearly all the major players in cardiac valve replacement have a keen interest in these technologies and clinical approaches.

It is important to note that, currently, a percentage of patients that have received transcatheter-delivered

A

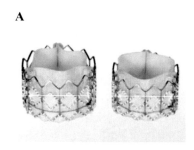

B

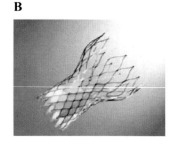

Fig. 33.4 (**A**) The Edwards Lifesciences SAPIEN transcatheter heart valve consists of a stainless steel balloon-expandable stent with an attached pericardial valve. It has been designed for transfemoral placement with the RetroFlex delivery system or for transapical placement with the Ascendra delivery system. Clinical studies are underway in the United States, Canada, and Europe. (**B**) The Corevalve® ReValving™ System by Medtronic, Inc. consists of a self-expandable nitinol stent with an attached pericardial valve. It is designed for both transarterial and transapical delivery and is currently in clinical trials in Europe

aortic valves have elicited conduction abnormalities which may include heart block. Most of the self-expanding or balloon-expanded valve prostheses exert radial forces on the interventricular septal wall and surrounding structures which is required to maintain proper position and to minimize paravalvular leaks. This force, coupled with the close anatomic proximity of the atrioventricular node, the bundle of His, and/or the left bundle branch with the basal annulus of the aortic valve (see Chapter 11), is the likely explanation for this phenomenon.

33.4 Mitral Valve

Mitral valve dysfunction can be related to several factors including diseased leaflets [7], annular changes [8], abnormal or damaged chordae [9], and ventricular dilatation [10] causing displacement of the papillary muscles. Due to this large variability in disease process, a wide variety of transcatheter devices are being investigated for the mitral valve. These transcatheter devices can be subdivided into five general types: (1) devices for Alfieri-type edge-to-edge repair; (2) indirect annuloplasty devices deployed into the coronary sinus; (3) direct annuloplasty devices placed on or near the mitral annulus; (4) devices for dimensional control of the left ventricle or left atrium; and (5) devices for mitral valve replacement [11, 12].

The edge-to-edge technique involves placing a stitch to join the anterior and posterior leaflets at the location of regurgitation [13–15]. This technique is most commonly used in patients with A2 or P2 prolapse, and the simplicity of the edge-to-edge technique has led to opportunities for percutaneous valve repair [16–18]. More recently, the MitraClip repair system was designed to use transcatheter clips to grasp the ventricular sides of the anterior and posterior mitral leaflets, leaving the clip in place upon deployment (Evalve, Inc., Menlo Park, CA).

For patients with annular dilatation, many devices are currently being developed to simulate a traditional annuloplasty procedure. These products are classified as either indirect, which typically involves a transvenous coronary sinus approach, or direct, which involves placing the device in direct contact with the mitral annulus. Percutaneous, transvenous mitral annuloplasty is a technology that implants a metal bar with flexible ends and a stiff midsection to reshape the posterior leaflet; it is a reversible procedure (Viacor, Inc., Wilmington, MA). The Monarc system features two self-expanding stents tethered together which reshape the posterior region of the annulus in 2–3 weeks (Edwards Lifesciences). Similar to the Monarc, Carillon XE (Cardiac Dimensions, Inc., Kirkland, WA) utilizes tethered stents in the coronary sinus to reshape the posterior annulus. These technologies rely on the proximity of the coronary sinus to the posterior aspect of the mitral annulus. Additionally, direct mitral annuloplasty is also being investigated; these devices are in direct contact with the mitral annulus either temporarily or permanently. MiCardia Corporation (Irvine, CA) and MitralSolutions, Inc. (Fort Lauderdale, FL) are both developing adjustable annuloplasty devices which are currently implanted surgically, but can be adjusted on the beating heart. The Mitralign device (Mitralign, Inc., Tewksbury, MA) places implants around the annulus and then cinches them closer together, thereby reducing the orifice area of the valve. QuantumCor, Inc. (San Clemente, CA) is developing a device which uses subablative temperatures applied to the annulus to constrict collagen and thereby reduce annular size. Nevertheless, the goal of these devices is to restore valve coaptation and thus eliminate mitral regurgitation.

Indirect approaches to mitral valve repair that influence left ventricular or left atrial dimensions are also under investigation. By changing left ventricular dimensions, products such as Coapsys and iCoapsys (Myocor ® Inc., Maple Grove, MN) are designed to improve mitral valve and left ventricular performance. The PS³ system (Ample Medical, Inc., Foster City, CA) shortens the left atrial dimension between the fossa ovalis and the great cardiac vein, and consequently the septal-lateral dimension of the mitral annulus [19].

As described for the aortic valve, it is possible to deploy a transcatheter mitral valve or affect a transcatheter repair using four different approaches: (1) transarterial (e.g., via the femoral artery); (2) transseptal via the right heart; (3) transatrial through the left atrial wall or a port in the atrial appendage; or (4) transapical through the left ventricular wall (Fig. 33.5). The human mitral valve is a very complex, dynamic, and highly variable structure. Therefore, complications in the deployment of a replacement valve or repair device into this position will potentially interact with the (1) valve leaflets themselves; (2) the chordae tendinae; and/or (3) the papillary muscles. As mentioned earlier, the valvular and subvalvular anatomy can be quite variable, with some individuals eliciting bifurcated or trifurcated papillary muscles, distinct chordae tendinae patterns, and numerous scallops of each mitral valve leaflet. Due to the complexity of the mitral valve apparatus and underlying disease processes, it is likely that a combination of the aforementioned devices will be required to provide percutaneous solutions for mitral valve repair.

A   B

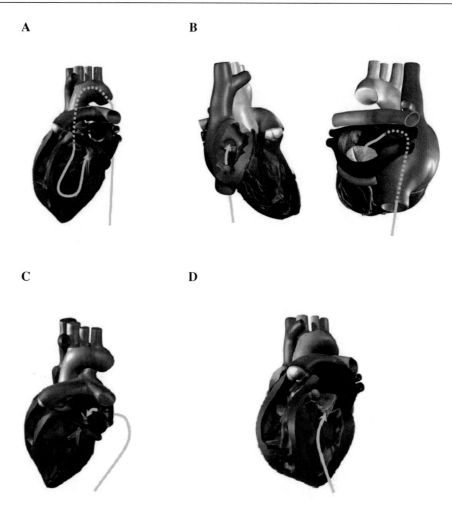

C   D

Fig. 33.5 Four potential approaches for the delivery of a transcatheter mitral valve or repair tool: (**A**) transarterially (e.g., via femoral artery access) retrograde through the aortic valve and up to the mitral valve via the left ventricular chamber; (**B**) transseptally from the right heart (transvenous access) into the left atrium, then to the mitral valve; (**C**) transatrially through the left atrial wall or through a port in the left atrial appendage, then to the mitral valve; or (**D**) transapically through the left ventricular wall. The latter two approaches would currently require a minimally invasive surgical procedure

33.5 Tricuspid Valve

As described for the mitral valve, the human tricuspid valve is a very complex, dynamic, and highly variable structure as well. The transcatheter approach to this valve structure would be similar to those described for the pulmonic valve (Fig. 33.1). It is envisioned that a transcatheter mitral valve or repair tool could be delivered either transvenously (via the superior or inferior venae cavae) into position or via a transapical puncture through the right ventricular wall. Furthermore, as described above for the repair and/or replacement of the mitral valve, nearly all options would also hold true for the tricuspid valve, which many surgeons feel is often overlooked when treating heart failure patients (for more detailed discussion, see Chapter 31). On the

other hand, the potential complications of damaging or altering the conduction system, as was described for the aortic valve replacement, would also be evident for procedures that involve the tricuspid septal annular structures, i.e., atrioventricular node, the bundle of His, and/or the right bundle branch of the conduction system (see Chapter 11).

33.6 Imaging

The development and use of transcatheter-delivered cardiac valves has transformed (and will continue to transform) heart valve procedures for those requiring open-heart surgery and/or cardiopulmonary bypass (see

Chapter 30) to a "percutaneous beating heart interventional procedure performed under image guidance" (fluoroscopy or echocardiography). Yet, these imaging modalities are considered to have advantages and disadvantages. For example, cardiac computed tomography (CT) imaging is considered extremely useful for identifying the relative degree of calcification that exists on a heart valve leaflet as well as the delivery anatomy, but is not useful as an intraoperative technique and it exposes the patient to considerable radiation dose.

Importantly, advanced imaging modalities will be required for pre-planning and intraoperative guidance of these interventions. More specifically, to date, there is no single imaging modality for intracardiac interventions without clinical limitations, which include low temporal or spatial resolution, excessive exposure to ionizing radiation, and interference with the clinical operator's freedom of movement. We believe that, in the near future, a combination of imaging modes will provide the information required to guide these complex interventions. Recently, our group set out to provide "a glimpse into the future" by demonstrating the unique direct visualization of transcatheter pulmonary valve implantation utilizing the Visible Heart® techniques (Figs. 33.6, 33.7, and 33.8) [20, 21].

We also suggest that, as cardiac repair and device implantation procedures become less invasive, we will need to study the deployment of these systems or techniques within beating heart models. Utilization of Visible Heart® methodologies provides unique visualization of cardiac device technologies. The preparation and images obtained can be used by design engineers and physicians to develop implant methodologies, as well as support clinical education and training. As more of these devices are implanted within the beating heart, unique means will be required to train individuals in the techniques to navigate and deploy them. For example, Fig. 33.9 shows the simultaneously obtained images of a stent being placed in the aortic position, including endoscopic views and time-synchronized images from fluoroscopy and ultrasound.

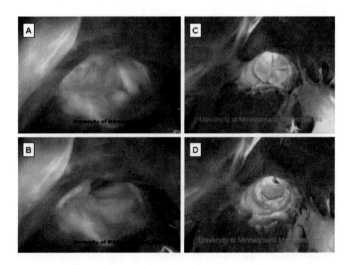

Fig. 33.6 Comparison of a human pulmonic valve (**A**) during diastole and (**B**) during systole to a transcatheter pulmonic valve placed in a human heart (**C**) during diastole and (**D**) during systole [21]

33.7 Training Systems

The complexity of intracardiac interventions has increased with the advent of transcatheter valve replacement and is expected to further escalate as clinicians become more comfortable with complicated cardiac repairs within the beating heart and as engineers invent new product solutions. Simulators designed to demonstrate the technical aspects of transcatheter-delivered valves have already been developed. Many state-of-the-

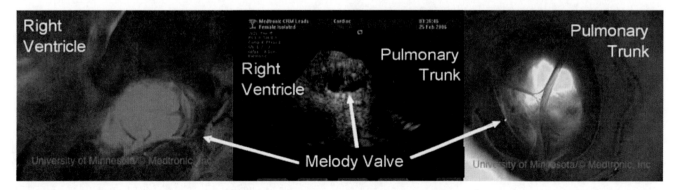

Fig. 33.7 Simultaneous endoscopic images on the left and right depict a deployed transcatheter pulmonary valve (Melody® Transcatheter Pulmonary Valve, Medtronic, Inc.) in the native right ventricular outflow tract, with the corresponding ultrasound image displayed in the center [21]

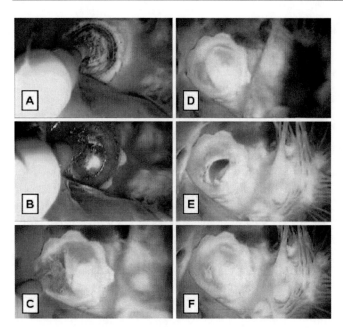

Fig. 33.8 Positioning (**A**), deployment (**B** and **C**), and function (**Panels D–F**) of a transcatheter aortic valve implanted into a surgically placed bioprosthetic aortic valve. It is interesting to note the lack of (or minimal) interactions between the implanted aortic valve and the native mitral valve [21]

art patient simulators enable pseudo-visualization via various imaging modes; for instance, one can practice using fluoroscopy for the valve implant without any exposure to radiation. The delivery systems for these transcatheter valves are often complex and require guidewires, introducers, and/or dilators; hence, prior practice on handling such tools is essential. Furthermore, for those physicians not familiar with performing such catheter-delivered and/or minimally invasive surgical approaches, these training sessions can be invaluable and highly educational. If such procedures are performed in a newly instrumented hybrid catheter lab/operating room, then the dynamics of team interactions could also be developed in such training sessions. More specifically, studies employing virtual reality simulation of such procedures have indicated that there is a documented learning curve, and catheter handling errors significantly decrease as assessed with measurable dynamic metrics with high test–retest reliability [22].

33.8 Summary

The use of transcatheter delivery systems to repair or replace cardiac valves is an area of intense research development. The potential to treat patients with valvular disease without the use of open-heart surgery will ultimately affect millions of individuals worldwide, improving the quality of life of these patients. The future of this field will likely see smaller delivery systems with greater intracardiac mobility, as well as replacement valves that better mimic healthy native valve function. Affecting the ultimate clinical success of these therapies will be adequate cardiac visual and function assessments prior to, during, and after the procedures. One can also foresee that simulation training will be employed even before such techniques are performed in animal models, as many procedures will require numerous tool components (e.g., introducers, dilators, balloon catheters, delivery catheters, etc.).

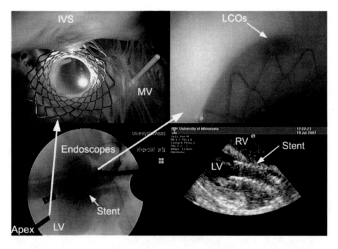

Fig. 33.9 The *top images* show endoscopic views of a prototype stent placed in the aortic position and the *bottom images* show time-synchronized images from fluoroscopy (*lower left*) and ultrasound (*lower right*). The *upper left image* shows the view from the ventricle; the interventricular septum (IVS) is at the top and the mitral valve (MV) is located on the *right*. The *upper right* image is a view from the aorta, specifically showing the interaction of the stent and left coronary artery ostium (LCOs): in this case, there would be minimal obstruction of flow into the left coronary artery. The fluoroscopic image clearly shows the stent as well as the endoscopes in the left ventricle and aorta. The stent is also clearly visible on the ultrasound image, projecting slightly into the left ventricle (LV). The right ventricle (RV) is located at the top of this image [21]

References

1. Andersen HR, Knudsen LL, Hasenkam JM. Transluminal implantation of artificial heart valves. Description of a new expandable aortic valve and initial results with implantation by catheter technique in closed chest pigs. Eur Heart J 1992;13:704–08.
2. Bonhoeffer P, Boudjemline Y, Saliba Z, et al. Percutaneous replacement of pulmonary valve in a right-ventricle to

pulmonary-artery prosthetic conduit with valve dysfunction. Lancet 2000;356:1403–05.

3. Cribier A, Eltchaninoff H, Bash A, et al. Percutaneous transcatheter implantation of an aortic valve prosthesis for calcific aortic stenosis: First human case description. Circulation 2002;106:3006–08.

4. Coats L, Tsang V, Khambadkone S, et al. The potential impact of percutaneous pulmonary valve stent implantation on right ventricular outflow tract re-intervention. Eur J Cardiothorac Surg 2005;27:536–43.

5. Khambadkone S, Bonhoeffer P. Nonsurgical pulmonary valve replacement: Why, when, and how? Catheter Cardiovasc Interv 2004;62:401–08.

6. Webb JG, Pasupate S, Achtem L, Thompson CR. Rapid pacing to facilitate transcatheter prosthetic heart valve implantation. Catheter Cardiovasc Interv 2006;68:199–204.

7. Roberts WC. Morphologic features of the normal and abnormal mitral valve. Am J Cardiol 1983;51:1005–28.

8. Yiu SF, Enriquez-Sarano M, Tribouilloy C, Seward JB, Tajik AJ. Determinants of the degree of functional mitral regurgitation in patients with systolic left ventricular dysfunction: A quantitative clinical study. Circulation 2000;102:1400–06.

9. Hickey AJ, Wilcken DE, Wright JS, Warren BA. Primary (spontaneous) chordal rupture: Relation to myxomatous valve disease and mitral valve prolapse. J Am Coll Cardiol 1985;5:1341–46.

10. Kono T, Sabbah HN, Rosman H, Alam M, Jafri S, Goldstein S. Left ventricular shape is the primary determinant of functional mitral regurgitation in heart failure. J Am Coll Cardiol 1992;20:1594–98.

11. Babaliaros V, Block P. State of the art percutaneous intervention for the treatment of valvular heart disease: A review of the current technologies and ongoing research in the field of percutaneous valve replacement and repair. Cardiology 2007;107:87–96.

12. Feldman T, Leon MB. Prospects for percutaneous valve therapies. Circulation 2007;116:2866–77.

13. Nakanishi K, Raman J, Hata M, Buxton B. Early outcome with the Alfieri mitral valve repair. J Cardiol 2001;37:263–66.

14. Alfieri O, Maisano F, De Bonis M, et al. The double-orifice technique in mitral valve repair: A simple solution for complex problems. J Thorac Cardiovasc Surg 2001;122:674–81.

15. Alfieri O, Maisano F. An effective technique to correct anterior mitral leaflet prolapse. J Card Surg 1999;14:468–70.

16. Alfieri O, Maisano F, Colombo A. Percutaneous mitral valve repair procedures. Eur J Cardiothorac Surg 2004;26:S36–37; discussion S37–38.

17. Alfieri O, De Bonis M, Lapenna E, et al. "Edge-to-edge" repair for anterior mitral leaflet prolapse. Semin Thorac Cardiovasc Surg 2004;16:182–87.

18. Alfieri O, Maisano F, Colombo A, Pappone C, La Canna G, Zangrillo A. Percutaneous mitral valve repair: An attractive perspective and an opportunity for teamwork. Ital Heart J 2004;5:723–26.

19. Rogers JH, Macoviak JA, Rahdert DA, Takeda PA, Palacios IF, Low RI. Percutaneous septal sinus shortening: A novel procedure for the treatment of functional mitral regurgitation. Circulation 2006;113:2329–34.

20. Quill JL, Laske TG, Hill AJ, Bonhoeffer P, Iaizzo PA. Direct visualization of a transcatheter pulmonary valve implantation within the Visible Heart® – A Glimpse into the Future. Circulation 2007;116:e548.

21. Iaizzo PA, Hill AJ, Laske TG. Cardiac device testing enhanced by simultaneous imaging modalities: The Visible Heart®, fluoroscopy, and echocardiography. Expert Rev Med Devices 2008;5:51–58.

22. Patel AD, Gallagher AG, Nicholson WJ, Cates CU. Learning curves and reliability measures for virtual reality simulation in the performance assessment of carotid angiography. J Am Coll Cardiol 2006;47:1796–802.

Chapter 34
Cardiac Septal Defects: Treatment via the Amplatzer® Family of Devices

John L. Bass and Daniel H. Gruenstein

Abstract The majority of patients with congenital heart disease present with defects comprised of vascular narrowing or absence (such as interruption or coarctation of the aorta or pulmonary arteries) or failure of structures to fuse or separate during development (total anomalous pulmonary venous connection, septal defects, fusion of valve cusps). Correction of these defects began with open-heart surgery but, more recently, many such repairs can be performed transvenously using catheter-delivered closure devices (e.g., Amplatzer closure devices). This chapter will review a brief history of such repairs and provide information on the design and animal testing of such systems.

Keywords Interventional cardiac catheterization · Atrial septal defect · Transcatheter closure · Patent ductus arteriosus · Muscular ventricular septal defect · Perimembranous ventricular septal defect

34.1 Introduction

Congenital heart disease affects eight of every thousand live births. The majority of these defects are comprised of vascular narrowing (such as interruption or coarctation of the aorta or pulmonary arteries), vessel absence, or failure of structures to fuse or separate during development (total anomalous pulmonary venous connection, septal defects, or fusion of valve cusps). Correction of these defects began with open-heart surgery, but this was originally limited to repairs that could be performed without stopping the patient's circulation (patent ductus arteriosus or coarctation of the aorta). The subsequent development of cardiopulmonary bypass allowed the

surgeon to safely visualize the inside of the heart, and more complex repairs were then developed. This was the true beginning of caring for children with congenital heart disease, thus dramatically extending and improving the quality of their lives. However, these advances also caused the art of diagnosis by physical examination to no longer be sufficient to provide details of anatomy needed by the surgeon. It then followed that the development of cardiac catheterization had a similar clinical explosion as the primary diagnostic tool. Still, surgeons had to be prepared to deal with the specific anatomy found during the operation, as some details were unexpected. This surgical license to make plans "on the fly" is critical to a successful operation and explains the historical liberation of surgery from restrictions by the Food and Drug Administration (FDA) and Institutional Review Boards.

Next, echocardiography developed to the point where it began to replace cardiac catheterization as the primary diagnostic tool for congenital heart disease (see also Chapter 20). Thus, the number of cardiac catheterizations diminished. Subsequently, the birth of interventional cardiac catheterization launched by Dr. Gruntzig's coronary angioplasty rescued cardiac catheterization. These techniques were applied to visualize congenital narrowing of the pulmonary arteries and coarctation of the aorta. Importantly, experimental testing preceded the use of such techniques in children with congenital heart disease [1, 2]. It was observed that no foreign materials were left behind with these procedures. Interventional cardiac catheterization was further expanded with Dr. Porstmann's use of an Ivalon plug to close the persistent patent ductus arteriosus (PDA) [3], as well as Dr. King's [4] and Dr. Rashkind's [5] devices for closure of secundum atrial septal defects (ASDs). Nevertheless, technical difficulties (i.e., limited retrievability and large delivery systems) and residual shunts plagued the development of these devices, and their application remained limited.

Two companies in particular, NuMED, Inc. (Hopkinton, NY) and AGA Medical Corporation (Plymouth, MN),

J.L. Bass (✉)
University of Minnesota, Department of Pediatric Cardiology, MMC 94, 420 Delaware St. SE, Minneapolis, MN 55455, USA
e-mail: bassx001@umn.edu

P.A. Iaizzo (ed.), *Handbook of Cardiac Anatomy, Physiology, and Devices*, DOI 10.1007/978-1-60327-372-5_34,
© Springer Science+Business Media, LLC 2009

focused their efforts on developing devices aimed at correcting congenital cardiac defects. In 2001, the Amplatzer Septal Occluder became the first device to receive FDA approval for closure of secundum ASDs, followed in 2003 by the Amplatzer Ductal Occluder. This, along with development of stents that could be applied to the larger vascular narrowing of congenital heart diseases, opened the floodgates for interventional cardiac catheterization in children. We consider that both NuMED, Inc. and AGA Medical Corporation deserve special recognition for choosing to focus their efforts on improving care for children with congenital heart disease, instead of the larger volume and remuneration of fixing adult problems with coronary artery stents or patent foramen ovale closure devices.

34.2 Amplatzer Devices

Amplatzer devices designed to close congenital cardiac defects are all quite similar; basically they all are self-expanding stents shaped to fit a given defect. These devices are composed of a Nitinol wire stent, with the ends of the wires bound together to form a closed frame fashioned with a plug to fill the defect and retention discs. The shape of the wire frame is tailored to fit the abnormal vascular or intracardiac communication. The retention discs are used to fix the device against vascular or cardiac walls. The central waist further holds the device in place by allowing for radial forces to be placed against the margins of the communication; this provides stable fixation of the device. Most available devices are concentric and designed to fill defects that are centrally located, and thus are surrounded by cardiac structures that will not be injured by the edges of the device. In general, subsequent occlusion occurs through thrombosis within the polyester baffles or by inserting suture inside of the wire frame. Importantly, within approximately 3 months, these devices will be covered with protein and cellular layers, thus reducing the potential for forming a surface thrombus and eliminating the risk of bacterial endocarditis [6].

Historically, the development of Amplatzer devices began when thin wire technology reached a point that allowed construction of a frame of nontoxic Nitinol wires. Like all stents, the collapsed device is long and narrow to fit through the delivery sheath. Uniquely, Nitinol metal has shape memory such that, as it exits the sheath, the device expands and assumes its original shape at body temperature. Each device has a microscrew fixed to the proximal end allowing attachment to a delivery cable. Hence, the device can be retrieved with the cable after deployment and removed or repositioned. Finally, the device is detached via unscrewing, once secure and effective position is confirmed.

34.2.1 Safety

Nickel-containing alloys, such as stainless steel, have been employed in human medicine for over 100 years. They have been used in surgical instruments as well as implants such as pacemaker wires, vascular clips, mechanical cardiac valves, orthopedic prostheses, Harrington rods, and inferior vena caval filters. Thus, this can be considered to demonstrate the relative lack of toxicity of nickel-containing metallic implants; no systemic effects were observed or have been reported. Yet, local fibrotic reactions surrounding stainless steel implants were thought to be due to local passivation of nickel ions into surrounding tissue, despite the absence of microscopically visible corrosion. Interestingly, the US Navy developed a new nickel-containing metal, Nitinol, in the 1960s. This alloy of nickel and titanium displayed superior corrosion resistance, and it still carries the name of its heritage—*NI*ckel *TI*tanium-*N*aval *O*rdnance *L*aboratory.

Nitinol has numerous properties besides corrosion resistance that make it desirable for use in medical devices, including super elasticity (pseudo-elasticity), thermal shape memory, high resiliency, and fatigue resistance. Originally, thin wire technology, more specifically the development of the "diamond-drawn" wire, provided a shape that could be used in endodontal appliances. The tendency for Nitinol to return to its nominal shape when deformed was especially useful in this application. Thus, this property also made Nitinol a valuable material in the production of endoluminal devices. Importantly, a Nitinol device stretched for introduction through a small delivery catheter will expand back to its original shape when deployed. This new alloy replaced most stainless steel devices, especially self-expanding stents. Furthermore, Nitinol's fatigue resistance prevents wire fractures and extends device durability. The absence of ferro-magnetic properties is compatible with magnetic resonance imaging.

Amplatzer devices have proven to be nontoxic [7]. In addition, such devices performed well in fatigue testing and, when immersed in a saline bath, they did not corrode. Nickel levels in patients before and after insertion of an Amplatzer device have been shown not to differ. Furthermore, devices examined 18 months post-implantation in humans and animals have not revealed any detectable surface corrosion. Nevertheless, it should be noted that the incidence of nickel allergy is approximately 10% in humans. With over 100,000 current implants of

Amplatzer devices worldwide over the past 13 years, no definitive case of a reaction has been reported in the literature.

34.3 Animal Models Mimicking Congenital Defects

Surgical repair of cardiac defects, such as those of the atrial or ventricular septums, specifically allowed the surgeon to evaluate the shape and surrounding structures on an individual basis. Yet, the initial diagnosis of an ASD was established only by typical findings on physical examination, electrocardiogram, and chest roentgenogram [8]. Associated abnormalities, such as anomalous pulmonary venous connection, were identified and dealt with by the surgeon at the time of the operative closure.

Animal models created to test experimental devices may not always account for associated anatomic details that can be encountered by the surgeon. It should be noted that, for most congenital heart defects, an exact animal model is not readily available. Nevertheless, by first creating a defect by dilation of a thin septum, sewing in an artificial vascular connection, or removing a portion of the thicker muscular septum, such models helped to address the ease and reliability of implantation and/or the efficacy of occluding the created defect. Such idealized "defects" are typically chosen according to the cardiologist's and radiologist's concepts from imaging and/or by examination of pathological specimens, but they do not always mimic the actual defect in humans.

34.4 Atrial Septal Defect

34.4.1 History

Atrial septal defects are congenital deficiencies in the wall separating the systemic and pulmonary venous returns as they enter the heart. This allows blood from the lungs to flow through the defect and increases the volume of blood passing through the pulmonary arteries. In most patients, after two decades of life with this flow pattern, this defect can permanently damage the pulmonary vasculature. Therefore, to prevent this and other problems such as associated cardiac arrhythmias, closure of ASDs is recommended during the first few years of life [9].

It is interesting to note that the University of Minnesota performed the first surgical closure of an ASD in 1954 [10]. This successful operative approach for correction of a congenital intracardiac defect remains as one of the safest open-heart operations performed, with a mortality rate under 0.5% [9]. Nevertheless, surgical closure includes morbidity from the imposed medial sternotomy (or an imposed right thoracotomy), the risk of exposure to blood products, a chest tube, 3–5 days hospitalization, 4–6 weeks of convalescence, and/or the chance of postpericardiotomy syndrome. Hence, consequences of these procedures spurred attempts to develop a method of transcatheter closure.

It is generally accepted that transcatheter closure to treat secundum ASDs is ideal. Atrial septal defects are typically surrounded by rims of tissue that a device can clasp, with no borders formed by or thus impeding the valves or the walls of the heart. King and Mills reported the first attempted transcatheter closure of a secundum ASD in 1974 [4]. This was followed by development of the Clamshell/CardioSEAL [11], Sideris Button [12], ASDOS [13], and Angel Wings [14] devices. Each of these devices not only provided an alternative to surgical closure, but also resulted in a number of new challenges. For example, large devices were required with the central post design; yet, most of these early designs were not self-centering and the center post could move within the defect. Further, these large devices required large delivery systems and, additionally, some were plagued by embolization (e.g., unbuttoning) [15]. It was also noted that frame fatigue and arm fracture occurred in up to 10% of some designs, with asymptomatic wire embolization found in several patients. It was concluded that most of these designs were difficult or impossible to recapture or retrieve after deployment. Hence, surgical removal was required if they were deployed in an improper position and residual shunt rates were significant [16].

34.5 Amplatzer Device Design

An ideal septal closure device should be: (1) easily delivered and implanted; (2) self-centering; (3) able to pass through a small delivery system; (4) recapturable and redeployable; (5) highly resilient (without fracturing); and (6) highly effective, i.e., without significant residual shunts. The materials used in device construction should also be biocompatible and nontoxic. It should be emphasized that durability is important, for the majority of patients are children and there is a long "lifetime" after implantation.

The Amplatzer ASD devices were designed to fulfill these requirements. For example, the Amplatzer Septal Occluder is a woven mesh of 72 Nitinol wires 0.003″–0.008″ in diameter with shape memory. There are two retention discs with a central waist within the defect

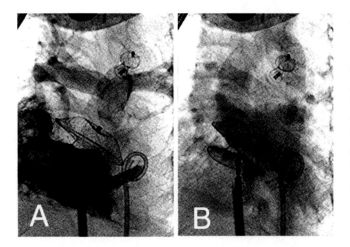

Fig. 34.1 Amplatzer Septal Occluder device. (**A**) Right atrial angiogram performed after deployment of the device in a secundum atrial septal defect, but before release. The right atrial disc is obscured by contrast with the waist within the atrial septal defect. (**B**) The levophase of the right atrial angiogram opacifying the left atrium. Contrast outlines the left atrial disc completely within the left atrium

(Fig. 34.1); the left atrial disc is 12–14 mm larger than the waist. The stenting action of the waist and the retention discs clasp the atrial septum, thus holding it in place. Additionally, fabric baffles sewn inside the discs and waist promote thromboses and overall occlusive abilities of the device. Importantly, the delivery systems are also relatively small (6–12 French delivery sheaths). These devices are all recapturable and redeployable with micro-screw/cable attachments. Available waist diameters range from 4 to 40 mm, thus allowing closure of quite large defects [16].

34.5.1 Animal Testing of the Amplatzer Device Designs

The Amplatzer Septal Occluder device was originally designed for occlusion of a secundum ASD. Initial animal studies were focused on reproducibly creating atrial septal communications, as a natural model of a secundum ASD did not exist. To do so, the flap of the foramen ovale in the experimental animal was perforated and dilated with a balloon to induce an atrial communication [6]; subsequently, devices were implanted and, in most cases, there were no complications or residual leaks. It was important to show that no thrombus formed on the devices. Afterward, human clinical trials confirmed that no retroaortic rim was required for stable device position and complete closure. Importantly, such patients could be discharged the morning after device placement, and remained on low-dose aspirin and endocarditis prophylaxis for 6 months after closure [16].

34.5.2 Required Testing for FDA Approval

A FDA-approved study to provide clinical evidence of the effectiveness of the Amplatzer Septal Occluder was originally initiated, based on both the prior success of animal studies and European trials in humans. Yet, the study design for this device was considered difficult. In general, most patients and their families wanted to avoid surgery despite the long history of safe surgical closure and the lack of long-term follow-up of this new device. Therefore, a blinded randomization was unsuccessful, as many patients and families chosen for the surgical group simply opted out of the trial, preferring to wait for final FDA approval. Subsequently, the overall study design was modified to allow device closure at some institutions with patients recruited to designated surgical centers. Note that this is not true randomization, but is representative of the difficulty of study design in the real world.

Afterward, the results of Phase II of the FDA trial also showed that the Amplatzer Septal Occluder was effective and safe compared with the surgical group. Importantly, at the end of 12 months, there was complete closure or a small (<2 mm) residual shunt in 98.5% of device patients, compared to 100% of surgically closed patients. Furthermore, there were no differences between groups in the incidence of major complications. It is noteworthy that minor complications were more common in surgical patients (27/442, 6.1% versus 29/154, 18.8%). Nevertheless, all patients were not truly randomized. There were differences between groups with the surgical patients being younger (18.1±19.3 versus 5.9±6.2 years, $p<0.001$) and smaller (42.3±27.3 kg versus 20.6±15.2 kg, $p<0.001$) [16]. In December 2001, the FDA granted premarket approval of the Amplatzer Septal Occluder, the first ASD closure device with FDA approval.

34.5.3 Continued Animal Research and Translation to Humans

After extensive successful clinical use, several reports of perforation of the heart by the device began to appear in a small number of patients with secundum ASDs [17]. Subsequently, a careful review of information from patients suffering from erosion after Amplatzer Septal Occluder placement suggested that individuals with "deficiency" of the superior and anterior rims of the atrial septum (Fig. 34.2) were at highest risk of this complication. In fact, the majority of patients with secundum ASDs have very little retroaortic rim, so many patients with ASDs may be at increased risk of erosion of the Amplatzer Septal Occluder through the superior, anterior

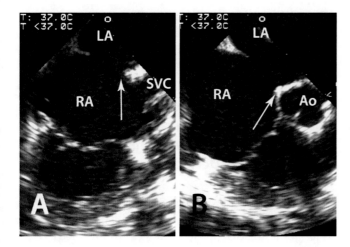

Fig. 34.2 Transesophageal images of an atrial septal defect with minimal superior and anterior (retroaortic) rims. In **A**, a bicaval view is recorded with almost no rim (*arrow*) by the superior vena cava (SVC). In **B**, a short axis view of the aorta (Ao) is recorded with minimal retroaortic rim (*arrow*). Atrial septal defects with minimal rims in these two areas are likely to bring the edges of right or left atrial retention discs in contact with the right or left atrial wall against the ascending aorta, and may have a higher risk of cardiac perforation. LA = left atrium; RA = right atrium

left, or right atrial wall. Importantly, the relationship of the ascending aorta to the anterior rim of the secundum ASD was not appreciated until the complication of erosion was reported. It should be noted that this original animal model did not truly mimic the anatomy of many patients with secundum ASDs. More recently, using stop flow to eliminate oversizing of the Amplatzer Septal Occluder device [17] has reduced the frequency of this complication (Personal communications with Ken Lock, AGA Medical Corporation).

34.6 Patent Ductus Arteriosus

Patent ductus arteriosus (PDA) is a failure of closure of a vascular channel that is present in the fetus that normally closes within the first 2 days after birth. When this vessel remains open, overcirculation of the lungs results. This, in turn, can damage the pulmonary vasculature, overwork the heart, and predispose these individuals to bacterial endocarditis. Closure is recommended to reduce the workload of the heart or when spontaneous closure is no longer likely (beyond 1–2 years of age) [18]. Much like operative closure of a secundum ASD, surgical closure of a PDA is a low-risk procedure that has been used for decades [19]. Therefore, any attempt to employ transcatheter closure methods must carry a risk at least as low as surgery. Furthermore, a PDA is similar to a secundum atrial defect in that the communication is surrounded by

normal vessels. It has been shown that concentric devices modified from the design of the Amplatzer Septal Occluder provided the opportunity for transcatheter closure in patients with these defects.

It is important to note that successful transcatheter closure of a small PDA was available before a specific device was developed. Specifically, coil occlusion of a PDA was first performed at the University of Minnesota in 1972. Such procedures included filling the aortic ampulla with stainless steel coils and their attached Dacron fibers, or "hanging" a coil across the narrowest part of a PDA; both procedures produced reliable closure. More specifically, the first embolization coils were not attached to delivery wires, and the coils sometimes embolized into the pulmonary circulation. These techniques were most effective when the narrowest diameters of the patent ductus were less than 3 mm [20]. Nevertheless, a retrievable device that would occlude larger ductuses was considered desirable.

The Amplatzer Ductal Occluder is shaped like a plug, sized to the aortic ampulla with an aortic retention disc designed to prevent embolization through the ductus (Fig. 34.3). These devices are typically delivered via a venous route and the delivery catheters are small (5–8 French) because of the small collapsed diameter. This simple modification of a self-expanding stent was found to be extremely successful in producing complete occlusion of even a large PDA. In the Phase II FDA trial, there was an observed complete closure of over 97% of defects at 6 and 12 months. There was only a 2.3% incidence of serious or major adverse events (including one embolization that required surgical removal and one death of a child, not

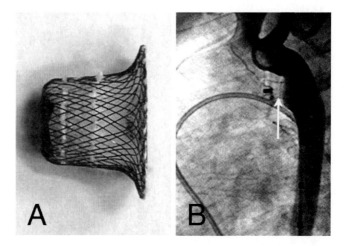

Fig. 34.3 Amplatzer Ductal Occluder Device. (**A**) Photograph of the device with clearly visible suturing of the baffle and stuffing to the ductal plug. (**B**) Aortogram immediately after device placement. The aortic disc is flat against the aortic wall with the plug within the ductal lumen. There is no flow through the ductus, and no obstruction of the aorta or left pulmonary artery (Arrow indicates the device plug filling the ductus arteriosus)

device-related, with a chromosomal trisomy) [21]. Premarket FDA approval of the Amplatzer Ductal Occluder device was received in January 2003.

34.6.1 Animal Testing of the Amplatzer Ductal Occluder and Translation to Human Use

A persistent PDA does not occur reliably in animals. Therefore, to test the efficacy of the Amplatzer Ductal Occluder, a synthetic tube was sewn between the descending aorta and the pulmonary artery in animals [22]. The Amplatzer Ductal Occluder device worked well, completely occluding this surgically created PDA which elicited endothelialization within 3 months. In these animal trials, there were no complications, the device was retrievable, and there were no residual hemodynamic abnormalities.

Subsequent to the successful animal studies, clinical trials were undertaken with a high rate of success in occluding various sizes of PDAs in patients [23]. Yet, with more extensive clinical use, a few reports began to surface of partial obstruction of the descending thoracic aorta by the retention disc of the Amplatzer Ductal Occluder device. This was the result of the angle (approximately 65°) of insertion of the naturally occurring PDA with the descending aorta. The superior portion of the retention disc was shown to be angled into the aorta by the plug within the PDA (Fig. 34.4), producing partial obstruction in smaller patients with larger PDAs. It

should be noted that the surgically created PDA in the animal model was sewn at a 90° angle to the aorta, and this complication was not predicted by the anatomically incorrect orientation.

34.6.2 Animal Trials Designed to Test Prototype-Angled Amplatzer Ductal Occluder Devices

To reduce the complexity of manufacturing the Amplatzer Ductal Occluder device and, at the same time, address the issues of the angle of the descending aorta with the PDA, a new device was designed with an angled retention disc; the wire count was also increased from 72 to 144 wires, thus eliminating the need for fabric in the device [24]. For animal testing of this new design in these trials, a synthetic tube was sewn between the pulmonary artery and aorta at the angle of the naturally occurring PDA. Subsequently, in all animals, the angled Amplatzer Ductal Occluder device was successful in occluding the created PDA (Fig. 34.5A); however, the initial human use of the device revealed shortcomings with these animal trials. Specifically, an angled Amplatzer Ductal Occluder was successfully placed in a young infant with initial success, which also avoided any protrusion of the device into the aorta; however, after 3

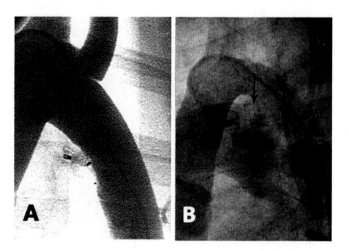

Fig. 34.5 In **A**, an aortogram is performed after placement and release of an angled ductal occluder device in a canine model with the artificial ductus sewn to mimic the natural angle of the human patent ductus arteriosus. (**A**) The angled aortic retention disc lies flat against the aortic wall with no protrusion into the aortic lumen. The "plug" of the device is compressed with immediate complete occlusion. In **B**, a similar angled patent ductus arteriosus device has been placed in a human infant. The angiogram is recorded 3 months after implantation. The device plug was initially compressed with minimal flow through the middle. After 3 months, the device has expanded the ductus (*arrows*) with increased interwire distance and "recanalization."

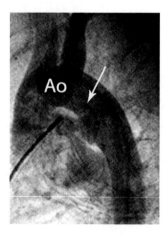

Fig. 34.4 An aortogram recorded in lateral projection after placement of an Amplatzer Ductal Occluder device, fully deployed before release. The aortic retention rim protrudes superiorly (*arrow*) into the aortic lumen (Ao). The angle of the patent ductus arteriosus is at an angle of approximately 65° instead of 90° in the animal model. This device is oversized, and can be retrieved using the delivery cable still attached to the device

months, the device expanded the PDA resulting in "recanalization" (Fig. 34.5B) [25]. This complication was considered to result from two unanticipated design problems. First, the hoop strength of the angled Amplatzer Ductal Occluder was sufficient to dilate the PDA in a young infant. This, in turn, resulted in an increase in the distance between the radial "spokes" of the device. In retrospect, it was considered that the animal model trial used a non-expandable "PDA" with small diameters that limited the distance between the wires of the device.

34.7 Muscular Ventricular Septal Defect

Muscular ventricular septal defects can be identified that occur in the lower, thicker ventricular septum. Closure of such defects is clinically recommended for the same indications as ASD and PDA—eliminating overwork of the heart and overcirculation of the lungs. However, unlike for the other two defects, surgery to close a muscular ventricular septal defect, in general, is not a simple or low-risk option. More specifically, the surgical closure of muscular ventricular septal defects can be at best difficult, e.g., the right ventricular aspect of the defect can be hidden from the surgeon's view by trabeculations within the right ventricular cavity. This, in turn, can result in a high incidence of residual leaks with a right ventricular approach. On the other hand, directly incising the left ventricle would allow clearer visualization of the defect margins, but left ventricular aneurysms or diminished left ventricular function sometimes result [26]. These surgical difficulties make the transcatheter closure of such ventricular defects an attractive alternative.

In general, the Amplatzer Muscular Ventricular Septal Occluder is very similar to the Amplatzer Septal Occluder. Like a secundum ASD, muscular ventricular septal defects are separated from cardiac valves by myocardium; the obvious difference is the thickness of the ventricular myocardium. Therefore, these devices were designed with greater distances between the disks to accommodate for the differences in myocardial thickness (Fig. 34.6). Greater stability was found to be produced by the radial force applied against the thicker muscular ventricular septum, and thus the retention disk diameters were decreased to 6–8 mm larger than the waist. From a design standpoint, it should be noted that initial attempts of transcatheter closure of muscular ventricular septal defects, using the Clamshell/CardioSEAL device, produced a 40% incidence of residual leaks [27]. These devices have a central post instead of a waist the size of the defect. Therefore, it was considered that any ventricular "retention" disk be sized at least twice the diameter

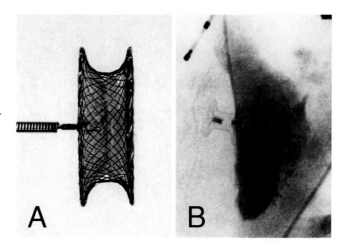

Fig. 34.6 Amplatzer Muscular Ventricular Septal Occluder. (**A**) Photograph of the device; the waist is wider than that of the Amplatzer Septal Occluder to allow for the thicker muscular ventricular septum. (**B**) Left ventricular angiogram 3 months after device placement showing complete occlusion of a mid-muscular ventricular septal defect

of the defect; residual leaks could result from migration of the central post within the defect. The self-centering Amplatzer Muscular Ventricular Septal Occluder is fixed within the defect by its waist. Another advantage of the Amplatzer device is the smaller maximum device diameter required to close a muscular ventricular septal defect, compared with central post devices.

34.7.1 Animal Trials Designed to Test Ventricular Closure Devices

Importantly, it was the successful animal trials to close surgically created muscular ventricular septal defects [28] that eventually led to human use [29], but clinical use in humans again demonstrated the shortcomings of these experimental models. In general, naturally occurring muscular ventricular septal defects in humans frequently are not circular (Fig. 34.7); at least 60% are twice as wide as they are tall [30]. The typical method of sizing muscular ventricular septal defects is to look at the vertical dimension of the defect using either echocardiography or angiography. Angiography, in particular, demonstrates only the vertical dimension and, because the shunt occurs primarily during systole, the defect is best outlined during contraction when the diameter of the muscular ventricular septal defect is smallest. Measuring the muscular ventricular septal defect from en face or 3D echocardiographic imaging accounts for the oval shape of the defect and can be timed in diastole. The frequency of residual shunts is reduced by using a device with the same circumference as the defect in diastole [30].

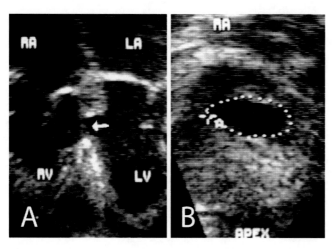

Fig. 34.7 Echocardiographic images of a mid-muscular ventricular septal defect. In **A**, an apical four-chamber view is recorded. There is "drop-out" of echoes from the mid-septum (*arrow*) with a short vertical dimension. In **B**, an en face view is recorded of the right ventricular surface of the ventricular septum in the same patient. The ventricular septal defect is outlined by the *dotted line*. The vertical dimension is significantly less than the horizontal one. If only the vertical dimension is considered in choosing the device size, there would be a significant residual shunt, or device embolization might be possible. LA = left atrium; LV = left ventricle; RA = right atrium; RV = right ventricle

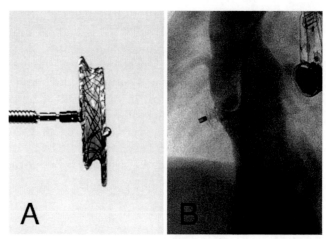

Fig. 34.8 Amplatzer Perimembranous Ventricular Septal Occluder device. (**A**) Photograph of the perimembranous device, in which the delivery cable is attached to the right ventricular disc. The asymmetric left ventricular disc is positioned with the minimal rim of the subaortic portion at the top of the device. This prevents interference with the aortic valve. (**B**) Left ventriculogram after device placement. The asymmetric left ventricular disc avoids distortion of the aortic valve. There is no flow through the device immediately after deployment

34.8 Perimembranous Ventricular Septal Defect

Amplatzer devices designed for closing secundum ASDs, PDA, and muscular ventricular septal defects are concentrically symmetrical, as there are typically no valves near the edges of the defects they are designed to close. In contrast, in perimembranous ventricular septal defects, both the aortic and tricuspid valves can be close to the defect margins. Early attempts were made to close perimembranous ventricular septal defects with the Clamshell and Sideris button devices. However, it was soon reported that distortions of the aortic valves resulted in aortic insufficiencies and, in some cases, the devices were found to have embolized [31]. It was considered that the flexibility of shaping the basic Amplatzer device frames could be advantageous to produce an eccentric, asymmetric device. More specifically, an Amplatzer Perimembranous Ventricular Septal Occluder (Fig. 34.8) was designed with a minimal rim of the left ventricular disk (0.5 mm) to sit beneath the aortic valve, a longer (5.5 mm) inferior left ventricular disk, and a short waist (1.5 mm) to keep the right ventricular disc away from the tricuspid valve. The subsequent animal trials showed that an eccentric design protected the aortic and tricuspid valves and yet closed perimembranous ventricular septal defects [32].

However, the difficulty with such systems was in the reliability of delivering the device in the proper orientation.

More specifically, advancing a pigtail catheter from the pulmonary artery through a patent ductus often results in the curl of the catheter oriented along the lesser curvature of the aorta. Therefore a sharply curved delivery sheath was designed to deliver these devices to the left ventricular apexes, mimicking this property. In addition, simply advancing the asymmetric device through this sheath did not always result in proper device orientation. Subsequently, a sharply curved delivery catheter was designed that forced attachment of the device with the longer left ventricular disk along the lesser curvature of the catheter (Fig. 34.9). When combined with the sharply curved delivery sheath positioned in the left ventricular apex, a device advanced to the tip of the delivery sheath assumed proper orientation [32]. This was confirmed in human trials, and complete closure occurred in 96% of patients. It should be noted that, in these trials, there were no serious complications, although the number of patients was small [29].

34.8.1 Animal Trials Designed to Test Perimembranous Ventricular Septal Occluders

Unlike all the previously described surgically created animal models of congenital cardiovascular defects, the perimembranous ventricular septal occluder device was tested in a naturally occurring animal model (Yucatan mini pig).

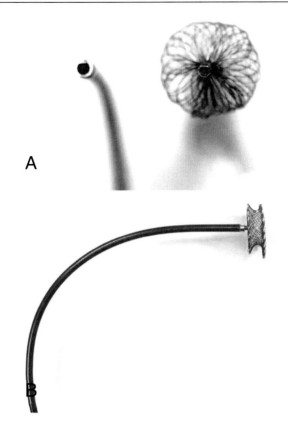

Fig. 34.9 Delivery system for an asymmetric device. (**A**) Photograph of the slot in the delivery catheter, flat at the upper margin. This matches a flattened area at the upper surface of the microscrew. The microscrew will only fit into the slot in the correct orientation. (**B**) The asymmetric perimembranous ventricular septal occluder is attached to the curved delivery catheter. The longer rim of the left ventricular disc is oriented along the lesser curvature of the delivery catheter

Morphologically the porcine defect closely resembles that in humans [33]. It was shown that the device and its unique delivery system were successful in occluding this congenital defect [32]. Nevertheless, after extensive use of these devices in humans, reports of complete heart block began to appear (Fig. 34.10). It should be noted that this did not occur in the animal trials, nor in the initial reports of use in humans [29]. More specifically, subsequent examination of pathological specimens in the animal models did not show any evidence to explain this complication [34]. It was considered that this could be a result of minor differences in the conduction system of these mini pigs as compared to humans, or it was a consequence of the extremely low incidence of complications associated with these devices. Therefore, caution must be taken when selecting an animal model that mimics a human defect; in this case, it did not foresee a complication when the device was taken to human trials. It should be noted that some of these reported problems may have resulted from implanting larger devices, as several European investigators

continue to implant this device, minimizing the device size without suffering the complication of complete heart block. Nevertheless, redesigning these devices and carefully avoiding oversizing during implant may reduce the incidence of complete heart block to an acceptable level.

34.9 Summary

The Amplatzer family of occluder devices provides successful methods for the transcatheter closure of congenital cardiovascular abnormalities. In general, the simple underlying device design allows for easy modification, thus enabling numerous different types of devices for treating a variety of abnormal communications. The device's unique characteristics include ease of delivery, a small delivery system, retrievability, safety, and effectiveness.

Despite the clinical success of these devices, the transition from an animal trial to the human condition demonstrated the failure of a model designed to ideally mimic the intricacies of human anatomy. Prior to such studies, many of these features had not been appreciated because surgical treatment was easily adjusted to account for them. For example, suture closure of a secundum ASD did not pin the atrial free wall between a stiff device rim and an aorta pulsating with systemic pressure. Likewise, suture ligation of the PDA is not affected by the angle between the PDA and aorta, or the ability of the PDA to expand when internal force is placed against it. Furthermore, surgical patches can be easily shaped to fit margins of an irregular muscular ventricular septal defect. Nevertheless, complete heart block is a known complication of surgical repair of perimembranous ventricular septal defects; importantly, this even led to the development of the cardiac pacemaker. The relative occurrence of complete heart block with device closure is not a surprise because of the known proximity of the penetrating bundle to ventricular septal defect margins, although it did not appear in preclinical trials. One must consider that there may be minor variations between the porcine model and humans (or even from patient to patient) in the relationship of the penetrating bundle and the ventricular septal defect that account for the variable occurrence of complete heart block. However, on the other hand, one should not consider this as a particular failure of the animal model design; ASD, muscular ventricular septal defect, and PDA devices are symmetrical, and a central defect was primarily created to test feasibility and efficacy of the device. The devices functioned perfectly in these models.

The variables of proximity of the ascending aorta to the anterior margin of a secundum ASD, the angle of the

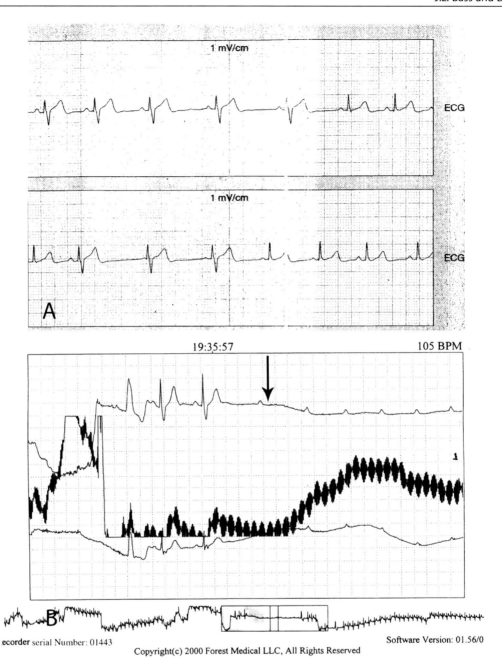

Fig. 34.10 Electrocardiographic recordings from a patient after insertion of a perimembranous ventricular septal occluder. In **A**, there is intermittent right bundle branch block 3 h after device insertion. In **B**, an episode of complete heart block is recorded on a Holter monitor recording 3 years after device placement. It is not clear if right bundle branch block heralded loss of atrioventricular conduction

PDA to the aorta, expansion of the PDA in younger patients, and frequent occurrence of oval muscular ventricular septal defects become significant only under certain conditions. In other words, the anatomic details of secundum ASD and PDA become more significant when interventional cardiologists oversize devices, either in fear of embolization or because of a perceived lack of risk with oversized devices. This is probably also true with perimembranous VSO devices, where a small aortic rim leads to the risk of embolization. It is likely that an oversized device increases the pressure against the conduction system in perimembranous ventricular septal defects and increases the risk of complete heart block.

There are notable limitations in creating any animal model for congenital heart disease. For example, tearing the interatrial septum to create an ASD, in general, does not produce large defects and there remains an anterior rim of atrial tissue. Furthermore, acutely creating larger communications between systemic and pulmonary circulations (a PDA or ventricular septal defect) is poorly tolerated, and acute congestive heart failure and pulmonary edema soon develop; long-term animal survival can be low. Likewise, testing of the abilities of such devices to close large defects in the animal models is also difficult, e.g., even the porcine congenital perimembranous ventricular septal defect is usually small or moderate in size when the animal comes to closure. Despite these limitations in designing animal models of congenital heart disease, preclinical testing of any such device is acutely effective in defining device function.

We consider here that when translating from a given animal model to human use, great care should be taken in defining the anatomy of the congenital heart defect to which the devices are applied. In particular, we suggest that careful review of pathological specimens should be supplemented by 3D imaging (echocardiographic, computed tomographic, or magnetic resonance imaging) to define proximity of important structures and relationships, such as between the inferior vena cava and interatrial septum or between the aorta and PDA. Nevertheless, prior surgical experience can also lend important insights as to the anatomy of such defects; note that some surgeons may be a bit reluctant to participate in creating "competition."

Devices whose central cores expand to fill an abnormal communication should not be oversized. When possible, device edges should be smooth and rounded rather than sharp, as they may have unanticipated contact with cardiac structures. Device closures of congenital cardiovascular defects have revolutionized the care of children with congenital heart disease. For many such transcatheter closures, the Amplatzer devices have been the first successfully employed nonsurgical treatments. Finally, animal testing is an integral part of developing new devices, and translation to humans requires careful thought.

References

1. Lock JE, Niemi T, Einzig S, Amplatz K, Burke B, Bass JL. Transvenous angioplasty of experimental branch pulmonary artery stenosis in newborn lambs. Circulation 1981;64:886–93.
2. Lock JE, Castaneda-Zuniga WR, Bass JL, Foker JE, Amplatz K, Anderson RW. Balloon dilation of excised human coarctations. Radiology 1982;143:689–91.
3. Porstmann W, Wierny L, Warnke H. Closure of ductus arteriosus persistens without thoracotomy. Fortsch Geb Rontgenstr Nuklearmed 1968;109:133–48.
4. King TD, Mills NL. Nonoperative closure of atrial septal defects. Surgery 1974;75:383–88.
5. Rashkind WJ. Transcatheter treatment of congenital heart disease. Circulation 1983;67:711–16.
6. Sharafuddin MJA, Gu X, Titus JL, Urness M, Cervera-Ceballos JJ, Amplatz K. Transvenous closure of secundum atrial septal defects. Preliminary results with a new self-expanding nitinol prosthesis in a swine model. Circulation 1997;95:2162–68.
7. Kong H, Wilkinson JL, Coe JY, Gu X, Urness M, Kim TH, Bass JL. Corrosive behaviour of Amplatzer devices in experimental and biological environments. Cardiol Young 2002;12:260–65.
8. Neal WA, Moller JH, Varco RL, Anderson RC. Operative repair of atrial septal defect without cardiac catheterization. J Pediatr 1975;86:189–93.
9. Latson LA. Atrial septal defect. In: Moller JH, Hoffman JIE, eds. Pediatric cardiovascular medicine. New York, NY: Churchill Livingstone, 2000:311–21.
10. Lewis FJ, Varco RL, Taufic, M. Repair of atrial septal defects in man under direct vision with the aid of hypothermia. Surgery 1954;36:538–56.
11. Rome JJ, Keane JF, Perry SB, Spevak PJ, Lock JE. Double-umbrella closure of atrial septal defects: Initial clinical applications. Circulation 1990;82:751–58.
12. Sideris EB, Sideris SE, Thanopoulos BD, Ehly RL, Fowlkes JP. Transvenous atrial septal defect occlusion by the buttoned device. Am J Cardiol 1990;66:1524–26.
13. Hausdorf G, Schneider M, Granzbach B, Kampmann C, Kargus K, Goeldner B. Transcatheter closure of secundum atrial septal defects with the atrial septal defect occlusion system: Initial experience in children. Heart 1996;75:83–88.
14. Das GS, Voss G, Jarvis G, Wyche K, Gunther R, Wilson RF. Experimental atrial septal defect closure with a new, transcatheter, self-centering device. Circulation 1993;88:1754–64.
15. Agarwal SK, Ghosh PK, Mittal PK. Failure of devices used for closure of atrial septal defects: mechanisms and management. J Thorac Cardiovasc Surg 1996;112:21–26.
16. Du Z-D, Hijazi ZM, Kleinman CS, Silverman NH, Larntz L. Comparison between transcatheter and surgical closure of secundum atrial septal defect in children and adults. J Am Coll Cardiol 2002;39:1836–44.
17. Amin Z, Hijazi ZM, Bass JL, Cheatham JP, Hellenbrand WE, Kleinman CS. Erosion of Amplatzer septal occluders after closure of secundum atrial septal defects: Review of registry of complications and recommendations to minimize future risk. Catheter Cardiovasc Interv 2004;63:496–502.
18. Gersony WM, Apfel HD. Patent ductus arteriosus and other aortopulmonary anomalies. In: Moller JH, Hoffman JIE, eds. Pediatric cardiovascular medicine. New York, NY: Churchill Livingstone, 2000:323–30.
19. Kirklin JW, Barratt-Boyes BG. Patent ductus arteriosus. In: Kirklin JW, Barratt-Boyes BG, eds. Cardiac surgery, 2nd ed. New York, NY: Churchill Livingstone, 1993:854.
20. Nykanen DG, Hayes AM, Benson LN, Freedom RM. Transcatheter patent ductus arteriosus occlusion: Application in the small child. J Am Coll Cardiol 1994;23:1666–70.
21. Pass RH, Hijazi Z, Hsu DT, Lewis V, Hellenbrand WE. Multicenter USA Amplatzer patent ductus arteriosus occlusion device trial: Initial and one-year results. J Am Coll Cardiol 2004;44:513–19.
22. Sharafuddin MJA, Gu X, Titus JL, et al. Experimental evaluation of a new self-expanding patent ductus arteriosus occluder in a canine model. J Vasc Intervent Radiol 1996;7:877–87.
23. Masura J, Walsh KP, Thanopoulous B, Chan C, Bass J, Goussous Y, Gavora P, Hijazi ZM. Catheter closure of moderate- to large-sized patent ductus arteriosus using the new Amplatzer duct occluder: Immediate and short-term results. JACC 1998;31:878–82.

24. Kong H, Gu X, Bass JL, Titus J, Urness M, Kim T-H, Hunter DW. Experimental evaluation of a modified Amplatzer duct occluder. Catheter Cardiovasc Interv 2001;53:571–76.

25. Ewert P. Challenges encountered during closure of patent ductus arteriosus. Pediatr Cardiol 2005;26:224–29.

26. Kirklin JK, Castaneda AR, Keane JF, Fellows KE, Norwood WI. Surgical management of multiple ventricular septal defects. J Thorac Cardiovasc Surg 1980;80:485–93.

27. Lock JE, Block PC, Mckay RG, Baim DS, Keane JF. Transcatheter closure of ventricular septal defects. Circulation 1988;78:361–68.

28. Amin Z, Gu X, Berry JM, et al. New device for closure of muscular ventricular septal defects in a canine model. Circulation 1999;100:320–28.

29. Bass JL, Kalra GS, Arora R, et al. Initial human experience with the Amplatzer Perimembranous ventricular septal occluder device. Catheter Cardiovasc Interv 2003;58: 238–45.

30. Berry JM, Krabill KA, Pyles LA, Lohr J, Steinberger J, Bass JL. Muscular ventricular septal defect geometry and Amplatzer device closure: A new en face view. Circulation 1999;100:18(I):I–30 (Abstract).

31. Rigby ML, Redington AN. Primary transcatheter closure of perimembranous ventricular septal defect. Br Heart J 1994;72: 368–71.

32. Gu X, Han Y-M, Titus JL, et al. Transcatheter closure of membranous ventricular septal defects with a new nitinol prosthesis in a natural swine model. Catheter Cardiovasc Interv 2000;50:502–09.

33. Ho SY, Thompson RP, Gibbs SR, Swindle MM, Anderson RH. Ventricular septal defects in a family of Yucatan miniature pigs. Int J Cardiol 1991;33:419–25.

34. Mackey-Bojack S, Urness M, Titus J, Bass J. HIS bundle pathology after insertion of the Amplatzer® perimembranous ventricular septal defect occluder in an animal model. Circulation 2005;112(17):II-547 (Abstract 2600).

Chapter 35
Harnessing Cardiopulmonary Interactions to Improve Circulation and Outcomes After Cardiac Arrest and Other States of Low Blood Pressure

Anja Metzger and Keith Lurie

Abstract Novel noninvasive technologies that harness the inherent physiological interactions between the heart, lungs, and brain have recently been shown to improve circulation and outcomes after cardiac arrest and other states of low blood pressure including hypovolemic shock. The impedance threshold devices (ResQPOD® and ResQGard®) and the intrathoracic pressure regulator (CirQlator™) are three new devices that create a negative intrathoracic pressure. The decrease in intrathoracic pressure creates a vacuum within the thorax relative to the rest of the body thereby enhancing venous blood return to the heart, increasing cardiac output and systemic arterial blood pressure, lowering right atrial and pulmonary artery pressures, lowering intracranial pressure, and increasing cerebral perfusion pressure. The animal and clinical data supporting the use of technologies that harness the intrathoracic pump are reviewed in this chapter.

Keywords Cardiac arrest · Cardiopulmonary resuscitation · Impedance threshold device · Active compression decompression CPR · Intrathoracic pressure regulator

35.1 Introduction

Cardiac arrest and life-threatening hypotension typically occur suddenly and without warning. This chapter will briefly review the traditional methods used in the treatment of sudden cardiac arrest and shock and will focus on novel noninvasive technologies that can be used to increase the chances for survival. These new approaches have been developed based on a greater understanding of the critical interactions between the heart, lungs, and brain. In the most general sense, the new technology takes advantage of the "other side of breathing," that is, the use of changes in pressures within the thorax to move blood in and out of the heart and to shift pressures via the spinal column within the brain. These recent discoveries have the potential for changing the way we think about the treatment of a wide variety of disease states including cardiac arrest, septic shock, traumatic brain injury, and/or stroke. To date, most of the research that utilizes these "natural" processes to augment circulation and lower intracranial pressure has focused on the treatment of cardiac arrest and hypovolemic shock. As such, this chapter will detail some of the most current clinical therapies that should be considered in treating such patients.

35.2 Sudden Cardiac Arrest

Despite the widespread practice of basic and advanced life support, the vast majority of patients in cardiac arrest never live to see hospital discharge. This clinical toll is enormous; more than 1,000 adults die each day in the United States alone from an out-of-hospital cardiac arrest. Furthermore, a similar number of patients die each day inside the hospital. Many of these patients have no warning and die in the prime of life. Sadly, little has changed in the practice of cardiopulmonary resuscitation (CPR) for nearly 50 years. Thus, it is not surprising that survival rates have remained relatively constant for decades, at ~5% nationwide for all patients with an

A. Metzger (✉)
University of Minnesota, Department of Emergency Medicine, 13683 47th St. N, Minneapolis, MN 55455, USA
e-mail: kohl0005@umn.edu

Conflict of Interest: Keith Lurie is the founder and Chief Medical Officer of Advanced Circulatory Systems, the company that manufactures the impedance threshold device. He is also a Professor of Emergency Medicine at the University of Minnesota (lurie002@umn.edu). Anja Metzger is employed by Advanced Circulatory Systems and is the Vice President of Research and Development.

P.A. Iaizzo (ed.), *Handbook of Cardiac Anatomy, Physiology, and Devices*, DOI 10.1007/978-1-60327-372-5_35,
© Springer Science+Business Media, LLC 2009

out-of-hospital cardiac arrest. For patients who present with ventricular fibrillation (VF), survival rates range from 10 to 45%, yet this is dependent on the city where they arrest. Since the frequency of VF is declining, and currently nearly 70% of all patients present with either pulseless electrical activity (PEA) or asystole, new approaches are desperately needed to decrease mortality from the "nation's #1 killer." While the differences in outcomes between regions are due to many factors, the intrinsic mechanical inefficiencies of standard manual cardiopulmonary resuscitation (standard CPR) limit the potential of even the most highly skilled rescuers. Moreover, the vast majority of the >300,000 cardiac arrests that occur annually in the United States happen in the home, and any delays to treatment severely limit the individual's chances for survival. As a result, even in regions with the most efficient emergency medical service (EMS) systems, less than 20% of all patients with an out-of-hospital cardiac arrest are discharged from the hospital with intact neurological function [1, 2].

It is critical to implement CPR when sudden cardiac arrest occurs. The purpose of manual standard CPR is to pump blood from the heart to the vital organs during the compression phase and to enhance the return of blood back into the heart during the chest wall recoil or decompression phase. Compression and decompression are illustrated in Fig. 35.1. Any such devices that can optimize this physiology are helpful adjuncts and have been shown to improve outcomes after cardiac arrest. Conversely, there are several common mistakes in standard CPR techniques that result in suboptimal CPR quality. These include: (1) not allowing full chest wall recoil; (2) inadequate compression force; (3) incorrect compression rate; (4) excessive ventilation rates; and (5) too high or too low tidal volume and inspiratory pressure. Taken together, it is clear that in order to perform high-quality standard CPR, before even thinking about new ways to augment circulation above and beyond the limits of standard CPR, new tools and technology are needed to optimize standard CPR.

The reality of commonly administered standard CPR, however, is that blood flow to the vital organs is severely reduced even under the best of circumstances [3, 4]. During standard CPR, chest compression results in an elevation of intrathoracic pressure and indirect cardiac compression. Both of these mechanisms result in forward blood flow out of the chest to perfuse the brain and other vital organs. However, the effectiveness of standard CPR is largely determined by the amount of blood return to the chest to refill the heart after each compression phase; this process is highly dependent on the degree of chest wall recoil. When the chest recoils, intrathoracic pressures fall relative to extrathoracic pressures, and venous blood then returns to the right heart.

35.3 The Impedance Threshold Device for Cardiac Arrest

Standard CPR by itself is inherently inefficient, in large part due to the lack of adequate blood return to the thorax during the chest wall recoil phase [3, 4]. Moreover, the coronary perfusion pressure, a critical determinant of CPR efficacy, is only marginally adequate, as the pressure gradient between the aorta, the right atrium, and left ventricle is often far from optimal. During the decompression (or passive relaxation) phase of CPR, a small decrease in intrathoracic pressure (relative to atmospheric pressure) develops, which promotes blood flow back to the heart. Myocardial perfusion predominantly occurs during this decompression phase. The impedance threshold device (ITD) (ResQPOD®, Advanced Circulatory Systems, Minneapolis, MN) was designed to improve venous return to the heart during the decompression phase of CPR [3–9]. In so doing, the ITD increases the coronary perfusion pressure during CPR, enhancing delivery of oxygenated blood to the heart and brain. The ITD shown in Fig. 35.2 works effectively with either a facemask or an endotracheal tube.

The concept underlying the ITD was first discovered when measuring intrathoracic pressures in patients undergoing a new type of CPR, active compression decompression (ACD) CPR [10]. If the endotracheal

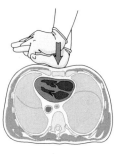

Compression

Compression of the chest results in direct mechanical compression of the heart and increases intrathoracic pressure, both of which circulate blood forward. The chest is compressed 1.5 –2"at a rate of 100/min.

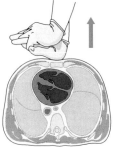

Decompression

Allow complete chest recoil after each compression to maximize the vacuum in the thoracic cavity to force blood flow back to the heart

Incomplete recoil reduces the vacuum created during chest wall decompression

Fig. 35.1 Compression and decompression phases of cardiopulmonary resuscitation

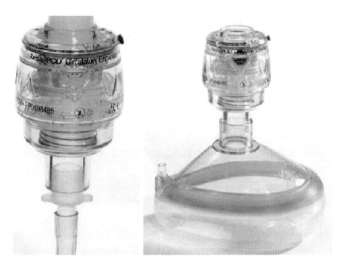

Fig. 35.2 Photograph of the impedance threshold device (ResQPOD®) shown on an endotracheal tube and a facemask

tube was transiently occluded during the active decompression phase, intrathoracic pressures became markedly more negative. This led to the idea of transiently blocking the airway or impeding inspiratory gas exchange during the chest wall decompression phase of CPR to create a greater pressure differential between the thorax and the rest of the body, thereby enhancing blood flow back into the thorax. As such, the ITD harnesses the kinetic energy of the chest wall recoil, thereby augmenting the "bellows-like" action of the chest with each compression–decompression cycle [8, 9]. The ITD contains pressure-sensitive valves that impede the influx of inspiratory gas during chest wall decompression, thereby augmenting the amplitude and duration of the vacuum within the thorax. This increased vacuum draws more venous blood back into the heart, resulting in increased cardiac preload, followed by improved cardiac output and thus vital organ perfusion. During chest compression, the one-way valve is open and does not cause any resistance to exhalation. When the resuscitation bag is squeezed during active rescuer ventilation, the one-way valve remains open and does not cause any resistance to gas exchange. In this manner, the ITD functions to lower intrathoracic pressure only during the decompression phase of CPR without compromising patient ventilation. The ITD consists of a valve body, a one-way pressure-sensitive silicone valve, and a safety check valve [5]. When a spontaneous pulse returns, the ITD is removed from the respiratory circuit. The safety check valve serves as a precautionary measure to prevent negative pressure pulmonary edema and potential barotrauma and to enable the patient to breathe if there is a return of spontaneous ventilation and the ITD is still in place. To date, beneficial animal and clinical data, described in detail below, form the basis for the Level

IIa recommendation for the ITD in the 2005 American Heart Association (AHA) guidelines. More recently, Aufderheide et al. reported outcomes from the use of the ITD in seven US EMS systems. His group showed that the changes in CPR practice resulted in a doubling of hospital discharge rates for all patients, regardless of presenting heart rhythm, from 8 to 16% [11]. Specifically the incorporated improvements included (1) emphasis on more compressions and fewer ventilations; (2) allowing complete chest wall recoil; (3) uninterrupted chest compressions during advanced airway management; and (4) the use of an ITD during basic life support and advanced life support. Importantly, patients who had an initial rhythm of VF had a hospital discharge rate of 28.1% compared with 17.2% in the historical control group.

One of the first animal studies performed with the ITD demonstrated that use of the active ITD increased 24-h survival and preserved neurological function after induced cardiac arrest in pigs [8]. There was a statistically significant increase in both of these key outcome parameters as shown in Fig. 35.3. There was improved neurological function in the overall study group, as well as in the subset of pigs that were resuscitated with defibrillation shock therapy and epinephrine. Blood gas data demonstrated that relative tissue oxygenation was considered adequate in both groups and no differences were observed between groups on autopsy. The intrathoracic pressures were significantly lower in the ITD group. Furthermore, subsequent studies have demonstrated that use of the ITD also lowers intracranial pressures more rapidly than in pigs treated with standard CPR alone. It is hypothesized that this observation helps to explain the markedly improved neurological outcomes in this porcine survival study [8].

The first randomized double-blinded prospective clinical trial showed that use of the ITD during standard CPR resulted in a doubling of systolic blood pressures. However, in that study nearly all of the patients received

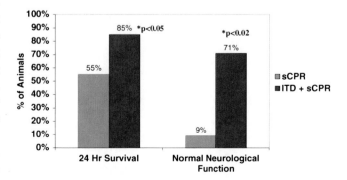

Fig. 35.3 Percentage of animals with 24-h survival and normal neurological function comparing standard CPR (sCPR) to impedance threshold device (ITD) + standard CPR after cardiac arrest in pigs

excessively high ventilation rates. Follow-up animal studies demonstrated that excessive ventilation (termed hyperventilation) during cardiac arrest actually inhibited venous return, compromised hemodynamics, and resulted in increased mortality. Nevertheless, these observations resulted in changes in the AHA recommendation on the frequency and quality of ventilations during CPR. In addition, frequent incomplete decompression of the chest was also witnessed and recorded in that study. Follow-up studies in animals demonstrated that incomplete chest wall recoil will result in positive intrathoracic pressures, decreased venous returns, and markedly poorer cardiac and cerebral blood flows; incomplete decompression is thus a key component in the deficiencies of standard CPR. These observations also demonstrate how important the cardio-pulmonary-cerebral interactions are during CPR.

In the first US double-blinded randomized survival study of the ITD, there was a nearly threefold increase in 1-h and 24-h survival rates in patients with an initial rhythm of PEA when comparing treatment with a sham versus active ITD. Figure 35.3 shows percent survival in all subjects initially presenting with PEA. It is important to emphasize that the results from this study were observed in the setting of real-world CPR, prior to the use of tools to help control ventilation frequency or the adequacy of compression rate, depth, and complete chest wall decompression. Figure 35.4 shows the percent survival in all subjects presenting with various types of cardiac rhythms.

The benefits of the ITD in patients with PEA can also be better understood by examining the hemodynamic tracing of one of the sub-study group patients as shown in Fig. 35.5. When CPR was discontinued, there was persistent regular electrical activity, but the aortic pressure was observed to be inadequate to generate a palpable pulse. This example of PEA demonstrates that, although there was a small rise in the arterial pressure with each cardiac contraction, this was functionally insufficient to cause a palpable pulse or effective vital organ blood flow. Importantly, without effective vital organ perfusion, return of spontaneous circulation is not possible. We speculate that the known increase in circulation and blood pressure associated with the use of the ITD in animals and in humans is enough to increase the aortic systolic and diastolic pressures to sufficient levels to allow for effective vital organ perfusion.

The number of patients in VF treated with the ITD in that study was too low to definitively determine if the ITD would benefit this patient subgroup. Nonetheless, hospital discharge rates were 6% in the control group and 14% with the active ITD in that study.

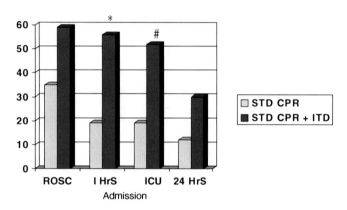

Fig. 35.4 Outcomes for all subjects initially presenting with pulseless electrical activity. *$p = 0.01$; #$p = 0.02$. 1 HrS = 1-h survival; 24 HrS = 24-h survival; ICU = ICU admission rate; ROSC = return of spontaneous circulation

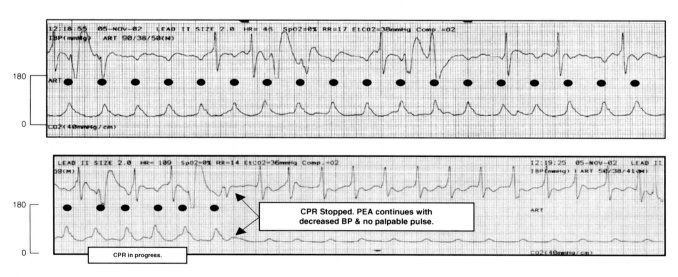

Fig. 35.5 Hemodynamic tracing of a patient with pulseless electrical activity (PEA). BP = blood pressure; CPR = cardiopulmonary resuscitation

One of the most important findings from the first clinical study when the ITD was used with standard CPR was that the overall quality of CPR was very poor. Based on the hemodynamic sub-study data collected in this clinical trial, hyperventilation was recorded in 100% of cases and incomplete chest wall recoil was recorded in approximately 50% of cases. These findings demonstrated the challenges of performing standard CPR with a pair of hands alone, and this resulted in a change in the initial design of the impedance threshold device; a timing light was added that flashes at 10 times/min to provide the rescuer with guidance on when to ventilate the patient and how to assure that compressions are performed 100 times/min (compress 10 times/light flash). Thus, in the future, equally promising is the possibility that the ITD will be even more effective once improved standard CPR is practiced and performed uniformly.

It is also important to emphasize that one of the very exciting advances in CPR research has been the recently rediscovered benefit of therapeutic hypothermia after successful resuscitation. Several studies have demonstrated a 50% increase in long-term survival rates and improved neurological function in survivors of cardiac arrest with VF who have received therapeutic hypothermia in the hospital shortly after resuscitation [12–14]. When hypothermia is applied to patients resuscitated after PEA, there should be a similar increase in long-term survival rates with good neurological function. Fortunately, a growing number of patients are now routinely treated with therapeutic hypothermia after successful resuscitation.

35.4 The Effects of Incomplete Chest Wall Recoil and Hyperventilation on the Quality of Standard CPR

The AHA recognized the inefficiencies of standard CPR in 2000 and 2005 when they issued a new guideline for performing CPR. This guideline reinforces the importance of the chest decompression phase in its teaching on the performance of CPR: "Release the pressure on the chest to allow blood to flow into the chest and heart. You must release the pressure completely and allow the chest to return to its normal position after each compression" [15].

As mentioned previously, Aufderheide et al. observed rescuers frequently leaning on the chest during the decompression phase, thereby maintaining some residual and continuous pressure on the chest wall during the decompression phase of CPR [11]. This prevented complete chest wall recoil. More specifically, airway pressures were consistently measured as positive during the decompression phase (>0 mmHg) in 6 out of 13 (46%) consecutive adults. This was caused by incomplete chest wall recoil alone or combined with prolonged, positive ventilations. With standard CPR and incomplete chest wall recoil, insufficient intrathoracic vacuum pressures are typical. In contradistinction, when active compression and decompression are performed in conjunction with the use of an ITD, significant intrathoracic vacuum results.

In 2005, Yannopoulos et al. conducted an animal study to address the question of the physiological impact of incomplete chest wall recoil [16]. Nine pigs in VF for 6 min were treated with an automated CPR device with compressions at 100/min, a compression depth of 25% of the anteropostero diameter, and a compression to ventilation ratio of 15:2. After complete (100%) chest wall decompression for 3 min during standard CPR, the decompression depth was reduced to 75% of complete decompression for 1 min of CPR and then restored for another 1 min of CPR to 100% decompression. Coronary perfusion pressure (CPP) was calculated as the diastolic aortic–right atrial pressure. Cerebral perfusion pressure (CePP) was calculated by measuring the area between the aortic pressure curves and the intracranial pressure curves. Figure 35.6 summarizes the results of this study including the differences in aortic systolic pressures, CPP,

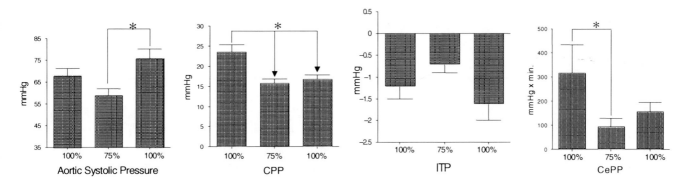

Fig. 35.6 Aortic systolic pressures, coronary perfusion pressures (CPP), intrathoracic pressures (ITP), and cerebral perfusion pressures (CePP) decrease when complete decompression is not allowed (75%). *$p < 0.05$

intratracheal pressure, and CePP. With 100–75–100% chest wall recoil, the CPP was 24.2 ± 2.0, 15.0 ± 1.2, 15.6 ± 1.3 mmHg ($p<0.05$); CePP was 320 ± 120, 95 ± 15, 150 ± 30 mmHg ($p<0.05$); diastolic aortic pressure was 26.8 ± 2.8, 18.9 ± 2.3, 18.2 ± 2.1 mmHg ($p<0.05$); intracranial pressure during decompression was 18.1 ± 2.8, 21.6 ± 2.3, 17.4 ± 2.6 mmHg ($p<0.05$); right atrial diastolic pressure was 2.7 ± 1.9, 3.9 ± 1.9, 2.7 ± 1.6 mmHg ($p<0.05$); and mean arterial pressure (MAP) was 41.4 ± 2.8, 32.5 ± 2.2, 36.6 ± 1.9 mmHg ($p<0.05$). The CPP and CePP never fully recovered after treatment with the 75% incomplete chest wall decompression. It is striking that a small reduction of chest wall recoil (1 cm), which can be a common occurrence during the performance of CPR, resulted in such marked reductions in both cerebral and coronary perfusion pressures.

The effect of incomplete chest wall recoil on reducing cerebral perfusion can be seen graphically in Figs. 35.7 and 35.8 [16]. Figure 35.7a represents, condensed in time, the sequential 100% chest recoil, 75% chest wall recoil, and return to 100% chest wall recoil. Tracings of intratracheal pressure, aortic pressure, and ICP (intracranial pressure) with 200 ms per division are indicated with arrows. Piston throw or compression depth (in cm) is also indicated to sequentially demonstrate the complete (100%) chest wall recoil (Fig. 35.7b), 75% chest wall recoil (Fig. 35.7c), and return to complete chest wall recoil (Fig. 35.7d). The positive area between the aortic pressure and intracranial pressure tracings represents cerebral perfusion (marked as black). Note how the area decreases, especially during decompression with incomplete chest wall recoil (75%), and that it partially recovers when full recoil is restored. Figure 35.8 shows the effect of positive pressure ventilation on CePP. The first tracing shows the aortic and ICP waveforms with full chest wall recoil after a ventilation cycle, while the second tracing shows the aortic and ICP waveforms with incomplete chest wall recoil after a ventilation cycle; positive pressure gradient (aortic–ICP) is colored black. Note the marked difference in total area during each compression–decompression cycle with and without a positive pressure breath. The bar graphic shows the mean four-beat area for all animals during and after a ventilation cycle. The mean $\pm$ SEM values during 100 and 75% decompression were also graphed. During positive pressure ventilation when there was incomplete chest wall recoil, intracranial pressure rose and the positive gradient disappeared. There was effectively no blood flow to the brain (Fig. 35.8, second panel). This study demonstrated that incomplete decompression has significant deleterious effects on both coronary perfusion pressure and cerebral perfusion pressure. The residual positive intrathoracic pressure during the decompression phase associated with incomplete chest wall recoil decreased forward blood flow, impeded venous return, increased intracranial pressure, and undermined the overall efficiency of CPR. These recent animal studies further underscore the fundamental hemodynamic importance of complete chest

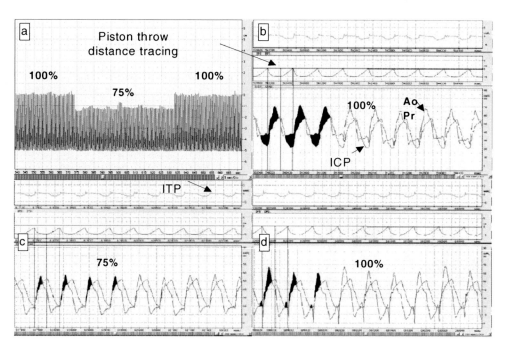

Fig. 35.7 Effect of incomplete chest wall recoil on reducing cerebral perfusion (see text for details). AoPR = aortic pressure; ICP = intracranial pressure; ITP = intrathoracic pressure; blue tracings = aortic pressures; pink tracings = intracranial pressures

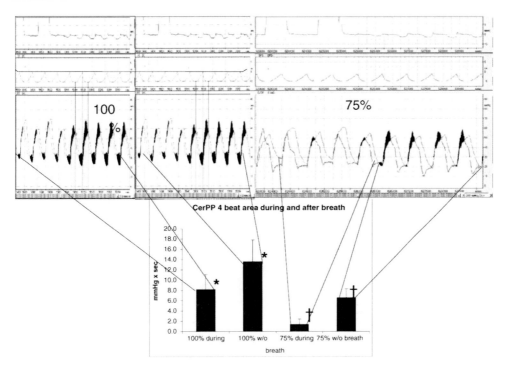

Fig. 35.8 Effect of incomplete chest wall recoil on reducing cerebral perfusion (see text for details). CerPP = cerebral perfusion pressure

wall decompression during CPR. Nevertheless, whether rescuers can be retrained to allow for complete chest wall decompression during standard CPR remains an important issue.

A change in CPR technique to allow for the palm of the compressing hand to lift off the chest at the end of decompression may be important to assure full chest wall recoil during standard CPR. Accordingly, Aufderheide et al. implemented a randomized prospective clinical trial using an independent group of 30 actively practicing, certified EMS providers, not aware of the ongoing trial, in a controlled setting using a recording CPR manikin. The purpose of the study was to evaluate three alternative CPR techniques to determine if they would improve complete chest wall recoil compared with standard CPR, while maintaining adequate compression depth and proper hand position placement. The three alternative CPR techniques were: (1) two-finger fulcrum technique (lifting the heel of the hand slightly but completely off the chest during the decompression phase of CPR, using the thumb and little finger as a fulcrum); (2) five-finger fulcrum technique (lifting the heel of the hand slightly but completely off the chest during the decompression phase of CPR, using all five fingers as a fulcrum); and (3) hands-off technique (lifting the heel and all fingers of the hand slightly but completely off the chest during the decompression phase of CPR).

In this study, during standard CPR using the traditionally taught hand position (standard hand position),

complete chest wall decompression was recorded in only 16.3% of all compression–decompression cycles, adequate depth of compression in 48.5%, and acceptable hand placement in 85.0% of compression–decompression cycles. When compared with standard CPR, the hands-off technique achieved the highest rate of complete chest wall recoil (95.0% versus 16.3%, $p<0.0001$) and was 129 times more likely to provide complete chest wall recoil [17]. Interestingly, there were no significant differences in the recorded accuracy of hand placement, depth of compression, or reported increase in fatigue or discomfort with its use, compared with the standard hand position (standard CPR). The hands-off technique was easily learned and applied by participating emergency technicians because it uses the same hand configuration as is currently recommended by the AHA.

35.5 Optimizing Outcomes with Standard CPR and the Impedance Threshold Device

Aufderheide and colleagues have recently analyzed and applied the combined lessons learned from the initial clinical trials on the ITD and standard CPR. They analyzed data from seven EMS systems that serve a population of more than 3 million patients and reported that, when CPR is performed correctly with the ITD and the mistakes described above are reduced or eliminated by rigorous training and correct ITD use, survival rates increased from 7.9 to 15.7% for all patients who presented with cardiac arrest; survival rates for those with an initial rhythm of VF increased from 17 to 28% [11]. Therapeutic hypothermia was not yet in use in these EMS systems and their associated hospitals when these data were obtained. Similar benefits from performing CPR according to the AHA 2005 Guidelines and use of the ITD have also recently been reported for patients in in-hospital cardiac arrest. For example, Thigpen reported that hospital discharge rates in one large Mississippi hospital increased from 17 to 28% with the administration of this new therapy [18]. Similar data from St. Cloud Hospital (Minnesota) are shown in Fig. 35.9; data from before the change in practice in July 2006 were compared to data after implementation of the new CPR techniques and the ITD. The survival rates after an in-hospital cardiac arrest nearly doubled. In summary, with greater attention to circulation, based on the newly discovered mechanisms underlying circulation during CPR, significant progress has been made by simply using a pair of hands and the ITD.

35.6 Active Compression Decompression CPR

It has been shown that, despite training, it is difficult to uniformly perform standard manual CPR correctly, allowing for the chest to fully recoil following each compression. This improper application results in significantly less blood flow back to the heart, and reemphasizes that perhaps another device is needed to alleviate this

widespread problem. It is generally accepted that correction of this basic flaw (incomplete chest wall recoil) through the use of a technique that ensures full chest wall recoil and user guidance has the potential to significantly improve the chances for survival after cardiac arrest. One such technique is active compression decompression (ACD) CPR and can be accomplished through the use of an ACD-CPR device.

ACD-CPR increases the naturally occurring negative intrathoracic pressure by physically lifting the chest wall and helping it return to its optimal decompressed position. During standard CPR, the chest wall's natural elasticity will partially recoil from compression. Several factors can contribute to less than optimal recoil: age, brittle or broken ribs, separated or broken sternum, barrel-shaped chest, chest concavity, and/or the tendency for rescue personnel to lean on the chest. These can cause incomplete chest wall recoil during performance of CPR. ACD-CPR helps ensure the chest re-expands to generate the negative intrathoracic pressure needed to allow passive filling of the heart.

The ACD-CPR technique can be performed with hand-held suction device (CardioPump® or ResQPump®) fixed on the anterior chest wall. During the compression phase, the chest is compressed and blood is forced out of the heart to perfuse the vital organs, as with standard CPR. When actively pulling up with the device, a vacuum is created within the thorax, drawing more blood back into the heart; this technique improves hemodynamics [19, 20]. In several reported studies, long-term survival rates of the patients in cardiac arrest improved as compared with patients receiving standard CPR alone [21, 22]. The ACD-CPR device is currently being used in many countries throughout the world including France, Israel, parts of China, Japan, and

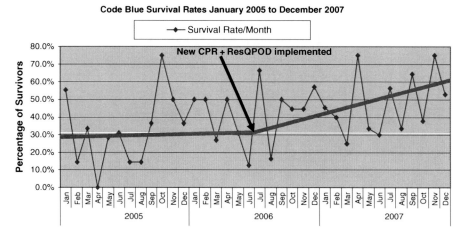

Fig. 35.9 *Code blue* survival rates in St. Cloud, Minnesota (Jan 2005–Dec 2007). CPR – cardiopulmonary resuscitation. Circulation, 2008; 118:S_1464

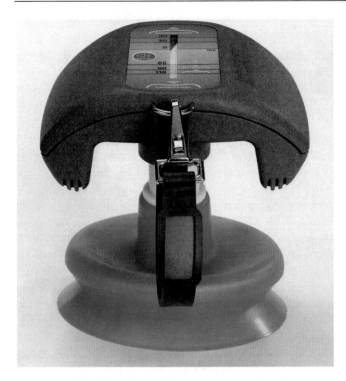

Fig. 35.10 The US version of the active compression decompression cardiopulmonary resuscitation device is the ResQPump®. The force gauge and metronome are used to guide the rescuer in the proper performance of the device

Germany (Fig. 35.10). To date, ACD-CPR is not currently practiced in the United States because the ResQPump® has not yet received regulatory approval from the Food and Drug Administration.

Recently, ACD-CPR + ITD has been evaluated in multiple animal and clinical trials and is currently recommended in the AHA Guidelines as an alternative to standard CPR. The device combination has been shown to quadruple blood flow to the heart and brain, compared with manual standard CPR alone. This device combination also significantly increases blood pressures and survival rates [15, 23].

Lurie et al. studied the effects of ACD-CPR and an ITD on blood flow; the results are summarized in Fig. 35.11. Animal studies demonstrated that left ventricle and cerebral blood flow were markedly improved with ACD-CPR + ITD [10, 24]. In these studies, coronary perfusion pressures were >20 mmHg, the minimum coronary perfusion pressure threshold needed to optimize the chances for survival in humans and in a porcine model of cardiac arrest [25, 26]. The device combination also optimized perfusion of the brain, which was found to be even greater than baseline levels after a prolonged arrest when comparing standard CPR to the combination of ACD-CPR + ITD [10]. The investigators believe that one of the reasons that the clinical trials with ACD-CPR + ITD have been successful is secondary to the marked increase in cerebral perfusion that can be achieved with this new approach. Importantly, these findings have been reproduced by several other investigators using both pediatric and adult pigs in cardiac arrest [4, 27]. Improved forward blood flow and vital organ perfusion with use of ACD-CPR + ITD was also shown to enhance drug efficacy during CPR [28]. Specifically, in hypothermic pigs, the effects of exogenous vasopressin were significantly enhanced with ACD-CPR + ITD, as reflected by higher coronary and cerebral perfusion pressures and improved cerebral metabolic profiles.

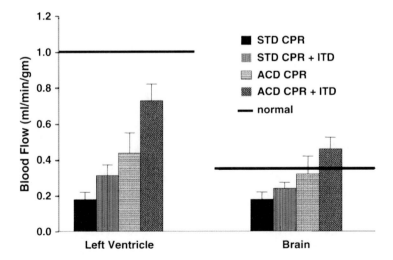

Fig. 35.11 Blood flow in a porcine model: the cumulative effect of ACD-CPR and ITD devices [9]. Solid horizontal line represents normal baseline values. ACD = active compression decompression; CPR = cardiopulmonary resuscitation; ITD = impedance threshold device; STD = standard

In general, the use of the combination of ACD-CPR and the ITD is synergistic. To date, four randomized clinical trials have been performed to evaluate the effectiveness and safety of the ACD-CPR + ITD in humans [23, 29–31]. The first blinded randomized clinical trial focused on hemodynamics in patients eliciting out-of-hospital cardiac arrest [30]. Eleven patients were treated with an active (functional) ITD and ten with a sham (placebo) ITD. In that study, end-tidal carbon dioxide levels rose more rapidly and reached higher levels with the active ITD. Additionally, systolic and diastolic blood pressures were nearly normal in the active ITD group (109/57 mmHg) versus the sham ITD group (89/35 mmHg, $p<0.01$). Finally, return of spontaneous circulation occurred more rapidly in the active ITD group compared with the sham ITD group. In part, based on these data, use of ACD-CPR + ITD was recommended as an alternative to standard CPR in the 2000 AHA Guidelines [15].

Another study has demonstrated that the ITD augments negative intrathoracic pressure when applied to a facemask [31]. This is important because it indicates that inspiratory impedance can be added during basic life support airway management (by first responders and perhaps even lay rescuers prior to intubation). Patients presenting with out-of-hospital cardiac arrest were randomized prior to endotracheal intubation to either a sham or active ITD, and intrathoracic pressure tracings were recorded. It was found that the addition of the active ITD to the facemask resulted in an immediate decrease in intrathoracic pressure during ACD-CPR. Each time the active ITD was used, there was a significant reduction in the decompression phase intrathoracic pressure. These studies demonstrated, for the first time, the degree of negative intrathoracic pressure achieved with ACD-CPR + ITD in humans. The average maximum negative intrathoracic pressure was –7.3 mmHg with the active ITD on an endotracheal tube versus –1.3 mmHg with the sham ITD. A second important finding was that it took up to five compression–decompression cycles to achieve the maximum negative intrathoracic pressure, as respiratory gases are expelled from the chest and prevented from re-entry. This mechanism plays a key role in the function of the ITD. Each time an active positive pressure ventilation was delivered, the decompression phase intrathoracic vacuum was lost and required regeneration. Thus, the less frequent the ventilation rate, the greater the blood flow back to the heart. A recent study using standard CPR with the ITD in pigs confirmed this important observation [32]. In general, this has become an important theme for all types of CPR, i.e., ventilations interrupt coronary perfusion pressure and should be reduced to the minimum required to maintain oxygenation and transpulmonary circulation.

It is generally accepted that ACD-CPR with an ITD improves short-term survival rates after cardiac arrest. A prospective controlled trial was performed in Mainz, Germany [30]; patients with out-of-hospital arrest of presumed cardiac etiology were sequentially randomized to ACD-CPR + ITD or standard CPR (control subjects) by the advanced life support team after intubation. Patients with an initial heart rhythm of VF (42% of the total), who could not be resuscitated by basic life support early defibrillation, were enrolled in this clinical trial, as well as patients with an initial rhythm of asystole or PEA. The primary end point was 1-h survival after a witnessed arrest. With ACD-CPR + ITD ($n = 103$), return of spontaneous circulation, 1-h, and 24-h survival rates were 55, 51, and 37% versus 37, 32, and 22% for standard CPR alone ($n = 107$; $p = 0.016$, 0.006, and 0.033), respectively (Fig. 35.12). One- and 24-h survival rates in patients with a witnessed arrest in VF were dramatically higher after ACD-CPR + ITD, 68 and 58% respectively versus 27 and 23% with standard CPR ($p = 0.002$ and 0.009), respectively, as shown in Fig. 35.13. Hospital discharge rates were 18% after ACD-CPR + ITD versus 13% in others ($p = 0.41$). Overall neurological function also trended higher with ACD-CPR + ITD versus control subjects ($p = 0.07$). Importantly, patients randomized >10 min after the call for help to the ACD-CPR + ITD group had a >3 times higher 1-h survival rate (44%) than other patients (14%) ($p = 0.002$). These time-related benefits were observed regardless of presenting rhythm. Interestingly, neurological outcomes in the survivors with delays to treatment with ACD-CPR + ITD were similar to those who were treated with ACD-CPR + ITD more rapidly.

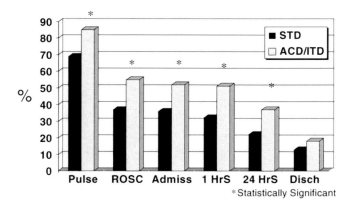

Fig. 35.12 Outcomes associated with comparison of standard cardiopulmonary resuscitation (STD) and ACD-CPR + ITD ($n = 210$) in Mainz, Germany. 1HrS = 1-h survival; 24HrS = 24-h survival; ACD = active compression decompression; Admis = hospital admission; CPR = cardiopulmonary resuscitation; Disch = hospital discharge; ITD = impedance threshold device; ROSC = return of spontaneous circulation

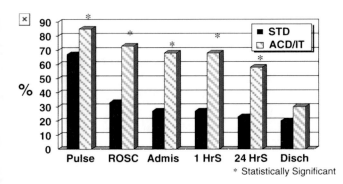

Fig. 35.13 Outcomes in patients randomized with either standard CPR (STD) or ACD-CPR + ITD with witnessed ventricular fibrillation in Mainz, Germany ($n = 70$). 1HrS = 1-h survival; 24HrS = 24-h survival; ACD = active compression decompression; Admis = hospital admission; CPR = cardiopulmonary resuscitation; Disch = hospital discharge; IT = impedance threshold device; ROSC = return of spontaneous circulation

Another prospective blinded study recently performed in France has also demonstrated significantly increased 24-h survival rates with use of ACD-CPR + ITD [23]. In one arm of this study, 200 patients were treated by advanced life support personnel with ACD-CPR and an active ITD, and another 200 patients were randomized to the control group and received treatment with ACD-CPR and a sham ITD. As in other studies from France, most of the patients had an initial rhythm of asystole [21, 22]. The group treated with ACD-CPR and an active ITD had a 24-h survival rate of 32% compared with a 24-h survival rate of 22% in the control population ($p<0.05$). Yet, because of the considered long EMS response times, survival rates in both groups were relatively very low; differences in neurological function in the survivors trended in favor of the ACD-CPR + ITD group. Only one out of eight survivors treated with the sham device had normal cerebral function at the time of hospital discharge versus six out of ten individuals in the functional ITD group ($p<0.07$).

Overall, the use of the ITD with either standard CPR or ACD-CPR results in significant increases in circulation and greater chances for meaningful survival after cardiac arrest. While these technologies represent a significant advance in the field, they are most effectively deployed in systems that are able to integrate the sequential interventions known to improve survival rates. These include early and effective bystander CPR, high-quality standard CPR or ACD-CPR together with ITD use, and post-resuscitation treatment protocols that ultimately include therapeutic hypothermia, cardiac revascularization procedures, and timely electrophysiology studies with appropriate treatment. This kind of comprehensive approach, which has been started in several US cities under a program named "Take Heart America," has been shown to markedly improve outcomes after out-of-hospital and in-hospital cardiac arrest.

35.7 Treatment of Life-Threatening Hypotension with the ITD in Spontaneously Breathing Patients

"Shock" can be defined as life-threatening hypotension and results in inadequate tissue perfusion. Hypovolemia caused by uncontrolled hemorrhage in trauma is the most common form or cause of shock, and is referred to as "hemorrhagic shock." Death following severe blood loss develops secondary to profound hypotension and vital organ ischemia. In other words, in the absence of a critical central blood volume, stroke volume and cardiac output are decreased and hypotension ensues.

Intravenous fluids and vasopressor agents have traditionally been the mainstay of therapy for patients with marked hypotension. While intravenous fluids and blood replacement, together with intravenous therapies such as epinephrine and other vasopressors, are often effective in the short term, providing a bridge to more definitive repair of the primary injury, they are also associated with significant clinical shortcomings such as the following: (1) they require intravenous or intraosseous access; (2) non-blood volume expanders can decrease the effectiveness of normal thrombus formation (by dilution of critical clotting factors); and (3) their use can ultimately reduce the oxygen carrying capacity of the blood. In addition, massive intravenous fluid replacement can cause pulmonary edema and peripheral edema (in some cases, cerebral edema), as well as hypothermia. Furthermore, vasopressors can also cause ischemia, especially to the gut. Vasopressors and fluids have been associated with "popping the clot" in the patient with significant blood loss secondary to sudden increases in blood pressure to normal or above normal values. Moreover, vasopressors like epinephrine can cause supraventricular and ventricular tachycardias, which can lead to a further compromise of the patient's already tenuous hemodynamic status. In addition, even the sinus tachycardia that is normally observed after epinephrine therapy can be detrimental in the setting of shock, as it results in a decreased amount of time for cardiac filling after each ventricular systole. This is an important issue, since blood flow back to the heart is markedly decreased because of the low central venous pressures. In this setting, one needs more time, and thus a slower heart rate, for effective refilling of the heart after each contraction.

As such, there is strong evidence that one of the primary mechanisms that contribute to reduced cardiac filling, stroke volume, and ultimately shock following an acute hemorrhage is the reduction in circulating blood volume and a subsequent reduction in cardiac filling pressure (i.e., lower central venous pressure or cardiac preload). Therefore, countermeasures designed to increase venous return and decrease cardiac filling without causing hemodilution and without "popping the clot" may be an effective therapy for the acute treatment of massive blood loss. It is important to recognize that the primary goal of any therapy used for the treatment of hemorrhagic shock is the restoration of sufficient vital organ perfusion to prevent death, even if the primary cause of the blood loss has not yet been established or repaired. Such therapies should act primarily to increase stroke volume rather than to increase peripheral resistance, as the latter may cause more harm than good. Ideally, a new therapy designed to improve vital organ perfusion in the setting of hemorrhagic shock should act primarily to optimize stroke volume, improve vital organ blood flow by a mechanism that is independent of increasing peripheral vascular resistance, and thus help to stabilize a permissive hypotensive state that provides adequate cerebral perfusion.

Building upon the work described above, two new technologies have been developed to treat clinically significant hypotension. One is termed the ITD for spontaneously breathing patients (ResQGard®) and the other is called the intrathoracic pressure regulator (ITPR, CirQlator™, Advanced Circulatory Systems, Inc., Minneapolis, MN). The ResQGard, shown in Fig. 35.14, functions in spontaneously breathing patients and can be considered as a natural extension of a normal physiological process, i.e., the transformation of the normal respiratory muscle function from a primary gas exchange function to the dual functions of gas exchange and augmentation of venous return which, in turn, will provide enhancement of cardiac stroke volume. At the present time, there are no clinical data on the ITPR, but some of the promising experimental animal data will be presented below. To avoid confusion, the differences between an ITD and the ITPR device are summarized in Fig. 35.14.

The ITD works by lowering intrathoracic pressures in the thorax with each inspiration, thereby enhancing venous blood flow back to the heart and lowering intracranial pressures. These mechanisms serve to enhance both cardiac output and blood pressure. There is also experimental data suggesting that use of the ITD will reduce the amount of vasopressor needed, since it

ITD	Intended Use:	
Inspiratory Impedance Threshold Device	Used in spontaneously breathing patients to assist in enhancing circulation and used in non-spontaneously breathing patients in cardiac arrest where CPR is being performed. Devices can be used on a facemask or an endotracheal tube.	For breathing patients For cardiac arrest
ITPR	Intended Use:	
Intrathoracic Pressure Regulator	Used in non-spontaneously breathing patients who are hypotensive and intubated, including those in cardiac arrest undergoing CPR. Device is directly attached to an endotracheal tube or other airway adjunct.	

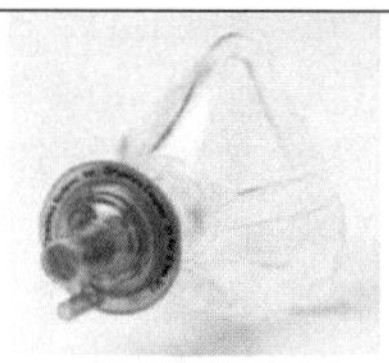

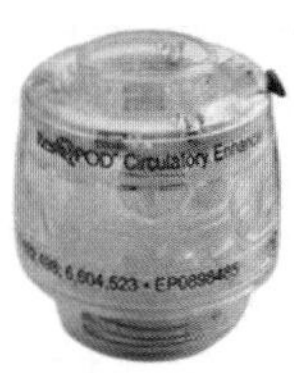

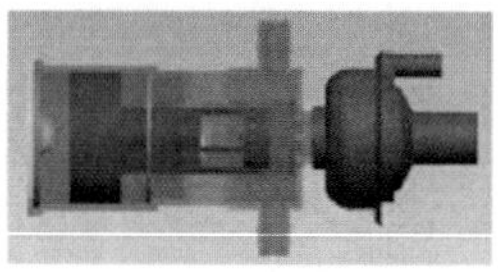

Fig. 35.14 Differences between an impedance threshold device (ITD) and the intrathoracic pressure regulator (ITPR)

increases overall cardiac output and circulation [28]. In this manner, the ITD provides an indirect drug enhancing effect, enabling the rescuers to use less of a vasopressor drug, and perhaps less fluid resuscitation, to obtain the same or greater hemodynamic effectiveness.

The spontaneously breathing version of the ITD is a small, disposable plastic airflow regulator that can be attached to a facemask, mouthpiece, or tracheal tube. The ITD attached to a facemask is shown in Fig. 35.15. The device has a spring-loaded diaphragm that requires a certain threshold (*cracking pressure*) to be achieved before it opens to allow airflow, thus functioning like a partial Mueller maneuver (inhaling against a closed glottis) to augment negative intrathoracic pressure with each inspiration [9]. In this manner, the device harnesses the patient's own respiratory pump to enhance circulation. In 1947, Cournand was the first to show that increases in mean airway pressure result in decreased systemic venous return, decreased pulmonary blood flow, and a resultant fall in cardiac output. Lower negative intrathoracic pressure during spontaneous inspiration, however, represents a natural mechanism for enhancing venous return and cardiac filling. Several natural physiologic reflexes, such as gasping and the Mueller maneuver, will augment negative intrathoracic pressure and thus increase cardiac output. Several investigators have shown that artificially induced negative pressure ventilation can be used to increase cardiac output [33, 34]. The ITD has been evaluated in both animals and humans for the treatment of cardiac arrest, hemorrhagic and heat shock, orthostatic hypotension, and during blood donation.

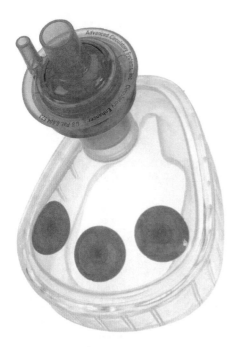

Fig. 35.15 Impedance threshold device on a facemask

In 2004, Lurie et al. demonstrated that spontaneous breathing through the ITD during hemorrhagic and heat shock in a porcine animal model resulted in an immediate sustained rise in systolic blood pressure in both conditions [35]. As shown in Fig. 35.16, the addition of the ITD (set to open at a "cracking pressure" of -12 cmH$_2$O after an acute hemorrhage) resulted in an immediate rise in systolic blood pressure that was sustained for 30 min. Upon removal of the ITD, the blood pressure decreased back to values identical with the controls. These studies showed a 30% increase in cardiac output when the ITD was employed in the pigs in shock. Subsequent studies have shown that use of the ITD in spontaneously breathing pigs after severe hemorrhage resulted in increases in cardiac output, blood pressure, cardiac chamber dimensions, transvalvular blood flow, and survival rates [36]. These studies also demonstrated how ITD use can augment cardiac output, improve hemodynamics, and increase survival in spontaneously breathing pigs under conditions of induced hypovolemic hypotension [37].

The ITD, with a cracking pressure of -6 cmH$_2$O, was first studied in normal volunteers by Convertino et al. at NASA in studies related to postflight orthostatic hypotension [38]. Inspiration through the ITD increased cardiac output by about 1.5 L/min in supine subjects and was well tolerated. The ITD use also resulted in increased stroke volume and was shown to aid in maintaining blood pressure in normal volunteers subjected to acute orthostatic stress, and later in patients presenting with symptomatic orthostatic hypotension. Use of the ITD in normal volunteers resulted in: (1) an immediate increase in cardiac stroke volume; (2) increases in both systolic blood pressure and heart rate; and (3) improved cardiac output (as shown in Fig. 35.17) [39]. It was also observed that total peripheral resistance was also reduced by ITD use.

Also highly relevant to discuss is how the ITD affects the work of breathing. To assess the work of breathing associated with use of the ITD, the power of breathing was measured in collaboration with NASA scientists in nine female and nine male subjects breathing through a facemask at two separate ITD conditions: (1) -6 cm H$_2$O and (2) control (0 cm H$_2$O). The results from this study demonstrated that breathing through the ITD was well tolerated by all subjects. Oxygen saturation levels were $>95\%$ in all subjects with the sham and -6 cm H$_2$O for the ITD group. For the sham and active ITD groups, respectively, peak inspiratory pressure was -1.13 ± 63 and -9.92 ± 6.2 cm H$_2$O ($p < 0.0001$); tidal volume was 958 ± 396 and 986 ± 389 mL (NS); and inspiratory time was 189 ± 81 and 296 ± 109 ms ($p = 0.002$). For the sham and active ITD groups, respectively, imposed work of breathing was 0.064 ± 0.04 and 0.871 ± 0.117 J/L ($p < 0.0001$); power of breathing was 0.88 ± 0.63 and 7.56 ± 3.55 J/min

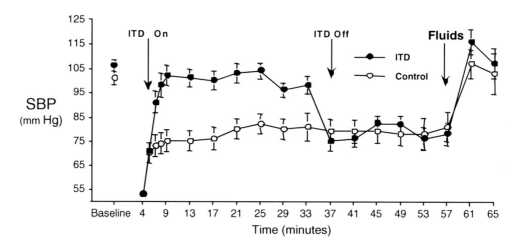

Fig. 35.16 Changes in systolic blood pressure (SBP) with and without impedance threshold device (ITD) breathing following controlled hemorrhage and shock in spontaneously breathing pigs

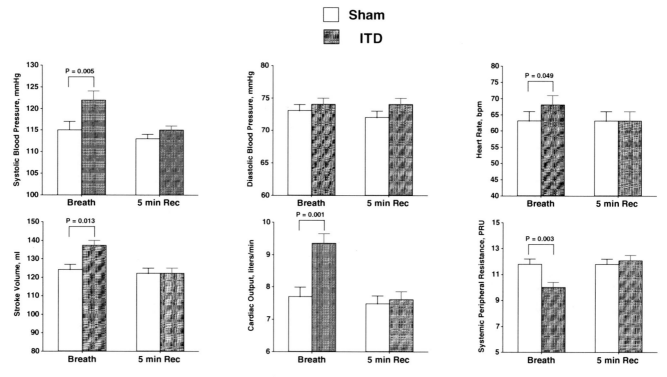

Fig. 35.17 Systolic and diastolic blood pressures, heart rate, stroke volume, cardiac output, and total peripheral vascular resistance during (Breath) and after (5 min Rec) spontaneous breathing on the impedance threshold device (ITD) at 0 cm H_2O resistance (sham control, *open bars*) and –6 cm H_2O resistance (*solid bars*) ($n = 20$)

($p < 0.0001$); peak inspiratory pressure was -1.13 ± 0.63 and -9.92 ± 6.2 cmH_2O ($p < 0.0001$); tidal volume was 958 ± 396 and 986 ± 389 mL (NS); and inspiratory time was 189 ± 81 and 296 ± 109 ms ($p = 0.002$). Interestingly, there were no significant observable differences between men and women in terms of work of breathing [40].

To put these data into perspective, one must understand the power of breathing for a normal individual, where power is work per unit time ($W = W \times f$, where f is respiratory frequency). The maximal power output for normal young adults is 613 cal/min (range 500–860) [41]. Thus, the amount of power output required during quiet breathing or use of the ITD seems rather minimal, amounting to less than 1.0% of maximum. Vigorous exercise requiring minute volume of 60 80 L requires ~80 J/min of power. The –6 cm H_2O ITD requires about 1–2 cal/min of respiratory power. For the ITD to be functional, the energy required for its operation should not exceed the energy available in the patient population where it is expected to be applied, for example in ill and injured patients with hypotension. It is known that critically ill patients who require mechanical ventilator support use about 1–2 cal/min for self-triggered ventilation and are generally able to sustain this level of effort for prolonged periods (hours to days) [41]. Therefore, we expect that most patients will be able to tolerate use of the ITD without excessive fatigue, given that it requires only a fraction of the respiratory power needed for a similarly ill group of patients to self-trigger a mechanical ventilator. We therefore conclude that, based on these measurements, the vast majority of conscious but hypotensive patients will be able to inspire through the ITD with a resistance of –7 cm H_2O and should thereby benefit hemodynamically from this device.

Most recently, the ITD was studied by Convertino et al. at the US Army Institute for Surgical Research using a lower body negative pressure chamber to decrease central blood volume, and thus induce a state of severe hypotension [42]. A photo of the lower body negative pressure chamber is shown in Fig. 35.18. The application of negative pressure to the lower body (below the iliac crest) results in a redistribution of blood away from the upper body (head and heart) to the lower extremities and abdomen. Thus, this research model provides a unique

method of investigating interventions such as the ITD under conditions of controlled, experimentally-induced hypovolemic hypotension. Absolute equivalence between the magnitude of negative pressure applied and the magnitude of actual blood loss cannot at this time be determined, but review of both human and animal data reveals ranges of effective blood loss (or fluid displacement) caused by lower body negative pressure. On the basis of the magnitude of central hypovolemia induced, Convertino et al. provide data to support that 10–20 mmHg negative pressure induces hemodynamic responses that are equivalent to those resulting from blood loss ranging from 400 to 550 ml; 20–40 mmHg negative pressure induces hemodynamic responses that are equivalent to those resulting from blood loss ranging from 550 to 1,000 ml; and >40 mmHg negative pressure induces hemodynamic responses that are equivalent to those resulting from blood loss approximating 1,000 ml or more [42]. Nine healthy and normotensive volunteers completed two counterbalanced protocols with (active) and without (sham) an ITD set to open at –6 cmH$_2$O pressure. Continuous noninvasive measures of systolic, diastolic, and mean arterial blood pressures were obtained during a lower body negative pressure protocol consisting of a 5-min rest period (baseline) followed by 5 min of chamber decompression at –15, –30, –45, and –60 mmHg, and additional increments of –10 mmHg every 5 min until the onset of cardiovascular collapse. The

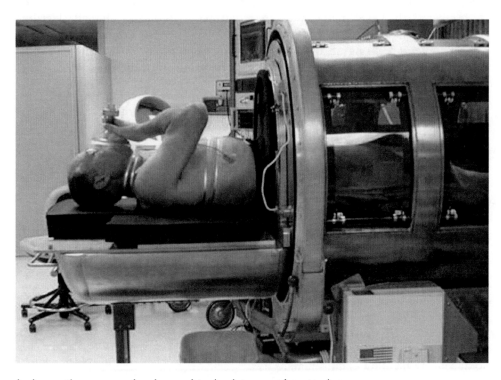

Fig. 35.18 Lower body negative pressure chamber used to simulate severe hypotension

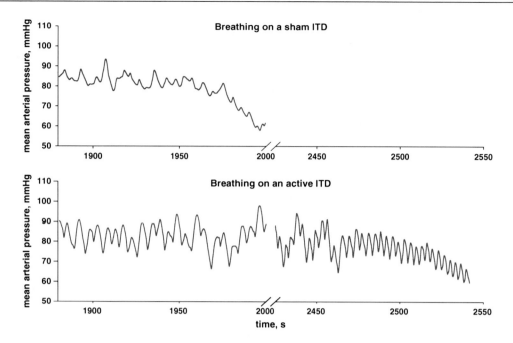

Fig. 35.19 Representative tracings of beat-to-beat mean arterial blood pressure obtained from the same subject while breathing on a sham impedance threshold device (ITD) (*top panel*) and active ITD (*bottom panel*) during the final 2 min of lower body negative pressure exposure prior to cardiovascular collapse

systolic blood pressure (79 ± 5 mmHg), diastolic blood pressure (57 ± 3 mmHg), and MAP (65 ± 4 mmHg) at the time of cardiovascular collapse were lower ($p<0.02$) when subjects breathed through the sham ITD than when they breathed through the active ITD at the same time point of lower body negative pressure (102 ± 3, 77 ± 3, 87 ± 3 mmHg, respectively). Elevated blood pressure was associated with a 23% increase ($p=0.02$) in lower body negative pressure tolerance using an active ITD (1639 ± 220 mmHg-min) compared with a sham ITD (1328 ± 144 mmHg-min). A representative tracing of such an investigation is shown in Fig. 35.19.

These results are the first to demonstrate, in humans, that the time to cardiovascular collapse associated with progressive reduction in central blood volume and subsequent development of severe hypotension can be significantly improved by inspiratory resistance induced by spontaneous breathing through an ITD. The results from the present experiment demonstrated an average elevation in systolic blood pressure of 23 mmHg when estimated central blood volume was reduced by more than 2 L [42].

Importantly, the use of an ITD also has a striking effect on cerebral artery blood flow. With each inspiration through the ITD, intracranial pressures are lowered and cardiac output is simultaneously increased. Specifically, the measurement with cerebral Doppler demonstrated that use of the ITD increased middle cerebral artery blood flow in spontaneously breathing adult humans as shown in Fig. 35.20 [43].

Our group recently performed another clinical trial which evaluated the use of the ITD to treat non-life-threatening hypotension (systolic blood pressure <95 mmHg) in the emergency room department. In this randomized double-blind clinical trial, patients received the current standard of care for hypotension, which currently consists of controlling the bleeding, reversing other potential causes of low blood pressure such as correcting hyperthermia, and administering fluids, oxygen, and/or blood products as appropriate. It was shown that use of

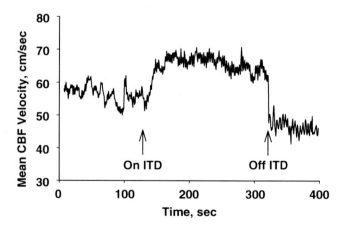

Fig. 35.20 Typical continuous recording of mean cerebral blood flow (CBF) velocity in a subject before, during (On ITD), and at the cessation (Off ITD) of spontaneous breathing on the impedance threshold device (ITD)

the ITD did not interfere with standard therapy. Once it was determined that the subjects met enrollment criteria based on the inclusion and exclusion criteria and informed consent was obtained, subjects were randomized to either a sham ITD or an active (functional) ITD. The sham and active ITDs appeared identical to the participating health care providers. The devices were kept in an opaque package, preventing anyone involved with the study from knowing whether any given device was a sham or active ITD based on visual inspection. Baseline blood pressure, heart rate, respiratory rate, oxygen saturation, and clinical findings (i.e., quality of the pulse and quality of respirations) were all initially recorded. The ITD was then placed and hemodynamic parameters were assessed every 2 min for a minimum of 6 min and up to 10 min. Standard therapies, including intravenous fluids, were administered as deemed clinically necessary, regardless of the effect of the ITD. It was observed that the active device was significantly more effective than the sham. The mean rise in systolic blood pressure for the active ITD group was 13.2 ± 7.8 mmHg ($n = 16$) versus 5.9 ± 5.5 mmHg for the sham ITD group ($n = 19$; $p = 0.003$). Mean fluids given during the study were 92 ± 170 ml for the active ITD group and 192 ± 200 ml for the sham ITD group ($p = 0.13$). In a subgroup of patients that received no fluids during device use, the maximum rise in systolic blood pressure (mean $\pm$ STD) was 12.8 ± 7.8 mmHg for the active ITD group and 5.6 ± 5.0 mmHg for the sham ITD group ($p = 0.04$). Mean arterial pressure was also statistically higher in the active ITD group (9.2 ± 7.8 versus 4.8 ± 3.3 mmHg, $p = 0.03$).

It is now the general consensus that the ITD harnesses the patient's own thoracic pump to enhance circulation, and thus offers a noninvasive means to treat many patients. However, the spontaneously breathing version of the ITD requires that patients be able to breathe on their own, and most patients in severe shock are usually intubated and require assisted ventilation. To fill this gap, the ITPR was developed. This technology was developed based on the same concept of lowering intrathoracic pressures to enhance circulation for patients with life-threatening hypotension that are dependent upon assisted ventilation.

35.8 ITPR Therapy: A Potential Novel Treatment of Severe Hypotension in Severely Ill Patients

The ITPR, which is described below, has at the time of this writing only been tested in animals. It combines a way to generate a controlled intrathoracic vacuum with a method to provide controlled positive pressure

ventilation. It can be used for the treatment of cardiac arrest and multiple forms of shock to buy time until more definitive therapy is available. The device can be used with a hand-held resuscitator bag or can be attached to a mechanical ventilator or anesthesia machine. While multiple designs are possible to embody this concept, the main function of the ITPR is to create a preset continuous and controlled expiratory phase-negative intrathoracic pressure that is interrupted only when positive pressure ventilation is needed to maintain oxygenation and provide gas exchange. The ITPR has been cleared for sale by the US Food and Drug Administration, with the approved indication of "a device to enhance circulation in patients requiring assisted ventilation."

It was recognized from the start that it would be important to develop a modification of the ITD for use in nonbreathing sicker hypotensive patients; this resulted in the concept of the ITPR. The ITPR employs an external vacuum source to lower intrathoracic pressures and thus enhance venous blood flow back to the heart in nonbreathing hypotensive patients. This refinement is based on the aforementioned breakthrough in our clinical understanding of the basic physiological principles of blood flow in hypotensive states. By transforming the chest into an active bellow during CPR, the combination of a relatively low level expiratory phase intrathoracic vacuum and intermittent positive pressure ventilation results in a significant augmentation of venous blood flow to the right heart, thereby increasing both stroke volume and cardiac output.

Contemporaneously, the decrease in intrathoracic pressures results in a decrease in intracranial pressures and thus provides an additional mechanism whereby the ITPR increases cerebral perfusion pressures; this is illustrated in Fig. 35.21. When the ITPR is turned on, the intrathoracic

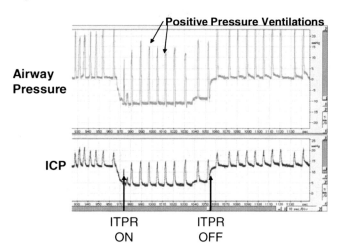

Fig. 35.21 Changes in airway pressure and intracranial pressure (ICP) when the intrathoracic pressure regulator (ITPR) is turned on and then off again

pressure between positive pressure breaths is lowered immediately, as is the intracranial pressure. Based on these findings, the ITPR may also ultimately have the potential for treatment of stroke and brain injury [16].

To date, the beneficial results of the ITPR have been studied in pigs in VF during CPR. In this setting, the ITPR was used to lower intrathoracic pressures and thus enhance venous return to the heart and increase overall efficacy [44]. Vital organ perfusion pressures and end-tidal carbon dioxide were significantly improved with ITPR-CPR and survival was 100% (10/10) with ITPR-CPR versus 10% (1/10) with standard CPR alone. Use of ITPR-CPR improved hemodynamics, vital organ perfusion pressures, and carotid blood flow in both VF and hypovolemic cardiac arrest. Figure 35.22 demonstrates the significant hemodynamic differences observed when using the ITPR during standard CPR in the animal models of cardiac arrest.

The physiological goals of the ITPR are to (1) lower intrathoracic pressures during the expiratory phase of ventilation and (2) provide positive pressure ventilation in patients requiring assisted ventilation. The first studies evaluating the effect of the ITPR on vital organ perfusion pressures were performed in normovolemic and hypovolemic pigs [45]. Six anesthetized animals received 5-min interventions with endotracheal pressure (a surrogate for intrathoracic pressure) set to 0, –5, 0, –10, 0, –10, 0, –5, 0 mmHg during euvolemia and then after a fixed hemorrhage of 50% of their total blood volume. Hemodynamic parameters were continuously measured and blood gases were obtained at the end of the first four 5-min intervals. Under both euvolemic and hypovolemic conditions, right atrial pressures and intracranial pressures decreased proportionally to the intrathoracic pressure, with more marked changes observed with hypovolemic conditions. In contrast, the increases in

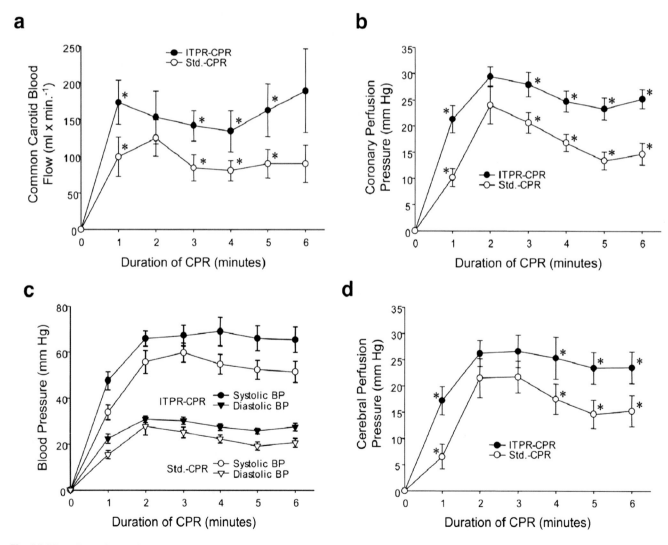

Fig. 35.22 Effect of intrathoracic pressure regulator (ITPR) CPR on carotid blood flow, coronary perfusion pressure, blood pressure, and cerebral perfusion pressure compared to standard CPR (Std-CPR). BP = blood pressure; CPR = cardiopulmonary resuscitation

Table 35.1 Basic hemodynamic parameters with endotracheal pressure set at 0, –5, and –10 mmHg with the ITPR for blood volumes after 0 and 50% blood loss

Blood loss	ETP	0	–5	–10
0%	MAP	89.9 ± 4.5	104.3 ± 7.3[*]	108.5 ± 6.1[*]
	RAP	1.8 ± 0.4	–0.8 ± 0.6[*]	–4.8 ± 0.4[*§]
	CPP	80 ± 3.9	94.2 ± 6.4[*]	103.3 ± 5.3[*§]
	CerPP	74 ± 4.8	90.3 ± 7.4[*]	95.1 ± 6[*]
	ICP	15.6 ± 0.6	14 ± 0.7	13.5 ± 0.6[*]
50%	MAP	28.8 ± 4.3	39.8 ± 5.9[*]	47.3 ± 7.3[*§]
	RAP	–2 ± 0.9	–5.7 ± 0.6[*]	–9.3 ± 0.3[*§]
	CPP	25.8 ± 5	38.5 ± 3.7[*]	48.3 ± 3.8[*§]
	CerPP	18.1 ± 4.4	32.9 ± 5.8[*]	43.1 ± 7.2[*§]
	ICP	10.7 ± 1.3	6.8 ± 1.4[*]	4.2 ± 1[*§]

[*] Statistically significant difference ($0.05 > p > 0.001$) when compared to the values with ETP of 0 mmHg; [§] statistically significant difference between values with –5 and –10 mmHg of ETP ($p < 0.05$). CerPP = cerebral perfusion pressure; CPP = coronary perfusion pressure; ETP = endotracheal pressure; ICP = intracranial pressure; MAP = mean arterial pressure; RAP = right atrial pressure.

MAP, CPP, and CePP were inversely proportional to the negative intrathoracic pressure both in normovolemic pigs and after hemorrhage. These data are consistent with findings in spontaneously breathing adult and pediatric swine models of shock and use of the ITD [35, 36]. The major hemodynamic parameters for 0, –5, –10 mmHg of endotracheal pressure are shown in Table 35.1. Based on the data available to date, we believe that the generation of intrathoracic pressures greater than –15 mmHg may be excessive and not beneficial with long-term use.

Our initial studies demonstrated that the ITPR can reproducibly decrease endotracheal pressure, intrathoracic pressure (as seen by the decrease in right atrial pressure), and ICP. The ITPR provided hemodynamic improvement with no significant acid–base changes during normovolemia. We have applied the ITPR in euvolemic anesthetized pigs for up to 6 h with an intrathoracic vacuum set to –9 mmHg without any obvious adverse effects on gas exchange or the overall metabolic state of the pigs. The long-term benefits of the ITPR after hemorrhage are much more dependent upon the degree of hypotension. During 50% hypovolemia, there was more acidosis associated with the generation of negative endotracheal pressure, as reflected by lower pH and higher $PaCO_2$ levels. However, despite the lower pH values which may be secondary to greater clearance of lactate, ITPR use increased blood pressure, pulse pressure, vital organ perfusion pressure, and end-tidal carbon dioxide levels, suggesting that there is an improved balance between the increase in circulation and the potential for metabolic acidosis with ITPR use; oxygenation saturation remained at 100% with ITPR use.

Studies on the potential benefits of longer-term generation-negative intrathoracic pressure have been explored in a preliminary manner. In pilot studies with spontaneously breathing pigs, in collaboration with researchers at the US Army Institute for Surgical Research, we applied the ITD to spontaneously breathing pigs in severe hemorrhagic shock in an uncontrolled model of severe blood loss [37, 46]. These splenectomized pigs were subjected to a 60% blood loss, followed by a 4 mm hole created in the abdominal aorta. Remarkably, use of the ITD in these pilot studies stabilized these pigs for about 60 min after the hemorrhage and injuries occurred. However, after 75 min we observed the development of a significant metabolic acidosis, as reflected by a more and more negative base excess; at that point, the pigs were hemodynamically stable. Shortly thereafter, the pigs became extremely agitated, hypotensive, and then died [37]. These pilot studies provided us with some fundamental insights related to the limitations of using the ITD, and by analogy the ITPR itself, in the setting of severe blood loss. While these devices can be used to "buy time," ultimately some fluid resuscitation and correction of the underlying cause of the blood loss is essential. Although some fluids were ultimately needed, we hypothesize that the ITD and ITPR, in this setting, were actually fluid sparing and would extend the window of opportunity to provide life-saving care in individuals with severe blood loss.

The ITPR is designed to provide a noninvasive means to increase MAPs in the setting of cardiac arrest and significant hypotension in apneic patients. The effect is rapid and can be turned on or off by the flip of a switch, unlike more long-lasting and sometimes harmful effects of fluid and drug administration. This switch-like effect is shown in Fig. 35.21. In another study, shown in Fig. 35.23, the intrathoracic pressures were varied between 0, –5 and –10 mmHg. With each change, there was a rapid adjustment in key hemodynamic variables and ICP. Based on the combined effects of the ITPR therapy shown in multiple pig studies, we believe that ITPR has the potential to become a first-line therapy for all patients in cardiac arrest, as well as provide benefit for many with hypotension from a wide variety of causes. This device can be applied quickly, often before intravenous access, intra-osseous access, or fluids may be available, and it safely and quickly increases systemic, coronary, and cerebral perfusion pressures. Moreover, based on our experience to date in noncardiac arrest models, use of the ITPR may be of significant benefit after traditional therapies have been administered, in that the ITPR may reduce: (1) the amount of volume needed for resuscitation from multiple etiologies; (2) the severity of secondary brain injury after an initial brain injury; and/or (3) the amount of vasopressor needed to maintain

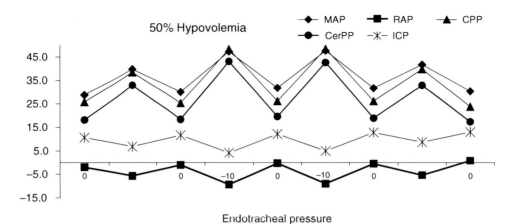

Fig. 35.23 Sequential changes in mean arterial pressure (MAP), coronary perfusion pressure (CPP), cerebral perfusion pressure (CerPP), right atrial pressure (RAP), and intracranial pressure (ICP) for sequential changes of endotracheal pressure (a surrogate for intrathoracic pressure) of 0, −5, 0, −10, 0, −10, 0, −5, 0 mmHg during 50% hypovolemia. Differences between the values of all parameters are statistically significant with $p<0.05$

"permissive hypotension." The ITPR approach may thereby become a useful therapy in the operating room and intensive care unit to help maintain vital organ perfusion. To date the ITPR has been used in patients with acute hypotension intra-operatively. It was well-tolerated and resulted in rapid increase in blood pressure in the absence of fluid administration or vasopressor therapy.

Studies to date have shown that the application of the ITPR therapy in cardiac arrest results in marked improvement in hemodynamics and survival rates. Application of the device in hypovolemic pigs enhances circulation, stroke volume, MAP, CPP, and CePP and decreases intracranial pressures. Studies in a porcine model of peritonitis (septic shock) have shown an augmentation in cardiac index and mean arterial pressure while simultaneously lowering pulmonary artery pressures during ITPR use. The longer-term potential consequences of the ITPR remain unknown. One known limitation is that, in order for this technology to be of clinical benefit, the thorax must be intact; otherwise, it is not possible to generate expiratory phase-negative intrathoracic pressures with the ITPR. Furthermore, it is not possible to lower the expiratory phase intrathoracic pressures and use positive end expiratory pressure concurrently, unless the ITPR is used as a pulsed therapy, which is currently under evaluation. Thus, the benefit of circulatory enhancement with the ITPR must be balanced clinically with the need to concurrently maintain at least minimally adequate ventilatory support. The animal studies to date have suggested that the ITPR can provide both circulatory and ventilatory support for up to at least 4 h in duration in severely compromised hypotensive animals and/or those suffering from cardiac arrest.

List of Abbreviations

ACD	active compression decompression
AHA	American Heart Association
CePP	cerebral perfusion pressure
CPP	coronary perfusion pressure
CPR	cardiopulmonary resuscitation
EMS	emergency medical services
ICP	intracranial pressure
ITD	impedance threshold device
ITPR	intrathoracic pressure regulator
MAP	mean arterial pressure
PEA	pulseless electrical activity
VF	ventricular fibrillation

References

1. Eisenberg MS, Horwood BT, Cummins RO, et al. Cardiac arrest and resuscitation: A tale of 29 cities. Ann Emerg Med 1990;19: 179–86.
2. Niemann JT. Cardiopulmonary resuscitation. N Engl J Med 1992;327:1075–80.
3. Lurie KG, Voelckel WG, Zielinski T, et al. Improving standard cardiopulmonary resuscitation with an inspiratory impedance threshold valve in a porcine model of cardiac arrest. Anesth Analg 2001;93:649–55.
4. Voelckel WG, Lurie KG, Sweeney M, et al. Effects of active compression-decompression cardiopulmonary resuscitation with the inspiratory threshold valve in a young porcine model of cardiac arrest. Pediatr Res 2002;51:523–27.
5. Lurie K, Voelckel W, Plaisance P, et al. Use of an inspiratory impedance threshold valve during cardiopulmonary resuscitation: A progress report. Resuscitation 2000;44:219–30.
6. Lurie KG, Lindner KH. Recent advances in cardiopulmonary resuscitation. J Cardiovasc Electrophysiol 1997;8:584–600.

7. Lurie KG, Mulligan KA, McKnite S, et al. Optimizing standard cardiopulmonary resuscitation with an inspiratory impedance threshold valve. Chest 1998;113:1084–90.

8. Lurie KG, Zielinski T, McKnite S, et al. Use of an inspiratory impedance valve improves neurologically intact survival in a porcine model of ventricular fibrillation. Circulation 2002;105:124–29.

9. Lurie KG, Zielinski T, Voelckel W, et al. Augmentation of ventricular preload during treatment of cardiovascular collapse and cardiac arrest. Crit Care Med 2002;30:S162–65.

10. Lurie KG, Coffeen P, Shultz J, et al. Improving active compression-decompression cardiopulmonary resuscitation with an inspiratory impedance valve. Circulation 1995;91:1629–32.

11. Aufderheide T. A tale of seven EMS systems: An impedance threshold device and improved CPR techniques double survival rates after out-of-hospital cardiac arrest. Circulation 2007;116:II-936.

12. Holzer M, Behringer W, Schorkhuber W, et al. Mild hypothermia and outcome after CPR. Hypothermia for Cardiac Arrest (HACA) Study Group. Acta Anaesthesiol Scand Suppl 1997;111:55–58.

13. Holzer M, Bernard SA, Hachimi-Idrissi S, et al. Hypothermia for neuroprotection after cardiac arrest: systematic review and individual patient data meta-analysis. Crit Care Med 2005;33:414–18.

14. Holzer M, Sterz F. Therapeutic hypothermia after cardiopulmonary resuscitation. Expert Rev Cardiovasc Ther 2003;1:317–25.

15. Guidelines 2000 for Cardiopulmonary Resuscitation and Emergency Cardiovascular Care. Part 2: Ethical aspects of CPR and ECC. Circulation 2000;102:I12–21.

16. Yannopoulos D, McKnite S, Aufderheide TP, et al. Effects of incomplete chest wall decompression during cardiopulmonary resuscitation on coronary and cerebral perfusion pressures in a porcine model of cardiac arrest. Resuscitation 2005;64:363–72.

17. Aufderheide TP, Pirrallo RG, Yannopoulos D, et al. Incomplete chest wall decompression: A clinical evaluation of CPR performance by EMS personnel and assessment of alternative manual chest compression-decompression techniques. Resuscitation 2005;64:353–62.

18. Thigpen KS, Simmons L, Hatten, K. Implementation of the 2005 cardiopulmonary resuscitation guidelines and use of an impedance threshold device improve survival from inhospital cardiac arrest. Ann Emerg Med 2008;51:475.

19. Cohen TJ, Tucker KJ, Lurie KG, et al. Active compression-decompression. A new method of cardiopulmonary resuscitation. Cardiopulmonary Resuscitation Working Group. JAMA 1992;267:2916–23.

20. Lindner KH, Pfenninger EG, Lurie KG, et al. Effects of active compression-decompression resuscitation on myocardial and cerebral blood flow in pigs. Circulation 1993;88:1254–63.

21. Plaisance P, Adnet F, Vicaut E, et al. Benefit of active compression-decompression cardiopulmonary resuscitation as a prehospital advanced cardiac life support. A randomized multicenter study. Circulation 1997;95:955–61.

22. Plaisance P, Lurie KG, Vicaut E, et al. A comparison of standard cardiopulmonary resuscitation and active compression-decompression resuscitation for out-of-hospital cardiac arrest. French Active Compression-Decompression Cardiopulmonary Resuscitation Study Group. N Engl J Med 1999;341:569–75.

23. Plaisance P, Lurie KG, Payen D. Inspiratory impedance during active compression-decompression cardiopulmonary resuscitation: A randomized evaluation in patients in cardiac arrest. Circulation 2000;101:989–94.

24. Lurie KG. Recent advances in mechanical methods of cardiopulmonary resuscitation. Acta Anaesthesiol Scand Suppl 1997;111:49–52.

25. Goetting MG, Paradis NA, Appleton TJ, et al. Aortic-carotid artery pressure differences and cephalic perfusion pressure during cardiopulmonary resuscitation in humans. Crit Care Med 1991;19:1012–17.

26. Paradis NA, Martin GB, Rosenberg J, et al. The effect of standard- and high-dose epinephrine on coronary perfusion pressure during prolonged cardiopulmonary resuscitation. JAMA 1991;265:1139–44.

27. Bahlmann L, Klaus S, Baumeier W, et al. Brain metabolism during cardiopulmonary resuscitation assessed with microdialysis. Resuscitation 2003;59:255–60.

28. Raedler C, Voelckel WG, Wenzel V, et al. Vasopressor response in a porcine model of hypothermic cardiac arrest is improved with active compression-decompression cardiopulmonary resuscitation using the inspiratory impedance threshold valve. Anesth Analg 2002;95:1496–502.

29. Plaisance P, Lurie KG, Vicaut E, et al. Evaluation of an impedance threshold device in patients receiving active compression-decompression cardiopulmonary resuscitation for out of hospital cardiac arrest. Resuscitation 2004;61:265–71.

30. Wolcke BB, Mauer DK, Schoefmann MF, et al. Comparison of standard cardiopulmonary resuscitation versus the combination of active compression-decompression cardiopulmonary resuscitation and an inspiratory impedance threshold device for out-of-hospital cardiac arrest. Circulation 2003;108:2201–05.

31. Plaisance P, Soleil C, Lurie KG, et al. Use of an inspiratory impedance threshold device on a facemask and endotracheal tube to reduce intrathoracic pressures during the decompression phase of active compression-decompression cardiopulmonary resuscitation. Crit Care Med 2005;33:990–94.

32. Aufderheide TP, Sigurdsson G, Pirrallo RG, et al. Hyperventilation-induced hypotension during cardiopulmonary resuscitation. Circulation 2004;109:1960–65.

33. Fritsch-Yelle JM, Convertino VA, Schlegel TT. Acute manipulations of plasma volume alter arterial pressure responses during Valsalva maneuvers. J Appl Physiol 1999;86:1852–57.

34. Shekerdemian LS, Bush A, Shore DF, et al. Cardiopulmonary interactions after Fontan operations: Augmentation of cardiac output using negative pressure ventilation. Circulation 1997;96:3934–42.

35. Lurie KG, Zielinski TM, McKnite SH, et al. Treatment of hypotension in pigs with an inspiratory impedance threshold device: A feasibility study. Crit Care Med 2004;32:1555–62.

36. Marino BS, Yannopoulos D, Sigurdsson G, et al. Spontaneous breathing through an inspiratory impedance threshold device augments cardiac index and stroke volume index in a pediatric porcine model of hemorrhagic hypovolemia. Crit Care Med 2004;32:S398–405.

37. Sigurdsson G, Yannopoulos D, McKnite SH, et al. Effects of an inspiratory impedance threshold device on blood pressure and short term survival in spontaneously breathing hypovolemic pigs. Resuscitation 2006;68:399–404.

38. Convertino VA, Ratliff DA, Crissey J, et al. Effects of inspiratory impedance on hemodynamic responses to a squat-stand test in human volunteers: Implications for treatment of orthostatic hypotension. Eur J Appl Physiol 2005;94:392–99.

39. Convertino VA, Ratliff DA, Ryan KL, et al. Hemodynamics associated with breathing through an inspiratory impedance

threshold device in human volunteers. Crit Care Med 2004;32:S381–86.

40. Idris A, Convertino, VA, Ratliff, MS et al. Imposed power of breathing associated with use of an impedance threshold device. Respir Care 2007;52:177–83.

41. Milic-Emili J, ed. The lung: Scientific foundations. New York, NY: Raven Press, 1991.

42. Cooke WH, Ryan KL, Convertino VA. Lower body negative pressure as a model to study progression to acute hemorrhagic shock in humans. J Appl Physiol 2004;96:1249–61.

43. Convertino VA, Cooke WH, Lurie KG. Inspiratory resistance as a potential treatment for orthostatic intolerance and hemorrhagic shock. Aviat Space Environ Med 2005;76:319–25.

44. Yannopoulos D, Nadkarni VM, McKnite SH, et al. Intrathoracic pressure regulator during continuous-chest-compression advanced cardiac resuscitation improves vital organ perfusion pressures in a porcine model of cardiac arrest. Circulation 2005;112:803–11.

45. Yannopoulos D, Metzger A, McKnite S, et al. Intrathoracic pressure regulation improves vital organ perfusion pressures in normovolemic and hypovolemic pigs. Resuscitation 2006;70:445–53.

46. Sigurdsson G, McKnite SH, Sondeen JL, et al. Extending the golden hour of hemorrhagic shock in pigs with an inspiratory impedance threshold valve. Paper presented at Critical Care in Medicine, 2005.

Chapter 36
End-Stage Congestive Heart Failure: Ventricular Assist Devices

Kenneth K. Liao and Ranjit John

Abstract Approximately 5 million Americans have congestive heart failure (CHF), and every year about 50,000 new cases are diagnosed. Advances in medical therapy, biventricular pacing, defibrillator implantation, and the ability to successfully perform surgery in high-risk patients have revolutionized the management of patients with CHF and greatly delayed CHF progression to end stage. Once patients develop end-stage CHF, treatment options are limited and typically ineffective, and the mortality is high. Heart transplant thus becomes the last resort for end-stage CHF patients. Ventricular assist devices (VAD), especially left ventricular assist devices (LVAD), have been increasingly used to support such ill patients as a bridge-to-transplant therapy in the last decade. More recently, these devices have been used as a destination therapy for end-stage CHF as well. A newer generation of VADs with better mechanics, smaller size, and longer durability has been developed in recent years.

Keywords Ventricular assist device · End-stage congestive heart failure · Axial flow pump · Centrifugal pump · Volume displacement pump

36.1 Introduction

Approximately 5 million Americans have congestive heart failure (CHF), and every year about 50,000 new cases are diagnosed. It is the most frequent cause of hospital admissions in patients older than 65 years, and it is the largest single expense for Medicare [1]. With current medical management, the 5-year mortality rate of CHF can be as high as 50%. Advances in medical therapy, biventricular pacing, defibrillator implantation, and the ability to successfully perform surgery in high-risk patients have revolutionized the management of patients with CHF and greatly delayed CHF progression to end stage. Once patients develop end-stage CHF, treatment options are limited and typically ineffective, and the mortality is high. Heart transplant thus becomes the last resort for end-stage CHF patients; it is a very effective therapy which offers excellent short-term and long-term survival benefits (over 90 and 50% survival rates at 1 and 10 years, respectively). Most patients enjoy a near-normal lifestyle after heart transplant [2]. However, donor hearts available for transplantation are limited to an average of 2,200 per year, compared to over 35,000 people per year who could benefit from such a therapy [1].

In addition to the scarcity of donor hearts, many patients die each year while waiting for ideal donor hearts. Ventricular assist devices (VAD), especially left ventricular assist devices (LVAD), have been increasingly used to support such ill patients as a bridge-to-transplant therapy in the last decade [3]. More recently, after the landmark REMATCH trial, the LVAD has been used as a destination therapy for end-stage CHF [4, 5]. A newer generation of VADs with better mechanics, smaller size, and longer durability has been developed in recent years [6–11]. Nevertheless, the ultimate goal of future VAD development is to produce a small, totally implantable, biocompatible, and durable heart pump that can physiologically function like a human heart.

A clinically effective VAD should be judged by various mechanical and physiological performances; it must: (1) provide sufficient cardiac output to allow patients to perform their usual daily activities; (2) have a low risk of thromboembolism, pump, or driveline infection, and a low incidence of device malfunction; (3) be easily implantable and removable; and finally (4) be small in size.

K.K. Liao (✉)
University of Minnesota, Division of Cardiovascular and Thoracic Surgery, Department of Surgery, MMC 207, 420 Delaware St. SE, Minneapolis, MN 55455, USA
e-mail: liaox014@umn.edu

P.A. Iaizzo (ed.), *Handbook of Cardiac Anatomy, Physiology, and Devices*, DOI 10.1007/978-1-60327-372-5_36,
© Springer Science+Business Media, LLC 2009

36.2 Classification of VADs

VADs can be classified based on their mechanics (volume displacement, axial flow, and centrifugal), therapeutic purposes (temporary, bridge-to-decision, bridge-to-recovery, bridge-to-transplant, and destination), sites of support (LVAD, right VAD or RVAD, and biventricular VAD or BiVAD), location of the pump (implantable, paracorporeal, and extracorporeal), and implanting approaches (sternotomy, thoracotomy, laparotomy, subcostal, and percutaneous).

36.3 VADs by Mechanics and Their Clinical Applications

36.3.1 Volume Displacement Pumps (Pulsatile Pumps)

The human left and right ventricles are volume displacement pumps. During each cardiac cycle, the ventricles generate over 60 cc of stroke volume. Each ventricle has a pair of inflow and outflow valves to maintain a unidirectional blood flow. The end result is that a human heart generates a pulsatile blood pressure and steady cardiac output. Its mitral and tricuspid valves function as the inflow valves, while aortic and pulmonary valves function as outflow valves. The current volume displacement VADs function exactly like human ventricles. They have a pump chamber that generates a stroke volume between 40 and 80 cc during each cardiac cycle, and have two artificial valves (either bioprostheses or mechanical valves).

The valves used inside VADs, i.e., bioprosthetic versus mechanical, can determine the durability of the VAD and the need for anticoagulation. Bioprostheses may have the advantage of not requiring anticoagulation therapy (thus reducing the risk of thromboembolism), but their limited lifespan inside the VAD may result in premature VAD failure (thus requiring VAD replacement). On the other hand, mechanical valves have the advantage of being durable, but they need adequate anticoagulation therapy to prevent clotting. Under- or over-anticoagulation treatment can increase the risks of thromboembolism or bleeding which can subsequently affect the patient's outcome.

Typically two mechanisms are used to eject blood in this type of VAD, one that uses compressed air to squeeze the blood-filled sac or to displace a flexible diaphragm within a hard shell to generate stroke volume, and another that uses a slow torque electrical motor to displace a flexible diaphragm inside the implantable unit within a hard shell to generate stroke volume. Compressed air seems to provide a simple and reliable way of either

moving the diaphragm or compressing the sac, with a pressure more comparable to a physiologically acceptable waveform. However, this design requires a bulky driving console, thus compromising the patient's mobility; in addition, the driving console makes a loud noise. If the diaphragm is propulsed by an electrical motor within a non-compressible metal chamber, the early systolic pressure generated by this pump is much higher than the pump driven by the compressed air. Such unphysiologically high pressure can speed the calcification process in the inflow bioprostheses and can cause early valve failure [12].

The blood and pump contact surface interaction plays an important role in determining the thrombogenicity of the pumps and therefore the need for anticoagulation. It is particularly important for the volume displacement pumps because of their relatively large contact surface area with blood as compared to the axial flow pumps. Initially, a smooth surface was pursued during VAD design and manufactured to avoid thrombosis but later it turned out that an evenly distributed textured surface generated less thrombosis. The textured surface promotes early platelet and fibrin deposition during initial contact with blood, which results in formation of stable pseudointima; the pseudointima subsequently prevents the formation of thrombosis [13].

Commonly used volume displacement pumps include the Thoratec HeartMate® XVE LVAD (Pleasanton, CA;

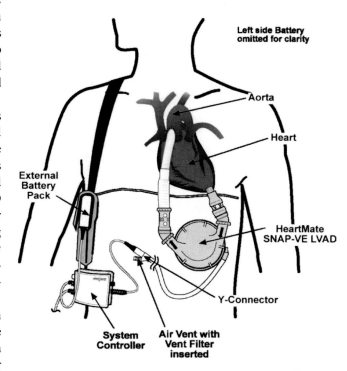

Fig. 36.1 Schematic of an internally implanted HeartMate® SNAP-VE left ventricular assist device (LVAD). The inflow cannula is inserted at the apex of the left ventricle. The outflow graft is connected directly to the ascending aorta. This LVAD utilizes an external battery pack and controller system

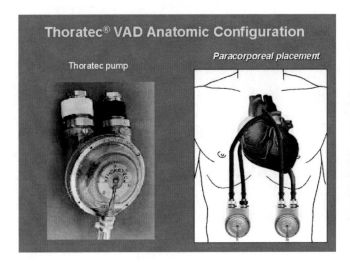

Fig. 36.2 Thoratec ventricular assist device (VAD) system. *Left insert:* the pump with both inflow and outflow valve housing connectors pointing upward and the compressed air driveline pointing downward. *Right insert:* the cannulas and grafts are implanted inside the body cavity while the pumps are connected outside the body cavity

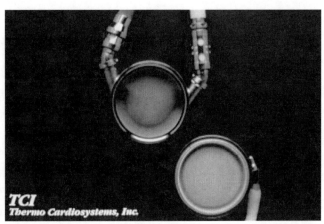

Fig. 36.3 Textured inner surface of HeartMate® XVE left ventricular assist device. The textured surface promotes formation of pseudointima which subsequently prevents thrombosis formation

Fig. 36.1) and VAD (Fig. 36.2) (Thermo Cardiosystems, Inc., Waltham, MA and the Texas Heart Institute, Houston, TX). The HeartMate® XVE is by far the mostly implanted and most studied LVAD worldwide. It is approved by the Food and Drug Administration (FDA) to be used both as a bridge-to-heart transplant and as destination therapy for end-stage congestive heart failure patients. It is driven by an electrical motor and can also be driven by compressed air when the electrical motor wears out. The HeartMate® XVE is implantable and powered through the driveline which exits from the abdominal wall; it can be either implanted in the abdomen or in the preperitoneal space. The inflow cannula is inserted into the left ventricle via an opening in the left ventricular apex, and the outflow graft is connected in the proximal ascending aorta. The device has a textured surface and a very low risk of thromboembolism (Fig. 36.3); furthermore, it does not need to be anticoagulated with coumadin or plavix (patients need aspirin only once a day). The HeartMate® XVE is a very attractive choice when the patient cannot take or tolerate anticoagulation. Additionally, it is the only implantable LVAD that has been approved as destination therapy for end-stage heart failure patients. Compared to maximal medical management including home inotropic therapy, the HeartMate® XVE significantly improves the quality of life and survival of end-stage congestive heart failure patients [5]. However, the disadvantages of this LVAD include its heavy weight and bulky size which mandates that the recipient body index must be larger than 1.5. In addition, the inflow valve failure or electrical motor failure is common after an average of 12 months of implantation [3–5, 14, 15].

The Thoratec® VAD [16] is used as an LVAD, RVAD, or BiVAD. It is implanted as a paracorporeal pump with the inflow cannula inserted in the left ventricle via the left ventricular apex and the outflow graft sewed to the ascending aorta when used as an LVAD, or the inflow cannula is inserted in the right atrium and the outflow graft is sewed to the pulmonary artery when used as an RVAD. It has numerous cannulation options. This device is made of a flexible sac housed in a plastic ball-shaped container. The sac material is composed of Thoralon which has a smooth surface to reduce the risk of thrombosis. The sac is squeezed by the compressed air via an air-driven console. The Thoratec® VAD has two mechanical valves—an inflow and outflow valve. It can be implanted in small or large size patients (weight between 17 and 144 kg), and can be used as short-term as well as long-term support. It is approved by the FDA to be used as a bridge-to-transplant and postcardiotomy support-to-recovery therapy. The disadvantages include inconvenience to patients being the paracorporeal pump is attached outside the body, and the need for patients to take anticoagulation therapy with coumadin to maintain an INR between 2.5 and 3.0 to prevent thromboembolism.

36.3.2 Axial Flow Pumps

Axial flow pumps are typically regarded as second-generation VADs, as compared to the first generation of volume displacement pumps. They incorporate continuous flow and rotary pump technology as the foundation of their design and manufacture, and have impellers inside the pumps that generate high-speed rotation in a blood system (Fig. 36.4). Depending on the motor

Fig. 36.4 HeartMate II left ventricular assist device. (**A**) Heartmate II pump and the high-speed rotor; the inflow cannula is connected to the pump. (**B**) Size comparison between the HeartMate VE and HeartMate II pumps; the inflow cannulas of both pumps are the same

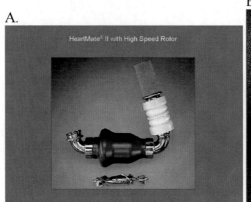

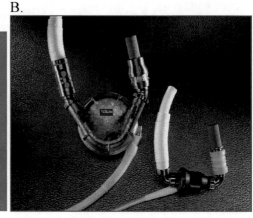

capacity and rotational speed, an axial flow pump can function either as a partial-flow or a full-flow support VAD. The speed of rotor can reach an RPM of 9000, and the pump can generate up to 10 L/min of flow at a mean pressure of 100 mmHg. Initially, serious doubts about such pumps were raised due to the concern of red blood cell destruction and heat generated by the high-speed motor inside the blood system. However, this theoretical concern was discarded when a hemopump was successfully used in a clinical setting without significant hemolysis [17]. The hemopump thus sets the stage for evaluation of other types of axial flow pumps that could be used for blood [6, 7, 9–11].

Common features of axial flow pumps include the following [6, 7, 9–11, 14, 15]: (1) the simpler design of continuous flow, rotary pump technology promises greater long-term mechanical reliability; (2) they do not require valves to create a unidirectional flow, nor do they require an external vent or a compliance chamber, thus making them more likely to be used as the platform for future development of a totally implantable VAD; (3) the inflow cannulas are inserted into the left ventricular apex or totally inside the left ventricle, and the outflow grafts are connected to the ascending or descending thoracic aorta; (4) the size of the pumps is small, 1/5–1/7 of the size of the volume displacement pumps, thereby extending therapy to underserved patient populations including women and even some children; and (5) these pumps are associated with minimal noise and greater patient comfort.

The HeartMate® II LVAD (Thoratec), the DeBakey MicroMed LVAD® (MicroMed Cardiovascular, Houston, TX), and Jarvik 2000 (Jarvik Heart, Inc., New York, NY) are the representatives of this group of VADs. Among them, the HeartMate® II and the DeBakey MicroMed LVAD have many similarities: (1) they are about the same size; (2) they consist of an internal blood pump with a percutaneous lead that connects the pump to an external system driver and power source; and (3) both pumps can generate up to 10 L/min of flow. To date, the accumulated clinical experience with axial flow pumps is small, compared with that of volume displacement pumps. However, initial results appear to be encouraging, with effective circulatory support and durability [6, 7, 9–11, 14, 15]. Diminished pulse pressure when utilizing an axial flow pump seemed to be tolerated well in patients, at least for the short term; the long-term consequences of axial flow pumps have yet to be evaluated. Hemolysis associated with axial flow pumps has been detectable, but is considered clinically insignificant. These pumps seem to activate platelets because of the physical strain on blood cells, yet such activation may be an important source of intravascular thrombosis and embolic complications. Intense anticoagulation regimens targeting platelet activation and clotting cascade have been employed to deal with the problems of thromboembolism. A combination of coumadin and plavix has been recommended for patients with the MicroMed LVAD.

Recently, several multicenter studies of the HeartMate II LVAD have shown improved clinical outcomes both as bridge-to-transplant and destination therapy, with markedly improved functional status and quality of life. An actuarial survival rate of 89% at 1 month and 75% at 6 months was reported. The HeartMate® II LVAD has proven to be safe and effective as bridge-to-transplant therapy. Compared to the HeartMate® XVE, the HeartMate II significantly reduced the device- and surgery-related complications. The lower incidence of postoperative bleeding and device-related infection may be due to its smaller size or the lack of need for a large pocket to house its pump and its smaller driveline. The absence of a large preperitoneal pocket (which was required with the larger pulsatile devices) has reduced: (1) the need for extensive dissection; (2) postoperative bleeding; and (3) LVAD pocket hematomas and the development of pocket infection. Based on the clinical trial outcomes [14, 15], the FDA recently approved HeartMate® II LVAD to be used as bridge-to-transplant therapy.

36.3.3 Centrifugal Pumps

Centrifugal pumps are considered the third generation of VADs. The technology used in these pumps can suspend and rotate blood flow in a magnetic field, avoiding any need for a contact point and thus eliminating the concern of wear of the rotor over a long period of time. Furthermore, such VADs have very little mechanical friction resistance to overcome; pulsatile flow can also be generated by a rapid variation of rotation speeds.

The VentrAssist LVAD (Ventracore, Chatswood, NSW, Australia) is a more recently developed third-generation centrifugal blood pump with hydrodynamic suspension (Fig. 36.5). It has only one moving part, an impeller, which consists of four small blades that are embedded with permanent magnets. The impeller blades spin when an electric current is sequentially switched between three pairs of oils contained within the pump's titanium housing. The impeller is suspended by a thin cushion of blood, within the gap of eight hydrodynamic bearings, one on each face of the four blades. Dynamic interplay between the eight hydrodynamic bearing forces, fluid forces, and gravitational forces prevents the spinning impeller from touching any part of the pump's housing.

The unique features of the VentrAssist design that have been incorporated to improve pump function, reliability, and durability include the following: hydrodynamic bearings, centrifugal design, diamond-like carbon coating, and biocompatible materials. The presence of hydrodynamic bearings has eliminated the frictional wear in the pump, and the diamond-like coating is believed to reduce the affinity for platelet deposition.

Recently published trials [18, 19] have supported the safety and efficacy of the VentrAssist LVAD as bridge-to-transplant therapy. Esmore et al. reported that 1 year after VentrAssist implantation in 33 bridge-to-transplant patients, >80% of patients achieved a successful outcome having been either transplanted or considered transplant eligible. Further, the incidence of adverse events was comparable to other currently used LVADs.

36.4 VAD Implantation Techniques

Implantation techniques for these three types of VADs are not significantly different from each other. The implantation for the later two VADs is probably easier because the need for tissue dissection is less for the smaller pumps and, subsequently, bleeding is reduced. A median sternotomy is performed and the patient is prepared for cardiopulmonary bypass. The pump is implanted in either the preperitoneal pocket below the posterior rectus sheath or inside the abdominal cavity (for the large pulsatile pump only). The inflow cannula is inserted through a cored out portion of the apex of the left ventricle, and the outflow graft is sewn to a longitudinal aortotomy in the proximal ascending aorta. Following appropriate connections, the patient is weaned off cardiopulmonary bypass and the pump is started. Optimizing pump speed is performed under echocardiographic guidance while monitoring patient hemodynamics. Adequate flow is achieved by adjusting pump speed and by ensuring adequate preload and appropriate inotropic support for right ventricular function. After meticulous hemostasis is achieved, the chest is closed with appropriately placed chest tubes.

36.5 Device Management

Standard postoperative care is used in the management of these patients. Device settings can be monitored and adjusted based on patient hemodynamics as well as echocardiographic findings. A combination of aspirin and warfarin is used as part of the anticoagulation protocol to maintain an INR between 2.0 and 2.5 for all the devices except the HeartMate® XVE, for which only aspirin is needed. The VAD flow is generally maintained above 4 L/min and the mean blood pressure is maintained over 60 mmHg. After LVAD placement, clinicians do not change defibrillator and biventricular pacing settings if patients had such a device implanted prior to VAD implantation. Finally, all patients undergo a standard postoperative rehabilitation program.

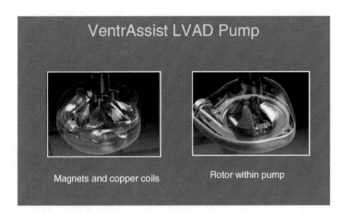

Fig. 36.5 VentrAssist left ventricular assist device (LVAD). The magnet and rotor within the pump are shown here

36.6 University of Minnesota VAD Experience

The University of Minnesota VAD and heart transplant program is one of the largest programs in the world. This program has been a participating center and leader in multiple NIH sponsored clinical trials, and six different types of VADs are used at our center currently. Since 1995, we have implanted 375 VADs for bridge-to-heart transplantation, bridge-to-bridge, bridge-to-recovery, and destination therapy. We developed an effective VAD implantation algorithm to successfully treat patients with refractory acute cardiogenic shock and multiorgan failure who would typically die [20] (Fig. 36.6). We also pioneered a minimally invasive LVAD exchange technique that avoided sternotomy [21] (Fig. 36.7). This minimally invasive LVAD implant and exchange technique made it possible for one patient to receive five LVAD exchanges, the most LVAD exchanges ever done in a single patient in the world to support one of the longest LVAD destination survivals in the world (Fig. 36.8).

36.7 Future

We have obtained abundant knowledge and experience from the use of earlier generations of VADs, and the future of ventricular assist devices is promising. The ideal future VAD should embody the following features:

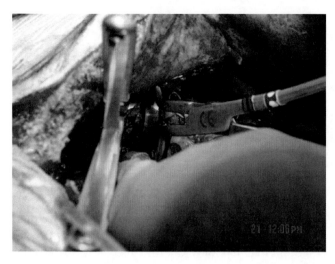

Fig. 36.7 Left ventricular assist device exchange is performed via laparotomy only, and sternotomy is avoided

1. It can provide adequate blood flow to meet the various physiological requirements.
2. It must be reliable and durable. For a VAD to be used as a destination therapy, 5–7 years has been suggested as an acceptable length of time for durability.
3. It must be biocompatible with the host and require no (or minimal) anticoagulation.

Fig. 36.6 Algorithm depicting the management of patients with refractory acute cardiogenic shock with multiorgan failure

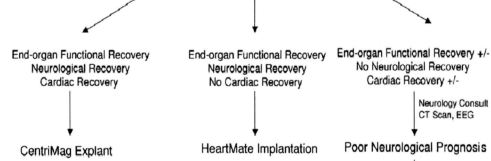

Fig. 36.8 The patient who received the fifth left ventricular assist device (LVAD) exchange. Photo was taken together with Dr. Kenneth Liao 3 weeks after his fifth LVAD exchange surgery

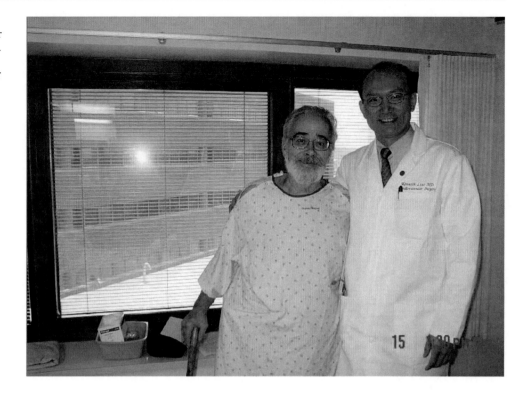

4. It must be small in size to minimize patient discomfort and ensure quality of life.
5. It should be easy to implant, preferably through a minimally invasive approach.

In the next 10 years, it is likely that we will see the birth of the "dream" VAD that meets the above-mentioned criteria. Perhaps one day implanting a VAD will be like implanting a prosthetic valve. Ultimately, the future of treating end-stage CHF lies in the cell therapy which can either reverse myocardium remodeling or regrow new myocardium.

References

1. Franco KL. New devices for chronic ventricular support. J Card Surg 2001;16:178–92.
2. Hosenpud JD, Bennett LE, Keck BM, Boucek MM, Novick RY. The registry of the international society for heart and lung transplantation: Eighteenth official report. J Heart Lung Transplant 2001;20:805–15.
3. Frazier OH, Rose EA, Oz MC, et al. Multicenter clinical evaluation of the HeartMate vented electric left ventricular assist system in patients awaiting heart transplantation. J Thorac Cardiovasc Surg 2001;122:1186–95.
4. Rose EA, Moskowitz AJ, Packer M, et al. The REMATCH trial: Rationale, design, and end points. Randomized Evaluation of Mechanical Assistance for the Treatment of Congestive Heart Failure. Ann Thorac Surg 1999;67:723–30.
5. Rose EA, Gelijns AC, Moskowitz AJ, et al. Long-term mechanical left ventricular assistance for end-stage heart failure. N Engl J Med 2001;345:1435–43.
6. Griffith BP, Kormos RL, Borovetz HS, et al. HeartMate II left ventricular assist system: From concept to first clinical use. Ann Thorac Surg 2001;71:116–120.
7. Frazier OH, Myers TJ, Westaby S, et al. Clinical experience with an implantable, intracardiac, continuous flow circulatory support device: Physiologic implications and their relationship to patient selection. Ann Thorac Surg 2004;77:133–42.
8. Esmore D, Kaye D, Spratt P, et al. A prospective, multicenter trial of the VentrAssist left ventricular assist device for bridge to transplant: Safety and efficacy. J Heart Lung Transplant 2008;27:579–88.
9. Goldstein DJ. Worldwide experience with the MicroMed DeBakey ventricular assist device as a bridge to transplantation. Circulation 2003;108:II272–77.
10. Westaby S, Banning AP, Jarvik R, et al. First permanent implant of the Jarvik 2000 Heart. Lancet 2000;356:900–03.
11. Wieselthaler GM, Schima H, Hiesmayr M, et al. First clinical experience with the DeBakey ventricular assist device continuous-axial-flow pump for bridge to transplantation. Circulation 2000;101:356–59.
12. Liao K, Li X, John R, et al. Mechanical stress: An independent determinant of early bioprosthetic calcification in human. Ann Thorac Surg 2008;86:491–5.
13. Rose EA, Levin HR, Oz MC, et al. Artificial circulatory support with textured interior surfaces. A counterintuitive approach to minimizing thromboembolism. Circulation 1994;90:II87–91.
14. Miller LW, Pagani FD, Russell SD, et al. Use of a continuous-flow device in patients awaiting heart transplantation. N Engl J Med 2007;357:885–96
15. Feller ED, Sorensen EN, Haddad M, et al. Clinical outcomes are similar in pulsatile and nonpulsatile left ventricular assist device recipients. Ann Thorac Surg 2007;83:1082–88.

16. Farrar DJ. The Toratec ventricular assist device: A paracorporeal pump for treating acute and chronic heart failure. Semin Thorac Cardiovasc Surg 2000;12:243–50.

17. Wampler RK, Baker BA, Wright WM. Circulatory support of cardiac interventional procedures with the Hemopump cardiac assist system. Cardiology 1994;84:194–201.

18. Esmore DS, Kaye D, Salamonsen R, et al. Initial clinical experience with the VentrAssist left ventricular assist device: The pilot trial. J Heart Lung Transplant 2008;27:479–85.

19. Esmore D, Kaye D, Spratt P, et al. A prospective, multicenter trial of the VentrAssist left ventricular assist device for bridge to transplant: Safety and efficacy. J Heart Lung Transplant 2008;27:579–88.

20. John R, Liao K, Lietz K, et al. Experience with the Levitronix CentriMag Circulatory support system as a bridge to decision in patients with refractory acute cardiogenic shock and multisystem organ failure. J Thorac Cardiovascular Surg 2007;134:351–58.

21. Liao K, Barksdale A, Park S, et al. Non-sternotomy approach for left ventricular assist device implantation, exchange or explantation. J Heart Lung Transplant 2007;26:S199.

Chapter 37
Cell Transplantation for Ischemic Heart Disease

Mohammad N. Jameel, Joseph Lee, Daniel J. Garry, and Jianyi Zhang

Abstract Cardiomyocyte regeneration may occur during physiological and pathological states in the adult heart; these data highlight the possibility that myocardial regeneration may occur via cardiomyocyte proliferation and/or differentiation of putative cardiac stem cells. To date, various cell types have been used for cardiac repair, including skeletal myoblasts, bone marrow-derived cells, mesenchymal stem cells, endothelial progenitor cells, umbilical cord blood stem cells, cardiac stem cells, and embryonic stem cells. This chapter will review each of these different stem cell populations in regard to the potential treatment of heart disease. It begins by examining the in vitro and in vivo animal studies, and then briefly discusses the cell therapy clinical trials that are currently underway for treating ischemic heart disease.

Keywords Embryonic stem cells · Adult stem cells · Skeletal myoblasts · Bone marrow-derived stem cells · Mesenchymal stem cells · Endothelial progenitor cells · Umbilical cord blood stem cells · Cardiac stem cells

37.1 Introduction

Although coronary interventions and associated medical therapies have improved post-infarction cardiac function in patients with coronary artery disease, approximately 45% still progress to end-stage heart failure [1]. To date, cardiac transplantation remains the only definitive therapy for replacing the lost muscle, but it is a widespread approach limited by the inadequate supply of donor hearts (approximately 2,200 donor hearts available each year in the United States). An alternative potential therapy for limiting post-infarction left ventricular (LV)

J. Zhang (✉)
University of Minnesota, Department of Medicine, 268 Variety Club Research Center, Minneapolis, MN 55455, USA
e-mail: zhang047@umn.edu

remodeling, and thus the development of congestive heart failure, is the focused replacement of infarcted myocardium with the new myocardium being generated from transplanted stem cells.

Recent studies have provided evidence to support the notion that cardiomyocyte regeneration may occur during physiological and pathological states in the adult heart; these data highlight the possibilities that myocardial regeneration may occur via cardiomyocyte proliferation and/or differentiation of putative cardiac stem cells [2]. Currently, various cell types have been used for cardiac repair, including skeletal myoblasts, bone marrow-derived cells, mesenchymal stem cells (MSCs), endothelial progenitor cells (EPCs), umbilical cord blood stem cells, cardiac stem cells, and embryonic stem cells (ESCs). In this chapter, we will review each of these different stem cell populations in regard to the potential treatment of heart disease. We will begin by examining the in vitro and in vivo animal studies, and then briefly discuss the cell therapy clinical trials that are currently underway for treating ischemic heart disease. We will conclude by summarizing selected techniques that have been used to enhance the beneficial effects of stem cell transplantation.

37.2 Cells for Myocardial Repair in Ischemic Heart Disease

37.2.1 Embryonic Stem Cells

Embryonic stem cells are considered to have tremendous therapeutic potential because they are pluripotent. They have the capacity to divide in an undifferentiated state while maintaining their ability to differentiate into cells belonging to all three embryonic germ layers. However, transplantation of these cells has certain limitations:

(1) they can form teratomas [3]; (2) they are immunogenic [4]; and (3) there are ethical concerns regarding their use.

37.2.1.1 Mouse Embryonic Stem Cells

The cardiogenic potential of mouse ESCs was first demonstrated in 1985 when these cells were cultured in suspension and formed 3D cystic bodies, termed embryoid bodies, which differentiated into cell types of the visceral yolk sac, blood islands, and myocardium [5]. Currently, such cells are separated from their feeder layer and then resuspended in leukemia inhibitory factor-free culture medium at a very low density [6]. Mouse ESCs are then cultured in small drops which are formed on the lid of tissue culture dishes. When kept in this hanging droplet setting for 2 days, the cells aggregate and form differentiating embryoid bodies [6]. Embryoid bodies are then transferred into ultralow attachment dishes where they further differentiate. Spontaneous contracting cells (cardiomyocytes) can be observed between 7 and 8 days of differentiation [6]. This process of cardiac differentiation can be further enhanced by the use of selective growth factors.

Importantly, mouse ESCs have been shown to engraft and regenerate myocardium after an induced myocardial infarction (MI) [7–9]. These cells can form cardiomyocytes that couple electrically with the host myocardium, endothelial cells, and blood vessels [7–9]. More recently, multipotent cardiac progenitor cells (CPCs) derived from mouse ESCs have been characterized from three independent laboratories [10–12]; Brachyury$^+$/Flk$^+$ and Isl1$^+$ CPC cell lines were shown to differentiate into cardiomyocytes, endothelial cells, and smooth muscle cells, while Nkx2-5/c-Kit CPCs could differentiate into cardiomyocytes and smooth muscle cells.

37.2.1.2 Human Embryonic Stem Cells

Human ESCs were first isolated from the human blastocyst in 1998 [3], and later it was shown that they could differentiate into cardiomyocytes [13]. Human ESCs also form embryoid bodies when cultured in suspension form; these are positive for cardiomyocyte markers such as myosin heavy chain, α-actinin, desmin, and troponin I [13]. Electrophysiological studies showed that most of the human ESC-derived cardiomyocytes resemble human fetal ventricular myocytes that can propagate action potentials [14]. Human ESCs can also differentiate into endothelial and smooth muscle cell lineages.

Initial in vivo studies have demonstrated that human ESC-derived cardiomyocytes can form new myocardium in the uninjured heart of athymic rats [15] or immunosuppressed pigs [14]. It was shown that the size of the graft could be increased fourfold by prior heat shock treatment of the cells [15]. When human ESCs are implanted in animal models that have a slow heart rate (such as in pigs or guinea pigs), they can form pacemakers when the native pacemaker (node) is dysfunctional, implying electrical integration with surrounding cardiomyocytes [14, 16]. However, when these cells are transplanted in the setting of MI, only 18% form myocardial grafts and these grafts also contain substantial noncardiac elements [17]. To enhance the yield and purity of cardiomyocytes from human ESC, Laflamme et al. developed a new technique to direct the differentiation of human ESC into cardiomyocytes using sequential treatment of high-density undifferentiated monolayer cultures with activin A and bone marrow morphogenic protein 4 [17]. This protocol has yielded greater than 30% cardiomyocytes, as compared to less than 1% with the embryoid body-based system which used serum to induce differentiation [17]. Furthermore, Percoll gradient centrifugation, which allows specific enrichment of human ESC-derived cardiomyocytes, resulted in cultures containing 82.6±6.6% cardiomyocytes [17]. Moreover, this laboratory used a prosurvival engraftment cocktail to improve graft survival in infarcted hearts. This cocktail included Matrigel to prevent anikis, a cell-permeant peptide from Bcl-XL to block mitochondrial death pathways, cyclosporine A to attenuate cyclophilin D-dependent mitochondrial pathways, a compound that opens ATP-dependent K$^+$ channels (pinacidil) to mimic ischemic preconditioning, insulin-like growth factor (IGF-1) to activate Akt pathways, and the caspase inhibitor ZVAD-fmk [17]. Importantly, transplantation of human ESC-derived cardiomyocytes, in combination with this prosurvival cocktail into infarcted hearts, resulted in myocardial grafts with improved ventricular function [17]. The other intriguing aspect of this study was that almost all noncardiac human ESC-derived cells died by the 4-week period [17].

37.2.2 Adult Stem Cells

37.2.2.1 Skeletal Myoblasts

Skeletal myoblasts are derived from satellite cells that lie in a quiescent state under the basal lamina of skeletal muscle fibers and yet can be rapidly mobilized, proliferate, and fuse to repair muscle after an injury [18]. Skeletal myoblasts form viable, long-term skeletal myotube grafts after transplantation into adult hearts [19]. In one study, it was shown that transplantation of autologous skeletal myoblasts in cryoinfarcted rabbit myocardium leads to myoblast engraftment at 3 weeks with subsequent improvement in systolic performance [18]. Importantly, as these cells are specified and committed to the skeletal muscle lineage, they do not differentiate into cardiomyocytes [20], and they are also not electromechanically coupled to each other or to the surrounding cardiomyocytes [21, 22].

37.2.2.2 Bone Marrow-Derived Stem Cells

The bone marrow contains many adult stem cells which have been used to treat hematological disorders for decades. It has recently been shown that bone marrow-derived stems can traverse cell lineage boundaries and, upon appropriate stimulation, transdifferentiate into hepatocytes, endothelial cells, skeletal muscle, and/or neurons [23–25]. Yet, the ability of bone marrow-derived cells to differentiate into cardiomyocytes remains controversial. For example, Bittner et al. were the first researchers to suggest that cardiac muscle cells may be derived from bone marrow cells [26]. Goodel et al. demonstrated that, following transplantation of murine bone marrow side population (SP) cells (c-kit$^+$, Sca-1$^+$, CD34$^-$/low), donor-derived cells with cardiomyocyte morphology as well as smooth muscle and endothelial cells were found in the heart following left anterior descending coronary artery ligation [27]. Orlic et al. [28] showed that transplantation of GFP-labeled Lin$^-$c-kit$^+$ cells (presumably containing both hematopoietic stem cells and mesenchymal stem cells) into the ventricular wall after left anterior descending coronary artery ligation resulted in improved function of the ventricle, and they detected a large number of GFP$^+$ cells that coexpressed myocardial proteins in the myocardium. In contrast to these findings, other laboratories using genetic mouse models to label cell populations (and their derivatives) have shown that lineage-negative, c-kit-positive cells did not differentiate into cardiomyocytes [29, 30]. On the other hand, more recently Anversa and colleagues have shown, using similar genetic techniques, that c-kit$^+$ bone marrow cells can engraft in the injured myocardium and differentiate into cells of the cardiogenic lineage, forming functionally competent cardiomyocytes and vascular structures [31].

37.2.2.3 Mesenchymal Stem Cells

Phenotype and Differentiation Potential

In the late 1980s and through the 1990s, Caplan's laboratory identified a subset of cells within the bone marrow which gave rise to osteoblasts and adipocytes and termed them mesenchymal stem cells (MSCs) [32]. MSCs are present in many different organs of the body including muscle, skin, adipose tissue, and bone marrow. They can be isolated from the bone marrow by a simple process involving Ficoll centrifugation and adhering cell culture in a defined serum-containing medium. In the early studies, MSCs were shown to be expanded for 4–20 population doublings only [33] with preservation of the karyotype, telomerase activity, and telomere length [34, 35]. Phenotypically, these cells were negative for CD31, CD34, and CD 45, unlike hematopoietic progenitors from bone marrow, and were positive for CD29, CD44, CD71, CD90, CD105, CD106, CD120a, CD124, SH2, SH3, and SH4 [36–38]. In the bone marrow, only 0.001–0.01% of the initial unfractionated bone marrow mononuclear cell population consists of MSCs [33, 36]. However, in a number of rodent studies, the adherent fibroblastic cells obtained from the unfractionated mononuclear class of the bone marrow are termed MSCs [39, 40].

MSCs were reported to have the potential to differentiate into any tissue of mesenchymal origin [32]. MSCs derived from rodent marrow aspiration have been shown to differentiate into cardiomyocyte-like cells in the presence of 5-azacytidine [41, 42]. The morphology of the cells changes from spindle-shaped to ball-shaped, and finally a rod-shaped form; thereafter, these cells fuse together to form a syncitium which resembles a myotube [43]. In addition, these cells exhibit markers of fetal cardiomyocytes [42]. Specific transcription factors of the myocyte and cardiac lineage including GATA4, Nkx2.5, and HAND 1/2 can be detected [41]. Yet, there are differences, as compared to native cardiomyocytes, to those derived from MSCs. First, the β-isoform of cardiac myosin heavy chain is more abundant than the α-isoform in these cells. Second, there is increased α-skeletal actin relative to α-cardiac actinin; myosin light chain 2v is also present. Third, both MEF2A and MEF2D isoforms replace MEF2C from early to late passage. Additionally, it was reported that these cells will beat spontaneously and synchronously, which is most likely due to the formation of intercalated discs, as has been shown when they are co-cultured with neonatal myocytes [44]. Finally, the differentiated cells will express competent α- and β-adrenergic and muscarinic receptors, as indicated by an increased rate of contraction in response to isoproterenol and a decreased rate of contraction induced by β-adrenergic blockers [45]. Yet, it should be noted that other studies suggest that bone marrow stem cells cannot differentiate to the cardiac myocytes [29, 30]. Finally, whether or not MSCs can differentiate into functional cells of the other three lineages will require further investigation.

Mesenchymal Stem Cells for Myocardial Repair

MSCs have several unique features that make them attractive candidates for cell transplantation. First, as they are easily accessible and expandable, MSCs could potentially become a so-called "off the shelf" allogeneic product, one which would be more cost-effective, easier to administer, and allow a greater number of cells to be transplanted. Additionally, they may also permit transplantation at the time of urgent interventions, e.g., to relieve ischemia and injury such as percutaneous or surgical revascularization procedures. Importantly, these cells appear to be hypoimmunogenic [46–48]. Additionally, these cells lack MHC-II and B-7 costimulatory molecule expression and thus limit T-cell responses [49, 50]. Yet, they are considered to directly inhibit inflammatory responses via paracrine mechanisms including production of transforming growth factor beta 1 and hepatocyte growth factor [51, 52]. Importantly, all the above properties taken together make them attractive candidates for cell transplantation.

It should be noted that MSC transplantation was tested in a study in which isogenic adult rats were used as donors and recipients to simulate autologous transplantation clinically. MSC intracoronary delivery in these rat hearts following an induced MI showed that there was a milieu-dependent differentiation of these cells, a fibroblastic phenotype within the scar, and cardiomyocyte phenotype outside the infarction area [53]. However, direct intramyocardial injection of autologous MSC into the scar resulted in the focal differentiation of these cells into "cardiac-like" muscle cells within the scar tissue. There was also noted increased angiogenesis and improved myocardial function [54]. In a different approach, the delivery of MSCs via direct left ventricular cavity infusion in a rat MI model resulted in the preferential migration and colonization of these cells in the ischemic myocardium (at 1 week) [55]. This MSC infusion also resulted in increased vascularity and improved cardiac function 2 months following delivery in a canine model of chronic ischemic disease [56]. However, it should be noted that Kloner's laboratory, using a rat model of post-infarction LV remodeling, found that the beneficial effects on left ventricular function were short term and were absent after 6 months [57].

Importantly, MSC transplantation has been reported to result in functional improvement in large animal models of MI. For example, the direct intramyocardial injection of 5-azacytadine-treated autologous MSCs was performed 4 weeks after MI in a swine model; these injected cells formed islands of cardiac-like tissue, induced angiogenesis, prevented thinning and dilatation of the infarct region, and ultimately improved regional

and global contractile function [58]. Similarly, allogeneic intramyocardial transplantation of MSCs in a porcine model of MI resulted in profound improvement in border zone energetic, regional contractile function [59]. These latter findings were hypothesized to be related to a paracrine mechanism, as evidenced by increased vascularity in the border zone, and spared native cardiomyocytes in the infarct zone [59]. Finally, the percutaneous delivery of allogenic MSCs 3 days after MI in a porcine model resulted in long-term engraftment (detected at 8 weeks), profound reduction in scar size, and near normalization of cardiac function [60].

37.2.2.4 Endothelial Progenitor Cells

Endothelial progenitor cells (EPCs) were first isolated from blood in 1997 [61]. They originate from a common hemangioblast precursor in the bone marrow [62]. However, many other cells including myeloid/monocyte ($CD14^+$) cells and stem cells from adult organs can also differentiate into cells with EPC characteristics. Thus, circulating EPCs are a heterogeneous group of cells originating from multiple precursors within the bone marrow and can be isolated in different stages of endothelial differentiation within peripheral blood. Therefore, the characterization of these cells can be challenging because they share certain surface markers of hematopoietic cells and adult endothelial cells. Typically, they express CD34 (a hematopoietic cell characteristic), CD-133 (a more specific marker of EPCs), and KDR (kinase insert domain-containing receptor), which is the receptor for vascular endothelial growth factor. Interestingly, in a study of sex-mismatched bone marrow transplant patients by Hebbel and coworkers, 95% of circulating endothelial cells in the peripheral blood of transplant patients had the recipient genotype, but 5% had the donor genotype [63]. It was found that the endothelial cells with the donor phenotype had delayed growth in culture, but had a high proliferative capacity with more than a 1000-fold expansion within 1 month, and were termed endothelial outgrowth cells. It was concluded that the endothelial outgrowth cells were of bone marrow origin [63]. In contrast, the cells with the recipient phenotype only had a 17-fold expansion within the same time period; these circulating endothelial cells most probably originated from the vessel wall [63].

EPCs have been used for treatment in different animal models of cardiovascular disease. The intravenous delivery of $CD34^+$ cells into athymic nude rats with MI was shown to promote angiogenesis in the peri-infarct region, leading to decreased myocyte apoptosis, reduced interstitial fibrosis, and improvement of left ventricular function

[64]. Similarly, intramyocardial implantation of CD34$^+$ selected human peripheral blood mononuclear cells into nude rats after MI resulted in neovascularization and improved LV function [65].

37.2.2.5 Umbilical Cord Blood Stem Cells

Human umbilical cord blood (UCB) is rich in stem and progenitor cells, which have high proliferative capacities [66–68]. Human UCB also contains fibroblast-like cells termed unrestricted somatic stem cells, which adhere to culture dishes, are negative for c-kit, CD34, and CD45, and differentiate both in vitro and in vivo into a variety of tissue types including cardiomyocytes [69]. Direct intramyocardial injection of these human unrestricted somatic cells into the infarcted hearts of immunosuppressed pigs resulted in (1) improved perfusion and wall motion; (2) reduced infarct size; and (3) enhanced cardiac function [70]. Further, intravenous injection of human mononuclear UCB cells, a small fraction of which were CD34$^+$, into NOD/SCID mice led to enhanced neovascularization with capillary endothelial cells of both human and mouse origin and reduced infarct sizes [71]. However, no myocytes of human origin were found, thus arguing against cardiomyogenic differentiation and regeneration of cardiomyocytes from donor cells. Finally, the direct intramyocardial injection of UCB CD34$^+$ cells into the peri-infarct rim in a rat model resulted in improved cardiac function [72]. To date, there have been no reported clinical studies of UCB transplantation.

37.2.2.6 Cardiac Stem Cells

Can the Heart Regenerate?

The innate ability of the cardiomyocytes to replicate has been a highly controversial issue for a long time. Previous studies have established that increases in cardiac mass in mammals during fetal life occur mainly due to cardiomyocyte proliferation. However, during the perinatal period, mammalian cardiomyocytes withdraw from the cell cycle, thus limiting their ability to divide and increase in number [73–75]. Thus, normal postnatal growth and adaptive increases in cardiac mass in adults, as a result of hemodynamic burden, are achieved mainly through the increase in cell size known as "hypertrophy" [73–75]. This belief was supported by the inability to identify mitotic figures in myocytes as well as the observation that regions of transmural infarction evolved into essentially avascular, thin collagenous scar. This paradigm of heart growth has been dominant over the past 50 years, and views the

heart as a post-mitotic organ consisting of a predetermined number of parenchymal cells that is defined at birth and preserved throughout life until the death of the organ and/or organism. However, recent studies have challenged this concept of the heart being a post-mitotic organ that is incapable of regeneration. It has been shown that the human heart contains cycling myocytes undergoing mitosis and cytokinesis under normal and pathological conditions [76–79]. The occurrence of these mitotic events is considered to support the hypothesis that cardiac progenitor cell populations reside in the adult heart and contribute to limited growth, turnover, and regeneration. This notion further supports that the adult heart belongs to the group of renewable adult tissues in which the capacity to replace cells depends on a resident stem cell population [80, 81].

Isolation of Cardiac Progenitor Cells

Cardiac progenitor cells (CPCs) have been isolated based on the expression (or absence) of specific cell surface markers, proteins, or tissue culture methods using the following strategies:

A. Isolation based on expression of the cell surface stem cell marker c-kit.
B. Isolation based on expression of the cell surface stem cell marker Sca-1.
C. Isolation based on the ability to efflux Hoechst 33342 dye (SP cells).
D. Isolation based on the expression of the islet-1 transcription factor.
E. Tissue culture of cardiac explants resulting in the spontaneous shedding of CPCs in vitro.

Isolation Based on Expression of the Cell Surface Stem Cell Marker c-kit

Beltrami et al. [82] isolated cells expressing the tyrosine kinase receptor for stem cell factor (also referred to as steel factor; c-kit) from the interstitial regions of the adult rat heart. The highest densities of these lineage negative (lin$^-$), c-kit$^+$ stem cells were in the atria and ventricular apex. These cells were identified to be self-renewing, clonogenic, and multipotent. Further, they had the ability to differentiate into cardiomocytes, endothelial cells, and smooth muscle cells. Moreover, the delivery of these c-kit-expressing clonogenic stem cells following myocardial injury resulted in both improved functional recovery and evidence of myocardial regeneration. Recently, the same laboratory expanded their analysis to include preclinical studies using large animal models. They have demonstrated that the canine model also harbors a c-kit-expressing stem cell population in the adult heart that is clonogenic, multipotent, and capable of activation following injury. In response to myocardial injury, these c-kit-expressing stem cells are activated by cytokines (including hepatocyte growth factor and insulin-like growth factor 1), and also home to areas of injury to participate in repair and regeneration. These preclinical studies have been further extended to the analysis of the human heart. A similar c-kit-expressing stem cell population (c-kit positive but negative for the expression of the hematopoietic and endothelial antigens including CD45, CD31, and CD34) has been isolated from the adult heart that was identified to be multipotent (capable of forming myocyte, smooth muscle cell, and endothelial cell lineages) in vivo and in vitro [83]. Moreover, studies have established that these human c-kit-expressing cardiac stem cells undergo both symmetrical and asymmetrical cell division [83]. Importantly, these studies are also currently being validated by other cardiac stem cell laboratories.

Isolation Based on the Expression of the Cell Surface Stem Cell Marker Sca-1

Resident murine CPCs have also been isolated on the basis of stem cell antigen-1 (Sca-1) expression [84]. These Sca-1-expressing CPCs were small interstitial cells that lacked hematopoietic lineage markers such as CD45, B220, TER119, or Flk-1, and they lacked c-kit expression, supporting the notion that they are distinct from the c-kit stem cell population. Using RT-PCR analysis, the Sca-1-expressing CPC population expressed the vascular marker CD31 and the cardiogenic transcription factors including Gata4, Mef2c, and TEF-1 (but lacked expression of Nkx2-5). A small percentage of these Sca-1-expressing CPCs activated cardiac genes, but did not exhibit spontaneous contractile properties in response to DNA demethylation with 5-azacytidine [84]. This laboratory further examined the ability of the Sca-1 CPCs to form cardiomyocytes independent of fusion to the differentiated host cardiomyocytes using genetic mouse models (Cre/Lox and the R26R genetic mouse models) for cellular labeling. Genetically tagged Sca-1 CPCs isolated from the αMHC-Cre transgenic mouse model and delivered into the R26R (all host cells are labeled with LacZ) injured the heart. Two weeks following injury, the animals were killed and hearts were examined for Cre and LacZ expression. Approximately half of the cells expressing αMHC-Cre did not express LacZ, suggesting that the Sca-1-expressing cells are capable of myocardial differentiation independent of fusion to existing (host) cardiomyocytes [84]. Additional studies from another laboratory (Matsuura and coworkers) have also isolated Sca-1$^+$

cells from adult murine hearts, and have demonstrated that they are capable of differentiation into beating cardiomyocytes in the presence of oxytocin but not 5-azacytidine [85]. These Sca-1 CPCs are heterogeneous, but a subpopulation is capable of effluxing Hoechst 33342 dye.

Isolation Based on the Ability to Efflux Hoechst 33342 Dye (SP Cells)

Recent efforts have utilized flow cytometry to identify an adult stem cell population that is capable of effluxing Hoechst 33342 dye. Due to their ability to efflux Hoechst 33342 dye, these cells were located as a side population using flow cytometry and were termed SP cells. Subsequently, these SP cells have been isolated from a number of lineages including adult bone marrow, skeletal muscle, lung, brain, liver, and mouse embryonic stem cells. These respective SP cell populations are multipotent when placed in a permissive environment. The ability of the SP cells to efflux the Hoechst dye is due to the presence of multidrug resistance proteins. Studies have demonstrated that Abcg2 is a member of the ATP [86] binding cassette (ABC) transporters (also known as multidrug resistance proteins), and is the molecular determinant for the SP cell phenotype. Both specific (FTC) and nonspecific (calcium channel blockers such as verapamil) blockers of Abcg2 prevent Hoechst 33342 dye exclusion. Abcg2-expressing SP cells participate in cardiac development and reside in the adult mouse heart. Following injury, these Abcg2-expressing cardiac SP cells increase in number and form fetal cardiomyocytes. In addition to serving as a marker for the SP cell population, Abcg2 has a cytoprotective function in response to oxidative stress. Moreover, recent studies have demonstrated that Hif2α is a direct upstream regulator of the Abcg2 gene. These results support the notion that CPCs in the adult heart likely play a protective role that promotes survival following injury.

To date, whole genome analyses using microarray platforms have examined the molecular signature of adult cardiac SP cells, adult bone marrow SP cells, adult skeletal muscle SP cells, and SP cells isolated from embryonic stem cells. As expected, cardiac SP cells express Abcg2, Sca-1, and c-kit. They also have induction of signaling pathways including the notch-signaling pathway and the Wnt-signaling pathway, which are characteristic of a number of other stem cell populations. Yet, the cardiac SP cells largely lack expression of hematopoietic markers (CD45 and TER119). Importantly, the cardiac SP cells appear to be a subpopulation of the Sca-1-expressing CPCs. Other groups have isolated so-called SP cells from mouse hearts based on their ability to exclude Hoechst 33342 dye [86, 87]. These cells express Abcg2, an ATP-binding cassette (ABC) transporter, and they are Sca-1$^+$ and c-kit low, and differentiate into cardiomyocytes after co-culture with rat cardiomyocytes.

Isolation Based on Expression of Islet-1 Gene

Recent studies by Laugwitz et al. have identified Isl-1-expressing cells as an important stem cell population during cardiac development [88]. The heart is derived from a primary heart field and a secondary heart field which segregate from a common progenitor at gastrulation. The primary heart field (which gives rise to the cardiac crescent) contributes to the left ventricle and atria, while the secondary heart field (which is derived from the pharyngeal mesoderm) gives rise to the right ventricle and the outflow tract. Utilizing a gene disruption strategy, embryos lacking Isl-1 are lethal and lack a secondary heart field (i.e., right ventricle and outflow tract), supporting the notion that Isl-1 is a critical regulator for cardiac development. Additional studies have further uncovered an Isl-1-expressing multipotent cardiac stem cell population that expresses Nkx2-5 and Flk-1 and gives rise to all the cardiac lineages (cardiomyocyte, smooth muscle, and endothelial cells) during heart development. While Isl-1-expressing cells are resident in the neonatal heart, there is no evidence of an Isl-1-expressing CPC population in the unperturbed or injured adult heart. Future studies will be necessary to define distinct and common molecular pathways that govern stem cell populations during cardiac development and regeneration of the adult injured heart. For more information on cardiac development, refer to Chapter 3.

Tissue Culture of Cardiac Explants with Spontaneous Shedding of CPCs In Vitro

In 2004, Messina et al. isolated undifferentiated cells that grew as self-adherent clusters (termed "cardiospheres") from subcultures of postnatal atrial or ventricular human biopsy specimens and also from murine hearts [89]. These cardiospheres varied in size (20–150 μm) and were observed to beat spontaneously in culture. The cardiosphere-forming cells had the properties of adult cardiac stem cells as they were clonogenic; they expressed stem and endothelial progenitor cell antigens/markers (c-kit, Sca-1, CD31 and Flk-1), were capable of long-term self-renewal, and could differentiate in vitro and in vivo into myocytes and endothelial cells [89]. Importantly, the expansion of the cardiosphere-forming cells resulted in more than one million human cardiospheres within a 1-month period. These studies were confirmed and expanded as Marban's group obtained ventricular tissue from percutaneous endomyocardial biopsies from

both humans and pigs. These ventricular biopsy specimens were cultured to form cardiospheres, which were further plated to yield cardiosphere-derived cells [90]. Cardiospheres and cardiosphere-derived cells expressed antigenic characteristics of stem cells at each stage of processing as well as proteins vital for cardiac contractile and electrical function [90]. Human and porcine cardiosphere-derived cells co-cultured with neonatal rat ventricular myocytes exhibited biophysical signatures characteristic of myocytes, including calcium transients synchronous with those of neighboring myocytes [90]. Moreover, the delivery of cardiosphere-derived cells following myocardial injury resulted in improved myocardial function compared to their respective controls.

Number of Cardiac Progenitor Cells

In 2005, Anversa and coworkers proposed that CPCs are undifferentiated multipotent cells that express the stem cell-related antigens, c-kit, MDR-1 (another ABC transporter), and Sca-1, in variable combinations [91]. Quantitative data in mouse, rat, dog, and human heart were provided that demonstrated there is approximately one CPC for every 30,000–40,000 myocardial cells. Interestingly, ~65% of all CPCs possess the three stem cell antigens, ~20% express two stem cell antigens, and ~15% express only one; roughly 5% each of these CPCs exclusively express c-kit, MDR1, or Sca-1 [91].

Importantly, none of these above-mentioned reports demonstrated a signature CPC phenotype; this cell population also has significant overlap in the expression of other surface markers. It remains to be determined whether these CPCs are actually the same stem cell type and that differing surface markers reflect differing developmental phases or qualitatively separate subpopulations. Nevertheless, it is believed that these CPCs may participate in myocyte turnover, the rate of which remains to be determined.

Origin of the Cardiac Progenitor Cell

To date, the primary origins of CPCs remain unclear. It is feasible that the cycling cardiomyocytes might be derived from uncommitted stem-like population cells that reside in the heart which expand and differentiate into cardiomyocytes in response to signals and cues in response to growth and/or injury. Alternatively, these stem-like cells may reside in extracardiac tissues such as the bone marrow, and are capable of being recruited into the circulation and induced to home to the heart by signals emanating from the injured heart.

Recently, Mouquet et al. demonstrated that cardiac SP cells are maintained by local progenitor cell proliferation under physiological conditions [92]. After MI, this cardiac SP is decreased by as much as 60% in the infarct and to a lesser degree in the noninfarct regions within 1 day. Cardiac SP pools are subsequently reconstituted to baseline levels within 7 days after MI, through both proliferation of resident cardiac SP cells and by homing of bone marrow-derived stem cells to specific areas of myocardial injury. These cells then undergo immunophenotypic conversion and adopt a cardiac SP phenotype (CD45$^+$ to CD45$^-$) [92]. Interestingly, bone marrow-derived stem cells accounted for approximately 25% of the SP cells in the heart under pathological conditions, as compared to <1% under physiological conditions [92]. In addition to these CD45$^+$ cells that Mouquet et al. reported, bone marrow also contains CD45$^-$, CXCR4$^+$, and Sca-1$^+$ cells within the nonadherent, nonhematopoietic mononuclear fraction, which will express early cardiac markers such as Nkx2.5 and GATA-4 [93]. These cells can also mobilize into the blood after MI and eventually home to the infarcted myocardium in mice. Cerisoli et al. [94] also demonstrated that (at least in pathological conditions) a subpopulation of the c-kit$^+$ CPC population may derive from cells that originate in the bone marrow which are capable of contributing to myocardial regeneration in a similar fashion as the CPCs that are resident in the adult heart.

Myocardial Regeneration from Cardiac Progenitor Cells

Anversa and coworkers demonstrated that the direct intramyocardial injection of c-kit$^+$ cells into an ischemic rat heart reconstituted well-differentiated myocardium, comprised of new blood-carrying vessels and cardiomyocytes with the characteristics of fetal cells; these cells were present in approximately 70% of the ventricle [82]. Later, it was also shown that intracoronary delivery of these cardiac stem cells in an ischemia/reperfusion rat model resulted in myocardial regeneration, infarct size reduction of 29%, and improvement of LV function [95]. Given intravenously after ischemia/reperfusion, Sca-1 cells also homed to injured myocardium and differentiated into cardiomyocytes [84]. The relative contributions of regenerated cardiomyocytes and preservation of injured native cardiomyocytes in these studies require clarification.

Wang et al. recently reported that heart-derived Sca-1$^+$/CD31$^-$ cells possess stem cell characteristics and play an important role in cardiac repair [96]. In that study, immunofluorescent staining and fluorescence-activated cell sorter analysis indicated that endogenous Sca-1$^+$/CD31$^-$ cells significantly increased in the infarct and peri-infarct areas at 3 and 7 days after MI. Western blotting confirmed elevated Sca-1 protein expression 7 days after MI. Sca-1$^+$/CD31$^-$ cells cultured in vitro were induced to express both endothelial cell and cardiomyocyte markers. Transplantation of Sca-1$^+$/CD31$^-$cells into a murine model of MI led to functional preservation and decreased remodeling after MI [96]. Immunohistochemical data indicated a significant increase of neovascularization, but a low level of cardiomyocyte regeneration at the infarct border zone. Despite the absence of significant cardiomyocyte regeneration, cell transplantation remarkably improved myocardial bioenergetics [96]. These findings provide evidence that Sca-1$^+$/CD31$^-$ cells possess both endothelial cell and cardiomyocyte progenitor cell characteristics. However, this study also reported that the regeneration rates of cardiomyocytes and/or endothelial cells from the engrafted stem cells were very low. Hence, trophic effects associated with the transplanted cells were most likely the primary basis of the beneficial effects of these cells [96]. Nevertheless, the expansion of these progenitor cells may have therapeutic applicability for the treatment of MI.

CPCs and early committed cells have been shown to (1) express c-Met and IGF-1 receptors and (2) synthesize and secrete the corresponding ligands, such as hepatocyte growth factor (HGF) and IGF-1 [97]. HGF mobilizes cardiac stem cells–early committed cells, and IGF-1 promotes their survival and proliferation [97]. Therefore, in a separate study, HGF and IGF-1 were injected in mice following MI and a growth factor gradient was introduced between the site of storage of primitive cells in the atria and the region bordering the infarct to facilitate homing. Importantly, the newly formed myocardium contained arterioles, capillaries, and functionally competent myocytes that increased in size over time. This regenerative response was associated with improved ventricular performance and overall increased survival. Surprisingly, this intervention rescued animals with infarcts that comprised as much as 86% of ventricular mass, which implied the elicited low ejection fractions. More recently, the above findings were replicated in a dog model, where HGF and IGF-1 were also used to stimulate resident cardiac stem cells after MI; noteworthy growth factor therapy again resulted in improvement of myocardial function [98].

Before they can be used therapeutically, CPCs have to be isolated from fragments of the myocardium and subsequently expanded in vitro. This was achieved in a pig model [99], where c-kit$^+$ cells were isolated and each cell was propagated to form approximately 400,000 cells. Another group performed autologous transplantation of CPCs in an ischemia/reperfusion swine model [100]. To accomplish this, each pig had an initial biopsy from the right ventricular septum at the time of injury. The biopsies weighed approximately 92 mg, and yielded mean cell counts of 14.2×10^6 cells after isolation and expansion (after 2.8 cell passages over 23 days). Intracoronary delivery was then performed 4 weeks after injury; engraftment primarily occurred in the MI border zone and islands of engrafted cells were present within the scar 8 weeks after coronary delivery [100].

Human cardiac progenitor cells have also been isolated from the myocardium, expanded in vitro, and then used for transplantation in animal models of ischemic myocardium. For example, Hosoda et al. isolated human CPCs from surgical samples [101], then these c-kit$^+$ human CPCs were injected into the hearts of immunodeficient mice and rats. Foci of myocardial regeneration were identified at 2–3 weeks which consisted of myocytes, resistance arterioles, and capillaries [101]. The presence of connexin 43 and N-cadherin in the developing human myocytes strongly suggested that the engrafted human cells were functionally competent. Two-photon microscopy was used to further demonstrate the functional integration of enhanced green fluorescent protein positive human myocytes with the surrounding myocardium [101]. More recently, Torella et al. [102] also isolated human CPCs from myocardial samples from all four chambers of the human heart; these were c-kit$^+$, MDR-1$^+$, and CD133$^+$. In these studies, one clone was shown to generate over 5×10^9 cells and form functional myocardium after injection into infarcted rat hearts [102].

Altogether, these studies provide early evidence of the rationale for the use of human cardiac progenitor cells in patients with ischemic heart disease. These cells appear to be excellent candidates for exogenous stem cell therapy, yet they must be harvested from patients and expanded ex vivo to generate numbers sufficient for transplantation. To date, there have been no reported clinical trials of human cardiac progenitor cell therapy.

37.3 An Update of Performed Clinical Trials of Stem Cell Treatment in Heart Disease

Skeletal myoblasts were the first cell type to be used in therapeutic clinical trials. These cells can be transplanted in an autologous fashion without immunosuppression, and have several advantages including a high proliferative potential that allows an initial biopsy to be easily expanded in vitro. They are also terminally differentiated, thus decreasing the chances of tumorigenesis, and are known to be resistant to ischemia, allowing them to

survive in scar or periscar areas where there is minimal perfusion. To date, there have been six phase I safety and feasibility studies of skeletal myoblast transplantation in patients with severe LV dysfunction caused by MI. Four of these studies [103–106] were surgical and entailed myoblast implantation at the time of coronary artery bypass grafting or left ventricular assist device implantation, and two were catheter-based trials [107, 108] using an endoventricular or coronary sinus transvenous approach. Although improvement of LV function was not the primary outcome of these studies, it did tend to be improved after transplantation. Engraftment of myoblasts has been documented in pathological specimens up to 18 months after transplantation [105, 109]. Yet, some concerns regarding the development of ventricular tachycardia have prompted the use of intracardiac defibrillators in protocols for skeletal myoblast transplantation. Future studies may utilize the use of skeletal muscle stem cells (i.e., satellite cells) as opposed to well-differentiated myoblasts.

Bone marrow cells have also received intense interest as a cell therapy for patients with cardiovascular disease. Importantly, the Transplantation of Progenitor Cells and Regeneration Enhancement in Acute Myocardial Infarction (TOPCARE-AMI) trial revealed significant improvement in LV ejection fraction as well as significantly enhanced myocardial viability and regional wall motion in the infarct regions following transplantation of bone marrow mononuclear cells or blood-derived progenitor cells [110, 111]. The BOOST (bone marrow cell transfer to enhance ST-elevation infarct regeneration) study [112] also resulted in an increase in LV ejection fraction at 6 months following cell transplantation, but surprisingly there was no statistical difference between the treated and placebo groups at 18 months. The Reinfusion of Enriched Progenitor Cells and Infarct Remodeling in Acute Myocardial Infarction (REPAIR-AMI) trial [113] randomized 204 patients with acute MI to receive either an intracoronary infusion of progenitor cells derived from bone marrow or a placebo medium into the infarct artery 3–7 days after successful reperfusion therapy. It was reported that the absolute increase in LV ejection fraction was significantly greater (2.5%) in the bone marrow cell group than in the placebo group at 4 months. However, other trials (i.e., ASTAMI- Autologous Stem Cell Transplantation in Acute Myocardial Infarction and STEMI-ST-elevation Acute Myocardial Infarction) [114, 115] have shown negative results with no improvement in ejection fraction with cell transplantation; differences in cell preparation [116] and numbers have been proposed as possible causes for these conflicting results. Bone marrow cells have also been used in the chronic heart failure setting. For example, in the Transplantation of

Progenitor Cells and Recovery of LV Function in Patients with Chronic Ischemic Heart Disease (TOP-CARE-CHD) trial [117], 75 patients with stable ischemic heart disease who had an MI at least 3 months previously were assigned to receive (1) no cell infusion; (2) infusion of circulating progenitor cells; or (3) bone marrow cell into the patent coronary artery supplying the most dyskinetic LV area. It was reported that the transplantation of bone marrow cells was associated with a moderate (2.9 percentage points), but significant improvement in LV function 3 months post-transplantation.

MSC transplantation has been used therapeutically in patients with acute MI 18 days after primary percutaneous intervention, and this resulted in significant improvement in LV ejection fraction up to 6 months following delivery [118, 119]. Furthermore, this was associated with a significant reduction in the size of the perfusion defect measured by positron emission tomography at 3 months following delivery [118, 119]. More recently, it has been demonstrated in a randomized double-blind placebo-controlled trial that intravenous delivery of allogenic human MSCs led to improved ventricular function after MI [120]. Yet, the degree of response to intravenous therapy occurred early after MI, and compared favorably with previous studies using intracoronary infusions of bone marrow cells [120].

The clinical application of EPCs is limited by the fact that it is difficult to expand them into sufficient numbers without either inducing a change in their phenotype or the development of cell senescence. Recently, Erb et al. randomized patients with chronically occluded coronary arteries to receive intracoronary progenitor cells or a placebo; they mobilized bone marrow cells using GCSF, harvested them from peripheral blood, and expanded them ex vivo. Subsequently, the intracoronary delivery of these cells led to improvement in coronary flow reserve and cardiac function at 3 months post-transplant [121]. Currently, clinical trials using CD34$^+$ cells from bone marrow that are enriched in EPC content are underway.

37.4 Mechanisms of Beneficial Effects of Stem Cell Treatment

Several studies using animal models have established that stem cell treatment leads to a functional benefit after MI. The initial results from the human clinical trials are also promising; however, to date, the mechanisms underlying the beneficial effects of stem cell transplantation remain somewhat unclear. The proposed mechanisms are discussed below.

37.4.1 Primary Remuscularization

First, the replacement of infarcted tissue by new myocardium generated by the transplanted cells is one explanation for the beneficial effects. This was observed in the case of human cardiac stem cells, which are able to form functional myocardium after transplantation into mice with MI; the transplanted cardiomyocytes were structurally integrated with the host myocardium and led to improvement in ventricular function [83]. This was also observed after the delivery of cardiomyocytes derived from human embryonic stem cells which were transplanted into mice with induced MIs [17]. To date, the ability of bone marrow cells to transdifferentiate into cardiomyocytes remains controversial with some reports suggesting that these cells can transdifferentiate into cardiomyocytes [31], while other reports refute this claim [29]. Other adult stem cells such as skeletal myoblasts and EPCs are not able to form cardiomyocytes, but have been found to still exert a beneficial effect, thus suggesting other mechanisms for improvement in LV function.

37.4.2 Attenuation of Adverse Remodeling

The human ventricle remodels after an injury (i.e., MI) and this process may consist of ventricular dilatation, wall thinning, increased chamber volume, and/or hypertrophy of the surrounding myocardium [122]. In general, this leads to increased wall stress and increased metabolic demand. Importantly, stem cell transplantation has been shown to reduce wall thinning and ventricular dilatation leading to functional improvement.

37.4.3 Improved Perfusion

Enhanced blood flow, as measured by microspheres, has been shown to increase after stem cell transplantation in a rat model following MI [123]. Increased blood flow can be due to new vessel formation (angiogenesis) or enlargement of preexisting collaterals (arteriogenesis). A number of the stem cell populations discussed in this chapter have been shown to promote or contribute to neovascularization after transplantation in the setting of MI. Yet, some groups have challenged this concept and have shown that stem cells home to the region of developing vascular collateralization, but do not anatomically incorporate into the vessel as either endothelial or smooth muscle cells [124]; however, the delivery of these cell populations still improves collateral flow.

37.4.4 Paracrine Effects

Stem cells may secrete factors that act through totally different repair pathways to ultimately promote cardioprotection. Evidence supporting such a hypothesis recently emerged from Dzau's laboratory; they showed that the injection of conditioned medium from Akt-overexpressing MSCs alone can decrease the infarct size and lead to functional improvement in an animal model of MI [125, 126]. Hypoxic Akt-transduced MSCs showed increased release of vascular endothelial growth factor (VEGF), FGF-2, IGF-1, HGF, and thymosin β4. It is likely that various factors acting in concert will ultimately exert numerous beneficial effect, as anti-VEGF and anti-FGF antibodies only partially decreased the conditioned medium-induced proliferation of endothelial and smooth muscle cells [127, 128].

37.4.5 Immunomodulation of the Infarct Environment

The inflammatory response after an MI has been recognized as a potential target for improving functional outcome after acute MI. Some stem cells may act, in part, by modulating the immune environment within the recently infarcted heart. For example, MSCs have been shown to directly inhibit the inflammatory responses via paracrine mechanisms including the production of transforming growth factor beta 1 and hepatocyte growth factor [51, 52].

37.4.6 Modulation of Extracellular Matrix Homeostasis

Remodeling of the ventricle is also known to involve modifications in the extracellular matrix which are thought to contribute to myocardial dysfunction. As such, MSC implantation in a rat model of MI significantly attenuated the increased expression of collagen types I and III, TIMP-1, and TGF-β, but had no effects on MMP-1 levels [129, 130]. This was associated with reduced LV dilatation and improved global ventricular function.

37.4.7 Stimulation of Endogenous Cardiac Progenitors Cells

Stem cell treatment could also lead to increased mobilization, differentiation, survival, and function of endogenous cardiac progenitor cells that are associated with the paracrine effects.

37.5 Techniques of Enhancing Efficacy of Stem Cell Therapy

Although stem cell transplantation improves LV function after MI, to date, the observed stem cell engraftment is still found to be minimal. Furthermore, the majority of transplanted cells that do engraft remain as spindle-shaped stem cells, and do not fully differentiate into the host cardiac cell phenotypes. Therefore, other techniques are considered necessary to enhance the efficacy of stem cell transplantation.

37.5.1 Mobilization

Granulocyte colony-stimulating factor, VEGF, stromal cell-derived factor-1 (SDF-1), angiopoeitin-1, placental growth factor, and erythropoietin are several factors that may be utilized as therapies to mobilize stem cells from the bone marrow to the systemic circulation. Once these stem cells are mobilized, they may participate in endogenous repair or alternatively be collected and expanded in vitro for future cell therapy uses. As an example, intracoronary infusion of peripheral blood stem cells mobilized by granulocyte colony-stimulating factor resulted in the improvement of LV function in patients with MI [131].

37.5.2 Homing

An important goal is to enhance the homing of stem cells to the injured region of the heart. It is known that factors that contribute to the homing of stem cells include stromal-derived growth factor (SDF-1) [132, 133], high mobility group box protein 1 [134], and integrins. It is also known that the microenvironment after acute MI is more favorable to cell homing as compared to the chronically infarcted myocardium. For example, Lu et al. [135] examined the local conditions requisite for cell homing and migration using a rat model of permanent coronary artery ligation, and concluded that the optimal time period for cell homing and migration is within the 2-week period following an MI.

37.5.3 Function and Survival

Assuming that the number of transplanted cells that survive is critical to therapeutic benefit, multiple research groups are exploring new methods to increase the survival of transplanted cells. As such, apoptosis can be decreased by the constitutive expression of Akt (a serine threonine kinase with potent prosurvival activity) or by heat shock prior to transplantation [136]. Furthermore, rat MSCs transduced to overexpress Akt1 (encoding the Akt protein) transplanted into ischemic myocardium were found to inhibit cardiac remodeling by reducing inflammation, collagen deposition, and myocyte hypertrophy in a dose-dependent fashion [137]. Similarly, MSCs transduced to express Akt were also studied in an ischemic porcine model, which showed an improvement in ejection fraction as compared to nontransduced MSCs. Recently, in order to determine the exact mechanisms of these beneficial effects, the effects of the apoptotic stimulus, H_2O_2, on MSCs transduced with Akt were studied in vitro. Specifically, Akt-MSCs were found to be more resistant to apoptosis and were related to higher levels of extracellular signal-regulated protein kinase activation and VEGF expression [138]. Yet, a significant concern also exists regarding the potential tumorigenicity of Akt-transduced cells, particularly when Akt is constitutively expressed, because Akt has been shown to be sufficient to induce oncogenic transformation of cells and tumor formation; therapeutic efforts are underway to target the Akt pathway for the treatment of malignancies [139]. Additional strategies that have been widely tested involve those to increase vasculogenesis with VEGF; transfection with VEGF and IGF-1 improved survival of transplanted bone marrow cells in a rat model of MI [140]. Furthermore, it was observed that the delivery of cells which had undergone adenoviral transduction and overexpressed VEGF also resulted in improved LV function and neovascularization [141], but the addition of VEGF protein alone to cells did not show any benefit in a rat model of fetal cardiomyocyte transplantation [142].

Enhanced expression of other gene products has also been examined and found to be effective, including cardiotrophin-1, heme oxygenase-1, an IL-1 inhibitor, and CuZn-superoxide dismutase. It was also shown that MSCs transfected with a hypoxia-regulated heme oxygenase-1 vector were found to be more tolerant to hypoxiareoxygen injury in vitro and resulted in improved viability in ischemic hearts [143]. Likewise, treatment with CuZn-superoxide dismutase has been shown to attenuate the initial rapid cell death following transplantation, leaving a twofold increase in the total number of engrafted cells at 72 h compared with controls [144].

To date, the use of viruses for gene expression cannot be translated into clinical studies due to the risk of mutagenesis, carcinogenesis, and induction of an immune response. Yet recently, Jo et al. [145] developed a nonviral carrier of cationized polysaccharide for the genetic engineering of MSCs. When genetically engineered by a spermine–dextran complex with plasmid DNA of adrenomedullin, MSCs secreted a large amount of adrenomedullin, an antiapoptotic and angiogenic peptide. Transplantation of these adrenomedullin gene-engineered MSCs improved cardiac function after MI significantly more than did nontransduced MSCs. Thus, this genetic engineering technology using the nonviral spermine–dextran (and other promising new methods) is an emerging strategy to improve MSC therapy for ischemic heart disease.

37.5.4 Use of Biomaterials to Design Microenvironment

The microenvironment in which the cells are injected is of extreme importance for their survival and subsequent beneficial effects. It has been shown that biomaterials can be designed to regulate quantitative timed release of factors, which direct cellular differentiation pathways such as angiogenesis and vascular maturation. Moreover, it is believed that smart biomaterials are capable of responding to the local environment, such as protease activity or mechanical forces, with controlled release or activation [146]. Specifically, cell sheet technology has been used to transplant a monolayer of MSCs in an ischemic myocardium with functional improvement [147]. Similarly, cardiac patches are 3D matrices composed of natural or synthetic scaffold materials that can house the cells to allow longer cell viability, and enhance differentiation and integration. These patches may also be designed to contain factors that enhance neovascularization to allow the patch to survive in ischemic tissue. For example, Zhang et al. showed that the controlled release of stromal cell-derived factor-1α (SDF-1α) in situ increased stem cell homing to the infarcted heart [148]. Likewise, PEGylated fibrinogen bound with recombinant mouse SDF-1α was mixed with thrombin to form a PEGylated fibrin patch which was placed on the surface of the infarct region of the LV after acute MI; 2 weeks after infarction, the myocardial recruitment of c-kit$^+$ cells was significantly higher in the SDF-1α PEGylated fibrin patch treated group. Moreover, the LV function was significantly improved compared with the control groups. Recently, Davis et al. [149] designed self-assembling peptide nanofibers for the prolonged delivery of IGF-1, a cardiomyoyte growth and differentiation factor, to the myocardium, using a "biotin sandwich" strategy.

Specifically, biotinylated IGF-1 was complexed with tetravalent streptavidin and then bound to biotinylated self-assembling peptides. After injection into rat myocardium, biotinylated nanofibers provided sustained IGF-1 delivery for 28 days, and targeted delivery of IGF-1 in vivo increased the activation of Akt in the myocardium. Therefore, cell therapeutic strategies using IGF-1 delivery by biotinylated nanofibers improved systolic function after experimental MI, demonstrating the importance of engineering the local cellular microenvironment and the impact of these and future interventions will need to improve the outcomes of cell therapy.

Importantly, many of these new biomaterials provide improved flexibility for regenerating tissues ex vivo, but emerging technologies such as self-assembling nanofibers can now establish intramyocardial cellular microenvironments following injection. This may allow percutaneous cardiac regeneration and repair approaches, i.e., injectable tissue engineering. It has been shown that materials can be made to multifunction by providing sequential signals with the custom design of differential release kinetics for individual factors. Thus, new rationally designed biomaterials no longer simply coexist with tissues, but can provide precision bioactive control of the microenvironment that may be required for cardiac regeneration and repair.

List of Abbreviations

CPCs	cardiac progenitor cells
EPCs	endothelial progenitor cells
ESCs	embryonic stem cells
HGF	hepatocyte growth factor
IGF-1	insulin-like growth factor
LV	left ventricular
MI	myocardial infarction
MSCs	mesenchymal stem cells
Sca-1	stem cell antigen-1
SDF-1	stromal cell-derived factor-1
SP	side population
UCB	umbilical cord blood
VEGF	vascular endothelial growth factor

References

1. Weir RA, McMurray JJ. Epidemiology of heart failure and left ventricular dysfunction after acute MI. Curr Heart Fail Rep 2006;3:175–80.
2. Anversa P, Nadal-Ginard B. Myocyte renewal and ventricular remodelling. Nature 2002;415:240–43.
3. Thomson JA, Itskovitz-Eldor J, Shapiro SS, et al. Embryonic stem cell lines derived from human blastocysts. Science 1998;282:1145–47.
4. Nussbaum J, Minami E, Laflamme MA, et al. Transplantation of undifferentiated murine embryonic stem cells in the heart: Teratoma formation and immune response. Faseb J 2007;21:1345–57.
5. Doetschman TC, Eistetter H, Katz M, et al. The in vitro development of blastocyst-derived embryonic stem cell lines: Formation of visceral yolk sac, blood islands and myocardium. J Embryol Exp Morphol 1985;87:27–45.
6. Wobus AM, Guan K, Yang HT, et al. Embryonic stem cells as a model to study cardiac, skeletal muscle, and vascular smooth muscle cell differentiation. Methods Mol Biol 2002;185:127–56.
7. Kolossov E, Bostani T, Roell W, et al. Engraftment of engineered ES cell-derived cardiomyocytes but not BM cells restores contractile function to the infarcted myocardium. J Exp Med 2006;203:2315–27.
8. Min JY, Yang Y, Converso KL, et al. Transplantation of embryonic stem cells improves cardiac function in postinfarcted rats. J Appl Physiol 2002;92:288–96.
9. Singla DK, Hacker TA, Ma L, et al. Transplantation of embryonic stem cells into the infarcted mouse heart: Formation of multiple cell types. J Mol Cell Cardiol 2006;40:195–200.
10. Kattman SJ, Huber TL, Keller GM. Multipotent flk-1 + cardiovascular progenitor cells give rise to the cardiomyocyte, endothelial, and vascular smooth muscle lineages. Dev Cell 2006;11:723–32.
11. Moretti A, Caron L, Nakano A, et al. Multipotent embryonic isl1 + progenitor cells lead to cardiac, smooth muscle, and endothelial cell diversification. Cell 2006;127:1151–65.
12. Wu SM, Fujiwara Y, Cibulsky SM, et al. Developmental origin of a bipotential myocardial and smooth muscle cell precursor in the mammalian heart. Cell 2006;127:1137–50.
13. Kehat I, Kenyagin-Karsenti D, Snir M, et al. Human embryonic stem cells can differentiate into myocytes with structural and functional properties of cardiomyocytes. J Clin Invest 2001;108:407–14.
14. Kehat I, Khimovich L, Caspi O, et al. Electromechanical integration of cardiomyocytes derived from human embryonic stem cells. Nat Biotechnol 2004;22:1282–89.
15. Laflamme MA, Gold J, Xu C, et al. Formation of human myocardium in the rat heart from human embryonic stem cells. Am J Pathol 2005;167:663–71.
16. Xue T, Cho HC, Akar FG, et al. Functional integration of electrically active cardiac derivatives from genetically engineered human embryonic stem cells with quiescent recipient ventricular cardiomyocytes: Insights into the development of cell-based pacemakers. Circulation 2005;111:11–20.
17. Laflamme MA, Chen KY, Naumova AV, et al. Cardiomyocytes derived from human embryonic stem cells in pro-survival factors enhance function of infarcted rat hearts. Nat Biotechnol 2007;25:1015–24.
18. Taylor DA, Atkins BZ, Hungspreugs P, et al. Regenerating functional myocardium: Improved performance after skeletal myoblast transplantation. Nat Med 1998;4:929–33.
19. Koh GY, Klug MG, Soonpaa MH, et al. Differentiation and long-term survival of C2C12 myoblast grafts in heart. J Clin Invest 1993;92:1548–54.
20. Dowell JD, Rubart M, Pasumarthi KB, et al. Myocyte and myogenic stem cell transplantation in the heart. Cardiovasc Res 2003;58:336–50.
21. Murry CE, Wiseman RW, Schwartz SM, et al. Skeletal myoblast transplantation for repair of myocardial necrosis. J Clin Invest 1996;98:2512–23.

22. Leobon B, Garcin I, Menasche P, et al. Myoblasts transplanted into rat infarcted myocardium are functionally isolated from their host. Proceedings of the National Academy of Sciences of the United States of America 2003;100:7808–11.

23. Ferrari G, Cusella-De Angelis G, Coletta M, et al. Muscle regeneration by bone marrow-derived myogenic progenitors. Science 1998;279:1528–30.

24. Krause DS, Theise ND, Collector MI, et al. Multi-organ, multilineage engraftment by a single bone marrow-derived stem cell. Cell 2001;105:369–77.

25. Mezey E, Chandross KJ, Harta G, et al. Turning blood into brain: Cells bearing neuronal antigens generated in vivo from bone marrow. Science 2000;290:1779–82.

26. Bittner RE, Schofer C, Weipoltshammer K, et al. Recruitment of bone-marrow-derived cells by skeletal and cardiac muscle in adult dystrophic mdx mice. Anat Embryol 1999;199:391–96.

27. Jackson KA, Majka SM, Wang H, et al. Regeneration of ischemic cardiac muscle and vascular endothelium by adult stem cells. J Clin Invest 2001;107:1395–402.

28. Orlic D, Kajstura J, Chimenti S, et al. Bone marrow cells regenerate infarcted myocardium. Nature 2001;410:701–05.

29. Murry CE, Soonpaa MH, Reinecke H, et al. Haematopoietic stem cells do not transdifferentiate into cardiac myocytes in myocardial infarcts. Nature 2004;428:664–68.

30. Balsam LB, Wagers AJ, Christensen JL, et al. Haematopoietic stem cells adopt mature haematopoietic fates in ischaemic myocardium. Nature 2004;428:668–73.

31. Rota M, Kajstura J, Hosoda T, et al. Bone marrow cells adopt the cardiomyogenic fate in vivo. Proceedings of the National Academy of Sciences of the United States of America 2007;104:17783–88.

32. Caplan AI. Mesenchymal stem cells. J Orthop Res 1991;9:641–50.

33. Prockop DJ. Marrow stromal cells as stem cells for nonhematopoietic tissues. Science 1997;276:71–74.

34. Phinney DG, Kopen G, Righter W, et al. Donor variation in the growth properties and osteogenic potential of human marrow stromal cells. J Cell Biochem 1999;75:424–36.

35. Pittenger MF, Mackay AM, Beck SC, et al. Multilineage potential of adult human mesenchymal stem cells. Science 1999;284:143–47.

36. Pittenger MF, Martin BJ. Mesenchymal stem cells and their potential as cardiac therapeutics. Circ Res 2004;95:9–20.

37. Majumdar MK, Keane-Moore M, Buyaner D, et al. Characterization and functionality of cell surface molecules on human mesenchymal stem cells. J Biomed Sci 2003;10:228–41.

38. Haynesworth SE, Baber MA, Caplan AI. Cell surface antigens on human marrow-derived mesenchymal cells are detected by monoclonal antibodies. Bone 1992;13:69–80.

39. Alhadlaq A, Mao JJ. Mesenchymal stem cells: isolation and therapeutics. Stem Cells Dev 2004;13:436–48.

40. Minguell JJ, Erices A, Conget P. Mesenchymal stem cells. Exp Biol Med 2001;226:507–20.

41. Fukuda K. Molecular characterization of regenerated cardiomyocytes derived from adult mesenchymal stem cells. Congenit Anom 2002;42:1–9.

42. Makino S, Fukuda K, Miyoshi S, et al. Cardiomyocytes can be generated from marrow stromal cells in vitro. J Clin Invest 1999;103:697–705.

43. Fukuda K. Use of adult marrow mesenchymal stem cells for regeneration of cardiomyocytes. Bone Marrow Transplant 2003;32(Suppl 1):S25–27.

44. Tomita S, Nakatani T, Fukuhara S, et al. Bone marrow stromal cells contract synchronously with cardiomyocytes in a coculture system. Jpn J Thorac Cardiovasc Surg 2002;50:321–24.

45. Hakuno D, Fukuda K, Makino S, et al. Bone marrow-derived regenerated cardiomyocytes (CMG Cells) express functional adrenergic and muscarinic receptors. Circulation 2002;105:380–86.

46. Bartholomew A, Sturgeon C, Siatskas M, et al. Mesenchymal stem cells suppress lymphocyte proliferation in vitro and prolong skin graft survival in vivo. Exp Hematol 2002;30:42–48.

47. Le Blanc K, Tammik L, Sundberg B, et al. Mesenchymal stem cells inhibit and stimulate mixed lymphocyte cultures and mitogenic responses independently of the major histocompatibility complex. Scand J Immunol 2003;57:11–20.

48. Tse WT, Pendleton JD, Beyer WM, et al. Suppression of allogeneic T-cell proliferation by human marrow stromal cells: Implications in transplantation. Transplantation 2003;75:389–97.

49. Zimmet JM, Hare JM. Emerging role for bone marrow derived mesenchymal stem cells in myocardial regenerative therapy. Basic Res Cardiol 2005;100:471–81.

50. Ryan JM, Barry FP, Murphy JM, et al. Mesenchymal stem cells avoid allogeneic rejection. J Inflamm 2005;2:8.

51. Le Blanc K, Tammik C, Rosendahl K, et al. HLA expression and immunologic properties of differentiated and undifferentiated mesenchymal stem cells. Exp Hematol 2003;31:890–96.

52. Di Nicola M, Carlo-Stella C, Magni M, et al. Human bone marrow stromal cells suppress T-lymphocyte proliferation induced by cellular or nonspecific mitogenic stimuli. Blood 2002;99:3838–43.

53. Wang JS, Shum-Tim D, Chedrawy E, et al. The coronary delivery of marrow stromal cells for myocardial regeneration: pathophysiologic and therapeutic implications. J Thorac Cardiovasc Surg 2001;122:699–705.

54. Tomita S, Li RK, Weisel RD, et al. Autologous transplantation of bone marrow cells improves damaged heart function. Circulation 1999;100:II247–56.

55. Barbash IM, Chouraqui P, Baron J, et al. Systemic delivery of bone marrow-derived mesenchymal stem cells to the infarcted myocardium: Feasibility, cell migration, and body distribution. Circulation 2003;108:863–68.

56. Silva GV, Litovsky S, Assad JA, et al. Mesenchymal stem cells differentiate into an endothelial phenotype, enhance vascular density, and improve heart function in a canine chronic ischemia model. Circulation 2005;111:150–56.

57. Dai W, Hale SL, Martin BJ, et al. Allogeneic mesenchymal stem cell transplantation in postinfarcted rat myocardium: short- and long-term effects. Circulation 2005;112:214–23.

58. Tomita S, Mickle DA, Weisel RD, et al. Improved heart function with myogenesis and angiogenesis after autologous porcine bone marrow stromal cell transplantation. J Thorac Cardiovasc Surg 2002;123:1132–40.

59. Zeng L, Hu Q, Wang X, et al. Bioenergetic and functional consequences of bone marrow-derived multipotent progenitor cell transplantation in hearts with postinfarction left ventricular remodeling. Circulation 2007;115:1866–75.

60. Amado LC, Saliaris AP, Schuleri KH, et al. Cardiac repair with intramyocardial injection of allogeneic mesenchymal stem cells after MI. Proceedings of the National Academy of Sciences of the United States of America 2005;102:11474–79.

61. Asahara T, Murohara T, Sullivan A, et al. Isolation of putative progenitor endothelial cells for angiogenesis. Science 1997;275:964–67.

62. Masuda H, Asahara T. Post-natal endothelial progenitor cells for neovascularization in tissue regeneration. Cardiovasc Res 2003;58:390–98.

63. Lin Y, Weisdorf DJ, Solovey A, et al. Origins of circulating endothelial cells and endothelial outgrowth from blood. J Clin Invest 2000;105:71–77.

64. Kocher AA, Schuster MD, Szabolcs MJ, et al. Neovascularization of ischemic myocardium by human bone-marrow-derived angioblasts prevents cardiomyocyte apoptosis, reduces remodeling and improves cardiac function. Nat Med 2001;7:430–36.

65. Kawamoto A, Tkebuchava T, Yamaguchi J, et al. Intramyocardial transplantation of autologous endothelial progenitor cells for therapeutic neovascularization of myocardial ischemia. Circulation 2003;107:461–68.

66. Lewis ID, Verfaillie CM. Multi-lineage expansion potential of primitive hematopoietic progenitors: Superiority of umbilical cord blood compared to mobilized peripheral blood. Exp Hematol 2000;28:1087–95.

67. Murohara T, Ikeda H, Duan J, et al. Transplanted cord blood-derived endothelial precursor cells augment postnatal neovascularization. J Clin Invest 2000;105:1527–36.

68. Mayani H, Lansdorp PM. Biology of human umbilical cord blood-derived hematopoietic stem/progenitor cells. Stem Cells 1998;16:153–65.

69. Kogler G, Sensken S, Airey JA, et al. A new human somatic stem cell from placental cord blood with intrinsic pluripotent differentiation potential. J Exp Med 2004;200:123–35.

70. Kim BO, Tian H, Prasongsukarn K, et al. Cell transplantation improves ventricular function after a MI: A preclinical study of human unrestricted somatic stem cells in a porcine model. Circulation 2005;112:I96–104.

71. Ma N, Stamm C, Kaminski A, et al. Human cord blood cells induce angiogenesis following MI in NOD/scid-mice. Cardiovasc Res 2005;66:45–54.

72. Hirata Y, Sata M, Motomura N, et al. Human umbilical cord blood cells improve cardiac function after MI. Biochem Biophys Res Commun 2005;327:609–14.

73. MacLellan WR, Schneider MD. Genetic dissection of cardiac growth control pathways. Annu Rev Physiol 2000;62:289–319.

74. Rubart M, Field LJ. Cardiac regeneration: Repopulating the heart. Annu Rev Physiol 2006;68:29–49.

75. Soonpaa MH, Field LJ. Survey of studies examining mammalian cardiomyocyte DNA synthesis. Circ Res 1998;83:15–26.

76. Beltrami AP, Urbanek K, Kajstura J, et al. Evidence that human cardiac myocytes divide after MI. N Engl J Med 2001;344:1750–57.

77. Quaini F, Urbanek K, Beltrami AP, et al. Chimerism of the transplanted heart. N Engl J Med 2002;346:5–15.

78. Anversa P, Kajstura J. Ventricular myocytes are not terminally differentiated in the adult mammalian heart. Circ Res 1998;83:1–14.

79. Nadal-Ginard B, Kajstura J, Leri A, et al. Myocyte death, growth, and regeneration in cardiac hypertrophy and failure. Circ Res 2003;92:139–50.

80. Anversa P, Sussman MA, Bolli R. Molecular genetic advances in cardiovascular medicine: focus on the myocyte. Circulation 2004;109:2832–38.

81. Sussman MA, Anversa P. Myocardial aging and senescence: Where have the stem cells gone? Annu Rev Physiol 2004;66:29–48.

82. Beltrami AP, Barlucchi L, Torella D, et al. Adult cardiac stem cells are multipotent and support myocardial regeneration. Cell 2003;114:763–76.

83. Bearzi C, Rota M, Hosoda T, et al. Human cardiac stem cells. Proceedings of the National Academy of Sciences of the United States of America 2007;104:14068–73.

84. Oh H, Bradfute SB, Gallardo TD, et al. Cardiac progenitor cells from adult myocardium: homing, differentiation, and fusion after infarction. Proceedings of the National Academy of Sciences of the United States of America 2003;100:12313–18.

85. Matsuura K, Nagai T, Nishigaki N, et al. Adult cardiac Sca-1-positive cells differentiate into beating cardiomyocytes. J Biol Chem 2004;279:11384–91.

86. Martin CM, Meeson AP, Robertson SM, et al. Persistent expression of the ATP-binding cassette transporter, Abcg2, identifies cardiac SP cells in the developing and adult heart. Dev Biol 2004;265:262–75.

87. Pfister O, Mouquet F, Jain M, et al. CD31⁻ but Not CD31⁺ cardiac side population cells exhibit functional cardiomyogenic differentiation. Circ Res 2005;97:52–61.

88. Laugwitz KL, Moretti A, Lam J, et al. Postnatal isl1⁺ cardioblasts enter fully differentiated cardiomyocyte lineages. Nature 2005;433:647–53.

89. Messina E, De Angelis L, Frati G, et al. Isolation and expansion of adult cardiac stem cells from human and murine heart. Circ Res 2004;95:911–21.

90. Smith RR, Barile L, Cho HC, et al. Regenerative potential of cardiosphere-derived cells expanded from percutaneous endomyocardial biopsy specimens. Circulation 2007;115:896–908.

91. Leri A, Kajstura J, Anversa P. Cardiac stem cells and mechanisms of myocardial regeneration. Physiol Rev 2005;85:1373–416.

92. Mouquet F, Pfister O, Jain M, et al. Restoration of cardiac progenitor cells after MI by self-proliferation and selective homing of bone marrow-derived stem cells. Circ Res 2005;97:1090–92.

93. Kucia M, Dawn B, Hunt G, et al. Cells expressing early cardiac markers reside in the bone marrow and are mobilized into the peripheral blood after MI. Circ Res 2004;95:1191–99.

94. Cerisoli F, Chimenti I, Gaetani R, et al. Kit-Positive Cardiac Stem Cells (CSCs) can be generated in damaged heart from bone marrow-derived cells. Circulation 2006;114:II-164.

95. Dawn B, Stein AB, Urbanek K, et al. Cardiac stem cells delivered intravascularly traverse the vessel barrier, regenerate infarcted myocardium, and improve cardiac function. Proceedings of the National Academy of Sciences of the United States of America 2005;102:3766–71.

96. Wang X, Hu Q, Nakamura Y, et al. The role of the sca-1⁺/CD31⁻ cardiac progenitor cell population in postinfarction left ventricular remodeling. Stem Cells 2006;24:1779–88.

97. Urbanek K, Rota M, Cascapera S, et al. Cardiac stem cells possess growth factor-receptor systems that after activation regenerate the infarcted myocardium, improving ventricular function and long-term survival. Circ Res 2005;97:663–73.

98. Linke A, Muller P, Nurzynska D, et al. Stem cells in the dog heart are self-renewing, clonogenic, and multipotent and regenerate infarcted myocardium, improving cardiac function. Proceedings of the National Academy of Sciences of the United States of America 2005;102:8966–71.

99. Bearzi C, Muller P, Amano K, et al. Identification and characterization of Cardiac Stem Cells in the Pig heart. Circulation 2006;114:II-125.

100. Johnston P, Sasano T, Mills K, et al. Isolation, expansion and delivery of cardiac derived stem cells in a porcine model of MI. Circulation 2006;114:II-125.

101. Hosoda T, Bearzi C, Amano S, et al. Human cardiac progenitor cells regenerate cardiomyocytes and coronary vessels repairing the infarcted myocardium. Circulation 2006;114:II-51.

102. Torella D, Elliso GM, Karakikes I, et al. Biological properties and regenerative potential, in vitro and in vivo, of human cardiac stem cells isolated from each of the four chambers of the adult human heart. Circulation 2006;114:II-87.

103. Menasche P, Hagege AA, Vilquin JT, et al. Autologous skeletal myoblast transplantation for severe postinfarction left ventricular dysfunction. J Am Coll Cardiol 2003;41:1078–83.

104. Herreros J, Prosper F, Perez A, et al. Autologous intramyo-cardial injection of cultured skeletal muscle-derived stem cells in patients with non-acute MI. Eur Heart J 2003;24:2012–20.

105. Pagani FD, DerSimonian H, Zawadzka A, et al. Autologous skeletal myoblasts transplanted to ischemia-damaged myocar-dium in humans. Histological analysis of cell survival and differentiation. J Am Coll Cardiol 2003;41:879–88.

106. Siminiak T, Kalawski R, Fiszer D, et al. Autologous skeletal myoblast transplantation for the treatment of postinfarction myocardial injury: Phase I clinical study with 12 months of follow-up. Am Heart J 2004;148:531–37.

107. Smits PC, van Geuns RJ, Poldermans D, et al. Catheter-based intramyocardial injection of autologous skeletal myoblasts as a primary treatment of ischemic heart failure: Clinical experi-ence with six-month follow-up. J Am Coll Cardiol 2003;42:2063–69.

108. Siminiak T, Fiszer D, Jerzykowska O, et al. Percutaneous trans-coronary-venous transplantation of autologous skeletal myoblasts in the treatment of post-infarction myocardial con-tractility impairment: The POZNAN trial. Eur Heart J 2005;26:1188–95.

109. Hagege AA, Carrion C, Menasche P, et al. Viability and differentiation of autologous skeletal myoblast grafts in ischaemic cardiomyopathy. Lancet 2003;361:491–92.

110. Assmus B, Schachinger V, Teupe C, et al. Transplantation of Progenitor Cells and Regeneration Enhancement in Acute Myocardial Infarction (TOPCARE-AMI). Circulation 2002;106:3009–17.

111. Schachinger V, Assmus B, Britten MB, et al. Transplantation of progenitor cells and regeneration enhancement in acute MI: final one-year results of the TOPCARE-AMI Trial. J Am Coll Cardiol 2004;44:1690–99.

112. Wollert KC, Meyer GP, Lotz J, et al. Intracoronary autolo-gous bone-marrow cell transfer after MI: The BOOST rando-mised controlled clinical trial. Lancet 2004;364:141–48.

113. Schachinger V, Erbs S, Elsasser A, et al. Intracoronary bone marrow-derived progenitor cells in acute MI. N Engl J Med 2006;355:1210–21.

114. Lunde K, Solheim S, Aakhus S, et al. Intracoronary injection of mononuclear bone marrow cells in acute MI. N Engl J Med 2006;355:1199–209.

115. Janssens S, Dubois C, Bogaert J, et al. Autologous bone marrow-derived stem-cell transfer in patients with ST-segment elevation MI: Double-blind, randomised controlled trial. Lan-cet 2006;367:113–21.

116. Seeger F, Tonn T, Krzossok N, et al. Cell isolation procedures matter: A comparison of different isolation protocols of bone marrow mononuclear cells used for cell therapy in patients with acute MI. Circulation 2006;114:II-51.

117. Assmus B, Honold J, Schachinger V, et al. Transcoronary transplantation of progenitor cells after MI. N Engl J Med 2006;355:1222–32.

118. Chen SL, Fang WW, Qian J, et al. Improvement of cardiac function after transplantation of autologous bone marrow mesenchymal stem cells in patients with acute MI. Chin Med J 2004;117:1443–48.

119. Chen SL, Fang WW, Ye F, et al. Effect on left ventricular function of intracoronary transplantation of autologous bone marrow mesenchymal stem cell in patients with acute MI. Am J Cardiol 2004;94:92–95.

120. Zambrano J, Traverse JH, Henry T, et al. Abstract 1014: The impact of intravenous allogeneic human mesenchymal stem cells (ProvacelTM) on ejection fraction in patients with myo-cardial infarction. Circ Suppl 2007;116:II-202.

121. Erbs S, Linke A, Adams V, et al. Transplantation of blood derived progenitor cells after recanalization of chronic

122. Pfeffer MA, Braunwald E. Ventricular remodeling after MI. Experimental observations and clinical implications. Circula-tion 1990;81:1161–72.

123. Reffelmann T, Dow JS, Dai W, et al. Transplantation of neonatal cardiomyocytes after permanent coronary artery occlusion increases regional blood flow of infarcted myocar-dium. J Mol Cell Cardiol 2003;35:607–13.

124. Ziegelhoeffer T, Fernandez B, Kostin S, et al. Bone marrow-derived cells do not incorporate into the adult growing vascu-lature. Circ Res 2004;94:230–38.

125. Gnecchi M, He H, Liang OD, et al. Paracrine action accounts for marked protection of ischemic heart by Akt-modified mesenchymal stem cells. Nat Med 2005;11:367–68.

126. Gnecchi M, He H, Noiseux N, et al. Evidence supporting paracrine hypothesis for Akt-modified mesenchymal stem cell-mediated cardiac protection and functional improvement. Faseb J 2006;20:661–69.

127. Kinnaird T, Stabile E, Burnett MS, et al. Marrow-derived stromal cells express genes encoding a broad spectrum of arteriogenic cytokines and promote in vitro and in vivo arter-iogenesis through paracrine mechanisms. Circ Res 2004;94: 678–85.

128. Kinnaird T, Stabile E, Burnett MS, et al. Local delivery of marrow-derived stromal cells augments collateral perfusion through paracrine mechanisms. Circulation 2004;109:1543–49.

129. Xu X, Xu Z, Xu Y, et al. Effects of mesenchymal stem cell transplantation on extracellular matrix after MI in rats. Cor-onary artery disease 2005;16:245–55.

130. Xu X, Xu Z, Xu Y, et al. Selective down-regulation of extra-cellular matrix gene expression by bone marrow derived stem cell transplantation into infarcted myocardium. Circ J 2005; 69:1275–83

131. Kang HJ, Lee HY, Na SH, et al. Differential effect of intra-coronary infusion of mobilized peripheral blood stem cells by granulocyte colony-stimulating factor on left ventricular func-tion and remodeling in patients with acute MI versus old MI: the MAGIC Cell-3-DES randomized, controlled trial. Circu-lation 2006;114:I145–51.

132. Ceradini DJ, Kulkarni AR, Callaghan MJ, et al. Progenitor cell trafficking is regulated by hypoxic gradients through HIF-1 induction of SDF-1. Nat Med 2004;10:858–64.

133. Askari AT, Unzek S, Popovic ZB, et al. Effect of stromal-cell-derived factor 1 on stem-cell homing and tissue regeneration in ischaemic cardiomyopathy. Lancet 2003;362:697–703.

134. Limana F, Germani A, Zacheo A, et al. Exogenous high-mobility group box 1 protein induces myocardial regeneration after infarction via enhanced cardiac C-kit + cell proliferation and differentiation. Circ Res 2005;97:e73–83.

135. Lu L, Zhang JQ, Ramires FJ, et al. Molecular and cellular events at the site of MI: from the perspective of rebuilding myocardial tissue. Biochem Biophys Res Commun 2004;320:907–13.

136. Zhang M, Methot D, Poppa V, et al. Cardiomyocyte grafting for cardiac repair: graft cell death and anti-death strategies. J Mol Cell Cardiol 2001;33:907–21.

137. Mangi AA, Noiseux N, Kong D, et al. Mesenchymal stem cells modified with Akt prevent remodeling and restore perfor-mance of infarcted hearts. Nat Med 2003;9:1195–201.

138. Lim SY, Kim YS, Ahn Y, et al. The effects of mesenchymal stem cells transduced with Akt in a porcine MI model. Cardi-ovasc Res 2006;70:530–42.

139. Cheng JQ, Lindsley CW, Cheng GZ, et al. The Akt/PKB pathway: Molecular target for cancer drug discovery. Onco-gene 2005;24:7482–92.

140. Yau TM, Kim C, Li G, et al. Maximizing ventricular function with multimodal cell-based gene therapy. Circulation 2005;112:I123–28.

141. Askari A, Unzek S, Goldman CK, et al. Cellular, but not direct, adenoviral delivery of vascular endothelial growth factor results in improved left ventricular function and neovascularization in dilated ischemic cardiomyopathy. J Am Coll Cardiol 2004;43:1908–14.

142. Schuh A, Breuer S, Al Dashti R, et al. Administration of vascular endothelial growth factor adjunctive to fetal cardiomyocyte transplantation and improvement of cardiac function in the rat model. J Cardiovasc Pharmacol Ther 2005;10:55–66.

143. Tang YL, Tang Y, Zhang YC, et al. Improved graft mesenchymal stem cell survival in ischemic heart with a hypoxia-regulated heme oxygenase-1 vector. J Am Coll Cardiol 2005;46:1339–50.

144. Suzuki K, Murtuza B, Beauchamp JR, et al. Dynamics and mediators of acute graft attrition after myoblast transplantation to the heart. Faseb J 2004;18:1153–55.

145. Jo JI, Nagaya N, Miyahara Y, et al. Transplantation of genetically engineered mesenchymal stem cells improves cardiac function in rats with MI: Benefit of a novel nonviral vector, Cationized Dextran. Tissue Eng 2007;13:313–22.

146. Davis ME, Hsieh PC, Grodzinsky AJ, et al. Custom design of the cardiac microenvironment with biomaterials. Circ Res 2005;97:8–15.

147. Miyahara Y, Nagaya N, Kataoka M, et al. Monolayered mesenchymal stem cells repair scarred myocardium after MI. Nat Med 2006;12:459–65.

148. Zhang G, Wang X, Wang Z, et al. A PEGylated fibrin patch for mesenchymal stem cell delivery. Tissue Eng 2006;12:9–19.

149. Davis ME, Hsieh PC, Takahashi T, et al. Local myocardial insulin-like growth factor 1 (IGF-1) delivery with biotinylated peptide nanofibers improves cell therapy for MI. Proceedings of the National Academy of Sciences of the United States of America 2006;103:8155–60.

Chapter 38
Emerging Cardiac Devices and Technologies

Paul A. Iaizzo

Abstract The primary goals of this last chapter are to: (1) discuss, in more detail, some of the technologies mentioned earlier in this book; (2) introduce readers to several additional technological advances associated with cardiovascular health care that have been recently introduced, are currently in clinical testing, or will soon be released; and (3) discuss future opportunities in the cardiac device arena. It should be noted that other areas of importance in cardiac treatment such as biological approaches to disease management (e.g., stem cell therapy), genomics (i.e., diagnostics and gene therapy), proteomics, and/or tissue engineering will also have a major impact on the future of cardiac clinical care, yet detailed discussions of these approaches are beyond the scope of this text. More specifically, in this last chapter, we will review several innovations in the following areas: (1) resuscitation systems and devices; (2) implantable therapies; (3) delivery systems; (4) invasive therapies; (5) procedural improvements; (6) less invasive surgical approaches; (7) post-procedural follow-ups; and/or (8) training tools.

Keywords Medical device development · Resuscitation devices · Implantable therapies · Catheter-delivered devices · Endocardial ablation devices · Device coating agents · Telemedicine · Implantable sensors · Cardiac imaging · Surgical tools · Less invasive surgery

38.1 Introduction

Since the first edition of this book was published in 2005, much has changed in the field of cardiac devices. In response, several new chapters were added and others were expanded in this second edition to accommodate the rapid growth and innovation in certain areas (e.g., cardiopulmonary resuscitation, imaging, cardiac care in the intensive care unit, transcatheter valves). In many of these updated chapters, the authors provided revised, yet brief, histories of cardiac device development and fairly thorough discussions of currently employed devices and/or assessment technologies. To appreciate how rapidly innovations in the area of cardiac disease are progressing, one can simply perform a search on the United States Patent & Trademark Office web site (www.uspto.gov). This search produces an impressive number of companies and/or individuals attempting to secure intellectual property protection in this clinical category. More specifically, the following are numbers of published patent applications, identified in May 2009 and July of 2004, citing the following key words:

CARDIAC (54,155 patent applications in 2009; 18,920 in 2004)

CARDIAC SURGERY (2,635 patent applications in 2009; 1,015 in 2004)

CARDIOLOGY (4,557 patent applications in 2009; 1,480 in 2004)

CARDIAC ELECTROPHYSIOLOGY (253 patent applications in 2009; 79 in 2004)

CARDIOVASCULAR STENTS (159 patent applications in 2009; 52 in 2004)

CARDIAC REPAIR (149 patent applications in 2009; 32 in 2004)

Note that this list likely does not include all issued patents, as some may be foreign, and many of these patents detail prospective future products. For example, in searching the same database mentioned above, the key word CARDIAC produces 51,714 issued patents in 2009 since 1976 (in 2004, there were 37,410 patents). There are several other places to locate information on emerging cardiac devices, such as the Food and Drug Administration web site (http://www.fda.gov/fdac/features/2001/301_home.htm), the Google™ patent search web site (http://www.google.com/patents?), or other web sites.

P.A. Iaizzo (✉)
University of Minnesota, Department of Surgery, B172 Mayo, MMC 195, 420 Delaware St. SE, Minneapolis, MN 55455, USA
e-mail: iaizz001@umn.edu

P.A. Iaizzo (ed.), *Handbook of Cardiac Anatomy, Physiology, and Devices*, DOI 10.1007/978-1-60327-372-5_38,

It should be mentioned that many novel ideas that eventually lead to new products, therapies, or training first occur through basic cardiac research. In order for emerging technologies to continue to advance at a rapid rate, it is imperative that laboratories performing basic research in such technological areas continue to receive necessary support. Furthermore, prototype testing and clinical trials are essential to insure that the best possible technologies are developed and eventually made available for general use. Yet, it is important to note that many critical lessons can be learned from trials that employ misdirected devices or technologies.

When considering the design of a medical device, there are typically a number of key processes or steps involved:

- A device sketch (e.g., on a cocktail napkin in a meeting with a clinician).
- The creation of an animation of device design, function, and/or placement.
- Device prototype development.
- Bench testing.
- Redesign: final design freeze.
- Animal testing.
- Redesign or clinical testing.
- Simulation systems of device implantation.
- Market release.

It should also be noted that some devices can be employed as lifesaving measures prior to approval for market release if a "Humanitarian Device Exemption" is obtained.

As cardiac devices become more and more beneficial and help people live longer lives, we foresee a need to design devices that: (1) have higher reliability and longevity; (2) can be upgraded, extracted, and/or replaced; and (3) enable easy data retrieval (i.e., remotely). More specifically, the retrieval of data and/or the reprogramming of implantable cardiac systems (e.g., sensor/pacing/defibrillation) should be accomplished without patient training or education; in other words, they should function as seamlessly and simply as possible (*you just implant them*). As these systems evolve, there will be interest from healthcare payers as well as the physicians and hospitals that monitor patients. Furthermore, data would ultimately and automatically be interfaced with "electronic health records." Such home monitoring may be perceived as the only possible way to manage the growing amount of data collected from "baby boomer" generation patients receiving such therapies, and may also result in (1) improved care; (2) a greater level of patient confidence; (3) improved understanding of disease-specific therapy; and/or (4) overall cost savings for both the healthcare industry and consumers. It should also be noted that, by 2014, there will be patient-owned medical records, as mandated in a Presidential order in 2004.

Within the last several years, we have witnessed a fair number of cardiac device recalls due to so-called *inherent failures*. However, this may be not so surprising, as the sophistication of such devices continues to increase, and more and more clinicians have begun to implant them. Perhaps, in the future, we will see that the use of implant simulators will partially decrease the incidences of failure due to so-called *user errors* (e.g., improper implantation). Nevertheless, it should be emphasized that human cardiac anatomy is highly variable and dynamic (i.e., ever changing, with reverse remodeling occurring with improving outcomes and survival), thus we need to consider that the implant environment continues to change post-therapeutically (post-implant).

Despite a number of known failed devices, all designs were required to pass rigorous bench testing, animal trials, and human clinical trials before approval for market release. It is of interest to note that each company often designs their own bench testing equipment because, in most cases, the device designs are novel or unique. In fact, many times this testing equipment also becomes proprietary. Nevertheless, it is likely that bench testing of cardiac devices with high sales volumes will likely become government regulated sometime in the near future.

To provide the reader with perspective on the design and testing issues facing the cardiac device industry, perhaps the following example will suffice. A pacing lead moves approximately 100,000 times every day, or 37,000,000 times annually, and this can occur in multiple locations and with numerous degrees of freedom. Furthermore, when considering failure of the lead insulation alone, one must consider failures due to abrasions, the association with the fibrous device pocket, the potential for lead-to-lead interactions, anatomical considerations (bones, ligaments, etc.), and/or other complications. It is also interesting to note that some features of lead implantation have received little attention or study, yet this may greatly influence lead failures, e.g., the design of the anchoring sleeves.

38.2 Resuscitation Systems and Devices

Even before the cardiac patient enters the emergency and/or operating room, there are many new technologies being developed to aid in his/her resuscitation. Such innovations range from improvements of existing tools (e.g., automated application of cardiopulmonary resuscitation) to novel mechanisms that accomplish better patient outcomes (e.g., impedance threshold valve). Furthermore, automated external defibrillators have become commonplace in the United States, with such units being purchased for use in schools, health clubs, emergency vehicles, shopping malls, and even personal homes. There are also relatively new defibrillator systems that can be worn externally by a patient (e.g., LifeVest™, LIFECOR, Inc., Pittsburgh, PA; http://www.lifecor.com/about_about.asp/about.asp), or those that are leadless and implanted subcutaneously (e.g., S-ICD, Cameron Health, San Clemente, CA; http://www.cameronhealth.com/). In summary, there have been rapid advances in both cardiopulmonary resuscitation and associated devices to improve patient outcomes (e.g., the use of active compression–decompression devices and mild hypothermia). As such, a new chapter dedicated to this topic was added to this textbook (Chapter 35).

38.2.1 External Defibrillators

Today, most Emergency Medicine Service units utilize a multi-tiered response system, with emergency medical technicians providing basic life support services, backed up by paramedics if advanced life support is needed. All of these personnel are trained in the use of automated external defibrillators. There are several companies that produce such devices, and their availability is no longer limited to hospital or emergency services settings. In fact, there is a rapidly growing home market, as many individuals are making the personal investment as a lifesaving precaution. Yet, such units may also have expanded features that not all individuals are sufficiently trained to utilize. For example, the LIFEPAK® 12 defibrillator/monitor series, manufactured by Medtronic, Inc. (Minneapolis, MN; http://www.medtronic.com/), allows for the recording of a standard 12-lead electrocardiogram (ECG) even in remote locations (Fig. 38.1). Nevertheless, with the same equipment, various personnel with different levels of expertise and training can provide lifesaving support, e.g., some units have incorporated push button turn controls with voice prompts.

In other words, these combination devices, such as the LIFEPAK® 12 defibrillator/monitor series, give paramedics access to sophisticated diagnostics and treatment in the field. This single piece of equipment monitors the ECG continuously, measures the level of oxygen in the bloodstream and, if necessary, provides defibrillation and/or pacing to help maintain the heart's rhythm. Thus, it allows paramedics to perform computerized 12-lead ECGs before the patient reaches the hospital. Such ECG data can be transmitted by wireless network to the emergency room physician from the ambulance while en route. With this information in hand, the team of doctors and nurses can be ready and waiting for the patient's arrival; importantly, they can administer treatment in as

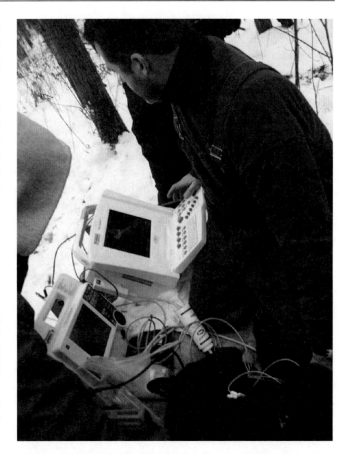

Fig. 38.1 A LIFEPAK® external defibrillator 12 (Medtronic, Inc.) and a Cyprus portable echocardiography unit (Acuson, Siemens, Malvern, PA) used externally (outside) on an overwintering black bear. In this case, research colleague Dr. Tim Laske was using these systems to monitor 12-lead ECGs via a connection to surface electrodes and echocardiography using a transthoracic probe

little as 15 min after the patient enters the emergency room, compared to an hour or more if the ECG is first done at the hospital. It is generally considered that any shortening of the time to treatment can significantly speed recovery and improve a patient's chances of returning to a fully productive life.

The following scenario has been provided by Physio-Control Corporation (Redmond, WA; http://www.physiocontrol.com/) to demonstrate the significance of such features—"by the time a given patient had arrived at the hospital, the symptoms had subsided, and the ECG in the hospital appeared normal, yet the attending doctors compared the ECG done in the ambulance with the one obtained from the patient's physical exam a month prior and then there was no question about the diagnosis, a progressing heart attack. With 12-lead ECGs on board, an ambulance becomes a mobile clinic and paramedics become the doctors' eyes and ears."

It is likely that more and more computerized data collection (e.g., pressures, flows) will be performed by paramedics and/or others prior to a patient entering the hospital setting, which will then be seamlessly integrated with hospital data to create a complete picture of a patient's medical condition from initial contact all the way through hospital discharge. Furthermore, it is possible that echocardiography will be performed in the field as such units are quite portable today (see Chapter 20). Many of these developments are currently available, and the challenge for healthcare providers in the coming years will be to provide the best possible care in the most cost-effective way. Perhaps we will see the day of the "family house call" once again, i.e., the healthcare provider visits the home and assesses and monitors all family members living there during one single visit (e.g., ECGs, electronic auscultations, pressure assessments, echocardiography, blood and genetic analyses). It should be noted that it was not that long ago, in the 1960s, that medical students were still instructed on how to perform a "traditional house call."

38.3 Implantable Therapies

Advances in micro-technologies have now made it possible to create implantable therapies that can be lifesaving, e.g., implantable defibrillators which have detected and treated thousands of episodes of sudden cardiac fibrillation. Recently, there has been a large push to implant vagal nerve stimulators for several proposed therapies including heart rate control, blood pressure control, dietary control, and/or even the reversal of depression. As mentioned above, the need for such devices will likely increase at an exponential rate, and will be directed specifically to all types of cardiac complications.

38.3.1 Left Atrial Appendage/Atrial Fibrillation Therapy

There are growing numbers of treatment for the side effects of atrial fibrillation which, in some patients, leads to crippling strokes. The focus of these devices is to modify the role of the left atrial appendage in pathologies associated with atrial fibrillation. More specifically, this tiny alcove of the heart that has been described to serve as a "starter heart" for the human embryo can be a site for blood to pool and subsequently form clots that can be expelled into the brain, causing strokes. Today, it is estimated that atrial fibrillation affects 5 million people worldwide and is thought to be responsible for up to 25% of all strokes. It has been reported that, due to aging of the population, the number of patients with atrial

fibrillation will likely increase by approximately 2.5-fold by the year 2050 [1].

At present, the most common treatment for atrial fibrillation is the administration of a strong anticoagulant drug called coumadin. From a device perspective, suggested approaches to treat this problem include tissue clamps, screens, and other methods to seal off the appendage (e.g., the Watchman and PLAATO devices). More specifically, one start-up company named Atritech Inc. (Plymouth, MN; http://www.atritech.net/) has promoted a solution to implant a tiny filter into the appendage, letting blood pass through but trapping clots inside the mini chamber; after some time, the body would then naturally seal off the chamber. Nevertheless, in the deployment or use of these devices, it is critical to appropriately visualize the procedure and assess its post-implant stability. Furthermore, if there is subsequent endothelial covering of the interface, this will allow for a reduction in anticoagulation therapy (e.g., the use of warfarin).

It should also be noted that more recent techniques to treat atrial fibrillation employ epicardial approaches via minimally invasive procedures. For example, there are numerous surgical tools available to: (1) epicardially dissect tissues (e.g., Cardioblate® Navigator Tissue Dissector, Medtronic, Inc.); (2) perform cardiac surface mapping, ablation, pacing, or sensing (e.g., Cardioblate® Maps Device, Medtronic, Inc.); and/or (3) create ablation lines or pseudo-Maze procedures (e.g., Cardioblate® Gemini, Surgical Ablation System, Medtronic, Inc.).

38.3.2 Cardiac Remodeling

Chronic cardiac remodeling is a well-known response of dilated cardiomyopathy and is thought to play a central role in disease progression [2–4]. Associated heart chamber dilation and/or wall thinning will elevate overall wall stress which is considered to trigger the local release of neurohormones, thereby adversely affecting myocardial molecular biology and physiology [5]. Therapeutic approaches to treat heart failure have been described primarily as a means to inhibit or even induce reverse remodeling (e.g., beta-adrenergic blockade). More recently, mechanical unloading using left ventricular assist devices (LVADs, see Chapter 36), extracorporeal pumps (see Chapter 30), or portable whole heart support systems (e.g., EXCOR®, Berlin Heart, Berlin, Germany; http://www.berlinheart.de/) have been employed as alternatives. Such interventions can profoundly unload a heart, leading to reverse remodeling and improved physiological performance [2]. The design of such pump systems has been ongoing, and the goal has been to transition from external or partially external to fully implantable pumps (e.g., internal pumps with small rechargeable battery packs). Furthermore, when system developers changed from pulsatile to continuous pumps, pump size was reduced by ~1/7, pump weight was reduced by ~1/4, and they were also quieter and more reliable (e.g., fewer moving parts). It should be noted that, today, approximately 600 LVADs are implanted in patients in the United States each year, and that 30% of all heart transplant patients had a prior LVAD.

Another approach for dealing with cardiac remodeling is to induce structural remodeling by imposing alteration on or within the heart. For example, the CorCap™ Cardiac Support Device (Acorn Cardiovascular Inc., St. Paul, MN; http://www.acorncv.com/healthcare_pro viders/corcap.cfm) is a fabric mesh multi-filament implant that is surgically positioned around the ventricles of the heart (to date, this device does not have FDA approval). This product is designed to reduce ventricular wall stress by supporting the heart muscle. Preclinical studies have shown that supporting the heart in this manner stops deterioration and also allows the muscle to heal or remodel [4]. More specifically, the deployment of this device is expected to improve the heart's ability to pump blood, provide relief of heart failure symptoms, improve quality of life, and ultimately extend survival for those who suffer from heart failure.

There are many other devices being developed and tested to structurally remodel the heart. Such devices may be used for individuals who have enlarged hearts due to failure (as above) or for patients who had congenital repairs performed when they were young, but now require structural remodeling due to heart growth and/or alterations due to disease. It is worth noting that there are approximately one million adults alive today in the U.S. who had congenital repairs when they were children; in 2007, there were ~900,000 children in the U.S. with congenital heart defects. In general, many of these patients will require repair or replacement of their pulmonary valves and/or remodeling of the outflow tracts concomitantly.

38.4 Catheter-Delivered Devices

Since the first edition of this textbook, there has been a boom in the delivery of specialized cardiac devices that can be introduced intravascularly or via intracardiac methods. Such devices include stents, septal occluder devices, valves, leads, and ablation tools (see also Chapters 7, 26, 27, and 32). Currently, the field of transcatheter-delivered valves is one of great interest and high competition within the medical device industry (see Chapter 33). In addition, there is a new dynamic in the clinical delivery of such systems, in that teams of cardiologists and cardiac surgeons are working together in hybrid catheter lab/operating rooms to perform multi-tiered treatments on patients (e.g., implanting pacing/defibrillation systems, valves, and/or bypass grafts). It is likely that, as *centers of excellence* are created to perform such procedures, older and older individuals will be receiving implantable devices and/or other cardiac therapies. It should be noted that there are also cardiac catheters on the market to deliver stem cell or gene therapies (see Chapter 37).

38.4.1 Stents

An intraluminal coronary artery stent is typically a small, self-expanding, wire mesh tube that is placed within a coronary artery to keep the vessel patent (open). Stents are commonly deployed: (1) during a coronary artery bypass graft surgery to keep the grafted vessel open; (2) after balloon angioplasty to prevent reclosure of the blood vessel; and/or (3) during other heart surgeries. For delivery, a stent is collapsed to a small diameter and put over a balloon catheter. Typically with the guidance of fluoroscopy, the catheter and stent are moved into the area of the blockage. When the balloon on the delivery catheter is inflated, the stent expands, locking it in place within the vessel, thus forming a scaffold which holds the artery open. Stents are intended to stay in the vessel permanently, keeping it open to improve blood flow to the myocardium and thereby relieving symptoms (usually angina). Note that a stent may be used instead of angioplasty. The type of stent to be deployed depends on certain features of the artery blockage, i.e., size of the artery and where the blockage is specifically located.

A key goal in the development of clinical stents is to reduce the incidence of restenosis, which generally occurs within 4–6 months following an angioplasty procedure. Before stents, the incidence of restenosis was about 35–45%. Restenosis is a renarrowing of the treated coronary artery, which is largely related to the development of neointimal hyperplasia (that which occurs within an artery after it has been treated with a balloon or atherectomy device). In general, restenosis can be considered as scar tissue that forms in response to a previous mechanical insult (see Chapter 7). Stents are now commonly coated with agents that are slowly released, further promoting the vessel from renarrowing and closing. Yet, it should also be noted that, typically, patients who have had a stent procedure must take one or more blood-thinning agents such as aspirin, ticlopidine, or clopidogrel.

Aspirin is typically used indefinitely, while one of the other two drugs is generally prescribed for 2–4 weeks. Therefore, goals for future stent technologies will continue to include the development of coatings that will minimize restenosis and/or the use of anticoagulation therapy. It is likely that other devices (e.g., implanted sensors or stented valves) would also benefit from employing such coatings.

It is interesting to note that, currently, there are a growing number of patients seen with clinical symptoms that received coronary stents 5 or more years ago, and now require coronary artery bypass graft procedures. Unfortunately, procedures in such patients can be considered as surgically difficult or less than ideal, for in many such cases there are limited or less than functionally ideal locations to perform the graft anastomoses due to the prior stent placements. It should also be noted that, in some patients, the stenting was performed so aggressively that there may be four or more stents placed end-to-end in a given vessel, thus spanning more than 7–8 cm in length; a graft cannot be easily placed into such stented vessels with currently available technologies.

38.4.2 Catheter-Delivered Leads

One of the continuing challenges in the area of intracardiac lead development is to downsize lead diameters and, at the same time, minimize the possibilities for fractures or failures. Similarly, there is growing practice in the placement of leads within the cardiac veins, as well as in the development of tools for cannulation of the coronary sinus. For example, the Attain™ Deflectable Catheter System (Medtronic, Inc.) features a percutaneous needle and syringe to access the venous insertion site, a guidewire

to access the vein, an adjustable hemostasis valve to reduce blood loss during the implant procedure, a deflectable catheter to cannulate the coronary sinus and deliver the pacing lead (e.g., 4 French), and slitters to remove the deflectable catheter. Additionally, the Attain Prevail™, a steerable coronary sinus cannulation tool is available from Medtronic (Fig. 38.2). These catheters need to be sterile and will likely be single use. It should be noted that such systems will likely aid in the delivery of leads for alternate site pacing, e.g., into the right ventricular outflow tract or to activate the His bundle.

38.4.3 Endocardial Ablation Devices

Ablation is used to prevent tachyarrhythmias by modifying or destroying abnormal tissue. Clearly identifying the site of origin of the tachyarrhythmia (or tissue that is essential for maintaining reentrant activity) is important to the success of ablation (see Chapters 26 and 29); the goal of ablation is to create scar tissue in a critical myocardial area. Since scar tissue is electrically inert, it cannot originate or conduct electrical impulses. Scar tissue is created in the myocardium either by surgical incision or application of energy. Various forms of energy have been employed and continue to be refined in the catheter-based approaches of ablation (Table 38.1). It is of interest to note that the use of cryoprobes has an advantage because the probe will adhere (freeze like a tongue on a flag pole in the winter) and it is easier to maintain its position during the application of the therapy. To date, surgical ablation is typically performed during an open-chest procedure, but it is likely that it could be performed using less invasive approaches with further enhancement of surgical methodologies (e.g., with a sub-xyphoid approach).

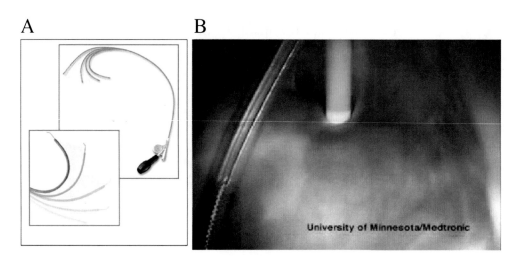

Fig. 38.2 (**A**) A steerable delivery catheter (Model 10600, Medtronic, Inc.) being used to deploy a lead. (**B**) Image was obtained in our laboratory in an isolated swine heart [6]

Table 38.1 Types of ablation energy

- Radiofrequency (RF) energy
- Direct current (DC) shock energy
- Laser energy
- Microwave energy
- Cryoenergy

There are multiple methods of delivering energy during ablation; radiofrequency delivery is the most common.

Currently, radiofrequency energy is used for almost all nonoperative ablation procedures. In the past, DC (direct current) shock energy was used for delivering energy to the endocardium. A standard defibrillator was connected to the ablation catheter to deliver the shock. DC shock had the following undesirable effects that occurred at the catheter tip during delivery of high energy: (1) excessive tip temperature and (2) irregular shaped lesions that then could be proarrhythmic. Radiofrequency ablation catheters use energy similar to electrocautery. Radiofrequency energy heats the catheter tip tissue interface with resultant injury to the underlying tissue. Some advantages of radiofrequency ablation are: (1) small amounts of energy are required; (2) output power is easily controlled; (3) it creates small, homogeneous lesions; and (4) it does not cause dangerous/unpleasant stimulation or sensory effects. The amount of heating produced during radiofrequency ablation at the electrode tip can result in local blood boiling. To avoid this problem, one type of ablation catheter controls the temperature at the tip by using a cooling fluid. There are numerous companies working on competing designs of such technologies. Thus, cardiovascular device companies continue to improve all design aspects of these catheter systems, i.e., improving the ease of positioning of the distal electrode.

Other methods to focally destroy cells endocardially are also emerging: (1) laser energy has been used to destroy arrhythmogenic tissue via a cautery-type process; (2) microwave energy has been investigated as a possible energy source; and (3) cryoablation freezes tissue at the catheter tip to destroy muscle fibers without harming connective tissues (Table 38.1). Visualization of the exact site where the lesion is to be created remains an area of intense research; advanced echocardiography systems as well as specialized catheters with built-in imaging possibilities are aggressively being pursued [7–9].

38.5 Novel Agents to Coat Devices

As described above, drug-coated stents have made a major impact in the field of interventional cardiology. There is little doubt that combined approaches which incorporate pharmaceutics with implantable devices will continue to expand as a means to improve clinical management of the heart. For example, steroid-eluting pacing leads have been on the market for years to manage acute inflammation associated with lead implantation (see Chapter 27). Steroid-elution technology is considered to reduce inflammation; by eluting a steroid at the lead tip, leads are designed to reduce the typical tissue inflammation. Reduced inflammation allows lower pacing system energy requirements. For example, by reducing tissue inflammation, it has been described that such leads allow the use of lower electrical settings for low, stable, acute, and chronic energy outputs. Nevertheless, it is likely that novel biologically engineered coatings will continue to be identified, and these need to be added without side effects of their own.

38.6 Implantable Sensors

Device and battery technologies continue to decrease in size and, at the same time, exhibit improved efficiencies. This, in turn, creates increasing possibilities for novel approaches to long-term assessment of various physiological parameters from unique aspects of the cardiovascular system.

One such device, the Chronicle® (Medtronic, Inc.), is intended to continuously sense and collect unique and valuable information such as intracardiac pressures, heart rate, and physical activity from a sensor placed directly in the heart's chamber. A patient can then periodically download this information to a home-based device that transmits this physiologic data securely over the Internet to a patient management network. Subsequently, physicians can access these data via a controlled web site at any time and review screens that present summaries from the latest downloads, trend information, and/or detailed records from specified times or problem episodes.

Other types of implantable sensors that will likely be available in the future include blood chemistries (respiratory gases, pH, heparin, polyanions, etc.), flows, cardiac outputs, temperatures, glucose levels, drug levels, and/or other physiologic data.

38.7 Procedural Improvement

With pressure on the healthcare system to continually reduce treatment costs and document the outcome benefits of a given therapy, much effort will continue to be focused on procedural improvements for cardiac care.

38.7.1 Cardiac Imaging

Our ability to image internal and external features of the heart continues to improve at a rapid rate and, as indicated in Chapters 20 and 22, the sophistication of such systems can be quite extreme. Yet, as the cost of computer hardware decreases while capabilities increase, opportunities to develop such technologies for widespread use continue to become more and more feasible.

Intracardiac echocardiography (ICE) offers many possible applications including guidance of radiofrequency ablation procedures and visualization of cardiac anatomy and physiology. Compared to standard 2D imaging, emerging 3D echocardiography may provide additional clinical utility. To assess this, in a recent study, our laboratory compared real-time 3D ICE images (RT3D ICE) to simultaneously captured real-time video images in an isolated four-chamber working swine heart [10]. These comparative images verified the ability of RT3D ICE to provide appropriate anatomic identification that could be applied to clinical practice. Stationary anatomical structures (i.e., coronary sinus ostium) are easily visualized with static 3D ICE images (Fig. 38.3). Moving structures (i.e., valves) were not easily distinguished on RT3D ICE when presented as still images, however, they were more easily identified during acquisition and full-speed playback.

Each imaging modality has advantages and disadvantages. For example, cardiac computed tomography imaging is considered as extremely useful for identifying the relative degrees of calcification that exist on a heart valve leaflet. Nevertheless, one should also consider that anesthesia use during image collection dramatically compromises cardiac function, i.e., when estimating the degree of mitral regurgitation in a patient, deep anesthesia may lead to an underestimation of the underlying compromised function. For additional details on cardiac imaging and new emerging approaches, see also Chapters 20, 22, and 29.

38.7.2 Specialized Surgical Tools

Cardiovascular device companies typically work closely with clinicians to develop not only new technologies but also modifications of existing devices and/or enhanced means to deploy them with better precision. One example of collaboration is the recently developed implant tool for the placement of epicardial leads during less invasive surgery. This malleable epicardial lead implant tool features a stainless steel shaft that can be shaped to maneuver and position a lead optimally on the posterior of the heart, either on the right or left ventricle (Fig. 38.4).

Note that a similar tool has also been developed for the placement of epicardial leads using robotic systems.

Another example of an innovative device that has been developed to fit a unique need is the device designed to trap plaque that may dislodge during interventional procedures; such plaque might otherwise migrate to smaller vessels, causing serious product deficits. The SPIDER™ Embolic Protection Device (ev3 Inc., Plymouth, MN; http://www.ev3.net/), FilterWire EZ™ Embolic Protection System (Boston Scientific, Natick, MA; http://www.bostonscientific.com/home.bsci), and the RX ACCUNET Embolic Protection System (Abbott Laboratories, Abbott Park, IL; http://www.abbott.com/) are examples of specially designed systems for capture and removal of dislodged embolic debris before it can harm the patient. Such devices (and there are many available on the market today) are considered important for providing protection while conforming to the requirements of the primary intervention. As an example, the SPIDER™ Embolic Protection Device has been recommended to provide distal embolization protection in patients during a general vascular procedure, including peripheral, coronary, and carotid interventions (Fig. 38.5).

38.7.3 Less Invasive Surgeries

In Chapter 32, the rapidly advancing field of less invasive cardiac surgery and some initial uses of robotics to perform epicardial procedures (e.g., bypass grafting and lead implantation) were described. Such approaches are becoming more practical because tools to perform such procedures are continually refined. For example, the Octopus®3 Tissue Stabilizer (Medtronic, Inc.) is the pioneering and market-leading suction device featuring: (1) malleable stabilizer pods that can be formed to the unique contours of the patient's anatomy; and (2) a unique tissue spreading mechanism that enhances stabilization of the anastomotic site and presentation of the coronary. Similarly, the Starfish® Heart Positioner (Medtronic, Inc.) has been shown to simplify cardiac positioning and thus minimize the associated hemodynamic deterioration [11].

As cardiovascular surgeries employ less invasive techniques, more novel devices and tools will be needed. For example, the HEARTSTRING® III Proximal Seal System (Boston Scientific) is a unique means to perform bypass procedures that meet the challenge of clampless hemostasis; another example is the Symmetry Bypass System (St. Jude Medical, St. Paul, MN; http://www.sjm.com/). Both of these devices allow the surgeon to successfully complete coronary artery bypass without cross-clamping or side biting.

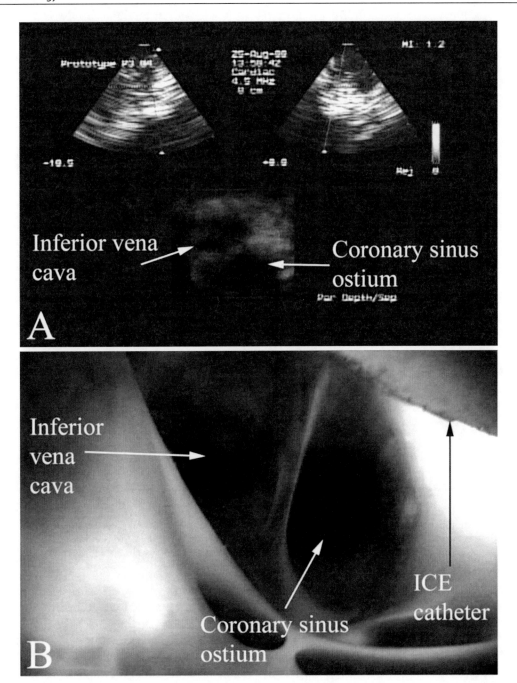

Fig. 38.3 Utilizing standard cardiac surgery procedures, the heart from a 70 kg swine was explanted to an isolated heart apparatus and reanimated. This preparation utilized a clear, crystalloid perfusate that allowed for intracardiac visualization. Following in vitro stabilization, the heart was instrumented with 6 mm videoscopes (Olympus Industrial, Tokyo, Japan) and a 12 Fr 3D ICE catheter (Duke University, Durham, NC) via access ports in the superior vena cava, left pulmonary vein, aorta, and right atrial appendage. Simultaneous ultrasound (Volumetrics Medical Imaging, Durham, NC) and intracardiac video images of the coronary sinus ostium and the tricuspid, mitral, and aortic valves were recorded to time-synchronized Beta video decks (Sony Beta SP, Tokyo, Japan). (**A**) RT3D ICE image and (**B**) intracardiac visualization. The inferior vena cava and coronary sinus ostium are very distinct in the three-dimensional ICE image [10]

38.8 Telemedicine

Telecommunication systems and devices, including the utilization of the Internet, have experienced unpredicted growth in the last decade. This explosion in technology has the potential to revolutionize the care of all types of cardiac patients. As noted above, some day each individual may have an instantaneously managed, personalized, and patient-owned health record that perhaps will be nothing more than an impeded chip within his/her

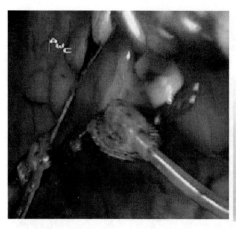
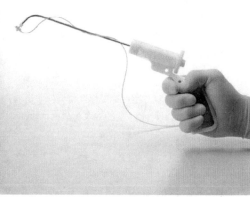

Fig. 38.4 (**Left**) The Model 5071 lead (Medtronic, Inc.) is designed for ventricular pacing and sensing. (**Right**) The Model 10626 (Medtronic, Inc.) is a single use device indicated to facilitate placement of the Model 5071 pacing lead. The lead has application where permanent ventricular dual-chamber pacing systems are indicated. Two leads may be used for bipolar pacing

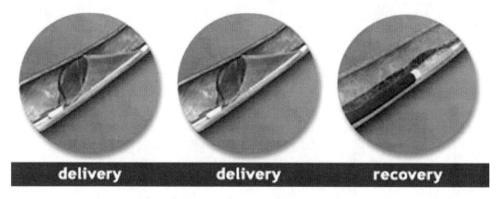

Fig. 38.5 The SPIDER™ Embolic Protection Device (ev3 Inc.) provides distal embolization protection in patients during general vascular use, including peripheral, coronary, and carotid interventions. It can be delivered by any guidewire of choice to initially cross the lesion; it has a Nitinol filter design that is HEPROTEC™ coated for patency up to 60 min. The radiopaque gold proximal loop is designed to provide visualization of filter to vessel apposition, and there are five filter sizes to appropriately match the vessel size

body that can be updated with sensed physiological parameters and uploaded via a wireless network.

38.8.1 Ambulatory Heart Monitors

Ambulatory heart monitors collect ECGs during daily patient activity. Today, a holter monitor typically collects several days of continuous ECG data. The patient wears the monitor and notes the time and type of symptoms experienced, which are then later correlated with the ECG. In contrast, an external event recorder has a memory buffer that can store several weeks of symptom data. Instead of keeping a diary, the patient activates the recorder when symptoms occur; this latter approach is quite convenient for evaluating symptoms that occur infrequently. A third type of device, an insertable loop recorder, is an implantable ECG recorder with a hand-held patient-controlled activator. The insertable loop recorder continuously records ECGs. When symptoms occur, the patient activates the recorder, and the recorder stores the ECG for a preprogrammed period of time before and after activation. An insertable loop recorder is useful for patients with even more infrequent symptoms and thus who remain undiagnosed after an initial workup. Such an approach is also recommended to the patient for whom an external event recorder is impractical. More specifically, the Reveal Plus (Medtronic, Inc.) is a second-generation insertable loop recorder; currently it features auto-activation, and is a high-yield, long-term, subcutaneous, leadless ECG monitor that offers continuous 14-month monitoring (search "CareLink" Remote Monitoring Network on http://www. medtronic.com). Such systems provide new diagnostic approaches for patients with transient symptoms that may suggest cardiac arrhythmias including: (1) unexplained syncope; (2) near syncope; (3) episodic dizziness; (4) unexplained recurrent palpitation; and/or (5) seizures and convulsions [12] (www.seizuresandfainting.com).

38.9 Training Systems

As technologies have become more advanced, so has the need to teach students, residents, and physicians how to use them. For example, our laboratory has developed a free access web site dedicated to the education of function cardiac anatomy and imaging (http://www.vhlab.umn.edu/atlas/).

38.9.1 Simulators or Simulator Mannequins

New products to enhance medical training and the implantation of medical devices are rapidly entering the marketplace. The most impressive new systems incorporate computerized mannequins, complex graphics, and sophisticated operator controls in state-of-the-art patient simulators. Students, residents, and/or physicians learn both medical concepts and manual procedures on life-size, interactive equipment that provides the benefits of anatomical correctness, unlimited repetition, scheduling convenience, and variable "health" conditions. Many major medical teaching centers have their own dedicated center for the incorporation of these systems into the training programs of all types of individuals. For example, at the University of Minnesota, Dr. Rob Sweet is the Director of the Simulation PeriOperative Resource for Training and Learning center (SimPORTAL; http://www.simportal.umn.edu/about.htm), which is the primary simulation training "portal," or point of entry, for the procedurally oriented departments within the Medical School. The group arranges for (or directly provides) space, equipment, and technical and logistical support for educational activities involving technical skills and team training via simulation. Furthermore, the Center for Research in Education and Simulation Technologies (CREST) at the University (http://www.crest.umn.edu/) also supplies research and evaluation capacity to support innovation in simulation equipment, tools, and processes as well as training curricula.

As an example of a specific system that is often incorporated into such facilities, the Human Patient Simulator (http://www.mbi.ufl.edu/facilities/hps.php) was developed by the University of Florida's College of Medicine to train anesthesiologists in routine and crisis situations. This interactive technology is considered to provide a realistic learning experience that is adaptable for a wide range of healthcare practitioners, including medical students, residents, nurses, and biomedical engineers. The simulator mannequin typically has palpable pulses, heart and lung sounds, simulated muscle twitch responses to nerve stimulation, and a body temperature. Thus, trainees can monitor its heart rate, cardiac rhythms, cardiac output, and blood pressure. Commonly equipped with interface software and an instructor's remote control, the simulator also gives accurate patient responses to over 60 different drugs, mechanical ventilation, and other medical therapies, and allows the instructor to introduce new conditions.

Another device that is currently available is the ultrasound training simulator, which allows students to perform sonographic examinations on a mannequin while viewing real-time sonographic images. The scanning motions and techniques which can be employed by the user realistically simulate the same skills necessary to examine a patient. It is considered that, by allowing trainees to practice on the simulator for as much time as needed to achieve initial competency, users should be able to perform more effectively in a shorter period of time in the actual clinical setting.

38.9.2 Endovascular Implant Simulators

A new generation of implant simulators that employ both visual and tactile feedback for practicing either right or left heart catheter-based procedures is currently available (e.g., AccuTouch® Endovascular Simulator (Immersion Medical, Gaithersburg, MD; http://www.immersion.com/medical/products/products). In addition, such devices can be used to simulate the placement of coronary stents (Procedicus VIST, Mentice AB, Gothenburg, Sweden; http://www.mentice.com/). More specifically, the VIST system allows for highly realistic simulation-based training of angiography, angioplasty, and coronary stenting using realistic 3D patient anatomy, real nested tools, tactile feedback, as well as different cases/scenarios and complications. This system consists of an interface device, a computer, and one or more displays (e.g., one for the simulated fluoroscopic image and another for the instructional system); the interface device is a virtual patient with an introducer in place. It is likely that such systems will become more realistic in the future. Through this training technique, various real-life tools and devices can be introduced and actual tools are used (and reused). All tools are active and can be manipulated at any time in the procedure. In the VIST system, the interface and tools (catheters, balloons, guidewires, etc.) interact with the simulator through a software package generating the fluoroscopic display, the forces that are reflected in the tools (for tactile feedback), the contrast flow, hemodynamics, and the results of the simulated intervention; a web-based user interface guides the user through the procedure and facilitates self-learning.

Many training centers around the world, in both academic and corporate settings, have been created, using various types of simulators, e.g., the Karolinska's training center uses a number of such devices (http://www.karolinska.se/templates/Page____75665.aspx?epslanguage = EN).

38.10 Summary

Within this book, and more specifically within this chapter, we have reviewed numerous areas of cardiology and cardiac surgery in which the development of innovative technologies continues to mature at a rapid rate. These areas include: (1) resuscitation systems and devices; (2) implantable therapies (e.g., pacemakers, implantable cardioverter defibrillators, stents, septal occluders, valves, annular rings, fibrin patches); (3) delivery systems/invasive therapies (e.g., angioplasty, ablations, catheters); (4) procedural improvements (e.g., mapping systems, 3D echocardiography, magnetic resonance imaging, training simulators); (5) less invasive surgical approaches (i.e., off-pump, robotics); (6) post-procedural follow-up/telemedicine (e.g., electrical, functional, adverse events); and (7) training tools. There is no doubt that continued improvement of these technologies, as well as advances in rehabilitation and other support services (e.g., patient education, training, home monitoring), will extend and/or save lives and enhance the overall quality of life for patients. Finally, it should be mentioned that much work has been done on the implantable replacement heart, yet such prosthetic systems have yet to be successfully used (e.g., The AbioCor™ Implantable Replacement Heart, Abiomed, Danvers, MA; http://www.abiomed.com/products/heart_replacement.cfm).

However, when a patient is at imminent risk of death, the implant of an artificial heart is designed to both extend life and provide a reasonable quality of life. After implantation, the device does not require any tubes or wires to pass through the skin; power to drive the prosthetic heart is transmitted across the intact skin, avoiding skin penetration that may provide opportunities for infection. Just like the natural heart, the replacement heart consists of two blood-pumping chambers capable of delivering more than 8 l of blood every minute.

In conclusion, it is exciting to think about the technologies that have been employed thus far as well as those that are being developed which will positively affect the overall health care of the cardiac patient. It continues to be an exhilarating era to be working in the field of cardiovascular sciences.

Web Site Sources

All web sites were accessed on July 24, 2008

http://www.uspto.gov
http://www.fda.gov/fdac/features/2001/301_home.htm
http://www.google.com/patents?
http://www.seizuresandfainting.com
http://www.vhlab.umn.edu/atlas/
http://www.berlinheart.de/englisch/
http://www.crest.umn.edu/
http://www.lifecor.com/about_lifevest/about.asp
http://www.cameronhealth.com/
http://www.medtronic.com/
http://www.physiocontrol.com/
http://www.atritech.net/
http://www.acorncv.com/
http://www.ev3.net/
http://www.bostonscientific.com/home.bsci
http://www.sjm.com/
http://www.abbott.com/
http://www.vhlab.umn.edu/atlas/
http://www.simportal.umn.edu/about.htm
http://www.crest.umn.edu/
http://www.mbi.ufl.edu/facilities/hps.php
http://www.immersion.com/
http://www.karolinska.se/templates/
http://www.heartreplacement.com

References

1. Santini M, Ricci RP. The worldwide social burden of atrial fibrillation: What should be done and where do we go? J Interv Card Electrophysiol 2006;17:183–88.
2. Cohn JN, Ferrari R, Sharpe N, International Forum on Cardiac Remodelling. Cardiac remodeling–Concepts and clinical implications: A consensus paper from an international forum on cardiac remodeling. J Am Coll Cardiol 2000;35:569–82.
3. Anversa P, Olivetti G, Capasso JM. Cellular basis of ventricular remodeling after myocardial infarction. Am J Cardiol 1991;68:7–16D.
4. Saaverda WF, Tunin RS, Paolocci N, et al. Reverse remodeling and enhanced adrenergic reserve from passive external support in experimental dilated heart failure. J Am Coll Cardiol 2002;39:2069–76.
5. Francis GS. Pathophysiology of chronic heart failure. Am J Med 2001;110:37S–46S.
6. Chinchoy E, Soule CL, Houlton AJ, et al. Isolated four-chamber working swine heart model. Ann Thorac Surg 2000;70:1607–14.
7. Fried NM, Tsitlik A, Rent K, et al. Laser ablation of the pulmonary veins using a fiberoptic balloon catheter: Implications for treatment of paroxysmal atrial fibrillation. Lasers Surg Med 2001;28:197–203.
8. Marrouche NF, Martin DO, Wazni O, et al. Phased-array intracardiac echocardiography monitoring during pulmonary vein

isolation in patients with atrial fibrillation: impact on outcome and complications. Circulation 2003;107:2710–6.

9. Haissaguerre M, Jais P, Shah DC, et al. Spontaneous initiation of atrial fibrillation by ectopic beats originating in the pulmonary veins. N Engl J Med 1998;339:659–66.

10. Hill AJ, McHenry BA, Laske TG, et al. Validation of real-time three-dimensional intracardiac echocardiography using Visible Heart™ methodologies. J Cardiac Failure 2003;9:S51.

11. Gründeman P, et al. Ninety degrees anterior cardiac displacement in off-pump CABG: The Starfish™ cardiac positioner preserves stroke volume and arterial pressure. Presented at ISMICS 2002, New York, NY.

12. Zaidi A, Crampton S, Clough P, Scheepers B, Fitzpatrick A. Misdiagnosis of epilepsy: Many seizure-like episodes have a cardiovascular cause (abstract). PACE 1999;22:814.

Index

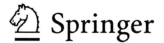 Springer

On the attached DVD-ROM, please find the "Companion" folder. Exit the program and search the DVD-ROM with Windows Explorer.